Atherosclerosis X

Atherosclerosis X

Proceedings of the 10th International Symposium on Atherosclerosis, Montréal, October 9–14, 1994

Chairman: J. Davignon

Editors:

F. Peter Woodford

Formerly Chief Scientific Officer to the Department of Health, London
Executive Editor, *Journal of Atherosclerosis Research,* 1961–63

J. Davignon

Clinical Research Institute of Montréal, Canada

A. Sniderman

Royal Victoria Hospital, Montréal, Canada

 1995

Elsevier

Amsterdam – Lausanne – New York – Oxford – Shannon – Tokyo

vi

Xth International Symposium on Atherosclerosis

M.D. Haust, Honorary Chairman
J. Davignon, Chairman
L. Campeau, Vice-chairman
A. Sniderman, Secretary

Xth International Symposium Organizing Committee

J. Davignon (Chairman)	R. Dufour	J. Lepage
D. Bouthillier	J. Griffith	E. Matteau
S. Brault	R. Jenkins	A. Sniderman
L. Campeau	R. Lambert	F. Theriault

Scientific Advisory Committee

G. Ailhaud, France	M.J. Halpern, Portugal	G. Rothblatt, USA
P. Alaupovic, USA	M. Hanefeld, Germany	E.M. Rubin, USA
P. Avogaro, Italy	L. Havekes, The Netherlands	A. Scanu, USA
G. Baggio, Italy	R.J. Havel, USA	E. Schaefer, USA
P.J. Barter, Australia	H. Hobbs, USA	C. Schwartz, USA
U. Beisiegel, Germany	H. Hoff, USA	S. Schwartz, USA
D.J. Betteridge, UK	S. Humphries, UK	J. Scott, UK
E. Bierman, USA	B. Jacotot, France	D. Seidel, Germany
B.H. Brewer, Jr., USA	I. Juhan-Vague, France	L. Simons, Australia
V. Blaton, Belgium	T. Kita, Japan	C.F. Sing, USA
G. Born, UK	R.S. Lees, USA	C.R. Sirtori, Italy
G. Camejo, Sweden	P. Libby, USA	O. Stein, Israel
L. Chan, USA	A.J. Lusis, USA	S. Stender, Denmark
S.B. Chen, China	M. Mancini, Italy	A. Tall, USA
G. Coetzee, South Africa	J. Marsh, USA	M.R. Taskinen, Finland
G. Descovich, Italy	Y. Matsuzawa, Japan	G. Thompson, UK
P. Douste-Blazy, France	S. Muntoni, Italy	G. Utermann, Austria
S. Eisenberg, Israel	M. Naruszewicz, Poland	D. Van Der Westhuysen, S. Africa
J.W. Farquhar, USA	K.R. Norum, Norway	A. Van Tol, The Netherlands
J.E. Fernandez-Britto, Cuba	M.F. Oliver, UK	M. Verstraete, Belgium
N. Fidge, Australia	J.R. Patsch, Austria	K. Weisgraber, USA
M.H. Frick, Finland	H.J. Pownall, USA	R. Zambahari, Malaysia
A.M. Gotto, Jr., USA	K. Pyörälä, Finland	
S.M. Grundy, USA	E.R. Quintão, Brazil	

International Finance Committee

C.A. Feldstein, Argentina
P.J. Nestel, Australia
G. Kostner, Austria
V. Blaton, Belgium
E.R. Quintão, Brazil
M.H. Tan, Canada
J. Frohlich, Canada
P. Aschner, Colombia
F. Ztoźický, Czech Republic
A. Kesäniemi, Finland

B. Jacotot, France
H. Greten, Germany
C.J. Miras, Greece
H. Jellinek, Hungary
J. Kisjanto, Indonesia
E. Leitersdorf, Israel
R. Paoletti, Italy
H. Orimo, Japan
J.G. Barranco, Mexico
K.R. Norum, Norway

R. Gamboa, Peru
M. Naruszewicz, Poland
A. Medina-Ruiz, Puerto Rico
M.J. Halpern, Portugal
N.N. Kipshidze, Georgia
A. Olsson, Sweden
A. Van Tol, The Netherlands
B. Howard, USA
V. Smirnov, Russia
G. Thompson, UK

National Finance Committee

M. Bélanger, Honorary Chairman
J. Davignon, Chairman
D. Bouthillier
B. Camuset

L. Campeau
L. Chartier
G. Lou

A. Piché
E. Simons
A. Van der Wee

International Program Committee

C. Assmann, Germany
K. Berg, Norway
M. Bihari-Varga, Hungary
J. Breslow, USA
M.S. Brown, USA
L. Carlsson, Sweden
R. Carmena, Spain
G. Crepaldi, Italy
J.L. De Gennes, France
J.C. Fruchart, France
J.L. Goldstein, USA
Y. Goto, Japan
H. Greten, Germany
G. Kostner, Austria
B. Lewis, UK
R. Mahley, USA
T. Miettinen, Finland
P.J. Nestel, Australia
R. Paoletti, Italy
D. Pometta, Switzerland
R. Ross, USA
M. Rosseneu, Belgium
J. Shepherd, UK
V. Smirnov, Russia

E. Smith, UK
Y. Stein, Israel
D. Steinberg, USA
G. Schettler, Germany
T.H. Van Berkel, The Netherlands
R. Wissler, USA
A. Yamamoto, Japan

National Program Committee

A. Sniderman
    Chairman
J. Davignon,
J.P. Després
J. Genest, Jr.
M. Hayden
R. Hegele
N. Kalant
E. Levy
P.J. Lupien
Y.L. Marcel
A. Minnich
S. Moore
G. Steiner

viii

Acknowledgements

The organizing committee gratefully acknowledges the generous financial support of the following:

Benefactors:

Bristol-Myers Squibb Pharmaceutical Group
Groupe Fournier
Merck
Parke-Davis
Sandoz

Major sponsor:

Boehringer Mannheim Canada

Sponsor:

Nordic Marion Merrell Dow

Supporters:

Astra Pharma
Becel
Dairy Bureau of Canada
Ciba-Geigy
Glaxo
Groupe Lipha
Japanese Atherosclerosis Society

Jouveinal
Miles Canada
Sankyo Pharmaceutical
Servier Canada
Schering-Plough
Sterling Winthrop
Wyeth Ayerst

Other contributors:

Bio Méga Boehringer Ingelheim Research
Cyanamid
Eli Lilly Canada, Inc.
Fonds de la Recherche en Santé du Québec
Heart & Stroke Foundation of Canada
Hoffmann-La Roche Ltd.
Kaneka America Corporation
Margarine Thibault
McGill University
McMaster University
Medical Research Council of Canada

Memorial University of Newfoundland
Ministère du tourisme du Québec
Queen's University
Université de Montréal
Université de Sherbrooke
Université Laval
University of British Columbia
University of Guelph
University of Western Ontario
Upjohn

Contents

Remnant metabolism

Modified lipoproteins and atherosclerosis

Chairman's Introduction

Jean Davignon

In introducing this volume of the proceedings of the Xth International Symposium on Atherosclerosis, I would like to emphasize the features that distinguish it from its predecessors. But first, let me acknowledge the tremendous help and advice as well as financial support given by industry, academia and government, by all my colleagues in Montreal and by the members of all the committees shown on earlier pages.

At the opening ceremony we were honored by contributions from Le Ministre Délégué à la Santé de France (M. Philippe Douste-Blazy), L'Honorable Ministre de la Santé du Canada (Mme. Diane Marleau), Le Président du Conseil de la Ville de Montréal (M. André Berthelet), Le Conseiller Spécial du Ministre de la Santé de la Province de Québec (le Docteur Pierre Duplessis), the President of the International Atherosclerosis Society, Dr Antonio Gotto and the Past President of the Society, Professor Gotthard Schettler. Also present were Dr Daria Haust (Honorary President of the Symposium), Dr Carl Breckenridge (president of the Canadian Atherosclerosis Society), Dr Serge Carrière (dean of the faculty of medicine of the University of Montreal), Dr Fernand Labrie (chairman of the Health Research Fund of the province of Québec), and Dr Bernard Leduc, representing the Medical Research Council of Canada.

The almost 3,000 registrants (a new record) came from over 50 countries on five continents: 46% from Europe, 27% from the American continent and 13% from Asia. The program was built up from the suggestions of the 114 members of national and international program committees, representing 26 countries. To cope with the increased number of topics and multidisciplinary nature of atherosclerosis research we expanded the number of plenary sessions to five, of workshops to 28 (each with seven speakers) and of state-of-the-art symposia to five, and invited young, promising researchers as speakers as well as established investigators. Scientists with known communication skills were engaged for the state-of-the-art reviews of both basic research and clinical trials. Particular emphasis was placed on genetics, molecular mechanisms and the clinical relevance of research findings; workshops 22–28 in particular were designed to be of major interest to cardiologists and vascular physiologists. Three workshops were devoted to recent advances, some of them spectacular, in therapeutics.

Considerable efforts were made to optimize the display of posters, of which 1,186 were accepted, and to synchronize them with related workshop topics. For a new Young Investigator Award competition (underwritten by Merck Frosst Canada), 371 poster abstracts were submitted, from which 25 finalists were selected, and from these the five winners were selected by the international board of judges on the basis of the quality of the full poster and its presentation (p 8). The poster abstracts were for the first time published as a volume (109) of the journal *Atherosclerosis*, which was available to many of the registrants, via their usual mailing of the journal, 2 weeks before the meeting as well as at the meeting itself. This facility was made possible through the close cooperation of the scientific editor (Dr F. Peter Woodford), another innovation for this Symposium, working from London with the publishers in Amsterdam and the printers in Eire. Dr

Woodford has also edited all the papers in these proceedings.

Besides the Young Investigator Awards there were two further meritorious awards: the Fredrickson Career Award was bestowed on Robert Wissler (p 11) and the Distinguished Achievement Award, the first of its kind, on Daria Haust (p 7).

Observing the Symposium in action brought to mind this passage in Milton's *Areopagitica*:

> "Where there is much desire to learn, there of necessity will be much arguing, much writing, many opinions; for opinion in good men is but knowledge in the making."

I hope that readers of this book will conclude that knowledge was indeed made, by good men and women, at the Xth International Symposium on Atherosclerosis.

Atherosclerosis X.
F.P. Woodford, J. Davignon and A. Sniderman, editors.

International symposia of the International Atherosclerosis Society: an overview

Gotthard Schettler
Past President, International Atherosclerosis Society
Ludolf-Krehl-Klinik, Heidelberg, Germany

The first International Symposium on Atherosclerosis was held in Athens in 1965 under the chairmanship of Costas Miras [1]. This small meeting was the "germ cell" for all the subsequent Symposia, and its mentor and superstar was undoubtedly "Mr Coronary", the unforgettable Paul Dudley White.

Four years later, Robert Wissler invited participants to the 2nd International Symposium. More than 200 scientists met in Chicago in November 1969, under the chairmanship of Louis N. Katz. This symposium was organized with the help of the International Society of Cardiology, the European Atherosclerosis Group and the American Heart Association. The subjects discussed were the pathogenesis of atherosclerosis, reactions of the arterial wall, thrombosis and atherosclerosis, lipids and lipoproteins, environmental and host factors, nutrition, advances in drug therapy affecting lipids, platelets, and autonomic nerve mediators. Some research lines for the future were proposed under the title "Progress in the control of atherosclerosis".

The keynote address [2] mentioned many of the problems we still face today, even though from one Symposium to the next significant, even epoch-making, advances have been made in many areas. In the field of prevention, however, success is only partial, especially in those Western countries where adoption of healthier diets and lifestyles has been only half-hearted. It is significant too that when countries of the former East European bloc, or rural areas in the Far East formerly on subsistence economies, have gained access in recent years to more Western food there has been a considerable increase in degenerative cardiovascular diseases, including stroke.

The 3rd International Symposium on Atherosclerosis was held in West Berlin in October 1973, and was sponsored by the American Heart Association, the British Atherosclerosis Group, the European Atherosclerosis Group, the International Society of Cardiology and the relevant ministries of the Federal Republic of Germany [3]. Dr Richard von Weizsäcker, the mayor of West Berlin, delivered a remarkable address on "The Responsibility of International Science". As a novelty, *workshops* were introduced at this symposium, as was a new topic, "Molecular principles of atherosclerosis". The number of participants exceeded 400.

The fourth Symposium was held in Tokyo in August 1976, under the chairmanship of K. Oshima. Stress was laid on the special characteristics of atherosclerosis in the Far East [4]. In Tokyo it was decided to form an *International Atherosclerosis Society* (IAS) in order to facilitate international co-operation in atherosclerosis research, and in particular to make it easier to seek funding for these international symposia. A vital contribution to the preparatory work was made by Dr Daria Haust as secretary of the Task Force charged with drawing up proposals for founding the International Atherosclerosis Society, together with the other members, Antonio Gotto, William Holmes and Rodolfo Paoletti. The first

Executive Committee elected in Milan in 1977 consisted of Antonio Gotto, Daria Haust and myself. The 1979 International Symposium therefore took place for the first time under the auspices of the IAS.

The IAS was conceived as an umbrella body for the existing national and regional groups concerned with atherosclerosis, in an attempt to serve as a catalyst, collator and co-ordinator, and in order to stimulate the formation of new national societies.

One of the most important objectives of the IAS [5] is to foster and encourage young investigators by establishing special scholarships, facilitating contacts between them, providing a forum for travel support to the international gatherings, and involving them in the organizational activities of the IAS.

The 5th International Symposium was held in Houston, Texas, in November 1979, under the Chairmanship of Antonio M. Gotto Jr. This meeting was greatly helped by the Baylor College of Medicine and The Methodist Hospital, Houston. Special awards were conferred on Mrs Mary Lasker of New York and Princess Lilian of Belgium for their longstanding support of biomedical research. From the *Proceedings* it is obvious that enormous progress had been made in the field of cardiovascular surgery [6]. Striking too were the results of clinical trials of new drugs and investigations of the interaction between vascular wall and platelets. Of course, plasma lipids and lipoproteins were again the subjects of extensive presentations and discussions. Discussions about the role of nutrition in the prevention of coronary heart disease were heated, but finally led to dietary recommendations which are still valid today. More than 1,400 scientists participated in this meeting.

A unanimous resolution was passed in Houston to hold the 6th Symposium again in West Berlin [7]. This Symposium took place in June 1982, when 1,400 scientists represented 42 nations. For the first time *poster sessions* were held. This form of presentation was very successful and gave rise to lively discussions.

The 7th International Symposium was held in Melbourne in October 1985, under the chairmanship of Paul Nestel. Since the previous Symposium, the volume of research activity had continued to rise rapidly, and this was reflected in the strength and breadth of scientific advances reported [8]. Nearly 1,000 scientists attended to present their work; there were four Plenary Sessions and 19 Workshops. Scientific interest focused on problems of nutrition and the atherosclerotic process and in this field, the host Australian Society documented some remarkable successes. Considerable progress had also been made in the use of new technologies, for a new era of research had been inaugurated by the molecular geneticists. In particular the work of Brown and Goldstein, for which they were awarded the Nobel Prize, turned out to be extremely fruitful for further research.

The 8th Symposium was held in Rome, in October 1988, under the chairmanship of Gaetano Crepaldi [9]. The pathology and therapy of genetic disorders were again discussed, as well as of diseases caused by environmental factors. At the center of attention were the results of cellular biology, molecular biology, human lipoprotein disorders, lipoprotein receptors, and the role of apoproteins. The effects of hemodynamic and rheological factors on atherosclerosis were also emphasized. As the main scientific interest of the chairman was diabetes, this disease as a promoter of atherosclerosis was presented in some detail. As with previous meetings, social events were also an important part of the Symposium, taking due note of the location in the Eternal City. Satellite Symposia took place elsewhere in Italy: Florence, Venice, Siena, Milan and Cagliari. A notable symposium on diabetes was held in Apulia.

The 9th Symposium has a special fate. Jerusalem had been chosen as the venue. Yechezkiel Stein had nearly completed the preparations, when the Gulf War with all its consequences on the host country broke out in early in 1991 and precluded the holding of the Symposium in Jerusalem. After several alternative sites had been considered, it was decided to move the Symposium to Chicago. It is amazing that Yechezkiel and Olga Stein and their staff managed to transfer all the organizational work to Chicago within a short time and without major hitch. Despite these adverse conditions, the Committee presented a diverse program including 9 hours for plenary sessions, 12 hours for sponsored symposia and 1,000 posters, and 18 hours for 22 workshops. Thus the activities at the Chicago Symposium reached the acme of all symposia held previously. If one compares the scientific contributions presented at that meeting [10] with those at the initial symposia, one is impressed by the enormous advances that had been made in cell biology, molecular biology and genetics, and also in the field of clinical research, long-term trials, therapeutic drugs and prevention of atherosclerosis.

The International Atherosclerosis Society currently has over 4,700 members in 38 countries. Four corporate sponsors (Bristol-Myers Squibb Company; Merck Sharp & Dohme; Parke-Davis Division, Warner-Lambert Company; and Sandoz Pharmaceuticals Corporation) have contributed to the President's Fund, which established the office of the Executive Director, allows publication of the Newsletter, and supports the Visiting Fellowship Program. Sandoz Pharmaceuticals Corporation has sponsored the Donald S. Fredrickson Award; the current recipient of this award, to be made at this symposium, is Robert W. Wissler.

And so we come to the 10th International Symposium on Atherosclerosis here in Montreal, under the chairmanship of Jean Davignon, which builds on the scientific and social traditions of the previous Symposia and will doubtless surpass them. One of Jean's many innovations was that the pre-conference abstracts were published as a volume of the journal *Atherosclerosis*, which has been the official journal of the IAS since 1980, although it was founded as an independent journal in the Elsevier stable some 20 years earlier at the instigation of Frits Böttcher in Leiden, The Netherlands, a pioneer in the analysis of lipids of the arterial wall. A second innovation is that the *Proceedings* of the Symposium are to be published by the same publishers as publish that journal. Both the abstracts and the *Proceedings* have benefited from the attentions of a Scientific Editor, Dr Peter Woodford, who was, interestingly, the first editor of the international journal *Atherosclerosis*, when it was published in English, French and German, more than 30 years ago.

References

1. Miras C, Howard A, Paoletti R. International Symposium on Atherosclerosis, Athens, 1965. Progress in Biochemical Pharmacology, vol 4. Basel: Karger, 1966.
2. Jones RJ. Atherosclerosis II. Proceedings of the Second International Symposium on Atherosclerosis, Chicago, Nov 2–5, 1969. New York, Heidelberg, Berlin: Springer-Verlag, 1970.
3. Schettler G, Weizel A. Atherosclerosis III. Proceedings of the Third International Symposium on Atherosclerosis, Berlin, Oct 24–28, 1973. New York, Heidelberg, Berlin: Springer-Verlag, 1974.
4. Schettler G, Goto Y, Hata Y, Klose G. Atherosclerosis IV. Proceedings of the Fourth International Symposium on Atherosclerosis, Tokyo, Aug 24–28, 1976. New York, Heidelberg, Berlin: Springer-Verlag, 1977.
5. Haust MD. A brief history and aims of the International Atherosclerosis Society (IAS). Atherosclerosis 1988;73:273–275.
6. Gotto AM Jr, Smith LC, Allen B. Atherosclerosis V. Proceedings of the Fifth International Symposium on Atherosclerosis, Houston, Nov 6–9, 1979. New York, Heidelberg, Berlin: Springer-Verlag, 1980.
7. Schettler G, Gotto AM Jr, Middelhoff G, Habenicht AJR, Jurutka KR. Atherosclerosis VI. Proceedings of the Sixth International Symposium on Atherosclerosis, Berlin, Jun 13–17, 1982. New York, Heidelberg, Berlin: Springer-Verlag, 1983.

6

8. NH Fidge, PJ Nestel. Atherosclerosis VII. Proceedings of the Seventh International Symposium on Atherosclerosis, Melbourne, Oct 6—10, 1985. Amsterdam, New York, Oxford: Excerpta Medica, 1986.
9. Crepaldi G, Gotto AM Jr, Manzato E, Baggio G. Atherosclerosis VIII. Proceedings of the Eighth International Symposium on Atherosclerosis, Rome, Oct 9—13, 1988. Amsterdam, New York, Oxford: Excerpta Medica, 1989.
10. Stein O, Eisenberg S, Stein Y. Atherosclerosis IX. Proceedings of the Ninth International Symposium on Atherosclerosis, Rosemont-Chicago, Oct 6—10, 1991. Tel Aviv: R & L Creative Communications Ltd, 1992.

©1995 Elsevier Science B.V. All rights reserved.
Atherosclerosis X.
F.P. Woodford, J. Davignon and A. Sniderman, editors.

Presentation of the 1994 Distinguished Service Award of the IAS and the establishment and naming of the M. Daria Haust Fellowship

Antonio M. Gotto Jr

President, International Atherosclerosis Society

It falls to me, on behalf of the International Atherosclerosis Society, to make not one but two presentations to our distinguished colleague Dr M. Daria Haust: first, the Society's Distinguished Service Award, and secondly the naming of the IAS Fellowship for young researchers in the field of atherosclerosis as the M. Daria Haust Fellowship.

Both presentations express the gratitude and admiration of the Society for Dr Haust's enthusiastic support of the Society and its goals. Together with William Holmes, Rodolfo Paoletti and me, Dr Haust served on the task force that founded the IAS in 1978, and has acted as Treasurer since that time. But it would be difficult to state briefly the many ways she has nurtured the IAS over these 16 years. A scientist of truly international stature, Dr Haust's leadership role in atherosclerosis research has helped this organization realize its global character.

Yet the IAS is but one of the numerous organizations that have benefited from her considerable knowledge and energy. Dr Haust, of Polish origin, began her career in medicine in Heidelberg, Germany, at Ruprecht-Karls University, where she received her Doctor of Medicine degree in 1951. She completed her residency in pathology at Kingston General Hospital and Queen's University in Kingston, Ontario where she also obtained a Master of Science degree in Medicine. In 1959, she became a Fellow of the Royal College of Physicians and Surgeons (Canada). From her initial appointment as Assistant Professor of Pathology at Queen's University, Dr Haust has established a reputation for excellence in research, practice, education, and service. She currently holds three professorships at the University of Western Ontario in London, Ontario — in Pathology, Pediatrics, and Obstetrics and Gynecology. Dr Haust's work in pediatric pathology is especially noteworthy; she is Director of Pathology at the Children's Psychiatric Research Institute in London, Ontario and serves as consultant to several Ontario hospitals. Dr Haust has lectured frequently in Canada and abroad, and her scholarly publications number well over 200. In addition to her work with the IAS, she has participated actively in many professional societies around the world, and is past president of the Society for Pediatric Pathology and of the Canadian Atherosclerosis Society.

In 1988, Dr Haust was awarded a Gold Medal from the IAS in recognition of her pioneering research in atherosclerosis, and she is of course Honorary Chairman of this Symposium. She has received numerous other honors, including the Special Recognition Award of the American Heart Association's Council on Arteriosclerosis and the Andreas Vesalius Medal "for scholastic and scientific contributions to medicine" by the University of Padova, Padua, Italy — both awarded in 1993.

Rarely does an individual make significant contributions to knowledge in such broad areas as has Dr Haust. What distinguishes her is a passion for achievement, measured in terms of commitment to medical progress and the alleviation of human suffering. It is therefore my great pleasure to announce the establishment of the M. Daria Haust Fellowship, which is intended to commend those who would emulate these ideals, and I hope I have succeeded in conveying why it has been named in her honor.

8

Presentation of the Young Investigator Awards for the best poster presentation at the Xth International Symposium on Atherosclerosis

Antonio M. Gotto Jr
President, International Atherosclerosis Society

The seven judges for this hard-fought competition were from six countries: Drs Giovanella Baggio (Italy), Ulrike Beisiegel (Germany; chair), Katherine Cianflone (Canada), Jean Dallongeville (France), Anna Kessling (UK), Henry J. Pownall (USA) and Edward J. Rubin (USA). Each of them scrutinized all poster abstracts that had been accorded a score of 7/10 or more by the preliminary specialist reviewers, and listed in rank order those they considered the best 20. These lists combined yielded the 25 finalists whose poster abstracts were asterisked in the published poster abstracts in *Atherosclerosis* volume 109 and whose posters were separately displayed in the exhibition hall. Six of the seven judges (Dr Rubin was unfortunately prevented from attending the Symposium) visited the posters on display, listened to their presentation and accorded them a score, which when combined yielded five winners out of the 371 submissions.

The judges asked me to say how instructive it was to hear the opinion of experts from very different fields from their own; for this reason the range of scores was often quite wide. However, the judges were agreed on two things: all the finalists' posters and their presentations were first-rate, and it was extremely difficult to select the best. The judges also wanted me to emphasize that in the run-up to the final they had considered all the poster abstracts submitted for the competition, not just those of the finalists; and if one of the finalists was a judge's colleague that judge had refrained from voting.

Finally, the judges wanted me to say that there were as many as *nine* close runners-up who were within a whisker of winning one of the awards. So for those who didn't make it this time, and who are still under 37 years of age, allow me to wish you good luck in the competition which we hope will be held at the XIth international symposium in 3 years' time.

Each of the five winners receives a certificate from the Society which they may like to frame and hang on the wall of their laboratory or clinic, plus 2,000 Canadian dollars which have been donated by our sponsor, Merck Frosst Canada. Here they are, then, not in order of merit (because this was impossible to determine), but in strict alphabetical order. The page reference is to *Atherosclerosis* vol 109 (September 1994).

Dr **A.K.M.J. Bhuiyan** (India), Department of Pathology, University of British Columbia at Vancouver, Canada, for the poster *Effect of diet on tissue levels of acyl-CoA binding protein*, p. 123.

Dr **J. Luoma**, University of Tampere, Finland, for *Expression of α_2-macroglobulin receptor/LDL receptor-related protein and scavenger receptor in human atherosclerotic lesions*, p. 115.

Dr **W.A. Mann**, University Hospital Eppendorf, Hamburg, Germany, for *Lipoprotein lipase can compensate for the defective function of apolipoprotein E variants in lipoprotein binding to cells*, p. 262.

Dr **A. von Eckhardstein**, Institute of Clinical Chemistry, Munster, Germany, for *Uptake, transfer, and esterification of cell-derived cholesterol in plasma of patients with familial HDL deficiency*, p. 232.

Dr **S. Wölle**, Warner Lambert Company, Parke Davis Pharmaceutical Research Division in Ann Arbor, Michigan, USA, for *Bovine scavenger receptor (SR) overexpression in murine liver blocks the diet-induced increase in apoB-containing lipoproteins*, p. 103.

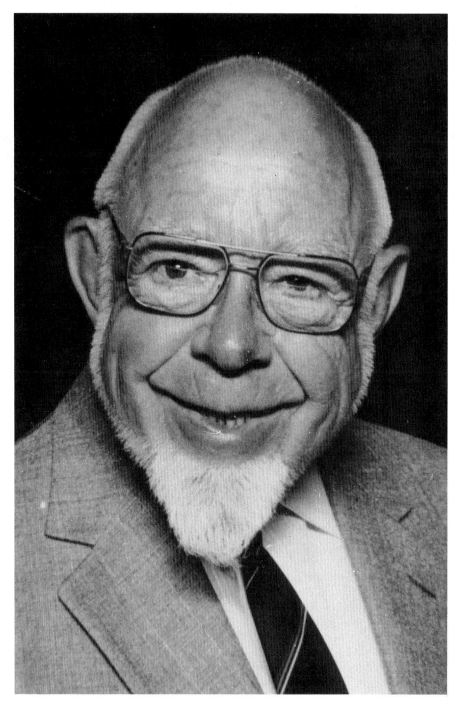

DR ROBERT W. WISSLER — 1994

Tribute to Dr Robert W. Wissler, the 1994 D.S. Fredrickson Career Awardee

M. Daria Haust

Department of Pathology, University of Western Ontario and CPRI, London, Ontario, Canada N6A 5C1

The D.S. Fredrickson Career Award was established by the International Atherosclerosis Society (IAS) at the IXth International Symposium on Atherosclerosis (ISA) held at Chicago-Rosemont, October 6–11, 1991.

As stipulated in the terms of reference, the recipient of this Award must be an outstanding scientist in the field of cardiovascular diseases in general, and in atherosclerosis in particular, and a renowned scholar. Dr Wissler not only fulfills these prerequisites, but in addition has been a devoted teacher, physician, organizer and administrator. Moreover, and as importantly, Dr Wissler as a man possesses qualities that command respect, admiration and warmth. Let us look therefore first at the man before considering his achievements in science and scholarly activities.

The man

It has been said: "Take closeness to the earth (soil), exposure to fresh air, affection and tranquillity at home, but also a firm hand in upbringing and early exposure to enquiry and learning, and you have the making of a very special human being". Whoever formulated the above must have known the early years of Dr Wissler's life.

Dr Robert W. Wissler was born on March 1, 1917 at his parents' home on South 17th Street in Richmond, Indiana. His father was a secondary school teacher and a senior administrator. His mother was also a teacher, but neither the home nor the upbringing of her two children were of secondary importance to her. "Mom raised chickens for the eggs and the occasional broiler" remembers Dr Wissler of these days. The family, including the only other child, his 9-year-older sister Eleanor, doted upon the little boy with the blond hair, called Bobby.

When he was 3 years old the family moved to live on a farm which was 18 miles west of Richmond (please note the address: the Lost Mile Road!). This location assumed quite a significance or a special sign of destination, because it was precisely halfway between Bobby's birth town (Richmond) and the place (Newcastle) where his future sweetheart and wife, Elizabeth Anne, was growing up! There was no electricity, inside plumbing or motor-driven vehicle on the farm; a windmill and the carriage horse, Old Billy, facilitated the daily life. The little boy, Bobby, thrived and the closely-knit family was happy on the farm. The family closeness extended to other members: grandparents, uncles, aunts and cousins, and the "get-togethers" on Sundays took place often (Fig. 1).

This was the time that brought Bobby close to nature and her creatures as he befriended "Old Billy", little calves and other animals. His teacher-parents introduced him to books early during this period.

When Bobby was 6 years of age the family moved to Hagerstown, Indiana, where he was enrolled in school. Soon he showed an eagerness to learn and a remarkable gift in all subjects. A "B" grade was an exception on his report cards. Of note is that in those

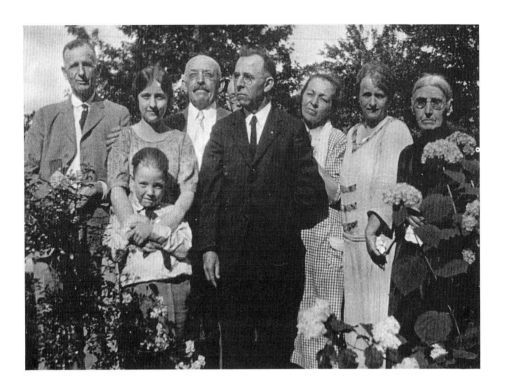

Fig. 1. Bobby (about 6 years old) in front of his sister Eleanor, is visiting Aunt Kate (Dad's sister) on a Sunday afternoon in Cambridge City, Indiana (with parents, grandma, uncles, aunts and cousins).

days even a "B" grade amounted to 90–95 percent with an "A" grade accounting for 95–100 percent! A report card of grade 3 indicates other also well-established trends and patterns that later will be so characteristic of Dr Wissler: appreciation of art and music, and self-discipline and dependability; he was not tardy even once through the entire year (Fig. 2).

The family moved back to Richmond, where Bobby entered grade 4, and went on to high school. He became involved in many extracurricular activities including those of the Boy Scouts of America (Fig. 3), while maintaining his scholastic achievements at the highest possible level and a remarkable self-discipline; in grade 12, e.g., he never once was tardy or absent (Fig. 4).

His high-school achievements earned Robert (Bob; no longer Bobby!) a 4-year, full tuition scholarship to the prestigious Earlham College founded in 1847, in Richmond. He majored in Biology and Chemistry, earning his first (an AB) degree in 1939 and a David Worth Dennis Award for excellence in chemistry.

The years in college were enormously stimulating and enriching in many ways, and enhanced the already existing foundation of a broad education as well as the enjoyment of life. "There was a rich mixture of drama, debating, band, orchestra, cross-country skiing, tennis playing, writing, and editing the school's newspaper and yearbook" remembers Dr Wissler fondly. Here, too, he met a fellow student, Miss Elizabeth (Betty) Anne Polk who graduated the same year (Fig. 5) and went on with him to the University

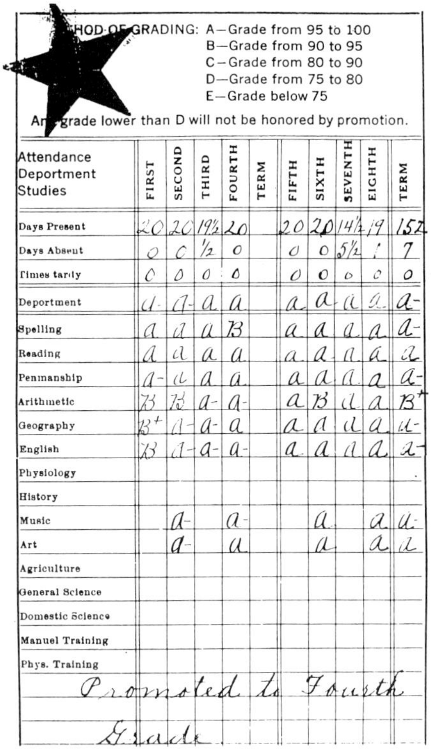
HOD OF GRADING: A—Grade from 95 to 100
B—Grade from 90 to 95
C—Grade from 80 to 90
D—Grade from 75 to 80
E—Grade below 75

A… grade lower than D will not be honored by promotion.

Attendance Deportment Studies	FIRST	SECOND	THIRD	FOURTH	TERM	FIFTH	SIXTH	SEVENTH	EIGHTH	TERM
Days Present	20	20	19½	20		20	20	14½	19	152
Days Absent	0	0	½	0		0	0	5½	1	7
Times tardy	0	0	0	0		0	0	0	0	0
Deportment	a-	a-	a	a		a	a	a	a	a-
Spelling	a	a	a	B		a	a	a	a	a-
Reading	a	a	a	a		a	a	a	a	a
Penmanship	a-	a	a	a		a	a	a	a	a-
Arithmetic	B	B	a-	a-		a	B	a	a	B+
Geography	B+	a-	a-	a		a	a	a	a	a-
English	B	a-	a-	a-		a	a	a	a	a-
Physiology										
History										
Music		a-		a-			a		a	a-
Art		a-		a			a		a	a
Agriculture										
General Science										
Domestic Science										
Manuel Training										
Phys. Training										

Promoted to Fourth Grade

Fig. 2. A grade 3 report card at school in Hagerstown, Indiana. Note the star (in upper left corner), the "value" of grades "A" and "B", and the absence of tardiness, in addition to the scholarship.

of Chicago. They were married a year later, had four children (and then also grandchildren) and have shared all the joys and sorrows of life in a long blissful union. They continued the tradition of their own upbringing in providing a loving, caring atmosphere at home, with close ties not only to their children but also to the relatives. Dr Wissler, a devoted family man, never omits to "sequester" off from his busy life time for family vacations, reunions with relatives and frequent visits with them. Amongst the latter is his, now 86-year-old, beloved sister, Eleanor, who so doted upon him in his youth (and later). She lives some 160 miles away and Dr and Mrs Wissler visit her often.

In the course of his professional life Dr Wissler travelled many times around the globe, lived in several countries (on sabbatical and study leaves), and made innumerable friends amongst foreigners, whom he also received in his laboratories as guests, or as graduate and postgraduate students. Thus, he became a true cosmopolitan. Nevertheless, he has been an American patriot in the pure meaning of that word. One never hears him speak on that subject nor does he ever boast about his country, but his deeds, quiet as they may be, attest to his love of his native land. At the time of the Korean War he served as a first lieutenant in the USPHS and proudly wore his uniform for 2 years.

Restriction upon space does not allow me to address other (and so many different) sides of Dr Wissler's personality, nor enlarge upon his lifelong love for the outdoors (his still competent tennis-playing often leaves younger players in awe), art, music and poetry.

14

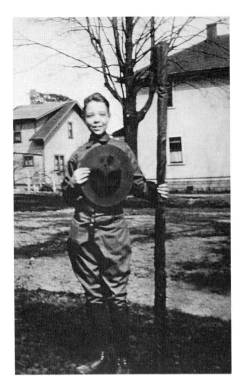

Fig. 3. This handsome 12-year-old Bobby, displaying the 6-foot army kite awarded to him as first prize for winning a city-wide kite contest in Richmond, Indiana (his native town), is dressed in his first Boy Scouts of America uniform. The prize is taller than the winner!

He himself is in a sense a poet, and his after-dinner speeches, addresses and Christmas letters are often delivered in rhymes. Gardening and photography also belong to his hobbies.

Dr Wissler has been devoting much time and energy to causes other than his profession. He served on various Committees/Boards of the Boy Scouts and his church in Chicago, and at the Earlham College.

Just where he finds the energies for all his activities is his secret — or perhaps he owes these to a special blessing from above.

The physician, scientist, scholar and teacher

The activities pertaining to this section are even more difficult to summarize on a few pages than were those in the preceding part. Again, the multitude and the versatility of these activities, and the associated honors and distinctions accorded Dr Wissler in recognition of his achievements, are truly overwhelming.

This chapter began at the University of Chicago School of Medicine which Dr Wissler entered in 1939 and which to this day remains his base, and Chicago his hometown. In the large city, the young man from a provincial town was attracted to nature, exploring the wonders of Lake Michigan and its beaches (Fig. 6).

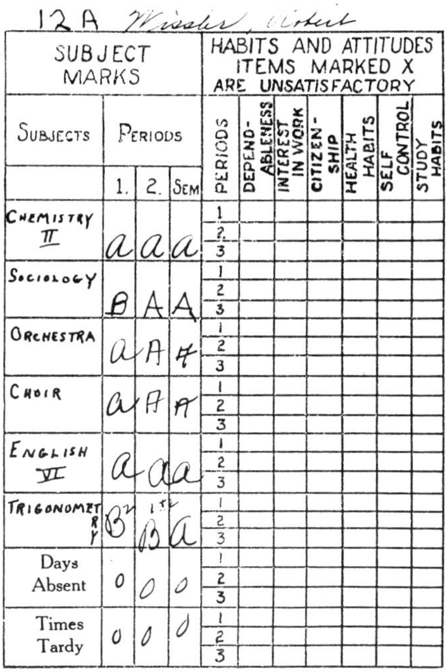

12 A *Wissler, Robert*

SUBJECT MARKS				HABITS AND ATTITUDES ITEMS MARKED X ARE UNSATISFACTORY								
SUBJECTS	PERIODS			PERIODS	DEPENDABLENESS	INTEREST IN WORK	CITIZENSHIP	HEALTH HABITS	SELF CONTROL	STUDY HABITS		
	1.	2.	SEM									
CHEMISTRY II	*a*	*a*	*a*	1 2 3								
SOCIOLOGY	*B*	A	A	1 2 3								
ORCHESTRA	*a*	*A*	*A*	1 2 3								
CHOIR	*a*	*A*	*A*	1 2 3								
ENGLISH VI	*a*	*a*	*a*	1 2 3								
TRIGONOMETRY	B		*a*	1 2 3								
Days Absent	0	0	0	1 2 3								
Times Tardy	0	0	0	1 2 3								

Fig. 4. This high school record earned Bob a 4-year full-tuition scholarship to Earlham College in Richmond, Indiana. Note: there were no examples of tardiness or of absent days.

In 1941 Bob withdrew from the School of Medicine and began working under the supervision of Dr Paul R. Cannon in the field of immunological and nutritional research sponsored by the Army and Navy. Later (1944) he received an award for his "civilian work with US Army." He enrolled in the graduate program at the University of Chicago, obtaining his MS degree in 1943, and continued as a graduate student in the Department of Pathology, receiving his PhD degree in 1946. The doctoral thesis was based on the results of his work on the effects of protein depletion upon the resistance of rabbits and rats to pneumococcal infection. In recognition of this work he received in 1947 the Howard Taylor Ricketts Graduate Student Award for Outstanding Research in Pathology and Bacteriology (Fig. 7).

Perhaps the association with and an appointment in the Department of Pathology during the years of graduate studies stimulated or motivated (now) Dr Wissler to complete his education in Medicine. He obtained his MD degree (with honors in Pathology) from the University of Chicago in 1948. Subsequently, he interned at the Chicago Marine Hospital of USPHS (1949–50) and completed the postgraduate training (residency and fellowship) at the University of Chicago Hospitals and Clinics (1950–53).

Dr Wissler's academic career actually began when he enrolled as a graduate student and was appointed as Instructor in the Department of Pathology (1943). Upon receiving his PhD degree he was promoted to Assistant Professor (1947), quickly progressing through the ranks and assuming chairmanship of the Department as full Professor in 1957. He held that post for 18 years (until 1972) and was awarded thereafter the Donald N. Pritzker Professorship of Pathology (1972–76) and the Donald N. Pritzker Distinguished

16

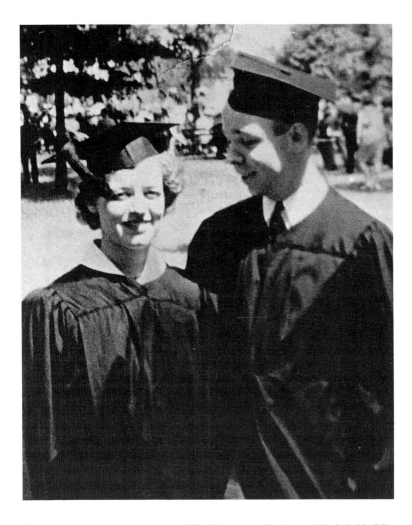

Fig. 5. Graduation from college, June 1939. Bob seems to be interested only in his fellow graduating student, Miss Elizabeth Anne Polk, who went on with him to the University of Chicago and whom he married a year later.

Service Professorship of Pathology (1977–87). Dr Wissler's status as an Emeritus Professor (active) conferred upon him in 1987, continues. Locally, Dr Wissler held also appointments as Professor at the Franklin McLean Memorial Institute (1953–80), Professor in the College of the University of Chicago (1965–80) and Cancer Coordinator for the Medical School (1965–75). He continues to be very active in academic affairs as a Professor on Graduate Committees at his University. It would be impossible to cite all the Committees of the University of Chicago or her Hospitals and Clinics on which Dr Wissler served, but their number amounts to approximately 25!

Notable are also academic appointments beyond Dr Wissler's own University: Visiting Scientist, Theodore Kocher Institute, University of Bern, Switzerland (1963); Faculty at

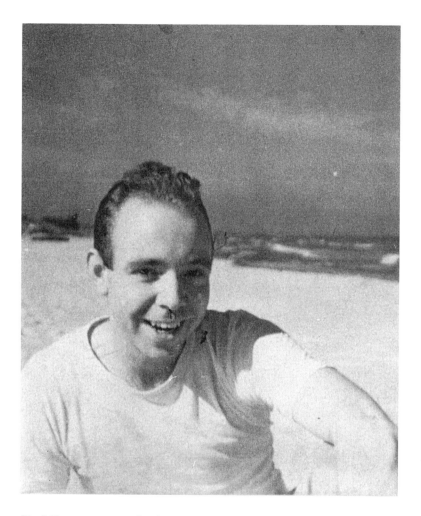

Fig. 6. The young man remains close to nature also in Chicago; here he discovers the wonders of Lake Michigan and its beautiful beaches.

Given Institute of Pathobiology, Aspen, Colorado (1964,71—73,78—81); Visiting Professor of Pathology, Nihon University School of Medicine, Tokyo, Japan (1974); and Visiting Scientist, Baker Institute for Medical Research, Melbourne, Australia (1985).

Equally impossible would be to make an attempt at listing all the committees of professional and related Societies at the city (Chicago), state (Illinois), national and international levels on which Dr Wissler served in his long and distinguished career as a Chairman, Member or Consultant. These are cited on three and a half single-typed pages! I shall provide a few examples, when he served as a President or Chairman of such Societies: American (Am) Association (Assn) for Accreditation for Laboratory Animal Care; Am Assn of Pathologists (Pathol) and Bacteriologists; Council on Arteriosclerosis of the Am Heart Assn; Council on Pathol of the Am Medical Assn; Am Society for Experimental Pathol; Scientific Advisory Board of the Armed Forces Institute of Pathol; Assn of Pathology Chairmen; Universities Associated for Research and Education in

18

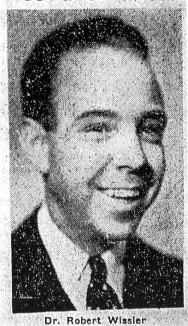

Dr. Wissler Is Awarded Prize For Outstanding Research Work

Dr. Robert Wissler, assistant professor of pathology at the University of Chicago, has been awarded the Howard Taylor Ricketts prize for outstanding research.

The award was announced recently by R. Wendell Harrison, dean of the Biological Sciences division at the university.

Dr. Wissler is the son of Mr. and Mrs. W. O. Wissler, 716 National road west. His father formerly was principal of Hibberd Junior High school and had taught in this district for many years.

Dr. Wissler received the prize for studies which demonstrate the effect of a protein deficient diet on pneumococcal infection. The title of his prize-winning research paper is "The Effects of Protein-Depletion and Subsequent Immunization upon the Response of Experimental Animals to Intradermal Pneumococcal Infection."

Nutrition Importance

His experiments pointed directly to the importance of nutrition in resistance against infectious agents and have bearing on the problem of infectious diseases as they are occurring in the hungry persons in the world today.

Dr. Robert Wissler

Thursday, June 19, 1947

Fig. 7. Dr Robert Wissler's research begins making news, as the press takes notice of the achievements of this young man with a PhD degree.

Pathology; Am Assn for Cancer Research (Chicago Chapter); Chicago Assn of Immunologists; Chicago Health Research Foundation; Chicago Heart Assn; Chicago Pathol Society, and others.

Dr Wissler has been also serving on National Boards (for Specialty Examinations) (Diplomate of National Board of Medical Examiners (Chairman); Diplomate of the Am Board of Pathol; Trustee of the Am Board of Pathol (President)) and on seven different Study Sections of the USPHS relating to Pathology and programs at the National Heart, Lung and Blood Institute (NIH).

His widely reaching, innovative research ensured Dr Wissler a place on Editorial Boards (as Associate Editor or Member) of eight scientific periodicals, and he still continues as a Member on one (Applied Pathology). He edited or co-edited nine monographs or Proceedings of major symposia. He was invited to teach at numerous Universities in the USA and abroad, deliver lectures or participate in other forms on scientific programs at innumerable national and international Congresses, Symposia and Conferences on a wide range of topics, and was the actual host himself to the second International Symposium On Atherosclerosis in Chicago, 2–5 November, 1969. Parenthetically, Dr Wissler has been a participant in all 10 of these Symposia; it was he who introduced the concept of International Symposia when a small international group of scientists gathered in Athens, Greece in 1966. It was also Dr Wissler who was instrumental in the establishment of the interdisciplinary Specialized Centers of Research in Atherosclerosis (SCOR) supported by the NIH, when he was the Chairman of the Long Range Planning Committee of the Council on Arteriosclerosis of the Am Heart Assn (1966–67). When this was realized, he directed one of these centers (Chicago) (1972–81). It was on his initiative, too, that the Multicenter Cooperative Study of the Pathobiological Determinants of Atherosclerosis in Youth (PDAY) was "created" in 1985 and has been supported since by the NIH. Naturally, Dr Wissler has been its first and only Program Director.

Dr Wissler published 318 full-length scientific communications and 10 are in press. Is there any wonder that he has been the recipient of Prizes, Awards, Special Lecturer Awards, Orations, Medals, Distinguished Achievement Awards, Gold Headed Cane Award, Gold Key Award and Honorary Memberships from Scientific Societies, Academies and Universities in the USA, Canada and other countries on 25 occasions, and holds honorary degrees from five world-renowned Universities or Colleges? These are:

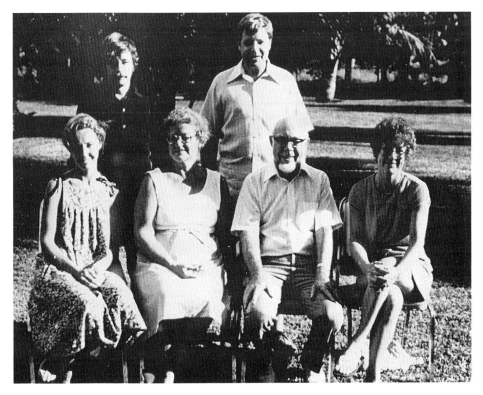

Fig. 8. Dr and Mrs Wissler with their family enjoy a vacation together on the West coast of Mexico in Ixtapa (1975). Mrs Elizabeth Wissler is the soul of the family. The daughter Barbara (seated on the right, next to Dr Wissler) is an exact image of her Mom when she was young (compare with Fig. 5).

20

Earlham College (DSc; 1959), Heidelberg University, Germany (MD, 1973), University of Medicine and Dentistry of New Jersey (DSc; 1982), University of Siena, Italy (MD and Surg; 1982) and Ohio State University (DSc; 1990).

Throughout his professional life Dr Wissler educated cadres of undergraduate students in medicine and in science, and supervised the work and training of innumerable graduate and postgraduate students. Many of the latter became themselves distinguished and prominent in science and medicine and may be found around the world.

Dr Wissler's achievements and impact in research may be broadly defined in three areas:

1. Experimental and (now) human atherosclerosis with emphasis on the pathogenesis of lesions and on their prevention or regression.
2. The basic mechanism of cellular immunity and its disorders.
3. Effects of nutrition on immune mechanisms and cancer.

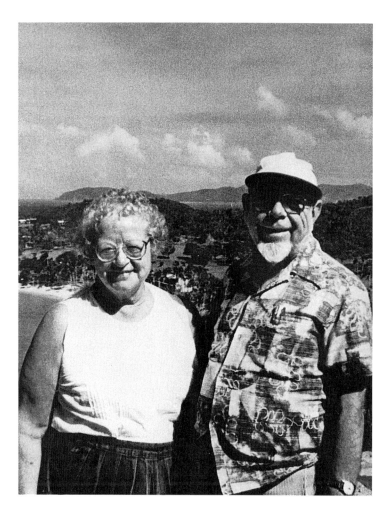

Fig. 9. Dr and Mrs Wissler celebrate their 50 years of marriage on the island of St. John (US-Virgin Island) in January 1990. Dr Wissler wrote: "Betty and Bob still enjoy each other's company most."

This abbreviated account on Dr Wissler's life and work would be incomplete without reference to Mrs Wissler. The old dictum "Behind every successful man is a special woman", does not reflect fully the role Mrs Elizabeth (Betty) Wissler plays in Dr Wissler's life and his stature as a scientist. Lovingly and selflessly, she has been standing by her husband at all times, and she has been the soul of her family (Fig. 8). There were periods when she typed Dr Wissler's manuscripts and lecture materials and assisted him, whenever there was a need, with other professional matters. She has always been sure not to overshadow her husband on social occasions, and being always modest while friendly and warm to his professional colleagues. And so hospitable! When invited to dinner on a professional visit to Chicago, one was certain to dine at Betty and Bob's home and be offered a dinner that was personally prepared by Betty. She remains his best, dearest and trusted friend (Fig. 9). May they live in that uniquely wonderful union for many more years, blessed by good health and the joys of life.

Acknowledgements

The author wishes to thank Mr Roger Dewar, RT for his skillful photographic work, and Mrs Cheryl Campbell and Mrs Joanne Weir for their competent typing of the manuscript.

Plenary Lectures

Atherosclerosis X.
F.P. Woodford, J. Davignon and A. Sniderman, editors.

The oxidative modification hypothesis of atherogenesis: strengths and weaknesses

Daniel Steinberg

University of California, San Diego, Department of Medicine, La Jolla, CA 92093–0682, USA

Abstract. The hypothesis that oxidative modification of LDL plays a pivotal role in atherogenesis is well supported by many lines of evidence but it cannot be considered proven, certainly not for the human disease. Oxidized LDL is taken up avidly by macrophages, partly via the acetyl LDL receptor, but partly also via one or more "oxidized LDL receptors". Recent studies in this laboratory suggest that the persistence of oxidized LDL receptors in evolution relates to their ability to recognize and phagocytose damaged or dying cells. If this is correct, interventions aimed at blocking these receptors could have deleterious consequences and should be approached cautiously.

Introduction

The oxidative modification hypothesis proposes that oxidative damage to low density lipoprotein (LDL) generates a series of modified forms of LDL (OxLDL) that are in a number of ways more atherogenic than native LDL. The implied corollary of the hypothesis is that the increase in atherogenicity associated with this oxidative modification is sufficiently important that inhibition of it will have a measurable beneficial effect on the progression of atherosclerosis.

The origin and development of the LDL oxidative modification hypothesis has been extensively reviewed elsewhere [1,2]. Here we present only a brief overview of the strengths and weaknesses and then present some very recent findings on the receptors that recognize OxLDL.

Strengths of the hypothesis

1. It rests on a well-defined, mechanistically plausible and testable theoretical footing.
2. It is consistent with a large number of phenomena demonstrated in cell culture and, to a more limited extent, in experimental animals. Beginning with the demonstration that OxLDL is taken up by macrophages more rapidly than native LDL (and taken up by way of a specific saturable pathway), a total of more than 15 properties of OxLDL have been reported that *in principle* could make it more atherogenic than native LDL.
3. Antioxidants have been shown to inhibit the development of early atherosclerotic lesions in animal models (LDL receptor-deficient rabbits, cholesterol-fed rabbits and cholesterol-fed monkeys). Moreover, several different antioxidants have been used (probucol, butylated hydroxytoluene, N,N′-diphenyl-phenylenediamine, and vitamin E).
4. Epidemiologic studies, observational and prospective, show that antioxidant intake (vitamin E, vitamin C, β-carotene) is associated with a lower risk of coronary heart disease.
5. It is supported, although not strongly, by the preliminary report of the results in a subset of men in the Physician's Health Survey, who had symptomatic coronary artery

disease at the beginning of the study and who had fewer coronary events on supplementary dietary β-carotene [3].

Weaknesses of the hypothesis

1. While we have learned a great deal about the mechanisms of LDL oxidation in in vitro systems, we still do not know where in the body LDL oxidation occurs, which cell types are involved, or which enzyme systems are involved.
2. While there are many biological properties of oxidized LDL that could, in principle, make it more atherogenic, very few of these have been evaluated in vivo.
3. While there is strong experimental evidence that antioxidants slow the development of the fatty streak, we still do not know whether antioxidants have any effect on the later lesions — the fibrous plaque or the complicated lesion. If the effects are indeed limited to fatty streak formation, some of the currently contemplated trials may be futile to the extent that their endpoints are clinical events in individuals with advanced disease. Perhaps the most logical clinical intervention trial would be one assessing early lesions, e.g., by measuring carotid intima/media thickness or the appearance of *new* coronary lesions.
4. While some epidemiologic studies provide highly significant data showing a negative correlation between antioxidant vitamin intake and risk of CHD, the results are not totally consistent. For example, in some studies vitamin C intake has been associated with decreased CHD and increased longevity, while in others it has had no effect. In any case, epidemiologic studies do not establish causal relationship; they only suggest clinical intervention trials that may settle the issue.
5. The only fully reported intervention study to date is the ATBC trial done in Finland [4]. Neither vitamin E (50 mg/d) nor β-carotene (20 mg/d) reduced CHD clinical events. The primary endpoint was the development of lung cancer, so it is technically not a test of the OxLDL hypothesis. Nevertheless, the failure to see an effect on CHD is sobering. Further studies are needed.

What degree of antioxidant protection is necessary to inhibit progression of atherosclerosis?

Most investigators assess antioxidant agents by isolating LDL from the recipient animal or patient and measuring its diene conjugation lag time under defined pro-oxidant conditions in vitro. Is that a sufficient basis on which to predict efficacy in preventing lesion formation? Possibly not. In a recent study in LDL receptor-deficient rabbits by Fruebis et al. [5], the efficacy of a probucol analog was compared to that of probucol itself. The effects of probucol on lesion formation were very much the same as those previously described by our laboratory — an approximately 50% inhibition — but the analog failed to show any effect, despite the very significant protection it afforded against LDL oxidation ex vivo (using diene conjugation lag time). The analog increased lag time approximately 3-fold yet showed no effect on lesion formation. Probucol caused an approximately 8-fold increase in lag time.

Sasahara et al. [6] treated cholesterol-fed Macaques with probucol and observed a significant inhibition of lesion progression in the thoracic aorta. The extent of protection correlated positively with the increase in lag time. However, there was a suggestion of a "threshold effect" in that only those monkeys with diene conjugation lag times > 400 min showed clear-cut protection. These results and those of Fruebis et al. are compatible with the concept of a "threshold of protection" but they could equally well reflect differences in the metabolic effects of the antioxidants over and above their ability to directly protect LDL. For example, probucol has been shown to have intracellular effects and vitamin E almost surely also has major intracellular effects.

Why have the scavenger receptors persisted in evolution?

Proteins persist in evolution because they confer some biological advantage. Participation of the scavenger receptors in atherosclerosis is obviously not an acceptable *raison d'être*! We have previously suggested [7] that the uptake of oxidized LDL by the scavenger receptor might be a "good guy" operation in the sense that oxidized LDL is cytotoxic and its removal might forestall endothelial damage that could otherwise lead to thrombosis. However, the scavenger receptor family appears to go back even to Drosophila [8] and so the function must be broader still.

Sambrano et al. [9] recently proposed that the essential function of the scavenger receptors may be to recognize and take up damaged and/or dying cells. The rationale was that a plasma membrane, made up of a phospholipid bilayer studded with protein, bears a loose family relationship to an LDL particle, which is surrounded by a phospholipid monolayer studded with protein. In both cases, oxidative damage could lead to the generation of related structures (e.g., aldehydic breakdown products of lipids, cross linking of proteins, masking of epsilon amino groups, etc.). To test the hypothesis, they first used oxidatively damaged red blood cells (OxRBC). The cells were exposed to copper and ascorbic acid for 90 min and then added to a culture of mouse peritoneal macrophages. Washed, untreated cells showed almost no binding. In contrast, the OxRBC bound very avidly. The critical point is that the binding of OxRBC was almost completely inhibited by OxLDL *but not at all by acetyl LDL* or by native LDL. Thus this function would seem to be one primarily not of the acetyl LDL receptor but of one or more OxLDL receptors.

There are a number of candidates for OxLDL receptor on the macrophage. Certainly the acetyl LDL receptor can bind and take up OxLDL [10] but it cannot account for all the uptake [11]. Ottnad et al. [12] have partially purified and characterized a mouse peritoneal macrophage membrane protein that has a significantly higher affinity for oxidized LDL than for acetyl LDL. It is a membrane protein of 94–97 kDa and was purified by conventional methods together with an OxLDL affinity column. Unlike the AcLDL receptor, it has a higher affinity for OxLDL than for AcLDL. Ottnad et al. also demonstrated an OxLDL-binding protein of the same molecular weight in RAW 246 cells, in foam cells recovered from the aortas of cholesterol-fed rabbits, in rabbit peritoneal macrophages and in rabbit subcutaneous carrageenan granulomas. This is most probably the same as the 95-kDa OxLDL ligand-binding protein in rat Kupffer cells demonstrated by de Rijke and van Berkel [13].

Endemann et al. [14], using expression cloning, isolated the mouse homolog of CD36 (muCD36) as an OxLDL-binding protein in mouse peritoneal macrophages. Its role in uptake of OxLDL by the mouse macrophage remains to be evaluated, but Endemann et al. were able to show that transfected cells expressing muCD36 degraded OxLDL 4 times faster than nontransfected cells. Using an antiserum against a fusion protein representing amino acids 169–244 of muCD36, we have shown that it has a molecular weight very like that of the human protein (approximately 88 kDa). Moreover, it separates from the 94–97 kDa receptor during the affinity chromatography step [12]. An intriguing possibility is that the Ottnad receptor and CD36 may act co-operatively in phagocytosis of damaged cells.

How does the macrophage recognize damaged cells?

Sambrano and Steinberg [15] have recently shown that the binding of apoptotic thymocytes to mouse peritoneal macrophages, like that of OxRBC, is inhibited by OxLDL but not by acetyl LDL. However, the inhibition was less complete, averaging only about 50% as compared to the 80–90% inhibition seen with oxidized RBC. Thus there may be more than one mechanism involved, and several studies in the literature suggest that recognition of damaged cells can occur in more than one way [16]. Taken together, our new findings suggest that there may be a broader generality to the role of the OxLDL receptor(s) in recognizing oxidatively damaged or apoptotic cells.

In part, the binding of OxRBC to macrophages probably depends on an increase in phosphatidylserine (PS) in the membrane [15]. Thus:
1. Oxidatively damaged RBC show an increase in phosphatidylserine on the outer leaflet.
2. The binding of OxRBC to macrophages increases progressively with increasing exposure of phosphatidylserine on the outer leaflet.
3. Phosphatidylserine-rich liposomes compete for binding of oxidized RBC and also compete for binding of oxidized LDL to macrophages.
4. A "ligand blot" using phosphatidylserine-rich liposomes (located by the use of fluorescent probes in the liposome or by the use of radioactive annexin V) picks up the same 94–97 kDa band that is picked up by blotting with ^{125}I-OxLDL.

We should quickly add that probably more than one mechanism is involved. Fadok et al. [16], for example, have shown that macrophages from the peritoneal cavity of the mouse recognize apoptotic lymphocytes by a mechanism different from that by which bone marrow macrophages recognize the same cells. In fact it would not be surprising to find that more than one mechanism has evolved for a function as vital as the removal of damaged cells (as during embryogenesis or following infection or tissue damage).

As described above, it appears that the acetyl LDL receptor may not be directly involved in the recognition of damaged cells even though the oxidized LDL receptor(s) is (are). In any case, it would be advisable to proceed cautiously with drugs that compete with these receptors or with other treatments that interfere with their function. If, of course, one could interfere not globally but selectively with receptors in *arterial cells*, that intervention would be less likely to cause unacceptable side effects.

Acknowledgements

This work was supported by a Specialized Center of Research on Arteriosclerosis grant (HL-14197) and by the Stein Institute for Research on Aging.

References

1. Steinberg D, Parthasarathy S, Carew TE, Khoo JC, Witztum JL. N Engl J Med 1989;320:915–924.
2. Steinberg D Witztum JL. J Am Med Assoc 1990;264:3047–3052.
3. Gaziano MJ, Manson JE, Ridker PM, Buring JE, Hennekens CH. Circulation 1990;82:III–201.
4. The Alpha-Tocopherol, Beta Carotene Cancer Prevention Study Group. N Engl J Med 1994;330:1029–1035.
5. Fruebis J, Steinberg D, Dresel HA, Carew TE. J Clin Invest 1994;94:392–398.
6. Sasahara M, Raines EW, Carew TE, Steinberg D, Wahl PW, Chait A, Ross R. J Clin Invest 1994;94: 155–164.
7. Steinberg D. Ann NY Acad Sci 1990;598:125–135.
8. Abrams JM, Lux A, Steller H, Krieger M. Proc Natl Acad Sci USA 1992;89:10375–10379.
9. Sambrano GR, Parthasarathy S, Steinberg D. Proc Natl Acad Sci USA 1994;91:3265–3269.
10. Freeman M, Ekkel Y, Rohrer L, Penman M, Freedman NJ, Chisolm GM, Krieger M. Proc Natl Acad Sci USA 1991;88:4931–4935.

11. Sparrow CP, Parthasarathy S, Steinberg D. J Biol Chem 1989;264:2599–2604.
12. Ottnad E, Parthasarathy S, Sambrano G, Ramprasad MP, Quehenberger O, Kondratenko N, Green S, Steinberg D. Proc Natl Acad Sci USA (in press).
13. de Rijke YB, van Berkel TJC. J Biol Chem 1994;269:824–827.
14. Endemann G, Stanton LW, Madden KS, Bryant CM, White RT, Protter AA. J Biol Chem 1993;268: 11811–11816.
15. Sambrano G, Steinberg D. Proc Natl Acad Sci USA (in press).
16. Fadok VA, Savill JS, Haslett C, Bratton DL, Doherty DE, Campbell PA, Henson PM. J Immunol 1991; 149:4029–4035.

Fredrickson Award Lecture: the PDAY study in perspective

Robert W. Wissler*

The University of Chicago, Department of Pathology, and the PDAY/RFEHA Administrative Center

Abstract. The unique features of the PDAY research program are summarized. The gross findings are briefly considered, especially those which contribute to the importance of early control of atherogenic risk factors, notably genetic variations, hyperlipidemia, smoking, glucose intolerance, obesity, and hypertension. The microscopic, chemical, and immunological discoveries which PDAY has fostered are summarized. Opportunities for future study utilizing material from approximately 3,000 cases are discussed. The implications of the results are reviewed for preventive pediatric cardiology, for preventive medicine in general, and for the health of the American population in particular.

The PDAY Research Program is now in its 9th year of funded support by the USA National Heart, Lung and Blood Institute (NHLBI) which followed the 10 years of planning and development of the structure and functional organization of the program, the integration of the five "core" centers and the integration of all 14 centers into a well organized group of nine collection centers and a number of study centers.

The proposal for this detailed, quantitative multicenter study of the chronological development of young people's lipid containing arterial lesions as related to risk factors was presented originally at an AHA "Committee on Lesions" meeting in 1975. The concept met with prompt and enthusiastic approval by that committee. This was after I had discussed the concept with Drs Henry McGill and Jack Strong in 1975. The plan was also carefully evaluated, critiqued, monitored, and the planning financially supported by the Board of Directors of Universities Associated for Research and Education in Pathology (UAREP). Furthermore, it received generous financial support for the rather complex planning process from the College of American Pathology (CAP) Foundation and from a number of anonymous donors. The more than 14 institutions bore much of the expense of travel and subsistence of the interested participants to the many planning meetings and to the research proposal review at the Dallas Fort Worth Airport in October of 1984 where the evaluation team assembled by Dr Gardner McMillan and ably led by Dr Una Ryan reviewed the applications. Special recognition also needs to be given to the late Dr Robert Stein[1], Dr Robert Kirschner[2], Dr Assad Daoud[3], Dr Charles Hirsch[4], and Dr Jack Frost[5] (for notes see page 36), who helped in many ways as we put in place the case and sample acquisition program at the nine cooperating forensic centers which were approved and funded throughout the USA. There are many other individuals whose voluntary services were and are of special value for the planning and the operation of the program.

Special contributions were made by Drs Margaret Oalmann and Gray Malcom on the LSU campus, Ed Herderick on the OSU campus, and a number of NIH leaders and staff members, including Dr Robert Levy, then director of the NHLBI, Dr Gardner McMillan,

* Donald N. Pritzker Distinguished Service Professor (Active Emeritus) and Program Director/(Coordinator) of PDAY (Pathobiological Determinants of Atherosclerosis in Youth — a USA multicenter research program)/ RFEHA (Risk Factors in Early Human Atherosclerosis).

at the time the director of the Atherosclerosis and Hypertension Section of the Cardiovascular Division of the NHLBI, and Dr Momtaz Wassef in his valuable guidance during the continuing PDAY/RFEHA programs. According to the guidelines of this type of "investigator-initiated multicenter study" the continuing input from the NHLBI staff is an important function. Dr Wassef has fulfilled that responsibility in an exemplary way.

The benefits of PDAY's unique features in perspective

This report includes the major contributions of the main centers as of August 31, 1994, the official cutoff date of the PDAY/RFEHA case collection program. By that date, standardized data and the available anatomically designated samples of arteries and other tissues and fluids from the more than 3000 cases had been acquired. They were collected according to the rigorous requirements of the protocol and the manual of procedures developed by Dr Oalmann's committee. This multicenter case acquisition activity has supplied the standardized arterial samples studied on each case and the results of the risk factor analyses [1–3]. More than a dozen approved and funded special pathobiological studies have been conducted at the 14 centers [4–7].

At present, we are sharing the risk factor and anthropometric data as well as many of the available samples with other investigators outside the PDAY centers. Their proposed protocols have been approved by the steering committee. An excellent example of this is furnished by the work of Dr James Hixson [8,9].

The available arterial samples including the core and other tissue samples are summarized in Table 1. This table illustrates the research potential of this program. It emphasizes the care in processing, and anatomical standardization that have gone into the procurement as well as the eight methods of preservation that were responsible for the quality of the arterial samples collected for the program. It is also important to note that quantitative risk factor data and anthropometric data are available on virtually all of the cases.

Tables 2 and 3 give overviews of the total number of cases collected during each of the separately funded collection periods as well as the results of an analysis of about 1,000 of these cases in which "core" sample lesions have been classified grossly and microscopically [7].

Some of the unique features of this program are listed here:

The autopsy population

- Geographically diverse cases widely dispersed in the United States.
- All cases are the result of sudden, unexpected, usually traumatic death.
- Absence of chronic debilitating diseases.
- Each 5-year age group from 15 to 34 is well represented.
- Similar numbers of black and white cases in each age group.
- Female cases well represented in each age and race group.

Quality of case samples

- Little postmortem autolysis — many with very short postmortem intervals.
- Protection of arterial intima often resulting in endothelial cell preservation.
- Standardization of the samples for both the gross and microscopic studies.
- Each "core" lesion classified and photographed close-up.
- All samples carefully marked for preserving orientation.

Table 1. Available PDAY/RFEHA samples which can be utilized for further research

Location of samples	Preservation (samples/artery)	Number available for distribution	Size of sample
Thoracic aorta	6 fixed[a]	>17000	5.0–10.0
(sample width, mm)	5 frozen[b]	>10500	5.0–20.0
Abdominal aorta	8 fixed[a]	>20150	2.5–5.0
(sample width, mm)	6 frozen[b]	>12000	5.0–15.0
LAD coronary artery	7 fixed pressure-perfusion	> 7560	5.0–10.0
(sample width, mm)			
Left circumflex	2 fixed	> 5350	5.0
coronary artery	5 frozen	>10700	5.0
Thoracic aorta (half)	Fixed and Sudan IV	> 2900	
	stained	> 2800	
Right coronary artery	Fixed and Sudan IV	> 2900	
(entire/7-12 cm)	stained	> 2800	
Serum (ml)	Frozen	> 1200	0.01–1.0
Liver (g)	Frozen	> 3000	10.0
Kidney[c]	Fixed	> 2850 (R)	
Spleen[c]	Frozen (OCT)	> 2850 (L)	
		> 1200	
Liver[c]	Frozen (OCT)	> 1200	
Heart[c]	Fixed	> 2800 (R vent)	
		> 2800 (L vent)	
Adipose tissue	Frozen	> 2800	

[a]Formalin (neutral buffered or formol sucrose), glutaraldehyde, Carnoy's.
[b]Snap frozen or frozen in OCT.
[c]Representative histological samples.

- Each sample through lesion-prone and lesion-resistant areas.
- High-resolution fat stains on each "core" sample and Gomori trichrome aldehyde fuchsin (GTAF) on each "core" sample (within 1 mm of each other).

The broad spectrum of available data

- Age, sex, race, toxicology, postmortem interval, obesity, height, and weight.
- Quantitative postmortem evaluation for smoking, blood lipids, hyperglycemia, and hypertension.
- Gross and microscopic lesion extent and severity, quantified by pathologist grading and independently by computer-assisted morphometry.

Table 2. Number of active PDAY and RFEHA cases by sex and race as of September 9, 1994

Sex	Race	Project		Total
		PDAY	RFEHA	
Male	White	707	353	1060
	Black	668	500	1168
Female	White	227	157	384
	Black	188	155	343
Total		1790	1165	2955

Table 3. Microscopic tabulation of all available samples from 915 cases in which intermediate lesions were classified

Sample No.	No micro lesion	Micro fatty streaks	Fatty plaques				Fibrous plaques	Total samples
			Intra-cellular lipid predom "1"	Extra-cellular lipid >50% "2"	MØ[a] foam cell >20% "3"	Rich in lympho-cytes "4"		
01	235	174	175	117	121	5	2	829
18	264	128	216	155	102	0	7	872
16	250	53	164	225	89	1	38	820
45	388	47	58	206	69	4	102	874

[a]Macrophage.

— Analyses of fatty acids in perirenal adipose tissue.
— Analyses of the lipids in standardized arterial samples (aorta and left circumflex coronary artery) including cholesterol and cholesteryl ester fatty acids.
— Many special study results, such as comparison of Lp(a) in blood and artery samples.
— Several genetic analyses focused on polymorphisms of apolipoproteins as related to lesion extent.

These and other special features have supplied and will continue to supply ongoing opportunities to study many risk factor/lesion component comparisons [10].

The main positive gross findings in perspective

The intensive interaction of investigators at the Southwest Foundation (McGill, Hixson, et al.), at LSU (Strong, Tracy, Oalmann, Malcom, Newman, et al.), OSU (Cornhill, Herderick, et al.), and at the statistical center at the U. of Texas Health Sciences Center at San Antonio (McMahan, Marinez), has made it possible to uncover many new relationships of lesions to risk factors which have implications regarding the relationships of individual and combined risk factors to the development of plaques. These have included:

— Very early and marked effect of hyperlipidemia and smoking both singly and in combination on lesion extent and severity [11]. This has been amply confirmed and extended in subsequent study of many additional cases and with much more emphasis on computer-assisted topography and quantitative evaluation of lesion extent and severity including micromorphometry at OSU.
— First demonstration that the Apo E phenotypes, which have been definitely implicated in more serious and accelerated clinical effects of atherosclerosis, affect the lesion extent and severity in these young people's arteries [8,12].
— Important discovery that the genetic deletion of Apo B amino acids, more common in black individuals, may be an important determinant of atherosclerosis development in young black people [9].
— Clear-cut evidence that hypertension has a strong influence early in life on coronary lesion development [13].
— Remarkable new evidence that glycated hemoglobin and obesity, as measured in young people at autopsy, affect the arterial lesion extent and severity in both the coronary arteries and in the aortas of young people [14]. These relationships were not the result of less favorable lipoprotein profiles or smoking.

Clearly these innovative studies with their informative results are just the beginning of the new discoveries of how the risk factors influence lesion development in youth. They have already been greatly amplified and more quantitatively expressed and more topographically defined by extensive computer-assisted gross and microscopic prevalence studies by Dr Cornhill's group at OSU. These extensive results are being prepared for publication.

Figure 1 illustrates the remarkable interaction among the core centers which has made these new studies possible.

Major microscopic discoveries in perspective

The pathobiological studies which have proved to be productive of new knowledge and which have led to publications have come from seven centers.

It is clear that these are concerned largely with both chemical and cellular components of these lesions as related to the anatomical site of the lesions as well as the risk factors which were present.

For example, in this laboratory very early results indicated that there was usually a greater number of monocyte-derived foam cells in the "lesion prone" (dorsal) part of the thoracic aorta sample while very few macrophages were identified in the abdominal aorta "lesion prone" samples where the lesions usually progress more rapidly [5,6]. Also, these early results indicated that the extent of apoB deposition and retention, as indicated by immunohistochemistry, was about the same in lesion-prone and lesion-resistant portions of the arterial intima in all core samples [5,6]. Lipid deposition and retention as revealed by Oil Red O staining was much more abundant in the lesion-prone areas.

Other major cellular pathobiological results of significance have been recently reviewed and will only be listed here [8]. They are as follows:
— Evidence for T-lymphocyte localization in these early lesions [14].
— Evidence for the presence of herpes viruses in the early lesions [15].
— Occasional presence of microthrombi in early atheromatous lesions [16].
— Feasibility and the use of digital imaging fluorescence microscopy for studying atherosclerosis [17,18].
— The effects of circulating immune complexes on the microarchitecture of coronary artery lesions in young people [19,20].
— The relation of cocaine abuse to mast cells in the arterial wall [21].
— The role of mast cells in atherogenesis [22].
— The localization of Lp(a) in the aortas of young people [23,24].
— The excess of epitopes of oxidized LDL in lesions of smokers [25].
— Arterial collagen as related to cholesterol in the lesions [26].
While these studies represent only a fraction of those under way at several centers both within and outside of the PDAY group, they do give some idea of the results of special studies which have been reported and critically evaluated.

The other major accomplishment at the time that this manuscript is being written is the development of a new, and we believe a very useful, microscopic classification of the "intermediate lesions" between the fatty streak and the fibrous plaque. We usually refer to these as "fatty plaques". They are fairly uniform, discrete raised lesions with no evidence of a fibrous cap either grossly, microscopically or by chemical analysis. This was the most common lesion encountered in this study. Table 3 includes important data about the frequency of these types of lesions. The new classification will help us understand the pathogenesis associated with each risk factor. The more detailed description of the method we are using and its results will soon be published [7].

35

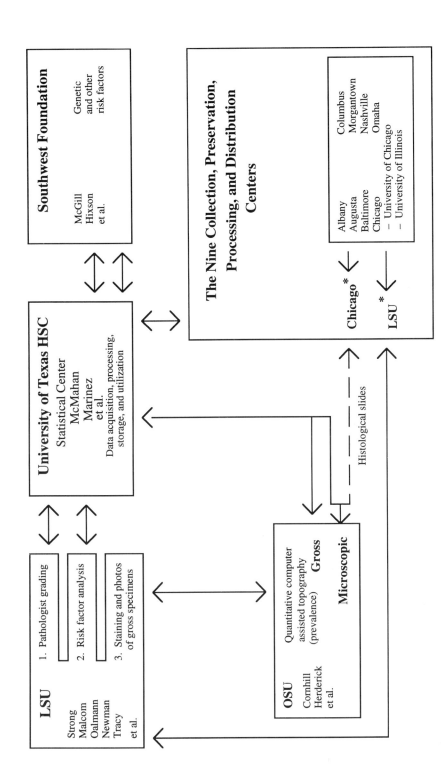

Fig. 1. Interaction among Core Centers to produce gross/risk factor studies.
*Two Core Centers responsible for the assembly and preservation of the frozen and fixed samples.

Benefits of this research program in perspective

This investigator-initiated multicenter study is unique. It may never be possible to repeat or extend it in the future. As more and more sudden-death victims are used for organ donors in an enlightened society, it may become impossible to gain access to arterial samples from young, healthy, sudden-death victims. Steps are being taken to preserve and distribute appropriate portions of this wealth of research material to qualified individuals who apply and who have a valid plan to make use of the samples and the data.

This study has demonstrated that a well-organized study of autopsy populations with careful planning can yield a wealth of new information. In this study the information gained from the tragically and often needlessly dead has strengthened the cardiovascular elements of the autopsy. It has benefited not only the image of Forensic Pathology Centers, but it has contributed widely to the pediatric medicine community in a way which may ultimately help to protect multitudes of young people from premature cardiovascular disease.

The fruits of this study are still being realized. The results to date, and those forthcoming, are likely to help support this nation's strong effort to develop preventive cardiology as an effective bulwark against accelerated atherosclerosis.

Personal acknowledgements by the author

I am not only deeply honored and proud of this award but I am also grateful for the work of a very large group of colleagues in the 14 PDAY/RFEHA centers. They have been remarkably supportive and helpful at all stages of this study.

To the extent to which this work and the results reflect the work at the University of Chicago I must hasten to acknowledge the contributions of Blanche Berger and Laura Hiltscher, my main technical assistants throughout this study, and a host of student assistants and postdoctoral fellows, as well as my long-time associate, Dr Dragoslava Vesselinovitch.

The preparation of this lecture and manuscript was aided greatly by the skillful editorial assistance of Gertrud Friedman and Mary C. Gorney and the excellent work of Taryn McFadden and Patti Dickson who spent many hours helping to prepare the text, the tables and the other components. Finally, I need to acknowledge the support of the grants which made our work possible, HL-33740 (PDAY) and HL-45715 (RFEHA).

Notes

1. Late, Chief Medical Examiner, Office of Cook County Medical Examiner, Chicago, IL.
2. Deputy Medical Examiner, Cook County, IL. Clinical Associate (Assoc. Professor), Department of Pathology, University of Chicago. Now: Deputy Chief Medical Examiner, Cook County, IL; Clinical Associate, Department of Pathology, University of Chicago.
3. Chief of Laboratory Services, Professor of Pathology, Albany Medical College, Albany County Coroner's Office, Pathologist. Now: Assistant Chief of Staff, Professor Emeritus, Pathology, Albany Medical College, Albany, NY.
4. Director of Forensic Medicine, Hamilton County Coroner's Office; Professor of Forensic Pathology, University of Cincinnati College of Medicine. Now: Chief Medical Examiner, New York City; Professor and Chairman, Department of Forensic Medicine; Professor of Pathology, New York University School of Medicine.
5. Deputy Chief Medical Examiner, State of West Virginia. Associate Professor of Pathology, West Virginia University Health Sciences Center. Now: Deputy Chief Medical Examiner, State of West Virginia; Professor of Pathology, West Virginia University Health Sciences Center.

Bibliography

1. Wissler RW. USA multicenter study of the pathobiology of atherosclerosis in youth. Ann NY Acad Sci 1991;623:26—39.
2. Cornhill JF, Herderick EE, Stary HC. Topography of human aortic sudanophilic lesions in blood flow in large arteries: applications to atherogenesis and clinical medicine. Monogr Atheroscler, Basel: Karger, 1990;15:13—19.
3. Strong JP, Oalmann MC, Malcom GT, Newman WP III, McMahan CA, and the Pathobiological Determinants of Atherosclerosis in Youth (PDAY) Research Group. Pathobiological Determinants of Atherosclerosis in Youth (PDAY): rationale, methodology, and selected risk factor findings. Cardiovasc Risk Factors 1992;88:1954—1960.
4. Wissler RW and the PDAY Research Group. Morphological characteristics of the developing atherosclerotic plaque. Animal studies and studies of lesions from young people. In: Weber PC, Leaf A (eds) Atherosclerosis: Its Pathogenesis and the Role of Cholesterol. (Atheroscler Rev, 23). New York: Raven Press, 1991;91—103.
5. Wissler RW, Komatsu A, Ko C, Kusumi Y, Vesselinovitch D. The cell populations and other components of the atheromatous lesions in young people. In: Hauss WH, Wissler RW, Bauch HJ (eds) New Aspects of Metabolism and Behavior of Mesenchymal Cells During the Pathogenesis of Atherosclerosis. Opladen: Westdeutscher Verlag, 1991;49—60.
6. Wissler RW and the PDAY Research Group. New insights into the pathogenesis of atherosclerosis as revealed by PDAY. Atherosclerosis 1994 (in press).
7. Wissler RW, Hiltscher L, Oinuma T, and the PDAY Research Group. Pathogenesis of atherosclerosis — the lesions of atherosclerosis in the young: from fatty streaks to intermediate lesions. In: Fuster V, Ross R, Topol E, (eds) Atherosclerosis and Coronary Artery Disease. New York: Raven Press, 1994 (in press).
8. Hixson JE, and the PDAY Research Group. Apolipoprotein E polymorphisms affect atherosclerosis in young males. Arterioscler Thromb 1991;11:1237—1244.
9. Hixson JE, McGill HC, Strong JP, McMahan CA, and the Pathobiological Determinants of Atherosclerosis in Youth (PDAY) Research Group. Apolipoprotein B insertion/deletion polymorphisms affect atherosclerosis in young black but not young white males. Arterioscler Thromb 1992;12:1023—1029.
10. Wissler RW, Vesselinovitch D, Komatsu A. The contribution of studies of atherosclerotic lesions in young people to future research. Ann NY Acad Sci 1990;598:418—434.
11. PDAY Research Group. Relationship of atherosclerosis in young men to serum lipoprotein cholesterol concentrations and smoking: a preliminary report from the Pathobiological Determinats of Atherosclerosis in Youth (PDAY) Research Group. J Am Med Assoc 1990;264:3018—3024.
12. Ordovas JM, Schaefer EJ. Apolipoprotein E polymorphisms and coronary heart disease risk. Cardiovasc Risk Factors 1994;4:103—107.
13. Strong JP, for the PDAY Research Group. Natural history and risk factors for early human atherogenesis. Clin Chem 1994 (in press).
14. Emeson EE, Robertson AL. T lymphocytes in aorta and coronary intimas — their potential role in atherogenesis. Am J Pathol 1988;130:359—369.
15. Yamashiroya HM, Ghosh L, Yang R, Robertson AL. Herpes viridae in the coronary arteries and aorta of young trauma victims. Am J Pathol 1988;130:71—79.
16. Spurlock BO, Chandler AB. Adherent platelets and surface microthrombi of the human aorta and the left coronary artery: a scanning electron microscopy feasibility study. Scanning Microsc 1987;1:1359—1365.
17. Jericevic Z, Wiese B, Homan R, Bryan J, Smith LC. Digital imaging fluorescence microscopy: statistical analysis of photobleaching and passive cellular uptake processes. In: Miller KR (ed) Advances in Cell Biology 1989;3:111—151.
18. Smith LC, Jericevic Z. Lipid distribution in human coronary lesions: analysis by digital imaging microscopy. Lenzi S, Descovitch G (eds) International Symposium on Atherosclerosis, Conference Proceedings. Amsterdam: Elsevier, 1990:148—155.
19. Wissler RW, Vesselinovitch D, Davis HR, Yamada T. The composition of the evolving atherosclerotic plaque. In: Strandness D, Didisheim P, Clowes A, Watson J (eds) Vascular Diseases: Current Research and Clinical Applications. Orlando: Grune and Stratton, 1987;241—256.
20. Wissler RW, Vesselinovitch D, Ko C. The effects of circulating immune complexes on atherosclerotic lesions in experimental animals and in younger and older humans. Transplant Proc 1989;21:3707—3708.
21. Kolodgie FD, Virmani R, Cornhill JF, Herderick EE, Smialek. Increase in athersclerosis and adventitial mast cells in young cocaine abusers: an alternative mechanism of atherosclerosis and thrombosis. J Col Cardiol 1991;17:1553—1560.

38

22. Atkinson JB, Harlan CW, Harlan GC, Virmani R. The role of mast cells in atherogenesis: a morphologic study of early atherosclerotic lesions in young people. Hum Pathol 1994;25:154–159.
23. Kusumi Y, Wissler RW and the PDAY Research Group. The localization of Lp(a) in the aortas of young people. The Ninth International Symposium on Atherosclerosis, 1991;44.
24. Kusumi Y, Yamada S, Liu P, Niihashi M, Kubo N, Sakurabayashi I, Sakurai I. Deposition of apo(a) free from LDL-like particle in arterial intima. Jpn Atheroscler J 1994 (in press).
25. Oyer CE. The greater extent of epitopes of oxidized low density lipoproteins in the early atherosclerotic lesions of smokers as compared to nonsmokers. Honors manuscript, the University of Chicago, 1993.
26. Miller EJ, Malcom GT, McMahan CA, Strong JP. Atherosclerosis in young white males: arterial collagen and cholesterol. Matrix 1993;13:289.

Pathobiological determinants of atherosclerosis in youth (PDAY research group)

Director
Program Director; R.W. Wissler, PhD, MD, University of Chicago.
Associate Directors: A.L. Robertson, Jr, MD, PhD, University of Illinois (1987–1992); J.P. Strong, MD, Louisiana State University (1992–present).

Steering committee
J.F. Cornhill, D.Phil, Ohio State University; H.C. McGill, Jr, MD, Southwest Foundation for Biomedical Research; C.A. McMahan, PhD, University of Texas Health Science Center (San Antonio); A.L. Robertson, Jr, MD, PhD, University of Illinois; J.P. Strong, MD, Louisiana State University Medical Center; R.W. Wissler, PhD, MD, University of Chicago.

Standard operating protocol and manual of procedures committee chairperson:
M.C. Oalmann, Dr P.H., Louisiana State University Medical Center.

Participating centers
University of Alabama (Birmingham), Department of Medicine — Principal Investigator (P.I.): S. Gay, MD, Coinvestigators: R.E. Gay, MD, G.-Q. Huang, MD (HL-33733); Department of Biochemistry — P.I.: E.J. Miller, PhD; Coinvestigators: D.K. Furuto, PhD, M.S. Vail, A.J. Narkates (HL-33728).
Albany Medical College (Albany, NY) — P.I.: A. Daoud, MD, Coinvestigators: A.S. Frank, PhD, M.A. Hyer, E.C. McGovern (HL-33765).
Baylor College of Medicine (Houston) — P.I.: L.C. Smith, PhD, Coinvestigator — F.M. Strickland, PhD (HL-33750).
University of Chicago (Chicago) — P.I.: R.W. Wissler, PhD, MD, Coinvestigators: D. Vesselinovitch, D.V.M., M.S., A. Komatsu, MD, PhD, Y. Kusumi, MD, G.M. Culen, D.P.M., A. Chien, B.A., A. Demopoulos, B.A., G. Friedman, B.A., R.T. Bridenstine, M.S., R.J. Stein, MD, R.H. Kirschner, MD, M. Bekermeier, ASCP, B. Berger, ASCP, L. Hiltscher, ASCP (HL-33740).
University of Illinois (Chicago) — P.I.: A.L. Robertson, Jr, MD, PhD, Coinvestigators: R.J. Stein, MD, E.R. Donoghue, MD, R.J. Buschmann, PhD, Y. Katsura, MD, T. Lyong An, MD, E. Choi, MD, N. Jones, MD, M.S. Kalelkar, MD, Y. Konakci, MD, B. Lifschultz, MD, V.R. Gumidyala, MD, R.M. Harper, B.S., F. Norris, H.T.L. (ASCP) (HL-33758).
Louisiana State University Medical Center (New Orleans) — P.I.: J.P. Strong, MD, Coinvestigators: G.T. Malcom, PhD, W.P. Newman III, MD, M.C. Oalmann, Dr P.H., P.S. Roheim, MD, A.K. Bhattacharyya, PhD, M.A. Guzman, PhD, A.A. Hatem, MD, C.A. Hornick, PhD, C.D. Restrepo, MD, R.E. Tracy, MD, PhD, C.C. Breaux, M.S., S.E. Hubbard, C.S. Zsembik, D.G. Gibbs, D.A. Trosclair (HL-33746).
University of Maryland (Baltimore) — P.I.: W. Mergner, MD, PhD, Coinvestigators: J.H. Resau, PhD, R.D. Vigorito, M.S., P.A., Q.-C. Yu, MD, J. Smialek, MD (HL-33752).
Medical College of Georgia (Augusta) — Co-P.I.: A.B. Chandler, MD, R.N. Rao, MD, Coinvestigators: D.G. Falls, MD, R.G. Gerrity, PhD, B.O. Spurlock, B.A., Associate Investigators: K.B. Sharma, MD, J.S. Sexton, MD, Research Assistants: K.K. Smith, HT (ASCP), G.W. Forbes (HL-33772).
University of Nebraska Medical Center (Omaha) — P.I.: B.M. McManus, MD, PhD, Coinvestigators: J.W. Jones, MD, T.J. Kendall, M.S., J.A. Remmenga, B.S., W.C. Rogler, B.S. (HL-33778).
Ohio State University (Columbus) — P.I.: J.F. Cornhill, D.Phil, Coinvestigators: W.R. Adrion, MD, P.M. Fardel, MD, B. Gara, M.S., E. Herderick, B.S., J. Meimer, M.S., L.R. Tate, MD (HL-33760).
Southwest Foundation for Biomedical Research (San Antonio) — P.I.: J.E. Hixson, PhD, P.K. Powers (HL-39913).

University of Texas Health Science Center (San Antonio) — P.I.: C.A. McMahan, PhD, Coinvestigators: H.C. McGill, Jr, MD, G.M. Barnwell, PhD, Y. Marinez, M.A., T.J. Prihoda, PhD, H.S. Wigodsky, MD, PhD (HL-33749).

Vanderbilt University — P.I.: R. Virmani, MD, Coinvestigators: J.B. Atkinson, MD, PhD, C.W. Harland, MD, L. Gleaves, R.A., C. Gleaves, H.T., P. Manik, R.A. (HL-33770).

West Virginia University — P.I.: S.N. Jagannathan, PhD, Coinvestigators: B.Caterson, PhD, J.L. Frost, MD, K.M.K. Rao, MD, P. Johnson, N.F. Rodman, MD (HL-33748).

Atherosclerosis X.
F.P. Woodford, J. Davignon and A. Sniderman, editors.

Microsomal triglyceride transfer protein: insights into lipoprotein assembly and abetalipoproteinemia

John R. Wetterau and Richard E. Gregg
Department of Metabolic Diseases, Bristol-Myers Squibb Pharmaceutical Research Institute, P.O. Box 4000, Princeton, NJ 08543-4000, USA

Abstract. The microsomal triglyceride-transfer protein (MTP) is found in the lumen of the endoplasmic reticulum of liver and intestine. MTP gene defects which result in an absence of MTP function cause abetalipoproteinemia, indicating that MTP is required for the assembly and secretion of chylomicrons and very low density lipoproteins. When HeLa cells, which normally do not make apoB-containing lipoproteins, were stably transfected with MTP, the cells were able to synthesize and secrete apoB53 particles in a manner similar to that of liver-derived cell lines. Thus, MTP plays a prominent role in facilitating the production of apoB-containing lipoproteins.

The microsomal triglyceride-transfer protein (MTP) is a soluble lipid-transfer protein which is found in the lumen of microsomes isolated from liver and intestine. MTP appears to be present in high concentrations within microsomes, possibly representing up to 0.5% of the soluble luminal contents, as suggested by the purification factor of the protein isolated from bovine liver microsomes [1]. In vitro, MTP accelerates the transfer of triglyceride (TG), cholesteryl ester (CE) and phosphatidylcholine (PC) between phospholipid surfaces [1]. The structure of MTP is unusual for an intracellular lipid-transfer protein. Previously characterized intracellular lipid-transfer proteins have been single polypeptides with molecular weights in the range of 8,000 to 35,000, while MTP is a heterodimer consisting of two proteins of molecular weights 55,000 and 97,000. The small subunit of MTP is the multifunctional enzyme, protein disulfide isomerase (PDI) [2]. In addition to being a component of MTP, PDI facilitates the correct folding of newly synthesized proteins within the lumen of the endoplasmic reticulum (ER) by promoting the proper formation of disulfide bonds. MTP expresses little or no disulfide isomerase activity unless the dimeric protein complex is disrupted. PDI is also the β subunit of the tetrameric enzyme, prolyl 4-hydroxylase ($\alpha_2\beta_2$).

The large subunit of MTP has been cloned and the cDNA sequenced from man, cow [3], and hamster [4]. There is 86% identity between the deduced aminoacid sequences of both the bovine and hamster protein with the human protein. The large subunit of MTP is not highly homologous to any previously characterized protein, though Shoulders et al. [5] proposed that there is a weak homology with *Xenopus laevis* lipovitellin 1, a member of the vitellogenin family of proteins. The absence of a KDEL ER retention sequence on the carboxy terminus of the MTP large subunit suggests that MTP is retained in the endoplasmic reticulum (ER) through its association with PDI, which does have a carboxy-terminal KDEL retention sequence.

Role of MTP in abetalipoproteinemia

Abetalipoproteinemia is an autosomal recessive disease which is characterized by a defect in the assembly and secretion of very low density lipoproteins (VLDL) and chylomicrons [reviewed in 6]. Affected individuals have virtually no plasma apoB, and total plasma cholesterol levels of approximately 25—50 mg/dl. Synthesis of the lipid and protein components of the apoB-containing lipoproteins are not impaired in abetalipoproteinemic subjects, which suggests that the defect lies in some factor necessary for the assembly of the lipoprotein particle. The tissue distribution, subcellular localization, and lipid-transport properties of MTP led to the hypothesis that MTP plays a role in the assembly of apoB-containing lipoproteins by transporting lipid from its site of synthesis in the ER membrane to developing lipoprotein particles in the ER lumen. Thus, MTP was a good candidate gene for abetalipoproteinemia.

To determine if defects in MTP may be a cause of abetalipoproteinemia, MTP activity in intestinal biopsies from control and from abetalipoproteinemic subjects was compared. MTP activity was readily detected in six control subjects and in two subjects who had genetic defects in the assembly of intestinal apoB-containing lipoprotein particles unrelated to abetalipoproteinemia (homozygous hypobetalipoproteinemia and Anderson's disease) [7]. In contrast, MTP activity was not detectable in intestinal biopsies obtained from four unrelated abetalipoproteinemic subjects. In addition, the unique large subunit of MTP could be detected by Western blot analysis in the biopsies from the eight control subjects, while it was not detectable in the biopsies from the four abetalipoproteinemic subjects.

The gene encoding the MTP large subunit in two of the abetalipoproteinemic subjects was sequenced to determine if mutations which explain the absence of MTP could be identified. A homozygous frameshift mutation was found in one subject while a homozygous nonsense mutation was found in the second (Table 1) [3]. These mutations predict primary translation products 9 and 66% the size of the wild-type protein, respectively, thus explaining the absence of MTP. In addition, Shoulders et al. [5] identified a homozygous point mutation that disrupts normal splicing of the MTP large-subunit message in another unrelated abetalipoproteinemic subject. From these studies, we concluded that an absence of functional MTP causes abetalipoproteinemia and that MTP is required for normal VLDL and chylomicron assembly (see Fig. 1).

Reconstitution of lipoprotein assembly in HeLa cells

MTP is a hepatic and intestinal specific factor required for the assembly of apoB-containing lipoproteins. To determine if it is sufficient to direct the synthesis of lipoproteins in cells which normally do not make them, Gordon et al. [8] investigated the ability of HeLa cells stably transfected with MTP (designated HLM-40 cells) to synthesize and secrete apoB-containing lipoproteins. HeLa cells were used for these studies because they

Table 1. Mutations in the gene encoding the large subunit of MTP from three subjects with abetalipoproteinemia

Subject[a]	Location	Change	Predicted number of amino acids in the translation product
1	bp 215	deletion of C	78
2	bp 1783	C→T, Arg→Stop	594
3	in intron 13, 5 bp 3′ of base 1867 of the cDNA	G→A	590

[a]Results from subjects one and two were reported in [3] while the results from subject 3 were reported in [5]. All subjects were found to be homozygous for the reported mutations.

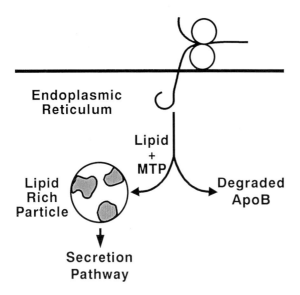

Fig. 1. Assembly of apoB-containing lipoproteins. Within the endoplasmic reticulum, apoB associates with phospholipid, triglyceride, and cholesterol to form a mature lipoprotein particle which is subsequently secreted. Lipid synthesis and MTP are required for this process. Abetalipoproteinemic subjects lack functional MTP, and as a result, are unable to assemble the lipoprotein particle.

have PDI levels and TG, CE, and PC synthesis rates similar to the human hepatocarcinoma-derived cell line, HepG2, which normally secretes apoB-containing lipoproteins. The HLM-40 cells had MTP activity levels approximately 25% that of HepG2 cells.

HeLa or HLM-40 cells were transfected with an expression vector that encoded apoB53, a truncated form of apoB, and then 48 h later, intracellular and secreted apoB were quantitated by Western blot analysis. Intracellular apoB was detected in both cell lines. However, when apoB secretion was compared, apoB was readily detectable in the media from HLM-40 cells which expressed MTP, while it could be detected only in trace quantities in the media from HeLa cells, and then only at the highest levels of the transfected apoB plasmid tested. ApoB secretion was estimated to be more than 30 times more efficient in HLM-40 cells than in wild-type HeLa cells.

In liver-derived cell lines, the amount of apoB secreted into the media is regulated by lipid synthesis and availability. To investigate the effect of lipid availability on apoB secretion in HLM-40 cells, we transiently transfected the cells with apoB and then cultured them for 24 h in Dulbecco's modified Eagle's media in the presence or absence of a 0.8 mM oleic acid, 50 µg/ml cholesterol, and 1 mM glycerol supplement. The cells grown in lipid-supplemented media secreted twice as much apoB as the cells grown in media alone. In addition, the secreted lipoproteins from cells grown in the presence of a lipid supplement were primarily found in the high density lipoprotein (HDL) and low density lipoprotein (LDL) fractions, in contrast to the cells grown in the absence of lipid supplements, where the apoB was found equally distributed between the HDL and d > 1.21 g/ml fractions after ultracentrifugal analysis. Secreted apoB53-containing particles with an HDL density were observed when McArdle RH-7777 cells, a cell line derived from rat liver, were transfected with apoB53 in control experiments. Thus, HeLa cells expressing MTP not only synthesize and secrete apoB-containing lipoproteins, but the density of the particles produced and the regulation of their secretion are similar to those observed for liver-derived cell lines.

Lipid-transport properties of MTP

Although studies of abetalipoproteinemia have clearly established that MTP is required for lipoprotein assembly, the role of MTP in the assembly process is not precisely known. Presumably, MTP transports lipid to nascent lipoprotein particles in the lumen of the ER. Kinetic analysis of MTP-mediated TG and CE transport indicated that MTP binds and shuttles lipid molecules between membranes [9]. Purified bovine MTP contains only a small amount of bound lipid [1], consistent with MTP shuttling only a few molecules at a time. It has not yet been determined if MTP has the capacity to couple all the lipid found in the final lipoprotein particle to apoB. Alternatively, MTP may be shuttling only a limited amount of lipid to apoB in a step which is part of a sequence of distinct steps leading to the assembly of the mature lipoprotein particle.

The availability of TG, CE, and PC has been implicated as being important for the efficient secretion of apoB from liver-derived cell lines. MTP has the ability to transport all three of these lipids. However, it is not known which transport properties of MTP are crucial for lipoprotein assembly. Consideration of fractional transfer rates shows that MTP displays a clear preference for neutral lipid, and in particular TG, transfer relative to PC transfer. However, because of the limited solubility of TG in a PC bilayer, the TG concentration in the in vitro lipid-transfer assays used to characterize MTP is low (typically less than 1% of the total lipid). Although a large fraction of the TG is transported, the actual mass of PC transferred exceeds that of TG or CE (Fig. 2). One needs to consider the absolute as well as the fractional transfer rates when considering possible roles of MTP in lipoprotein assembly.

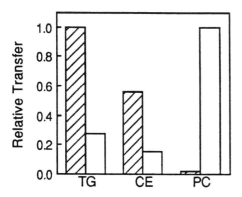

Fig. 2. MTP-catalyzed transport of triglyceride (TG), cholesteryl ester (CE), and phosphatidylcholine (PC) from donor to acceptor phospholipid vesicles. When neutral lipid transfer was assayed, both donor and acceptor vesicles contained 0.5 mol% TG or CE, while PC transfer was measured in the absence of neutral lipid. For the hatched bars, the transfer rates were expressed as the percent donor lipid transferred per hour (fractional transfer rate), while for the open bars, the transfer rates were expressed as the moles of lipid transferred per hour (absolute transfer rate). The rates were then normalized to the lipid species with the fastest transfer rate. Data for the figure were obtained from [1].

MTP regulation

Because of the central role of MTP in lipoprotein assembly, it is reasonable to speculate that its levels may affect the rate of lipoprotein production or the nature of the lipoproteins produced. To determine the extent to which MTP levels may vary in vivo, the regulation of MTP by various diets which affect lipid and lipoprotein metabolism was investigated in hamsters [4]. A 31-day high-fat diet increased MTP large-subunit mRNA levels in the intestine (226% of control) and liver (155% of control). Hepatic MTP mRNA levels were also elevated (155% of control) by a high-sucrose diet. When the animals from all four of the dietary treatments investigated were combined, there were highly significant positive correlations between MTP large-subunit mRNA levels and plasma lipid levels. This suggests that MTP may play a role in regulating plasma lipid levels or alternatively, that common factors may be regulating MTP mRNA levels and plasma lipid levels.

To investigate the mechanisms by which MTP gene expression may be regulated in vivo, Hagen et al. [10] characterized the regulatory elements for the MTP large-subunit genes from human and hamster. The two promoters share over 70% sequence homology for the first 200 bp upstream of the transcription start site. Using luciferase reporter-gene constructs and cell-culture models, the hepatocyte and enterocyte cell-specific elements were found to be contained in the first 600 bp of both promoters. Consensus recognition sequences for the liver-specific factors HNF-1 and HNF-4, and the activator protein AP-1, were found within −123 to −85 bp upstream of the transcription start site. Deletion analysis indicated that this region is crucial for promoter expression. A conserved liver-cell-specific repressor element was found between bp −240 and −140 of the human promoter. They reported that the promoter is positively regulated by cholesterol and negatively regulated by insulin. An insulin-response-negative element was found 120 bp upstream of the transcription start site.

In conclusion, MTP is a liver- and intestine-specific lipid-transfer protein that is required for lipoprotein assembly. The gene for the large subunit of MTP can be transcriptionally regulated by metabolically relevant mediators, and mutations in this gene are the proximal cause of abetalipoproteinemia.

References

1. Wetterau JR, Zilversmit DB. Chem Phys Lipids 1985;38:205–222.
2. Wetterau JR, Combs KA, Spinner SN, Joiner BJ. J Biol Chem 1990;265:9800–9807.
3. Sharp D, Blinderman L, Combs KA, Kienzle B, Ricci B, Wager-Smith K, Gil CM, Turck CW, Bouma M-E, Rader DJ, Aggerbeck LP, Gregg RE, Gordon DA, Wetterau JR. Nature 1993;365:65–69.
4. Lin MCM, Arbeeny C, Bergquist K, Kienzle B, Gordon DA, Wetterau JR. J Biol Chem (in press).
5. Shoulders CC, Brett DJ, Bayliss JD, Narcisi TME, Jarmuz A, Grantham TT, Leoni PRD, Bhattacharya S, Pease RJ, Cullen PM, Levi S, Byfield PGH, Purkiss P, Scott J. Hum Mol Genet 1993;2:2109–2116.
6. Gregg RE, Wetterau JR. Curr Opin Lipid 1994;5:81–86.
7. Wetterau JR, Aggerbeck LP, Bouma M-E, Eisenberg C, Munck A, Hermier M, Schmitz J, Gay G, Rader DJ, Gregg RE. Science 1992;258:999–1001.
8. Gordon DA, Jamil H, Sharp D, Mullaney D, Yao Z, Gregg RE, Wetterau JR. Proc Natl Acad Sci USA 1994;91:7628–7632.
9. Atzel A, Wetterau JR. Biochemistry 1993;32:10444–10450.
10. Hagan DL, Kienzle B, Jamil H, Hariharan N. J Biol Chem (in press).

Role of the plasminogen/plasmin system in the vessel wall

Peter Carmeliet and Désiré Collen

The Center for Molecular and Vascular Biology, University of Leuven, Leuven, B-3000, Belgium

Abstract. Indirect evidence suggests a crucial role for the plasminogen/plasmin system in many proteolytic processes in the vessel wall including blood clot dissolution (thrombolysis), atherosclerosis, restenosis, hemostasis, aneurysm formation and neovascularization. The implied role of the fibrinolytic system in vivo is, however, deduced from correlations between fibrinolytic activity and (patho)physiological phenomena, which does not allow us to definitively establish a causal role of this system in these processes. The previously generated and phenotyped transgenic mice with loss of gene function of the primary fibrinolytic system components (Carmeliet et al. J Clin Invest 1993;92:2746–2760, Nature 1994;368:419–424) are currently being examined for their role in thrombosis, restenosis and atherosclerosis.

The plasminogen/plasmin system

The fibrinolytic or plasminogen/plasmin system comprises an inactive proenzyme, plasminogen, that is activated to the proteolytic enzyme plasmin by two physiological plasminogen activators, tissue-type plasminogen activator (tPA) and urokinase-type plasminogen activator (uPA) [1]. Inhibition of the fibrinolytic system may occur at the α_2-antiplasmin level of plasmin, mainly by α_2-antiplasmin or at the level of the plasminogen activators by specific plasminogen activator inhibitors (PAIs), of which PAI-1 appears to be the principal inhibitor [2]. tPA is believed to be primarily responsible for removal of fibrin from the vascular tree through its specific affinity for fibrin [1]. uPA binds to a cellular receptor (uPAR) and might participate in pericellular proteolysis via degradation of matrix components or via activation of latent proteinases or growth factors [3]. Cell-specific clearance of plasminogen activators (PA) by LDL receptor-related protein (LRP) or gp330 protein might constitute a mechanism to modulate pericellular proteolysis.

Thrombosis/thrombolysis

Deficient fibrinolytic activity, e.g. resulting from increased plasma PAI-1 levels or reduced plasma tPA or plasminogen levels, might participate in the development of thrombotic events (for references see [4]). Elevated plasma PAI-1 levels have indeed been correlated with a higher risk of deep venous thrombosis and of thrombosis during hemolytic uremic syndrome, sepsis, surgery and trauma. PAI-1 plasma levels were also elevated in patients with ischemic heart disease, angina pectoris and recurrent myocardial infarction. A possible causal relationship between high PAI-1 levels and the occurrence of thrombosis was inferred from observations that PAI-1 specific antibodies enhance endogenous thrombolysis and reduce thrombus extension in rabbits and that PAI-1 inhibits endogenous fibrinolysis and contributes to thrombus stabilization in dogs. However, the acute-phase

Address for correspondence: D. Collen, MD, PhD, Center for Molecular and Vascular Biology, Campus Gasthuisberg, Herestraat 49, University of Leuven, Leuven, B-3000, Belgium. Tel.: +32-16-34-57-72. Fax: +32-16-34-59-90.

reactant behavior of PAI-1 does not allow one to deduce whether increased PAI-1 levels are a cause or consequence of thrombosis. To date, genetic deficiencies of tPA or uPA have not been reported in man, but quantitative and qualitative deficiencies of plasminogen have been associated with increased thrombotic tendency. Microscopic analysis of tissues from uPA deficient mice [5] revealed occasional minor fibrin deposits in liver and intestines. No spontaneous fibrin deposits were observed in tPA deficient mice. Mice with a combined deficiency of tPA and uPA, however, revealed extensive fibrin deposits in several normal and inflamed organs with ischemic necrosis, possibly resulting from thrombotic occlusions [5]. Although mice with a single deficiency of tPA or uPA had only a minor spontaneous thrombotic phenotype, they were significantly more susceptible to development of venous thrombosis after local injection of proinflammatory endotoxin in the footpad. The increased susceptibility of tPA deficient mice to endotoxin and the severe spontaneous thrombotic phenotype of the combined tPA:uPA deficient mice could be explained by their significantly reduced rate of spontaneous lysis of ^{125}I-fibrin-labeled plasma clots, injected via the jugular vein and embolized into the pulmonary arteries [5]. On the contrary, PAI-1-deficient mice were virtually protected against development of venous thrombosis following a similar dose of endotoxin, which is consistent with their ability to lyse plasma clots at a significantly higher rate than wild-type mice [6]. The increased susceptibility of uPA deficient mice to endotoxin might be due to their impaired macrophage function. Indeed, thioglycollate-stimulated macrophages (which express increased cell-associated uPA) from uPA-deficient mice, but not from tPA-deficient or PAI-1-deficient mice, lacked plasminogen-dependent breakdown of ^{125}I-labeled fibrin (fibrinolysis) or ^{3}H-labeled subendothelial matrix (mostly collagenolysis) [5].

Restenosis

Vascular reconstructions including coronary angioplasty, endarterectomy, bypass surgery, vascular stents and heart transplantation have become widely used treatments for patients with atherothrombotic disease. However, chronic restenosis in 30–50% of patients, necessitating costly and complicated reinterventions, remains a major limitation of these procedures. Elastic recoil, adventitial remodeling and thrombosis have been implicated in this process. Restenosis might, however, also result from excessive accumulation of smooth muscle cells (SMC) and deposition of matrix in the intimal layer as part of a hyperactive wound-healing process subsequent to vascular trauma. Recently, evidence has been provided for a significant role of the plasminogen/plasmin system in vascular remodeling [4,7,8]. In an uninjured vessel, expression of tPA by endothelial cells (EC) and, to a variable extent, of PAI-1 by SMC suggests a primary role in maintaining vascular patency or hemostasis, respectively. Expression of uPA and its cellular receptor appears to be undetectable whereas low levels of the PA-clearance receptor LRP are detected on SMC. Vascular trauma results, however, in activation of the plasminogen/plasmin system and net plasmin proteolysis. Following transient reduction of tPA in the vessel wall as a result of EC damage, tPA and uPA activity in the vessel wall are significantly increased coincident with the time of medial SMC proliferation and migration. Whereas tPA immunoreactivity is confined to SMC in the media adjacent to and migrating through the internal elastic membrane and to SMC in the neointima, uPA might be produced by infiltrating macrophages, SMC or EC. In vitro, treatment of cultured EC, SMC and macrophages with basic fibroblast growth factor (bFGF), platelet-derived growth factor (PDGF), tumor necrosis factor (TNFα), angiotensin II and thrombin, growth factors that are released after injury, induce expression of uPA, its cellular receptor and occasionally of tPA. Induction of uPA:uPAR expression has also been observed after wounding of EC and SMC in vitro. Plasmin-independent effects by tPA on proliferation of SMC and of uPA on migration of EC further support a role of the plasminogen system in vascular wound healing. Control of excessive plasmin proteolysis may result from inhibition by PAI-1, released by platelets or adjacent endothelium following thrombosis, or by SMC following injury. In vitro, PAI-1 expression is induced in EC, SMC and macrophages in response to similar molecules that promote plasmin production (PDGF, thrombin, angiotensin II, TNFα and IL-1β), suggesting tight control of this proteolytic system. In addition, plasmin-mediated activation of latent transforming growth factor-β (TGF-β), which induces expression of PAI-1 by SMC, EC or macrophages, may constitute another paracrine proteinase inhibitor-control mechanism. Interestingly, balloon injury-induced production of PAI-1 is significantly higher in hypercholesterolemic than in normocholesterolemic rabbits.

Local increase of plasmin proteolysis in the injured vessel may serve several functions: it might aid in dissolution of mural thrombus (a possible mediator of restenosis) or participate in passivation of the injured vessel lumen. Alternatively, pericellular proteolysis might participate in the migration and/or proliferation of SMC, EC and macrophages during vascular wound healing. In fact, tPA has been suggested as mediating, at least in part, the migratory response of SMC to PDGF. Plasmin proteolysis might also be involved in the characteristic tissue remodeling associated with vascular wound healing via activation of latent TGF-β or matrix-degrading proteinases. Finally, the plasminogen/plasmin system might affect neovascularization of stenotic or occluded vessels. To date, the effect of pro- or antifibrinolytic treatment has been inconclusive. In one study, the antifibrinolytic drug tranexamic acid reduced migration of smooth muscle cells in rat carotid artery and in another study, administration of uPA to patients did not affect restenosis. An inhibitory effect of heparin on tPA production has been proposed as a possible mechanism for the reduction of neointima formation in injured rat carotid artery.

In a recent analysis (unpublished data) of neointima formation following vascular trauma in mice with deficiencies of tPA, uPA or PAI-1, we have observed that deficiency of tPA does not affect the degree or rate of neointima formation or neointimal cell accumulation, whereas deficiency of uPA delayed and deficiency of PAI-1 accelerated neointima formation and neointimal cell accumulation. Interestingly, an inverse relationship between neointima formation and thrombosis was observed in these knock-out mice, suggesting that the role of the fibrinolytic system in neointima formation is probably related to its effects on cell proliferation or migration more than on clot lysis. Our data also suggest that uPA- rather than tPA-mediated plasmin proteolysis contributes to vascular wound healing and restenosis in mice. Further study is required to elucidate whether loss of plasminogen activator gene function affects cellular migration or proliferation. Another unresolved question is whether deposition or composition of the matrix are affected by these genetic manipulations, as suggested by our previous observations [4] of impaired degradation of ^{3}H-proline-labeled subendothelial matrix by uPA-deficient but not by tPA-deficient macrophages.

Atherosclerosis

The plasminogen/plasmin system may also be involved in the development and/or progression of atherosclerosis [9—13]. Current evidence suggests that impaired fibrinolysis is correlated with coronary heart disease. Epidemiological studies indeed revealed a positive association of plasma PAI-1 activity not only with reinfarction but also with the

48

degree of coronary artery disease. Furthermore, known risk factors for atherosclerosis including obesity, non-insulin-dependent diabetes, hyperinsulinemia, hypertriglyceridemia and hypertension, all possibly related to an insulin-resistance syndrome, have been correlated with increased plasma PAI-1 levels. In situ analysis of the atherosclerotic plaque also revealed increased expression of PAI-1 in intimal SMC and macrophages, coincident with expression of tissue factor, thrombin and fibrin. Lipids including VLDL, LDL, oxidized or acetylated LDL and Lp(a) might also contribute to impaired plasmin proteolysis by induction of PAI-1 and suppression of tPA expression by EC and liver cells. Genetic analysis of postinfarction patients has recently revealed a polymorphism in the PAI-1 promoter that might confer responsiveness to VLDL and render these individuals more prone to thrombotic complications. Collectively, these data suggest that impaired fibrinolysis might contribute to the progression of atherosclerosis via a prothrombotic action. The role of the plasminogen/plasmin system in atherosclerosis may, however, be more complex. Increased plasmin proteolysis in plaques has indeed been observed and elevated plasma tPA levels have been correlated with later myocardial infarction and long-term mortality among patients with coronary atherosclerosis. Since most interest has, however, hitherto been focused on PAI-1, knowledge of the role of tPA, uPA, its cellular receptor and of the PA-clearance receptor LRP is only fragmentary [7]. Possible roles of plasmin proteolysis in lesion development might include effects on cell proliferation, migration, matrix remodeling or possibly on plaque rupture [13]. In a preliminary analysis of cholesterol feeding-induced atherosclerosis, we have observed that tPA-deficient mice develop fatty streak lesions to the same extent as their wild-type littermates. However, whether, to what extent and at what stage the fibrinolytic system might affect atherosclerotic lesions remains to be further analyzed. This could be achieved by cross-breeding tPA-, uPA- and PAI-1-deficient mice with other atherosclerosis-prone transgenic mice such as the apolipoprotein E-deficient mouse.

An interesting but unresolved issue is whether the atherothrombotic activity of the plasminogen homolog lipoprotein(a) might, at least in part, be attributed to an inhibitory role on plasmin formation [11,12]. A significant correlation between high levels of apo(a), lower in situ plasmin activity and active TGF-β levels was observed in atherosclerotic vessels of the transgenic mice overexpressing apo(a). Whether reduced TGF-β activation (resulting from reduced plasmin activity) might constitute a growth stimulus for vascular smooth muscle cells can be further examined in tPA-, uPA- and PAI-1-deficient mice and the recently obtained uPA receptor-deficient mice (unpublished data).

Conclusion

In conclusion, targeting of the principal fibrinolytic system components has not only confirmed its role in maintaining vascular patency but has also yielded novel insights into the healing process of vascular trauma that ultimately leads to restenosis. These knock-out mice will be of further use in elucidating the role of the plasminogen/plasmin system in other proteolytic processes in the vessel wall such as neovascularization or atherosclerosis.

References

Because of space limitation, only selected review articles and the original gene targeting references have been included. A more complete reference list is available in [7].

1. Collen D, Lijnen HR. Blood 1991;78:3114–3124.
2. Schneiderman J, Loskutoff DJ. Trends Cardiovasc Med 1991;1:99–102.
3. Blasi F, Vassalli JD, Dano K. J Cell Biol 1987;104:801–804.

4. Carmeliet P, Collen D. Fibrinolysis 1994;8(suppl 1):269–276.
5. Carmeliet P, Schoonjans L, Kieckens L, Ream B, Degen J, Bronson R, De Vos R, van den Oord JJ, Collen D, Mulligan R. Nature 1994;368:419–424.
6. Carmeliet P, Stassen JM, Schoonjans L, Ream B, van den Oord JJ, De Mol M, Mulligan RC, Collen D. J Clin Invest 1993;92:2756–2760.
7. Carmeliet P, Collen D. Role of the plasminogen/plasmin system in thrombosis, restenosis and athero-sclerosis. Evaluation in transgenic mice. Trends Cardiovasc Med (in press).
8. Jackson CL, Reidy MA. Ann NY Acad Sci 1992;667:141–150.
9. Hamsten A, Erikson P. Fibrinolysis 1994;8(suppl 1):253–262.
10. De Bono D. Br Heart J 1994;71:504–507.
11. Nachman RL. Blood 1992;79:1897–1906.
12. Liu AC, Lawn RM. Trends Cardiovasc Med 1994;4:40–44.
13. Fuster V, Stein B, Ambrose JA, Badimon L, Badimon JJ, Cheseboro JH. Circulation 1990;82(suppl II): II.47–II.59.

Hypoalphalipoproteinemia: from a mutation to drug development

Cesare R. Sirtori and Guido Franceschini

Center E. Grossi Paoletti and Institute of Pharmacological Sciences, University of Milan, 20133 Milan, Italy

Abstract. The mutant apolipoprotein A-I-Milano (A-I$_M$) was described in a family with marked hypoalphalipoproteinemia (HDL-cholesterol 7–15 mg/dl), frequent hypertriglyceridemia and absence of cardiovascular disease. It is characterized by a Cys for Arg replacement at position 173 and is transmitted as an autosomal dominant trait. A-I$_M$ very rapidly associates with and dissociates from lipids in vitro; the A-I$_M$ dimer (A-I$_M$/A-I$_M$) has a prolonged half-life in plasma and direct fibrinolytic properties, quantitatively and mechanistically similar to those of direct thrombolytics. Current animal studies with a recombinant A-I$_M$ dimer indicate that the protein, injected before and after procedures determining arterial stenosis, can maintain arterial patency, thus presenting as a possible candidate drug for the prevention or management of arterial disease.

Interest in a potential use of human apolipoproteins for therapy is steadily growing. Apolipoproteins, due to their chemical stability, water solubility and capacity to bind at the same time lipids and other chemicals pose, in fact, an attractive option for potential therapeutic use. Apolipoproteins or their segments have been proposed for a variety of clinical indications, ranging from the activation of sperm motility [1] to the treatment of gout or related conditions [2], of neurodegenerative disorders [3], obesity [4], the acquired immunodeficiency syndrome [5] and endotoxin shock [6]. The prevention and possibly the treatment of atherosclerosis seem, however, to be the area of most immediate, potentially most exciting use of apolipoproteins. The well-founded specific knowledge about the role of apolipoproteins in the determination of vascular damage or in preventing it [7] does, in fact, provide a very useful background to any approach to therapy involving extractive or recombinant apolipoproteins.

Along this line, a number of industrial initiatives are already considering the development of apolipoproteins for the direct management of initial or advanced arterial lesions or for the prevention of the rapid vascular changes resulting in, e.g., early closure of arterial by-passes or restenosis of coronary angioplasties [8]. Among apolipoproteins considered for potential therapeutic use, a genetic mutant of apolipoprotein A-I (apo A-I), discovered in Italy, carries now considerable hope as a recombinant protein for the management of conditions resulting from rapid atherosclerosis progression, ranging from development from initial to advanced arterial plaques, down to the prevention of restenosis after angioplasty.

Apo A-I-Milano — background

The apo A-I-Milano (A-I$_M$) is the first described genetic mutant of human apolipoproteins. The original clinical observation dates back 20 years, to the clinical evaluation of a 43-year-old man with a history of gastritis, who presented with a severe hyperlipoproteinemia (total plasma cholesterol up to 402 mg/dl and triglycerides sometimes above

---

Address for correspondence: Prof Cesare Sirtori, Institute of Pharmacological Sciences, Via Balzaretti 9, University of Milan, 20133 Milan, Italy.

1,000 mg/dl) [9]. Reports from his personal physician indicated that treatment with clofibrate had proved ineffective, possibly resulting in a worsening of the biochemical data.

The clinical findings were uninformative, except for the presence of a gerontotoxon (not found in any other member of the large kindred). Further biochemical evaluation of his plasma lipid profile disclosed a remarkably low HDL-cholesterol level (not routinely measured at the time): this ranged from a minimum of 7 mg/dl to a maximum of 12–13 mg/dl. On electrophoresis the α band was essentially invisible [9,10]. An initial screening of close family members (father, mother and three children) showed that the father had a very similar biochemical picture, but in the absence of significant hyperlipidemia, and so had two of the three children; the mother had a perfectly normal lipoprotein pattern and died at age 70 of a stroke. Extensive investigations on the original carrier failed to detect any notable abnormalities in the vascular system or any lipid deposits at the parenchymal or mucosal level, thus ruling out a possible diagnosis of Tangier disease. Attempts to correct the hyperlipidemia by the use of metformin, polyunsaturated phospholipids or different dietary interventions also had no significant effect.

A considerable effort into the determination of the molecular basis for the lipoprotein abnormality led to the definition, in 1980, of a major change in the amino acid composition of apo A-I, i.e., the presence of a cysteine residue, replacing one arginine [11]. This leads to no change in the molecular weight of the protein, determined by SDS PAGE, but to the possibility that the abnormal protein may form dimers with itself (A-I_M/A-I_M) or complexes with apo A-II (A-I_M/A-II). The proportion of monomeric A-I_M vs. dimer and complex is highly variable among carriers [12] and may relate both to sex and to HDL-C levels [13].

With definition of the molecular origin of the abnormality, interest rose as to the mode of genetic transmission and the possible "beneficial" role of the mutation in maintaining normal cardiovascular health despite dramatic reduction of the putative protective lipoprotein fraction.

The mode of *genetic transmission* of A-I_M was established by a population study in Limone sul Garda, a small community on Lake Garda in Northern Italy, characterized by a high level of consanguinity due to the lack of incoming roads up to 1953. In this small community (about 1,000 citizens) there has been no isolation of harmful genes in spite of the high intermarriage rate. A survey of the whole population, carried out in 1981, established the presence of 33 carriers (the number has increased to 37 in the past 12 years) and that the mutation is transmitted as an autosomal dominant trait, starting from an original mating couple in 1780 [10]. Careful analysis of the genealogic tree by the use of church registers failed to identify any homozygous carrier while, in addition, there were apparently no records of sudden deaths among the carriers (with the exception of a 54-year-old hypertensive, heavy smoker, who died around 1950). There was clear evidence, by examining the lifespan of the carriers in the past 2 centuries, of a tendency to relative longevity. Among the 45 A-I_M carriers, most are characterized by mild to severe hyper-triglyceridemia, HDL-C levels in the range of 10–25 mg/dl, some with elevation of LDL-cholesterol; none follows a specific diet and about one-third are smokers.

The molecular error was recognized as a Cys for Arg substitution at position 173, i.e., in one of the 11 amphipathic helical segments characterizing apo A-I and allowing its interaction with plasma and lipids [14]. A series of in vitro studies comparing A-I_M with wild type A-I indicated that the mutant protein is characterized by enhanced spatial flexibility in solution, resulting in an accelerated interaction with phospholipids and a more rapid release of these after in vitro binding [15]. More recent in vivo kinetic studies in A-I$_M$ carriers and noncarriers receiving either labeled A-I or A-I$_M$ [16] have provided additional major findings:

— the A-I$_M$ monomer disappears faster from plasma than wild-type A-I;
— the A-I$_M$/A-I$_M$ dimer by contrast is characterized by a very slow turnover (half-life more than double that of A-I), possibly consistent with a precursor–product relationship between the dimer and the resulting monomer.

Evaluation of the potential use of A-I$_M$ in therapeutics and more recent supporting evidence

The growing number of contributions showing the dramatic effectiveness of infusions of HDL fractions or of extractive apo A-I on atheromatous lesions have certainly strengthened the working hypothesis that increasing HDL/A-I levels may provide a beneficial effect on atheroma formation and possibly induce a regression. Studies have ranged from direct repeated injections of lipoproteins of d > 1.125 (HDL+VHDL) in cholesterol-fed rabbits to the infusion of isolated human A-I in these same animals. Infusions of HDL+VHDL can both prevent atheroma formation and also induce regression after the dietary lesions have been established [17,18]. Contrasting data have on the other hand been provided on the impact of immunogenicity on the antiatherogenic activity of HDL/apo A-I. German investigators clearly showed, in rabbits, that only the homologous HDL is effective in plaque removal vs. no activity of human HDL [19]; in contrast, a US study showed that the human A-I is as effective as rabbit HDL on plaque removal in cholesterol-fed rabbits [20]. Finally, mice transgenic for human apo A-I display a remarkable resistance to the dietary induction of atherosclerotic lesions [21]; if mice deficient in apo E (a condition resulting in severe atheroma formation) are made transgenic for human A-I, then atherosclerosis is prevented [22].

Availability of the *recombinant A-I$_M$ monomer and A-I$_M$/A-I$_M$ dimer* proteins prompted an extensive evaluation of their in vivo and in vitro properties. The clinical use of the A-I$_M$ dimer seemed more promising, in view of the prolonged plasma half-life and of the possible precursor–product relationship with A-I$_M$ in man [16]. To the investigators' surprise, in vitro evaluation of the A-I$_M$/A-I$_M$ dimer (Fig. 1) showed an unexpected *potent fibrinolytic activity*. The dimer was, therefore, selected for extensive development, involving establishment of the most appropriate cultural techniques in engineered *Escherichia coli*, toxicological and immunological evaluation, as well as application to a variety of tests of experimental atherosclerosis, prior to clinical studies.

Expression and major findings with the recombinant A-I$_M$ dimer

The *E. coli* K12 strains were used as appropriately modified. Plasmid pUC9 was used for subcloning of an 821-bp BamHI fragment of a cDNA copy of a human apo A-I; a second vector was obtained by using a 822 bp BamHI fragment of human apo A-I$_M$ DNA (produced by site-directed mutagenesis of apo A-I cDNA). Appropriate plasmids were created with a transposon containing a *tac* promoter, a derivative of an *OmpA* signal sequence, a kanamycin resistance marker and two transcription terminators. By appropriate characterization of the product, it could be established that the final BC 0050 (*xyl-7, ara-14*, T4^R) *E. coli* strain can produce 4.4 g/l of apo A-I$_M$ in the supernatant after 22 h of induction [23]. The monomer can be later converted to the dimer and purified according to conventional methods. Characterization by different biochemical procedures identified the A-I$_M$/A-I$_M$ dimer as essentially identical to the product directly isolated from plasma.

Two major in vitro properties of the recombinant A-I$_M$ dimer (Fig. 1) have become

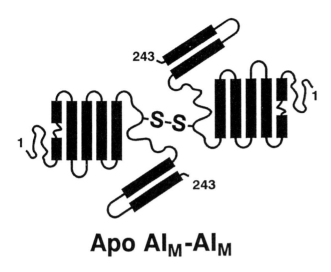

Apo AI$_M$-AI$_M$

Fig. 1. Spatial structure of the A-I$_M$ dimer.

clearly apparent: a) an enhanced capacity to remove cholesterol from cultured cells and b) a direct fibrinolytic activity, also exerted by promoting plasminogen autoactivation.

The in vitro addition of recombinant A-I$_M$/A-I$_M$ complexed with egg phosphatidyl-choline (EPC) results in an *enhanced removal of membrane cholesterol* from cultured fibroblasts. Comparison of A-I$_M$ EPC liposomes with similar liposomes complexed with wild-type A-I showed a significantly higher activity; EPC *per se* has a negligible capacity for cholesterol removal.

A series of investigations was carried out on the effects of A-I$_M$ dimer on the *human fibrinolytic system*. These were stimulated by prior observations of a moderate activity of human A-I or of isolated HDL on the fibrinolysis activated by urokinase [24]. In the case of the A-I$_M$ dimer, fibrinolytic activity was evaluated in terms of: a) autoactivation of plasminogen and b) potentiation of specific activators, tPA and uPA, in the presence of a chromogenic substrate.

Addition of apo A-I to a mixture of Glu-plasminogen did not enhance the amount of released plasmin. In contrast there was a concentration-dependent increase of plasmin upon addition of the A-I$_M$ dimer in the 11.7–93.9 µg/ml range, which suggested that the dimer can influence plasminogen autoactivation. Furthermore, in a system quite similar to that already employed for extractive HDL/A-I [24], i.e., by incubating plasminogen with tPA or uPA, the addition of apo A-I (130 µg/ml) increased plasmin formation by only ~35 and ~60% respectively in the absence or presence of fibrin, but the A-I$_M$ dimer at the same final concentrations was far more effective. Plasmin release was raised, in fact, several-fold (in the absence and presence of fibrin) over that by controls, the effect being concentration-dependent. The potentiating effect of the A-I$_M$ dimer was of similar magnitude to the plasminogen activation induced by tPA (Fig. 2). Interestingly, the addition of ε-aminocaproic or tranexamic acid to the incubation mixture completely abolished the capacity of A-I$_M$/A-I$_M$ to stimulate plasminogen activation, which strongly suggests that the lysine-binding sites on plasminogen may be involved in the interaction with the A-I$_M$ dimer.

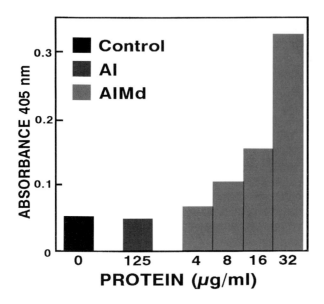

Fig. 2. Effect of plasminogen activation on a chromogenic substrate (S-2251) induced by different concentrations of apo A-I or of apo A-I_M dimer (courtesy of Dr J. Chmielewska).

In vivo studies

The limited availability up till now of a highly purified recombinant A-I_M dimer has somewhat restricted the in vivo evaluation. However, at least two studies should be mentioned.

In a *peripheral angioplasty* model in cholesterol-fed rabbits, A-I_M/A-I_M liposomes (50 mg per injection) or an equivalent amount of EPC were given five times according to a schedule of evenly spaced injections before and after the surgical procedure. Forty-two days after the angioplasty, vehicle-treated rabbits showed the expected >80% stenosis of the operated artery, vs. less than 40% involvement in A-I_M dimer-treated animals [Shah PK, personal communication].

In the second model, a *carotid constriction* was applied to cholesterol-fed rabbits according to Booth et al. [25]. In this case too the dimer was injected i.v. five times, evenly spaced before and after application of the restricting collar. A more than 50% reduction of lesion development was observed.

Conclusions

Studies on the A-I-Milano mutation and the subsequent development of its potential use in therapy offer an interesting example of how the current rapid progress in recombinant DNA technology allows the direct evaluation on in vitro and in vivo models of hypotheses raised from clinical observations. The case of recombinant apolipoproteins, in particular of the A-I_M dimer, capable of removing lipid deposits from arterial plaques is of special interest, because rapidly emerging clinical technologies permit a direct, noninvasive evaluation of arterial wall conditions. Such is the case of B-mode ultrasound for carotid and major peripheral arteries [26] and of two-dimensional echocardiography [27] or fat-suppressed "breath-hold" nuclear magnetic resonance [28] for the evaluation of coronaries. When these techniques achieve world-wide application, the need for direct correction of initial or more advanced arterial lesions will prompt the use of recombinant proteins capable of removing atheromatous lesions, most likely apolipoproteins.

Among these, the A-I$_M$ dimer offers an attractive choice because of: a) combined lipid-mobilizing and fibrinolytic activities; b) long half-life in plasma; c) better patent protection in a very competitive and struggling field. These 20 years of studies have, in any case, provided an exciting opportunity for establishing a direct link between a genetic observation, evaluation of the phenotypic expression and translation into a usable therapeutic tool.

References

1. Pousette A, Leijonhufvud PK, Akerlöf E. Scand J Clin Lab Invest 1993;213:39—44.
2. Terkeltaub RA, Dyer CA, Martin J, Curtiss LK. J Clin Invest 1991;87:20—26.
3. Nathan BP, Bellosta S, Sanan DA, Weisgraber KH, Mahley RW, Pitas RE. Science 1994;264:850—854.
4. Fujimoto K, Fukagawa K, Sakata T, Tso P. J Clin Invest 1993;91:1830—1833.
5. Owens RJ, Anantharamaiah GM, Kahlon JB, Srinivas RV, Compans RW, Segrest JP. J Clin Invest 1990;86: 1142—1150.
6. Levine DM, Parker TS, Donnelly TM, Walsh A, Rubin AL. Proc Natl Acad Sci 1993;90:12040—12044.
7. Maciejko JJ, Holmes DR, Kottke BA, Zinsmeister AR, Dinh DM, Mao SJT. N Engl J Med 1983;309:385—389.
8. Shah PK, Amin J. Circulation 1992;85:1279—1285.
9. Franceschini G, Sirtori CR, Capurso A, Weisgraber KH, Mahley RW. J. Clin Invest 1980;66:892—900.
10. Gualandri V, Franceschini G, Sirtori CR, Gianfranceschi G, Orsini GB, Cerrone A, Menotti A. Am J Human Genet 1985;376:1083—1097.
11. Weisgraber KH, Bersot TP, Mahley RW, Franceschini G, Sirtori CR. J. Clin Invest 1980;66:901—907.
12. Franceschini G, Frosi TG, Manzoni C, Gianfranceschi G, Sirtori CR. J Biol Chem 1982;257:9926—9930.
13. Bekaert ED, Alaupovic P, Knight-Gibson CS, Franceschini G, Sirtori CR. J Lipid Res 1993;34:111—123.
14. Weisgraber KH, Rall SC Jr, Bersot TP, Mahley RW, Franceschini G, Sirtori CR. J Biol Chem 1983;258: 2508—2513.
15 Franceschini G, Vecchio V, Gianfranceschi G, Magani D, Sirtori CR. J Biol Chem 1985;260:16321—16325.
16. Roma P, Gregg RE, Meng MS, Ronan R, Zech LA, Franceschini G, Sirtori CR, Brewer HB Jr. J Clin Invest 1993;91:1445—1452.
17. Badimon JJ, Badimon L, Galvez A, Dische R, Fuster V. Lab Invest 1989;60:455—461.
18. Badimon JJ, Badimon L, Fuster V. J Clin Invest 1990;85:1234—1241.
19. Beitz J, Beitz A, Antonov IV, Misharin AY, Mest HJ. Prostagland Leukotr Ess Fatty Acids 1992;47:149—152.
20. Trachtenberg JD, Cochrane H, Sun S, Sauther M, Lassere M, Choi E, Li AP, Callow AD. Circulation 1993;88:1-522.
21. Rubin EM, Krauss RM, Spangler EA, Verstuyft JG, Clift SM. Nature 1991;353:265—267.
22. Paszty C, Maeda N, Verstuyft J, Rubin EM. J Clin Invest 1994;94:899—903.
23. Calabresi L, Vecchio G, Longhi R, Gianazza E, Palm G, Wadensten H, Hammarström A, Olsson A, Karlström A, Sejkitz H, Sirtori CR, Fanceschini G. A molecular characterization of native and recombinant apolipoprotein A-I-Milano dimer. The introduction of an interchain disulfide bridge remarkably alters the physicochemical properties of apolipoprotein A-I. J Biol Chem (in press).
24. Saku K, Ahmad M, Glas-Greenwalt P, Kashyap ML. Thromb Res 1985;39:1—8.
25. Booth RFG, Martin JF, Honey AC, Hassall DG, Beesley JE, Moncada S. Atherosclerosis 1989;76:257—268.
26. Poli A, Tremoli E, Colombo A, Sirtori M, Pignoli P, Paoletti R. Atherosclerosis 1988;70:253—261.
27. Yoshida K, Yoshikawa J, Hozumi T, Yamaura Y, Akasaka T, Fukaya T, Kato H. Circulation 1990;81: 1271—1276.
28. Manning WJ, Li W, Boyle NG, Edelman RR. Circulation 1993;87:94—104.

Atherosclerosis X.
F.P. Woodford, J. Davignon and A. Sniderman, editors.

Smooth muscle lineage diversity and atherosclerosis

Mark W. Majesky[1] and Stavros Topouzis[2]

Departments of [1]Cell Biology and [2]Pathology, Baylor College of Medicine, One Baylor Plaza, Houston, TX 77030, USA

Abstract. Dramatic differences in the incidence and severity of atherosclerotic plaques are commonly found in different segments of the same disease-prone artery. Aortic homografts transplanted from thoracic to abdominal positions (and vice versa) provide evidence for intrinsic differences in growth and extracellular matrix (ECM)-producing properties of smooth muscle cells (SMCs) in different aortic segments. What is the basis for SMC diversity within a common artery wall? Recent lineage analysis studies in the avian and mammalian embryo indicate that at least two distinct SMC lineages contribute to formation of the major outflow tract arteries. SMCs in the thoracic aorta originate in the neural crest, whereas abdominal aortic SMCs arise from lateral plate mesoderm. Coronary artery SMCs originate from yet a third precursor population in intracardiac mesenchyme. A mixture of SMC types of diverse developmental lineages within a common vessel wall raises new questions about the potential for SMC type-specific responses to growth factors and cytokines involved in human atherogenesis.

Atherosclerotic plaques that arise in different locations within major, disease-prone arteries clearly differ in their incidence and rate of progression to advanced, complicated lesions [1]. The variation in lesion formation between different arterial segments is often attributed to differences in blood flow dynamics and shear stress forces acting upon the endothelium in an arterial site-specific manner. Endothelial cells respond to variations in fluid shear stress with changes in the production or release of factors that act upon underlying smooth muscle cells (SMCs) to modulate their growth and extracellular matrix (ECM) production. It is generally assumed that SMCs in different segments of the same artery respond in essentially similar ways to growth factors and cytokines released by endothelial cells (or other cell types). However, intrinsic differences in the growth and ECM-producing properties of SMCs from different segments of a common vessel wall have been reported [2,3] that may play important, possibly even determining, roles in the variability of plaque properties and distribution found in human arteries [1–3].

What is the basis for intrinsic SMC diversity in different segments of the major outflow tract arteries? Recent lineage analysis studies of arterial SMC origins in the avian and mammalian embryo demonstrate that more than one type of SMC is present in the walls of large outflow tract vessels [4,5]. Therefore, the commonly held view that a single type of multifunctional SMC makes up the tunica media of the artery wall may be too simplistic. A mixture of unique SMC types within a common vessel wall raises important new questions about the potential of different SMC populations to carry out distinct functions in vivo and about their ability to respond in a SMC type-specific way to growth factors and cytokines involved in the origins and progression of atherosclerotic vascular disease.

Address for correspondence: Mark W. Majesky, PhD, Department of Pathology, Baylor College of Medicine, 1 Baylor Plaza, Houston, TX 77030-3498, USA. Tel.: +1-713-798-5837; Fax: +1-713-798-8920.

Arterial smooth muscle diversity

A historical perspective

The concept that only a single type of SMC is present in the artery wall arose from the regularity of ultrastructural appearance of cells in the mammalian tunica media. Pease and Paule [6] examined the ultrastructure of the rat aorta and concluded that only one type of cell can be found in the tunica media and that is "a form of smooth muscle cell". They remarked that aortic SMCs differed in appearance from SMCs found in small, muscular pial arteries of the rat. Although structurally distinct in subtle ways from their counterparts in smaller arteries, the aortic SMC population in the rat nevertheless appeared homogeneous by ultrastructural criteria.

In the early 1960s, many investigators maintained that both fibroblasts and SMCs were present in the tunica media, the former accounting for collagen, elastin and other ECM proteins found in artery walls while the latter served as the contractile element. In 1968, Wissler proposed that both functions — contraction and ECM synthesis — were carried out by a single, "multifunctional" type of SMC. The ability to isolate pure cultures of arterial SMCs and directly test their ability to synthesize in vitro the matrix proteins found in the vessel wall quickly led to acceptance of the idea that SMCs themselves were the source of these ECM proteins [7]. Therefore, SMCs could indeed synthesize both contractile and ECM proteins and thus the postulate that a second cell type (fibroblast) was present in the wall seemed unnecessary.

In 1979, Chamley-Campbell et al. proposed that the two principal functions of arterial SMCs in vivo, contraction and ECM synthesis, were embodied in different but interconvertible phenotypic states that they termed "contractile" and "synthetic" [8]. Thus, SMCs adapted to cell culture, as well as SMCs at sites of arterial wound repair, express a "synthetic" phenotype whereas fully differentiated SMCs in normal vessel wall display a "contractile" phenotype. Recent work suggests that the conversion of SMCs from one phenotype to the other may depend upon the nature of the contacts made by SMCs with specific components of the ECM.

Evidence for arterial SMC diversity

There is little doubt that phenotypic modulation is an important adaptive property of vascular SMCs and that the concept can explain much of the variation in gene expression patterns of SMCs in vitro compared to their counterparts in the mature, fully differentiated vessel wall. However, a global reliance on the model of SMC phenotypic modulation to explain the full range of variation in arterial SMC properties may ignore important exceptions to this general rule.

Indeed, our own studies comparing PDGF ligand and receptor gene expression between neointimal SMCs and normal medial SMCs from rat carotid artery cannot easily be explained by phenotypic modulation of a single type of SMC [3]. Consideration of alternative explanations for our data led us to suggest that the walls of large elastic arteries, such as the rat common carotid artery, might be composed of more than one type of SMC [3]. Our proposed scheme is analogous to the fiber-type diversity found in most skeletal muscles where fast fibers, slow fibers and fast/slow (mixed) fiber types are combined together within a common muscle bundle. All myofiber types are similar in ultrastructural appearance but they differ in the expression of myosin heavy-chain genes, the rate of myosin ATPase activity and hence their rate of contraction [9]. Different myofiber types have been shown to originate from different types of myoblasts that arise within the somites in a distinct temporal sequence and then migrate in separate "waves" to the developing limb bud musculature [9]. Myocardial cells are also recognized to be of many types, segregated into different regions of the heart with unique developmental origins and functional properties. Since the structural, functional and regulatory demands on vascular SMCs are no less intricate than for skeletal or cardiac myocytes, it seems reasonable to ask if a similar type of diversity might exist for SMCs in the vessel wall.

Developmental origins of vascular SMC

In vertebrates, SMCs in most blood vessels are of mesodermal origin. In contrast, SMCs in the great vessels of the cardiac outflow tract originate in the neural crest, a neural ectoderm-derived structure unique to the vertebrate embryo. This was first shown by LeLievre and LeDouarin [4] who transplanted quail premigratory neural crest into chick embryo hosts whose neural crest at equivalent levels had been surgically removed (chick–quail chimeras). Kirby and co-workers [5] then showed that the smooth muscle-forming potential of the neural crest is localized to a region between the mid-otic placode and the caudal limit of somite three. This region is now called the "cardiac neural crest" (CNC). Ablation studies in which the CNC and nodose placode (a source of surrogate ectomesenchyme) are destroyed by surgical means results in severe malformation of the aortic arch arteries in the chick embryo [5]. LeLievre and LeDouarin termed the SMCs that originate in the CNC ectomesenchymal (Ect) SMCs to indicate their derivation from neural ectoderm and to distinguish them from mesoderm-derived mesenchymal (Mes) SMCs [4]. These pioneering studies revealed that SMCs that form the walls of the outflow tract arteries (thoracic aorta, brachiocephalic and common carotid arteries, pulmonary trunk and ductus arteriosus) are a mixture of SMC types derived from two distinct embryological lineages, neural ectoderm and mesoderm (Fig. 1).

Properties of Ect and Mes SMCs in the chick embryo aorta

The chick–quail chimera mapping studies [4] revealed that the upper thoracic aorta is composed primarily of Ect SMCs whereas the abdominal aorta contains only Mes SMCs. On the basis of this rigid anatomical distribution, as well as the ability to surgically ablate the premigratory CNC, the properties of Ect and Mes SMCs have been described both in vivo and in vitro.

Kirby and co-workers showed that proper formation of the septum dividing the truncus arteriosus into the aorta and pulmonary artery depends upon Ect SMCs [5]. The failure of these cells to arrive in the truncal cushion tissue after surgical ablation of the CNC results in persistent truncus arteriosus [5]. Rosenquist et al. found that Ect SMCs play a critical role in the initiation and downstream propagation of elastogenesis in the developing outflow tract vessels [10]. They found that thermal ablation of the CNC resulted in delayed downstream deployment of elastin synthesis and in the impaired assembly of the elastic fibers that were produced [10]. The developmental defects in the heart and great vessels after ablation of the CNC in the chick embryo are highly reminiscent of the clinical anomalies found in the DiGeorge Syndrome in humans [5].

In our laboratory, we have examined the growth and adhesion properties of Ect and Mes SMCs in vitro [11]. We found that both SMC types express similar levels of desmin, α-smooth muscle actin, calponin and tropoelastin in vitro, thus confirming their SMC identity. Although similar in expression of these SMC markers, Ect and Mes SMCs differed dramatically in their growth responses to transforming growth factor-β1 (TGF-β1) [11]. Confluent Ect SMCs exhibited increased DNA synthesis after TGF-β1 addition

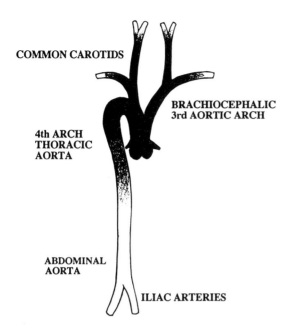

COMMON CAROTIDS

BRACHIOCEPHALIC
3rd AORTIC ARCH

4th ARCH
THORACIC
AORTA

ABDOMINAL
AORTA

ILIAC ARTERIES

Fig. 1. Distribution of two SMC types in the chick embryo aorta. Lineage analysis studies show that two different SMC types form the walls of the major outflow tract arteries in the chick embryo. Ectomesenchymal SMCs (Ect, black) originate in the neural crest and construct the proximal walls of the major outflow tract vessels. Mesenchymal SMCs (Mes, white) originate in lateral plate mesoderm and form the walls of the abdominal aorta as well as more distal portions of the outflow tract vessels. In between, a mixed population of Ect and Mes SMCs is found (gray), the precise extent and composition of which is presently unknown.

(0.01–10 ng/ml) while Mes SMCs had no response or were growth-inhibited by TGF-β1. Radioligand binding and receptor cross-linking studies showed that Ect and Mes SMCs have similar levels of ^{125}I-TGF-β1 receptors on their cell surface. However, the extent of receptor-mediated increases in expression of a number of TGF-β1-responsive genes is consistently greater in Ect than in Mes SMCs. In preliminary transfection studies using a luciferase reporter gene driven by the TGF-β1 response elements from the human PAI-1 promoter, we observed much greater increases in reporter activity after TGF-β1 stimulation in Ect than in Mes SMCs. Thus Ect and Mes SMCs in vitro appear to differ in signal transduction pathways leading to activation of transcription factors involved in the control of TGF-β1-dependent changes in gene expression. This possibility is consistent with the findings of Wrenn et al. [12] who showed that protein kinase C activation and intracellular levels of 1,2-diacylglycerol were increased after stimulation of Ect SMCs with TGF-β1 whereas Mes SMCs showed no evidence of either response.

The fact that two different SMC lineages combine to form the tunica media raises the question of whether Ect and Mes SMCs intermix freely in vivo or prefer to segregate into "zones" or "patches" during morphogenesis of the artery wall. We have begun to examine this question by analysis of the proteins that mediate cell–cell adhesion in vertebrate tissues. Using RT-PCR and direct sequencing of the reaction products, our results to date suggest that Ect SMCs express a different repertoire of cadherins (a family of calcium-dependent cell–cell adhesion molecules) at their cell surface from Mes SMCs. These intriguing results suggest that Ect and Mes SMCs may not freely interact during vessel wall morphogenesis and raise the possibility that an even greater regional heterogeneity of SMC populations might exist than had been previously anticipated.

Acknowledgements

We thank Marcia Smith-Anderson and Xiu-Rong Dong for help with chick embryo cultures and molecular cloning studies. We also thank Joey Barnett, Jeffrey Wrana, Joan Massague, Robert Schwartz, Dave Loskutoff and Daniel Rifkin for cDNA probes and reagents, Victor Koteliansky and Jean-Paul Thiery for help with cadherin cloning and sequencing, and Tim McQuinn and Michael Schneider for helpful discussions. This work was supported by NIH Grant HL-47655, AHA Grant 91G-181 and The Moran Foundation.

References

1. DeBakey ME, Lawrie GM, Glaeser DH. Ann Surg 1985;201:115–131.
2. Haimovici H, Maier N, Strauss L. Arch Surg 1958;76:282–288.
3. Majesky MW, Giachelli CM, Reidy MA, Schwartz SM. Circ Res 1992;71:759–768.
4. LeLievre CS, LeDouarin NM. J Embryol Exp Morphol 1975;34:125–154.
5. Kirby ML, Waldo KL. Circulation 1990;82:332–340.
6. Pease DC, Paule WJ. J Ultrastr Res 1960;3:469–483.
7. Ross R, Klebanoff SJ. J Cell Biol 1971;50:159–171.
8. Chamley-Campbell JH, Campbell GR, Ross R. Physiol Rev 1979;59:1–61.
9. Stockdale FE. Dev Biol 1992;154:284–298.
10. Rosenquist TH, Beall AC. Ann NY Acad Sci 1990;588:106–119.
11. Topouzis S, Majesky MW. J Cell Biochem 1994;18(A):294.
12. Wrenn RW, Raeuber CL, Herman LE, Walton WJ, Rosenquist TH. In Vitro Cell Devel Biol 1993;29A: 73–78.

©1995 Elsevier Science B.V. All rights reserved.
Atherosclerosis X.
F.P. Woodford, J. Davignon and A. Sniderman, editors.

Immunity, inflammation, and the role of T lymphocytes in atherosclerosis

Göran K. Hansson and Sten Stemme

Gothenburg University, Department of Laboratory Medicine, Sahlgrenska University Hospital, S-41345 Gothenburg, Sweden

Abstract. The presence of substantial numbers of T lymphocytes and activated macrophages in atherosclerotic plaques suggests that components of the immune system may play an important role in the development of the disease. This is supported by the detection of local cytokine secretion and of circulating antibodies to modified lipoproteins and other antigens present in the lesion. This contribution provides a brief overview of our current knowledge of immune mechanisms in atherogenesis.

It has been known for several decades that a mononuclear cell infiltrate is invariably present in the atherosclerotic plaque. This led to speculations of a role for immune and inflammatory mechanisms in atherogenesis, but its specificity and consequences have been obscure. Recent research has renewed this idea and new evidence has appeared that supports a role for immune mechanisms in atherosclerosis.

The earliest morphological evidence of disease in hypercholesterolemic animal models of atherosclerosis is the attachment of monocytes to the intact endothelium [1]. This is followed by the subendothelial accumulation of macrophages, which differentiate into lipid-laden foam cells [1–3] and of T lymphocytes, which enter the intima together with monocytes [3]. This stage is also recognized in early human lesions [4] and is later followed by the migration and proliferation of smooth muscle cells, which form a fibrous cap around the lipid-rich, inflammatory lesion [2,5].

Evidence for a local activation of T lymphocytes in atherosclerotic plaques

By the use of monoclonal antibodies in an immunohistochemical mapping of gene expression in human plaques it was found [6] that the HLA class II gene HLA-DR is expressed by many smooth muscle cells, although these cells do not normally express this gene. Since HLA-DR is induced by the T-cell cytokine γ-interferon the obvious conclusion was that activated T cells present in the lesion induced HLA-DR expression on smooth muscle cells by release of this cytokine [6]. This was confirmed by an immunohistochemical analysis of the cellular composition of advanced human atherosclerotic plaques. 10–20% of all cells were found to express T cell-specific antigens such as CD3, with approximately two-thirds of the T cells expressing CD4 and one-third the CD8 antigen [5].

The presence of T cells and monocyte-derived macrophages makes it possible that antigen presentation and immune activation may occur in atherosclerotic plaques. In support of this, it was shown that many T cells express interleukin-2 receptors and HLA-DR [7]. Flow cytometric analysis of T cells isolated from plaques revealed a total dominance of the memory T cell phenotype and expression of the VLA-1 (very late activation) antigen [8]. Cytokines that are released by activated T cells have been found in plaques by immunohistochemistry [7] and PCR [9] and the "aberrant" expression of

62

HLA-DR in the plaque [6] provides indirect evidence for a local γ-interferon secretion.

Mechanisms for recruitment of immunocompetent cells to the vessel wall in atherosclerosis

In the cholesterol-fed rabbit, the two earliest detectable vascular events are expression of endothelial adhesion molecules and intimal complement deposition. Focal expression of VCAM-1 (vascular cell adhesion molecule-1) can be found as early as 1 week after the start of the atherogenic diet [10,11] and is followed by the entry of MHC-class-II-expressing monocyte-macrophages and other leukocytes a couple of weeks later [11]. VCAM-1 is a ligand for VLA-4, a cell-surface protein expressed by lymphocytes and monocytes [12]. It is not expressed by granulocytes and it is therefore possible that the expression of VCAM-1 on atherosclerotic endothelia selectively recruits mononuclear cells to the forming lesion. This could explain the lack of granulocytes in atherosclerotic lesions.

VCAM-1 is not expressed constitutively by endothelial cells but is inducible by proinflammatory cytokines including interleukin-1 (IL-1), tumor necrosis factor (TNF) and γ-interferon [11,13]. It is likely that the production of such cytokines in the underlying atheroma contributes to the continued expression of VCAM-1 on the surface of the forming plaque but it is less likely that IL-1, TNF or γ-interferon will be present in sufficient concentrations at the pre-lesion stage. Surprisingly, VCAM-1 expression is also induced by lysophosphatidylcholine, which may be present in lipoproteins and generated during lipoprotein oxidation and cell-membrane injury [14]. In the hypercholesterolemic state, lysophosphatidylcholine might therefore perhaps induce VCAM-1 expression on the endothelium.

Humoral immune reactions and effector mechanisms in atherosclerosis

The vascular reaction in early hypercholesterolemia is characterized not only by de novo gene expression in vascular cells but also by an infiltration and accumulation of plasma proteins. There is a deposition of lipoproteins but also a prominent infiltration and deposition of immunoglobulins and complement factors. IgG deposits on intracellular filaments and extracellular collagen fibers are due to specific interactions between the Fc part of the immunoglobulin molecule and protein components of these filaments [15]. The intracellular accumulation of IgG in injured endothelial cells is particularly striking and can be used to detect damaged endothelial cells [16].

Several complement factors are detectable in the atherosclerotic intima, including C1 and C3b [17]. The accumulation of C5b-9 is particularly important since it is indicative of an activation of the complement cascade. C5b-9 deposits are found in the rabbit aorta within 2 weeks after initiation of a cholesterol-rich diet and increase with the progression of the disease process [18]. These deposits represent membrane-anchored attack complexes with the capacity to perforate cellular membranes and might effectuate cytolytic processes in the atherosclerotic artery. Peptide fragments such as C3a and C5a, which are released during activation of the complement cascade prior to the formation of the C5b-9 complex, exhibit chemotactic and leukocyte-activating properties and could be important for the recruitment of leukocytes to the lesion [19]. The initiation of the cascade reaction might occur at the IgG deposits at sites of cell injury but also on cholesterol deposits. The latter may, at least in vitro, activate the complement cascade through the alternative pathway in a reaction that is amplified by oxidative modification of the cholesterol molecule [20].

The search for "athero-antigens"

The presence of activated T cells and macrophages strongly suggests that an immunologic reaction is taking place in the atherosclerotic plaque. The antigens that elicit this response are not yet known, and both microorganisms and autoantigens have been proposed to play a role. The most interesting candidates at present are oxidized LDL and heat-shock proteins.

Autoantibodies to oxidized LDL lipoproteins are common in man [21]; their titer appears to correlate with the progression of atherosclerosis [22]. Aminoacid conjugates such as malondialdehyde-lysine serve as B-cell epitopes [23] and are found in significant amounts in plaques [24,25]. It is likely that the B-cell response is dependent on T-cell help and it has therefore been proposed that CD4+ cells in the plaque initiate an autoimmune response to oxidized LDL. This hypothesis is supported by the recent observation that CD4+ T cells cloned from human plaques respond to oxidized LDL in an HLA class II-restricted fashion [26]. The T-cell epitopes on the oxidized LDL particle have not yet been identified.

Many inflammatory and autoimmune diseases, including atherosclerosis, are associated with antibody production against heat-shock proteins. These are intracellular chaperones that stabilize the conformation of other proteins. They are synthesized in excessive amounts during cell injury and induce T cell-dependent antibody production [27]. Several heat-shock proteins are found in atherosclerotic lesions [28] and the titer of autoantibodies to heat-shock protein 60 appears to correlate with the extent of carotid atherosclerosis [29]. In cholesterol-fed rabbits, immunization with heat shock protein 60 aggravates atherosclerosis, which suggests that this autoimmune response may be of pathogenic significance [30].

Very few B cells are found in the plaque [5] and it is therefore likely that B-cell activation and antibody production occur in regional lymph nodes. T cells might "patrol" peripheral tissues (including plaques), recognize antigen, home to lymph nodes, and activate B cells [31]. Advanced cases of atherosclerosis may, however, be complicated by periadventitial inflammation which can result in large inflammatory infiltrates. Microscopically, these lesions are dominated by B lymphocytes and macrophages together with oxidized lipid components and antibodies to oxidized LDL [32,33] and it is possible that they represents an autoimmune response to oxidized LDL [33].

Immunologic effector mechanisms, cytotoxicity, and antigen elimination

Cellular immune responses may initiate inflammatory reactions, cell-mediated cytotoxicity and cytokine-dependent regulatory loops in the atherosclerotic plaque. T cell-dependent induction of antibody production to plaque antigens such as oxidized LDL could represent a mechanism for antigen elimination. Immune complexes consisting of LDL and anti-LDL antibodies are readily taken up by Fc receptor-bearing macrophages, which may transform into cholesterol-laden foam cells [34]. In addition, if antigens are fixed on cell surfaces, they could bind antibodies. Both the complement cascade and Fc receptor-bearing macrophages and cytotoxic lymphocytes would attack antibody-coated target cells. The presence of membrane-bound C5b-9 complexes in experimental plaques [18] indicates that complement lysis takes place. It is not clear, however, whether this occurs as the result of antibody binding to specific antigens on the surface of cells or is due to an "innocent bystander" attack after alternative complement activation on the extracellular cholesterol deposits [20].

64

Cytokines and the regulation of gene expression in the atherosclerotic plaque

Several reports demonstrate the presence of immune-regulatory cytokines in the atherosclerotic plaque. Proinflammatory cytokines including IL-1, TNF, IL-6, and γ-interferon are secreted in the plaque [35], probably by T lymphocytes, macrophages, endothelial cells and smooth muscle cells. The pathogenetic consequences of such a paracrine cytokine secretion could include activation of macrophages and endothelial cells [35], modulation of cholesterol uptake [36] and an inhibition of vascular contractility [37–39] and cell proliferation [37,40]. Most of these mechanisms have been identified and characterized in cell culture studies. There is, however, in vivo evidence in experimental animal models for cytokine control of endothelial activation [41] and inhibition of smooth muscle proliferation [42].

It will be important to establish the role of other potential regulatory mechanisms by in vivo studies of cytokine action on the vessel wall. Finally, it will be critically important to clarify to what extent the immune response is beneficial or detrimental for the atherosclerotic patient. However, in view of the complexity of the immune system and of the disease process, it appears unlikely that this question will have a simple answer. It is more probable that certain phases and components of the vascular immune response may accelerate the atherosclerotic process, while others may modulate or control it.

Acknowledgements

This work is supported by the Swedish Medical Research Council (project 6816) and the Swedish Heart-Lung Foundation.

References

1. Gerrity RG. Am J Pathol 1981;103:181.
2. Faggiotto A, Ross R. Arteriosclerosis 1984;4:323.
3. Hansson GK, Seifert PS, Olsson G, Bondjers G. Arterioscler Thromb 1991;11:745.
4. Munro JM, van der Walt JD, Munro CS, Chalmers JAC, Cox EL. Hum Pathol 1987;18:375.
5. Jonasson L, Holm J, Skalli O, Bondjers G, Hansson GK. Arteriosclerosis. 6, 131 (1986).
6. Jonasson L, Holm J, Skalli O, Gabbiani Hansson GK. J Clin Invest 1985;76:125.
7. Hansson GK, Holm J, Jonasson L. Am J Pathol 1989;135:169.
8. Stemme S, Holm J, Hansson GK. Arterioscler Thromb 1992;12:206.
9. Geng YJ, Holm J, Nygren S, Bruzelius M, Stemme S et al. Arterioscler Thromb 1994 (in press).
10. Cybulsky MI, Gimbrone MA. Science 1991;251:788.
11. Li H, Cybulsky MI, Gimbrone MA, Libby P. Arterioscler Thromb 1993;13:197.
12. Elices MJ, Osborn L, Takada Y, Crouse C, Luhowskyj S et al. Cell 1990;60:577.
13. Bevilacqua MP, Pober JS, Mendrick DL, Cotran RS, Gimbrone MA. Proc Natl Acad Sci USA 1987;84:9238.
14. Kume N, Cybulsky MI, Gimbrone MA. J Clin Invest 1992;90:1138.
15. Hansson GK, Starkebaum GA, Benditt EP, Schwartz SM. Proc Natl Acad Sci USA 1984;81:3103.
16. Hansson GK, Schwartz SM. Am J Pathol 1983;112:278.
17. Seifert PS, Kazatchkine MD. Atherosclerosis 1988;73:91.
18. Seifert PS, Hugo F, Hansson GK, Bhakdi S. Lab Invest 1989;60:747.
19. Hansson GK, Lagerstedt E, Bengtsson A, Heideman M. Exp Cell Res 1987;170:338.
20. Seifert PS, Kazatchkine MD. Mol Immunol 1987;24:1303.
21. Ylä-Herttuala S, Palinski W, Rosenfeld ME, Parthasarathy S, Carew TE et al. J Clin Invest 1989;84:1086.
22. Salonen JT, Ylä-Herttuala S, Yamamoto R, Butler S, Korpela H et al. Lancet 1992;339:883.
23. Palinski W, Ylä-Herttuala S, Rosenfeld ME, Butler SW, Socher SA et al. Arterioscl Thromb 1990;10:325.
24. Palinski W, Rosenfeld ME, Ylä-Herttuala S, Gurtner GC, Socher SA et al. Proc Natl Acad Sci USA 1989;86:1372.
25. Ylä-Herttuala S, Palinski W, Butler SW, Picard S, Steinberg D et al. Arterioscler Thromb 1994;14:32.

26. Stemme S, Faber B, Holm J, Bondjers G, Witztum JL et al. Proc Natl Acad Sci USA 1994 (in press).
27. Kiessling R, Grönberg A, Ivanyi J, Söderström K, Ferm M et al. Immunol Rev 1991;121:91.
28. Xu Q, Kleindienst R, Waitz W, Dietrich H, Wick G. J Clin Invest 1993;91:2693.
29. Xu Q, Willeit J, Marosi M, Kleindienst R, Oberhollenzer F et al. Lancet 1993;341:255.
30. Xu Q, Dietrich H, Steiner HJ, Gown AM, Schoel B et al. Arterioscler Thromb 1992 (in press).
31. Mackay CR, Marston WL, Dudler L. J Exp Med 1990;171:801.
32. Parums DV, Chadwick DR, Mitchinson MJ. Atherosclerosis 1986;61:117.
33. Parums DV, Brown DL, Mitchinson MJ. Arch Pathol Lab Med 1990;114:383.
34. Griffith RL, Virella GT, Stevenson HC, Lopes-Virella MF. J Exp Med 1988;168:1041.
35. Libby P, Hansson GK. Lab Invest 1991;64:5.
36. Geng YJ, Hansson GK. J Clin Invest 1992;89:1322.
37. Hansson GK, Jonasson L, Holm J, Clowes MM, Clowes AW. Circ Res 1988;63:712.
38. Geng YJ, Hansson GK, Holme E. Circ Res 1992;71:1268.
39. Hansson GK, Geng YJ, Holm J, Hårdhammar P, Wennmalm Å et al. J Exp Med 1994;180:733.
40. Hansson GK, Hellstrand M, Rymo L, Rubbia L, Gabbiani G. J Exp Med 1989;170:1595.
41. Pober JS, Cotran RS. Physiol Rev 1990;70:427.
42. Hansson GK, Holm J, Holm S, Fotev Z, Hedrich HJ et al. Proc Natl Acad Sci USA 1991;88:10530.

Osteoprogenitor cells and mechanism of plaque calcification

Linda L. Demer, Kristina Boström, Karol E. Watson and William P. Stanford

University of California, Los Angeles, Department of Medicine, Division of Cardiology, 47–123 Center for Health Sciences, Los Angeles, California, USA

Abstract. The mechanism of calcium mineral deposition in atherosclerotic plaque is not known. Evidence to support a regulatory mechanism includes: (1) expression of bone morphogenetic protein, a potent osteoinductive factor, (2) expression of bone matrix proteins, and (3) formation of hydroxyapatite mineral and matrix vesicles in calcified human atherosclerotic lesions. In addition, fully-formed bone tissue, including marrow-like elements, occurs frequently in advanced plaque. In smooth muscle cell cultures, a subpopulation of cells have been isolated that undergo osteoblastic differentiation in response to oxysterols and transforming growth factor beta. These cells share features with pericytes and we speculate that they are neural crest-derived multipotent cells.

Calcium mineral deposits occur frequently in atherosclerotic lesions. More than 80% of clinically significant coronary atherosclerotic plaques contain calcium deposits large enough to be detectable by intravascular ultrasound. Such deposits increase the risk of clinical events, possibly because of increased lesion stiffness or increased susceptibility to plaque rupture along the plane separating the mineral from the more compliant noncalcified regions where solid shear stress is concentrated.

The mechanism of mineral formation in the artery wall is not known. Although it occurs in the absence of hypercalcemia, it is widely considered a passive chemical process rather than an active one. Some evidence suggests that the process is regulated and resembles osteogenesis. The mineral in atherosclerosis is hydroxyapatite or bioapatite bone mineral, rather than merely amorphous calcium phosphate, and matrix vesicles have been demonstrated by electron microscopy [1]. Furthermore, the mineral often takes the form of mature, actively remodeling bone, including marrow-like elements. This ossification occurs not only in the aorta, but also in femoral and coronary artery atherosclerosis. The source of the osteoprogenitor cells that produce and remodel the bone tissue and of the marrow stromal-like cells is unknown.

Bone-related factors in the artery wall

To test the hypothesis that atherosclerotic calcification occurs by a regulated mechanism similar to osteogenesis, we looked for expression of the potent osteogenic differentiation factor bone morphogenetic protein-2 (BMP-2, previously BMP-2a [2,3]) in calcified atherosclerotic lesions, using in situ hybridization and immunohistochemistry (cDNA probe and monoclonal antibody kindly provided by Genetics Institute). Both message RNA and protein were found in association with areas of calcium mineral deposition [4,5]. The similarity with osteogenesis has been confirmed by recent reports of Giachelli

Address for correspondence: Linda L. Demer, University of California, Los Angeles, Department of Medicine, Division of Cardiology, 47–123 Center for Health Sciences, 10833 Le Conte Avenue, Los Angeles, CA 90024-1679, USA.

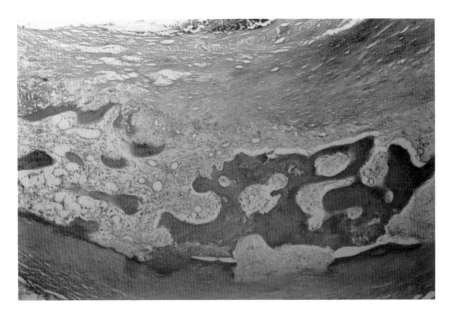

Fig. 1. Human atherosclerotic plaque containing bone and marrow.

et al., Ikeda et al. and others [6,7] demonstrating bone-related proteins colocalized with calcification in human atherosclerotic lesions.

Bone morphogenetic protein may serve as the initiating factor in the osteogenic differentiation of artery wall cells. It may also indicate activation of latent embryonic programs. Embryonic development of many tissues in addition to bone is regulated by bone morphogenetic proteins. In particular, BMP-2 is virtually identical to the drosophila developmental protein, decapentaplegic (dpp), which regulates whole body dorsal-ventral patterning. In the mouse embryo, it is found in embryonic limb buds, heart, whisker follicles, tooth buds and craniofacial mesenchyme [8]. Bone morphogenetic proteins are believed to act, in part, through regulation of homeobox genes whose downstream effectors are thought to be adhesion molecules.

One of the cell-substratum adhesion molecules found in bone and plaque is osteopontin. Both actin-positive cells and macrophages appear to produce osteopontin in the artery wall. Both are also associated with regions of calcification. Interestingly, the promoter for osteopontin contains a binding site for Egr-1, which is regulated by bone morphogenetic protein.

In vitro model of atherosclerotic calcification

In bone-cell culture, calcium mineral deposits form within nodules arising from the monolayer culture. Similar nodules form in cultures of retinal and renal pericytes and limb bud cells [9]. The nodules formed by retinal pericytes and limb bud cells also produce calcium mineral. Although smooth muscle cell cultures also produce nodules after 1 or 2 weeks, the phenomenon is not often observed because the cultures usually are not allowed to grow beyond confluence. In practice, cultures that do produce nodules are considered senescent, and they are discarded. Bjorkerud observed that the nodules contain matrix and foam cells with some similarity to atheromatous lesions [10].

In our laboratory Boström isolated cells from the aortic media that produce nodules and hydroxyapatite mineral in vitro [4]. Cultures were enriched for these cells by using trypsin to remove the monolayer surrounding the nodules. Cultures obtained by using the nodules as explants or by dispersing nodule-derived cells using collagenase were greatly enriched for nodules. Recognizing that this could represent enrichment of a subpopulation of cells, we returned to the primary cultures and used dilutional cloning to generate cultures cloned from single cells. Approximately 90 clones have been derived from four aortas and about one-third of the clones have been shown to produce calcified nodules [5]. In general, although the cloned cultures vary slightly in degree of nodule formation and surface ganglioside expression from one passage to the next and from one culture condition to the next, they retain their distinction from non-nodule-forming cells. Non-nodule-forming cells generally remain free of nodules over many passages. We have operationally defined the cloned cells that produce calcified nodules as calcifying vascular cells.

Bone-related proteins in in vitro model

No single marker identifies cells as osteoblasts in vitro. Osteoblast-like cells, usually harvested from skull bone or osteosarcomas, are considered osteoblastic only if they satisfy many of a set of criteria. Watson demonstrated that calcifying vascular cells meet the criteria of synthesis of alkaline phosphatase, particularly in the nodules, osteonectin, osteopontin, osteocalcin (considered a bone-specific protein) and collagen I (the primary collagen in bone) [5]. Many clones were also positive for cAMP response to parathyroid hormone. These features support a close relation between calcifying vascular cells and osteoblasts.

Factors that induce vascular calcification in vitro

The colocalization of calcium deposits and plaque, and the colocalization of cholesterol and calcium deposits within plaque [11], suggest a mechanistic relation. Two factors present in atherosclerotic lesions that may contribute to osteoblastic differentiation are transforming growth factor-beta (TGF-β) and oxysterols. Both were found to promote osteogenic differentiation in calcifying vascular cells in vitro [5].

Progenitor cells

Calcifying vascular cells do not stain with antibodies directed against CD2, CD11c, or Factor VIII-related antigen, distinguishing them from lymphocytes, monocytes and endothelial cells. They are positive for α and β smooth muscle actin and for the epitope of monoclonal antibody (mAb) 3G5, a surface ganglioside [12], specific for pericytes in the vasculature. This profile matches that of microvascular pericytes and is distinct from that of non-nodule-forming smooth muscle cells.

The growth characteristics and morphology of calcifying vascular cells also closely resemble those of microvascular pericytes, stellate-shaped cells that envelop and share basement membrane with the endothelial cells in the microvasculature. Furthermore, in tissue sections of normal bovine and atherosclerotic and nondiseased human aorta, a subset of subendothelial cells stain positively with mAb 3G5.

The similarities with pericytes are intriguing in that pericytes are osteoprogenitor cells [13]. Histologists have long postulated the existence of cells in loose connective tissue of the adult that retain the multipotentiality of embryonic mesenchymal cells. The pericyte has been postulated to be that multipotent cell [14]. In the liver and kidney, pericytes are believed to be responsible for the fibrotic response to injury and to platelet-derived growth factor and TGF-β [15].

Pericytes are believed to derive from the neural crest, which consists of stellate, multipotent cells [15]. As they migrate, neural-crest cells respond with progressive commitment to factors they encounter in their environment [16]. Removal from their original environment, the basement membrane of the neural crest, appears to induce both migration and commitment to differentiation. Phenotypes derived from neural-crest cells include melanocytes, glial cells, differentiated neurons, chondroblasts, osteoblasts, smooth muscle cells and fibroblasts.

Speculation

We speculate that calcifying vascular cells represent immature, neural crest-derived mesenchymal cells, similar to pericytes, and that they and other types of pericytes retain varying degrees of multipotentiality in the adult, allowing versatile repair. We also speculate that, when stimulated, these cells produce extensive extracellular matrix contributing to the fibrocellular component, as well as to the bone-like matrix in atherosclerosis, in a process recapitulating embryonic endochondral ossification.

Acknowledgements

This work was sponsored in part by the Streisand Research Fund of the Lincy Foundation, the Oberkotter Foundation, and NIH grants HL-30568, HL-07412, and HL-43379. We are grateful to the Immunology Department of Genetics Institute, Inc. for providing anti-BMP-2 monoclonal antibody and BMP-2 cDNA probe and to Dr. Larry W. Fisher for supplying antiosteopontin antibody.

References

1. Anderson HC. Arch Pathol Lab Med 1983; 107:341–348.
2. Urist MR. Science 1965;150:893–899.
3. Wozney JM, Rosen V, Celeste AJ, Mitsock LM, Whitters MJ, Kriz RW, Hewick RM, Wang EA. Science 1988;242:1528–1534.
4. Boström K, Watson, KE, Horn S, Wortham C, Herman IM, Demer LL. J Clin Invest 1993;91:1800–1809.
5. Watson KE, Boström K, Ravindranath R, Lam T, Norton B, Demer LL. J Clin Invest 1994;93:2106–2113.
6. Giachelli CM, Bae N, Almeida M, Denhardt DT, Alpers CE, Schwartz SM. J Clin Invest 1993;92(4): 1686–1696.
7. Ikeda T, Shirasawa T, Esaki Y, Yoshiki S, Hirokawa K. J Clin Invest 1993;92(6):2814–2820.
8. Lyons KM, Pelton RW, Hogan BL. Development 1990;109(4):833–844.
9. Schor AM, Allen TD, Canfield AE, Sloan P, Schor SL. J Cell Sci 1990;97:449–461.
10. Bjorkerud S, Bjorkerud B, Joelsson M. Arterioscler Thromb 1994;14(4):644–651.
11. Hirsch D, Azoury R, Sarig S, Kruth HS. Calcif Tiss Intl 1993;52(2):94–98.
12. Nayak RC, Berman AB, George KL, Eisenbarth GS, King GL. J Exp Med 1988;167:1003–1015.
13. Brighton CT, Lorich DG, Kupcha R, Rielly TM, Jones AR, Woodbury RA. Clin Orthop Relat Res 1992; 275:287–299.
14. Ross MH. In: Ross MH, Reith EJ, Romrell LJ (eds) Histology: a Text and Atlas. Baltimore: Williams & Wilkins, 1989;103.
15. Parola M, Pinzani M, Casini A, Albano E, Poli G, Gentilini A, Gentilini P, Dianzani M. Biochem Biophys Res Comm 1993;194:1044–1050.
16. LeDouarin NM, Ziller C, Couly G. Dev Biol 1993;159:24–49.

State-of-the-art Symposia

Familial approach of cardiovascular risk factors: the "Fleurbaix Laventie Ville Santé" study

M.A. Charles[1], F. Thomas[1], A. Fontbonne[1], J.M. Borys[2], D. Boute[2], C. Toursel[2], P. Fossati[3] and E. Eschwège[1]

[1]INSERM Unit 21, Villejuif, France; [2]Association Fleurbaix Laventie Ville Santé, Fleurbaix, France; and [3]Department of Endocrinology and Metabolism, University Hospital, Lille, France

In 50 years of cardiovascular epidemiology, much has been learned about the clinical and biological factors that increase the probability of developing cardiovascular diseases. The deleterious effect of high cholesterol level, high blood pressure and tobacco smoking is common knowledge. Information and intervention campaigns are starting to show favorable effects [1,2].

However, much remains to be learned. The progress of genetic modeling and molecular biology opens a new area for epidemiologists. Indeed, it becomes evident that if we want to understand the pathophysiology of atherosclerosis and cardiovascular diseases better, we have to take into account both the genetic predisposition of the subjects and the interactions between the genes and the environment.

Special attention needs to be given to children, as the development of atherosclerosis may start in childhood [3]. Moreover, the changes in lifestyle necessary for the prevention of cardiovascular diseases are probably easier to implement with children than with adults.

The "Fleurbaix Laventie Ville Santé" survey was specially designed to study the interactions between genetic and environmental factors in the determination of cardiovascular risk. It includes three-generation families enrolled on a geographical basis, hence avoiding the usual bias of genetic analyses related to recruitment of families through a proband with the disease of interest. The family study is cross-sectional but a 5-year follow-up is planned at school for all the children. The effect of the environment is assessed through a detailed nutritional and lifestyle survey performed for each member of the family. Moreover, this cross-sectional study is the basis of a controlled intervention study in which nutritional education is given at school to all children. A second nutritional survey will be done 5 years after the first to evaluate the effect of the education given to children on their own dietary habits and those of the whole family.

Methods

The choice of Fleurbaix and Laventie

Fleurbaix and Laventie are two small towns of northern France with respectively 2,235 and 4,410 inhabitants. This total of 6,645 subjects was considered the right population size as it allowed the potential inclusion of all eligible inhabitants in the study.

The population is stable (70% of the inhabitants were born in the two towns) and young (58% of the subjects are under the age of 40 years). For most families, members of three generations live in Fleurbaix or Laventie or the immediate surrounding areas.

An additional great asset of these two towns was a team of general practitioners who are used to working together and eager to take an active part in epidemiologic studies.

The support given by the local and "regional" authorities, the school administrative body and teachers was another element of the choice.

The population of the study

The population of the study was defined as family members of the children in the highest age-groups of preschool or in primary school (all grades) in Fleurbaix and Laventie.

A family tree was sent to the parents of children attending these schools. The family trees asked for names and addresses of brothers, sisters, parents, paternal and maternal grandparents, uncles, aunts, great-uncles and -aunts.

Clinical and biological examinations

Children are clinically examined at school by school doctors specially trained for the study. It comprises measurement of height, weight, waist, hip and brachial circumference of four different skinfolds (biceps, triceps, subscapular, sub-iliac). The skinfolds are measured in triplicate with Harpenden's compasses and averaged. Systolic and diastolic blood pressures are measured in the left and right arms in the sitting position after a 5-min rest with a mercury sphygmomanometer and an adapted cuff. The pubertal development is recorded by the Tanner classification. The child's health record booklet is reviewed and birthweight as well as presence or history of any significant disease is recorded.

The biological examination of the children is also performed at school. For each school on a defined day, all the children are asked to arrive fasting. After the biological test, the children are invited to a free breakfast. The biological test consists of the determination of blood glucose, cholesterol and triglyceride on capillary blood with a Reflotron® device [4]. The Reflotron® needs 30 μl of capillary blood and gives a result in about 3 min. Systematic quality checking of the device is performed at the beginning of each examination day.

A 5-year follow-up of all children based on the same clinical and biological examinations is currently under way.

Adults, teenagers and children not attending school in Fleurbaix or Laventie, but eligible for the study because relatives of one of the children, are contacted by phone and appointments are arranged for examination either by their general practitioner or by one of the doctors in consultation centers set up specially for the study in town halls. Industrial doctors collect the data from the active population.

In addition to the clinical examination as given to the children, the teenagers (12–18 years) are questioned about their lifestyles (tobacco and alcohol consumption, physical activity) plus reproductive history for girls. In the clinical examination of adults, an interview about cardiovascular diseases and risk factors (diabetes, high blood pressure, dyslipidemia, obesity) as well as a vascular examination (pulses and bruits) are added.

The biological test is done in the doctor's office with a Reflotron® device which is systematically checked every week. As for the children, blood glucose, triglycerides and cholesterol measurements are performed.

Nutritional and lifestyle survey

The method of recording everything eaten during 3 days (2 weekdays and 1 weekend day) is used for adults. The same method is used for children but the food intake is recorded for only 1 weekday and the information is completed by a questionnaire about frequency of consumption. A dietitian checks the validity of the records with each of the family members on the following days.

In addition, questionnaires about eating behavior, weight history and lifestyle (tobacco and alcohol consumption, physical activity) are also completed individually, and one questionnaire about food consumption and preparation at the family level is given to the mother.

Ethics

The study has received the approval of the ethical committee of Lens. All adult participants signed an informed consent. The consent of the parents was necessary for participation of the children. The computer files has been declared to the "Commission Nationale Informatique et Liberté" which checks the absence of nominative information in the files and protects subjects from disclosure of the content to any unauthorized person.

Results

Participation rates

The study began in 1993 with the identification of the families. All the 825 children attending school in Fleurbaix and Laventie in the grades concerned received clinical examination at school. Ninety-five percent (782) of these children consented with their parents to the biological examination and 97% (755) of all these possible biological tests have in fact been carried out. The 825 children belonged to 579 different families and 519 (90%) complete family trees have been obtained. Five hundred and one families were contacted for the dietary survey and 417 (83%) gave their consent and essentially completed all the questionnaires.

The second year (1993–1994) of examinations of the children has just been completed with similar participation rates. Examinations of the adults were started in 1994 and around 300 subjects have already been seen. Three more years will be necessary to examine all the adults of the consenting families.

These high participation rates have been obtained thanks to special communication efforts made to inform the population of Fleurbaix and Laventie, the medical team, school teachers and town leaders about the study. Press releases, exhibitions in the town halls and shops, and drawing contests for the children were part of the communication plan.

Description of the children examined during the first year

The population of children examined during the first year includes 825 children, 435 boys and 390 girls, between 6 and 11 years of age. Table 1 gives the distribution by sex, age

Table 1. Distribution of children by age, sex and Tanner stage

	Age (years)								Total
	4	5	6	7	8	9	10	11	
Boys	0	52	76	65	84	73	59	26	435
Girls	1	40	98	59	58	58	69	7	390
Total	1	92	174	124	142	131	128	33	825
Tanner >1	0	0	0	0	0	2	23[a]	12	37

[a]One girl had missing value for Tanner stage in this group.

Table 2. Sex differences (mean (SE)) for clinical and biological parameters after adjustment for age by multiple linear regression

	Boys	Girls	p
Weight (kg)	26.2 (0.2)	26.5 (0.3)	0.43
Height (cm)	128.2 (0.3)	127.2 (0.3)	0.01
BMI	15.7 (0.1)	16.1 (0.1)	0.03
Waist circ. (cm)	56.8 (2.3)	55.8 (2.5)	0.003
Hip circ. (cm)	65.9 (2.7)	67.7 (3.0)	<0.001
WHR	0.864 (0.002)	0.828 (0.002)	<0.001
Brachial circ. (cm):	19.3 (1.0)	19.7 (1.1)	0.005
Skinfolds (mm)			
Subscapular	57 (1)	71 (1)	<0.001
Sub-iliac	57 (2)	71 (2)	<0.001
Triceps	95 (2)	114 (2)	<0.001
Biceps	52 (1)	65 (2)	<0.001
SBP (mmHg)	112.8 (0.5)	113.0 (0.5)	0.71
DBP (mmHg)	72.6 (0.4)	73.6 (0.5)	0.14
Blood cholesterol (g/l)	1.78 (0.20)	1.83 (0.21)	0.09
Blood glucose[a] (mg/dl)	87.6 (6.6)	88.1 (7.1)	0.61

[a]One girl with insulin-dependent diabetes (blood glucose: 290 mg/dl) excluded.

and Tanner stage.

The results presented are restricted to the 787 children (424 boys, 363 girls) with a Tanner stage equal to 0, as we had too few children to study the effect of puberty.

Mean age was 8.1 years (range: 5.2–11.8) for boys and 7.8 years (range: 4.9–11.4) for girls. Table 2 shows the sex differences in clinical and biological parameters after adjustment for age. Because of the high threshold of sensitivity of the Reflotron® for triglyceride measurement (0.7 g/l), a class variable was used for the comparison of triglyceride concentrations. Figure 1 gives the percentage of children with triglyceride concentrations above 0.7 g/l and Table 3 the characteristics of the distribution of triglyceride concentrations by sex and age-groups.

Although there was no significant difference in weight between prepubertal boys and girls, girls were significantly shorter, had thicker skinfolds and a less centralized fat

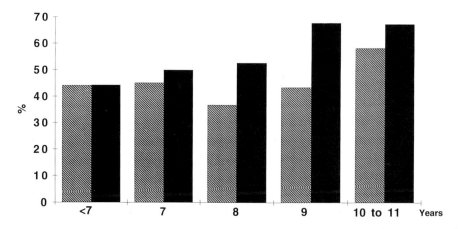

Fig. 1. Percentage of boys (hatched bar) and girls (solid bar) with triglyceride concentrations >0.7 g/l by age.

Table 3. Triglyceride concentrations (g/l) in boys and girls by age-group

		<7	7	8	9	10–11
	Age (years)					
Boys	maximum[a]	2.02	1.19	1.34	1.56	1.86
	median	0.70	0.70	0.70	0.70	0.75
	75th percentile	0.88	0.81	0.77	0.88	0.92
Girls	maximum[a]	1.70	1.88	1.46	1.39	2.55
	median	0.70	0.71	0.74	0.80	0.79
	75th percentile	0.88	0.82	0.86	0.95	0.97

[a]Minimum is 0.70 g/l in all age-groups.

distribution as shown by the lower waist to hip ratio. Blood glucose concentration was similar in prepubertal boys and girls. Cholesterol concentrations tended to be higher in girls and there was a higher percentage of girls with triglyceride concentration over 0.7 g/l than boys, especially after the age of 8 years. Overall, in prepubertal children, after appropriate adjustment for age by logistic regression, the sex difference in triglyceride was significant ($p = 0.009$).

Conclusion

The "Fleurbaix Laventie Ville Santé" study is the first epidemiologic study of cardiovascular risk factors to include three-generation families. It was specially designed to study the interactions between environmental and genetic risk factors.

The first data on prepubertal children show interesting differences between sexes. Boys have higher waist to hip ratios than girls. Thus, the difference observed in adults is already present in children before the beginning of morphologic changes related to pubertal secretion of sex hormones, despite a recent report [5] showing in females in early puberty that sex hormones have some influence on fat distribution. However, the literature on waist to hip ratio in children is scarce and additional information would be of interest.

Concerning triglyceride concentration, an opposite relationship was observed in children from what is found in adults, where it is higher in men than women. In children, triglyceride concentrations rise sharply in girls after the age of 8 years. The same phenomenon seems to start later in boys. The age of appearance of this phenomenon and the sex gap could suggest a relationship with the adrenal secretion of androgens. These possible hormonal factors, as well as other factors influencing triglyceride concentrations such as nutritional factors [6], are reasons why the tracking of this variable over years is less important than for other parameters such as cholesterol concentrations [3].

These cross-sectional data and the results from the 5-year follow-up in children will allow the study of the interrelationships between cardiovascular risk factors and the comparison with those observed in adults as well as the changes related to the effect of puberty.

With the information from parents, grandparents and their sibs, the influence of genetic factors and their interaction with the environment and especially nutritional factors will be studied. The existence of a familial aggregation of risk factors will be tested, and analyses of segregation will be performed to try to identify major genetic factor(s) and mode(s) of transmission.

The high participation rate and the enthusiasm of all participants encouraged us to start planning a second phase of the study in which venous blood samples will be collected. A more thorough study of biological risk factors will thus be possible and DNA will be stored anonymously for more genetic analyses.

References

1. Vartianen E, Puska P, Pekkanen J, Tuomilehto K, Jousilahti P. Br Med J 1994;306:23−27.
2. Jackson R, Beaglehole R. Int J Epidemiol 1987;3:377−382.
3. Webber LS, Cresanta JL, Voors AW, Berenson DS. J Chron Dis 1983;36:647−660.
4. Price PC, Koller PU. J Clin Chem Clin Biochem 1988;26:233−250.
5. De Ridder GM, Bruning PF, Zonderland ML, Thijssen JHH, Boonfrer JMG, Blankenstein MA, Huisveld A, Erich WBM. J Clin Endocrinol Metab 1990;70:888−893.
6. West CE, Sullivan DR, Katan MB, Halferkamps IE, Van Der Torre HW. Am J Epidemiol 1990;131:271−282.

Lp(a) and coronary heart disease

E.J. Schaefer, J.L. Jenner, L.J. Seman, J.R. McNamara, J.H. Contois, J.J. Genest, Jr., P.W.F. Wilson and J.M. Ordovas
Lipid Metabolism Laboratory, Jean Mayer USDA Human Nutrition Research Center on Aging at Tufts University, Boston, MA 02111, USA

Abstract. Lipoprotein(a) [Lp(a)] is an LDL-like particle with an additional protein known as apo(a). Apo(a) exhibits genetically determined size heterogeneity which is inversely associated with plasma levels of Lp(a). High Lp(a) plasma levels have been associated with increased coronary heart disease (CHD) risk in both case-control and prospective studies. This association may be due to direct deposit of Lp(a) in the artery wall, or to interference with clot lysis in vitro because of inhibition of plasminogen activation. Lp(a) levels should be measured in all patients with established CHD, and in those patients with levels >30 mg/dl as assessed by immunoassay and >10 mg/dl as assessed by Lp(a)-cholesterol, consideration should be given to drug therapy for men with niacin, and for women with hormone replacement.

Lipoprotein(a), originally described by Berg [1], is an LDL-like particle with an additional protein known as apo(a) attached to the apoB moiety by a disulfide bond. Apo(a) has been found to have a very interesting structure, in that it contains a variable number of kringle 4-like domains which have 75—85% homology with the kringle 4 domain of plasminogen [2]. Lp(a) is highly heritable and different molecular weight isoforms of apo(a) exist with over 30 isoform types. Decreased apo(a) molecular weight isoforms have been associated with elevated levels of Lp(a). Both Lp(a) levels and isoforms are highly heritable [3,4]. Lp(a) can be deposited directly in the artery wall. Moreover, it has been reported to interfere with clot lysis in vitro because of inhibition of plasminogen activation. Many studies have shown higher levels of Lp(a) in patients with coronary heart disease or stroke than in control subjects. Both niacin therapy [5] and hormonal replacement with estrogen [6] have been shown to lower Lp(a) levels significantly.

Measurement of Lp(a)

Lp(a) has been assessed by a variety of methods. The initial method was to subject plasma or serum to ultracentrifugation and then test for the presence of lipoproteins with pre-beta mobility in the 1.006 g/ml infranate by electrophoresis. Lp(a) is the only lipoprotein with pre-beta mobility in the 1.006 g/ml infranatant. This was a crude test for the presence of Lp(a). Subsequently, immunoassays were developed that were specific for Lp(a) and these studies clearly documented that most individuals had Lp(a) circulating in their plasma. Such studies also clearly showed that there was a very wide range of Lp(a) concentrations in human plasma, with over 1000-fold differences in actual values. Initial assessment was based on radioimmunoassay [7]. Subsequently, enzyme-linked immunoassays were developed. These assays have been calibrated to the mass of the entire Lp(a) particle, rather than to a specific protein constituent. Standardization of Lp(a) has been difficult

---

Address for correspondence: Dr Ernst J. Schaefer, Lipid Metabolism Laboratory, Jean Mayer USDA Human Research Center on Aging, Tufts University, 711 Washington Street, Boston, MA 02111, USA.

because Lp(a) contains two separate proteins and the molecular weight of apo(a) varies between individuals. Automated immunoturbidometric assays have recently been developed with a high throughput which allows laboratories to measure Lp(a) much more quickly in large numbers of samples. The difficulty with this methodology is that its sensitivity is less than optimal. As an alternative to immunoassays, most recently Seman et al. [8] have developed an Lp(a)-cholesterol assay in which Lp(a) is determined in whole plasma after absorption to wheat germ agglutinin in 4% agarose. The Lp(a) is then eluted off with N-acetyl-D-glucosamine, and the cholesterol in Lp(a) is measured. This assay correlates with an ELISA assay with an r value of 0.99.

Population studies

A number of investigators have measured Lp(a) in populations. We have applied the Strategic Diagnostics ELISA to the Framingham Offspring Study, and mean values were 14 mg/dl in men, 15 mg/dl in women, and in men with premature CHD 20 mg/dl ($p < 0.01$). Coefficients of variation for this assay both between and within runs have always been <5%. No significant correlations of Lp(a) with other factors have been noted, except for a very weak inverse correlation with triglyceride levels [9]. We have also applied the Lp(a) INCSTAR assay to the Framingham Offspring Study. We obtained mean values of 20 mg/dl in men and 21 mg/dl in women. The advantage of such an assay is the high throughput that can be obtained when the assay is set up on an automated instrument. The disadvantage is the low sensitivity, so that on many occasions one cannot measure a detectable Lp(a) level in patients.

Association of Lp(a) with coronary heart disease

It has long been known that patients and families with premature coronary heart disease are more likely to have elevated Lp(a) levels than controls. Moreover, our own family studies indicate that approximately 15–20% of CHD cases and their families have elevated levels of Lp(a), making Lp(a) excess among the most common of the lipid disorders associated with premature CHD [10]. Our data indicate that this familial disorder is as common in CHD patients as familial combined hyperlipidemia or familial hypertriglyceridemia associated with low levels of HDL-cholesterol. Elevated Lp(a) is among the most common lipid abnormalities observed in CHD patients [11,12].

Prospective studies

One question is whether an elevated Lp(a) will be a risk factor in prospective studies. There have been to date seven prospective studies of Lp(a) and coronary heart disease. Rhoads et al. [13] in 1986 showed that an elevated Lp(a) as assessed by lipoprotein electropheresis was a risk factor for premature coronary heart disease. Rosengren et al. [14] in 1990 documented that an elevated Lp(a) was an independent risk factor in CHD patients. This finding could not be duplicated by Jauhiainen et al. [15] in 1991, but in this study samples were stored at –20°. Subsequently, Ridker et al. [16] in the Physicians' Health Study reported no significant association between Lp(a) and CHD as assessed prospectively in male US physicians on a clinical trial, where they received aspirin together with beta-carotene therapy, in some cases. The lack of association was possibly because these subjects were already on aspirin. In 1994 we reported [17] that Lp(a) was an independent risk factor in the prospective Lipid Research Clinic's trial with cholestyramine. In the LRC studies, mean levels of Lp(a) were approximately 24 mg/dl in cases and 19−20 mg/dl in controls. Also, Bostom et al. [18] has noted that an elevated Lp(a) as assessed by electrophoresis is elevated in female participants in both the original cohort as well as the Framingham Offspring Study. It should be noted that in this study, as in a previous study by Rhoads et al. [13], Lp(a) was assessed by electrophoresis following ultracentrifugation at density 1.006, a relatively insensitive method. Even more recently, Cremer et al. have reported [19] that elevated Lp(a) was a significant risk factor for premature CAD in the prospective GRIPS study. Other significant risk factors included elevated LDL-cholesterol, family history, fibrinogen, HDL-cholesterol, and age. Hypertension and smoking were also significant risk factors in this study.

Screening and treatment of elevated Lp(a) levels

The question that remains is: should Lp(a) be measured, and if so, when? In our view, Lp(a) is clearly associated with premature coronary heart disease, with close to 20% of kindreds with premature coronary heart disease being afflicted with familial Lp(a) excess. There is clear evidence that dietary modifications have no significant effect on Lp(a) levels. It has been reported that niacin or nicotinic acid therapy at a dose of 3 g per day will cause significant reductions in Lp(a) levels of approximately 25% [5]. In addition, it has been reported that hormonal replacement, specifically with estrogen or estrogen and progestin, will also decrease Lp(a) levels in women [6,20]. In our view, Lp(a) levels should be measured in all patients with established coronary heart disease; in those patients with levels >30 mg/dl as assessed by immunoassay and >10 mg/dl as assessed by Lp(a)-cholesterol, consideration should be given to drug therapy for men with niacin, and for women with hormonal replacement. One can justify these approaches, since both niacin and estrogen replacement have been shown to reduce the risk of coronary heart disease in men with established CHD or in normal women. In future three parameters will be measured in our laboratory as part of a lipoprotein profile for CHD risk assessment: HDL-cholesterol following precipitation of other lipoproteins, Lp(a)-cholesterol utilizing the lectin wheat germ agglutinin system, and direct LDL-cholesterol by a method that causes a removal of non-LDL lipoproteins by immunoprecipitation. This direct LDL-cholesterol assay allows investigators and physicians to sample their patients in the nonfasting state, something which we hope will be available in the future for both HDL- and Lp(a)-cholesterol. In our view, either niacin or estrogen replacement therapy is indicated in patients with established heart disease and elevated Lp(a) levels. Niacin and estrogen replacement therapy have been associated with decreased all-cause and CHD mortality.

Acknowledgements

Supported by NIH grant HL 39326 from the National Institutes of Health, and contract 53-3K06-5-10 from the USDA Department of Agriculture Research Service.

References

1. Berg K. Acta Pathol Microbiol Scand 1963;59:369−382.
2. McLean JW, Tomlinson JE, Kuang WJ, Eaton DL, Chen EY, Fless GM, Scanu AM, Lawn RM. Nature 1987;330:132−137.
3. Lamon-Fava S, Jimenez D, Christian JC, Fabsitz RR, Reed T, Carmelli D, Castelli WP, Ordovas JM, Wilson PWF, Schaefer EJ. Atherosclerosis 1991;91:97−106.
4. Rodriguez CR, Seman LJ, Ordovas JM, Jenner JL, Genest JJ Jr, Wilson PWF, Schaefer EJ. Chem Phys Lipids 1994;67−68:389−398.

82

5. Carlson LA, Hamsten A, Asplund A. J Intern Med 1989;226:271–276.
6. Soma MR, Osnago-Gadda I, Paoletti R, Fumagalli R, Morrisett JD, Meschia M, Crosignani P. Arch Intern Med 1993;153:1462–1468.
7. Albers JJ, Adolphson JL, Hazzard WR. J Lipid Res 1977;18:331–338.
8. Seman LJ, Jenner JL, McNamara JR, Schaefer EJ. Clin Chem 1994;40:400–403.
9. Jenner JL, Ordovas JM, Lamon-Fava S, Schaefer MM, Wilson PWF, Castelli WP, Schaefer EJ. Circulation 1993;87:1135–1141.
10. Genest JJ Jr, Martin-Munley SS, McNamara JR, Ordovas JM, Jenner JL, Myers RH, Silberman SR, Wilson PWF, Salem DN, Schaefer EJ. Circulation 1992;85:2025–2033.
11. Genest J Jr, Jenner JL, McNamara JR, Ordovas JM, Silberman SR, Wilson PWF, Schaefer EJ. Am J Cardiol 1991;67:1039–1145.
12. Genest JJ Jr, McNamara JR, Ordovas JM, Jenner JL, Silberman, SR, Anderson KM, Wilson PWF, Salem DN, Schaefer EJ. J Am Coll Cardiol 1992;19:792–802.
13. Rhoads GG, Dahlen GH, Berg K. J Am Med Assoc 1986;256:2540–2544.
14. Rosengren A, Wilhelmsen L, Eriksson E, Risberg B, Wedel H. Br Med J 1990;301:1248–1251.
15. Jauhiainen M, Koskinen P, Ehnholm C, Frick MH, Manttari M, Manninen V, Huttunen J. Atherosclerosis 1991;89:59–67.
16. Ridker PM, Hennekens CH, Stampfer MJ. J Am Med Assoc 1993;270:2195–2199.
17. Schaefer EJ, Lamon-Fava S, Jenner JL, McNamara JR, Ordovas JM, Davis CE, Abolafia JM, Lippel K, Levy RI. J Am Med Assoc 1994;271:999–1003.
18. Bostom AG, Gagnon DR, Cupples LA, Wilson PWF, Jenner JL, Ordovas JM, Schaefer EJ, Castelli WP. A prospective investigation of elevated lipoprotein(a) detected by electrophoresis and cardiovascular disease in women: The Framingham Heart Study. Circulation 1994;90 (in press).
19. Cremer P, Nagel D, Labrot B, et al. Eur J Clin Invest 1994;24:444–453.
20. Sacks FM, McPherson R, Walsh BW. Arch Intern Med 1994;154:1106–1110.

Pharmacologic modulation of the atherogenic LDL profile in dyslipidemia

M.J. Chapman[1], E. Bruckert[2], M. Guérin[1], S. Dejager[1] and P.J. Dolphin[3]
[1]INSERM Unit 321 and [2]Service d'Endocrinologie-Métabolisme, Hôpital de la Pitié, Paris, France; and [3]Dalhousie University, Halifax, Canada

The Framingham Heart study has clearly established that elevated plasma levels of low-density lipoproteins (LDL) significantly increase the risk of premature coronary heart disease [1]. However, quantitative elevations in plasma LDL do not alone account for the atherogenicity associated with these particles. On the one hand, circulating LDL do not appear to be of uniform atherogenic potential in different patients presenting with familial hypercholesterolemia, and indeed some 20% of heterozygous FH subjects do not suffer a myocardial infarction before age 60 despite high LDL concentrations [2]. On the other, plasma LDL level does not appear to be predictive of the age of coronary death [2]. The atherogenic risk associated with these cholesterol-rich lipoproteins therefore appears to be linked to their structure, composition and metabolism as much as to their plasma concentration.

LDL are pseudomicellar particles containing a hydrophobic core consisting of cholesteryl esters, triglycerides, and fat-soluble vitamins, surrounded by a polar coat composed of free cholesterol, phospholipids and a specialized, multifunctional protein component, apolipoprotein B100. This high molecular weight protein is of hepatic origin, and affects not only the molecular structure of LDL particles, but also their intravascular metabolism and cellular degradation.

In plasma, LDL are distributed over the density range from 1.019 to 1.063 g/ml as a continuum of particles. However, substantial evidence now attests to the qualitative heterogeneity of LDL particles within this density interval. Indeed, the occurrence of several subspecies of LDL particles which vary markedly in their physicochemical, hydrodynamic, immunological and structural properties is typical of normolipidemic and dyslipidemic subjects [3–5]. Although as many as 15 distinct LDL particle subspecies have been identified [4], LDL particles may be grouped into three major subclasses on the basis of their physicochemical properties, namely light, large LDL displaying the highest ratio of cholesterol molecules to apoB protein (~2750:1), intermediate LDL, and small, dense LDL of low cholesterol:protein ratio (~2100:1) (Fig. 1).

The distribution of LDL mass as a function of density varies between normolipidemic subjects, but is frequently quasi-symmetrical [5]. The plasma profile of LDL particles results from a dynamic equilibrium between the processes of production from hepatic VLDL precursors, of intravascular transformation, and of tissue catabolism [6–8]. Key factors in these processes are lipoprotein lipase, hepatic lipase, the cholesterol ester transfer protein (CETP), and the cellular LDL receptor, whose points of impact on the metabolism of the apoB-containing lipoproteins are summarized in Fig. 2.

How then do the qualitative features of LDL profile relate to the atherogenic potential of these particles? The major pathway for removal of LDL from plasma is represented by the cellular LDL receptor [7]. In man, LDL receptors are primarily expressed in the liver, and up to two-thirds of LDL degraded per day are catabolized by this route. The LDL-

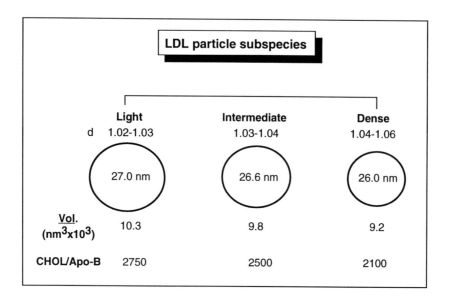

Fig. 1. Major physicochemical characteristics of the three principal subpopulations of LDL particles in normolipidemic subjects. CHOL: no. of cholesterol molecules (in free and esterified forms) per particle; ApoB, no. of protein copies per particle.

receptor pathway is nonatherogenic, as a series of feedback mechanisms control the levels of both receptor activity and endogenous cholesterol synthesis: in this way, cellular cholesterol homeostasis is assured. The LDL receptor is, however, exquisitely sensitive to both the conformation of apoB100 and to LDL particle structure. Indeed, we have

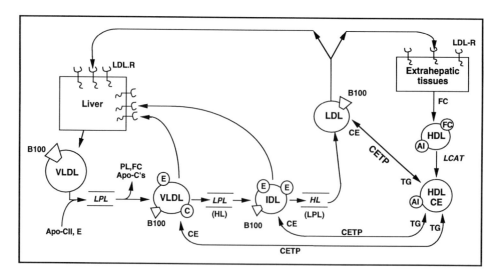

Fig. 2. Formation, intravascular metabolism and tissue catabolism of LDL. FC, free cholesterol; CE, cholesteryl ester; PL, phospholipid; TG, triglyceride; CETP, cholesterol ester transfer protein; HL, hepatic lipase; LCAT, lecithin:cholesterol acyltransferase; A-I, apolipoprotein A-I.

shown that small LDL possess a lower binding affinity for the LDL receptor than light LDL [9] and as a consequence, display a longer residence time in plasma in vivo [10]. Such dense LDL are therefore exposed to biological modifications [11] which may lead to their catabolism by pathways more atherogenic than that of the LDL receptor, among which is the macrophage scavenger pathway [11]. It is especially relevant in this context that dense LDL in both normal, as well as in dyslipidemic subjects exhibit diminished resistance to oxidative stress in vitro [12,13]. Oxidized LDL are avidly bound, internalized and degraded by macrophages; the accumulation of cholesterol derived from oxidized LDL leads to their transformation into foam cells, the latter representing a key cellular component of atheromatous lesions [12]. Clearly, then, dense LDL are of enhanced atherogenic potential.

The three most common forms of atherogenic dyslipidemia are hypercholesterolemia, combined hyperlipidemia and hypertriglyceridemia. While hypercholesterolemia and combined hyperlipidemia are characterized by elevated plasma LDL concentrations, all three forms feature either a predominance, or an elevated concentration, or both, of small, dense LDL particles [5,13–15]. Such LDL profiles have been referred to as "pattern B" by Austin [16]. In addition to their association with premature vascular disease, small, dense LDL represent a qualitative marker for a number of other lipid risk factors, which include increases in plasma levels of triglyceride-rich lipoproteins and apoB, and reductions in HDL and apoA-I [16].

The pharmacological modulation of the quantity and of the quality of small, dense LDL represents an important potential therapeutic approach in patients presenting atherogenic dyslipidemia. In a clinical study initiated recently, we have begun to evaluate the effect of a third-generation fibrate, fenofibrate, on the atherogenic LDL profile in primary combined hyperlipidemia. Male outpatients have been selected on the basis of clinical and biological criteria described earlier [13]; briefly, after stabilization on a normocaloric diet and after drug washout for 8 weeks, patients with a total plasma triglyceride level of 200 mg/dl or more and total cholesterol > 250 mg/dl were included in the study. All patients gave informed consent; the protocol was approved by the Human Subjects Review Committee. A secondary hyperlipidemia was excluded. It is important to note that our working definition of primary combined hyperlipidemia is as defined by Arad et al. [17], a definition which is quite distinct from that proposed for Familial Combined Hyperlipidemia [18].

As indicated above, a major feature of combined hyperlipidemia is the predominance of dense LDL (d 1.039–1.063 g/ml), which typically account for ~45% or more of total LDL mass in such patients [13]. Furthermore, the plasma concentrations of dense LDL may be up to 3-fold greater than those in matched control subjects (250 vs. 85 mg/dl, respectively) [13].

In our open-study protocol, preliminary data for five patients at inclusion confirmed that dense LDL predominated (~60% of total LDL mass), with lesser proportions of intermediate (d 1.029–1.039 g/ml; 24%) and of light d 1.019–1.029 g/ml (16%) LDL subfractions. After 8 weeks of fenofibrate therapy (200 mg/day; micronized fenofibrate), the proportions of dense LDL were reduced to ~48% with an equivalent increase (to ~34%) in the proportion of the intermediate subfraction; the proportion of light LDL was unchanged. Moreover, total plasma LDL concentrations were reduced upon treatment by ~20%.

The susceptibility of individual LDL subfractions (Nos. 1–5; see [13]) to copper-mediated oxidation was then evaluated in vitro by determination of the time course of production of conjugated dienes [19]. Conjugated dienes represent an intermediate product

86

in the free radical-mediated oxidation of polyunsaturated fatty acids in the lipid esters (phospholipids, cholesteryl esters and triglycerides) of LDL [19]. By this criterion, fenofibrate treatment resulted in a marked increase in the resistance to oxidation of all LDL subfractions.

These preliminary findings suggest that fenofibrate may modulate both the qualitative and quantitative features of an atherogenic LDL profile and particularly those dominated by dense LDL. They are consistent with the recent findings of Caslake et al. [10], in which fenofibrate therapy in hypercholesterolemic patients enhanced formation of LDL with high affinity for the LDL receptor. Such LDL particles were catabolized rapidly by the receptor-dependent pathway, leading to a 30% reduction in LDL-cholesterol levels [10].

The mechanisms underlying the modulation of atherogenic lipoprotein phenotypes by fenofibrate are summarized in Fig. 3. Evidence is available to implicate five major mechanisms: (1) reduction in hepatic LDL production, (2) optimization of hepatic VLDL size, leading to intravascular formation of LDL with high affinity for the cellular LDL receptor, (3) marked induction of lipoprotein lipase activity, (4) down-regulation of hepatic lipase gene expression and activity, and (5) reduction in neutral lipid exchange (cholesteryl esters and triglycerides) as a result of decreased plasma levels of apoB-containing lipoprotein acceptors [10,20,21]. The pharmacologic action of fenofibrate thus affords new insight into the mechanisms underlying atherogenic lipoprotein phenotypes, and more specifically, into the mechanisms which control formation of atherogenic, dense LDL.

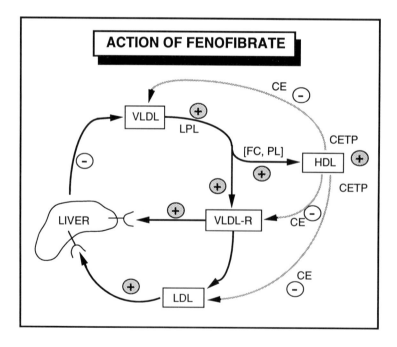

Fig. 3. Mechanisms of action of fenofibrate on atherogenic, apoB-containing lipoproteins. CE, cholesteryl ester; FC, free cholesterol; CETP, cholesterol ester transfer protein; LPL, lipoprotein lipase; PL, phospholipid; VLDL-R, VLDL remnants.

Acknowledgements

The authors are indebted to Misses V. Soulier and L. Bonheur for production of the typescript and figures.

References

1. Anderson KM, Castelli WP, Levy D. J Am Med Assoc 1987;257:2176—2180.
2. Heiberg AG, Slack J. Br Med J 1977;2:493—495.
3. Lee DM, Alaupovic P. Biochemistry 1970;9:2244—2252.
4. Chapman MJ, Laplaud PM, Luc G, Forgez P, Bruckert E, Goulinet S, Lagrange D. J Lipid Res 1988;29:442—458.
5. Luc G, Chapman MJ, De Gennes JL. Atherosclerosis 1988;71:143—156.
6. Havel RJ. J Lipid Res 1984;25:1570—1576.
7. Brown MS, Kovanen PT, Goldstein JL. Science 1981;212:628—635.
8. Grundy SM. J Lipid Res 1984;25:1611—1618.
9. Nigon F, Lesnik P, Rouis M, Chapman MJ. J Lipid Res 1991;32:1741—1753.
10. Caslake MJ, Packard CJ, Gaw E, Murray E, Griffin BA, Vallance BD, Shepherd J. Arterioscler Thromb 1993;13:702—711.
11. Steinberg D, Parthasarathy S, Carew TE et al. N Engl J Med 1989;320:915—924.
12. De Graaf J, Hak-Lemmers HLM, Hectors MPC, Demacker PNM, Hendricks JCM,, Stalenhoef AFH. Arterioscler Thromb 1991;11:298—306.
13. Dejager S, Bruckert E, Chapman MJ. J Lipid Res 1993;34:95—105.
14. Eisenberg S, Gavish D, Oschry Y, Fainaru M, Deckelbaum RG. J Clin Invest 1984;74:470—482.
15. Guérin M, Dolphin PJ, Chapman MJ. Arterioscler Thromb 1994;14:679—685.
16. Austin MA. Curr Opin Lipidol 1993;4:125—132.
17. Arad Y, Ramakrishanam R, Ginsberg HN. J Lipid Res 1990;31:567—582.
18. Goldstein JL, Schrott GG, Hazzard WR, Bierman EL, Motulsky AG. J Clin Invest 1973;52:1544—1568.
19. Esterbauer H, Striegl G, Puhl H, Rotheneder M. Free Rad Res Comm 1989;6:67—75.
20. Shepherd J. Postgrad Med J 1993;69(suppl 1):S34—S41.
21. Staels B, Peinado-Onsurbe J, Auwerx J. Biochim Biophys Acta 1992;1123:227—230.

Postprandial lipemia in type II diabetic patients

E. Cavallero[1], A. Piolot[1], S. Braschi[1], C. Corda[2] and B. Jacotot[1]

[1]*Service Médecine 5, Hôpital Henri Mondor, 94010-Créteil; and* [2]*Laboratoire Fournier SCA, 21121-Daix, France*

Abstract. Lipoprotein abnormalities, mainly high VLDL-triglycerides (VLDL-TG) and low HDL-cholesterol (HDL-C) levels, increase the risk of atherosclerotic ischemic disease in type II diabetic patients. The study of postprandial lipemia unmasks atherogenic changes in plasma lipoproteins in these patients. Preliminary results indicate that beneficial effects could be obtained by fenofibrate treatment in diabetic patients with moderate hypertriglyceridemia, not only in the level of fasting triglycerides (TG) but also in the postprandial lipemia and lipoprotein composition.

Atherosclerotic cardiovascular diseases are the major causes of morbidity and mortality in non-insulin-dependent diabetes (NIDD) [1,2]. Among the risk factors of ischemic diseases, dyslipidemias are very frequently observed in NIDD. The most prevalent lipid change is a moderate increase of TG, often associated with a reduction of HDL-C [3]. The increase of LDL-cholesterol (LDL-C), a major risk factor in the general population, is less frequently observed in diabetics. Several epidemiological studies have demonstrated the relation between increased TG and cardiovascular ischemic disease in diabetic subjects [4,5]. During the last decade, some studies evidenced the atherogenicity of TG-rich lipoproteins, particularly in the postprandial state. Thus, chylomicron remnants and other TG-rich particles were able to induce lipid accumulation in macrophages in vitro [6]. On the other hand, the link between TG-rich lipoproteins and HDL metabolism has been demonstrated, since efficient catabolism of chylomicrons and TG-rich lipoproteins contribute to the intravascular formation of HDL [7].

Recently, the role of insulin resistance (I-R) was stressed to explain the physiopathological mechanism of hyperTG and HDL-C deficiency in NIDD. Several epidemiological studies have demonstrated a significant relationship between hyperinsulinemia and incidence of cardiovascular ischemic diseases [8]. The plasma level of insulin, which is directly correlated with the degree of I-R, is also positively related to plasma TG [9]. I-R is associated with decreased insulin-related inhibition of adipose tissue lipolysis, increased plasma free fatty acids (FFA) and increased hepatic synthesis of VLDL-TG and secretion of VLDL. Hyperinsulinemia probably also reduces and delays the secretion of lipoprotein lipase (LPL) from adipose tissue and muscle. These mechanisms determine a loss of lipid homeostasis and different degrees of lipid intolerance, whereas the increase of fasting TG is generally moderate in patients with NIDD.

In a previous study, we have explored postprandial lipemia after a fat-load test to unmask atherogenic changes of the plasma lipoproteins in diabetics. Thus, type II diabetic patients under adequate nutritional and hypoglycemic therapy display a wider and delayed blood TG response after the fat load than do nondiabetic subjects, despite a fasting TG frequently below 2 g/l (mean 1.8 g/l) [10,11]. Net TG enrichment and cholesteryl ester (CE) depletion occurred within the postprandial HDL fraction that was correlated with the magnitude of postprandial lipemia, as described by Patsch in non-diabetic subjects [12]. Gradient ultracentrifugation analysis of fasting and postprandial samples shows denser LDL and HDL in diabetics than in controls, with reduced shift of these particles to lighter species. Increased postprandial lipemia and subsequent increase in net lipid transfer between lipoproteins may explain these abnormalities. It is known that small dense LDLs may also partially contribute to the increased cardiovascular risk. Increased postprandial lipemia has also been shown in obese severe hyperTG [13] or moderate hyperTG hyperglycemic type II diabetics [14].

With respect to the role of the dyslipidemia as a risk factor of cardiovascular disease in NIDD, it is important to try to normalize lipid levels. The improvement of glycemic balance and the reduction of excess weight can partially reduce the lipid abnormalities. However, postprandial lipid and lipoprotein levels and composition are not completely normalized to those of a control nondiabetic group. On the other hand, fibrates are able to reduce the plasma level of TG-rich lipoproteins, probably by two mechanisms: (a) decrease of hepatic synthesis of VLDL-TG and secretion of VLDL; (b) stimulation of plasma LPL activity. These drugs can also increase HDL-C. Postprandial lipemia can be reduced in NIDD by fibrate treatment [15]. We have therefore studied the effect of fenofibrate on postprandial lipemia in 30 type II diabetic men undergoing intensive nutritional treatment, increased physical activity and optimized hypoglycemic therapy (biguanide alone or biguanide + sulfonylurea), with body mass index < 27, and HbA_{1C} < 6.5, (N = 3.6–4.5). We used two fat-load tests during a 26-h exploration period (standardized breakfast and dinner with 32.5 g of lipids/m^2 body surface). Compared to a control group of 12 nondiabetic subjects, most of the patients showed a greater postprandial lipemia after the first load; moreover, 12 h after the second load, several patients presented a much higher level of fasting TG.

In the diabetic patients, we evaluated in a double-blind placebo-controlled study the effect of 4 months of fenofibrate therapy (200 mg o.d.) on postprandial lipemia. Before treatment, the postprandial lipemia was not different between the fenofibrate and placebo groups (Fig. 1). After 4 months of treatment, the fasting plasma TG were markedly

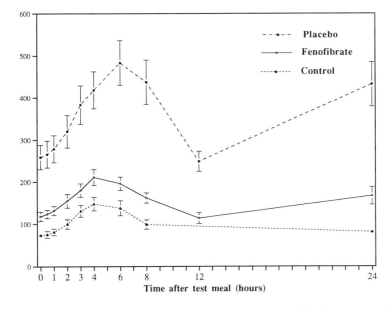

Fig. 1. Postprandial triglycerides in patients under fenofibrate or placebo treatment and in control subjects.

decreased in the fenofibrate group, and this group exhibited a lower postprandial lipemia than the placebo group. There was a significant reduction of the area under the curve and of the magnitude of TG during the postprandial state in the fenofibrate group, and indeed these values were similar to those of nondiabetic control subjects.

Lipoprotein mass and chemical composition were modified by fenofibrate treatment. Fasting and postprandial TG-rich lipoprotein mass, particularly of chylomicrons, VLDL and IDL, was lower than in the placebo group. This was associated with reduced TG content within HDL_2 and HDL_3, mainly in the postprandial state. From a general point of view, lipoprotein mass levels and composition in diabetic patients after fenofibrate treatment were closer to those of nondiabetic subjects than diabetic patients on placebo. Fenofibrate treatment did not alter either the glycemic balance or the area under the curve of insulin and C-peptide.

The present study indicates that type II diabetic patients show moderately raised fasting TG and postprandial lipemia with associated lipoprotein abnormalities despite optimized glycemic and metabolic control. A dramatic reduction of TG, particularly during the postprandial state, can be obtained by fenofibrate treatment. This treatment influences the lipoprotein levels and composition in an antiatherogenic direction.

References

1. Wilson PWF, Kannel WB, Anderson KM. Atherosclerosis 1985;13:1—11.
2. Pyorala K, Laakso M, Uusitupa M. Diabetes Metab Rev 1987;3:463—524.
3. Fontbonne A, Eschwege E, Cambien F et al. Diabetologia 1989;32:300—304.
4. Steiner G. In: Vranic M, Hollenberg CH, Steiner G (eds) Comparison of type I and type II diabetes. Plenum Publishing, 1985;277.
5. Reaven GM. Am J Med 1987(suppl 34);83:31—40.
6. Gianturco SA, Lin AHY, Hwang SC et al. J Clin Invest 1988;82:1633—1640.
7. Eisenberg S. J Lipid Res 1984;25:1017—1058.
8. Vusitupa MIJ, Niskanen LK, Siitonen O et al. Circulation 1990;82:27—36.
9. Olepsky JM, Farquhar JW, Reaven GM. Am J Med 1974;57:60.
10. Cavallero E, Jacotot B. In: Stein Y, Stein O, Eisenberg S (eds) Atherosclerosis IX. R & L Creative Comm, 1992;479—483.
11. Cavallero E, Dachet C, Neufcour D et al. Metabolism 1994;43:270—278.
12. Patsch JR, Prasad S, Gotto A et al. J Clin Invest 1987;80:341—347.
13. Georgopoulos A, Margolis S, Bachorik P, Kwiterovich PO. Metabolism 1988;37:866—871.
14. Lewis GF, O'Meara NM, Soltys PA et al. J Clin Endocrinol Metabol 1991;72:934—944.
15. Syvanne M, Hilden H, Taskinen MR. Arterioscler Thromb 1993;13:286—295.

LDL particle size: effects on apoprotein B structure, receptor recognition, and atherosclerosis

Narmer F. Galeano[1], Steven C. Rumsey[1], Peter Kwiterovich, Jr.[2], Daniel Preud'Homme[3], Yves Marcel[4], Ross Milne[4], Mary T. Walsh[5] and Richard J. Deckelbaum[1,3]

[1]*Department of Pediatrics, Columbia University, New York, USA;* [2]*The Children's Medical and Surgical Center, The Johns Hopkins Hospital, Maryland, USA;* [3]*Institute of Human Nutrition, Columbia University, New York, USA;* [4]*Heart Institute, University of Ottawa, Ontario, Canada; and* [5]*Biophysics Institute, Boston University Medical Center, Massachusetts, USA*

Abstract. We questioned the effects of LDL particle size vs. lipid composition on apoprotein B (apoB) structure and function. We examined apoB structure (by circular dichroism and monoclonal antibody immunoreactivity) and affinity for the LDL receptor in LDL of different sizes and lipid compositions. Both large and small LDL, but not triglyceride-rich LDL of normal size, had decreased affinity for the LDL receptor on human fibroblasts, and this was associated with modified circular dichroism (CD) spectra and immunoreactivity of monoclonal antibodies recognizing the LDL-receptor-binding region of apoB. In addition, small LDL had increased oxidation susceptibility in vitro and enhanced binding to non-LDL-receptor-binding sites. Thus, deviation from an optimal size of LDL may produce changes in apoB structure and affinity for the LDL receptor. Decreased affinity for the LDL receptor, increased affinity for low-affinity cell-binding sites and enhanced susceptibility for oxidation may all be contributing factors in the atherogenicity of small/dense LDL.

Although higher plasma levels of triglycerides (TG) have been linked to accelerated atherosclerosis, the association diminishes after correction for LDL-cholesterol levels and disappears when HDL levels are considered [1]. In humans, LDL are produced after lipolysis of VLDL, with the final lipid composition of LDL depending upon the composition of VLDL and the intravascular particle remodeling due to the activity of cholesterol ester transfer protein (CETP) coupled with lipolysis [2]. The complex interrelation of these processes contribute to the heterogeneity in LDL size and lipid composition described in hypertriglyceridemia [3,4]. Our recent studies suggest that the lipoprotein particle abnormalities observed in LDL isolated from subjects with hypertriglyceridemia (HTG-LDL) and other dyslipidemias result in alterations of apoB structure, which then affect the binding of LDL to the LDL receptor and to non-LDL receptor sites on the cell surface.

Lipoprotein abnormalities in hypertriglyceridemia

Plasma levels of triglycerides depend upon the relationship between the synthesis of triglyceride-rich particles (chylomicrons and VLDL) and their catabolism and removal from the intravascular compartment. Hypertriglyceridemia (HTG) results either from overproduction of VLDL, impaired clearance of triglyceride-rich lipoproteins, or both.

Independent of the mechanism of hypertriglyceridemia, a number of common abnormalities in lipoprotein structure and composition have been described [3–6].

Address for correspondence: Narmer F. Galeano, MD, Department of Pediatrics, Columbia University, 630 West 168th Street, New York, NY 10032, USA; Tel: +1-212-305-7082; Fax: +1-212-305-8995.

Compared to VLDL from normolipidemic subjects, HTG-VLDL (d < 1.006) are larger and have relatively lower protein and higher free and esterified cholesterol, but little difference in phospholipid content. LDL populations from HTG subjects are polydisperse, but with an overall smaller mean particle diameter of the major LDL fractions. HTG-LDL is relatively enriched in protein but relatively poor in both free and esterified cholesterol and phospholipids. These modifications in size and composition are inversely related to the total triglyceride plasma levels and return towards normal with treatment of hyper-triglyceridemia. HTG-HDL are also enriched in protein and triglycerides and depleted in esterified cholesterol, and generally smaller than normal. The observed changes in both particle size and lipid composition were attributed, over a decade ago, to the increased availability of triglyceride-rich lipoproteins promoting transfer of triglycerides from VLDL to LDL and HDL, as mediated by the activity of neutral lipid transfer protein [2,3,7], now known as CETP [8]. At the same time, cholesteryl ester depletion from LDL and HDL is enhanced by the greater availability of triglyceride-rich particles [3]. Hydrolysis of TG by lipases then results in smaller/denser LDL and HDL [4,7,8].

Small/dense LDL and coronary artery disease

Small LDL have been significantly associated with an elevated risk for coronary artery disease [9,10]. It has been suggested that a gene contributing to the presence of small LDL is located in chromosome 19, which is near to or at the LDL-receptor locus; haplotypes at the apoAI-CIII-AIV and Mn superoxide dismutase gene are also linked to the presence of small LDL [11]. Other factors such as age, gender and diet also appear to modify LDL size. Predominance of small LDL is independent of age, sex and weight, but is correlated with elevated plasma TG levels [9,10] and low levels of HDL-cholesterol. Small LDL is described in specific lipid disorders such as hyperapobeta-lipoproteinemia, familial combined hyperlipidemia, and in patients with the so-called Syndrome X (which includes insulin resistance, increased VLDL levels, low levels of HDL, and hypertension). Small LDL are often triglyceride-rich. Thus, although small/dense LDL may not be an independent risk factor for coronary artery disease, its presence may explain increased coronary artery disease risk with increasing plasma triglycerides, at least in some subjects.

Effects of LDL particle size vs. lipid composition on apoB structure and function

Realizing that particle size often changes with changes in LDL-lipid composition, we initially sought to differentiate between the effects of particle size vs. lipid composition on apoB conformation, and how any changes in apoB conformation would affect LDL binding to the cell surface. We first systematically studied the effects of particle size on apoB conformation and LDL–cell interaction utilizing small/dense LDL isolated from hypertriglyceridemic donors [6]. Using an approach of analyzing native LDL obtained from normal and dyslipidemic donors together with in vitro remodeling of LDL (by incubating LDL with lipid emulsions and CETP), we were able to prove that enriching LDL with triglyceride, depleting it of free cholesterol, or adding surface phospholipid had no effect on apoB secondary structure, or configuration of the apoB-receptor binding domain. Changes in these lipids also had no effect on LDL binding to the LDL receptor in cultured fibroblasts if they were not accompanied by changes in LDL size. In contrast, reduction in LDL particle size (with or without changes in lipid composition) consistently showed marked changes in apoB structure as determined by circular dichroism (decreased α-helix contribution), as well as decreased immunoreactivity to monoclonal antibodies targeting near or at the apoB-receptor recognition domain. In parallel to these structural changes in apoB, LDL affinity to its receptor progressively decreased to one-fourth of normal values as LDL size progressively decreased. (When different subpopulations of small/dense LDL were isolated from the same donor, the smallest LDL fraction showed the poorest LDL-receptor binding.) Our in vitro remodeling approaches, which use artificial lipid emulsions rather than VLDL to remodel LDL, suggested that previous reports describing LDL-triglyceride composition as a major modulator of LDL binding to the LDL receptor might be due to contamination of their remodeled LDL with VLDL-derived C-apoproteins or lipase. In our experiments, LDL size affected the LDL-receptor binding even when triglyceride composition was unchanged [6]. Thus, small LDL size, and not triglyceride content, predicted apoB structure and apoB affinity to the LDL receptor.

We have also initiated studies on large LDL. A major question was whether LDL had an optimal size for binding to the LDL receptor. In fact, large LDL particles from hypertriglyceridemic subjects show lower binding to the LDL receptor. This decreased binding is also accompanied by alterations in apoB secondary structure and configuration of the apoB-receptor binding domain (as determined by monoclonal antibody immunoreactivity) [12,13]. We have also found, using LDL isolated from homozygous FH subjects (with defined LDL-receptor defects), that large LDL from these patients has lower affinity for the LDL receptor than their normal-sized subfractions.

Our data also help to understand a frequent observation on LDL subpopulations in HTG. In these persons the major LDL populations most often consist of large and small particles, with normal-sized particles in the minority [4]. It may be that the normal-sized particles in HTG are cleared more efficiently via the LDL receptor than either the large or small LDL.

Effects of small LDL-particle size on non-LDL-receptor binding to the cell surface

Although most of the LDL are cleared via the LDL receptor, it has been calculated that at least 30% is cleared by non-LDL-receptor mechanisms, and the non-receptor clearance may be of particular importance in extra-hepatic tissues. Our initial studies on LDL-receptor binding were performed using competitive displacement assays. When we utilized direct binding assays of normal and small [^{125}I]LDL from normal and dyslipidemic subjects, we had a surprising finding. Scatchard analysis showed that small LDL occupy only 10–60% of available binding sites on the cell surface [6]. These observations suggested that small dense LDL might have higher binding affinity to non-LDL-receptor sites on the cell surface. In comparing the binding properties of normal [^{125}I]LDL and small TG-rich [^{125}I]LDL with normal LDL made triglyceride-rich by in vitro remodeling with triglyceride emulsions and CETP, we found that small dense LDL had lower total-cell binding, lower LDL-receptor high-affinity binding, but greater ($\times 1.5$–2.5) low-affinity binding to normal fibroblasts. At higher LDL concentrations (100 µg/ml) non-LDL-receptor cell binding of small LDL was up to 3.5 times that of normal-size LDL. Impressively, we found that in LDL-receptor-negative fibroblasts, non-LDL-receptor binding of small LDL was up to 4–14 times that of normal LDL [14]. These results may in fact explain a previous report, in which the non-LDL-receptor clearance rate for HTG-LDL was 2.5-fold that of the normal LDL [15]. Of additional interest, we have confirmed in our laboratory that, compared to normal-sized LDL, small LDL were considerably more susceptible to oxidation (2.5-fold higher lag phases in presence of $CuCl_2$), and that increased LDL-triglyceride content alone, or large LDL size, does not affect LDL oxidizability (Preud'Homme D et al., unpublished data).

Conclusions

We have provided evidence that both large and small LDL have lower binding to the LDL receptor in cultured cells than normal-sized LDL, and that this is associated with changes in apoB conformation. We also found that changes in the LDL lipid core, especially triglyceride enrichment, in the absence of change in LDL size does not affect apoB secondary structure or binding to the LDL receptor. Our conclusions are supported by data of Nigon et al. [16] who found that, even in normal LDL, both lighter and denser fractions of LDL had lower LDL-receptor affinity than the LDL of normal density (1.029–1.035 g/ml). Our data and those of others raise the hypothesis that changes in the surface curvature ratio of LDL may determine modifications in the structure of the apoB molecule, particularly on flexible epitopes such as the LDL-receptor binding region [6]. Of interest, a recent preliminary report has suggested that in small LDL, decreased phospholipid content at the particle surface would induce unfolding of apoB in order to cover the surface deficit [17].

Our studies raise important hypotheses relevant to what occurs in vivo. We suggest that LDL has an optimal size or optimal binding to the LDL receptor. LDL particles that deviate from normal or optimal size will show decreased clearance by tissues rich in LDL receptors, e.g. liver, and thus may be more available for clearance and uptake in other tissues, e.g. the arterial wall. Moreover, the increased adherence to non-LDL-receptor sites on the cell surface will allow modifications of small dense LDL, which further enhance their atherogenic potential, e.g., by local LDL oxidation.

Acknowledgements

This work has been supported in part by NIH grants HL 40404 and HL 21006.

References

1. Hulley SB, Rosenman RH, Bawol RD, Brand RJ. N Engl J Med 1980;302:1383–1389.
2. Deckelbaum RJ, Olivecrona T, Eisenberg S. In: Carlson LA, Olsson AD (eds). Treatment of hyper-lipoproteinemia. New York: Raven Press, 1984;85–93.
3. Deckelbaum RJ, Granot E, Oschry Y, Rose L, Eisenberg S. Arteriosclerosis 1984;4:225–231.
4. Eisenberg S, Gavish D, Oschry Y, Fainaru M, Deckelbaum RJ. J Clin Invest 1984;74:470–479.
5. Vakakis N, Redgrave TG, Small DM, Castelli WP. Biochim Biophys Acta 1983;751:280–285.
6. Galeano NF, Milne R, Marcel YL, Walsh MT, Levy E, Nguyen TD, Gleeson A, Arad Y, Witte L, Al-Haideri M, Rumsey SC, Deckelbaum RJ. J Biol Chem 1994;269:511–519.
7. Barter PJ. Curr Opin Lipidol 1990;1:518–523.
8. Tall AR. J Lipid Res 1993;34:1255–1274.
9. Austin MA, Breslow JL, Hennekens CH, Buring E, Willet WC, Krauss RM. J Am Med Assoc 1988;260:1917–1921.
10. Coresh J, Kwiterovich PO, Smith HH, Bachorik P. J Lipid Res 1993;34:1687–1697.
11. Austin M. Curr Opin Lipidol 1993;4:125–132.
12. Walsh MT, Galeano NF, Arad Y, Marcel Y, Milne R, Deckelbaum RJ. Circulation 1991;84:II–456.
13. Arad Y, Rumsey SC, Galeano NF, Al-Haideri M, Walsh MT, Marcel YL, Milne R, Kwiterovich PO, Deckelbaum RJ. Circulation 1992;86:I-551.
14. Galeano NF, Rumsey SC, Preud'Homme D, Gleeson A, Deckelbaum RJ. Circulation 1993;88:I-366.
15. Shepherd J, Caslake MJ, Lorimer AR, Vallance BD, Packard CJ. Arteriosclerosis 1985;5:162–168.
16. Nigon F, Lesnik P, Rovis M, Chapman J. J Lipid Res 1991;32:1741–1753.
17. McNamara JR, Small DM, Schaefer EJ. Circulation 1993;88:I-133.

Interactions of triglyceride-rich lipoproteins (TGRLP) with arterial cells and their role in atherosclerosis

Sandra H. Gianturco and William A. Bradley

University of Alabama at Birmingham, 690 Diabetes Research and Education Building, Birmingham, AL 35294-0012, USA

Abstract. A potential cellular mechanism for the atherogenicity of TGRLP, mediated by a unique TGRLP receptor of human monocytes and macrophages, is described. Plasma chylomicrons and hypertriglyceridemia VLDL, unlike normal VLDL, are rapidly internalized, degraded, and cause lipid accumulation in these cells in vitro after binding to specific, high-affinity (Kd ~2–6 nM) sites. Two membrane-binding proteins (MBP) of apparent molecular masses of 200 and 235 kDa from human monocytes and macrophages share the ligand specificity and the same lack of regulation exhibited by the cellular binding site. The MBPs are related, cell-surface proteins which upon reduction yield a single species that retains full ligand-binding activity. This receptor pathway may be involved in nutrition of circulating monocytes and accessible macrophages and, in the face of elevated TGRLP, may be involved in atherosclerotic changes, including foam-cell formation and endothelial-cell dysfunction.

Other presentations in this symposium have addressed significant epidemiologic relationships of elevated plasma triglycerides and abnormalities in the interrelated metabolism of triglyceride-rich lipoproteins (TGRLP) and HDL and the development of premature atherosclerosis [1,2]. Here we focus on a potential cellular mechanism for the atherogenicity of TGRLP, mediated by a TGRLP receptor of human monocytes and macrophages [3]. As this receptor is also expressed on endothelial cells, it may be relevant to atherogenic changes that occur in the artery wall involving these two reticuloendothelial-cell types. In atherosclerosis monocytes are converted into foam cells, and endothelial cells express a variety of dysfunctions, including a phenotypic conversion into a multinucleated 'giant cell' morphology over atherosclerotic lesions in humans [4]. TGRLP which bind to the TGRLP receptor include plasma chylomicrons and HTG-VLDL (VLDL from hypertriglyceridemic patients), and these TGRLP, unlike normal VLDL, cause rapid, receptor-mediated lipid accumulation in human monocytes and macrophages in vitro after uptake and degradation [3] and induce giant cell formation in cultured porcine and human coronary artery endothelial cells [5]. Since TGRLP which bind to this receptor induce these potentially atherogenic cellular changes in vitro, this suggests that the receptor may mediate similar changes in vivo when faced with elevated levels of atherogenic TGRLP, as in some forms of hypertriglyceridemia and in prolonged postprandial lipemia known to be associated with increased coronary artery disease [6].

To demonstrate a specific, high-affinity binding site, direct 4° binding studies were conducted in both human blood-borne and THP-1 monocytes and macrophages differentiated 1–7 days using both iodinated HTG-VLDL and a modified VLDL, alone and in the presence of excess unlabeled VLDL. VLDL were modified by incubation with trypsin to remove immunochemically detectable apoE, whose presence would confound results because of its binding to the LDL receptor, LRP, or the VLDL receptor, when expressed. After treatment, trypsin was removed by affinity chromatography and the VLDL were reisolated by gradient flotation. It is important to note that although all apoE is removed, the trp-VLDL retain essentially all apoB immunoreactivity, in fragments of 100 kDa and smaller. Trp-VLDL no longer bind to the LDL receptor because there is no apoE [7], but they retain full (or enhanced) binding to the TGRLP receptor [3]. HTG-VLDL S_f 100–400 and trp-VLDL bind to both freshly isolated blood-borne monocytes and THP-1 monocytes and macrophages 1–7 days after adherence, with similar high affinities (Kd in the nanomolar range) and specificities [3]. Chylomicrons also bind with high affinity, but normal VLDL and LDL have low affinity, as does acetyl LDL [3].

Ligand-blotting experiments identified two membrane-binding proteins (MBP) of apparent molecular masses of 200 and 235 kDa [3] from both human blood-borne and THP-1 monocytes and macrophages that shared the ligand specificity and other critical characteristics of the cellular binding site. Like the cellular binding site, these proteins did not appear to be affected by the state of differentiation of the cells, unlike receptors whose activity decreases (the LDL receptor) or increases (LRP and the acetyl LDL receptor) upon differentiation. Both the cellular binding site and the MBPs were unaffected by changes in media sterol content, unlike the LDL receptor [3].

As in murine macrophages [8], pretreatment and/or coincubation of cells or ligand blots with heparin had no effect on binding or triglyceride accumulation by TGRLP in human THP-1 monocyte-macrophages or on binding to MBP 200 and 235. Since heparin pretreatment removes surface-bound lipoprotein lipase (LpL) and coincubation causes release of surface-bound lipase and thereby enhances triglyceride accumulation induced by TGRLP, these studies indicate that macrophage-derived LpL is not necessary for the observed interactions. Moreover, the MBPs and the high-affinity cell site are expressed in monocytes and in adherent macrophages prior to expression of LpL. Competitive binding studies in cells and in ligand-blotting experiments demonstrate that LpL inhibits binding of ^{125}I-VLDL to cells and to MBP 200 and 235.

Moreover, neither the cellular binding site nor MBP-binding activities were susceptible to heparinase treatment, indicating that the cellular binding site and the MBPs are not composed of or assisted by heparin sulfate proteoglycans. The MBPs are, however, sensitive to 4° cell-surface proteolysis under conditions where the cells remain intact and >95% viable, which indicates that MBPs are expressed on the cell surface and are therefore capable of interacting with extracellular ligands. The MBPs appear to be related proteins, as MBP 235 and 200 are quantitatively converted upon reduction into an active binding species of intermediate apparent molecular mass on SDS-PAGE, termed MBP 200R, with full retention of binding activity [9]. This distinguishes the MBPs from the LDL receptor and the acetyl-LDL receptor, both of which lose activity under strong reducing conditions. Quantitative ligand-blotting analyses show that MBP 200, MBP 235, and MBP 200R have similar saturation binding characteristics to the cell site, with nanomolar Kds [9]. Studies of temperature sensitivity demonstrate that MBP 235 activity is converted into MBP 200 activity, which can then be reduced to MBP 200R activity by 2-mercaptoethanol or dithiothreitol. These studies suggest that the two binding activities share a common large protein backbone (MBP 200R). MBP 200R has been purified in our laboratory, and the peptide sequences obtained by microsequencing were unique. Characterization of the cDNA for this protein is under way; transfection studies in receptor-negative cells are required to demonstrate whether or not it functions as a receptor for TGRLP.

In summary, the TGRLP receptor is distinct from members of the LDL-receptor gene superfamily and the acetyl LDL (scavenger) receptor in a number of respects, including ligand specificity, expression during differentiation, apparent molecular masses of the candidate receptor proteins and their retention of binding activity after reduction. The cellular binding site and the candidate receptors, MBP 200 and 235, share a number of characteristics, including ligand specificity, TGRLP binding that is independent of apoE and of lipoprotein lipase, lack of regulation by sterol or by state of differentiation [3]. The expression of these MBPs on monocytes, endothelial cells and macrophages and their recognition of plasma chylomicrons suggest that they may be involved in nutrition of circulating monocytes and accessible macrophages, as in bone marrow. Excessive uptake, as in hypertriglyceridemia or excessively pronounced and prolonged postprandial lipemia, may lead to atherogenic changes in monocytes, macrophages, and endothelial cells.

Acknowledgements

This work was supported in part by National Institutes of Health grants HL 44480 and HL 46304. We thank Marilyn Robinson for her expert editorial assistance in preparation of the manuscript. We gratefully acknowledge the work of Drs M.P. Ramprasad and Ran Li in purification and characterizing the MBPs and the technical skill of Caryl Reese, Ruiling Song, and Dana Stinson in performing cell studies and lipoprotein isolation and characterization.

References

1. Austin M. Atherosclerosis 1994;109:259 (abstract).
2. Patsch JR. Atherosclerosis 1994;109:259 (abstract).
3. Gianturco SH, Ramprasad MP, Lin AH-Y, Song R, Bradley WA. J Lipid Res 1994;35:1674—1687.
4. Repin VS, Dolgov VV, Zaikina OE, Novikov ID, Antonov AS, Nikolaeva MA, Smirnov VN. Atherosclerosis 1984;50:35—52.
5. Parks JM, Grammer JR, Bradley WA, Gianturco SH and Booyse FM. Circulation 1993;88(4—2):1227A.
6. Patsch J R, Miesenbock G, Hopferwieser T, Muhlberger V, Knapp E, Dunn, JK, Gotto AM, Jr. Arterioscler Thromb 1992;12:1336—1345.
7. Gianturco SH, Gotto AM Jr, Hwang S-LC, Karlin JB, Lin AH-Y, Prasad SC and Bradley WA. J Biol Chem 1983;258:4526—4533.
8. Gianturco SH, Lin AH-Y, Hwang S-LC, Young J, Brown SA, Via DP, Bradley WA. J Clin Invest 1988; 82:1633—1643.
9. Ramprasad MP, Li R, Bradley WA, Gianturco SH. Surface localization and characterization of the human THP-1 monocyte-macrophage membrane binding proteins for triglyceride-rich lipoproteins. Circulation (in press).

Workshops

Spontaneous development of hypercholesterolemia and advanced coronary atherosclerosis in the familial hypercholesterolemic (FHC) swine

Margaret Forney Prescott[1], Judith Hasler-Rapacz[2], Jean Von Linden-Reed[1] and Jan Rapacz[2]

[1]*Atherosclerosis Research, Pharmaceuticals Division, Ciba-Geigy Corporation, Summit, NJ 07091, USA; and* [2]*Department of Genetics and Meat and Animal Science, University of Wisconsin, Madison, WI 53706, USA*

Abstract. The familial hypercholesterolemic (FHC) strain of swine spontaneously exhibits elevations in total cholesterol, LDL, apolipoproteins B, C-III, E and triglycerides, decreases in HDL and apoA-I, and develops stenotic atherosclerotic lesions which resemble advanced human plaques. Coronary lesions contain necrotic cores, fibrous caps, cholesterol clefts, calcification, and neovascularizition. As these pigs age, plaque hemorrhage, fissuring, myocardial infarction and ischemia are commonly observed. FHC was first identified in swine bearing the apoB mutant allele, Lpb5. Recent studies, however, demonstrate that neither spontaneous hypercholesterolemia nor the development of coronary artery disease occurs exclusively in animals bearing the Lpb5 allele, demonstrating the polygenic nature of disease development. Thus, because of their development of dyslipidemia resembling human type IIb as well as their spontaneous development of advanced atherosclerotic lesions resembling complex human plaques, the FHC swine represent a unique model for the study of coronary artery disease and restenosis.

Elevated levels of total cholesterol (TC), triglycerides (TG), apolipoproteins B and C-III and reduced levels of HDL-cholesterol and apolipoprotein (apo) A-I have been associated with development of coronary atherosclerosis [1—4]. To date, the familial hypercholesterolemic (FHC) swine developed by Rapacz and Hasler-Rapacz [5] is the only animal model which has been shown to spontaneously develop both hypercholesterolemia [5—7] and advanced coronary atherosclerotic lesions which resemble complex human lesions [8,9].

Apolipoprotein and lipid profiles in the FHC swine

The FHC swine carries components of at least six domestic breeds and exhibits spontaneous hypercholesterolemia when fed a low cholesterol (60 mg/day), low fat (6%) diet [5—7]. FHC was first identified in swine which bore the apoB mutant allele Lpb5 and spontaneously developed elevations in TC, LDL and apoB [5,10,11]. Selective breeding, however, has allowed identification of a new cholesterol subphenotype in which TC, TG, LDL, apolipoproteins B, C-III and E are elevated and HDL and apoA-I are decreased (Table 1) [7,12,13].

Abnormalities in the LDL particles from FHC swine may play a role in the development of their hypercholesterolemia. Buoyant cholesteryl ester-enriched LDL particles account for approximately 70% of the total plasma LDL protein in Lpb5 swine

Address for correspondence: Dr M. Prescott, Atherosclerosis Research, Ciba-Geigy Corporation, 556 Morris Avenue, Summit, NJ 07901, USA.

Table 1. Concentrations of plasma lipids and apolipoproteins in FHC hypercholesterolemic swine vs. normo-cholesterolemic swine

	Normocholesterolemic swine	FHC swine
	mg/dl (mean $\pm$ SD)	
TC	105 $\pm$ 12.0	316 $\pm$ 62.2[a]
LDL	67 $\pm$ 18.4	275 $\pm$ 63.1[a]
HDL	33.5 $\pm$ 1.9	22.3 $\pm$ 2.2[a]
ApoB	48 $\pm$ 5.7	152 $\pm$ 32.5[a]
ApoC-III	3 $\pm$ 0.1	10 $\pm$ 4.2[b]
ApoE	5 $\pm$ 0.7	17 $\pm$ 3.4[a]
ApoA-I	62.4 $\pm$ 9.3	42.6 $\pm$ 4.8[a]
TG	29 $\pm$ 5.7	48 $\pm$ 10.8[b]

Significance FHC vs. normocholesteromic = [a]$p < 0.001$, [b]$p < 0.01$.

[7,11,14]. LDL from Lpb5 swine has been shown to have a lower affinity for the LDL receptor in vitro [10,15], and in vivo it was catabolized more slowly than LDL from non-Lpb5 normocholesterolemic swine [14]. Although studies using the original Lpb5/5 progenitors indicated that LDL receptors functioned normally [10], recent studies suggest that the hypercholesterolemia found in some of the FHC swine may be due to a defect in LDL-receptor activity [16]. This finding is in agreement with earlier segregation data indicating that more than one major gene contribute to the dyslipidemia observed in the FHC swine [5]. Recent studies demonstrating that spontaneous hypercholesterolemia is not exclusive to the Lpb5 genotype [9] support the hypothesis that the familial dyslipidemia observed in the FHC swine is polygenic in origin. Quantitative pedigree analysis suggests that at least two major gene loci contribute to the dyslipidemia [13,16].

Development of complicated atherosclerotic lesions

Complicated lesions resembling advanced human atherosclerosis are common in the major coronary arteries as well as the aortic bifurcation and the iliac, femoral, and carotid arteries [8]. Stenotic lesions are most frequently observed in the left anterior descending, right coronary and left circumflex coronary arteries [9]. Such lesions occur as early as 14 months of age. Eccentric lesions are most common, but concentric lesions are frequently observed. Advanced lesions contain necrotic cores, fibrous caps, cholesterol clefts, calcification, neovascularization, and intraplaque hemorrhage (Figs. 1A and B). Lesion fissuring, myocardial infarction and ischemia have also been observed [9]. Thus the coronary lesions correspond closely to the advanced human atherosclerotic lesions described as Stage IV, V, and VI [17]. The most frequent and advanced lesions are found in those FHC swine in which lipid values (TC, LDL, apoB, apoC-III, apoE) increase with age [12].

Conclusions

The FHC swine is the first animal model shown to develop advanced atherosclerosis spontaneously in the same vascular sites which are prone to lesion development in humans. Complex lesions containing necrotic cores, fibrous caps, calcification, neovascularization and intraplaque hemorrhage closely mimic advanced human atherosclerosis. Development of advanced coronary artery disease with ischemia and

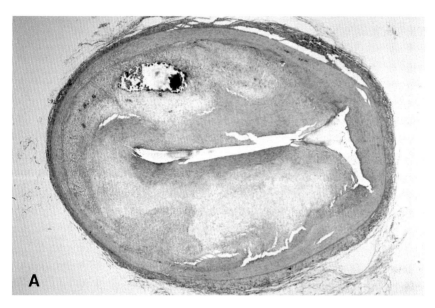

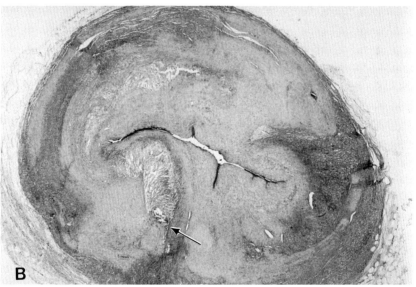

Fig. 1. A: Right coronary artery of a 24-month-old FHC female swine. A complex stenotic lesion contains several necrotic core areas, one of which is extensively calcified (3.75 ×). B: Right coronary artery of a 60-month-old FHC female swine. A complex, occlusive lesion contains several necrotic core areas, cholesterol clefts, inflammatory cell infilltration and intraplaque hemorrhage (arrow) (2.5 ×).

myocardial infarction has previously only been reported in animal models employing the combination of vascular injury and a cholesterol-enriched diet. Thus the FHC swine represent a unique model for the study of atherosclerosis or restenosis.

References

1. Castelli WP, Garrison RJ, Wilson PWF, Abbott RD, Kalousdian S et al. J Am Med Assoc 1986;256: 2835–2838.
2. Genest J, McNamara JR, Ordov MJM, Jenner JL, Siberman SR et al. J Am Coll Cardiol 1992;19:792–802.
3. Kwiterovich PO, Coresh J, Smith HH, Bachorik PS, Derby CA, Pearson TA. Am J Cardiol 1992;69: 1015–1021.
4. Hodis HN, Mack WJ, Azen SP, Alaupovic P, Pagoda JM et al. Circulation 1994;90:42–49.
5. Rapacz J, Hasler-Rapacz J. In: Lenzi S, Descovich GD (eds) Atherosclerosis and Cardiocascular Diseases. Editrice Composition, Bologna, Italy, 1984;99–108.
6. Rapacz J, Hasler-Rapacz J. In: Lucis AJ, Sparkes RS (eds) Genetic Factors in Atherosclerosis: Approaches and Model Systems. Monographs in Human Genetics. Basel: Karger, 1989;139–169.
7. Hasler-Rapacz JO, Nichols TC, Griggs DA, Bellinger DA, Rapacz J. Arterioscler Thromb 1994;14:923–930.
8. Prescott MF, McBride CH, Hasler-Rapacz J, Von Linden J, Rapacz J. Am J Pathol 1991;139:139–147.
9. Prescott MF, Hasler-Rapacz J, Von Linden J, Rapacz J. Ann NY Acad Sci (in press).
10. Rapacz J, Hasler-Rapacz J, Taylor KM, Checovich WJ, Attie AD. Science 1986;234:1573–1577.
11. Lee DM, Mok T, Hasler-Rapacz J, Rapacz J. J Lipid Res 1990;13:839–847.
12. Hasler-Rapacz JO, Rapacz J, Hu L, Rapacz Jr JM, Von-Linden-Reed J, Prescott MF. (submitted).
13. Rapacz J, Dentine MR, Hasler-Rapacz J, Rapacz Jr JM. Proc XXVI Int Conf Animal Genetics. Prague 1994;B34.
14. Checovich WJ, Fitch WL, Krauss RM, Smith MP, Rapacz J et al. Biochemistry 1988;27:1934–1941.
15. Lowe SW, Checovich WJ, Rapacz J, Attie AD. J Biol Chem 1988;263:15467–15473.
16. Aiello RJ, Nevin DN, Ebert DL, Uelmen PJ, Kaiser ME et al. Arterioscler Thromb 1994;14:409–419.
17. Stary HC. Virchows Archiv A (Pathol Anat) 1992;421:277–290.

The hyperlipidemic and diabetic hamster, a novel animal model

Maya Simionescu[1], Doina Popov[1], Anca Sima[1], Mirela Hasu[1], Gabriela Costache[1], Silviu Faitar[1], Alexandra Vulpanovici[1], Camelia Stancu[1], David Stern[2] and Nicolae Simionescu[1]

[1]Institute of Cellular Biology and Pathology, Bucharest, Romania; and [2]Department of Physiology and Cellular Biophysics, Columbia University, New York, New York, USA

Abstract. Male hamsters were subjected to a hyperlipidemic diet combined with streptozotocin-induced diabetes (HD); for comparison, other animals were rendered either diabetic or hyper-lipidemic only. At intervals ranging from 2 to 24 weeks, the animals were examined for changes in plasma constituents and structural modifications of relevant tissues. The plasma of the HD group was characterized by a gradual increase in glycemia, cholesterol and lipid peroxides, and the appearance of glycalbumin and irreversibly glycated albumin. Progressive intimal atherosclerotic lesions of a fibrolipid type appeared at an accelerated rate in the cardiac valves and aorta. Coronaries showed pronounced focal proliferations of smooth muscle cells. Concomitantly, characteristic diabetic microangiopathy occurred in myocardium, kidney and retina.

Numerous observations on humans and experimental animals have shown that diabetes mellitus confers an excess risk for atherosclerosis. Previously, we have shown that male hamsters fed a fat-rich diet develop atherosclerotic plaques [1] which in many respects are similar to those described in humans [2]. Using the ability of streptozotocin (SZT) to produce free radical-mediated damage of pancreatic β-cells [3], we tried to induce diabetes in hyperlipidemic hamsters, thus making available an animal model with combined hyperlipidemia and hyperglycemia and the associated vascular lesions characteristic of atherosclerosis and diabetes.

Materials and Methods

Experimental protocol

180 male Golden Syrian hamsters were subjected to three different experimental conditions : (i) diet-induced hyperlipidemia (H), (ii) streptozotocin-induced diabetes (D) and (iii) a combination of both states, hyperlipidemia and diabetes (HD). The HD and D hamsters' response to STZ injection varied. At time intervals of 2, 4, 6, and 12 weeks the most responsive animals, with extreme loss in body weight (up to 30%) and high glycemia, were selected for examination, while the most resistant were used for later time points of 18 and 24 weeks.

Methods of investigation

Plasma assays were used to measure glucose, cholesterol, peroxides (expressed as thiobarbituric acid reactive substances (TBARS)), apolipoprotein B, glycalbumin (gAlb) and irreversibly glycated albumin as advanced glycosylation endproducts-albumin (AGE-Alb).

    For tissue examination by light and electron microscopy, animals were anesthetized, and through a catheter placed in the abdominal aorta (and using vena cava as outlet) the vasculature was perfused with phosphate-buffered saline followed by a mixture of

106

buffered aldehydes. After 10 min, the heart right atrium and left ventricle, coronary arteries, sigmoid and mitral valves, thoracic aorta, retina, and kidney were dissected. All specimens were treated with buffered 1% OsO_4 and uranyl acetate, dehydrated and embedded in Epon 812.

Results and Discussion

Plasma assays

In the HD hamsters, while the values of mean glycemia and peroxides increased progressively up to 3-fold at 24 weeks, plasma cholesterol reached concentrations 9 times higher than normal (Fig. 1). In parallel with increasing glycemia, about 85% of animals had high levels of gAlb (~3 times normal) reaching maximal values at 6–12 weeks. The remaining 15% of animals, resistant up to 24 weeks, showed only a slight augmentation in plasma gAlb. Compared with normal hamster plasma albumin, albumin fluorescence rose to 2.5–6 UF (units of fluorescence) at 6 weeks, and to 1.8–4 UF in the animals that resisted up to 24 weeks; this was due to the presence of AGE-Alb in the HD hamsters.

Pathology of blood vessels

The H animals, starting with the second to third week of diet, developed in the lesion-prone areas of the aortic valves, aortic arch and coronaries, detectable fatty streaks which later evolved into advanced fibro-lipid plaques [1] which obstructed some small branches of coronary arteries [4]. Usually, microvessels did not show significant alterations.

The D animals displayed characteristic diabetic microangiopathy, particularly prominent in myocardium, kidney and retina. In addition, large vessels such as aorta and coronaries, as well as aortic valves, became the sites of marked lipid deposition, complex

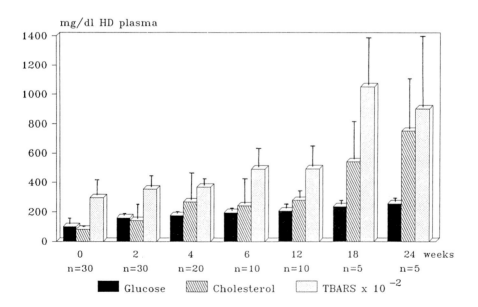

Fig. 1. Hyperlipidemic-diabetic hamsters (HD): plasma assays for glucose, cholesterol and TBARS (expressed as nmol MDA/ml).

stromal proliferation and calcification. Although in several aspects these modifications were similar to those found in the H animal, in the D hamsters such alterations which appeared in advanced diabetes exhibited certain peculiarities which will be detailed in a separate paper (manuscript in preparation).

The HD hamsters exhibited a combined pathology: macroangiopathy of atherosclerotic nature and microangiopathy of diabetic type. In the intima of aortic valves, aorta and coronary arteries, atherogenic alterations evolved faster than in the H animals. Under a morphologically intact, often attenuated endothelium, there was an early accumulation of modified reassembled lipoproteins (MRLp), the most evident in the standard electron microscopic preparation being extracellular liposomes [5,6]. MRLp were commonly interspersed within a network of highly hyperplasic multilayered basal lamina (Fig. 2), and regions of proliferated extracellular matrix (especially microfibrils and elastin bundles). The local endothelial cells were enriched in biosynthesis-associated organelles (endoplasmic reticulum, Golgi complex, Weibel-Palade bodies) and in elements of the intracellular digestive apparatus (endosomes, multivesicular bodies, lysosomes), and cytoskeletal elements (microfilaments and microtubules) were well represented. The increased number of Weibel-Palade bodies may be correlated with the data showing [7] that the rise in plasma concentration of von Willebrand factor in diabetic patients may have a causative role in the development of vascular complications. At 2–4 weeks, the regions with MRLp showed monocytes adherent, migrating through endothelial junctions or already becoming subendothelial macrophages loaded with lipid droplets (Fig. 3). The foam cells continued to accumulate rather rapidly; at 6 weeks, they could form protruding clusters that led to marked deformation of the aorta and aortic valves. In coronaries, the plaques contained focal proliferations of smooth muscle cells (Fig. 4). After 18 weeks, advanced lesions were characterized by marked stromal proliferation, calcification and deposition of cholesterol crystals. In the advanced plaques, calcium deposits may be extended through the intima and media, generating necrotic cores. The early presence of calcification centers observed in the HD animals was similar to the reported data in human pathology [8]. Overlying endothelial cells, though continuous, were often flattened and could contain lipid droplets and even cholesterol crystals. A notable change observed was an early gradual thickening of the left ventricular wall that in time became heart hypertrophy.

The ultrastructural alterations detected in the microvessels of the myocardium, kidney

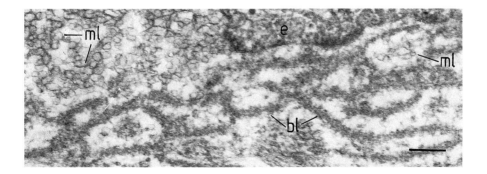

Fig. 2. A subendothelial area (aortic valve), displaying a hyperplasic, multilayered basal lamina (bl) containing within its network modified and reassembled lipoproteins (ml). e, endothelium. Bar: 13 nm. All electron micrographs are from HD hamsters.

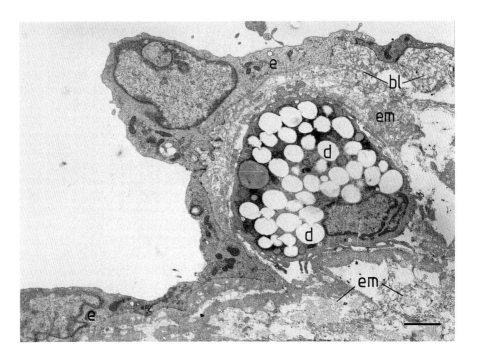

Fig. 3. Sigmoid valve showing an intact endothelium (e), proliferated basal lamina (bl) and extracellular matrix (em) and a macrophage-derived foam cell filled with lipid droplets (d). Bar: 0.3 μm.

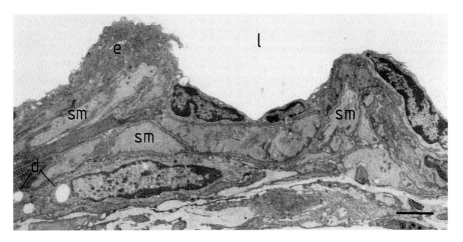

Fig. 4. Atherosclerotic fibro-muscular plaques in a small coronary artery. Under morphologically intact endothelium (e), pronounced proliferation of smooth muscle cells (sm), some containing lipid droplets (d). l, lumen. Bar: 2.5 μm.

and retina were characterized especially by the polymorphic proliferation of basal lamina and of the various components of the extracellular matrix. Such changes were noticed earlier and were more severe than those found in the D hamsters. Of special relevance,

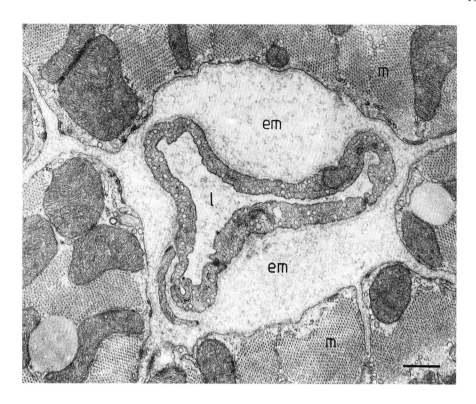

Fig. 5. Irregularly narrowed myocardial capillary surrounded by a hyperplasic extracellular matrix (em). l, lumen, m, myocyte. Bar: 0.5 μm.

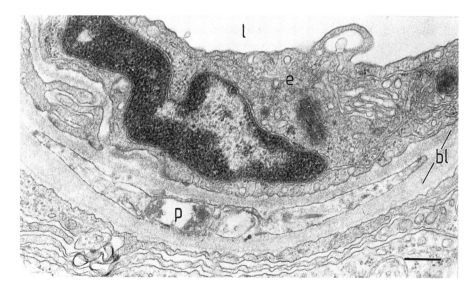

Fig. 6. Retinal capillary displaying cytolysis of a pericyte (p). e, endothelial cell; bl, basal lamina; l, lumen. Bar: 0.4 μm.

both in kidney glomeruli and myocardium, was the relatively large number of irregularly narrowed or collapsed capillaries, surrounded by thickened basal laminae and extracellular matrix (Fig. 5), frequently containing membranous debris. The myocardial microvascular endothelia occasionally showed patent transendothelial channels and open intercellular junctions. Retinal capillaries displayed characteristic pericyte disruption and basal laminae proliferation (Fig. 6). The cardiomyopathic, cytolytic, nephropathic, and retinopathic modifications detected in the HD hamsters at 24 weeks were similar to those reported for diabetic animals [9].

This novel HD animal model may be useful to elucidate some of the mechanisms by which the metabolic disturbances of diabetes could lead to more severe atherosclerosis. Diabetes and myocardial lesions may act independently of the traditional risk factors, and therefore could be mediated by other conditions such as the hemostatic abnormalities of heart microvessels [10]. The HD hamster may also be an adequate model for testing the effect of various drugs on these combined diseases.

Acknowledgements

This work was supported by the Romanian Academy and the USA, NIH-Fogarty International Research Collaboration Award — TW00118. The authors are grateful for the excellent technical assistance of M. Misici, E. Stefan and N. Dobre.

References

1. Nistor A, Bulla A, Filip DA, Radu A. Atherosclerosis 1987;68:159—173.
2. Wissler RW. Am J Med 1991;91(suppl 1B):3S—9S.
3. Jackson RL, Ku G, Mao SJT, Sheetz MJ, Robinsen KM, Thomas CE. In: Born GVR, Schwartz CJ (eds) New Horizons in Coronary Heart Disease. London: Current Science, 1993;20:1—13.
4. Sima A, Bulla A, Simionescu N. J Submicrosc Cytol Pathol 1990;22:1—16.
5. Simionescu N, Vasile E, Lupu F, Popescu G, Simionescu M. Am J Pathol 1986;123:109—125.
6. Simionescu N, Sima A, Dobrian A, Tîrziu D, Simionescu M. In: Vollmer/Roessner (eds) Current Topics in Pathology 87. Berlin: Springer Verlag, 1993;1—45.
7. Katayama M, Hirai S, Kato I, Titani K. Clin Biochem 1994;27:123—131.
8. Born GVR. In: Born GVR, Schwartz CJ (eds) New Horizons in Coronary Heart Disease. London: Current Science, 1993;22:1—11.
9. Nathan DM. N Engl J Med 1993;328:1676—1685.
10. Burchfiel CM, Reed DM, Marcus EB, Strong JP, Hayashi T. Am J Epidemiol 1993;137:1328—1340.

Lessons concerning human lipoprotein metabolism from the study of the WHHL rabbit

Toru Kita, Makoto Tanaka, Hideo Otani, Noriaki Kume and Masayuki Yokode

Department of Geriatric Medicine, Faculty of Medicine, Kyoto University, 54 Kawahara-cho Shogoin, Sakyo-ku, Kyoto 606, Japan

Abstract. The Watanabe heritable hyperlipidemic (WHHL) rabbit has a genetic defect identical with that in familial hypercholesterolemia (FH) in humans. In the homozygous form, this defect leads to a nearly complete deficiency of LDL receptors [1,2]. As a result, the plasma level in these rabbits is elevated 10–20 times above normal [3,4]. LDL deposits are oxidatively modified in the arterial wall, producing xanthoma and atheromas, as in FH patients. We can therefore use WHHL rabbits as animal models for studying human FH. We have previously demonstrated that in this model serum LDL particles are elevated by overproduction and undercatabolism. In this study, we show that the rate of production and secretion of apoB-containing lipoproteins is the same in normal and WHHL rabbit hepatocytes. The cholesteryl ester content of hepatocytes regulates the degradation of apoB protein itself. Even when LDL receptors are not available in WHHL rabbit hepatocytes, the latter takes up LDL-cholesterol via a non-LDL-receptor pathway. Therefore, as long as the hepatic content of cholesteryl ester in WHHL rabbits is the same as that of normal rabbits, the production and secretion of apoB-containing lipoproteins is unchanged.

Materials and Methods

Animals

Homozygous WHHL rabbits were raised in Kyoto by mating heterozygous WHHL females with homozygous WHHL males. Male Japanese White rabbits and WHHL rabbits were anesthetized with pentobarbital and parenchymal hepatocytes were isolated by in situ perfusion of the liver with collagenase, as described by Tanaka et al. [5].

Lipoproteins

LDL from human and rabbits (p = 1.019–1.063) were isolated by sequential ultracentrifugation from plasma of healthy human subjects and Japanese White rabbits.

Anti-rabbit apoB monoclonal antibody and ELISA were described by Tanaka et al. [5].

Results and Discussions

Effect of cholesterol on apoprotein B secretion in rabbit hepatocytes

To investigate the effect of cholesterol on apoB secretion, we incubated normal rabbit hepatocytes with increasing amounts of LDL or pravastatin (an inhibitor of HMG-CoA reductase) and measured the amount of apoB secreted into culture media by ELISA. In the absence of pravastatin, LDL caused a significant and dose-dependent increase in apoB secretion: in culture media containing LDL at 50 and 500 µg/ml, apoB secretion from normal hepatocytes was increased by 33 and 167% respectively. In WHHL hepatocytes, apoB secretion increased by 49% at the concentration of 500 mg/ml LDL but there was no increase at 50 µg/ml LDL.

112

We examined the effect of pravastatin on apoB secretion by normal and WHHL hepatocytes. When the cells were cultured in the absence of LDL, the HMG-CoA reductase inhibitor (10 µg/ml) suppressed apoB secretion by 66% in normal rabbit and 62% in WHHL rabbit respectively.

De novo cholesterol synthesis, cholesterol content and apoB secretion

To investigate the relationship between de novo cholesterol synthesis and apoB secretion, we incubated hepatocytes with increasing concentrations of pravastatin. ApoB secretion from rabbit hepatocytes was decreased in parallel with the decrease of de novo cholesterol synthesis. There were parallel changes in the cellular content of cholesteryl ester and the net secretion of apoB with a correlation coefficient of 0.8. No significant changes were observed in the cellular content of free cholesterol, triglyceride or phospholipid. These findings were similar in WHHL rabbit hepatocytes.

Intracellular turnover and secretion of apoB

To study the mechanism by which LDL and pravastatin regulate apoB secretion, we examined intracellular turnover and secretion of apoB by pulse-chase experiment. The net secretion of apoB from normal and WHHL rabbit hepatocytes was lowered by incubation with pravastatin. Moreover pravastatin accelerated intracellular degradation of apoB, while LDL slowed the rate of intracellular degradation.

Effect of LDL and pravastatin on cellular apoB mRNA level

Northern blot hybridization analysis and a quantitative solution hybridization RNase protection assay indicated that there were no significant changes in apoB mRNA levels in normal and WHHL hepatocytes incubated with pravastatin or with 500 µg/ml LDL. Therefore apoB regulation is not at the transcriptional level.

LDL degradation, cellular cholesteryl ester level and apoB secretion in WHHL hepatocytes

The concentration of LDL apoB in plasma in vivo was 168 and 16 mg/dl in WHHL and normal rabbits respectively [6]. Cultured WHHL and normal rabbit hepatocytes were therefore incubated in media containing ^{125}I-LDL at these concentrations, namely 1,680 and 160 µg protein/ml respectively, for 24 h. The rate of apoB degradation was similar in the two types of hepatocytes, as were the levels of cellular cholesteryl ester and apoB secretion rate.

In summary, the cellular cholesteryl ester content in hepatocytes regulates the intracellular degradation of apoB protein in normal and WHHL rabbits. Intracellular regulation of apoB production is at the posttranslational, not transcriptional level.

When incubated with a high concentration of LDL, WHHL hepatocytes could take up a substantial amount of LDL through a receptor-independent pathway. Therefore at a high plasma level of LDL in vivo, the rate of apoB secretion by WHHL hepatocytes could be the same as from normal hepatocytes.

Acknowledgements

This research was supported by Ministry of Education, Science, and Culture of Japan Research Grants (05404039, 05557052, 05044163 and 06354011), a Research Grant for

Health Sciences from Japanese Ministry of Health and Welfare, Grant for Cardiovascular Diseases (5A-2) from Japanese Ministry of Health and Welfare, the HMG-CoA Reductase Research Fund, and Japanese Foundation of Metabolism and Diseases.

References

1. Watanabe Y. Atherosclerosis 1980;36:261–268.
2. Kita T, Brown MS, Watanabe Y, Goldstein JL. Proc Nat Acad Sci USA 1981;78:2269–2272.
3. Kita T, Brown MS, Bilheimer DW, Goldstein JL. Proc Nat Acad Sci USA 1982;79:5693–5697.
4. Goldstein JL, Kita T, Brown MS. N Engl J Med 1983;309:288–296.
5. Tanaka M, Jingami H, Otani H, Cho M, Ueda Y, Arai H, Nagano Y, Doi T, Yokode M, Kita T. J Biol Chem 1993;268:12713–12718.
6. Have RJ, Kita T, Kotite L, Kane JP, Hamilton RL, Goldstein JL, Brown MS. Arteriosclerosis 1982;2: 467–474.

Rabbit models of atherosclerosis and restenosis

N.M. Caplice, P.A. Fennessy, J.A. Manderson, G.R. Campbell and J.H. Campbell

Centre for Research in Vascular Biology, Department of Anatomical Sciences, University of Queensland, Brisbane, Queensland 4072, Australia

Abstract. Since the early egg-white feeding studies of Ignatowski in 1908 rabbits have been used as a model for atherosclerosis. They have many advantages over other species as they are easily handled and inexpensive, they breed well and reliably develop lipid-rich plaques on exposure to cholesterol. However, the plaques generally consist of a subendothelial accumulation of macrophage-derived foam cells with little contribution by smooth muscle, and thus do not resemble, histologically, the human disease. In this report an improved rabbit model for primary lesion development is described. This involves the formation, prior to cholesterol feeding, of a myointimal thickening closely resembling the human diffuse intimal thickening — the site of predilection for lesion formation. Secondly, a new model for restenosis is described in which balloon dilatation (aided by fluoroscopy and intravascular ultrasound) is performed on a pre-existing plaque induced by combined endothelial injury and cholesterol diet.

Rabbits have long been used as a model for atherosclerosis [1]. Vesselinovitch [2] has listed the following requirements for the ideal animal model to be used in atherosclerosis research:
1. Available and inexpensive.
2. Easy to maintain and manipulate.
3. Proper size.
4. Available as genetically pure-bred lines.
5. Reproduce easily in captivity.
6. Develop lesions with relative ease.
   a. Nutritional manipulation conducive to development of advanced plaques.
   b. Practical length of time for the development of severe disease.
7. Low incidence of spontaneously developed disease.
8. Similar to human anatomy, physiology, and biochemistry.
9. Similar to human atherosclerosis regarding:
   a. Serum lipoprotein and lipid metabolism (lack of loading of reticuloendothelial system);
   b. Pathogenesis of lesions (e.g., hypercholesterolemia and hypertension);
   c. Topography of lesions (sparing of small arteries);
   d. Lesion components;
   e. Clinical complications (e.g., ischemia, myocardial infarction, thrombosis and gangrene).

Unfortunately, no single animal model fulfills all of these requirements. Thus it has been necessary to study several animal species including mice, rats, rabbits, birds, dogs, pigs

Address for correspondence: Dr Julie H. Campbell, Centre for Research in Vascular Biology, Department of Anatomical Sciences, University of Queensland, Brisbane, Queensland 4072, Australia.

and nonhuman primates, utilizing cholesterol feeding and balloon injury techniques to investigate different aspects of this human disease.

Rabbits are one of the most extensively studied animals of this group. With a normal diet most strains of rabbit do not develop atherosclerosis, but may develop degenerative lesions of the arterial intima resembling Monckberg's medial sclerosis [3]. Severe hyper-cholesterolemia can be readily achieved by diet alone; it results from the rabbit's inherently poor catabolic system for cholesterol. This is associated with widespread cholesterol deposition throughout the reticuloendothelial system which resembles the lipid storage diseases in humans. Lesions develop in the arterial intima of the aorta and great arteries, composed predominantly of lipid-laden foam cells, but lesions rarely display features of advanced atherosclerosis such as calcification, central necrosis, luminal ulceration or thrombosis [4]. Lesions of similar morphology to human atherosclerotic plaques can be obtained either by feeding animals a 0.1% cholesterol diet [5] or an intermittent hypercholesterolemic diet over a longer period of time (up to 2 years) [6] or by combining cholesterol feeding with balloon injury to the vessel wall [7]. In developing a more relevant model to the human disease, we have utilized a modification of the latter procedure.

A primary atherosclerotic plaque model

In humans, atherosclerosis develops in those arteries which have pre-existing myointimal thickenings either diffusely along the vessel or as "intimal cushions" at branch points [8]. These thickenings begin to develop shortly after birth, and by the second decade of life diffuse intimal thickenings can be up to 5 times the thickness of the media in vessels such as the left descending coronary artery. Atherosclerosis rarely develops in vessels where the endothelium lies directly on the internal elastic lamina. Therefore, in order to model as closely as possible the human disease, the right carotid artery of the rabbit is de-endothelialized with a 2F Fogarty balloon catheter. This results in smooth muscle cells from the inner part of the media undergoing phenotypic change characterized by a decrease in the volume fraction of myofilaments ($V_v$myo) from $67.9 \pm 3.6\%$ to $42.7 \pm 3.3\%$, followed by migration through fenestrations in the internal elastic lamina, and pro-liferation. During the development phase of the thickening (the first 2 weeks) the $V_v$myo of the smooth muscle cells is low ($38.8 \pm 1.0\%$). However, after 6 weeks this starts to increase ($55.1 \pm 3.4\%$), approaching the level in smooth muscle cells of the media by 12 weeks ($64.7 \pm 2.9\%$). At this stage the myointimal thickening closely resembles the diffuse intimal thickening of human large and medium-size arteries [9]. Starting at week 14, the rabbits are fed a 1% cholesterol-enriched diet for 6 weeks, the plasma cholesterol levels rising from 1.10 ± 0.45 mmol/l to 10.68 ± 0.98 mmol/l. This remains high (10.16 ± 1.97 mmol/l) after a further 6 weeks on normal chow because of enhanced cholesterol synthesis in the liver. The lesions which develop in the preformed intimal thickenings resemble human atherosclerotic plaques with a central core of extracellular lipid and foam cells and a thick fibrous cap of proliferated smooth muscle cells and matrix (Fig. 1). In contrast, the lesions which develop in the aorta consist of simple subendothelial accumu-lations of lipid-filled macrophages with little smooth-muscle involvement (Fig. 2) — reminiscent of human juvenile fatty streaks.

A restenosis model

The historical rabbit models of restenosis after angioplasty have been developed using the conventional method of endothelial denudation with a Fogarty balloon catheter [10]. These

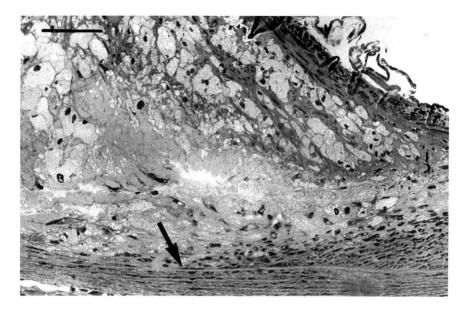

Fig. 1. Atherosclerotic plaque in rabbit carotid artery after balloon de-endothelialization and a 6-week 1% cholesterol diet. Stained with 1% toluidine blue. Note fibrous cap and lipid-filled macrophages. Arrow = internal elastic lamina. Scale bar = 200 μm.

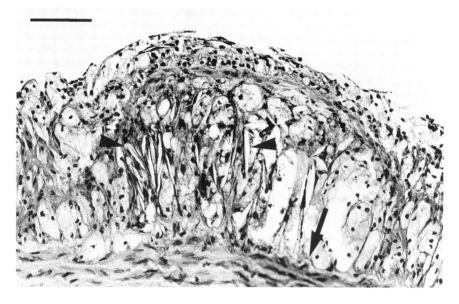

Fig. 2. Lesion in thoracic aorta from rabbit fed a 1% cholesterol diet only. Stained with 1% toluidine blue. Note abundance of lipid-filled macrophages and cholesterol crystals (arrowheads). Arrow = internal elastic lamina. Scale bar = 100 μm.

studies have concentrated on injury to the carotid, iliac and less commonly the aortic arteries. The intimal thickening resulting from balloon injury consists predominantly of vascular smooth muscle cells which have migrated from the media through fenestrations in the internal elastic lamina. This lesion does not resemble the restenotic plaque seen in humans, which has far more complex histology. The myointimal thickening generated from a normal rabbit vessel will therefore have cellular and growth factor responses which are different from a human angioplasty lesion derived from pre-existing primary plaque. This difference in primary substrate between the rabbit and human suggests that normal vessel denudation may be too simple a model for studying the restenotic process.

In an attempt to circumvent this problem and approximate the human restenotic plaque, several workers have initially created primary lesions using a hyperlipidemic diet [11]. Following the creation of a fatty plaque, lesions are then subjected to balloon angioplasty which results in rupture of the fatty neointima, platelet deposition and fibrin formation. Subsequently restenosis occurs in up to 25% of these vessels at the site of previous angioplasty [12]. Histological analysis of these lesions shows marked concentric luminal restenosis comprising loose, acellular, lipid-rich connective tissue with smooth muscle cells filling the spaces created by rupture of the media. Approximately 50% of ballooned lesions have organized thrombus apparent in the neointima, a feature which is uncommon after balloon injury of normal rabbit vessels [12]. Areas of thrombus formation are rich sources of platelet-derived growth factor and may act as a source of mitogenic stimulus for restenotic plaque progression [13].

In our laboratory we have sought to create a rabbit restenotic model which mimics the histological features of the human lesions as much as possible. We have used the iliac artery, as it is approximately the same size and has similar morphological structure to human coronary arteries. A fatty fibrocellular primary plaque is created using a combination of endothelial denudation with a conventional angioplasty balloon and follow-up feeding with a 1% cholesterol diet for 4 weeks. This primary lesion has an abundance

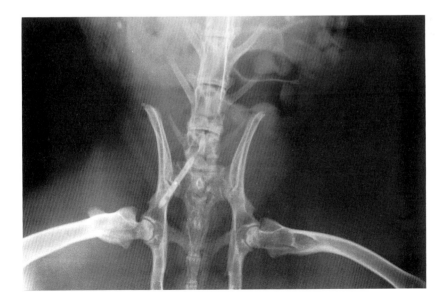

Fig. 3. Radiograph showing inflated angioplasty balloon in the right iliac artery of the rabbit.

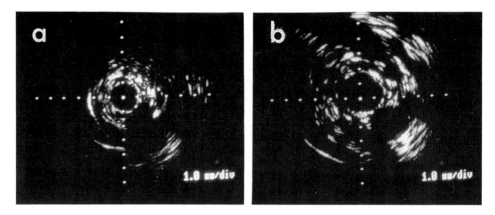

Fig. 4. Intravascular ultrasound of a) primary atherosclerotic plaque in the iliac artery of the rabbit and b) same lesion after dilatation. Note the increase in lumen diameter.

of foam cells in a lipid-rich core with a fibrocellular cap. At 4 weeks the lipid diet is stopped and under fluoroscopic and intravascular ultrasound guidance the primary plaque is dilated using a human angioplasty balloon catheter (see Figs. 3 and 4). An appropriate size of balloon catheter is selected using the intravascular ultrasound measurement of the reference vessel and lesion luminal diameters before angioplasty. In a group of 18 rabbits we found the mean balloon size selected was 2.42 ± 0.12 mm. This technique avoids inappropriate sizing of balloons which may either achieve an insufficient dilatation of the lesion or alternatively excessive medial injury. As this type of balloon sizing is common

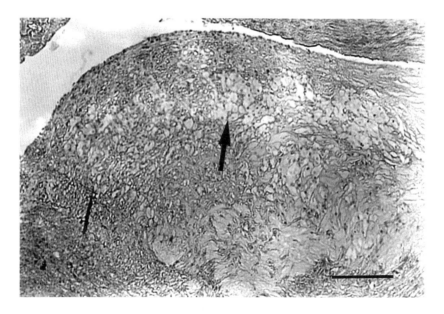

Fig. 5. Restenotic plaque in rabbit iliac artery 4 weeks after dilatation of a primary atherosclerotic plaque. Stained with hematoxylin. Note the fibrocellular intima with central lipid deposition (arrow). Scale bar = 200 μm.

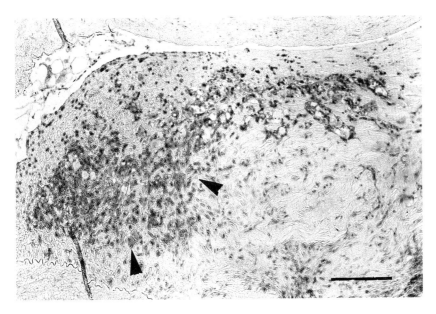

Fig. 6. Restenotic plaque in rabbit iliac artery 4 weeks after dilatation of primary atherosclerotic plaque. Immunostained with antimacrophage antibody (Ram 11). Note the central area of immunostaining within the intima which is rich in lipid-laden macrophages (arrowheads). Scale bar = 200 µm.

practice in humans [14] it seems appropriate that similar methodology be used in rabbit models. After balloon dilatation the luminal diameter across the lesion is again measured using intravascular ultrasound to ensure a successful result. Rabbits are then sacrificed at different times after balloon injury. The cellular and growth factor responses within the vessel are then analyzed (see Figs. 5 and 6).

The creation of a primary lesion with endothelial denudation and a lipid-rich diet followed at 4 weeks by balloon angioplasty closely mimics the human restenotic lesion. This rabbit model should be used more frequently in the future as it helps to separate the cellular and growth factor changes which occur in primary lesions from those which are peculiar to balloon injury and restenosis.

Acknowledgements

This work was supported by grants from Servier Laboratories, the National Health and Medical Research Council of Australia and the National Heart Foundation of Australia. The technical and photographic assistance of Nicole Smith is gratefully acknowledged.

References

1. Ignatowski A. Izvest Imper Voennomed Akad, St Petersburg 1908;16:154−173.
2. Vesselinovitch D. Arch Pathol Lab Med 1988;112:1011−1017.
3. Haust MD, Geer JC. Am J Pathol 1970;60:329−346.
4. Gross DR. Boston: Martinus Nijhoff 1985;537−547.
5. Prescott MF, Sawyer WK. Drug Development Research 1993;29:88−93.
6. Constantinides P, Booth J, Carlson G. Arch Pathol 1960;70:712−724.
7. Tsukada T, Rosenfeld M, Ross R, Gown AM. Arteriosclerosis 1986;6:601−613.
8. Velican C, Velican D. Atherosclerosis 1976;23:345−355.

120

9. Manderson JA, Mosse PRL, Safstrom JA, Young SB, Campbell GR. Arteriosclerosis 1989;9:289—298.

10. Baumgartner HA, Struden A. Pathol Microbiol 1966;29:393—405.

11. Weidinger FF, McLenachan JM, Cybulsky MI, Fallon JT, Hollenberg NK, Cooke JP, Ganz P. Circulation 1991;84:755—767.

12. Hanke H, Strohschneider T, Oberhoff M, Betz E, Karsch KR. Circ Res 1990;67:651—659.

13. Wilcox JN, Emerik G, Hultgren B, Hitchkiss A. In: Biology of Vascular Cells Sixth International Symposium, Paris, August, 1990.

14. Hodgson JMcB, Reddy KG, Suneja R, Nair RN, Lesnefsky EJ, Sheehan HM. J Am Coll Cardiol 1993;21: 35—44.

The atherosclerosis-prone JCR:LA-corpulent rat

J.C. Russell

Department of Surgery, 275 Heritage Medical Research Center, University of Alberta, Edmonton, Alberta T6G 2S2, Canada

Abstract. The JCR:LA-corpulent rat is one of a number of strains incorporating the autosomal recessive gene originally isolated by Koletsky and later designated as cp (corpulent) that is unique to a closed, outbred colony, in contrast to the congenic inbred character of other cp strains. In common with other cp strains, rats that are homozygous cp (cp/cp) are obese from an early age, highly insulin-resistant, and hypertriglyceridemic. The cp/cp rats are hyperinsulinemic and have a marked hypersensitivity to insulinotrophic agents such as GIP and arginine. They also have an insulin resistance that is extreme in males and results in a total absence of insulin-mediated glucose turnover. This forces the diversion of large amounts of diet-derived glucose to the liver and conversion to triacylglycerol with secretion as VLDL, leading to hypertriglyceridemia. The JCR:LA-cp strain is unique among rat strains in the spontaneous development of both atherosclerosis and ischemic myocardial lesions in cp/cp male rats. Treatments that improve insulin sensitivity and reduce insulin levels inhibit or prevent the cardiovascular disease. This strain of rat strongly mimics the obese, insulin-resistant segments of the human population and provides an extremely valuable animal model for studies of mechanisms of atherogenesis and putative treatments.

Effective study of the complex mechanisms underlying atherosclerosis will require good animal models exhibiting vascular disease. Since atherosclerosis quite clearly is an end-stage process with many contributing causes and a polygenetic basis for susceptibility, more than one animal model will be needed. The development of atherosclerotic disease is highly correlated with the marked elevation of low-density lipoprotein (LDL) cholesterol that is characteristic of genetic defects in the LDL receptor. The Watanabe Heritable Hyperlipidemic (WHHL) rabbit has proven to be an invaluable model in unravelling the causes of hypercholesterolemia. Kita has already discussed this model (see pp. 111–113). Atherosclerosis in the human population is also highly correlated with both type 1 (insulin-dependent) diabetes and the syndrome characterized by abdominal obesity, insulin resistance, and hypertriglyceridemia. There are two genetic models of obesity in rats, one due to the fatty (fa) and the other to the corpulent (cp) genes originally isolated by Zucker and Zucker and by Koletsky, respectively [1,2]. There are also a number of obese strains of mice (e.g., ob/ob and db/db). The rats are larger and have been the subject of ongoing studies of metabolic abnormalities. The cp gene has been bred into a number of different strains of rat, most being inbred, allowing for the creation of congenic strains. The JCR:LA-cp strain is unique among the obese rodent strains in that the obese males spontaneously develop atherosclerotic lesions and ischemic myocardial lesions. The development of disease does not occur in the fatty Zucker or in any of the other corpulent strains.

Development of the JCR:LA-cp rat

The autosomal recessive cp gene arose as a mutation in a cross between a Sprague-Dawley and an SHR rat by Koletsky [2]. The resultant obese, hypertensive rats developed a fulminant atherosclerosis. Stock of this "obese SHR" rat was given to Hansen at the National Institutes of Health. He was obliged by breeding difficulties to cross the Koletsky strain to two in-house strains, the SHR/N and LA/N. He then backcrossed repeatedly to the parent strains to obtain two congenic strains, the SHR/N-cp and LA/N-cp. At the fifth backcross, nucleus breeding stock of the LA/N-cp strain was sent to the University of Alberta in 1978. This noncongenic colony included an approximately 3% genetic contribution from the original Koletsky strain. It has been developed and maintained as a closed, outbred colony using the Poiley method [3] for some 8 years to prevent genetic drift. The strain was originally referred to as LA/N-cp, but this was changed to JCR:LA-cp in response to a request by the National Academy of Sciences, Washington, to correctly describe the outbred colony and distinguish it from the fully congenic LA/N-cp.

Metabolic abnormalities

Rats that are homozygous for the cp gene (cp/cp) are obese and exhibit extensive metabolic abnormalities that have a marked sexual dimorphism. Animals that are heterozygous (cp/+) or homozygous normal (+/+) are lean and indistinguishable from each other or the parent LA/N strain. The obesity is extreme, with cp/cp male rats weighing over 850 g at 9 months of age (vs. approximately 450 g for a +/+ male). The fat is present subcutaneously, especially over the trunk, but is most prominent within the three major abdominal fat depots: omental, perirenal, and epididymal. The obesity is associated with a significant hyperphagia, cp/cp males having a peak food consumption at 3 months of age of 35 g/day compared to 18 g/day for +/+ animals. The development of the obese phenotype persists in animals fed as little as 12 g/day from 4 weeks of age, reflecting a profound disturbance of carbohydrate and lipid metabolism.

The central metabolic defect in the cp/cp rat appears to be a profound insulin resistance in the peripheral tissues. This effect is characteristic of the cp/cp male rats, with the cp/cp females being only mildly affected. It is evident in a total failure of the cp/cp male rat to increase glucose turnover in response to insulin while under euglycemic insulin clamp conditions [4]. In confirmation of this, the muscle of cp/cp male rats shows no increase in the uptake of radiolabeled glucose in response to insulin. The insulin resistance is also reflected in an impaired glucose tolerance that is much more marked in the cp/cp male than in the cp/cp female. This leads to transient postprandial hyperglycemia, but not to a frank diabetes with glucosuria. It is accompanied by a severe hyperinsulinemia that is secondary to an extreme pancreatic hypersecretion of insulin. This is associated with a physiologically normal, but greatly exaggerated, insulin-secreting response to the seratogogues arginine and GIP (gastric-inhibiting polypeptide) [5]. In contrast, the fatty Zucker rat has a more modest insulin-secreting response, but is responsive to arginine and GIP, inappropriately, at very low glucose levels. An unresolved major question is whether the insulin resistance is a consequence of established hyperinsulinemia due to β-cell hypersensitivity or whether the hypersensitivity/hypersecretion is an adaptive response to peripheral insulin resistance.

The peripheral inability to take up glucose forces the liver to take up the larger flow of glucose from the carbohydrate-based diet. As shown in Fig. 1, this leads, in the cp/cp rat, to a greatly enhanced flow of glucose to hepatic fatty acid synthesis. The resulting triglycerides are packaged into very low density lipoprotein (VLDL), secreted into the plasma, and taken up by the peripheral tissues. The flow of VLDL is such that the animals exhibit a very severe VLDL hyperlipidemia that is greater in the cp/cp female than in the cp/cp male [6,7], despite the more modest insulin resistance and hyperin-

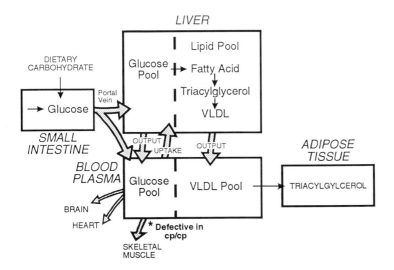

Fig. 1. Principal pathways of carbohydrate and lipid flow illustrating the diversion of diet-derived glucose to hepatic lipid synthesis and release due to peripheral insulin resistance.

sulinemia in the former. This suggests that the metabolic disorder may have sex-linked elements in addition to those described above that are not yet recognized.

Pathology of the JCR:LA-cp rat

Lean rats of both sexes are normal, with no evidence of pathological states other than those usually associated with aging in rats. The colony at the University of Alberta is also demonstrated virus antibody-free. The cp/cp females are clinically normal, except for their extreme obesity and related difficulties in grooming and an increased tendency to develop renal calculi and hydronephrosis. The cp/cp male rats, in contrast, spontaneously develop atherosclerotic lesions on the arch of the aorta and major arteries. Figure 2 illustrates an advanced raised lesion on the arch of the aorta of a 9-month-old cp/cp male rat. Lesions are evident from 3 months of age (a young adult rat) and increase in severity up to 9 months of age (a middle-aged rat). The advanced lesions may be seen on transmission electron microscopy to contain foam cells, smooth muscle cells, and lipid debris within the intimal space (Fig. 3). Areas of extensive desquamation and adherent macrophages are also common, and large fibrin deposits also occur in older animals. We have examined fatty Zucker rats and found no similar lesions whatsoever in 9-month-old fa/fa rats [8].

The vascular lesions seen in the cp/cp male rats are accompanied by myocardial lesions that are apparently of ischemic origin. These have been categorized by stage as follows: Stage 1, areas of cell necrosis; Stage 2, areas of cell "drop-out" and lysis, with chronic inflammatory cell infiltration; Stage 3, small foci of chronic inflammatory cells; Stage 4, old, mature collagen lesions. These vary in age and maturity, from hours to a day for Stage 1 lesions, to many months for Stage 4 lesions. From both a pathophysiological and practical point of view, the Stage 2 and Stage 4 lesions are the important indicators of the extent of disease. Figure 4 shows a typical Stage 2 lesion, and Fig. 5, a typical, mature Stage 4 lesion.

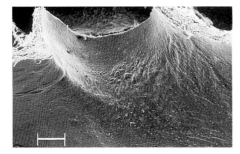

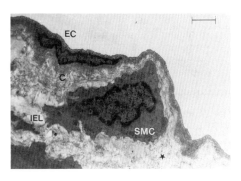

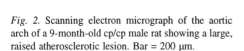

Fig. 2. Scanning electron micrograph of the aortic arch of a 9-month-old cp/cp male rat showing a large, raised atherosclerotic lesion. Bar = 200 μm.

Fig. 3. Transmission electron micrograph of a raised intimal lesion on the arch of the aorta of a 14-month-old cp/cp male rat showing smooth muscle cell (SMC) in a subendothelial position, amorphous material (A), and collagen (C). The internal elastic lamina (IEL) and an endothelial cell (EC) are also visible. Bar = 1 μm.

Therapeutic interventions

Atherosclerosis in particular, and cardiovascular disease in general, have been a very difficult challenge in terms of treatment and prevention as well as of understanding. A good animal model should mimic the response of humans to known therapeutic measures and facilitate the assessment and development of new strategies. The cp/cp male rat has been subjected to a number of treatments, and the extent of atherosclerosis and frequency of myocardial lesions have been found to be decreased markedly by some treatments and not at all by others. In general terms, treatments that improve insulin/glucose metabolism and decrease plasma insulin levels are protective, while those that merely reduce plasma lipid levels have no effect. Interestingly, castration of either sex does not alter the disease pattern, with males continuing to develop myocardial lesions and females still being spared, despite their degree of hyperlipidemia becoming equal [9]. Thus, the end-stage disease is sex-linked, but non-sex-hormone-dependent. Lastly, agents that inhibit

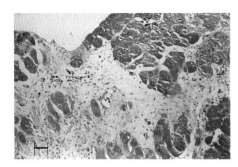

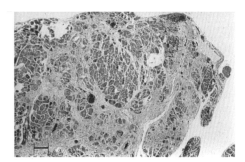

Fig. 4. Section of the heart of a 9-month-old cp/cp male rat showing a Stage 2 lesion with cell lysis and chronic inflammatory cell infiltration, hematoxylin and eosin. Bar = 200 μm.

Fig. 5. Section of heart of a 9-month-old cp/cp male rat showing a mature scarred Stage 4 lesion, Masson's trichrome. Bar = 200 μm.

vasospasm are protective against myocardial lesions, possibly by compensating for a defect in the endothelium-dependent relaxation mechanism [10]. These results with a limited range of agents and treatments are encouraging and confirm the usefulness of this animal model for the study of disease affecting humans.

Summary and Conclusions

The JCR:LA-cp rat has been shown to provide a unique animal model for the study of atherosclerosis, its mechanistic antecedents, and its serious sequelae. It provides a useful complement to the BB rat as a model for mild type 2 diabetes and its complications and to the WHHL rabbit. The strain promises to be particularly useful in the future for basic studies of proposed preventative and therapeutic measures against cardiovascular disease.

Acknowledgements

The development of this strain has been supported financially principally by the Heart and Stroke Foundation of Alberta. Numerous people have contributed to the development of the strain and our understanding of its nature, in particular Dorothy Koeslag, Sandra Graham, Roger Amy and Peter Dolphin.

References

1. Zucker LM, Zucker TF. J Hered 1961;52:275–278.
2. Koletsky S. Exp Mol Pathol 1973;19:53–60.
3. Poiley SM. Animal Care Panel 1960;10:159–161.
4. Russell JC, Graham S, Hameed M. Metabolism 1994;43:536–543.
5. Pederson PA, Campos RV, Buchan AMJ, Chisholm DB, Russell JC, Brown JC. Int J Obesity 1991;15:461–470.
6. Dolphin PJ, Stewart B, Amy RM, Russell JC. Biochim Biophys Acta 1987;919:140–148.
7. Vance JE, Russell JC. J Lipid Res 1990;31:1491–1501.
8. Amy RM, Dolphin PJ, Pederson RA, Russell JC. Atherosclerosis 1988;69:199–209.
9. Russell JC, Amy RM, Graham S, Wenzel LM, Dolphin PJ. Atherosclerosis 1993;199:113–122.
10. McNamee CJ, Kappagoda CT, Kunjara R, Russell JC. Circ Res 1994;74:1126–1132.

Are tree shrews and Beijing ducks good models for the study of antiatherogenicity of serum HDL?

K.Q. Wang[1], B.S. Chen[1], Z.G. Li[1], Y.C. He[1], X.J. Wu[1], M.P. She[1], R.Y. Xia[1] and Y.Z. Lu[2]

[1]*Institute of Basic Medical Sciences, Chinese Academy of Medical Sciences, Beijing; and* [2]*Institute of Medical Biology, Chinese Academy of Medical Science, Kunming, China*

Abstract. Tree shrews and Beijing ducks, both of which have a high proportion (70%) of HDL in the serum lipoproteins, do not develop atherosclerosis on a high-cholesterol, high-fat diet. They have high LCAT but very low CETP activities, high HDL-C and apoA-I. Their lipid and lipoprotein patterns change differently from those of human and rabbit during feeding experiments. The cholesterol and its esters are carried mainly by HDL and metabolized essentially through the HDL-receptor pathway rather than the LDL-receptor pathway. This unusual metabolism makes tree shrews and Beijing ducks good models of antiatherosclerosis by HDL.

Anitschkow's discovery in the 1920s that rabbits develop atherosclerosis on a diet supplemented with cholesterol has provided a model of atherosclerosis ever since. Studies of the mechanisms by which cholesterol, or rather lipoproteins, promote atherosclerosis have elucidated the role of serum lipoprotein and apoliproteins in the development and regression of atherosclerosis as well as the causes of the familiar hyper- and hypo-β-lipoproteinemia. However, few models have been found for the study of antiatherosclerosis. In the late 1970s we discovered that both tree shrews (TS) and Beijing ducks (BD) have a high proportion of serum HDL (>70% of serum lipoproteins) and do not develop atherosclerosis on an atherogenic diet [1,2]. These findings led us to perform experiments to confirm our discoveries and to elucidate the mechanisms of antiatherosclerosis by HDL in TS and BD.

Serum lipids and lipoproteins of TS

Cholesterol, VLDL, LDL levels and α- and β-lipoprotein (Lp) percentages were determined on about 100 normal TS and those fed a high-cholesterol, high-fat diet. Agarose electrophoresis and ultracentrifugation showed TS serum α-Lp to be >70% of lipoproteins and serum cholesterol similar to that in humans (158 mg/dl). No atherosclerosis developed after feeding the atherogenic diet for 32 weeks (Fig. 1). These experiments provided for the first time in vivo evidence supporting the proposal of Miller et al. [3] and Gordon et al. [4] in the 1970s that HDL is a negative risk factor for coronary heart disease.

Chemical and physical properties

Pooled TS serum samples were separated into VLDL, LDL and HDL by discontinuous density gradient ultracentrifugation according to Wang et al. [5]. The profile of optical density values showed that HDL was the major lipoprotein of TS and it did not decrease

Address for correspondence: K.Q. Wang, Institute of Basic Medical Sciences, Chinese Academy of Medical Sciences, 5 Dongdansantiao, Beijing 100005, China.

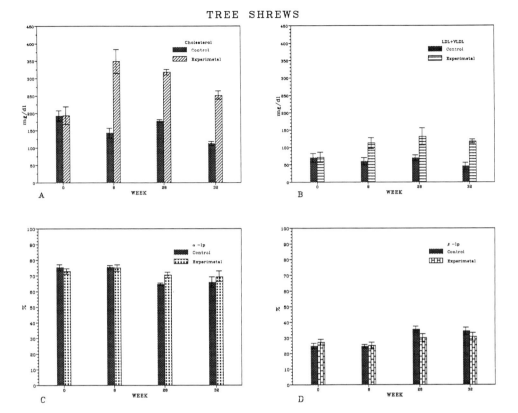

Fig. 1. Changes of concentrations of total cholesterol and LDL, and the percentages of α- and β-Lp, in control and experimental (fed high-cholesterol, high-fat diet) tree shrews. A: change of total cholesterol; B: change of α-Lp percentage; C: change of LDL + VLDL; D: change of β-Lp percentage.

on feeding the atherogenic diet. The HDL were further divided into three subfractions: HDL-1, HDL-2 and HDL-3, which were all delipidated according to Scanu et al. [6]. ApoHDLs of the subfractions showed many apolipoproteins on immunoelectrophoresis, with apoA-I as the major one. Each subfraction was examined by electron microscopy with negative staining. They ranged in size from about 98 to 120 ng, HDL-1 being the largest. The flotation rates of TS LDL, HDL-1, HDL-2 and HDL-3 were 6.3, 3.0, 2.8 and 1.9 respectively. ApoA-I of TS HDL was further purified by HPLC. Its amino acid composition showed Asp at the N-terminus and almost equal numbers of the polar amino acids Glu, Asp, Arg and Lys as in human apoA-I. Dichroism of HDL showed a strong negative peak between 204 and 240 nm, indicating that apoA-I of TS may form an amphipathic α-helix easily.

Pathology

The aortas of TS were examined visually for atherosclerotic plaques at the end of the experiment after staining with Oil Red O, and also by electron microscopy. No plaques were found in the intima of the aorta; only TS no. 107 showed fatty streaks. Meanwhile about 70% of the experimental TS developed gallstones consisting of pure cholesterol. Thus, most of the cholesterol fed had been metabolized in the liver and excreted, probably through the bile.

Serum lipid and lipoprotein levels, α-Lp and β-Lp percentages of Beijing duck and rabbit

We carried out the same kind of experiments on BD and rabbit as on TS and confirmed our previous findings that BD was rich in HDL (>70%) and did not develop AS. During the experiments its serum lipid and lipoproteins changed very differently from those of rabbit but similarly to TS (Figs. 2 and 3). The α-Lp% of both TS and BD remained constant — in fact that of BD had a tendency to increase. In contrast VLDL, LDL and lipid levels in experimental rabbits were about 10 times those of controls while their α-Lp percentage decreased tremendously.

Metabolism of apoA-I of Beijing duck HDL in vivo and its transfer among lipoproteins in vitro

^{125}I-HDL studies indicated that the half-life of BD HDL in vivo was about 41 h, and its

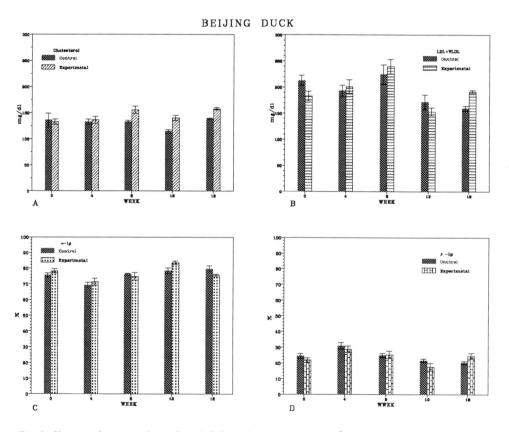

Fig. 2. Changes of concentrations of total cholesterol and LDL, α- and β-Lp percentages of control and experimental groups of Beijing ducks. A: change of total cholesterol; B: change of LDL + VLDL; C: change of α-Lp percentage; D: change of β-Lp percentage.

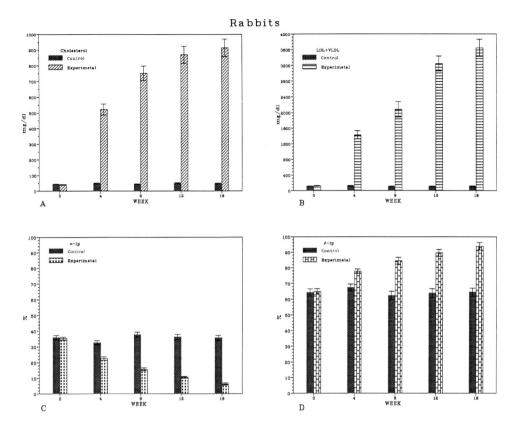

Fig. 3. Changes of concentrations of total cholesterol and LDL, α-Lp and β-Lp percentage of control and experimental groups of rabbits. A: change of total cholesterol; B: change of LDL + VLDL; C: change of α-Lp percentage; D: change of β-Lp percentage.

distribution among the main organs was in the order liver > kidney > spleen > lung > intestine > muscles > aorta, which suggests that liver is the main organ for metabolizing HDL and that kidney also plays an important part. ApoA-I transferred in vitro only from VLDL and LDL to HDL, not the reverse.

LCAT and CETP activities, and cholesterol metabolism

The LCAT and CETP activities in TS and BD serum were assayed and compared with those of human and rabbit serum. The LCAT activities of TS and BD serum were, at an average of 52 and 90 U/l, both higher than in human serum (35 U/l), whereas CETP in BD was very low (<1% of ^{3}H-labeled cholesteryl ester in HDL transferred to VLDL and LDL), compared with human (18%) and rabbit (26%). During the feeding experiments the LCAT activity of BD underwent little change (remaining about 100 U/l), while the rabbit showed great increases in both LCAT (average of 25 U/l to 50 U/l) and CETP (26 to 56%) activities. BDs higher HDL-C (86 mg/dl) and apoA-I (144 mg/dl) show that most of its cholesterol and esters are also carried by HDL.

HDL receptor in the liver membrane of Beijing duck

We have previously proposed the HDL-receptor pathway for metabolizing cholesterol and its esters. Recently Wu and Wang [7] have obtained evidence of HDL receptors existing on the liver cell membrane by using ^{125}I-labeled apoE-free HDL. Our results showed a specific, saturable and high-affinity HDL receptor, with $K_d = 9.6$ µg/ml, B_{max} of 8.9 µg/mg cell membrane protein and $K_d = 7.4$ µg/ml and B_{max} of 5.8 µg/mg hepatocyte protein. ApoA-I was found to be the main ligand of the receptor. To confirm the presence of the HDL receptor we first identified the liver membrane receptor protein by ligand blotting and then isolated and purified the protein by multiple SDS-PAGE processes. Its chemical and physical properties showed that this hepatocyte membrane protein is a glycoprotein consisting of 689 amino acids, about 89 kDa, and four isoforms on IEF.

The results combine to support strongly our hypothesis that exogenous cholesterol in BD and TS is carried mainly by HDL and metabolized in the liver through an HDL-receptor pathway in situ instead of being transferred to VLDL and LDL and metabolized via the LDL-receptor pathway (Fig. 4). This unique mechanism for metabolizing lipoproteins and cholesterol makes both species useful models for studying the antiatherogenicity of HDL. Furthermore, we propose that the way in which cholesterol is transported and metabolized may be used to predict or determine whether a species will develop atherosclerosis or not. A species which like TS and BD metabolizes cholesterol via a HDL-receptor pathway will not be susceptible to atherosclerosis, whereas those which utilize the LDL-receptor pathway will be susceptible, like rabbit, dog, pig, chicken and human beings.

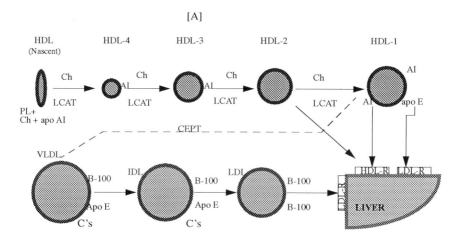

Fig. 4. Schematic illustration of the metabolic pathway of cholesterol and its esters in lipoproteins of Beijing duck. A: Upper row, the HDL-receptor pathway for metabolizing HDL-cholesterol and its esters postulated by Wang et al. Nascent HDL comprises phospholipid, cholesterol (Ch) and apoA-I. Under the action of LCAT the Ch is esterified to cholesteryl ester, and the nascent HDL becomes spherical in shape (HDL-4). With further esterification of the HDL-cholesterol by LCAT, the particles acquire more cholesteryl ester and increase in size from HDL-4 to HDL-1. The latter and HDL-2 are metabolized through the HDL-receptor pathway in the liver. B: Lower row, the LDL-receptor pathway for metabolizing LDL and its cholesteryl ester postulated by Brown and Goldstein. In this pathway HDL-1 cholesteryl esters are transferred back to VLDL, IDL and finally LDL, which is metabolized in the liver through LDL receptors.

Acknowledgements

The research was supported by grant 75-62-02-11 from the National Science and Technology Committee and Chinese Ministry of Public Health.

References

1. Wang KQ, Chen BS, Wang JM. Physiol Sci 1982;2:23—24.
2. She MP, Wang KQ et al. Soshiran 1983;1:66—73.
3. Miller GJ, Miller NE. Lancet 1975;I:16—19.
4. Gordon T et al. Am J Med 1977;62:707—712.
5. Wang KQ et al. In: Ralph A. Bradshaw et al. (eds) Proteins in Biology and Medicine. New York: Academic Press, Inc. 1982;82—308.
6. Scanu AM et al. Biochemistry 1969;8:3309—3316.
7. Wu XJ, Wang KQ. Chinese Med Sci J 1994;9:81—86.

132

Cynomolgus monkeys for the study of hormonal influences on atherogenesis

Thomas B. Clarkson and Ginger Tansey

Comparative Medicine Clinical Research Center, Bowman Gray School of Medicine of Wake Forest University, Winston-Salem, North Carolina, USA

Abstract. Little evidence exists that hormones play an important role in the progression of coronary artery atherosclerosis in males, but do appear to be a principal modulator of coronary atherosclerosis in females. Studies in women may suffer from selection bias; therefore the use of cynomolgus monkeys has been proposed as advantageous. Pre- and postmenopausal female cynomolgus monkeys share characteristics of lipoprotein profiles, reproductive biology, vasoconstrictor responses, and responses to oral contraceptives, while avoiding problems of selection bias and compliance.

There is little evidence supporting an important role of hormones in the progression of coronary artery atherosclerosis in males; however, estrogen appears to be a principal modulator of coronary atherogenesis of females. Consequently, we shall limit this brief review to females and ovarian hormones.

Women during their reproductive years are protected against the progression of coronary artery atherosclerosis. That ovarian hormones provide this protection is supported by loss of protection after surgical or natural menopause, and by studies showing that postmenopausal women taking estrogen replacement therapy have less CHD than women not taking hormone therapy [1].

Need for a primate model

The reduced rates of CHD in women on ERT may be biologically real or they may be artifactual; i.e., related to selection bias. Support for the argument that the association of reduced CHD is a result of selection bias is summarized in Table 1 [2].

These controversies about the observational studies in women and the effects of ERT on CHD make randomized trials in cynomolgus monkeys useful. The advantages and disadvantages of using cynomolgus monkeys are presented in Table 2.

Characteristics of female cynomolgus as an animal model

Cynomolgus monkeys fed an atherogenic diet develop atherosclerosis with many similarities to atherosclerosis in human beings [3,4]. In addition to these lipoprotein/atherosclerosis characteristics, there are reproductive biological similarities. The cynomolgus female has a 28-day menstrual cycle like that of women [5]. Plasma hormone concentrations have been measured throughout the cynomolgus menstrual cycle, and the duration of the follicular and luteal phases and plasma estradiol and progesterone concentrations across the cycle are remarkably similar to those of women [5,6].

Address for correspondence: Dr Thomas Clarkson, CMCRC, Bowman Gray School of Medicine of Wake Forest University, Medical Center Blvd, Winston-Salem, NC 27157-1040, USA.

Table 1. CHD is lower amongst postmenopausal estrogen users. Is the association real or an artifact of selection bias?

Estrogen users vs. nonusers
Younger
Exercise more
Have higher incomes
More highly educated
Leaner
Etc.

Derived from refs. [1,2,16], Rosenburg et al., 1979; Ravnikar et al., 1987; Criqui MH et al., 1988

Table 2. Randomized trials with cynomolgus monkey models

Disadvantages	Advantages
Nonhuman rather than human primates	Avoid selection bias
Certain measures difficult e.g., quality of life	Compliance not an issue
	Better control possible e.g. diet
	Pathological endpoints possible

Male–female differences

CAA was found to be more extensive in males than in premenopausal females [7]. Like premenopausal women, premenopausal cynomolgus females have significantly higher plasma concentrations of HDL-C than their male counterparts, and gender differences in the extent of CAA are like those of human beings during the reproductively active years [7]. Plaque extent in male and female cynomolgus monkeys is presented in Fig. 1 as the mean percent lumen stenosis. Males had significantly lower concentrations of high density lipoprotein cholesterol (HDL-C) and higher systolic blood pressures than premenopausal nonpregnant females [8]. The magnitude of the male/female difference in CAA was similar to that among New Orleans Caucasians [9].

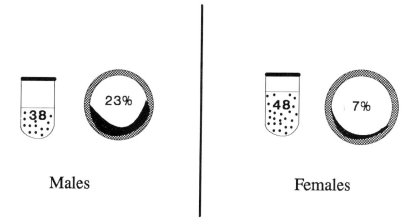

Fig. 1. Plaque extent in male vs. female cynomolgus monkeys (mean percent lumen stenosis) and plasma HDL-C concentrations (mg/dl). Modified from [7].

Premenopausal–postmenopausal differences

Women who have undergone either natural or surgical menopause have rather large increases in the rates of progression of CAA. Surgically menopausal cynomolgus monkeys share this pathophysiologic process; the comparison of plasma HDL-C concentrations and CAA of pre- and postmenopausal cynomolgus monkeys is presented in Fig. 2. Postmenopausal cynomolgus monkeys, like women, have lower plasma concentrations of HDL-C, increased LDL accumulation, more pronounced vasoconstrictor responses, and coronary artery atherosclerotic plaques that are much larger than those in premenopausal monkeys fed the same atherogenic diet for the same length of time [10].

Premenopausal estrogen effects

Estrogen defiency

Psychosocial stress has effects on the progression of CHD. Cynomolgus monkeys form complex social dominance hierarchies in competitive interactions. Those in the lower half of the dominance hierarchy within a social group are subordinate and those in the upper half of the hierarchy are dominant. A monkey's relative rank is stable over time [11].

The chronic stress of social subordination resulted in impaired ovarian function [8]. The subordinate animals had both fewer normal menstrual cycles and deficient luteal-phase progesterone concentrations that correlated with low periovulatory plasma estradiol concentrations. The chronically stressed, subordinate animals also had lower HDL-C concentrations and after necropsy were found to have more atherosclerosis than the socially dominant monkeys (Fig. 3).

We have analyzed CAA data from 77 premenopausal female monkeys, all fed the same atherogenic diet for the same length of time. Thirty of the animals had been housed in single cages and the other 47 lived in social groups. About half of each of these groups were treated with oral contraceptives. There were no differences in plasma lipids or lipoprotein concentrations between groups. The females housed in single cages had significantly more CAA than the socially housed monkeys (plaque area 0.13 mm^2 vs. 0.03 mm^2, p = 0.01) [12]. The chronically stressed (socially subordinate) monkeys had more extensive CAA than the dominant animals. The single-caged monkeys had more extensive

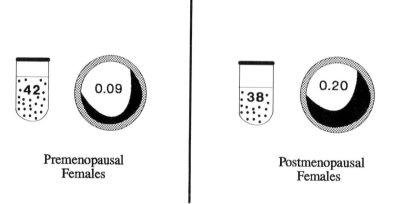

Premenopausal
Females

Postmenopausal
Females

Fig. 2. Comparison of pre- and postmenopausal cynomolgus females: plasma HDL-C concentrations (mg/dl) and mean percent lumen stenosis of coronary arteries. Modified from Adams MR et al. Arteriosclerosis 1987;7:378–384.

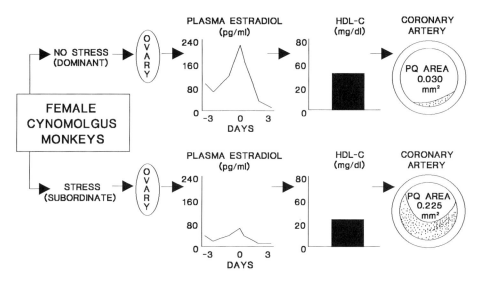

Fig. 3. Chronically stressed (socially subordinate) female cynomolgus monkeys compared to their dominant counterparts had more ovarian dysfunction, lower HDL-C concentrations, and greater coronary artery plaque (PQ) area. A probable mechanism is reduced arterial uptake of LDL. Reprinted with permission from [6].

atherosclerosis than the dominant monkeys, but did not differ significantly from the subordinates. The mechanism for this effect of social isolation is unknown, but it appears unrelated to impaired ovarian function. We speculate that this form of social isolation may trigger sympathetic nervous system arousal. Although the single-caged females not treated with oral contraceptives did not appear to be estrogen-deficient, exogenous estrogen therapy (either premenopausally with oral contraceptives or postmenopausally with estrogen replacement) may confer cardiovascular protection. In fact, the oral contraceptive-treated females housed in single cages had somewhat less CAA than the untreated single-caged females, although this was not statistically significant [12].

Estrogen treatment

Studies over the past 13 years have concerned the effects of exogenous hormone treatment on cardiovascular risk factors, physiologic characteristics, and atherosclerosis of cynomolgus females. In all studies, the doses usually taken by women were extrapolated to monkey doses on a caloric basis to account for both the smaller body and the higher metabolic rate of the monkeys.

During the late 1970s there arose serious concern about whether the lower HDL-C concentrations of women taking oral contraceptives (OCs) put them at the same increased risk for CHD as other women with low HDL-C concentrations. Fortunately, the plasma lipoprotein response of cynomolgus to OCs was strikingly similar to that of women [13]. Premenopausal monkeys receiving OC treatment actually had less CAA than untreated premenopausal female monkeys (Fig. 4). Among monkeys at higher risk of CAA because of their deleterious lipid profile at baseline (a TPC:HDL-C ratio >4.5), the protective effect of the OCs on CAA was even more pronounced [14].

To elucidate the mechanism of decreased atherosclerosis among the OC-treated groups, we examined the effects of OC treatment on LDL uptake in the artery wall [15]. This was

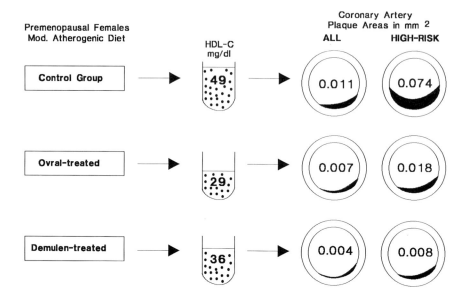

Fig. 4. Premenopausal cynomolgus monkeys given oral contraceptive treatment had reduced HDL-C concentrations but less coronary artery plaque than untreated controls. This was true even of high-risk animals (those with TC:HDL-C ratios >4.5 before treatment). Modified from [14].

conducted after only 16 weeks of consumption of an atherogenic diet, so that we could focus on mechanisms of early atherogenesis. Three groups of premenopausal females — one untreated, one treated with Triphasil (Wyeth-Ayerst), and one treated with Ovral (Wyeth-Ayerst) — were studied. Radiolabeled LDL coupled with tyramine cellobiose was used to measure intracellular accumulation of LDL and LDL degradation products in arteries. The amount of LDL accumulation in the coronary arteries of the treated groups was significantly less than in the control group. Estrogen may be acting to inhibit atherogenesis, at least in part, by inhibiting the arterial uptake and/or metabolism of plasma LDL.

Postmenopausal estrogen effects

Coronary artery atherosclerosis

Evidence exists that for postmenopausal women, estrogen replacement therapy is protective against CHD [1]. However, the mechanisms for this protection are unclear. Barrett-Connor and Bush [16] have suggested that somewhat less than half the protection can be explained by improvements in lipid risk factors (e.g., higher HDL-C and lower LDL-C concentrations).

Surgically postmenopausal cynomolgus were treated or not treated with estrogen; a third group was treated with estrogen and physiologic amounts of progesterone (Fig. 5) [17]. Circulating plasma estradiol concentrations averaged about 220 pg/ml among the estrogen-treated monkeys, which is similar to late follicular or periovulatory phase concentrations in women. Mean plasma progesterone concentrations were about 9 ng/ml during the month-long progesterone treatment phase in group 3, which is within the normal range during the midluteal phase in women. Estrogen replacement inhibited the

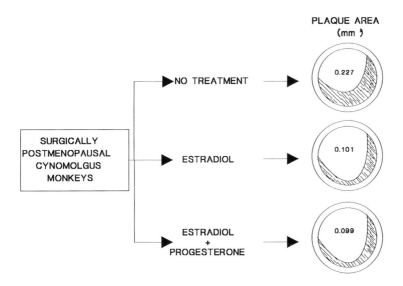

Fig. 5. In a trial designed to mimic physiologic hormone replacement therapy in women, surgically postmenopausal cynomolgus monkeys given 17β-estradiol with or without cyclic progesterone had less coronary artery atherosclerosis than untreated controls. Reprinted with permission from Douglas P (Ed) Coronary Heart Disease in Women, pp. 283–302, W.B. Saunders Co., Philadelphia, 1993.

progression of CAA, and physiologic progesterone replacement did not affect this. TC and HDL-C concentrations were not significantly different between groups, although within treatment groups these parameters were predictive of atherosclerosis extent [10].

To understand the mechanism of postmenopausal estrogen replacement effects on atherogenesis better, we performed an LDL uptake study [18]. Postmenopausal (ovariecto-mized) female cynomolgus were fed an atherogenic diet for 18 weeks with or without hormone replacement. Radiolabeled LDL coupled with tyramine cellobiose was injected to evaluate intracellular accumulation of LDL and LDL degradation products in arteries. Hormone replacement therapy resulted in lower LDL accumulation in the coronary arteries, suggesting that hormone replacement may inhibit atherosclerosis by suppressing accumulation and/or degradation of LDL in the artery wall.

Postmenopausal estrogen effects

Coronary vasomotion

Angina pectoris is more common in postmenopausal women than in premenopausal women, and appears to be at least as frequent in postmenopausal women as in men [19]. The angina frequently occurs in the absence of clinically significant CAA, as only about 26–37% of women with chest pain have angiographically defined coronary artery disease (Syndrome X) [20]; it is postulated that vasospasm may be one cause [21]. Using quantitative coronary angiography, coronary artery constriction or dilation is measured after intracoronary artery infusion of acetylcholine (ACH). Normally functioning coronary arteries without atherosclerosis dilate in response to ACH; however, atherosclerotic coronary arteries of both human beings [22] and nonhuman primates [23] exhibit a paradoxical constriction.

138

Chronically stressed (socially subordinate) premenopausal female monkeys have impaired vascular reactivity (greater vasospasm potential), in addition to impaired ovarian function compared to dominant animals [6,24], which suggests that estrogen is instrumental in preventing vasospasm.

Further studies have focused on the effects of exogenous estrogen administration on vascular reactivity. ACH responses in atherosclerotic coronary arteries were measured in surgically postmenopausal monkeys before and 20 min after intravenous infusion of physiologic doses of ethinyl estradiol. The estrogen treatment prevented the vasoconstriction seen before treatment [25]. Estrogen's effects on vasomotion seem to be independent of plaque size and lipoproteins [26].

Conclusions

Cynomolgus monkeys in the study of hormone effects on atherogenesis have proven useful for several reasons. Their lipoprotein characteristics and atherosclerotic responses are similar to those in women. In addition, they share similarities in their reproductive biology, particularly in plasma hormone concentrations. Surgically postmenopausal cynomolgus reflect the changes that human women undergo after surgical or natural menopause.

Estrogen defiency occurs in socially subordinate cynomolgus, and is reflected in the increased rate of CAA in these females. Estrogen replacement therapy resulted in less CAA and less accumulation of LDL in arterial walls. Estrogen appears to inhibit atherogenesis by inhibiting arterial uptake and/or metabolism of plasma LDL. Estrogen treatment prevents vasoconstriction in atherosclerotic coronary arteries. The advantages of using cynomolgus monkeys also include reduction of selection bias and avoidance of problems with compliance.

Acknowledgements

The research described in this review was supported in part by Grants P01 HL45666 and R01 HL38964 from the National Heart, Lung, and Blood Institute; and Contract HD-32800 from the National Institute of Child Health and Human Development; all of which are part of the National Institutes of Health, Bethesda, Maryland, USA.

References

1. Stampfer MJ, Colditz GA. Prev Med 1991;20:47—63.
2. Derby CA, Hume AL, Barbour MM, McPhillips JB, Lasater TM, Carleton RA. Am J Epidemiol 1993;137: 1125—1135.
3. Kramsch DM, Hollander H. Exp Mol Pathol 1968;9:1—22.
4. Stary HC, Malinow MR. Atherosclerosis 1982;43:151—175.
5. Williams RF, Hodgen GD. Am J Primat 1982;1(suppl 1):181—192.
6. Adams MR, Kaplan JR, Koritnik DR. Phys Behav 1985;35:935—940.
7. Hamm TE Jr., Kaplan JR, Clarkson TB, Bullock BC. Atherosclerosis 1983;48:221—233.
8. Kaplan JR, Adams MR, Clarkson TB, Koritnik DR. Atherosclerosis 1984;53:283—295.
9. Tejada C, Strong JP, Montenegro MR, Restrepo C, Solberg LA. Lab Invest 1968;18:509—526.
10. Adams MR, Kaplan JR, Manuck SB, Koritnik DR, Parks JS, Wolfe MS, Clarkson TB. Arteriosclerosis 1990;10:1051—1057.
11. Shively CA, Kaplan JR. Am J Primat 1991;23:239—245.
12. Shively CA, Clarkson TB, Kaplan JR. Atherosclerosis 1989;77:69—76.
13. Koritnik DR, Clarkson TB, Adams MR. In: Blye et al. (eds) Contraceptive Steroids: Pharmacology and Safety. New York: Plenum Press, 1986:303—319.

14. Clarkson TB, Shively CA, Morgan TM, Koritnik DR, Adams MR, Kaplan JR. Obstet Gynecol 1990;75: 217–222.
15. Wagner JD, Adams MR, Schwenke DC, Clarkson TB. Circ Res 1993;72:1300–1307.
16. Barrett-Connor E, Bush TL. J Am Med Assoc 1991;265:1861–1867.
17. Clarkson TB, Adams MR, Williams JK, Wagner JD. In: Douglas PS (ed) Cardiovascular Health and Disease in Women. Philadelphia: W.B. Saunders, 1993:283–302.
18. Wagner JD, Clarkson TB, St. Clair RW, Schwenke DC, Adams MR. J Clin Invest 1991;88:1995–2002.
19. Eaker ED, Castelli WP. In: Eaker et al. (eds) Coronary Heart Disease in Women: Proceedings of an NIH Workshop, New York: Haymarket Doyma, Inc., 1987:120–130.
20. Chaitman BR, Bourassa MG, Lam J, Hung J. In: Eaker et al. (eds) Coronary Heart Disease in Women: Proceedings of an NIH Workshop. New York: Haymarket Doyma, Inc., 1987:222–228.
21. Tofler GH, Stone PH, Muller JE, Braunwald E. In: Eaker et al. (eds) Coronary Heart Disease in Women: Proceedings of an NIH Workshop. New York: Haymarket Doyma, Inc., 1987:215–221.
22. Ludmer PL, Selwyn AP, Shook TL, Wayne RR, Mudge GH, Alexander RW, Ganz P. N Engl J Med 1987; 315:1046–1051.
23. Williams JK, Vita JA, Manuck SB, Selwyn AP, Kaplan JR. Circulation 1991;84:2146–2153.
24. Williams JK, Adams MR, Herrington DM, Clarkson TB. J Am Coll Cardiol 1992b;20:452–457.
25. Williams JK, Shively CA, Clarkson TB. Circulation 1994;90:983–987.
26. Williams JK, Adams MR, Klopfenstein HS. Circulation 1990;81:1680–1687.

140

Public health action programs: past and future

Sergio Muntoni

Center for Metabolic Diseases and Atherosclerosis, The ME.DI.CO. Association, Cagliari, Italy

Abstract. Cardiovascular diseases are the leading cause of premature death and disability in the developed world. Broad consensus exists on their preventability through reduction of risk factors at both the individual and population level. This implies involvement of policy-making institutions, because of the manifold implications (agriculture, industry, environment) of such public health action programs. Their implementation can result only from merging of biomedicine and politics. Other basic issues of a public action program are a strong scientific-ethical basis, great cost saving, institutionalization, allocation of funds, use of mass media, and transferability to other communities.

Among a host of preventable chronic illnesses, atherosclerotic cardiovascular diseases (CVD) and, in particular, coronary heart disease (CHD) and stroke deserve priority, not only because they continue to be the leading cause of premature death and disability in the developed world and are going to be the same in the developing countries [1], but also because our knowledge about how to prevent them is more advanced than for other diseases. Moreover, preventive efforts against CVD can be expected to yield wider health benefits inasmuch as several other chronic diseases share some multipotent risk factors and can, therefore, be simultaneously influenced by the same preventive measures [1].

Strategies for CVD prevention

As far as CVD prevention is concerned, two main strategies have been recommended: population strategy and individual (high-risk) strategy, the latter comprising primary and secondary prevention [1].

The high-risk strategy fits into a medical model of patient care, where the physician assumes guidance of his individual patient. However, as in high-incidence countries the levels of main risk factors are inappropriately high in the majority of people, most cases of CVD occur among the large number of individuals in whom risk factors are moderately elevated, rather than the small number with high values. Therefore, only a mass approach can help the entire community [1].

A population strategy poses several problems and presents manifold implications. Among these, the six basic ones are highlighted below.

Scientific-ethical basis

Any program aimed at influencing behavior and health must rest on a solid scientific-ethical basis, as far as its effectiveness and safety are concerned. Community-based prevention of CVD meets this requirement, inasmuch as it is based on measures consisting in the removal of "unnatural factors" and the restoration of "biological normality", to which humans are genetically adapted [2]. Such measures include reduction of excessive

Address for correspondence: Sergio Muntoni MD, Center for Metabolic Diseases and Atherosclerosis, The ME.DI.CO. Association, 23/29 viale Merello, 09123 Cagliari, Italy. Fax: +39-70-284-849.

intake of saturated fat and salt, quitting smoking, and avoiding physical inactivity, severe obesity, and some forms of stress. The encouraging reduction in CVD mortality in some countries has resulted largely from the public assuming healthier living habits, rather than from medical treatment [3]. This preventive approach is far from having yielded the maximum benefit, and a further 60–80% reduction in heart attacks should be a not unreasonable goal [3]. The success of a health care system should be measured not only in terms of prolongation of life, but also in improvement of its quality, compression of morbidity and extension of active life expectancy. This can be attained through a balance between the curative and preventive approaches, within the framework of a comprehensive health care system [3]. In actual fact, curative medicine, when not combined with disease prevention, by reducing mortality contributes beyond its own aims to create an aging and chronically-ill society. A mass strategy based on simple measures aimed at reducing the excessive levels of "unnatural" factors can result in extension of active life expectancy, without causing any harm to single individuals in the community. It is therefore also ethical in its nature.

Cost-effectiveness

Besides safety and efficacy, a strong reason in favor of the mass strategy is its cost-effectiveness. Sound evidence exists that reduction of morbidity and extension of active life together with great cost saving can be obtained through population-based education programs [3]. The attainment of this dual goal can be defined as "health promotion" in the sense proposed by Fries et al. [4], i.e., improvement in both physical and financial health. The central goal remains improvement in health habits, from which reduction in need and demand for medical services ensues.

Political responsibility

While the scientific background for CVD prevention and health promotion at the community level is provided by biomedical research and knowledge, decisions regarding public health must be taken by policy-makers, all the more when action is aimed at promoting lifestyle changes in the community. Decisions regarding health care are taken by ministries of health, but decisions that profoundly influence the underlying causes of disease (such as those related to agriculture, industry, environment) are taken by other government departments, either at national or regional level [1]. This is the key issue of the process, when the biomedical and the political components merge into a public health action program and adopt the comprehensive strategies of CVD control and health promotion.

Fund allocation

As great cost saving can be realized by implementation of mass prevention programs, the necessary funds should be regarded as investment at high interest rate, for future benefit in both economic and human terms [1]. The costs should be borne by those who will ultimately have savings, that is to say those now paying the health costs: insurers, industry, and government [4], particularly the latter, because health promotion is mainly the government's responsibility. Whether and in what amount funds will be allocated depends on health policy choices, sensitivity and culture of the politicians, and suitable legislative instruments.

Communication

As public health interventions are aimed at changing individual behavior, they must make use of modern communication media and techniques, on which the "era of persuasion", originated by the information revolution, is based [5]. Good examples exist of mass media campaigns that have been successful. Their results suggest generalization of this extensive type of community approach [5].

Transferability

The possibility of extending or transferring a preventive program to other regions or, reciprocally, to adopt an already operating program from another region, should be considered when planning a regional program. This seems the best way to develop a national program [1].

Public health action programs

Past and present

Numberless programs of CVD prevention have been and/or are being carried out in almost every part of the world. Surveying them is far from the scope of this report, not only because of the great heterogeneity and wide variety of their aims and design, but also because most of them do not meet the requirements for public health action programs we are dealing with. In fact, a great number of CVD prevention programs were designed as either pilot and demonstration projects or intervention trials, often in limited areas and featured as research activities rather than national or regional campaigns supported by the respective governments.

Nearly all current public health action programs share some common features. They generally adopt the strategy of influencing lifestyle of the population as a whole, although most of them also include in their design the detection and treatment of people at high risk [6]. Most local or regional projects were designed to be reproduced in other areas of the country, according to WHO recommendations [1]. On the other hand, local programs are likely to be more effective if they operate in the context of a national commitment to improve public health [6].

Future

Present knowledge of the manifold issues of CVD prevention and health promotion calls for implementation of comprehensive, community-based public education strategies. Public intervention that combines consideration of high-risk individuals with broad educational efforts appears to be the best choice. This implies involvement of both biomedical and political authorities, with many questions on how to take the initiative and to carry out the intervention.

The first step is taken, in general, by individuals who have sound knowledge of the scientific justification, supported by reliable studies and international consensus, for comprehensive public health intervention. As a rule, a public health strategy for primary prevention of chronic diseases has to be developed through three phases [7].

Phase 1 consists of observational studies that allow comparison between different areas, contribute to isolation of the environmental, modifiable risk factors, and provide baseline data for evaluation of future intervention.

Phase 2 is an intermediate step for testing and validating the intervention methods in a given area versus a reference area. In my opinion, Phase 2 can be skipped to jump directly to Phase 3 when an already accomplished public health action program is reproduced in another area or extended to the whole country, provided that no major ethnical, cultural, geographic and economic differences exist between the populations involved.

Phase 3 is the point of arrival at public health action through either Phase 2 accomplished in the same area, or transfer of Phase 3 from another area. While Phases 1 and 2 typically belong to biomedical research, Phase 3 is the result of merging of biomedical and policy-making components into a public health program at a national, regional or local level.

In order to attain permanent health benefits, a successful community-oriented prevention program should explicitly include institutionalization, otherwise it will have to be discontinued when the initial government grant ends. This implies that both the biomedical and political components realize and accept the political dimension of the program [8]. "The primary determinants of disease are mainly economic and social, and therefore its remedies must also be economic and social. Medicine and politics cannot and should not be kept apart" [9].

Acknowledgements

This work has been developed within research contract No. 93.00774.PF41, National Research Council (CNR), Targeted Project "Prevention and control of disease factors" (FAT.MA.), Subproject SP6 "Community medicine".

References

1. World Health Organization. Primary prevention of coronary heart disease. Copenhagen: World Health Organization, 1985.
2. Rose G. Br Med J 1981;282:1847—1851.
3. Leaf A. J Am Med Assoc 1993;269:616—618.
4. Fries JF, Koop E, Beadle CE, Cooper PP, England MJ, Greaves RF, Sokolov JJ, Wright D. N Engl J Med 1993;329:321—325.
5. Farquhar JW, Fortmann SP, Flora JA, Maccoby N. In: Holland WW, Detels R, Knox G (eds) Oxford Textbook of Public Health 2. Oxford, New York, Toronto: Oxford University Press, 1991;331—344.
6. Longfield J, Rayner M. Preventing cardiovascular disease in Europe. London: HMSO, 1993.
7. Stern MP. Diabetes Care 1991;14:399—410.
8. Abelin T. In: Holland WW, Detels R, Knox G (eds) Oxford Textbook of Public Health 3. Oxford, New York, Toronto: Oxford University Press, 1991;557—589.
9. Rose G. The Strategy of Preventive Medicine. Oxford, New York, Tokyo: Oxford University Press, 1992.

The Victoria Declaration on heart health: its international implications

John W. Farquhar

Stanford Center for Research in Disease Prevention, Stanford University School of Medicine, Palo Alto, CA 94304-1825, USA

Introduction

The Victoria Declaration is a policy blueprint and a consensus document for prevention of cardiovascular disease (CVD) on a global scale [1]. It was issued by the Advisory Board of the first International Heart Health Conference, which consisted of representatives of 21 international health organizations and agencies (Victoria, BC, Canada, 1992). I was the Chair of the Board and Dr David Maclean of the Faculty of Medicine, Dalhousie, Nova Scotia, was Vice-Chair. The initial organizing and many continued contributions have been derived from Canadian scientists and from the Canadian Ministry of Health. These efforts continue a tradition of innovative Canadian contributions to health policy, such as the pioneering Lalonde Report of 1974 and the Canadian Heart Health Initiative of 1992 [2,3]. The Declaration is addressed, among others, to governments, the research community, health professionals, voluntary health organizations and the private sector. Its 64 recommendations span population groups, risk-factor reduction issues and strategies for prevention. For implementation, emphasis is placed on international collaboration and assistance to support developing countries in the development of infrastructures for health promotion and disease prevention.

Background

The hallmark of the document is the endorsement of a public health approach as a key strategy; this is based on the recognition that CVD risk is highly prevalent in populations and that we now have enough knowledge to act to stem the CVD epidemic. This knowledge derives from the past 40 years of productive basic, clinical and epidemiologic research confirming the relevance of risk factors for CVD. Considerable experience has also been gained in developing and applying methods of intervention in clinical settings, schools, worksites and communities. In addition to education and clinical care, regulatory changes affecting both the tobacco and food industry have added many strategies for reducing CVD.

In many countries, including Canada, these strategies for primary and secondary prevention have resulted in impressive declines in mortality rates for CVD, particularly in the middle-aged population. For example, the United States, which started with very high CVD rates, the adjusted death rates for coronary heart disease have fallen by 52% since 1967 and stroke death rates by 72% since 1940 [4]. Unfortunately, many countries in Eastern Europe and Asia, including China, have shown comparable dramatic increases during the past two decades. A major premise of the Victoria Declaration was founded on optimism derived from strategies that influenced the recent large CVD decline from relatively high death rates in some countries. The premise was that adoption of the Declaration's policy recommendations could aid developing countries to avoid the very large increases in CVD rate increases experienced by developed countries in the fourth to seventh decades of this century.

Policy recommendations

The Victoria Declaration's policy recommendations emphasize the issues of diet, tobacco, and physical activity on a public health basis integrated into clinical identification and management of hypertension, abnormal blood lipid levels, abdominal obesity and diabetes.

Many of the public health recommendations for blood lipid control centered on population — wide strategies in nutrition and exercise form a supportive background for clinical activity. The 11 recommendations on blood lipids included recommendations for increased professional education and for an increase in quality control of laboratory procedures.

The Board recommended decisive actions towards the eradication of smoking habits, realizing that the power of the tobacco industry underlies a continued growth of the smoking epidemic in developing countries. One recommendation favors high and uniform taxation worldwide, and proposes an international ban on tobacco advertising and of coercive export trade policies for tobacco.

Recommendations on the topic of diabetes recognized its increasing prevalence, the growing understanding of the insulin-resistance syndrome and the central role of exercise as well as diet in achieving weight control. The two major recommendations were directed toward professional associations and health professionals.

Needs of population subgroups based on age, gender and economic status were addressed. Among the young, for example, the need for a broad approach involving governments, international efforts and schools was described. The critical role of a combined regulatory and educational strategy was put forth for tobacco control, recognizing young people as the main entry point for nicotine addiction worldwide.

Although all 64 recommendations were on policy, the declaration also recommended research on policies themselves, on topics such as community organizing, social marketing and advocacy.

Impact of the Victoria Declaration

The declaration has been translated into 10 languages and it has been widely endorsed by professional organizations, by ministries of health of many countries, and international bodies such as the World Health Organization. A 35-member international Implementation Committee has been created to advocate, establish appropriate partnerships and encourage activities to make the recommendations a reality. A review of accomplishments will take place at the Second International Heart Health Conference (Barcelona, May 28 — June 1, 1995). The Advisory Board for this conference will extend the Victoria Declaration into the issues of economic development and health. This topic will address the phases of economic development that at first lead to great health benefits, which themselves often accelerate economic development in a pattern of reciprocal benefit. Continued development moves rapidly to a phase of increased affluence, which paradoxically often leads to diminished health and blunted economic development as various chronic diseases emerge. Evidence for the relationship between economic development and health will be sought in both phases and recommendations will be made to foster favorable interactions.

These efforts will create a follow-up document for this conference as the "Barcelona Report", as part of a planned Victoria Declaration Publication Series.

146

Summary

The Victoria Declaration represents a goal and a framework to move our present knowledge and skills in primary and secondary prevention of cardiovascular disease into rapid international adoption. Many strategies will be required to achieve this goal, but none is more central than the need for health professionals to go beyond their usual clinical and research roles to help mobilize the forces needed for this world-wide approach.

References

1. Victoria Declaration on Heart Health. Advisory Board for the International Heart Health Conference, (Victoria BC, 1992), Health Canada, Ottawa, 1993.
2. Lalonde, M. A new perspective on the health of Canadians. Department of Health & Welfare, Ottawa, 1974.
3. The Canadian Heart Health Initiative. Health Promotion Magazine (special issue) 30:4. Health and Welfare Canada, Ottawa, Spring 1992.
4. 1993 Heart and Stroke Facts, American Heart Association, Dallas, 1992.

Strategies to improve patient compliance

Harvey D. White[1] and Hitesh Patel[2]

[1]Director of Coronary Care and Cardiovascular Research; and [2]Cardiology Registrar, Green Lane Hospital, Auckland, New Zealand

Abstract. Poor compliance limits the effectiveness of therapies and drives up medical costs. Compliance at 1 year in routine clinical practice is often only 50%. It is usually higher in clinical trials because of patient selection, ongoing education and close monitoring. The LIPID Study (Long-term Intervention with Pravastatin in Ischaemic Disease) has randomized 9014 patients in Australia and New Zealand to pravastatin or placebo following admission for myocardial infarction or unstable angina. The follow-up period is 7 years with a primary endpoint of coronary heart disease mortality. Compliance at 4 years is 88%.

Thirty months after attendance at the Green Lane Hospital risk-factor clinic, ongoing care by general practitioners had maintained the results achieved by the clinic. Cholesterol levels were lower than at discharge from the clinic, both in patients with vascular disease (6.1 vs. 6.4 mmol/l) and those without (6.8 vs. 7.5 mmol/l). Compliance can be improved with major efforts by physicians and nurses. Better compliance is likely to improve patient care and lower health costs.

Patient compliance with dietary advice and prescribed medications is often poor [1–4]. The first prescription may not be collected in up to 14% of cases, and 30% of patients given repeat prescriptions may not collect the drugs from their pharmacist [2,3]. In the long term, 50% of patients may be noncompliant [4]. In asymptomatic conditions such as hypertension or dyslipidemia, patient compliance may be very low. Compliance with fibrates has been reported as being 27% at 19 months despite a low incidence of side effects [5]. Compliance with the HMG-CoA reductase inhibitors has been reported as being 50% at 1 year [5]. The effectiveness of treatment is a function of compliance [6]. Noncompliance may also be dangerous if drugs are taken erratically, and may result in more visits and unnecessary, expensive investigations or treatments.

Several factors are associated with noncompliance (Table 1). Although elderly patients require special care, they tend to be more compliant [7,8]. Noncompliance increases if there are family problems and if the patient lives alone or is unemployed [9]. Complexity

Table 1. Factors associated with poor compliance

Younger age
Living alone, family problems
Unemployed
Asymptomatic conditions
Adverse effects or fear of adverse effects
Frequency and complexity of drug regime
Number of drugs
Cost

Address for correspondence: Dr Harvey White, Cardiology Department, Green Lane Hospital, Epsom, Auckland 1003, New Zealand. Tel.: +64-9-638-9909. Fax: +64-9-631-0703.

of dosing [10] and adverse events [11] are also associated with noncompliance. The cost of the drugs themselves is not usually a major factor [12]. Income and level of education appear to be unrelated to compliance [13].

Compliance with national guidelines

National and international guidelines have played a major role in making physicians aware of the importance of hypercholesterolemia and have also assisted physicians with diagnosis and management [14]. Efforts to improve compliance with guidelines were assessed in a trial randomizing 33 third-year physician residents to one of three approaches: control, chart reminders, or patient-specific chart reminders [15]. Feedback consisted of the patients' most recent lipid results with explicit recommendations on the next step to take. Surprisingly, after 5 weeks there were no differences between the three groups. Compliance in the intensive reminder group was only 47%. Although this trial raises questions about the effectiveness of education, there were small numbers of participants, the trial was not performed in the community and had a short follow-up period.

Compliance of New Zealand doctors

In 1988 the National Heart Foundation of New Zealand published guidelines for screening and management of dyslipidemia [16] which recommended that specific dietary advice should be given to all patients with cholesterol levels >6 mmol/l. Drug treatment was considered appropriate if levels were ≥7.5 mmol/l after 6 months of dietary treatment in those without other risk factors and >7 mmol/l in those with other cardiac risk factors or coronary heart disease. In August 1991 we sent questionnaires to all New Zealand doctors

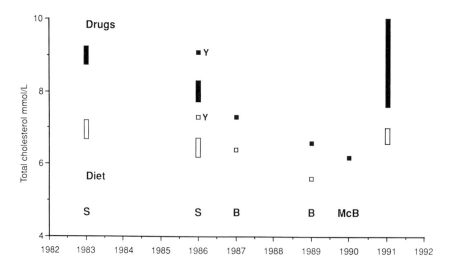

Fig. 1. Median thresholds for starting dietary (open symbols) and drug therapy (solid symbols) in asymptomatic patients of New Zealand general practitioners and physicians in 1991 (vertical bars) compared with a survey of New Zealand general practitioners in 1986 (Y) [24] and previous surveys of American general practitioners and physicians (B) [25], (S) [26] and (McB) [27]. The 1991 New Zealand study and the study by Schucker et al. (S) [26] reported a median range denoted as a vertical bar; the other studies reported a mean value (represented by a square symbol) and standard error (not shown).

and received 1798 responses, a response rate of 64%. Only 25% of doctors stated that they measured blood lipids in all their adult patients, 92% in patients with coronary heart disease, 86% in those with hypertension and 60% in smokers. Amongst doctors, 73% had measured their own cholesterol levels. The median threshold for dietary intervention in patients without risk factors was >6.5 mmol/l. The threshold was lower in patients with other risk factors or coronary heart disease (Fig. 1). The median threshold for initiation of drug treatment in patients without risk factors was the same as the guidelines. However, for patients with coronary heart disease or risk factors the level was actually lower (6.5 mmol/l) than the guidelines recommended.

More recently, updated guidelines have been published emphasizing the importance of absolute risk assessment in the individual patient before initiation of pharmacologic therapy (Table 2) [17]. Following publication of these guidelines, the National Heart Foundation of New Zealand initiated a program in which the authors of the guidelines ran a series of small-group teaching sessions with physicians. The idea was for these physicians to teach general practitioners who would in turn teach other general practitioners. It is estimated that approximately 25% of general practitioners took part in these sessions. A follow-up questionnaire is planned to evaluate the usefulness of the sessions.

Compliance in clinical trials

Compliance in clinical trials is usually much higher than the rates reported from routine

Table 2. Management of dyslipidemia − National Heart Foundation of New Zealand guidelines

Assessment of patient risk	If cholesterol level	Dietary advice[a], exercise, no smoking	Dietary treatment[a], exercise, no smoking	Consider medication
Very high risk 10-year coronary event risk >30%[b] Retest against goals every 3 months during first year	≤6.5 mmol/l >6.5 mmol/l		Yes Yes	Yes Yes (after 6-month diet)
High risk 10-year coronary event risk 20−29%[b] Retest against goals every 3 months during first year	≤6.5 mmol/l >6.5 mmol/l		Yes Yes	Yes (after 6-month diet)
Moderate risk 10-year coronary event risk 10−19%[b]	≤7.5 mmol/l >7.5 mmol/l		Yes Yes	Yes (after 6-month diet)
Mild risk 10-year coronary event risk 5−9%[b]	5.2−6.5 mmol/l >6.5 mmol/l	Yes Yes	Yes (if no response to dietary advice)	
Low risk 10-year coronary event risk <5%[b]		Yes		

[a]Dietary advice emphasizes the National Heart Foundation nutrition policy for the general population. Dietary treatment requires more stringent goals and targets, and referral to a qualified dietitian may be necessary.
[b]Based on data from the Framingham study.

clinical practice. This may be due to a number of reasons including selection of patients, use of run-in periods and close follow-up with continuing education by nurses and physicians.

The LIPID study (Long-term Intervention with Pravastatin in Ischaemic Disease) is a large randomized trial of lipid-modifying drug therapy in secondary prevention. The cholesterol entry range was 4–7 mmol/l and the follow-up period is 7 years. At 86 sites in Australia and New Zealand, 9014 patients have been randomized to pravastatin 40 mg/day or to placebo. The aim is to determine if cholesterol reduction with pravastatin reduces mortality from coronary heart disease in patients with a history of acute myocardial infarction or unstable angina pectoris. The trial is expected to have 77% power (p < 0.05) for coronary heart disease mortality and 68% power for total mortality, assuming that there will be an 18% long-term cholesterol difference between the two randomized groups after allowance for patient discontinuation, and that each 1% reduction in cholesterol will lead to a 1% reduction in coronary deaths. Importantly, the trial will provide valuable data on the effects of cholesterol lowering in a group of women at high risk (17% of the study population) and in patients over the age of 65 years (34% of the study population). These groups have been underrepresented in previous studies.

Compliance is being very carefully monitored and at 4 years is approximately 88%, with only 3.4% of patients having begun other cholesterol-lowering treatment. It is hoped to maintain this high level of compliance through to the completion of the trial in 1997. It is interesting that a large proportion of the patients who have dropped out of the LIPID trial had a high incidence of associated risk factors, i.e., the very patients who would be most likely to benefit from treatment. It is important to note that this is a double-blind trial, and neither doctors nor patients know if they are on active or placebo medications. A special meeting was held in 1993 with Dr Jeffrey Probstfield as guest speaker running workshops with the study nurses and doctors to try to improve the already high rate of compliance. Table 3 lists the potential strategies that the workshop participants thought would be useful to improve compliance. Subsequently, special newsletters and patient sessions have been conducted. The recommencement rate of study drugs is approximately 1.6%.

Steps to improve compliance in clinical practice

A logical first step is to identify noncompliant patients. Although it is not possible to

Table 3. Compliance strategies proposed by the investigators at the 4th annual LIPID scientific meeting

Patient-orientated strategies
    Attempt to get patients who have discontinued to recommence
    Identify at-risk patients and attempt to prevent subsequent discontinuation
    Study-nurse allocated adequate time to spend with individual patients
    Adopt a flexible approach with respect to appointments, etc.
    Increase cardiologist time spent with the participant
    Involve spouse/significant other
    Organize patient parties
Center management strategies
    Cardiologist to spend adequate time with study nurse: regular meetings reviewing patients and strategies
    Dietary advice to be reinforced
    Review and act on feedback on tablet counts and participant visits
GP relationships
    Provide information on the study and the validity of the question at GP meetings and via the local media

Table 4. Signs and symptoms of potential noncompliance

Missed visits
Difficulty in reaching by phone or failure to return calls
Rescheduling twice for an appointment (change in behavior)
Complaints about office visits
Impatience during clinic visits
"Distance" during interview
Humor dealing with negative aspects of the trial or study medication
Sarcasm about trial or study medication
Any expression by participant that he/she may discontinue study medication
Unusual or unexplained change in adherence to study medication
Lack of concern by participant about adherence rate
Failure to achieve therapeutic goal
Reassignment to new primary care manager
Reassignment to other new clinic personnel
Any illness with increased attention to "trial-related disease"
Hospitalization for any reason
Any major change in lifestyle that is imminent (before the next visit)

After Probstfield et al. [28].

predict accurately which patients may not comply, there are some signs of potential noncompliance (Table 4). Directly asking the patient in a nonconfrontational and nonjudgemental manner has the highest yield. In some studies, but not in others [5,15,18,19], education has been shown to be very important in determining patient compliance with diet and drug therapy for dyslipidemia. Intuitively it would seem that for patients to comply, they must understand what the medication is for, why it may be beneficial and why they need to take it frequently and regularly. Compliance at 1 year was much higher in patients in the Wellness Program, which involved an intensive lecture and follow-up individual counseling, than in a control population [5]. The main reason identified for discontinuation of treatment was failure of patients to realize that therapy was lifelong. At 1 year 63% of patients were still taking niacin, 64% cholestyramine, 84% gemfibrozil and 87% lovastatin. The patients were highly selected, being retired military personnel or their spouses, and these results may be difficult to duplicate in routine practice.

The color, size, taste and any possible adverse effects of medication all contribute to compliance. Patients prefer white or pale-colored pills which are small. Once or twice-daily therapy results in better compliance than therapy taken 3 or 4 times per day [20]. Substitution of generic drugs for brand-name drugs may have an important impact on compliance because of potential confusion about the color, shape and size of the pill, as well as the name. Patients may also choose not to comply because of denial or failure to accept the presence of a risk factor or disease [21].

Compliance devices are useful for patients who simply forget. Calendar blister packs, medication containers which can store and deliver a whole week's supply of pills, alarm systems and computerized pill bottles which record whenever the bottle is opened are all helpful for such patients [22]. The most useful practical aid is an individualized reminder chart listing each medication, when they are to be taken and what they are for. Because handwritten information may be incomplete or difficult to read, as well as time-consuming to produce, computer-generated charts have been produced. These have been shown to increase compliance from 47 to 83% on short-term follow-up [3]. Possible ways to improve compliance are listed in Table 5.

Table 5. Possible ways to improve compliance

Ask the patient at each visit
Try to assist patients to accept responsibility for their own treatment
Education about disease and risk for the individual patient, benefit/risk of intervention
Realistic expectations: patient goal, physician goal
Importance of continuing diet and/or medication even when the cholesterol level is "normal"
Ongoing discussion about contradictory information in the media, results of new trials
Written instructions, pamphlets, videos
Simplification of drug regimen
Reminder systems
Drug-count devices, calendar packs
Computer programs
Patient-doctor relationship: personal, caring, listening, patient feels free to ask questions, time spent after
    writing prescription
Involvement of nurses
Involvement of family or friends

Thirty-month follow-up of patients attending a risk factor clinic

Patients who had attended the Green Lane Hospital risk factor clinic at least twice for dietary advice and, if thought appropriate, given pharmacologic treatment were followed up 30 months after discharge from the clinic. Generally, patients were discharged if they had achieved a goal cholesterol of <7.5 mmol/l without vascular disease or <7 mmol/l with vascular disease. Cholesterol levels were lower at follow-up than at discharge from the clinic, both in patients with vascular disease (6.1 vs. 6.4 mmol/l) and those without (6.8 vs. 7.5 mmol/l).

The physician's role

The physician has an important role in improving patient compliance, which correlates closely with the quality of the relationship between patient and physician [23]. Several factors have been identified which influence patient compliance (Table 6) [10,23]. The patient should trust and respect the physician, and all communication must be in language that is easily understood. Patients are more likely to retain minimal information and especially the first piece of advice [10,23].

Table 6. Important factors in the physician's role for improving compliance

The physician's interest in modifying the risk factor
The physician's choice of an appropriate, uncomplicated regimen
The physician's willingness to change the medication if adverse effects occur
Monitoring whether patients are complying, i.e., asking them directly, getting them to describe their pills and
    when they take them

Conclusion

Clearly, compliant patients will benefit more from nonpharmacologic and pharmacologic treatment than noncompliant patients. Many factors are associated with noncompliance, and remedies will vary according to which factor is important in the individual patient. A major goal to improve patient care is to rapidly adopt the lessons from clinical trials into clinical practice, but this cannot be achieved unless patients comply with advice and medications. Surprisingly, there are no cost-effectiveness studies evaluating whether programs to improve patient compliance may reduce costs. More attention needs to be paid to compliance by clinicians and other health providers, with the objectives being to improve patient health care and reduce costs.

References

1. Hunninghake DB, Stein EA, Dujovne CA, Harris WS, Feldman EB, Miller VT, Tobert JA, Laskarzewski PM, Quiter E, Held J, Taylor AM, Hopper S, Leonard SB, Brewer BK. N Engl J Med 1993;328: 1213–1219.
2. Berg JS, Dischler J, Wagner DJ, Raia JJ, Palmer-Shevlin N. Annals of Pharmacotherapy 1993;(suppl):5–19.
3. Raynor DK, Booth TG, Blenkinsopp A. Br Med J 1993;306:1158–1161.
4. Burgess MM. Can Med Assoc J 1994;141:777–780.
5. Wirebaugh SR, Whitney EJ. Pharmacy Therap 1993;18:559–571.
6. Lipid Research Clinic's Program Group. J Am Med Assoc 1984;251:351–364.
7. Weingarten MA, Cannon BS. Family Practice 1988;5.
8. Klein LE. Hypertension 1988;II:61–64.
9. Griffith S. Br J Gen Pract 1990;40:114–116.
10. Morgan TO, Nowson C, Murphy J, Snowden R. Drugs 1986;31(suppl 4):174–183.
11. Larrat EP, Taubman AH, Willey C. Am Pharmacy 1990;82:18–23.
12. Clark LT. Am Heart J 1991;121:664–669.
13. Greenberg RN. Clin Therap 1984;6:592–599.
14. Schucker B, Wittes JT, Santanello NC, Weber SJ, McGoldrick D, Donato K, Levy A, Rifkind BM. Arch Intern Med 1991;151:666–673.
15. Headrick LA, Speroff T, Pelecanos HI, Cebul RD. Arch Intern Med 1992;152:2490–2496.
16. National Health Foundation of New Zealand Advisory Group. NZ Med J 1988;101:629–631.
17. Mann JI, Crooke M, Fear H, Hay DR, Jackson RT, Neutze JM, White HD, on behalf of the Scientific Committee of the National Heart Foundation of New Zealand. NZ Med J 1993;106:133–142.
18. Morisky DE, Levine DM, Green LW et al. Am J Public Health 1983;74:153–162.
19. Sackett DL et al. Am Heart J 1977;94:666–667.
20. Greenberg RN. Clin Ther 1984;6:590–599.
21. Boza RA, Milanes F, Slater V, Garrigo L, Rivera CE. Postgrad Med 1987;81:163–169.
22. Wright EC. Lancet 1993;342:909–913.
23. Neal WW. Am J Cardiol 1989;63:17B–20B.
24. Yates K, Jackson R, Tester P et al. NZ Med J 1988;101:76–78.
25. Bostick RM, Luepker RV, Kofron PM, Pirie PL. Arch Intern Med 1991;151:478–484.
26. Schucker B, Wittes JT, Cutler JA et al. J Am Med Assoc 1987;258:3521–3526.
27. McBride PE, Plane MB, Underbakke G. Am Heart J 1992;123:817–824.
28. Probstfield JL, Russell ML, Insull W, Yusuf S. In: Shumaker, Schron, Okene (eds) The Handbook of Health Behavior Change. New York: Springer, 1990:376–400.

154

Approach to improve patient compliance

Donald B. Hunninghake

Director, Heart Disease Prevention Clinic, University of Minnesota, Minneapolis, MN 55455, USA

Atherosclerosis is a multifactorial disease, and effective reduction in cardiovascular risk may require several interventions. Low-fat diet, weight control, sodium restriction, exercise and drugs to control dyslipidemia, blood pressure and diabetes may be indicated. General population measures focus on lifestyle changes, while high-risk patients may require both lifestyle modifications and drug therapy. Effective compliance is essential for successful implementation of either lifestyle modification or drug therapy.

This discussion will focus primarily on compliance with lipid-lowering drugs, but the same general principles are applicable to all interventions. The increased use of lipid-lowering drugs has occurred very recently, and there is little information on compliance in clinical practice. One must either extrapolate compliance information for other drugs or follow the general recommendations that have been made for maintaining compliance to lipid-lowering drugs [1,2]. A single study on compliance in a specialized type of clinical practice is available [3], but compliance has been assessed in many clinical trials [4–9]. Much of the information in this chapter is based upon hypotheses generated from personal experience in both clinical trials and clinical practice.

Some general estimates of compliance to lipid-lowering drugs are indicated in Table 1. In the clinical trials, compliance is usually assessed by pill count. Generally, compliance is best for the HMG-CoA reductase inhibitors and least for the resins and niacin. Compliance to resin and niacin is inversely related to the total daily dosage. In actual clinical practice, the only estimate of compliance is provided by Prescription Monitoring Services. These services provide data only on persistency or continued use of the drug. It is disappointing that only 50–60% of patients are continuing to take a reductase inhibitor at 1 year. Continued administration of the fibric acids and resins is even lower. There are no data available on niacin since this is available without a prescription.

The data obtained from the Wellness Program probably represents the maximum compliance that could be obtained in clinical practice under ideal conditions [3]. The patients were from a military population that is very disciplined; they received extensive education before initiating therapy; they were monitored regularly and the staff were fairly

Table 1. Estimates of compliance[a]

| | Compliance (%) | Persistency (%) | |
	Clinical trials	Prescription monitor	Wellness program
HMGRI	80–95	50–60[b]	87[c]
Fibric acids	80–90	30–40	84
Resins	60–70	20–30	64
Niacin	50–60	—	63

[a]Data after 12 months of therapy.
[b]Rates have gradually been improving.
[c]Wirebaugh SR, Whitney EJ. Pharmacy and Therapeutics 1993;18:559–571.

skilled in the administration of these drugs. In the Wellness Program, the rate of discontinuance of drug was 4, 1, 15 and 22% respectively for lovastatin, gemfibrozil, cholestyramine and niacin, and the corresponding discontinuance rates initiated by the patient were 2, 7, 15 and 6%, respectively, Overall, the discontinuance rates presumed to be due to adverse effects were about one-third for lovastatin and 50% for the other drugs.

Compliance or persistency rates are generally much higher in clinical trials and wellness programs than in clinical practice. In clinical trials, the participants are volunteers who receive frequent and intense monitoring, the patient education is quite extensive, the staff is frequently very experienced, there is a definite duration to the trial, and there is no direct cost to the patient. However, in clinical practice the monitoring is frequently erratic or irregular, there tends to be more limited patient education and the staff may also be less experienced. Therapy may also be for a lifetime and the cost to the patient quite considerable. In the Wellness Program reported in Table 1, there was minimal cost to the patient. Cost may be an important consideration, but frequently is not a major deterrent to compliance. Also, adverse effects are frequently overestimated as the cause for poor compliance. It appears that the remedial approaches for achieving better compliance should focus on patient education, monitoring and staff/clinic activities.

The consequence of poor or noncompliance is that the beneficial effects of treatment in reducing cardiovascular events will not be realized. This may create some personal costs for the patient including guilt, fear, decreased quality of life, or disability if an event occurs. There are also societal costs in that the costs generated for screening, diagnosis, and initiation of therapy are wasted if therapy is not persistent. Also, there is now considerable evidence that medical care costs may be decreased with risk-factor management, especially in secondary intervention. Thus, the overall utilization of medical care and resources may be increased if compliance is not effective, and this could increase health-care costs.

Physician/health professionals barriers

The personal beliefs and attitudes of the health professional are transmitted to the patient both verbally and nonverbally. Thus, if the health professional has ambivalent feelings regarding the benefits or type of therapy indicated, this will be transmitted to the patient. Many health professionals are still unconvinced of the benefits of risk-factor management. There is often a lack of sense of urgency to treat since the atherosclerotic process is viewed as a slow process and intervention is not critical. There is also not a clear sense of the role of cholesterol in the development of the atherosclerotic process. In practice, information in terms of correlation of cholesterol with atherosclerosis is frequently not presented to the patient. Additionally, there may be lingering doubts about the safety of the interventional procedures.

Many patients and some health professionals do not understand that drug administration should be for a lifetime. This is a common cause of drug discontinuance. It is essential that patients understand that the medication must be administered lifelong and that the lipid values will return to their former levels when medication is discontinued. A regular system of monitoring or follow-up visits is essential; it is practically impossible to maintain effective compliance without regular, systematic follow-up visits. Additionally, inadequate instruction of the patient on the purpose and goals of therapy, follow-up procedures and control of side effects is frequent.

Other factors associated with better compliance in clinical trials have been identified. One is the patient's perception of the staff. If the patient develops good feelings toward the staff in terms of sensing that they are caring, trustworthy and understanding, compliance is better. Also, compliance tends to be inversely correlated with clinic waiting time. Patients who spend an inordinate amount of time waiting in the clinic are more likely to feel that drug therapy is less important and their compliance will be less. Simplified regimens for drug administration are also indicated. The available data suggest that taking medication once a day is best, but most patients do well with a twice-daily administration. Also, patients may be taking a number of other medications. Generally, if a patient has to take more than three or four different medications at one time, compliance will be drastically reduced.

Patient barriers

Major patient barriers include lack of education and understanding of the rationale of drug therapy. Additionally, the patient must understand the regimen for taking the drug and that drug administration must be continued indefinitely. Patients also receive many inconsistent messages from the media and health professionals regarding the need for treatment. Cost may be a consideration and safety concerns are frequent. Safety concerns are increased by inability to interpret the frequency and severity of adverse effects that are enumerated in the package insert.

Patient education is crucial. Written instructions are very helpful. The patient is frequently overwhelmed by the decision either to take or not to take drugs and the rest of the conversation may not be heard or understood or is quickly forgotten. In addition to the specific regimen for taking the drug, they must understand what they are being treated for, why, the specific goals of therapy, the expected outcomes, and why a specific drug was selected. They should also receive a reasonable assessment of the risks, how to identify and manage side effects and how and who to contact if the need arises. Patients should be active participants and should be responsible for maintaining their own record of lipid values, drug doses, weight and diet adherence. They should also participate in the titration of drug dosages for the resins and nicotinic acid.

General strategies

Cholesterol lowering is not a medical emergency. With the potential exception of the reductase inhibitors, which are generally well tolerated, drug therapy should generally be initiated with a small dose and then the dose should gradually be increased. The initial experience of the patient with the drug will generally determine whether or not they will continue to take the medication. Especially for drugs which are more difficult to take, such as the resins and niacin, it is essential that the dose of drug be gradually increased. For these drugs, the patient will never tolerate higher doses unless they have been able to tolerate the dose which is currently being administered. It is also helpful if the patient is given the responsibility for titrating the dose, but the parameters must be provided to the patient. Even for drugs such as the fibric acids, which are generally well tolerated, some individuals will discontinue because of gastrointestinal complaints. If therapy is initiated with a small dose and gradually increased, the likelihood of developing gastrointestinal complaints is decreased.

Compliance is important, and this message should be conveyed to the patient in a nonthreatening manner. An evaluation of compliance should be made at each clinic visit. This is especially important if the patient has not achieved the expected response to the medication. If compliance is low, attempts to help the patient should be made, rather than utilizing a condemning attitude. Involvement of a supportive staff member and other support persons, such as a spouse or a friend, may be helpful. For those patients who are good compliers, it is essential to make the clinic visits interesting. One way of doing this is to provide regular updates about what is new in the area.

Compliance is frequently poor or medication is discontinued during a variety of stressful situations. Patients should be encouraged to reduce the dose or discontinue medication during severe intercurrent illnesses. Compliance is frequently reduced when there has been a significant change in lifestyle. This may include either divorce, death of a spouse or family member or any change in employment status which may include retirements, unemployment, or job change. Compliance is also reported to be less in patients with certain behaviors such as smoking. However, it is probably better to adopt a positive attitude and assume that all patients can comply rather than starting out with a defeatist attitude.

It may not always be possible, but a team approach to compliance is generally better. In office practice, it is important to define the role of other staff members in the office. For example, the physician may provide the overall risk assessment, the rationale for therapy, and the goals. The office nurse or other staff member may then educate regarding the initiation and monitoring of the various therapies. In many localities, the pharmacist also provides education for the patient. If dietary therapy is utilized, the dietitian or nutritionist may also provide helpful insight.

Specific approaches

Written instructions are essential for administration of the resins and niacin. With the resins, it is crucial to give the patient specific instructions to initiate therapy with a small dose, preferably the equivalent of one packet per day. The initial goal should then be for the patient to determine the amount and type of vehicle that will be used. Instructions must also carefully delineate when to take the resin and the frequency, and how to make the decision as to when to increase the dose. Some general instructions on how to handle side effects may also be included. Niacin is generally available without a prescription, and so the specific manufacturer's preparation which is desired should be indicated. Instructions must also include the recommendations for tablet size, and therapy should be initiated with a small dose. The time of administration is crucial with nicotinic acid, and the recommendation should be that the medication is taken during or after meals. There are often a number of specific comments that should be made regarding side effects, and it is essential, for instance, that the patient understands that the initial flushing that is observed does not represent an allergic reaction.

At the present time, most physicians are comfortable with monotherapy in terms of lipid-lowering drugs. However, in a number of situations, combination therapy may actually be better tolerated, be more cost-effective and be associated with fewer side effects. Effective compliance will eventually require establishment of disease-management systems for the treatment of atherosclerosis. Cholesterol lowering is one of the components of disease management. System programs for the patient will include educational programs, pharmacy counseling, and other consumer programs to aid the patient. The physician and other health professionals will benefit from patient-management support systems and various educational conferences. In some situations, the hospitals can also be active participants with their cardiac-care and lipid-management programs. For managed-care systems, it will be important to perform outcome studies to document the benefits of cholesterol treatment which will facilitate acceptance of lipid-management programs.

158

References

1. Cramer JA, Spilker B (eds) Patient compliance in medical practice and clinical trials. New York: Raven Press, 1991.
2. National Cholesterol Education Program. Circulation 1994;89:1329—1445.
3. Wirebaugh SR, Shapiro ML, McIntyre TH, Whitney EJ. Pharmacotherapy 1992;12:445—450.
4. Bradford RH, Shear CL, Chremos AN, Dujovne C, Downtown M, Franklin RF, Gould AL, Hesney M, Higgins J, Hurley DP, Lanendorfer A, Nash DT, Pool JL, Schnaper H. Arch Intern Med 1991;151:43—49.
5. Pravastatin Multicenter Study Group II. Arch Intern Med 1993;153:1321—1329.
6. Frick MH, Elo O, Haapa K, Heinonen OP, Heinsalmi P, Helo P, Huttunen JK, Kaitaniemi P, Koskinen P, Manninen V, Mänttäri M, Norola S, Pasternack A, Pikkarainen J, Romo M, Sjöblom T, Nikkilä EA. N Engl J Med 1987;317:1237—1245.
7. Illingworth DR, Stein EA, Mitchel YB, Dujovne CA, Frost PH, Knopp RH, Tun P, Zupkis RV, Greguski RA. Arch Intern Med 1994;1546—1595.
8. McKenney JM, Proctor JD, Harris S, Chinchili VM. J Am Med Assoc 1994;271:672—677.
9. Lipid Research Clinics Program. J Am Med Assoc 1984;251:351—364.

Progress in assessment of CAD markers: the epidemiology of coronary artery calcification

Patricia A. Peyser[1], Rachel B. Kaufmann[1], Julie E. Maher[1], Lawrence F. Bielak[1], Patrick F. Sheedy II[2] and Robert S. Schwartz[2]

[1]*Department of Epidemiology, The University of Michigan, Ann Arbor, MI 48109; and* [2]*Mayo Clinic, Rochester, MN 55905, USA*

Abstract. Coronary artery calcification (CAC), a marker for atherosclerosis, can be accurately and noninvasively identified by electron beam computed tomography (CT). Population-based studies in asymptomatic adults have established that CAC presence is associated with established risk factors. However, 12% of asymptomatic adults have CAC but do not have many established risk factors. The quantity of CAC predicts the presence of CAD and maximum stenosis better than any combination of risk factors. CAC, measured by electron beam CT, has potential to identify those with early CAD, predict severity of their disease, and allow the identification of factors associated with incidence, prevalence, and progression of CAD.

While coronary artery disease (CAD) is a major cause of morbidity and mortality, the proportion of the population with CAD is unknown because many have asymptomatic disease. A large number of individuals destined to die suddenly from CAD or experience myocardial infarction will have no warning symptoms. Previous population studies have been unable to identify individuals with mild, non-flow-limiting plaques because a sensitive, specific, noninvasive tool was lacking.

It is well known that calcium deposits in coronary arteries are almost always located within atherosclerotic plaques, although not all plaques are calcified. Aging and degenerative smooth muscle or mesenchymal cells initiate atherosclerotic calcification by releasing extracellular vesicles [1]. The presence of coronary artery calcification (CAC) in asymptomatic individuals indicates pathologic changes in the arteries before symptoms or morbid events occur and indicates the presence of preclinical coronary atherosclerosis.

The presence, quantity, and location of CAC has been detected noninvasively with electron beam CT (EBCT) in postmortem hearts, clinical patients undergoing coronary angiography, and asymptomatic individuals from the general population. Recent studies have evaluated the validity and reliability of EBCT measures of CAC, estimated the proportion of individuals with CAC, and identified CAD risk factors associated with CAC.

Electron beam CT (EBCT)

EBCT examinations produce cross-sectional images of the heart in 100 ms, stopping cardiac motion in living subjects and producing high-resolution CT images with little motion unsharpness and artifact. Total radiation dose to the skin is approximately 10 mGy (1.0 rad). In our studies, a single EBCT examination of the heart consists of 40 contiguous 3-mm-thick transverse two-dimensional scans obtained from the root of the aorta through

Address for correspondence: Patricia A. Peyser PhD, The University of Michigan, 109 Observatory, Ann Arbor, MI 48109, USA.

160

the entire heart using a model C-100 Ultrafast CT scanner (Imatron, South San Francisco, CA). Electrocardiographic triggering of scans is used so that all images are obtained at the same phase in the cardiac cycle. No iodine contrast media is used. All examinations are reviewed for gaps, overlaps, and overall technical quality by a radiologist. Image processing software computes the area of all foci identified by a radiologic technologist that consist of at least two adjacent pixels within a coronary artery with CT number above 130 Hounsfield Units (HU). Each examination result is scored by a single technologist because a study of interobserver and intraobserver reliability showed that it is not necessary for several observers to evaluate an examination independently [2]. After scoring is completed, the examination result is reviewed, evaluated, and interpreted by a radiologist. The examination provides information about presence, quantity, and location of CAC.

Postmortem studies of validity

Recent studies of hearts and coronary arteries obtained at postmortem examination have compared the quantity of CAC detected by EBCT and histologic calcium area in 50 hearts from males 30–69 years of age with varied histories of CAD symptoms [3,4]. The quantity of calcium detected by EBCT in all epicardial arteries was highly correlated with histopathologic calcium in these arteries (r = 0.96) regardless of age or CAD symptom status [3]. In these same hearts, the prevalence of CAC in an artery was strongly related to the percentage of stenosis. The prevalence of CAC detected by histomorphometry was 4, 28, 61 and 93% in arteries with maximum stenosis of 0–25, 26–50, 51–75 and 76–100%, respectively [4]. These studies suggest that EBCT can accurately detect CAC and that presence of CAC measured by EBCT predicts histomorphometric presence of CAD.

Studies of validity and repeatability in living subjects

A study of 160 patients (27 females) under age 60 who had an EBCT examination and coronary angiography indicated that defining CAC as a focus at least 2 mm^2 in size with CT number above 130 HU throughout the focus provided an accurate indication of the presence of CAD ($\geq$ 10% stenosis). The sensitivity was 82%, specificity was 85%, and overall accuracy was 83% [5]. In these same patients, the quantity of CAC in the heart (total area in mm^2) explained 55% of the variability in the largest stenosis size on angiography, and no CAD risk factor studied contributed any further information [6].

A study of 256 subjects who had two EBCT examinations separated by several minutes' time reported that foci at least 2 mm^2 in size seen on the first examination appeared on the second examination 50% of the time or more [5]. The total quantity of CAC in the heart with CT number above 130 HU was highly repeatable between the two examinations, the intraclass correlation coefficient being equal to 0.96 (p < 0.001). EBCT measures of CAC in living subjects are highly repeatable and accurate for detecting CAD.

Studies of prevalence of CAC and associated risk factors in asymptomatic individuals from the general population

A study was initiated to 1) describe the prevalence of CAC in asymptomatic adults from the general population, 2) identify which established risk factors for CAD were associated with CAC in females and males, and 3) determine the proportion of asymptomatic individuals with CAC who did not fit the high-risk profile based on established risk factors. The sample included 740 asymptomatic individuals (378 females), ages 20–59, identified through the Rochester Family Heart Study which has been described in detail elsewhere [7]. None of these individuals had signs or symptoms of CAD, hypertension, or diabetes mellitus. All of the individuals had an EBCT examination of the heart, a physical examination, and fasting blood drawn for measurement of lipids and lipoproteins.

The prevalence of CAC, defined as any focus at least 2 mm^2 in size with CT number above 130 HU in any of the four epicardial arteries, was higher in males (31%) than in females (7%) (p < 0.001). Figure 1 shows that the prevalence of CAC increased with age in both females and males. The low prevalence of CAC in males under age 30 and females under age 40 is consistent with recent autopsy data of calcification [8].

The association between presence of CAC and selected risk factors was investigated in these asymptomatic females and males. When all the risk factors were considered simultaneously, age, body mass index, and systolic blood pressure were all positively associated with CAC in females (p < 0.05). In males, age, the ratio of waist to hip circumferences, and cholesterol/HDL-C were all positively associated with CAC (p < 0.05). The association found between CAC and measures of lipid metabolism, blood pressure, and body size is consistent with the associations found between CAD endpoints and these risk factors as well as hypothesized mechanisms of the roles of these risk factors in atherogenesis.

Finally, the asymptomatic females and males were stratified on the basis of their risk factor status. Individuals were considered high-risk if they had LDL-C levels above 220 mg/dl or at least two of the following risk factors: total cholesterol at least 240 mg/dl, HDL-C below 35 mg/dl, age at least 45 for males or at least 55 for females, and current cigarette smoking. Elevated HDL-C was a negative risk factor, such that a value of 60 mg/dl or greater decreased the total number of risk factors by one. Family history of premature CAD was not included in assigning risk groups and no one in the sample had hypertension or diabetes. As shown in Fig. 2, 12% of the asymptomatic sample had CAC but were considered to be low-risk. These individuals would not be identified by standard screening techniques yet may represent the proportion of the asymptomatic general population at undetected increased risk for CAD events. These individuals also provide the opportunity to search for previously unidentified risk factors for atherosclerosis including genes, since a recent study in inbred mice provides the first evidence that coronary calcification is determined in part by genetic factors [9].

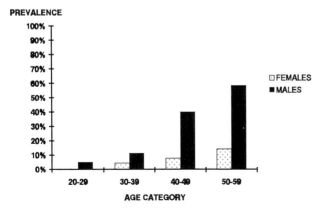

Fig. 1. The age- and sex-specific prevalence of CAC in 740 asymptomatic adults.

162

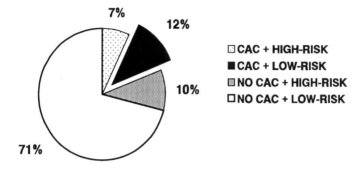

7%

12%

10%

71%

☐ CAC + HIGH-RISK
■ CAC + LOW-RISK
▦ NO CAC + HIGH-RISK
☐ NO CAC + LOW-RISK

Fig. 2. The proportion of asymptomatic adults classified by risk status (see text) and presence of CAC.

Conclusions

EBCT provides reliable measures of CAC. These measures of CAC have high sensitivity and specificity for identifying angiographically defined CAD. While additional studies will need to address the relationship between CAC and future clinical events, EBCT currently provides the opportunity to identify individuals with early CAD and predict the severity of their disease. Through follow-up studies of changes in the presence and quantity of CAC, factors associated with the incidence and progression of CAD will be identified.

Acknowledgements

The research in asymptomatic adults from the general population was supported by NIH HL 46292.

References

1. Anderson HC. Rheum Dis Clin North Am 1988;14:303–319.
2. Kaufmann RB, Sheedy PF, Breen JR, Kelzenberg JR, Kruger BL, Schwartz RS, Moll PP. Radiology 1994;190:347–352.
3. Mautner GC, Mautner SL, Froehlich J, Feuerstein IM, Proschan MA, Roberts WC, Doppman JL. Radiology 1994;192:619–623.
4. Mautner SL, Mautner GC, Froehlich J, Feuerstein IM, Proschan MA, Roberts WC, Doppman JL. Radiology 1994;192:625–630.
5. Bielak LF, Kaufmann RB, Moll PP, McCollough CH, Schwartz RS, Sheedy PF. Radiology 1994;192:631–636.
6. Kaufmann RB, Moll PP, Sheedy PF, Schwartz RS. J Am Coll Cardiol 1994;23:401A (Abstract).
7. Turner ST, Weidman WH, Michels VV, Reed TJ, Ormson CL, Fuller T, Sing CF. Hypertension 1989;13:378–391.
8. Pathological Determinants of Atherosclerosis in Youth (PDAY) Research Group. Arterioscler Thromb 1993;13:1291–1298.
9. Qiao JH, Xie PZ, Fishbein MC, Kreuzer J, Drake TA, Demer LL, Lusis AJ. Arterioscler Thromb 1994;14:1480–1497.

Economic aspects of cardiovascular disease prevention

John P.D. Reckless

School of Postgraduate Medicine, University of Bath, Royal United Hospital, Bath, UK

Abstract. Prevention of CHD is important, for it is a major cause of death and morbidity. Both population and high-risk strategies are required and are cost-effective. Lipid-lowering drug therapy is cost-effective when targeted towards high-risk individuals, either as secondary prevention for those with existing clinical macrovascular disease, or for primary prevention in those with severe inherited dyslipidemia or those with multiple CHD risk factors, especially when accompanied by a poor family history.

Coronary heart disease (CHD): rates and costs

Annually 1.5 million Americans have a myocardial infarct, 30% die, 300,000 have coronary surgery, and CHD health care cost $109 billion in 1992 [1]. Five-year postinfarct costs were $51,200 and for coronary surgery $32,500 [1]. Direct and indirect costs for sickness and death from cardiovascular disease <65 years in wealthier countries were 1.6% of Gross National Product in 1985. CHD caused 43% of all deaths and cerebrovascular disease 25% more. CHD is the commonest UK cause of death, 1987 direct costs being £481 million, and accounting for 2.5% of NHS expenditure.

CHD prevention strategies

Population and high-risk strategies are complementary and not mutually exclusive. Most westernized individuals have ≥1 CHD risk factors, so healthy life style, weight reduction, improved diet, exercise and smoking cessation are appropriate. An individual approach to such moderate-risk people is expensive and inappropriate and lipid-lowering drugs are rarely needed. Stroke risk increases from a low pressure threshold, but costs and adverse events outweigh drug benefits until blood pressure is moderately raised. Similarly, most CHD events are associated with "average" cholesterol values, but relative risk for CHD is greatest at high cholesterol. Population approaches are inadequate for high-risk individuals with personal CHD, severe inherited hyperlipidemia or multiple risk factors.

Outcome and cost-effectiveness

Demands and expectations for health care are rising: in the USA, coronary artery surgery doubled from 1981 to 1985 in 65- to 74-year-olds and tripled above age 75 [2]. Greater scrutiny for cost-effectiveness will help obtain value for money. One can measure surrogate (e.g., blood pressure, cholesterol), intermediate (related to morbidity) or final (death or disease prevented) endpoints [3,4]. Direct costs include primary care and hospital costs, offset by benefits of disease prevention or delay. Indirect costs relate to income and employment, sickness benefits and pensions, but may not be analyzed to avoid discrimination by gender or unemployment. Funded US programs may cost $20–50,000

Address for correspondence: John P.D. Reckless, School of Postgraduate Medicine, University of Bath, Royal United Hospital, Bath BA1 3NG, UK. Tel.: +44-225-824527. Fax.: +44-225-824529.

per life year saved, while costs >$100,000 are not usually appropriate [5]. Analyses may include wellbeing, morbidity and mortality, and life years can be quality-adjusted (QALYs). Costs (and benefits) delayed into the future may be considered in discounted monies (usually 6% p.a.). Differences in income and health care expenditure prevent comparison between countries on a currency basis. UK cost-effective programs average £2–7,000 per QALY saved.

Management programs for hypertension and hyperlipidemia

Economic benefits from stroke prevention in the UK have been demonstrated with savings in excess of drug costs [3]. A blood pressure program in North Karelia, Finland led to $7 million in increased earnings, program costs of $5.2 million and hospital cost savings.

UK cholesterol levels are high (mean 5.9 mmol/l) but economic and resource constraints modify the approach, making it important to target resources carefully [3]. Cholesterol mass screening is more costly than opportunistic or targeted approaches, which can be applied when people visit their primary care physician.

Cost-effectiveness of cholesterol lowering

Cost-utility measures for cholesterol lowering may assess a whole program or drug use alone [3,6–8]. Single interventions are easier to measure but benefits cost less in a multifactorial approach. Nonfatal (and fatal) coronaries result in loss of good-quality life and residual years may be reduced in quality. Benefits relate to cholesterol lowering from dietary and lifestyle change, and additional (incremental) effects from drug therapy.

Cholesterol management costs have been calculated [3] for 29 million England and Wales adults. Costs were averaged over 10 years included sampling, measurement, and staff costs. Treatment and review frequency depended on cholesterol level, subsequent lipid profiles, global CHD risk and presence of modifiable risk factors. The overall QALY cost was £550 (Table 1) but was lower for males than females for the same risk, reflecting relative female CHD protection. Costs are greater for young patients because of their lower CHD risk. Costs averaged over a lifetime rather than 10 years reduces but does not remove the greater cost of treating younger people. Costs fall to £120/QALY for diet and lifestyle only, while incremental cost for drug use is higher at £3,060. QALY

Table 1. Costs (£/QALY) for cholesterol lowering in adult general practice (England and Wales) [3]

Group	Age		
	20–39	40–64	20–64
Overall cost			
Male	4720	185	370
Female	27050	545	1090
All	8000	280	550
Diet-only cost; no drug use			
Male	1010	40	80
Female	5800	120	235
All	1710	60	120
Incremental cost, drug addition			
Male	26580	1050	2080
Female	153100	3080	6140
All	45300	1550	3060

costs are less if lower drug use is targeted at high-risk people and treatment duration is limited, and treatment is initiated later in life.

Similar calculations for lifetime QALY costs were made for the UK Department of Health [7] (Table 2). Overall cost for 25- to 69-year-old adults was £2,979, with a diet-only figure of £176. Reducing 4% drug use to 1% of the population reduces lifetime QALY costs to £960, yet nearly 90% of life years would still be saved. Groups at high risk (smokers, hypertensives, those with CHD) have good economic performance, emphasizing the importance of targeted treatment.

German calculations [8] considered treatment for moderately or markedly elevated cholesterol levels with fibrate or statin respectively, to achieve a target LDL-cholesterol <4.15 mmol/l. Costs (1988 US $) per life year saved in men were $15,650 to 21,610 for treatments initiated from age 35–39 to 60–64 years, and in women $58,090 to 52,720. Cost nadir was $15,600 for men aged 45–49, and $45,740 for women aged 55–59 years.

Drug treatment for cholesterol lowering

Instead of integrated approaches using combinations of diet, lifestyle change and drugs, incremental drug treatment costs can be considered alone. Oster and Epstein [9] using Framingham data calculated that CHD reduction by 16 g/day of cholestyramine was more cost-effective at high cholesterol, for younger patients and for individuals with multiple risk factors. It might not be cost-effective over age 65, and lifelong treatment may be less effective than shorter treatment duration. However, it is difficult to stop treatment in successfully treated individuals. Similar Netherland's results [10] for cholesterol lowering from 8 mmol/l with 12 g/day cholestyramine showed relative costs to be lowest when drug therapy was initiated at age 45–55, and when multiple risk factors were present. These studies used cholestyramine efficacy data of 6.6 and 8.2%, respectively, derived from the Lipid Clinics Program [11]. Poor drug compliance occurs in "intention-to-treat" trials, but cholesterol lowering of 30% occurs in clinical practice in resin-tolerant patients.

Goldman [6] examined lovastatin (20 mg/day) in respect of age, gender, prior CHD and other risk factors in 35- to 84-year-olds. Assuming 19% cholesterol reduction, cost-effectiveness (1989 US$) was best for secondary prevention (Table 3), and in younger men (35–64 years) there were savings rather than costs per life year saved. In older people life-year costs were $3,300–15,000. For cholesterol <6.5 mmol/l, lovastatin 20 mg/day was still cost-effective in men and in women >55 years. Primary prevention was cost-effective for cholesterol ≥7.8 mmol/l when there were additional risks, and for treatment initiated in middle age. For age 45–74 years in men with ≥1 risk, cost per life

Table 2. Costs of cholesterol management in different risk groups (UK) [7]

Group	Cost £/QALY
Males and females, age 25–69 years	
Whole group	2979
Whole group with half of drug use (2%)	1688
Whole group with quarter of drug use (1%)	960
Whole group with no drug use (diet only)	176
Males, age 40–69 years	
Whole group	1957
Whole group, diet only	44
With personal CHD	223
Without personal CHD	2598

Table 3. Cost per year of life saved, for treatment with Lovastatin 20 mg/day, in presence of other risk factors (USA) [6]

BP mmHg	Smoker	Weight % of ideal	CHD	35–44 years	45–54 years	55–64 years	65–74 years
Male, cholesterol >7.8 mmol/l							
<95	No	<110	No	330000	110000	58000	58000
≥105	No	<110	No	190000	69000	37000	37000
≥105	Yes	≥130	No	24000	13000	15000	23000
Males (mean risk factors) Cholesterol >6.5 mmol/l			Yes	[a]	[a]	1600	10000
Females (mean risk factors) Cholesterol >6.5 mmol/l			Yes	4500	3500	8100	12000

[a]Savings, rather than costs.

year was usually <$50,000. Below 45 years several other risks were necessary for effectiveness. It is of note that cost-effectiveness is better in the smoker than nonsmoker because of the former's greater risk, contrasting with surgery for CHD where a smoker has a higher perioperative risk, and less survival improvement.

Relative drug costs and efficacy

Relationships were similar for cholestyramine and simvastatin [10], the latter being more cost-effective related to drug cost and assumed cholesterol-lowering abilities of 6.2 and 27%, respectively.

Schulman [12] examined USA costs ($US 1,989) and efficacy of cholestyramine, colestipol, gemfibrozil, lovastatin, nicotinic acid and probucol. Annual costs were from $139 for 3 g/day nicotinic acid to $1,881 for 80 mg/day lovastatin. Adjusted for side effects and monitoring, nicotinic acid had the lowest 5-year cost per 1% LDL-cholesterol fall at $134, lovastatin 20 mg/day was $177, and cholestyramine was $347. Resins were only considered to lower cholesterol by 9%, although resin-tolerant patients may achieve 30%. Side effects were considered in the calculations, but nicotinic acid is difficult to initiate and maintain, with substantial potential side effects. Bezafibrate, ciprofibrate and fenofibrate, available outside the USA, may cost less, lower cholesterol a little more than gemfibrozil, and lower fibrinogen. Triglycerides and HDL alterations need to be considered also.

Absolute drug costs vary in different markets, but relative costs are more constant. Cholesterol lowering is underestimated in intention-to-treat trials compared to patient use where only tolerable and effective agents are continued. These comparisons may not consider triglyceride, HDL or other changes, and choice of drug is also influenced by the target cholesterol to be achieved.

References

1. Hay JW. Proceedings of the Xth International Symposium on Drugs Affecting Lipid Metabolism, 1990. New York: Elsevier.
2. Anderson GM, Newhouse JP, Roos LL. N Engl J Med 1989;321:1443–1448.
3. Reckless JPD. Bailliére's Clin Endocrinol Metab 1990;4:947–972.
4. McBride PE, Davis JE. Circulation 1992;85:1939–1941.

5. Goldman L, Gordon DJ, Rifkind BM, Hulley SB, Detsky AS, Goodman DS, Kinosian B, Weinstein MC. Circulation 1992;85:1960—1968.
6. Goldman L, Weinstein MC, Goldman PA, Williams LW. J Am Med Assoc 1991;265:1145—1151.
7. Standing Medical Advisory Committee. Report to the Secretary of State for Health, 1990. Department of Health, London.
8. Assmann G, Schulte H. In: Lewis B, Assmann G (eds) The Social and Economic Contexts of Coronary Prevention. Curr Med Literat, London, 1990;37—55.
9. Oster G, Epstein AM. J Am Med Assoc 1987;258:2381—2387.
10. Martens LL, Rutten FFH, Erkelens DW, Ascoop CA. Am J Cardiol 1990;65:27F—32F.
11. Lipid Research Clinics Program. J Am Med Assoc 1984;251:351—374.
12. Schulman KA, Kinosian B, Jacobson TA, Glick H, Willian MK, Koffer H, Eisenberg JM. J Am Med Assoc 1990;264:3025—3033.

168

Mechanisms of hepatic uptake and endocytosis of chylomicron remnants

Richard J. Havel[1], Joachim Herz[2], Shahida Shafi[1], Hiroshi Mokuno[1], André Bensadoun[3], Sandra Brady[1], Leila Kotite[1] and Harshini deSilva[4]

[1]Cardiovascular Research Institute, University of California, San Francisco, CA 94143-0130; [2]Department of Molecular Genetics, University of Texas, Southwestern Medical School, Dallas, TX 75235-9046; [3]Division of Nutrition, Cornell University, Ithaca, NY 15853; and [4]Department of Biology, University of North Carolina, Charlotte, NC 28223, USA

Abstract. Hepatic uptake and endocytosis of chylomicron remnants (CR) are mediated, in part, by distinct interactions with surface proteins. Depletion of hepatic lipase reduces initial uptake but increases endocytosis of CR into hepatocytes. Initial uptake of CR is normal in LDL receptor-knockout mice and is only slightly inhibited by pre-injection of an amount of the LDL receptor-associated protein (RAP) that abolishes uptake of activated α_2-macroglobulin. RAP almost abolishes endocytosis of CR into hepatocytes of normal rats and mice. In LDL receptor-knockout mice, endocytosis of CR is markedly delayed, which suggests that endocytosis via other RAP-sensitive receptors requires extracellular processing.

Earlier studies by Jäckle et al. [1] have shown that the uptake of chylomicron remnants (CR) into the liver of estradiol-treated rats, which express large numbers of low density lipoprotein (LDL) receptors on the basolateral surface of hepatocytes, is followed by prompt endocytosis, as with LDL itself. By contrast, in livers of normal rats endocytosis is delayed following initial hepatic uptake [2]. These observations have led to the suggestion that the initial uptake in normal rats is mediated, at least in part, by interaction of CR with macromolecules distinct from the LDL receptor. In estradiol-treated rats, both initial uptake and endocytosis appear to be mediated by the LDL receptor, which has a high affinity for CR [1,3]. The initial uptake of CR in normal rats could be mediated by a "chylomicron remnant" receptor, or by other macromolecules.

Previous studies by Griglio, Sultan and their associates [4] have shown that prior administration of antiserum to rat hepatic lipase reduces the rate of uptake of CR into rat liver. We have confirmed and extended these observations in studies of the initial uptake and endocytosis of CR in isolated, perfused rat livers [5]. Both inhibition of hepatic lipase with specific antiserum and depletion of hepatic lipase by prior perfusion of livers with heparin reduced initial uptake by 50–65%. By contrast, however, the rate of endocytosis of the CR taken up was increased in both cases by more than 40%. We found that the triglycerides of CR were normally rapidly and extensively hydrolyzed following initial uptake and that this hydrolysis was largely inhibited by hepatic lipase antiserum and to a much lesser extent by heparin pretreatment. These observations led us to suggest that the initial uptake of CR by normal rat liver is mediated to a substantial extent by hepatic lipase on hepatic cell surfaces, leading to hydrolysis of component triglycerides and phospholipids [6], and that this processing is followed by transfer to one or more endocytic receptors that then mediate the endocytic step. Such processing may not be

Address for correspondence: Dr R.J. Havel, Cardiovascular Research Institute, University of California, San Francisco, CA 94143-0130, USA.

required in estradiol-treated rats in which the initial uptake as well as endocytosis are mediated by the LDL receptor.

Earlier observations in experimental animals [7] and humans [8] have led to the suggestion that a receptor other than the LDL receptor (putative CR receptor, recognizing apoE) can mediate the endocytosis of CR when the LDL receptor is genetically deficient or suppressed. The discovery by Herz et al. [9] of an LDL receptor-related protein (LRP) that binds apoE-enriched lipoproteins [10] has provided a candidate CR receptor because it is highly expressed in liver and has the properties of a typical recycling endocytic receptor [9,11]. LRP, however, is a multifunctional receptor for many proteins [12] and may have emerged early in evolution [13], so that it cannot be considered to be solely a CR receptor. An LRP-associated protein (RAP) which has a high affinity for LRP inhibits the binding of LRP to all of its known ligands [14]. We have therefore used RAP as a probe to study the mechanism of endocytosis of CR into hepatocytes.

RAP is itself avidly taken up by the liver of rats and mice and rapidly undergoes endocytosis into hepatocytes [15]. We have therefore preadministered a sufficient amount to intact rats or into the circulation of isolated rat livers to ensure that LRP is saturated with RAP during the uptake and endocytosis of remnants derived from chylomicrons (in intact rats) or of apoE-enriched chylomicrons in isolated, perfused livers [15]. In both cases, RAP somewhat reduced the rate of initial uptake of chylomicron-derived particles, consistent with the participation of hepatic lipase in the initial uptake process. In perfused livers, however, we found that rapid endocytosis of apoE-enriched chylomicrons was virtually abolished. We also found that RAP bound, albeit weakly, to the LDL receptor expressed at high levels in the liver of estradiol-treated rats. Moreover, prior administration of a saturating amount of RAP to estradiol-treated rats greatly reduced the initial uptake and endocytosis of human LDL injected intravenously. Thus, although RAP-sensitive processes appear to mediate the rapid endocytosis of CR into rat hepatocytes, these experiments in rats could not assign a specific function to a receptor other than the LDL receptor, such as LRP.

In subsequent experiments, we have evaluated the initial uptake and endocytosis of CR by the livers of normal mice and mice totally lacking LDL receptors (LDL receptor-knockouts) [16]. Initial uptake of remnants derived from chylomicrons occurred at a normal rate into livers of the knockout mice after intravenous injection of small chylomicrons, but the rate of endocytosis appeared to be markedly reduced. As in rats, prior administration of RAP reduced the initial uptake of remnants derived from chylo-microns only moderately, indicating that RAP-insensitive processes predominate in the initial uptake step. Although it was difficult to demonstrate appreciable accumulation of CR within endosomes from the liver of mice lacking LDL receptors, component cholesteryl esters of CR were gradually hydrolyzed in the liver, albeit much more slowly than in normal mice.

These results in rodents lead to the following conclusions: 1) The initial hepatic uptake of CR is mainly independent of endocytic receptors such as the LDL receptor and LRP, and involves cell surface-bound hepatic lipase; 2) CR normally undergo endocytosis mainly via the LDL receptor, and this occurs promptly after the CR particle encounters the LDL receptor; and 3) in the absence of the LDL receptor, endocytosis occurs sluggishly after initial uptake, which suggests that receptors such as LRP cannot interact effectively with CR immediately after they bind to other sites on liver cell surfaces (such as to hepatic lipase).

Given the confirmation in LDL receptor-knockout mice that lack of the LDL receptor does not lead to appreciable accumulation of CR [16] and that overexpression of RAP in such mice (but not in normal mice) produces gross accumulation of particles resembling CR that contain apoB48 [17], it appears that LRP or a receptor with remarkably similar properties can mediate the endocytosis of CR, albeit inefficiently as compared with the LDL receptor. CR appear to require either additional apoE [10] or apoE in a special conformation to interact effectively with LRP. We thus suggest that hydrolysis of triglycerides or phospholipids of CR may promote acquisition of additional apoE, known to be present on the microvillous surface of hepatocytes [18], to alter the conformation of the endogenous apoE of CR [19], or both, so as to produce high-affinity binding of CR to such a receptor. Similar proposals have been made previously [18,20]. The role of processing in promoting endocytosis of CR in normal animals is less clear, given the efficient endocytosis of CR by the LDL receptor. LRP may thus be viewed as a backup receptor that can prevent gross accumulation of CR when the LDL receptor is suppressed or genetically deficient.

Acknowledgements

This research was supported by grants from the U.S. Public Health Service (HL-14237 — Arteriosclerosis SCOR), HL-20948, and the Perot Family Foundation.

References

1. Jäckle S, Brady SE, Havel RJ. Proc Natl Acad Sci USA 1989;86:1880–1884.
2. Jäckle S, Runquist E, Brady S, Hamilton RL, Havel RJ. J Lipid Res 1991;32:485–498.
3. Kita T, Goldstein JL, Brown MS, Watanabe Y, Hornick CA, Havel RJ. Proc Natl Acad Sci USA 1982;79: 3623–3627.
4. Sultan F, Lagrange D, Jansen H, Griglio S. Biochim Biophys Acta 1990;1042:150–152.
5. Shafi S, Brady SE, Bensadoun A, Havel RJ. J Lipid Res 1994;35:709–720.
6. Griglio S, Sultan F, Lagrange D. Diabète & Metab 1992;18:150–155.
7. Havel RJ, Hamilton RL. Hepatology 1988;8:1689–1704.
8. Rubinsztein DC, Cohen JC, Berger GM, van der Westhuyzen DR, Coetzee GA, Gevers W. J Clin Invest 1990;86:1306–1312.
9. Herz J, Hamann U, Rogne S, Myklebost O, Gausepo H, Stanley KK. EMBO J 1988;7:4119–4127.
10. Kowal RC, Herz J, Goldstein JL, Esser V, Brown MS. Proc Natl Acad Sci USA 1989;86:5810–5814.
11. Lund H, Takahashi K, Hamilton RL, Havel RJ. Proc Natl Acad Sci USA 1989;86:9318–9322.
12. Wilnow TE, Goldstein JL, Orth K, Brown MS, Herz J. J Biol Chem 1992;267:26172–26180.
13. Yochem J, Greenwald I. Proc Natl Acad Sci USA 1993;90:4572–4576.
14. Warshawsky I, Bu G, Schwartz AL. J Biol Chem 1994;269:3325–3330.
15. Mokuno H, Brady S, Kotite L, Herz J, Havel RJ. J Biol Chem 1994;269:13238–13243.
16. Ishibashi S, Brown MS, Goldstein JL, Gerard RD, Hammer RE, Herz J. J Clin Invest 1993;92:883–893.
17. Willnow TE, Sheng Z, Ishibashi S, Herz J. Science 1994;264:1471–1474.
18. Hamilton RL, Wong JS, Guo LS, Krisans S, Havel RJ. J Lipid Res 1990;31:1589–1603.
19. Brasaemle DL, Cornely-Moss K, Bensadoun A. J Lipid Res 1993;34:455–465.
20. Brown MS, Herz J, Kowal RC, Goldstein JL. Current Opinion in Lipidology 1991;2:65–72.

Dissection of the chylomicron remnant clearance pathway

Thomas E. Willnow, Shun Ishibashi and Joachim Herz

Department of Molecular Genetics, University of Texas Southwestern Medical Center, Dallas, TX 75235, USA

Abstract. At least two independent endocytic receptors mediate the uptake of chylomicron remnants into the hepatocytes. Apolipoprotein (apo) E is required for the binding of the remnants to these receptors and apoE-deficient patients and mice accumulate these lipoprotein particles in their circulation. Two apoE-specific receptors are known to be expressed in the liver. One is the low density lipoprotein (LDL) receptor, the other is the LDL receptor-related protein (LRP). Much circumstantial evidence has accumulated over the last few years which has implicated LRP in the chylomicron remnant clearance process. We have applied gene disruption and gene transfer in mice to distinguish the contributions of LDL receptor and LRP to remnant clearance. LDL receptor-deficient mice (LDLR-/-, generated by homologous recombination in embryonic stem cells) do not accumulate chylomicron remnants in their circulation. Because LRP-deficient embryos die in utero, it has not been possible to assess the relative contribution of LRP to remnant uptake. To circumvent this problem we overexpressed receptor-associated protein (RAP), a dominant negative regulator of LRP activity, in the livers of normal and LDLR-/- mice using adenoviral gene transfer. In the LDLR-/- animals RAP overexpression resulted in massive accumulation of chylomicron remnants. Wild-type mice were largely protected from this RAP-induced hyperlipemia. These findings suggest that both LDL receptor and LRP participate in the endocytic uptake of remnants into the hepatocytes.

The transport of lipids through the circulation to the peripheral tissues and back to the liver involves two distinct pathways [reviewed in 1]. An endogenous pathway starts in the liver with the secretion of very low density lipoproteins (VLDL) from the hepatocytes. These VLDL particles transport triglycerides from the liver to the peripheral tissues. The action of lipoprotein lipase converts the VLDL particles to intermediate density lipoproteins (IDL) and eventually to the cholesterylester-rich low density lipoproteins (LDL). The LDL receptor is responsible for the hepatic uptake of the IDL and LDL particles which closes the loop of this endogenous lipid transport pathway [2]. In humans virtually all liver-derived VLDL are characterized by the presence of apoB100 on the particle, whereas in some animal species substantial amounts of apoB48 are present in the VLDLs.

The exogenous pathway originates in the intestine, where dietary lipids are transported across the intestinal epithelium and packaged into large triglyceride-rich particles, the chylomicrons. These in turn are secreted into the mesenteric lymph from where they are drained into the venous circulation. Like VLDL, the chylomicrons are stripped of their triglycerides through the action of lipoprotein lipase in the peripheral tissues. This new particle, which is significantly reduced in size and relatively enriched in cholesterol, is now being called a chylomicron remnant. It contains primarily two apolipoproteins, a structural component, apoB48, and apoE, which contains a positively charged receptor-

Address for correspondence: Joachim Herz, Department of Molecular Genetics, University of Texas Southwestern Medical Center, 5323 Harry Hines Blvd., Dallas, TX 75235-9046, USA. Tel.: (214) 648 5633; fax: (214) 648 8804.

binding site. These chylomicron remnants are rapidly cleared from the circulation by the liver.

The LDL receptor not only binds apoB100, the sole apolipoprotein present in LDL, but has an even higher affinity for apoE. Nevertheless, human patients and animals which genetically lack functional LDL receptors accumulate only the end product of the endogenous pathway, LDL, in their circulation [3–5]. The hepatic uptake of the chylomicron remnants that depends upon the apoE present on the particles is apparently not significantly impaired in the absence of the LDL receptor. These observations suggest that another lipoprotein receptor besides the LDL receptor is active in the liver. This receptor would be specific for apoE and unable to recognize apoB100, as it apparently cannot clear LDL, which accumulates in the circulation. The LDL receptor-related protein (LRP) has been postulated as functioning as such a chylomicron-remnant receptor, on the basis of its striking structural similarity to the LDL receptor [6].

However, LRP mediates not only the binding and cellular uptake of lipoproteins. It has been recognized as a multifunctional receptor which functions in a number of diverse biological processes, including the regulation of plasminogen activation, the clearance of α_2-macroglobulin/proteinase complexes and the cellular uptake of toxins of microbial and plant origin [reviewed in 7]. Probably because of this multifunctional nature mice that are genetically deficient for LRP die in utero early during gestation [8]. This precludes any analysis of the effect of LRP deficiency on the metabolism of lipoproteins in vivo. In contrast, LDL receptor-deficient mice develop normally and are viable [5].

The activity of LRP can be modulated in vitro by the addition of a small protein of approximately 39 kDa to the medium of cultured cells [9–11]. This protein was discovered because it copurifies with LRP and binds very tightly to the receptor. It was subsequently found to inhibit the binding of all currently known ligands to LRP. Although a physiological regulatory function for this receptor-associated protein (RAP) has not yet been directly demonstrated, this is the basis for an attractive hypothesis [12]. While RAP binds to LRP with high affinity, it interacts only weakly with the LDL receptor [13].

Because of these discriminating inhibitory properties of RAP, we decided to test directly the consequences of the overexpression of RAP in intact mice that were either wild-type or deficient for the LDL receptor. We reasoned that overexpression of RAP might selectively inhibit LRP, and therefore remnant-receptor activity, while LDL receptor activity might be relatively unaffected. In this case we would not expect to observe major changes of the plasma lipoprotein profile of wild-type mice, because the LDL receptor could be expected to compensate for the loss of LRP function. In contrast, a block of LRP activity in LDL receptor-deficient mice should result in the accumulation of chylomicron remnants in the circulation of the animal, if LRP were indeed the hypothetical remnant receptor. In pursuing this goal, we aimed at a highly liver-specific expression of RAP which could be temporarily induced to high levels in adult animals of any desired genotype, rather than following a traditional transgenic approach in which an expression construct is injected into the nucleus of fertilized mouse eggs. The latter approach could be expected to result at best in an incomplete inhibition of LRP, because some LRP function is required for normal development.

The use of recombinant adenoviruses to express exogenous genes efficiently in the liver of laboratory animals has previously been shown by several investigators [14]. In particular, the effect of various viruses carrying different genes on the metabolism of plasma lipoproteins has been characterized [5,15,16]. These experiments have demonstrated that the infection of mouse hepatocytes with a wild-type adenovirus or with a recombinant virus expressing an irrelevant marker gene (e.g., β-galactosidase or luciferase), albeit causing a mild hepatocellular inflammation, does not elicit any changes in the metabolism of lipoproteins per se. In contrast, transfer of the human LDL-receptor cDNA into the livers of LDL receptor-deficient mice resulted in the complete, transient reversal of the hypercholesterolemic phenotype. These findings demonstrate the exceptional usefulness of recombinant adenoviruses for the transient, high-level overexpression of foreign genes in vivo.

To achieve RAP overexpression we constructed a recombinant adenovirus in which the RAP cDNA was driven by the strong cytomegalovirus promoter (AdCMV-RAP). This virus was tested in cultured cells in vitro and found to block the cellular degradation of ^{125}I-α_2-macroglobulin, a ligand for LRP, in a dose-dependent manner. The inhibition of LRP took place on the cell surface. This was shown by incubation of an iodinated monoclonal antibody directed against RAP with cultured cells that had been infected with various doses of recombinant virus. Degradation of the monoclonal was directly proportional over a wide range to the amount of virus used to infect the cells (Fig. 1).

Injection of AdCMV-RAP into wild-type or LDL receptor-deficient mice resulted in the induction of circulating RAP in the plasma of the animals. RAP protein concentration was variable over a wide range up to approximately 500 μg RAP/ml plasma. This recombinant protein was biologically active and completely inhibited the plasma clearance of ^{125}I-labeled α_2-macroglobulin in mice of either genotype expressing RAP at levels exceeding 40 μg/ml plasma.

We then investigated the effect of RAP overexpression in vivo on the lipoprotein profile of the two mouse strains. As expected, RAP overexpression led to an increase of

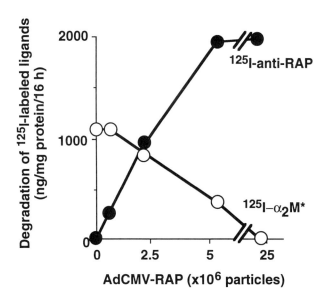

Fig. 1. Degradation of ^{125}I-labeled α_2-macroglobulin and of a monoclonal antibody directed against RAP by AdCMV-RAP-infected CV-1 cells. 2.5×10^5 CV-1 cells grown in 12-well plates were infected with the indicated number of recombinant adenovirus particles. Thirty-six hours later the medium was changed and the indicated ^{125}I-labeled ligands (5 μg/ml methylamine-activated α_2-macroglobulin, specific activity 680 cpm/ng; 5 μg/ml anti-RAP monoclonal antibody, specific activity 600 cpm/ng) were added. After another 16 h the medium was removed from the cells and the amount of trichloroacetic acid-soluble radioactivity present in the culture medium was determined. Values shown are the average of duplicate experiments.

174

only approximately 50% of the total plasma cholesterol concentration (from ~100 mg/dl to ~150 mg/dl) in wild-type mice, most of which was contained in the VLDL/chylomicron remnant fraction. In contrast, LDL receptor-deficient animals showed a marked elevation of their total plasma cholesterol (from ~250 mg/dl to >1,000 mg/dl). This was primarily contained in apoB48/apoE-containing particles which were indistinguishable from chylomicron remnants. Simultaneously, the HDL fraction was significantly reduced or absent.

That LRP in fact mediates both α_2-macroglobulin and chylomicron remnant uptake in the liver is further supported by the dose–response correlation with which RAP blocked α_2-macroglobulin turnover and cholesterol clearance in the virus-injected knockout mice. In both cases, maximal inhibition was obtained at RAP concentrations >40 µg/ml and the two inhibition curves are virtually superimposable. The effect of RAP overexpression was specific for LRP and did not extend to other endocytic receptors expressed on the sinusoidal surface of the hepatocytes. This was verified by measuring the activity of the asialoglycoprotein receptor in control virus-injected and in RAP-overexpressing mice. Irrespective of the genotype of the animal (wild-type or LDL-receptor knockout) RAP overexpression did not affect the asialoglycoprotein receptor at any level, which indicates that the RAP effect was restricted and did not generally affect endocytosis.

In summary, our results lend further strong support to the hypothesis that LRP functions as a chylomicron-remnant receptor in vivo. Under physiological circumstances both LDL receptor and LRP appear to be equally effective mediators of chylomicron remnant uptake into the liver.

References

1. Havel RJ, Kane JP. In: Scriver CR, Beaudet AL, Sly WS, Valle D (eds) The Metabolic Basis of Inherited Disease. New York: McGraw-Hill, 1989;1129–1138.
2. Goldstein JL, Brown MS. In: Scriver CR, Beaudet AL, Sly WS, Valle D (eds) The Metabolic Basis of Inherited Disease. New York: McGraw-Hill Publishing Co, 1989;1215–1250.
3. Kita T, Goldstein JL, Brown MS, Watanabe Y, Hornick CA, Havel RJ. Proc Natl Acad Sci USA 1982;79:3623–3627.
4. Rubinsztein DC, Cohen JC, Berger GM, van der Westhuyzen DR, Coetzee GA, Gevers W. J Clin Invest 1990;86:1306–1312.
5. Ishibashi S, Brown MS, Goldstein JL, Gerard RD, Hammer RE, Herz J. J Clin Invest 1993;92:883–893.
6. Herz J, Hamann U, Rogne S, Myklebost O, Gausepohl H, Stanley KK. EMBO J 1988;7:4119–4127.
7. Krieger M, Herz J. Ann Rev Biochem 1994;63:601–637.
8. Herz J, Clouthier DE, Hammer RE. Cell 1992;71:411–421 and Cell 1992;73:428.
9. Herz J, Goldstein JL, Strickland DK, Ho YK, Brown MS. J Biol Chem 1991;266:21232–21238.
10. Moestrup SK, Gliemann J. J Biol Chem 1991;266:14011–14017.
11. Williams SE, Ashcom JD, Argraves WS, Strickland DK. J Biol Chem 1992;267:9035–9040.
12. Herz J. Curr Opin Lipid 1993;4:107–113.
13. Mokuno H, Brady S, Kotite L, Herz J, Havel RJ. J Biol Chem 1994;269:13238–13243.
14. Stratford-Perricaudet LD, Makeh I, Perricaudet M, Briand P. J Clin Invest 1992;90:626–630.
15. Herz J, Gerard RD. Proc Natl Acad Sci USA 1993;90:2812–2816.
16. Willnow TE, Sheng Z, Ishibashi S, Herz J. Science 1994;264:1471–1474.

Role of lipases and LDL receptor-related protein in human chylomicron remnant metabolism

Ulrike Beisiegel[1], Annette Krapp[1], Wilfried Weber[1], Alexander Mann[1], Jörgen Gliemann,[2] Anders Nykjaer[2], Gunilla Olivecrona[3] and Michael Hayden[4]

[1]Medical Clinic, University Hospital Hamburg, Germany; [2]Department of Medical Biochemistry, University of Aarhus, Denmark; [3]Department of Medical Biochemistry and Biophysics, University of Umea, Sweden; and [4]Department of Medical Genetics, University of British Columbia, Canada

Abstract. The LDL receptor-related protein (LRP) has been described as a chylomicron-remnant receptor. Ligands for LRP in lipoprotein catabolism are apolipoprotein E and lipoprotein lipase (LpL). LpL was found to be associated with remnant particles [1]. In vitro binding studies showed that LpL can mediate the binding of human chylomicrons to proteoglycans and LRP. The binding site has been localized at amino acids 390–421 in the C-terminal at portion of LpL. Hepatic lipase (HL), expressed in the liver, might also be involved in the promotion of chylomicron catabolism. We found that HL mediates the binding of lipoproteins to proteoglycans and LRP just like LpL.

Chylomicron remnant catabolism

It is known that chylomicrons need to be catabolized by LpL to become a ligand for cellular receptors, which then mediate their uptake into the cells. Lipolysis changes the surface structure and exposes apoE in such a way that the chylomicron remnants (CR) can be recognized by cellular receptors. The LDL receptor has been described as mediating the binding and uptake of lipoproteins via apoE, as well as the LRP [2].

Since substantial binding in vitro was obtained only when apoE was added to the lipoproteins we suggested that additional structures might be necessary for effective catabolism. As a second ligand structure LpL, which had been found to be associated with the particles after lipolysis [1], might be involved in receptor binding. It was shown [3] that as a first step LpL mediates the binding of chylomicrons to proteoglycans, whereby the ligands accumulate on the surface of the cells and can more easily interact with specific receptors [4]. Uptake itself seems to be mediated mainly by the LDL receptor and LRP. ApoE, as well as HL and LpL, can bind to the proteoglycans on the liver cells. HL is believed to play a role in chylomicron remnant catabolism and our data support this by demonstrating that HL also mediates the binding and uptake of chylomicrons and β-VLDL by human hepatoma cells. Our current concept for the catabolism of chylomicrons is therefore that an efficient uptake of these particles in the liver can be achieved only when apoE is exposed at the surface and LpL or HL, or both enzymes are present on the particle. Our in vitro data showed that all three ligand proteins are heparin-binding proteins and able to interact directly with LRP. We therefore propose LRP as the main receptor for chylomicron remnant catabolism.

Address for correspondence: Dr Ulrike Beisiegel, Medical Clinic, University Hospital Hamburg, Martinistr. 52, D-20246 Hamburg, Germany. Phone: +49-40-47176873, Fax: +49-40-47174592.

ApoE-mediated binding of lipoproteins

We showed that human apoE binds to LRP in human hepatoma cells. A semiquantitative analysis with cross-linking showed that all isoforms and mutants are able to bind to LRP. The mutants do not, however, mediate the binding of β-VLDL in the same way as apoE-3. This might be due to a reduction in binding to the LDL receptor as described for apoE-2. Analysis of the heparin-binding capacity of these mutants, however, indicated that a reduced binding to the proteoglycans on the cell surface is responsible for the reduced cellular binding (Table 1). Addition of LpL to the apoE-containing particles was able to overcome the defective binding of all isoforms and mutants studied. This is in our opinion mainly due to the compensation of the heparin-binding defect. We propose that the difference in the expression of type III hyperlipidemia in patients with the genotype apoE 2/2 might be due to the amount of LpL associated with the remnant lipoproteins.

Interaction between lipoprotein lipase and LRP

LpL mediates the binding of lipoproteins to cells, and in our experiments the binding of human chylomicrons to human hepatoma cells and hepatocytes. The LpL binds to the lipoproteins and to proteoglycans of the cell surface. In addition we proposed a direct interaction between LpL and LRP [5]. The LRP binding can be demonstrated for the LpL monomer, while effective mediation of lipoprotein binding needs an intact dimer of the enzyme [6]. We consider the mediation of lipoprotein binding as a physiologically relevant mechanism for chylomicron remnant uptake in the liver. To study this mechanism it was important to discriminate between the effect of enzyme activity and structural binding activity, both being dependent on the dimeric form.

To inhibit the activity we used Orlistat (La Roche, Basel; earlier tetrahydrolipstatin = THL) and found that in vitro the increase of lipoprotein binding to cells was independent of the enzymatic activity. We also used bacterial lipase, which is able to hydrolyze chylomicrons, but has a structure different from that of LpL. The bacterial lipase did not increase the binding of lipoproteins to cells (Fig. 1).

To determine the structural site which is involved in the LRP binding we employed the chymotrypsin-cleaved LpL prepared by G. Olivecrona [7] which lacks the 58 C-terminal amino acids of the human LpL. The c-LpL is not able to bind to LRP (Fig. 1) and therefore at least part of the binding site must be in the C terminus [3,6]. The production of a C-terminal peptide of the LpL, comprising the amino acid sequence 378–448, revealed that this fragment is able to bind to LRP, and to inhibit the LpL-mediated binding of lipoproteins to cells [Nykjaer et al.; J Biol Chem, 1994, manuscript in revision]. Moreover, CNBr fragments of bovine LpL were used and it was shown that

Table 1. ApoE: heparin binding and mediation of β-VLDL binding

ApoE isoforms and mutants	β-VLDL binding[a]	Heparin binding[b]
ApoE-3	× 14	100%
ApoE-2 (158 Arg-Cys)	× 3	58%
ApoE-1 (158 Arg-Cys; 127 Gly-Asp)	× 9	37%
ApoE-1 (146 Lys.Glu)	× 2	21%

[a]The apoE-mediated increase of binding is given compared to the binding of ^{125}I-β-VLDL alone. Binding experiments were done on LDL-receptor-deficient fibroblasts.
[b]The heparin binding was determined on heparin columns and the binding of apoE was set at 100%.

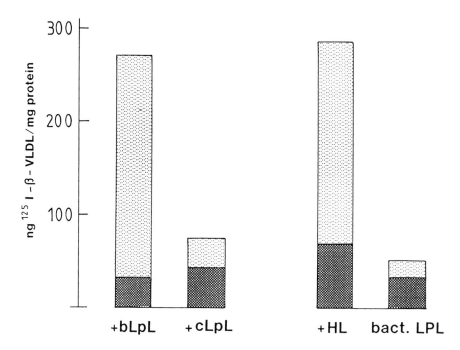

Fig. 1. Heparin-releasable binding of ^{125}I-β-VLDL to HepG₂ cells. Experiments were performed at 0°C for 30 min. The incubation was in the absence (dark bars) or presence of 0.5 mg of lipase (light bars). The lipases were: bLpL = bovine LpL, cLpL = chymotrypsin-cleaved LpL, HL = hepatic lipase, bact.LpL = bacterial LpL (*Pseudomonas fluorescens*). The bound β-VLDL was released by heparin after extensive washing.

a fragment containing amino acids 380–425 also bound to LRP. In addition to the binding studies with the LpL fragments we used mutant human LpL produced in M. Hayden's laboratory [8]. In agreement with data obtained from the fragment experiments a deletion in the C-terminus of amino acids 421–430 did not destroy the effect of the LpL protein on cellular binding of lipoproteins. A deletion of amino acids 404–414, which is in the proposed binding site, showed reduced binding. These studies show that the direct interaction between LpL and LRP is mainly due to aminoacid residues 390–421. Point mutations in this region seem also to inhibit the binding of LpL to LRP [9].

Interaction between hepatic lipase and LRP

HL activity has been inferred as involved in chylomicron remnant catabolism. It is located on proteoglycans of the liver cell surface, and in the lipase family the HL is most homologous to the LpL. These facts suggest that HL might be an additional candidate as a ligand for the receptor-dependent uptake of chylomicron remnants. Pancreatic lipase, another member of the lipase family, is less homologous to LpL and did not mediate the binding of lipoproteins to cells, nor does it bind to LRP.

In experiments similar to those we did with LpL [2], we studied the interaction of HL and LRP. HL increased the binding of lipoproteins (human chylomicrons and rabbit β-VLDL) to different cell types, similarly to the LpL effect (Table 2). This increase in binding is also due to the interaction with proteoglycans, but it leads to an uptake of the particles via LRP. A direct interaction between HL and LRP was demonstrated on purified LRP [Nykjaer et al.; J Biol Chem, 1994, manuscript in revision]. The C termini of LpL

178

Table 2. Uptake of lipoproteins in Hep3b cells mediated by HL and LpL

Ligand	No addition ng/mg cell protein	0.05 µg HL ng/mg cell protein	0.2 µg LpL ng/mg cell protein
Human chylomicrons	9	87	98
Rabbit β-VLDL	52	83	102

One experiment (37°C, 90 min) for each ligand out of a series of experiments is shown. All experiments showed a similar increase of ligand uptake for the two enzymes. The actual amount of uptake differed considerably, however.

and HL are very similar and we plan to study C-terminal mutants of the HL to localize the binding site in this enzyme too. Substitution of amino acids 390–393 in LpL by the corresponding HL sequence preserved the binding activity of the protein, while a deletion of these four amino acids in the LPL molecule reduced the binding by around 50%. We conclude therefore that HL interacts directly with the LRP, and the binding site might be localized in the C-terminus as shown for the LpL. The role of HL in chylomicron remnant catabolism in vivo needs to be verified.

Acknowledgements

This work was supported by a grant of the Deutsche Forschungsgemeinschaft (SFB 232, C1). For technical assistance we thank Nicolette Meyer and Juliane Bergmann.

References

1. Felts J, Itakura H, Crane RT. Biochem Biophys Res Commun 1975;66:764–772.
2. Willnow TE, Sheng Z, Ishibashi S, Herz J. Science 1994;264:1471–1474.
3. Eisenberg S, Sehayek E, Olivercrona T, Vlodavsky I. J Clin Invest 1992;90:2013–2021.
4. Beisiegel U, Krapp A, Weber W, Olivecrona G. The role of α_2M receptor/LRP in chylomicron remnant metabolism. Ann New York Acad Sci 1994;(in press).
5. Beisiegel U, Weber W, Bengtsson-Oivecrona G. Proc Natl Acad Sci USA 1991;88:8342–8346.
6. Nykjaer A, Bengtsson-Olivecrona G, Lookene A, Moestrup SK, Petersen CM, Weber W, Beisiegel U, Gliemann J. J Biol Chem 1993;213:185–194.
7. Lookene A, Bengtsson-Olivecrona G. Eur J Biochem 1993;213:185–194.
8. Hanfang Z, Krapp A, Ma Y, Ginzinger D, Beisiegel U, Hayden M. Abstract AHA, Supplement to Circulation, 1994.
9. Chapell DA, Inoue I, Fry G, Pladet MW, Bowen SL, Iverius P-H, Lalouel J-M, Strickland DK. J Biol Chem 1994;269:18001–18006.

Role of apoE on the surface of hepatocytes in chylomicron remnant catabolism

Nobuhiro Yamada, Hitoshi Shimano and Yoshio Yazaki

3rd Department of Internal Medicine, University of Tokyo, Hongo, Tokyo, Japan

Abstract. To investigate the role of apolipoprotein E (apoE) in hepatic uptake of chylomicron remnants, we used transgenic mouse lines with integrated rat apoE gene under control of metallothionein promoter. Plasma clearance of injected ^{125}I-labeled human chylomicrons was 5 times faster in transgenic mice than in controls. Immunohistochemistry demonstrated that apoE was specifically localized at the basolateral surface of hepatocytes of fasted transgenic mice. After injection of a large amount of chylomicrons, the density of the cell-surface apoE was markedly reduced and vesicular staining was observed in the cytoplasm, which suggests that the cell-surface apoE was used for hepatic endocytosis of chylomicrons and remnants.

ApoE, as well as apoB100, is a major component of mammalian lipoproteins and functions in the metabolism of plasma lipoproteins through its interaction with LDL receptor, mainly in the liver. ApoE is also thought to be a specific ligand for putative hepatic chylomicron remnant receptor (apoE receptor). ApoE is expressed in many tissues and plays a crucial role in transport and redistribution of lipids in peripheral tissues such as brain, peripheral nerve, and arterial wall [1]. Several lines of evidence suggest that lipoproteins with several molecules of apoE have a higher affinity for LDL receptors than those without apoE [1–5]. Recently, we established lines of transgenic mice with high plasma levels of rat apoE, which is overproduced in the liver under the control of the metallothionein promotor [5]. Homozygotes for line 4-20, the highest liver expresser, exhibited a marked reduction in plasma cholesterol and triglyceride levels, with elimination of very low density lipoprotein (VLDL) and a marked decrease in LDL. These decreases were due to enhanced plasma clearance of lipoproteins containing apoB, which were enriched with apoE. Kinetic studies of plasma lipoproteins in these animals demonstrated that hepatic overexpression of apoE markedly enhances plasma turnover of VLDL and LDL through interactions with LDL receptors and possibly with LDL receptor-related proteins (LRP) [6]. We also performed oral challenge with retinal palmitate as a marker for chylomicron remnant metabolism and the data suggested that hepatic overexpression of apoE markedly enhances clearance of chylomicron remnants [6]. In the present study, we directly measured plasma clearance of ^{125}I-labeled human chylomicrons. For further study of the mechanism by which hepatic overexpression of apoE enhances hepatic uptake of chylomicrons, the distribution of apoE in hepatocytes and changes in its distribution after injection of lipoproteins were investigated by immunohistochemistry [7].

Address for correspondence: Nobuhiro Yamada, 3rd Department of Internal Medicine, University of Tokyo, Hongo, Tokyo, Japan 113. Fax: +81-3-3392-1870.

Materials and Methods

Animals

Transgenic mice MAE 4-20, which overexpress rat apoE under the control of the metallothionein promotor, MAE 4-20, were established as described previously (5). This line has three copies of integrated genes, and the inheritance pattern of the transgene was compatible with a single autosomal integration site. Homozygous and heterozygous lines 4-20 aged 16–20 weeks were used in this study. The animals were maintained on normal chow and given water supplemented with 20 mM $ZnSO_4$ for more than 1 week to induce the expression of rat apoE from the transgene. Prior to intravenous injection of lipoproteins for kinetic studies and immunohistochemistry, the animals were fasted for 12 h.

Lipoproteins and iodination

Chylomicrons were prepared from the pleural effusion of a patient with malignant lymphoma and chylothorax. VLDL and LDL were prepared from plasma drawn from normolipidemic volunteers. Chylomicrons were separated by ultracentrifugation at 40,000 rpm in a Beckman SW28 rotor for 0.5 h, followed by repeat ultracentrifugation at 20,000 rpm for 16 h. For separation of VLDL, and LDL, plasma was ultracentrifuged in a 50.2 Ti rotor at 45,000 rpm at 12°C at KBr densities of 1.006 and 1.063 for 16 h and 20 h, respectively. The floating lipoproteins were re-ultracentrifuged in a 40.3 rotor. Chylomicrons and VLDL were iodinated with ^{125}I by the iodine monochloride method with slight modification. Turnover studies of iodinated chylomicrons and VLDL were performed as previously described [6].

Immunohistochemical procedures for light microscopy

Animals fasted for 12 h were anesthetized with pentobarbital. Lipoproteins (0.3 mg protein of chylomicrons or VLDL, or 0.5 mg protein of LDL/100 µl phosphate-buffered saline [PBS]) or saline as a control were injected through the tail vein. Seven minutes after injection, the livers were perfused with ice-cold saline through a portal vein and resected. Small aliquots from the right lobes of the resected livers were immediately fixed in 4% paraformaldehyde in PBS (pH 7.4). Other portions of the samples were used for preparation of membrane pellets. Paraformaldehyde-fixed, paraffin-embedded sections were subjected to immunohistochemistry. For apoE immunostaining, two primary antibodies were used: a rabbit anti-rat apoE polyclonal antibody, which detects both rat and mouse apoE's, and rabbit polyclonal antibody to rat apoE-specific synthetic oligopeptide, which does not cross-react with mouse apoE [5].

Results

Effects of apoE overexpression on lipoprotein metabolism

Expression of the transgene and secretion into the plasma were confirmed by the detection of rat apoE in the plasma of the transgenic animals on immunoblot analysis using rat apoE-specific antibody. The level of rat apoE in homozygotes was twice that in heterozygotes, suggesting expression from both integrated rat apoE genes. When the mice were given water supplemented with 20 mM zinc sulfate for 1 week, the plasma level of rat apoE was increased to 17.4 mg/dl by 1.6-fold. The mouse apoE level of pooled nontransgenic mice (n = 16) was estimated as 4.56 mg/dl. This overexpression of apoE caused marked alterations in plasma lipids. Homozygotes exhibited 43% lower serum cholesterol after zinc administration than zinc-treated nontransgenic littermates (controls) (p < 0.01). Plasma triglyceride levels were also compared among animal groups. In homozygotes, remarkable decreases were observed both before and after the zinc treatment (by 64%, p < 0.005, and 68%, p < 0.01, respectively). These data indicated that the overexpression of rat apoE in the transgenic mice, remarkably and dose-dependently, reduces both plasma cholesterol and triglyceride levels.

Kinetics of ^{125}I-chylomicrons and ^{125}I-VLDL

^{125}I-labeled chylomicrons were injected intravenously and plasma clearances were compared in transgenic mice and controls. The injected chylomicrons were much more rapidly cleared in transgenic mice than in controls. In the first 5 min, 59 and 22% of apoB in injected chylomicrons were removed in transgenic and control mice, respectively. In one experiment, livers were resected 10 min after the injection and the total counts in the liver were measured after extensive perfusion. The total count in the liver of transgenic mice was 72% of total injected count and was 3 times higher than in controls (n = 2). Thus, injected chylomicrons were taken up primarily by the liver and the rapid plasma clearance in transgenic mice was attributed mainly to enhanced hepatic uptake. In contrast, plasma clearance of ^{125}I-labeled human VLDL was similar in transgenic and control mice. It is possible that the human VLDL used was sufficiently apoE-rich and that there was no space for additional incorporation of rat apoE to enhance plasma clearance.

Immunohistochemical localization of apoE in liver of transgenic mice

For determination of the direct involvement of hepatic overexpression of apoE in enhanced chylomicron remnant clearance, livers of transgenic mice were immunohistochemically studied with rat apoE-specific antibody. This antibody detects only the transgene product rat apoE, and not mouse or human apoE. A marked immunostaining of apoE was found peripherally near the basolateral surface of every hepatocyte, while minimal in the cytoplasm. There was no marked basolateral staining in the liver of control animals. As a test of whether the basolateral hepatic apoE was used for hepatic uptake of chylomicron remnants, a large amount of chylomicrons (0.3 mg protein) was injected intravenously in a bolus and the changes in apoE distribution were studied. Seven minutes after the injection of chylomicrons, the liver was resected and stained. Sinusoidal immunostaining of apoE was markedly lower than before injection. Instead, immunostaining was observed in a vesicular pattern in the cytoplasm. This change in the immunostaining pattern suggests that in the process of hepatic uptake of large amounts of injected chylomicrons, basolateral apoE was consumed and reduced, while endosomes containing apoE-rich lipoproteins appeared in a vesicular pattern in the cytoplasm. In contrast, injection of VLDL and LDL had no effect on the sinusoidal staining of apoE, although slight vesicular staining appeared in the cytoplasm.

Discussion

Overexpression of apoE in transgenic mice caused dramatic changes in plasma lipids and lipoprotein profile [5]. The lowering effects of overexpressed apoE on plasma lipoprotein lipid levels were dose-dependent. A decrease in plasma cholesterol level was observed at the plasma apoE level of zinc-treated heterozygotes. Decreases in plasma VLDL- and LDL-cholesterol levels were already observed at the plasma apoE level of untreated heterozygote animals, and the greater the plasma apoE level, the more prominent decreases in plasma VLDL- and LDL-cholesterol levels were observed. At the same plasma apoE level, decreases in plasma triglycerides were much more remarkable than those in plasma cholesterol. Supporting the significant reduction in plasma lipoprotein lipids in transgenic mice, a marked reduction in plasma apoB level of treated homozygotes was observed, which indicates the elimination of most of the lipoproteins containing apoB. VLDL particles, which are synthesized in the liver, can be associated with overexpressed apoE in the liver and achieve a high affinity for LDL receptor, resulting in a rapid plasma clearance of VLDL through receptor-mediated pathways. Reduction in LDL-cholesterol could be caused by reduced production in a metabolic cascade from VLDL whose clearance was enhanced.

We have established that hepatic overexpression of apoE markedly enhances plasma clearance of chylomicron remnants. A high apoE content in chylomicron remnants would be essential to an efficient receptor-mediated endocytosis. The chylomicrons used in this study were prepared from pleural effusions of a patient with chylothorax and were relatively poor in apoE. A key question is whether apoE molecules overexpressed by the liver were transferred to chylomicron remnants from other apoE-rich lipoproteins in the plasma or directly from the liver. To address this question, hepatic localization of apoE was investigated.

It was reported that rat apoE molecules are localized at the basolateral surface of rat hepatocytes, on the microvillous extensions into the space of Disse [8]. Our present immunohistochemical data from both transgenic and control mice were consistent with this. The reduction in basolateral apoE density after injection of chylomicron strongly suggests that hepatic apoE molecules aggregating at the sinusoidal front of hepatocytes were consumed for apoE enrichment of chylomicrons and remnants. Enrichment of chylomicrons and remnants with apoE may be immediately followed by hepatic uptake through LDL receptors, since several lines of evidence indicate that LDL receptors play a major role in plasma clearance of chylomicron remnants in rodents [9]. LRP, which is a likely candidate as chylomicron remnant receptor, appears to be similarly localized and involved in hepatic uptake of chylomicrons and remnants.

These results, even if under nonphysiological conditions, might imply an interesting mechanism of transport of intestinally absorbed lipids to the liver. Daily food intake results in episodic appearance of intestinal lipoproteins in the circulation. These intestinal chylomicron particles are subjected to lipolysis by lipoprotein lipase (LPL) and probably to competitive transfer of apoE and apoCs from other apoE- and apoC-rich lipoproteins. Meanwhile, apoE is produced continuously in the liver. The apoE molecules that escape attachment to nascent VLDL are stored at the sinusoidal front of hepatocytes, ready for the influx of chylomicron remnants. Postprandially, chylomicron remnants flowing through the portal vein encounter abundant apoE molecules on the cell surface of hepatocytes or newly secreted apoE molecules in the sinusoidal space and become highly apoE-rich. Subsequently, these apoE-rich particles are endocytosed through the interaction of apoE with hepatic lipoprotein receptors. If the initial capture of the remnant particles were mainly by the cell-surface apoE, the rapid plasma clearance of chylomicron remnants can be well explained by this initial sequestration in the sinusoidal space. This system would be very suitable for the removal of steep episodic influx of intestinal lipoproteins, which lack apoE, into plasma. The system is specific for chylomicron remnants and not for hepatic lipoproteins such as VLDL and LDL.

References

1. Mahley RW. Science 1988;240:622—630.
2. Yamada N, Shames D, Stoudmier J, Havel RJ. Proc Natl Acad Sci USA 1986;83:3479—3483.
3. Yamada N, Shames D, Havel RJ. J Clin Invest 1987;80:507—515.
4. Yamada N, Shimano H, Mokuno H, Ishibashi S, Gotohda T, Kawakami M, Watanabe Y, Akanuma Y, Murase T, Takaku F. Proc Natl Acad Sci USA 1989;86:665—6696.
5. Shimano H, Yamada N, Katsuki M, Shimada M, Gotoda T, Harada K, Murase T, Fukazawa C, Takaku F, Yazaki Y. Proc Natl Acad Sci USA 1992;89:1750—1754.
6. Shimano H, Yamada N, Katsuki M, Yamamoto K, Gotoda T, Harada K, Shimada M, Yazaki Y. J Clin Invest 1992;90:2084—2091.
7. Shimano H, Namba Y, Ohsuga J, Kawamura M, Yamamoto K, Shimada M, Gotoda T, Harada K, Yazaki Y, Yamada N. J Clin Invest 1994;93:2215—2223.
8. Hamilton RL, Wong JS, Guo LSS, Krisans S, Havel RJ. J Lipid Res 1990;31:1589—1603.
9. Choi SY, Fong LG, Kirven MJ, Cooper AD. J Clin Invest 1991;88:1173—1181.

184

Regulation of apoprotein E secretion

G.S. Getz, S.Q. Ye, B. Thurberg and C.A. Reardon

University of Chicago, Department of Pathology MC6079, 5841 S. Maryland Ave, Chicago, IL 60637, USA

Apoprotein E (apoE) is an important ligand for at least three related receptors involved in lipoprotein metabolism: the LDL receptor; the LDL receptor-related protein; and the more recently described VLDL receptor. The ligand efficacy of the apoprotein depends not only on its presence on the surface of the lipoprotein, but also on its surface concentration, as well as on its conformation on this surface. Studies involving the resistance of transgenic mice overexpressing apoE to elevations in serum cholesterol levels on a high fat/high cholesterol diet [1] and the enhanced clearance of apoE-enriched chylomicron remnants in rabbits and marmosets [2] have suggested that for lipoproteins to be taken up via apoE, their surface concentration needs to be enriched in the apoprotein. On the other hand, the lower apoE concentration in the heterozygous apoE knockout mice is associated with a normal lipoprotein phenotype [3]. Thus, clearance of lipoprotein particles may depend as much on the presentation of apoE to lipoprotein particles as on the apoprotein concentration on the particle. These two sets of apparently paradoxical observations may be reconciled by the fact that apoE is much more efficient when presented in close proximity to the cell surface receptors responsible for lipoprotein clearance i.e., on or near the cell surface. This presentation begins to emphasize the potential role of cell-surface apoE.

We have previously demonstrated that the human hepatoma cell, HepG2, releases about twice as much apoE in the presence as in the absence of high, but physiological, concentrations of human LDL [4]. This effect is not unique to LDL, as HDL and chylomicrons [5] were also able to stimulate apoprotein output. We further demonstrated that the effect of lipoproteins on apoE secretion occurs posttranslationally in a post-Golgi compartment.

The identity of the post-Golgi compartment from which LDL released additional apoE was not clear. A reasonable possibility was the cell surface. Hamilton and colleagues had noted, using an immunochemical approach, that there is an easily demonstrable association of apoE with the cell surface of hepatocytes [6]. A more recent study examining hepatic apoE distribution following clearance of chylomicron remnants in transgenic mice overexpressing apoE reinforced this conclusion [7]. Studies by two groups using heparin and heparinase treatment of hepatoma cells has led to the conclusion that apoE might be associated with heparan sulfate proteoglycans on the cell surface [8,9]. The relationship between the effects of heparin and lipoprotein were not clear. Consequently, Dr Ye set out to investigate three questions: could LDL release apoE from a cell surface compartment; what is the relationship between the effects of lipoprotein, phospholipid vesicles and heparin; and what is the apoprotein and domain specificity of this cell-surface binding?

Release of apoE from the cell surface by LDL

To show the cell-surface association of apoE, we took advantage of the fact that at 4°C no endocytosis or exocytosis occurs. Cells were pulse-labeled with [^{35}S] methionine at 37°C for 60–120 min and the labeled cells were shifted to 4°C for a further 60 min in the absence or presence of LDL. In view of the fact that during the 4°C chase no further apoE can be exocytosed from the cell interior, the apoE released during the chase with LDL was presumed to have come from a pool already on the cell surface. Since we have no information on the residence time of apoE on the cell surface, it is not possible to quantitatively relate the LDL effect observed at 37°C to that observed at 4°C. The absolute amount of apoE released by LDL at 4°C is a small proportion of the release observed at 37°C. However, the response to differing concentrations of LDL is very closely parallel whether the incubation is performed at 37°C or 4°C. A parsimonious interpretation is that the LDL effect at 37°C is mostly attributable to a release of surface apoE which is continuously being deposited there from the cell interior. Thus, the 4°C results represent a snapshot of what occurs at 37°C.

Lipoprotein, phospholipid vesicles and heparin release apoE from the cell surface

The same experimental strategy was used to show that heparin and phospholipid vesicles also release apoE from the surface of HepG2 cells. Our results confirm the observations made by others that heparin releases apoE from a heparan sulfate proteoglycan complex. The source of the apoE released by LDL and phospholipid vesicle is not clear. To ascertain whether the same pool was the source of the apoE released by each of the three agents, we employed the agents in sequence over the 1st and 2nd hour of the chase period (Fig. 1). If each of these agents acted on an independent pool of apoE, the combined use of any two agents should release an amount of apoprotein equal to that of each used separately. This appears to be the case when phospholipid vesicles and heparin were used together in the first chase but only when maximal concentrations of each was employed.

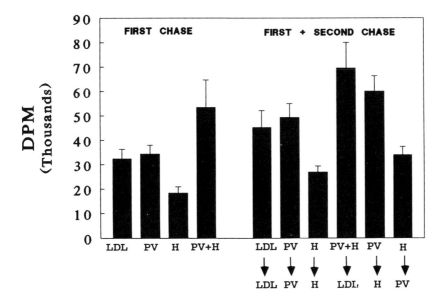

Fig. 1. Sequential use of different apoE-releasing agents. HepG2 cells were pulsed with 250 µC/ml [^{35}S]-methionine for 2 h and chased with serum-free media supplemented with 10 mM methionine first for 1 h with LDL (400 µg/ml), phospholipid vesicles (PV) (5 mg/ml), heparin (H) (30 mg/ml) or PV + H, followed by a second chase for 1 h with either LDL, PV or H. The ^{35}S-labeled apoE in the chase medium was immuno-precipitated and analyzed by SDS-polyacrylamide gels and fluorography. The radiolabeled bands were excised from the gel and counted.

This suggests that the apoE released by phospholipid vesicles and heparin are in two distinct pools. When the same agent was added during the second chase (e.g., PV→PV), additional apoE was released, representing approximately one-third the amount released during the first chase. When heparin was used in a second chase after an initial chase with phospholipid vesicles, the total apoE released was similar to the sum of the two release agents used independently. This was, however, not the case when the first chase agent was heparin followed by phospholipid vesicles. The explanation for this discrepancy is not obvious. A possible interpretation is that once apoE is released from the proteoglycan site, the apoprotein may move from the phospholipid site to the proteoglycan site from which it is not readily releasable, even by heparin. Since LDL contains phospholipids and also apoB that like apoE can bind to proteoglycans, we suggest that LDL can release apoE from both cell-surface pools, but only incompletely.

Many cell types have releasable apoE on their surface

The association of apoE with the cell surface is not unique to HepG2 cells. ApoE can be released from the surface of rat ovarian granulosa cells [10] and human JEG choriocarcinoma cells by lipoproteins. Lipoproteins, phospholipid vesicles and heparin also release human apoE expressed in transfected McA-RH7777 rat hepatoma cells, CHO cells, and J774 mouse macrophage cells [11]. However, the relative proportions of apoE distributed between the proteoglycan complex and the plasma membrane phospholipid site vary from cell type to cell type. For example, unlike HepG2 cells, McA-RH7777 cells appear to bind approximately equal proportions of apoE in proteoglycan and phospholipid sites, while heparin is much less effective as a release agent than is either phospholipid or LDL in transfected CHO cells.

How specific are these effects for apoE?

Phospholipid vesicle, LDL and heparin are effective in releasing apoA-I and apoC-III also from the HepG2 cell surface at 4°C. Heparin was less effective than the two lipid agents. Given that these apoproteins lack the previously identified heparin-binding sites, it was surprising that heparin had an influence. At this point, we cannot exclude the possibility that a multi-apoprotein complex is associated with heparan sulfate proteoglycans, which is capable of being released by heparin. However, these agents do not influence the secretion of all hepatic proteins since they had no effect on the release of albumin into the HepG2 cell medium.

ApoE does not bind to the cell surface via its LDL receptor-binding site

One possible explanation for the release of apoE from the cell surface by LDL is that apoE is attached to cell-surface receptors that recognize it as ligand and that LDL displaces it from these sites. The following facts argue against this interpretation. HDL and phospholipid vesicles have the same effect as LDL, although neither is a ligand for apoE receptors. ApoA-I and C-III are also displaced by LDL, yet neither is a ligand for the LDL receptor. We observed that a mutant of apoE (Arg^{145}→Cys) defective in LDL-receptor binding capacity expressed in transfected CHO cells was released by LDL.

What apoprotein domains are responsible for cell-surface association?

The fact that LDL and phospholipid vesicles release apoE, apoC-III and apoA-I argues that no single sequence accounts for their association with the cell surface. Other genetically engineered constructs reinforce this conclusion. A chimeric protein, generated by exon shuffling between apoA-I and apoE and which contains the third-exon-encoded amino acids (N-terminus) of apoA-I and the fourth-exon-encoded amino acids of apoE (C-terminus), when transfected into McA-RH7777 cells, produced a protein that accumulated on the cell surface and was released by LDL, phospholipid vesicles and heparin, like the other proteins described. The reciprocal chimeric protein containing the fourth-exon-encoded sequences of apoA-I behaves similarly. Finally, a truncated mutant of apoE (residues 1–201) which lacks the major lipid-binding domain and one of the heparin-binding sites still responded to phospholipid vesicles and heparin as release agents for surface apoproteins.

Conclusion and significance

It is becoming generally believed that cell-surface apoE may provide the additional apoprotein ligands to neighboring lipoproteins to facilitate their uptake by nearby receptors. This has been particularly applied to the uptake of chylomicron remnants — this being designated the secretion–recapture hypothesis. It has been suggested that most of this recycling of apoE is through a heparan sulfate proteoglycan pool. Our recent studies suggest that there is an additional surface pool for which interaction with phospholipid is important. The two pools together produce a larger cell-surface density of apoE, perhaps allowing for the translation of lipoprotein particles along the outer plane of the membrane until an endocytosis-competent receptor is encountered. The role of the phospholipid pool of cell-surface apoE in the uptake of lipoprotein remnants needs to be investigated further.

Our results also extend this concept to apply to other apoproteins. The presence of cell-surface apoproteins may be important in refashioning the lipoproteins in proximity to the cell surface for whatever functions may be important to the local lipoproteins: whether for endocytosis, the promotion of lipid efflux from the cell, or the modification or transfer of effluxed lipid. Clearly, further examination of these possibilities is needed.

Acknowledgements

This work was supported by HL 15062 (Specialized Center of Research in Atherosclerosis) from the National Institutes of Health.

References

1. Shimano H, Yamada N, Katsuki M, Shimade M, Gotoda T, Harada K, Murase T, Fukazawa C, Takaki F, Yazaki Y. Proc Natl Acad Sci USA 1992;89:1750–1754.
2. Hussain MM, Mahley RW, Boyles JK, Fainaru JM, Brecht WJ, Linquist PA. J Biol Chem 1989;264: 9571–9582.
3. Plump AS, Smith JD, Hayek T, Aalto-Setala K, Walsh A, Verstuyft JH, Rubin EM, Breslow JL. Cell 1992; 71:343–353.
4. Ye SQ, Olson LM, Reardon CA, Getz GS. J Biol Chem 1992;267:21961–21966.
5. Graig WY, Nutrik R, Cooper AD. J Biol Chem 1988;263:13880–13890.
6. Hamilton RL, Wong JS, Guo LS, Krisans S, Havel RJ. J Lipid Res 1990;31:1589–1603.
7. Shimano H, Manba Y, Ohsuga J, Kawamura M, Yamamoto K, Shimada M, Gotoda T, Harada K, Yazaki KY, Yamada N. J Clin Invest 1994;93:2215–2223.
8. Ji ZS, Brecht WJ, Miranda RD, Hussain MM, Innerarity TL, Mahley RW. J Biol Chem 1993;268:10160–10167.
9. Lilly-Stauderman M, Brown TL, Balasubramaniam A, Harmony JAK. J Lipid Res 1993;34:190–200.
10. Wyne K. University of Chicago, Ph.D. Thesis.
11. Mazzone T, Pustelnikas L, Reardon CA. J Biol Chem 1992;267:1081–1087.

Remnant lipoproteins and coronary artery disease progression

Fredrik Karpe, Per Tornvall and Anders Hamsten
Atherosclerosis Research Unit, King Gustaf V Research Institute, Department of Medicine, Karolinska Institute Karolinska Hospital, S-171 76 Stockholm, Sweden

Abstract. The relations between triglyceride-rich lipoproteins, alimentary lipemia and coronary heart disease (CHD) have remained obscure and much debated. It has recently been shown that the increase in the number of triglyceride-rich apoB100-containing lipoprotein particles after fat intake is far greater than that of apoB48-containing lipoproteins. Interestingly, the increase in VLDL is confined to the larger VLDL particles, whereas the plasma concentration of small VLDL does not change in response to oral fat intake. Furthermore, the alimentary lipemia-induced transfer of cholesteryl esters from HDL is to a large extent confined to the apoB100-containing triglyceride-rich lipoproteins. Conversely, 80% of the postprandial increase in triglycerides is accounted for by lipoproteins containing apoB48. On the basis of the respective plasma levels and compositional characteristics of postprandial triglyceride-rich lipoproteins and the magnitude of the responses to fat intake observed for chylomicron remnants and VLDL, it could be hypothesized that chylomicrons and their remnants contribute to atherogenesis by impeding the normal LPL-mediated catabolism of cholesterol-enriched VLDL. This should be taken into consideration when the association between postprandial lipoproteins and development of coronary atherosclerosis is evaluated.

The issue of whether chylomicron remnants are atherogenic has been much debated. A number of reports discussed later point to an association between impaired metabolism of postprandial triglyceride-rich lipoproteins and the presence of coronary artery disease (CAD). For the purpose of standardization the levels of plasma lipids and lipoproteins are generally measured in the fasting state, despite the fact that most of our lives are spent between regular meals. For obvious reasons no consensus has been reached on how postprandial lipoproteins could be quantified in the clinical setting. A large body of studies from the 1950s and 1960s focused on plasma levels of triglycerides after a fat meal in case-control studies. Unfortunately, interest declined when it was found that the peak postprandial triglyceride level was closely reflected by fasting plasma concentrations [1]. A few fairly recent studies then used vitamin A supplementation of the test meal leading to retinyl ester (mainly retinyl palmitate, RP) incorporation into chylomicrons and their remnants as a means of tracing intestinal lipoproteins in plasma. It was shown that postprandial plasma concentrations of RP were higher in CAD patients than in healthy subjects [2,3]. With the discovery of the truncated apolipoprotein (apo) B variant, apoB48, which in humans is carried only in intestinally-derived triglyceride-rich lipoproteins, a specific marker for chylomicrons and their remnants was found [4]. The simultaneous quantification of apoB48 and apoB100 in subfractions of triglyceride-rich lipoproteins after fat intake has led to a better understanding of the metabolism of postprandial triglyceride-rich lipoproteins and of their relation with CAD.

Address for correspondence: Fredrik Karpe, Atherosclerosis Research Unit, King Gustaf V Research Institute, Department of Medicine, Karolinska Institute Karolinska Hospital, S-171 76 Stockholm, Sweden. Tel.: +46-8-7293203. Fax: +46-8-311298.

Metabolism of chylomicrons and their remnants

Chylomicrons are secreted by the intestine after fat feeding. Chylomicron particles contain apoB48 as the structural protein, which in humans is formed exclusively in the intestine after tissue-specific editing of the apoB100 mRNA [5]. However, there is evidence that the intestine may secrete small amounts of full-length apoB100 [6]. The significance of this finding has not been established. Once the chylomicron particle reaches the plasma compartment, it acquires apoCs, in particular apoC-II, to enable efficient unloading of its massive triglyceride content after attaching to lipoprotein lipase (LPL) bound to the endothelium [7]. In plasma the chylomicrons and their remnants mix with endogenous lipoproteins. Exchange of lipoprotein core lipids is enhanced and, essentially, a flow of cholesteryl esters from high density lipoprotein (HDL) and low density lipoprotein (LDL) is balanced by a counterflow of triglycerides leaving the expanding pool of triglyceride-rich lipoproteins. The half-life of chylomicrons is very short. It has been estimated to approximate 5 min [7]. Chylomicron remnants do, on the other hand, seem to remain in plasma for longer periods of time. The bulk of the remnants is taken up by the liver using apoE as a ligand. The presence of apoE2 allele/alleles results in a delayed uptake of chylomicron remnants. Indeed, patients with type III hyperlipidemia who are homozygous for the apoE2 allele have a severely retarded elimination of chylomicron remnants [8].

VLDL metabolism in the postprandial state

Very low density lipoprotein (VLDL) particles are secreted continuously from the liver. In contrast to chylomicrons and their remnants, they are characterized by their apoB100 content [5]. The secretion rate of VLDL is partly determined by the availability of triglycerides, whereas the generation of the apoB100 protein seems to be constant [5]. This means that immature triglyceride-poor VLDL particles will be degraded intracellularly instead of being secreted. The triglyceride substrate for the VLDL secretory pathway derives essentially from three sources, all of which can be regulated by food intake. First, free fatty acids (FFA) generated by lipolysis in adipose tissue through the action of hormone-sensitive lipase provide a major source of liver triglycerides. Second, hepatic uptake of poorly lipolysed remnant particles from either VLDL or chylomicrons can contribute. Similarly, a defective uptake of FFA in adipose and muscle tissues after LPL-mediated lipolysis of chylomicrons and VLDL may lead to excessive delivery of FFA to the liver, in particular in the postprandial phase [9]. Third, the liver has the capacity of de novo synthesis of triglycerides, which is most evident in carbohydrate overfeeding. The second point might be of specific importance, since it has been shown that LPL is released from endothelium by high ambient concentrations of FFA both in vitro [10] and in vivo [12]. It is therefore hypothesized that the targeting of chylomicron- and VLDL-derived FFA to adipose tissue in the postprandial state under these circumstances can be diverted to the liver. Accordingly, after a fat meal, LPL increased in plasma in both healthy and hypertriglyceridemic men, but the increment was most pronounced in the hypertriglyceridemic subjects [9]. Concomitantly, chylomicron-derived FFA were elevated in plasma, despite the fact that total plasma FFA levels were unchanged. One interpretation of these findings is that LPL might have a regulatory role in lipolysis, by means of localization rather than activity. If the lipase is dissociated from the endothelium by accumulating FFA, these fatty acids could be shunted to the liver and provide the substrate for an enhanced VLDL secretion [12]. Hypertriglyceridemic subjects might be particularly susceptible to this mechanism.

After a fat meal, chylomicrons and VLDL are mixed in the blood and thus compete for the same lipolytic pathway [13]. It has been shown that endogenous triglyceride-rich lipoproteins accumulate in human plasma after fat intake [14–16], but the mechanism behind this phenomenon is not obvious since both an enhanced synthesis and an attenuated lipolysis of VLDL have to be considered. Importantly, the increase in the number of triglyceride-rich apoB100 containing lipoprotein particles after fat intake is far greater than that of apoB48 containing lipoproteins. Schneeman et al. [16] showed that 80% of the increase in particle number was accounted for by particles containing apoB100. Similar results were obtained independently and by Karpe et al. [15] and Cohn et al. [14]. Interestingly, the increase was confined to the population of large VLDL particles, whereas the plasma concentration of small VLDL did not change in response to oral fat intake [15]. Conversely, 80% of the postprandial increase of triglycerides was accounted for by lipoproteins containing apoB48 [17]. The increase of cholesterol in the triglyceride-rich lipoprotein fraction was, on the other hand, accounted for by VLDL [16], i.e., up to 90% of the increase of cholesterol in the triglyceride-rich lipoprotein fraction after a fat meal was explained by the elevation of VLDL particle number. Cholesteryl esters are transferred from HDL, and perhaps from LDL, to VLDL in exchange for triglycerides. The exchange mechanism is dependent on the concentration of acceptor lipoprotein particles and on the concentration of cholesterol ester transfer protein (CETP). Several reports testify that the transfer of cholesteryl esters from HDL to the triglyceride-rich lipoprotein fraction is enhanced during alimentary lipemia [18,19]. As a result HDL is depleted of cholesterol whereas HDL particle concentration measured as apoA-I-containing lipoprotein particles with and without apoA-II is unaffected by a fat meal [20]. Furthermore, Mann et al. [21] have shown that the exchange of cholesteryl esters is enhanced with increasing plasma triglyceride levels in normotriglyceridemic plasma, in contrast to hypertriglyceridemic plasma, in which the excess of acceptor lipoprotein is sufficient to allow CETP to be the rate-limiting factor for the exchange of core lipids. It is therefore likely that the massive increase in the number of potential acceptor lipoprotein particles for cholesteryl esters in the postprandial state determines the amount of cholesterol recovered in the VLDL fraction of fasting plasma samples. Accordingly, the contribution of cholesterol-rich chylomicron remnant particles is limited in alimentary lipemia, compared with the VLDL remnants. This should be taken into consideration when an evaluation of the association between postprandial lipoproteins and development of coronary atherosclerosis is attempted.

Remnants of triglyceride-rich lipoproteins and CAD

Quantification of postprandial triglyceride-rich lipoproteins is a major methodological challenge. Many researchers have made use of the chylomicron-specific transport route for vitamin A. After ingestion, vitamin A is to a large extent incorporated into chylomicron particles as retinyl esters, mainly retinyl palmitate (RP) [22]. In human plasma, only minor amounts of RP are exchanged between lipoproteins. Instead, a major proportion of RP stays within the chylomicron until it is taken up by the liver. In fact, there were no signs of exchange of RP between chylomicrons and VLDL in a Type I hyperlipidemic patient [23]. The high specificity of RP as a marker for chylomicrons and chylomicrons remnants was also indicated by the minute amounts of retinoids present in the LDL fraction after vitamin A ingestion [24]. However, a few studies have questioned the applicability of RP as a means of quantifying intestinally derived triglyceride-rich lipoproteins. First, Krasinski et al. [25] have shown that the postprandial RP pattern in plasma does not always coincide with the postprandial triglyceride pattern and that a substantial proportion of the plasma RP at late time-points after oral fat intake is found in the LDL fraction. Second, we have found that the postprandial elevations of apoB48 and RP in fractions of triglyceride-rich lipoproteins do not coincide, and that there are many more RP molecules per apoB48 molecule in the largest (Sf >400 fraction) particles compared with the smaller ones (Sf 60—400 and Sf 20—60 fractions) [26]. Third, separation of apoB100-containing lipoproteins from apoB48 lipoproteins by immuno-affinity chromatography indicates that RP is found in VLDL (apoB100-containing lipoproteins), in particular at late time points after oral fat intake [17]. It should therefore be emphasized that RP is a marker of chylomicrons and their remnants with only limited specificity. These recent findings suggest that the interpretation of clinical studies using RP measurements after a fat load is confounded by the transfer of RP to apoB100-containing lipoproteins.

A second and nowadays neglected way of quantifying postprandial triglyceride-rich lipoproteins is the simple determination of plasma triglycerides. Peak plasma triglycerides after fat intake have been shown to reflect above all the fasting plasma level, but the triglyceride concentration measured at late time points after an oral fat load seems to be a potential discriminator for the presence of CAD [27]. It could therefore be argued that plasma triglycerides measured at late time-points after fat intake might reflect a kind of fat intolerance that is of clinical importance.

In humans, specific quantification of chylomicron and chylomicron remnants can be achieved only by direct determination of the plasma concentrations of apoB48. A method for specific quantification of apoB48 and apoB100 has been described by Poapst et al. [28]. Zilversmit et al. [29] also evaluated the quantification of apoB48 and apoB100 using sodium dodecyl sulphate polyacrylamide gel electrophoresis (SDS-PAGE), gel scanning and radio-iodination. We have adopted a similar approach [30], which clearly shows that overloading of apoB100 on the analytical SDS-PAGE gel is the principal cause of analytical problems.

As previously discussed in detail it has become apparent that the apoB100-containing triglyceride-rich lipoproteins constitute an overwhelming majority of the apoB-containing lipoproteins present in the postprandial state [15,16,26,30]. Chylomicrons and chylomicron remnants account for 10 or at most 20% of the total increase of triglyceride-rich lipoprotein particles after fat intake. In addition, it has become apparent that the postprandial state modulates both the metabolism and composition of the apoB100-containing lipoprotein particles [15]. It is therefore justified to include VLDL remnants in discussing the importance of remnant lipoproteins in CAD progression. Two studies suggest an association between elevated postprandial levels of chylomicron remnants and the presence of CAD. First, Simons et al. [31] showed that the enrichment of apoB48 relative to apoB100 in the Sf > 60 lipoprotein fraction sampled 4 h after fat intake was significantly greater among CAD patients than with controls. Unfortunately, the results of this study are difficult to interpret since there was also a significant difference in baseline plasma triglycerides. The difference found in the 4-h sample, which would coincide with the peak plasma triglyceride level, is therefore just as likely to reflect the baseline difference between the groups. Second, we have shown that the postprandial concentrations of small chylomicron remnants (apoB48 in the Sf 20—60 lipoprotein fraction) after a mixed-meal type of oral fat tolerance test correlates with the 5-year progression of coronary atherosclerosis in young postinfarction patients as determined by repeated coronary angiography [32]. Unfortunately, the patients in this study were highly selected. First, females and patients with severe hyperlipoproteinemia were not investigated. Second, a certain number of patients died in the course of the follow-up period. It is also evident from this study that apoB48-containing lipoproteins constitute only a very small fraction of the total population of triglyceride-rich lipoproteins in plasma. Interestingly, an investigation of a similar patient group [33] revealed that both the triglyceride concentration in small dense LDL and the number of cholesteryl ester molecules in small VLDL particles were linked to the severity of coronary lesions in a larger group of unselected young postinfarction males. Similarly, Phillips et al. [34] have suggested that 'VLDL remnants' are linked to progression of CAD. Furthermore, the MARS study, which is an angiographic, randomized, double-blind, placebo-controlled 2-year trial of lovastatin monotherapy, indicates that triglyceride-rich lipoproteins are specifically linked to progression of mild to moderate coronary lesions [35].

In all, future clinical studies of the association between postprandial lipoproteins and CAD should include more than measurement of chylomicron remnants. In terms of the production of potentially atherogenic remnant lipoproteins after fat intake, the apoB100-containing lipoproteins seem to be of major importance. Furthermore, hypertriglyceridemia, in particular prolonged alimentary lipemia, has been hypothesized to be a hypercoagulable condition [36].

Acknowledgements

This study was supported by grants from the Swedish Medical Research Council (8691), the Swedish Heart-Lung foundation the King Gustaf V 80th Birthday Fund, the Professor Nanna Svartz´ Fund, the Nordic Insulin Foundation and the Swedish Margarine Industry Fund for Research on Nutrition.

References

1. Nestel PJ. J Clin Invest 1964;43:943–949.
2. Simpson HS, Williamson CM, Olivecrona T, Pringle S, Maclean J, Lorimer AR, Bonnefous F, Bogaievsky Y, Packard CJ, Shepherd J. Atherosclerosis 1990;85:193–202.
3. Groot PHE, van Stiphout WAHJ, Krauss XH, Jansen H, van Tol A, van Ramshorst E, Chin-On S, Hofman A, Cresswell SR, Havekes L. Arterioscler Thromb 1991;11:653–662.
4. Kane JP, Hardman DA, Paulus HE. Proc Natl Acad Sci USA 1980;77:2465–2469.
5. Chan L. J Biol Chem 1992;267:25621–25624.
6. Hoeg JM, Sviridov DD, Tennysson GE, Demosky Jr SJ, Meng MS, Bojanovski D, Safonova IG, Repin VS, Kuberger MB, Smirnov VN, Higuchi K, Gregg RE, Brewer Jr HB. J Lipid Res 1990;31:1761–1769.
7. Patsch J. Baillière's Clin Endocrinol Metab 1987;1:551–580.
8. Hazzard WR, Bierman EL. Metabolism 1976;25:777–801.
9. Karpe F, Olivecrona T, Walldius G, Hamsten A. J Lipid Res 1992;33:975–984.
10. Saxena U, Witte LD, Goldberg IJ. J Biol Chem. 1989;264:4349–4355.
11. Peterson J, Bihain BE, Bengtsson-Olivecrona G, Deckelbaum RJ, Carpentier YA, Olivecrona T. Proc Natl Acad Sci USA 1990;87:909–913.
12. Sniderman AD, Cianflone K. Arterioscler Thromb 1993;13:629–636.
13. Brunzell JD, Hazzard WR, Porte Jr D, Bierman EL. J Clin Invest 1973;52:1578–1585.
14. Cohn JS, McNamara JR, Cohn SD, Ordovas JM, Schaefer EJ. J Lipid Res 1988;29:925–936.
15. Karpe F, Steiner G, Olivecrona T, Carlson LA, Hamsten A. J Clin Invest 1993;91:748–759.
16. Schneeman, BO, Kotite L, Todd KM, Havel RJ. Proc Natl Acad Sci USA 1993;90:2069–2073.
17. Cohn JS, Johnson EJ, Millar JS, Cohn SD, Milne RW, Marcel YL, Russel RM, Schaefer EJ. J Lipid Res 1993;34:2033–2040.
18. Eisenberg S. J Lipid Res 1985;26:487–494.
19. Dullaart RPF, Groener JEM, van Wijk H, Sluiter WJ, Erkelens DW. Arteriosclerosis 1989;9:614–622.
20. Karpe F, Bard J-M, Steiner G, Carlson LA, Fruchart J-C, Hamsten A. Arterioscler Thromb 1993;13:11–22.
21. Mann CJ, Yen FT, Grant AM, Bihain BE. J Clin Invest 1991;88:2059–2066.
22. Goodman DS. Fed Proc 1980;39:2716–2722.

23. Sprecher DL, Knauer SL, Black DM, Kaplan LA, Akeson AA, Dusing M, Lattier D, Stein EA, Rymaszewski M, Wiginton DA. J Clin Invest 1991;88:985−994.
24. Wilson DE, Chan I-F, Ball M. Metabolism 1983;32:514−520.
25. Krasinski SD, Cohn JS, Russel RM, Schaefer EJ. Metabolism 1990;39:357−365.
26. Karpe F, Bell M, Björkegren J, Hamsten A. Quantification of postprandial triglyceride-rich lipoproteins in healthy men by retinyl ester labelling and simultaneous measurement of apolipoproteins B-48 and B-100. Arterioscler Thromb (in press).
27. Patsch JR, Miesenböck G, Hopferwieser T, Mühlberger V, Knapp E, Dunn JK, Gotto AM, Patsch W. Arterioscler Thromb 1992;12:1336−1345.
28. Poapst M, Uffelman K, Steiner G. Atherosclerosis 1987;65:75−88.
29. Zilversmit DB, Shea TM. J Lipid Res 1989;30:1639−1646.
30. Karpe F, Hamsten A. J Lipid Res 1994;35:1311−1317.
31. Simons LA, Dwyer T, Simons J, Bernstein P, Mock P, Poonia NS, Balasubramaniam S, Baron D, Branson J, Morgan J, Roy P. Atherosclerosis 1987;65:181−189.
32. Karpe F, Steiner G, Uffelman K, Olivecrona T, Hamsten A. Atherosclerosis 1994;106:83−97.
33. Tornvall P, Båvenholm P, Landou C, de Faire U, Hamsten A. Circulation 1993;88(part 1):2180−2189.
34. Phillips NR, Waters D, Havel RJ. Circulation 1993;88:2762−2770.
35. Hodis HN, Mack WJ, Azen SP, Alaupovic P, Pogoda JM, LaBree L, Hemphill LC, Kramsch DM, Blankenhorn DH. Circulation 1994;90:42−49.
36. Hamsten A. Thromb Res 1993;70:1−38.

Measurement of remnant-like particle-cholesterol in human serum with a mixed immunoaffinity gel

K. Nakajima[1] and H. Nakamura[2]

[1]*Japan Immunoresearch Laboratories Co., Ltd.; and* [2]*First Department of Int. Med. National Defence Medical College, Gunma, Japan*

Abstract. A simple, rapid assay method has been developed for the determination of serum remnant-like particles using an immunoaffinity gel mixture of anti apoB100 and apoA-I antibodies coupled to sepharose 4B. A monoclonal antibody to apoB100 (JI-H) with unique epitope was used to absorb LDL and VLDL from serum and a monoclonal antibody to apoA-I to remove HDL and chylomicrons. Lipoproteins not bound to the mixed gel were characterized as chylomicron- and VLDL-remnant-like particles and were quantified by assay of cholesterol. Serum levels of remnant-like particle-cholesterol (RLP-C) were determined in normolipidemic subjects and patients with familial dysbetalipoproteinemia, coronary heart disease and related diseases.

Monoclonal antibodies against apolipoproteins have been very useful in studies of lipoprotein structure, heterogeneity and function and it is very likely that some Mabs will selectively detect lipoprotein subpopulations of clinical interest. However, isolation of such a subpopulation from unfractionated blood plasma has not yet been reported. Here we describe the use of an immunoaffinity gel — a mixture of anti apoB100 and apoA-I Mabs coupled to Sepharose 4B — to separate a subpopulation of triglyceride-rich particles in the unbound fraction enriched in apoE. This subpopulation includes all of the apoB, as well as some of the apoB100 of the triglyceride-rich lipoproteins which are not recognized by the unique anti-apoB100 Mab named JI-H [1,2]. By adding an anti-apoA-I affinity gel to the anti-apoB100 gel, we were able to adsorb almost all of the apoA-I-containing lipoproteins onto the mixed gel.

Because characteristics of the lipoproteins that did not bind to the anti-apoB100 immunoaffinity gel suggested that they resemble chylomicron and VLDL remnants, we have called them remnant-like particles (RLP) [2]. For the quantification of RLP, assay of total cholesterol was shown to be the most accurate and easy to handle. A very sensitive assay for cholesterol is used because RLP-cholesterol varies from 5–200 mg/dl.

Materials and Methods

419 healthy volunteers, 139 subjects with diabetes and 120 with coronary artery disease (at least one lesion with >50% stenosis by coronary angiography) were studied, as well as a total of 1,153 subjects undergoing routine examinations. In normolipidemic and hyperlipidemic patients, all sera or EDTA plasmas were obtained in the postabsorptive state (9–15 h after the last meal), separated by immediate centrifugation at 2,000 × g for 30 min at 4°C, and subsequently kept at 4°C until analyzed within 5 days.

5 mg of anti-apoB100 and anti-apoA-I (IgG) were each coupled to 1 ml of CNBr-

Address for correspondence: Katsuyuki Nakajima, Japan Immunoresearch Laboratories Co., Ltd., 351-1 Nishi-Yokote cho, Takasaki Gunma 370, Japan.

Sepharose 4B gel. Serum samples (100 μl) were applied to 1 ml (1.0 × 2.5 cm) columns of mixed gels and the unbound fraction was eluted with 3.5 ml of 10 mM phosphate buffer (pH 7.2). The bound lipoproteins were then eluted with 1.0 M acetic acid/0.5 M NaCl. The unbound and bound fractions were separated by ultracentrifugation at a density of 1.21 g/ml and both were analyzed by SDS-polyacrylamide gel electrophoresis.

10 μl of serum or plasma was added to 600 μl of mixed gel suspension solution which contained 50 μl of apoB100 gel (250 μg of IgG) and 50 μl of apoA-I gel (250 μg of IgG).This reaction mixture was gently shaken for 60 min at room temperature to assure complete mixing. Then the test tubes were allowed to stand for 10 min and 30 μl or an adequate amount of the supernatant (unbound lipoproteins) was withdrawn to assay cholesterol with a diagnostic kit (Merko test). High-performance liquid chromatography (HPLC) was carried out according to Hara and Okazaki [3].

The electrophoretic mobilities of plasma lipoproteins and the fractions bound and unbound to the immunoaffinity gel were determined using 1% agarose gel (CIBA-Corning) in 0.074 M barbital buffer (pH 8.6) for 90 min at 25°C and 60 V. Agarose gels were stained with Sudan Black B (0.1%) in 60% ethanol and washed three times with 50% ethanol.

The size of lipoprotein particles was measured by a negative staining procedure. The grids were exposed to 3% phosphotungstic acid (pH 7.1) for 2 min. The samples were photographed with a JEOL-100CX (JEOL, Tokyo, Japan) electron microscope.

Results

Characterization of monoclonal antibodies and binding capacity of anti-apoA-I and anti-apoB100 immunoaffinity mixed gels

Mab anti-apoA-I (H-12) (IgG_1) reacted against a protein band with the molecular weight of apoA-I from serum, chylomicrons and HDL. The K_a value of anti-apoA-I was 4.2 × 10^8 l/mol. Mab anti-apoB100 (JI-H) (IgG_1) reacted with the apoB100 protein from serum, VLDL and LDL. The K_a value of anti-apoB100 was 5.5 × 108 l/mol, with equal reactivity to LDL and VLDL. The apoB specificity of JI-H was studied by immunoblotting using two VLDL samples that contained apoB100 and apoB48. JI-H reacted with apoB100, but not with apoB48, suggesting that this epitope is masked in the remnant-like particles.

The binding capacity of the anti-apoA-I and anti-apoB100 immunoaffinity mixed gels was determined by immunoaffinity chromatography. 1 ml of immunoaffinity mixed gels was used in a column (1.0 × 2.5 cm) for immunoadsorption capacity tests. The capacity was determined by running increasing amounts of HDL or LDL and measuring cholesterol and apolipoprotein (apoA-I and apoB100) bound after each run. Subsequent runs were performed with a column ratio of serum/mixed gels of 1:10 (volume) in which the amounts of apoA-I or apoB100 applied were <50% of the total column capacity.

Identification of unbound lipoproteins

From the electron photomicrographs obtained in normal and hyperlipidemic subjects, the unbound fraction seemed to consist mainly of particles (diameter 30–80 nm) in the range of very low density lipoproteins. HPLC analysis of unbound lipoproteins in 2 normal, 1 hypertriglyceridemic and 5 diabetic patients confirmed that they consisted mainly of lipoproteins of VLDL size. Figure 1 is the elution profile of RLP in a Type III patient, showing CM- as well as VLDL-sized particles. Agarose electrophoresis of unbound lipoproteins (d < 1.006 g/ml) showed β or slow pre-β mobility, while bound (d < 1.006

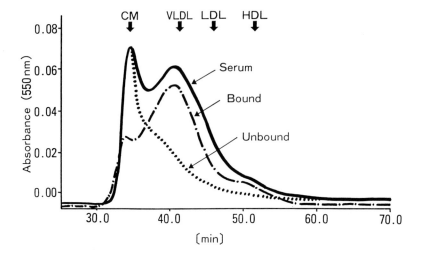

Fig. 1. Elution profiles of serum lipoprotein-cholesterol (solid line), unbound (RLP) (dotted line), and bound (dashed line) from a Type III patient by HPLC using a G5000 PW column (Toso). Elution times for chylomicrons (CM), VLDL, LDL are indicated by arrows.

g/ml) and normal (d < 1.006 g/ml) VLDL showed fast pre-β mobility.

These unbound lipoproteins of d < 1.006 g/ml in both Type III and other hyper-lipidemic patients were found to be enriched in apoE (Table 1) and contained essentially all of the apoB48 as well as some of the apoB100 of triglyceride-rich lipoproteins. It was concluded that they consist of chylomicron and VLDL remnant-like particles (RLP).

Immunoadsorption assay method

60 min for the antigen–antibody reaction was found to be a sufficient incubation time at room temperature. Shaking conditions were found to be optimal at a speed of 60 times/min. RLP-C values were stable when sera or plasmas were stored for 5 days at 4°C, but after 1 week in storage, there was a gradual increase of RLP-C. Serial 5- and 10-fold

Table 1. Composition of RLP (unbound VLDL) and bound VLDL to immunoaffinity mixed gels from three patients with Type III hyperlipoproteinamia

	Unbound VLDL (RLP)	Bound VLDL
Free cholesterol (FC)	8.6 ± 1.9	14.7 ± 3.2
Cholesteryl ester (CE)	10.8 ± 2.5	11.0 ± 2.8
Triglyceride	62.8 ± 4.6	49.1 ± 5.0
Phospholipid	13.0 ± 3.2	19.4 ± 4.6
Protein	4.8 ± 0.9	5.8 ± 1.0
Mass ratio		
CE:apoB × 10⁻³	4.3 ± 0.15[a]	3.5 ± 0.13
ApoE:apoB	8.3 ± 0.39[a]	4.4 ± 0.29
Diameter (Å)	452 ± 60	346 ± 32

Values are mean ± SD (weight %).
[a]p < 0.01, [b]p < 0.001 by Student's t-test vs. Mass ratios of bound VLDL.

dilution of sera from 5 diabetic patients showed the linearity of the RLP-C assay. The mean values and within-run assay coefficients of variation for the RLP-C assay were 10.3 mg/dl (4.5%), 46 mg/dl (3.7%) and 107.3 mg/dl (3.5%). Between-day assay coefficients of variation were 5.0%, 3.3% and 4.6%, respectively. The lowest concentration of cholesterol that could be measured in this RLP-C assay was 1.5 mg/dl.

RLP-C concentrations in healthy subjects and patients with coronary heart disease (CHD)

The mean ($\pm$ SD) serum concentration of RLP-C in 419 male and female healthy subjects (ages 10–80) with serum TG levels < 150 mg/dl was 2.1 $\pm$ 2.9 mg/dl. The upper value of the RLP-C range was statistically determined (95% percentile range) to be 5 mg/dl by an iterative truncation analysis. An abnormal RLP-C concentration (> 5 mg/dl) was found in 12.5% of 1153 Japanese subjects who underwent a physical check-up. An abnormal concentration was twice as frequent in men as in women and the frequency of abnormal values tended to increase with age. Among the group of 120 patients with coronary heart disease (at least one lesion with > 50% stenosis by coronary angiography) whose serum TG level was less than 150 mg/dl, the prevalence of an abnormal RLP-C concentration was much higher (44.7%) than in healthy subjects with similar TG levels (5.2%). High serum RLP-C levels in patients with various diseases are shown in Fig. 2. Probucol treatment showed a significant decrease of serum RLP-C in diabetic patients (Fig. 3).

Discussion

To ensure that we were not overloading the gel, we routinely applied serum at < 50% of the total gel capacity in this study. Because analysis of the unbound lipoproteins by SDS-PAGE showed apoB100 to be the predominant apolipoprotein component, we used the Mab anti-apoB100 gel to characterize the unbound fraction in detail. The K_a and reactivity with normal VLDL of anti-apoB100 (JI-H) was sufficiently high for useful immunoad-

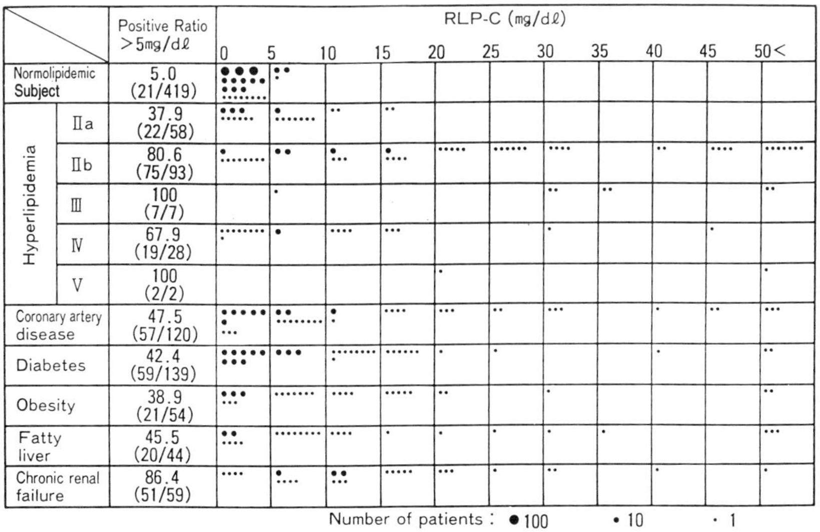

		Positive Ratio >5mg/dℓ	RLP-C (mg/dℓ) 0	5	10	15	20	25	30	35	40	45	50<
Normolipidemic Subject		5.0 (21/419)	•••• :••										
Hyperlipidemia	IIa	37.9 (22/58)	:••:	•.......	••	••							
	IIb	80.6 (75/93)	•........	••	•:...	•:...	••••••	•••••••	••••		••	••••	••••••••
	III	100 (7/7)		•					••	••			••
	IV	67.9 (19/28)	:........	•	••••	•••			•			•	
	V	100 (2/2)			•						•		
Coronary artery disease		47.5 (57/120)	•••••• •••	:•:........	•	••••	•••	••	•••	•	••	•••	
Diabetes		42.4 (59/139)	••••••• •••	•••	:.........	•••••••	•	•		•		••	
Obesity		38.9 (21/54)	:••	••••••••	••••	••••••	••		•			••	
Fatty liver		45.5 (20/44)	:•.	•••••••••	••••	•	•	•	•	•		•••	
Chronic renal failure		86.4 (51/59)	••••	•:...	:•:	••••••	•••	•	••		•	•	

Number of patients : • 100   • 10   · 1

Fig. 2. Serum RLP-C levels in hyperlipidemia, coronary artery disease, diabetes mellitus, obesity, fatty liver and chronic renal failure.

198

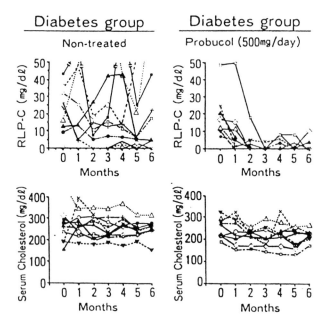

Fig. 3. Probucol effect on serum RLP-C levels for 6 months in diabetic patients. Untreated control patients (n = 8) with initial serum RLP-C levels exceeding 5 mg/dl.

sorption [2]. We found that this unbound VLDL fraction was related primarily to the differential immunoreactivity of Mab JI-H and consisted mainly of chylomicrons and VLDL remnant-like particles [1,2]. We added an anti-apoA-I immunoaffinity gel to eliminate HDL and any chylomicrons that contained this protein and selected cholesterol as the marker of RLP because of the sensitivity of the cholesterol assay and the wide use of cholesterol measurement to estimate atherosclerotic risk.

Yamada et al. [4] have reported that apoE-rich VLDL are normally removed rapidly into the liver of rabbits by receptor-mediated endocytosis, whereas RLP detected by our method tended to accumulate in the blood. We have found, however, that the unbound particles, although rich in apoE, do not have a very high affinity for the LDL receptor [1] while RLP from fasting diabetic patients significantly increases incorporation of ^{14}C-oleate into lipids in mouse peritoneal macrophages [5]. The factors that regulate the plasma concentration of RLP in health and disease are currently unclear, but may include those that influence the conformation of apoE on the particles or receptor for it or the activity of hepatic lipase [6].

Reference values for RLP-C based on 419 healthy normolipidemic subjects proved less than 5 mg/dl. Older subjects have somewhat higher serum levels of RLP-C than younger subjects. Although males and females of the same age range had similar values, in a random population men had a higher percentage of abnormal values than women. In normotriglyceridemic healthy subjects, 5.2% had an abnormal RLP-C level, whereas almost 50% of the normotriglyceridemic patient group with CHD had an abnormal level. This observation strongly suggests that the RLP-C level may vary independently of serum triglyceride and also cholesterol concentration; it responded dramatically to the lipid-lowering drug probucol (Fig. 3).

RLP-C levels are particularly high in familial dysbetalipoproteinemia [2,7,8] and very high levels would strongly suggest this diagnosis, which should be confirmed by apoE phenotyping or genotyping [9].

Triglyceride-rich lipoproteins probably contain both atherogenic and nonatherogenic particles [10]. The RLP-C assay reported here provides a measure of particles with β or slow pre-β mobility by agarose electrophoresis that are most likely to be atherogenic [1,2]. Further studies are needed to evaluate the relationship of serum RLP-C levels to CHD risk.

Acknowledgements

We thank Dr R. Havel, University of California, San Francisco and Dr N. Yamada, Tokyo University for valuable discussions.

References

1. Campos E, Nakajima K, Tanaka A, Havel RJ. J Lipid Res 1992;33:369—380.
2. Nakajima K, Saito T, Tamura A et al. Clin Chim Acta 1993;53—71.
3. Hara I. Okazaki M. Methods Enzymol 1986;129:57—78.
4. Yamada N, Shames DH, Stoudemire JB, Havel RJ. Proc Natl Acad Sci USA 1986;83:3479—3483.
5. Shimoyama M, Kanatani K, Saito T et al. J Jap Atheroscler Soc 1991;19:542.
6. Murase T, Itakura H. Atherosclerosis 1981;39:293—300.
7. Havel RJ, Kane JP. Proc Natl Acad Sci USA 1973;70:2015—2019.
8. Nakajima K, Saito T, Tamura A et al. J Atheroscler Thromb 1994;1:30—36.
9. Utermann G, Hees M, Steinmez A. Nature 1977;269:604—607.
10. Havel RJ. Clin Exp Hypertension 1989;11:887—900.

Postprandial remnant-like particles and coronary artery disease

K. Ikewaki[1,2], H. Shige[1], K. Nakajima[3] and H. Nakamura[1]

[1]First Department of Internal Medicine, National Defense Medical College, Tokorozawa, Saitama; [2]Mitsuke City Hospital, Niigata; and [3]Japan Immunoresearch Lab. Co., Ltd., Gunma, Japan

Abstract. The objective of this study was to assess the role of postprandial remnant-like particles (RLP) in coronary artery disease (CAD). 15 angiographically defined normolipidemic CAD patients underwent a fat-loading test. Postprandial RLP-C (cholesterol) were increased (levels >5 mg/dl) in 93% of CAD patients but in only 80% of control subjects. Multivariate analysis revealed that postprandial RLP was the major factor contributing to CAD in our study subjects. In a second study, eicosapentaenoic acid administered to seven normolipidemic CAD patients reduced postprandial RLP-C levels. We suggest that the determination of postprandial RLP-C is a novel method to assess potential susceptibility to CAD and the effect of lipid-lowering drugs on postprandial lipid metabolism.

Although the lipid profile in the fasting state has been used to determine the risk of cardiovascular disease, people spend much of their time in the postprandial state. After a meal, triglyceride-rich apoB-containing lipoproteins are secreted from intestine and liver, both of which are then hydrolyzed by the action of lipoprotein lipase to generate remnant lipoproteins. Remnant lipoprotein particles have been shown to deposit on the arterial wall [1]. Type III hyperlipoproteinemia due to dysfunctional apoEs (apoE2 or variant apoE), in which cholesterol-rich remnants accumulate in the plasma, predisposes to premature atherosclerosis [2]. Furthermore, it has recently been conclusively shown in apoE knockout mice that the accumulation of remnants causes atherosclerotic lesions [3,4]. Despite the potential importance of remnant lipoproteins, methods of analyzing postprandial lipemia have been poorly developed, mainly because of the complexity of apoB-containing lipoprotein fractions. We have developed a simple, rapid method for the determination of serum remnant-like particles (RLP) utilizing anti-apoB100 and anti-apoA-I antibodies linked to immunoaffinity gels [5]. We have now investigated postprandial RLP metabolism in normolipidemic CAD patients using this method.

Postprandial RLP metabolism in normolipidemic CAD patients

Fifteen angiographically defined normolipidemic CAD patients underwent a fat and vitamin A loading test. Chylomicron and chylomicron remnants were isolated by ultra-centrifugation. Plasma and lipoprotein lipids, retinyl palmitate, and RLP-C concentrations were determined up to 12 h after the fat ingestion. Peaks of plasma triglyceride and retinyl palmitate concentrations were delayed and their concentrations were significantly higher in CAD patients than in control subjects. Postprandial RLP-C are shown in Fig. 1. RLP-C levels were markedly higher in the CAD group, in whom RLP were not completely removed from the circulation 12 h after the fat ingestion. Postprandial RLP-C were present at levels > 5 mg/dl in 93% of CAD patients, whereas the majority of control

Address for correspondence: Katsunori Ikewaki MD, First Department of Internal Medicine, National Defense Medical College, 3-2 Namiki, Tokorozawa, Saitama, Japan.

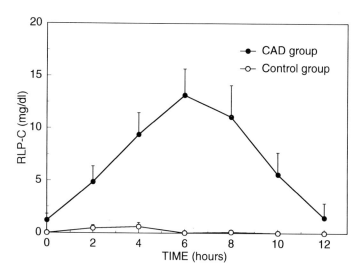

Fig. 1. Postprandial RLP-C levels in CAD group (n = 15, closed circles) and in control group (n = 15, open circles) after fat ingestion. Data are given as the mean ± SEM.

subjects (80%) remained RLP-negative. Multivariate analysis revealed that postprandial RLP-C was the major factor contributing to CAD in our study subjects (partial correlation coefficient 0.76).

Effect of eicosapentaenoic acid (EPA) on postprandial RLP metabolism

EPA was administered to 7 normolipidemic CAD patients. Postprandial RLP-C levels were significantly decreased by EPA (Fig. 2), even though the steady-state (fasting) triglyceride levels were unchanged, which indicates that EPA preferentially improved the postprandial lipemia in these subjects.

Discussion

It has been proposed that postprandial lipemia may contribute to the development of coronary atherosclerosis, but the atherogenicity of remnant lipoproteins has not been established. Nakajima et al. [5] have reported an increased level of RLP-C in patients with diabetes, obesity, and CAD. RLP have been shown to be rich in cholesterol, apoE, and apoB48, consistent with chylomicron remnants [5–7]. In the present study, we found that RLP-C accumulates after a fat meal in the CAD patient group despite normal fasting lipid levels, indicating that impaired metabolism of remnant lipoproteins may result in the development of CAD. Simons et al. [8] correspondingly reported that the postprandial apoB48/apoB100 ratio was higher in CAD patients and an independent risk factor for CAD. In the current study, we studied chylomicron remnant metabolism using vitamin A as a tracer and observed both high levels of chylomicron remnant and delayed clearance, consistent with the hypothesis of impaired remnant metabolism. In the second study, we investigated the effect of EPA on postprandial RLP metabolism. Interestingly, although EPA did not modulate the steady-state (fasting) triglyceride levels, postprandial RLP metabolism was found to be accelerated by EPA, which suggests that EPA may preferentially correct the impaired postprandial remnants metabolism.

202

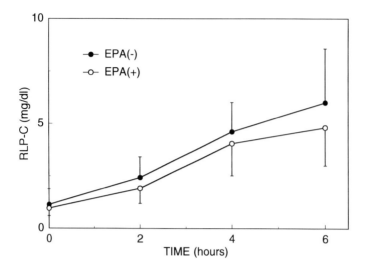

Fig. 2. Effect of eicosapentaenoic acid on postprandial RLP-C levels in 7 normolipidemic CAD patients. Data are given as the mean ± SEM.

References

1. Zilversmit DB. Circulation 1979;60:473–485.
2. Mahley RW. Science 1988;240:622–630.
3. Zhang SH, Reddick RL, Piedrahita JA, Maeda N. Science 1993;258:468–471.
4. Plump AS, Smith JD, Hayek T, Aalto-Setala K, Walsh A, Verstuyft JG, Rubin EM, Breslow JL. Cell 1993; 71:343–353.
5. Nakajima K, Saito T, Tamura A, Suzuki M, Nakano T, Adachi M, Tanaka A, Tada N, Nakamura H, Campos E, Havel RJ. Clin Chim Acta 1993;223:53–71 (see also previous paper).
6. Campos E, Nakajima K, Tanaka A, Havel RJ. J Lipid Res 1992;33:369–380.
7. Schneeman BO, Kotite L, Todd KM, Havel RJ. Proc Natl Acad Sci USA 1993;90: 2069–2073.
8. Simons LA, Dwyer T, Simons J. et al. Atherosclerosis 1987;65:181–188.

Free radicals and oxidative modification of LDL: role of natural antioxidants

H. Esterbauer, S. Gieseg, A. Giessauf, O. Ziouzenkova and P. Ramos

Institute of Biochemistry, University of Graz, Schubertstr. 1, A-8010 Graz, Austria

LDL oxidation is a lipid peroxidation process, so that initiation-preventing and chain-breaking antioxidants should have a major impact not only on the oxidation resistance of LDL but perhaps also on the development of atherosclerosis. The most frequently used assay to assess in vitro oxidation resistance of LDL is the measurement of conjugated dienes with copper ions as pro-oxidant. Vitamin E supplementation and an oleate-rich diet increase the oxidation resistance of LDL, whereas β-carotene supplementation has no effect. Ascorbate has a dual effect: it inhibits LDL oxidation by recycling vitamin E, but it probably also acts as a preventative antioxidant by scavenging initiating radicals.

Antioxidants in LDL

An LDL particle contains in total approximately 2,200 cholesterol molecules (free and esterified), and the total number of fatty acids bound in the different lipid classes is on average 2,600, roughly half of which are polyunsaturated fatty acids, mainly linoleic acid (1,100 mol/mol), arachidonic acid (150 mol/mol) and docosahexaenoic acid (29 mol/mol) [1]. LDL is therefore not only rich in cholesterol but also in polyunsaturated fatty acids known to be highly susceptible to free-radical-initiated lipid peroxidation. Nature protects LDL by a number of antioxidants [1], by far the major one being α-tocopherol, of which on average about seven molecules are present in each LDL particle. Other potential antioxidants in LDL are γ-tocopherol, carotenoids (β-carotene, α-carotene, lycopene, cryptoxanthin, cantaxanthin, lutein, zeaxanthin, phytofluene), retinoids and ubiquinol-10. However, these are present in amounts some 10–300 times lower than α-tocopherol. Reported values for ubiquinol-10 (in mol/mol LDL) range from 0.09 [1], 0.32 [2], 0.54 ubiquinol + ubiquinone [3] to 0.5–1.2 [4]. Tribble et al. [5] reported 0.12 for buoyant and 0.07 mol ubiquinol/mol in dense LDL. Some investigators [4] assume that ubiquinol-10 is more important for protecting LDL against oxidation than α-tocopherol. It seems reasonable that other components of LDL can scavenge free radicals, including lipid radicals, and thereby affect the oxidation resistance of LDL. For example, plasmalogens were reported to act as antioxidants; an LDL particle contains on average 24 molecules of ethanolamine plasmalogen and 2 molecules of choline plasmalogen.

Mechanism of oxidation of LDL

LDL oxidation can be initiated in vitro by incubation with macrophages, smooth muscle cells and endothelial cells, or in cell-free systems utilizing a variety of pro-oxidants. Such powerful pro-oxidants are: lipoxygenase, peroxidase/H_2O_2, myeloperoxidase/H_2O_2/Cl$^-$, hemoglobin/H_2O_2, peroxynitrite, hypochlorite, native ceruloplasmin, UV-B-light, azo-compounds decomposing to free radicals (AAPH, AMVN), and Cu^{++} ions. The mechanism of initiation of LDL oxidation in vivo is largely a matter of speculation, and even in model systems the true nature of the initiating radicals X• is in many instances uncertain.

LDL oxidation possesses the general characteristics of lipid peroxidation reactions and three consecutive time phases can in most instances clearly be detected, i.e., the lag phase, propagation phase and decomposition phase. Thus it begins when an initiating radical X• abstracts a hydrogen atom from one of the polyunsaturated fatty acids LH contained in the LDL lipids (Fig. 1A). The rate of initiation R_i is essential for the whole peroxidation process. Once formed, the carbon-centered lipid radical L• reacts very quickly with molecular oxygen yielding a lipid peroxyl radical LOO•, which then abstracts with a certain rate constant k_p (p = propagation) a hydrogen atom from an adjacent LH to yield a lipid hydroperoxide and a new L• radical. It is this latter reaction, termed propagation, that causes the lipid peroxidation chain. The antioxidants in LDL, especially vitamin E (TOH) and ubiquinol-10, compete with chain propagation by scavenging LOO• radicals.

It is generally assumed that the tocopheroxyl radical TO• formed by the reaction of LOO• with TOH has only a very low reactivity and is not able to initiate a new chain by abstracting a hydrogen atom from LH according to LH + TO• → L• + TOH. However, one cannot ignore several observations [4] which suggest that under certain conditions (e.g., low rate of initiation) tocopherol-mediated propagation (TMP) may occur. A consistent finding of many laboratories is that at "normal" rates of initiation, producing lag times of about 10 min to several hours, the antioxidants in LDL slow down the propagation and thereby inhibit lipid peroxidation. If no recycling (e.g., by ascorbate) takes place the antioxidants are consumed in the sequence ubiquinol-10, vitamin E, oxycarotenoids and β-carotene. When LDL has lost most of its antioxidant compounds the propagation phase commences and the lipids in LDL are rapidly oxidized to lipid hydroperoxides (Fig. 1B). At this stage the only competing reaction is the termination by radical-radical combination: LOO• + LOO• → nonradical products (NRP) + O_2. This Russel mechanism leads to keto- and hydroxy fatty acids containing conjugated double bonds as end products. The propagation phase is finally followed by the decomposition phase, where the lipid hydroperoxides break down to a wide range of products including aldehydes, hydrocarbon

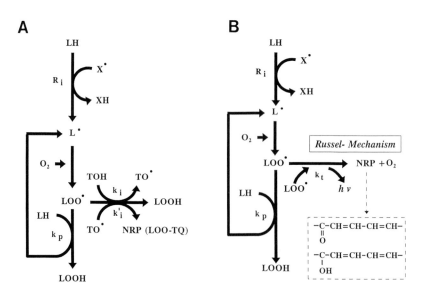

Fig. 1. Scheme showing the major events during inhibited (A) and uninhibited (B) oxidation of LDL. For abbreviations see text.

gases, epoxides, alcohols and others. Such a three-phase sequence has been demonstrated for the oxidation of LDL initiated by macrophages and copper ions and is probably common to all processes of LDL oxidation regardless of the method of initiation.

How to measure oxidation resistance of LDL

Oxidation resistance, susceptibility to oxidation, prone to oxidation are semantic terms which have never been clearly defined and up to now no general and broad consensus exists as to how oxidation resistance and/or protective effects of antioxidants should be measured [6]. In the recent literature, it appears that most laboratories consider oxidation resistance as a kinetic parameter described by the progress of the lipid peroxidation process. One such model to measure kinetic parameters that has become popular is copper-mediated oxidation (0.1 μM LDL in PBS, 10–50 μM Cu^{++}) in conjunction with continuous measurement of the conjugated diene absorption at 234 nm [1,6]. This model of LDL oxidation is highly reproducible, easy to perform and suitable for routine measurements. The oxidation indices which can readily be obtained from such measurements are: length of lag time where propagation is inhibited, rate of oxidation during the lag time, maximum rate of oxidation during propagation, and maximum amount of conjugated diene formed. About 25 papers have been published since 1993 using the measurement of conjugated dienes during copper-catalyzed oxidation for assessment of the oxidation resistance of LDL.

Effect of vitamin E, β-carotene and ascorbate on oxidation resistance of LDL

By means of the conjugated diene assay it can be shown that the LDL oxidation resistance varies widely amongst different subjects. We have found [1,7] that in healthy individuals the lag phase ranged from 33 to 138 min. This variation is caused partly by variations in the α-tocopherol content of LDL, but also depends on not yet clearly defined variables. In most studies, including ours [1,7], the α-tocopherol content or total antioxidant content (including carotenoids) were in themselves not predictive of the lag phase in healthy, not

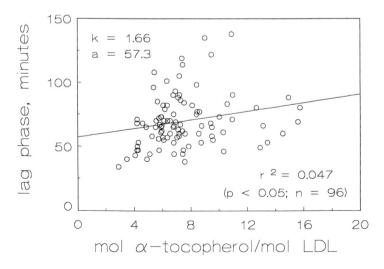

Fig. 2. Scatter plot showing the relationship between lag phase and α-tocopherol content of LDL from subjects not supplemented with vitamin E.

vitamin E-supplemented subjects (Fig. 2). Our screening revealed the relationship: lag (min) = $1.57x + 59.9$ ($r = 0.22$, $p < 0.05$, $n = 96$, x = mol α-tocopherol/mol LDL). This relationship is in close agreement with the report by Frei et al. [2].

To dissociate the effect of vitamin E from the protective effect of the other antioxidants, LDL from given donors was loaded with α-tocopherol by incubating plasma samples with increasing concentrations of α-tocopherol prior to the isolation of LDL. The α-tocopherol of a given LDL could be increased in this way several-fold, whilst all other properties of the LDL were probably not affected [1,7]. The oxidation resistance of such α-tocopherol-loaded LDL samples always increased strictly linearly ($r^2 = 0.96$) with the α-tocopherol content according to the equation $y = kx + a$, where y is the lag phase in minutes and x is mol α-tocopherol/mol LDL, k is an efficiency constant of α-tocopherol and a is a vitamin E-independent variable.

Values for the constants k and a in different subjects revealed wide individual variation $k = 4.39 \pm 3.05$ (SD) (range 0.7 to 17), and $a = 35.99 \pm 35.86$ min (range −68.6 to +108.6 min). This suggests large individual differences in the protective effects of vitamin E, persons with a large k value being good responders whereas those with low values respond only slightly. This relationship found for LDL loaded in vitro with vitamin E is also valid for oral vitamin E intake [8]. Daily doses of 150, 225, 800 or 1,200 IU RRR-α-tocopherol over 3 weeks increased the LDL α-tocopherol content to 138 ± 12, 158 ± 32, 144 ± 12 and $215 \pm 47\%$ of baseline values (= 100%), and the oxidation resistance (= lag phase) increased in parallel to 118 ± 17, 156 ± 22, 135 ± 23 and $175 \pm 21\%$ of baseline (= 100%). The increase of the lag phase was linearly correlated ($y = kx + a$) with the α-tocopherol content, with r^2 0.56–0.95. Mino et al. [9] found a strict linear correlation between the lag phase (T-inhibition) and the α-tocopherol content of LDL and HDL with AAPH-induced oxidation, and a similar observation was made by Thomas et al. [10].

The α-tocopherol content of a given LDL is, because of the strong individual variation of k and a, itself not predictive of the lag phase in Cu^{++}-initiated oxidation. However, on the basis of a large number of different LDL samples with different α-tocopherol contents (baseline values, supplemented in vitro or by oral intake) for which the oxidation resistance was determined, a statistical prediction is possible [7]. We now find a statistical correlation between lag phase (y) and LDL α-tocopherol content in mol/mol LDL (x) with the equation: $y = 2.94 x + 52.4$, $r^2 = 0.46$, $p < 0.001$, $n = 206$. On statistical average therefore, the lag phase with 6.88 mol vitamin E/mol LDL should be 72 min, and this agrees very well with the experimentally determined value of 67.5 ± 15.1 ($n = 76$). Statistically, vitamin E (α- + γ-tocopherol) contributes about 30% to the lag phase, whereas 70% is due to the vitamin E-independent variable. A similar relationship was found by Frei et al. [2].

It should be emphasized again that some subjects' LDL (with low or negative a value) depend solely on the protection by α-tocopherol. The contribution of vitamin E to the lag phase can range from less than 10% up to 100%. The finding that oral supplementation with vitamin E increased the oxidation resistance of LDL as measured by the lag phase has been confirmed by a number of other laboratories [11–15]. Supplementation studies with animals and humans further revealed that an oleate-rich diet increases oxidation resistance of LDL as measured by lag time and rate of propagation, whereas a linoleate-rich diet has the opposite effect [15–17].

Analysis of patients' LDL performed since 1993 show a decreased LDL oxidation resistance in patients with coronary artery disease [18,19], hypertensive patients [20,21], uremic patients [22] and cystic fibrosis patients [23,24]. De Graaf et al. [25] reported that dense LDL is more susceptible to copper oxidation than buoyant LDL, and Tribble et al.

Table 1. Effect of ascorbate on copper-mediated LDL oxidation

Time of ascorbate addition	Stage of oxidation	% residual vitamin E	Lag phase (min)	prolongation (min)
0	lag	100	146	80
12	lag	7	140	75
18	lag	0	148	83
36	lag	0	116	57
66	lag end	0	108	43
114	1/2 dienes	0	66	0
Control without ascorbate			65 ± 5	

Ascorbate added to 10 μM at the indicated minutes after initiation of oxidation by Cu^{++}.
LDL 0.1 μM, Cu^{++} 1.66 μM.

[5] found a highly significant correlation between oxidation resistance of LDL subfractions and their ubiquinol-10 and vitamin E content. Jialal et al. [26] and Lavy et al. [27] reported that loading LDL in vitro with β-carotene increases its oxidation resistance. However, all studies [28–30] on oral intake of β-carotene (15–60 mg/day over 2 weeks to 2 months) revealed that β-carotene enrichment of LDL does not increase its resistance to oxidation initiated by copper ions, AAPH or other pro-oxidants. In our study (unpublished), supplementation with daily doses of 30 mg of β-carotene over 2 weeks increased the LDL β-carotene about 5 times above baseline values, but without any effect on the oxidation resistance of LDL. Similarly, we were not able to increase oxidation resistance by increasing β-carotene in vitro 17-fold above baseline.

In vitro, ascorbate is a very potent inhibitor of LDL oxidation initiated either by AAPH or copper ions. One of the mechanisms involved is probably the well-known recycling of vitamin E in LDL mediated according to: TO• + ascorbate → TOH + ascorbyl radical. However, at least in copper-mediated oxidation, additional protective mechanisms must be considered. In our in vitro experiments in which ascorbate was added to a concentration of 10 μM at different stages of oxidation, there was an equal protective effect (prolongation of lag phase) in conditions when LDL was fully depleted of α-tocopherol (Table 1). This clearly indicates that ascorbate can protect, independently of vitamin E, perhaps by acting as a preventative antioxidant by scavenging initiating radicals X•.

Recent animal studies [31,32] with the synthetic antioxidant probucol demonstrate that the antioxidant resistance of LDL as measured by the lag time must be increased several-fold to reach a significant reduction in lesion size.

Acknowledgements

The authors' work has been supported by the Austrian Science Foundation project No. 7102 MED. Pilar Ramos is supported by a Lise-Meitner-Fellowship No. MO152-CHE from the Austrian Science Foundation.

References

1. Esterbauer H, Gebicki J, Puhl H, Jürgens G. Free Rad Biol Med 1992;13:341–390.
2. Frei B, Gaziano JM. J Lipid Res 1993;34:2135–2145.
3. Kontush A, Hübner C, Finckh B, Kohlschütter A, Beisiegel U. FEBS Lett 1994;341:69–73.
4. Bowry VW, Stocker R. J Am Chem Soc 1993;115:6029–6044.

208

5. Tribble DL, van den Berg JJM, Motchnik PA, Ames BN, Lewis DM, Chait A, Krauss RM. Proc Natl Acad Sci USA 1994;91:1183–1187.
6. Esterbauer H, Jürgens G. Curr Opin Lipid 1993;4:114–124.
7. Esterbauer H, Puhl H, Waeg G, Krebs A, Dieber-Rotheneder M. In: Packer L, Fuchs J (eds) Vitamin E in Health and Disease. New York: Marcel Dekker, 1992;649–671.
8. Dieber-Rotheneder M, Puhl H, Waeg G, Striegl G, Esterbauer H. J Lipid Res 1991;32:1325–1332.
9. Mino M, Miki M, Miyake M, Ogihara T. Ann NY Acad Sci 1989;570:296–310.
10. Thomas MJ, Thornburg T, Manning J, Hooper K, Rudel LL. Biochem 1994;33:1828–1834.
11. Abbey M, Nestel PJ, Baghurst PA. Am J Clin Nutr 1993;58:525–532.
12. Jialal I, Grundy SM. Circulation 1993;88:2780–2786.
13. Rifici VA, Khachadurian AK. J Am Coll Nutr 1993;12:631–637.
14. Reaven PD, Witztum JL. Arterioscler Thromb 1993;13:601–608.
15. Reaven PD, Grasse BJ, Tribble DL. Arterioscler Thromb 1994;14:557–566.
16. Reaven P, Parthasarathy S, Grasse BJ, Miller E, Steinberg D, Witztum JL. J Clin Invest 1993;91:668–676.
17. Abbey M, Belling GB, Noakes M, Hirata F, Nestel PJ. Am J Clin Nutr 1993;57:391–398.
18. Cominacini L, Garbin U, Pastorino AM, Davoli A, Campagnola M, De Santis A, Pasini C, Faccini GB, Trevisan MT, Bertozzo L, Pasini F, Lo Cascio V. Atherosclerosis 1993;99:63–70.
19. Chiu HC, Jeng JR, Shieh SM. Biochim Biophys Acta 1994;1225:200–208.
20. Maggi E, Marchesi E, Ravetta V, Falaschi F, Finardi G, Bellomo G. J Hypertension 1993;11:1103–1111.
21. Keidar S, Kaplan M, Shapira C, Brook JG, Aviram M. Atherosclerosis 1994;107:71–84.
22. Maggi E, Bellazzi R, Falaschi F, Frattoni A, Perani G, Finardi G, Gazo A, Nai M, Romanini D, Bellomo G. Kidney Int 1994;45:876–883.
23. Kleinveld HA, Naber AH, Stalenhoef AFH, Demacker PNM. Free Rad Biol Med 1993;15:273–280.
24. Winklhofer-Roob BM, Puhl H, Khoschsorur G, Esterbauer H, Shmerling DH. Free Rad Biol Med 1994 (in press).
25. De Graaf J, Hendriks JCM, Demacker PNM, Stalenhoef AFH. Arterioscler Thromb 1993;13:712–719.
26. Jialal I, Norkus EP, Cristol L, Grundy SM. Biochim Biophys Acta 1991;1086:134–138.
27. Lavy A, Amotz B, Aviram M. Eur J Clin Chem Clin Biochem 1993;31:83–90.
28. Princen HMG, Van Poppel G, Vogelezang C, Buytenhek R, Kok FJ. Arterioscler Thromb 1992;12:554–562.
29. Reaven PD, Khouw A, Beltz WF, Parthasarathy S, Witztum JL. Arterioscler Thromb 1993;13:590–600.
30. Reaven PD, Ferguson E, Navab M, Powell FL. Arterioscler Thromb 1994;14:1162–1169.
31. Sasahara M, Raines EW, Chait A, Carew TE, Steinberg D, Wahl PW, Ross R. J Clin Invest 1994;94:155–164.
32. Fruebis J, Steinberg D, Dresel HA, Carew TE. J Clin Invest 1994;94:392–398.

Nitric oxide and macrophage-mediated oxidation of low-density lipoprotein

Wendy Jessup

Cell Biology Group, Heart Research Institute, 145 Missenden Road, Sydney, NSW 2050, Australia

Abstract. We have studied the capacity of nitric oxide radical (NO•) to regulate cell-free and cell-mediated oxidation of LDL. Macrophages stimulated with γ-IFN and lipopolysaccharide to induce NO• synthase activity demonstrated a nitric oxide-dependent loss of their ability to promote LDL oxidation. This could be reproduced by exposure of uninduced cells to some synthetic NO• donors. Macrophage "foam" cells containing oxidized LDL could not generate NO• in response to IFN/LPS or suppress their ability to further oxidize LDL. This suggests that intimal NO• may limit lipoprotein oxidation in vivo. However, the bioavailability of NO• may be depressed in lesions where oxidized LDL is present.

Background

Many studies have implicated lipoprotein oxidation as a contributory, if not essential, factor in the development of atherosclerotic lesions. The significance of such oxidative modifications is less clear, although formation of "high-uptake" forms of LDL which can accelerate lipid loading of macrophages is often cited as a likely atherogenic event. The site of LDL oxidation appears to be predominantly within the intima, on the basis of the detection of immunocytochemical and biochemical parameters of oxidation in this tissue and their general absence from the circulating lipoprotein pool. It is quite likely that endothelial cells and monocyte-derived macrophages which are present in the intima, together with components of the extracellular matrix, have a profound influence on such local oxidation of lipoproteins. In vitro studies have confirmed that the exposure of LDL to cells and to matrix can accelerate its oxidation. The biochemical mechanisms by which cell-mediated lipoprotein oxidation can proceed are of interest as a potential target for pharmacological intervention. However, the precise way in which cells can promote lipoprotein oxidation still remains unclear [1].

The ability of cells to produce and release nitric oxide radical (NO•) by an arginine-dependent pathway through the action of nitric oxide synthase (NOS) is known. A constitutive form of the enzyme is present in endothelial cells which produces short bursts of NO•, active as a vasodilator (EDRF), in response to stimuli such as bradykinin and acetylcholine. An inducible form of NOS can also be found in several cell types (including macrophages) following their exposure to stimuli such as TNF or γ-IFN/LPS. While NO• is a weak reductant, it can react with superoxide anion radical ($O_2^{•-}$) to form peroxynitrite anion ($ONOO^-$); this decomposes to form a very strong oxidant indistinguishable from hydroxyl radical (OH•). The contribution of cell-free and cell-derived NO•, both alone and in the presence of $O_2^{•-}$, to LDL oxidation were therefore studied.

Exposure of LDL to nitric oxide in cell-free systems

When LDL was exposed to aqueous nitric oxide solutions under aerobic conditions at pH 7.4 and 37°C, only very minor oxidation could be detected using highly sensitive assays for lipid hydroperoxide generation and antioxidant consumption [2]. These small alterations in the composition of the LDL particle did not cause any detectable changes in its electrophoretic mobility, apoB integrity, or rate of endocytosis by macrophages. Inclusion of an initial anaerobic incubation of the NO• and LDL did not alter the results, nor did either treatment affect the subsequent sensitivity of LDL to oxidation in the pro-oxidant Ham's F-10 medium. These results clearly show that NO• alone is not capable of causing significant oxidative damage to LDL lipids or protein.

However, while neither NO• nor O_2•$^-$ [3] is an efficient oxidizer of LDL, together these radicals can react to generate much more powerful oxidants derived from the intermediate peroxynitrite. Thus a sydnonimine, SIN-1, can generate peroxynitrite as it decomposes spontaneously in solution by base-catalyzed hydrolysis to generate both NO• and O_2•$^-$ simultaneously. Incubation of LDL with SIN-1 at 37°C and pH 7.4 produced rapid consumption of all antioxidants and the generation of substantial amounts of cholesteryl ester hydroperoxides [2,4]. Addition of superoxide dismutase (SOD) decreased the oxidative alterations to the LDL particle. Solutions of authentic peroxynitrite had a similar pro-oxidant effect and generated a high-uptake form of LDL [5]. It would be expected that exposure of LDL in vivo to conditions in which NO• is released in the presence of O_2•$^-$ will also accelerate its oxidative modification.

Macrophage-mediated oxidation in the presence of modulators of NOS activity

Macrophages which have been activated by incubation with γ-interferon and bacterial lipopolysaccharide contain an active nitric oxide synthase (NOS) enzyme which utilizes L-arginine as a substrate and can generate NO• at a sustained rate for several days. The activity of the enzyme can be determined by the accumulation of stable end-products of NO• (nitrite and nitrate) in the culture supernatant. We anticipated that activated macrophages might be very potent agents of LDL oxidation, particularly when O_2•$^-$ output was stimulated simultaneously. However, the reverse proved to be the case. The ability of activated macrophages synthesizing NO• to mediate LDL oxidation was profoundly *inhibited* compared with inactivated cells [2,6]. That this effect was closely related to induced NO• synthesis was demonstrated by its dependence on L-arginine and its reversal by both competitive (the arginine analogue N^G-monomethyl arginine) and noncompetitive (diphenyl iodonium) inhibitors of NOS. Moreover, stimulation of superoxide secretion by activation of the respiratory burst oxidase had no impact on the NO•-dependent inhibition of macrophage-mediated oxidation [1,2]. This suggests that even under favored conditions these cells do not generate peroxynitrite, or at least that any peroxynitrite which the cells may generate does not access the sites of LDL oxidation.

The mechanism by which NO• generation limits cell-mediated oxidation is not yet understood. It is not the consequence of the formation of a stable antioxidant activity in the extracellular medium, since Ham's F-10 medium "conditioned" by exposure to activated cells for 24 h supported LDL oxidation by inactivated cells as well as fresh medium (W. Jessup, unpublished observation). Nor does nitric oxide synthesis inhibit release of endogenous low-molecular-weight thiols, a possible stimulant of LDL oxidation, by the cells (W. Jessup and D. van Reyk, unpublished observation). Treatment of unstimulated macrophages with a range of synthetic NO• donors had variable effects on simultaneous LDL oxidation. Thus glyceryl trinitrate (GTN) and diethylamine NONOate had no effect on cell-mediated oxidation, while S-nitroso acetyl penicillamine (SNAP), sodium nitroprusside (SNP) and, to a lesser extent, spermine NONOate were inhibitory. At this stage it is not possible to discriminate between intracellular and extracellular sites of action, since some of these compounds also had a lesser, but significant, effect on cell-free oxidation.

Modulation of nitric oxide output and LDL oxidation in lipid-loaded macrophages

"Foam" cells were generated in tissue culture by incubation of macrophages with either acetylated (AcLDL; nonoxidized) or copper-oxidized LDL (OxLDL), and their ability to synthesize NO• was compared with that of nonloaded cells. Following exposure to γIFN/LPS, nitric oxide production (measured by nitrite secretion) was similar in nonloaded cells and those which had endocytosed acetylated LDL, despite substantial cholesterol and cholesteryl ester accumulation by the latter. However, oxidized LDL-loaded cells produced 68–99% less nitrite than nonloaded cells [7,8]. OxLDL had no direct effect on NOS activity when added directly to the enzyme in vitro, but has recently been shown to suppress de novo synthesis of enzyme protein [9].

The suppression of NOS induction in cells containing oxidized LDL was inversely correlated with their ability to oxidize LDL. Thus when the various model foam cells were activated by γIFN/LPS, those preloaded with OxLDL oxidized added extracellular native LDL much more extensively than nonloaded or AcLDL-loaded cells [8]. This further confirms the association between nitric oxide production and inhibition of lipoprotein oxidation by cells, and indicates that in situations in the intima in which NOS-containing cells come into contact with OxLDL, the protective effect of NO• synthesis on LDL oxidation may be lost.

Significance of these observations in human atherosclerosis

Of the cells present in the human intima, only endothelial cells can consistently be shown to generate NO•. This is likely to be the major source of nitric oxide in this tissue under normal circumstances, its sustained production playing an important role in the maintenance of vascular tone. Most observations of inducible NOS activity in macrophages (including those above) have been performed in rodent cells, whereas reports of human

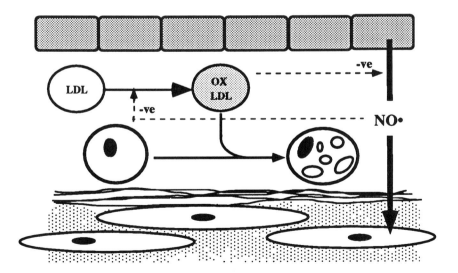

Fig. 1. Proposed balance between nitric oxide availability and lipoprotein oxidation within the intima.

monocyte/macrophage NO• output are only occasional. We propose that normal intimal levels of NO• may play an important role in the suppression of local lipoprotein oxidation (Fig. 1). This in turn may limit foam-cell formation and further progression of the lesion. A delicate balance between the ability of NO• to inhibit LDL oxidation on the one hand, and the ability of OxLDL to inhibit NO• synthesis on the other, is suggested, which should favor NO• synthesis in normal intima. However, in circumstances where antioxidant mechanisms are overwhelmed and some lipoprotein oxidation products are generated, the balance would shift to limit NO• formation and to favor further oxidation. Together these events could produce a "catalytic" enhancement of LDL oxidation through progressive loss of NO• availability and subsequent relatively uninhibited cell-mediated lipoprotein oxidation. This model is consistent with many observations of reduction in the availability of endothelium-derived relaxing factor (EDRF) in hypercholesterolemic and atherosclerotic vessels and its reversal by dietary Vitamin E supplementation.

Acknowledgements

This work was supported by the National Heart Foundation of Australia and the National Health and Medical Research Council of Australia. The participation of Elaine Bolton, Roger Dean, Steven Gieseg, Detlef Mohr, Roland Stocker, David van Reyk and Philippa Zuker in the studies described is acknowledged.

References

1. Jessup W. Biochem Soc Trans 1993;21:321–325.
2. Jessup W, Mohr D, Gieseg SP, Dean RT, Stocker R. Biochim Biophys Acta 1992;1180:73–82.
3. Jessup W, Simpson JA, Dean RT. Atherosclerosis 1993;99:107–120.
4. Darley-Usmar VM, Hogg N, O'Leary VJ, Wilson MT, Moncada S. Free Rad Res Commun 1992;17:9–20.
5. Hogg N, Darley-Usmar VM, Graham A, Moncada S. Biochem Soc Trans 1993;21:358–362.
6. Jessup W, Dean RT. Atherosclerosis 1993;101:145–155.
7. Bolton EJ, Jessup W, Stanley KK, Dean RT. Atherosclerosis 1994;106:213–223.
8. Jorens PG, Rosseneau M, Devreese A-M, Bult H, Marescau B, Herman AG. Eur J Pharmacol 1992;212: 113–115.
9. Yang X, Cai B, Sciacca RR, Cannon PJ. Circ Res 1994;74:318–328.

Atherosclerosis X.
F.P. Woodford, J. Davignon and A. Sniderman, editors.

Biological effects of minimally oxidized lipoproteins

Judith A. Berliner, Mahamad Navab, Andrew Watson, Brian J. Van Lenten, Feng Liao, Aldons J. Lusis, Farhad Parhami, Devon Vora, Mary C. Territo and Alan M. Fogelman
Departments of Pathology and Medicine, University of California, Los Angeles, California, USA

Abstract. Mild oxidation of LDL by lipoxygenase or by cocultures of aortic endothelial cells and smooth muscle cells causes the modification of phospholipids to a product that activates endothelial cells to synthesize cAMP by stimulating Gs and inhibiting Gi activities. This elevation in cAMP increases the synthesis of monocyte-binding molecules and chemotactic factors. The active phospholipids in MM-LDL can be destroyed by incubation with Platelet Activating Factor Acetyl Hydrolase, an enzyme present in HDL.

The entry of monocytes into the vessel wall is an important event in atherogenesis [1]. It represents the beginning of fatty streak formation in animals fed a high-cholesterol diet and is the mechanism by which the atherosclerotic lesion expands. The latter is shown by analysis of regression experiments in which the major change noted is a decrease in lesion-associated monocytes [2]. Our group has shown that treatment of endothelial cells with minimally oxidized LDL (MM-LDL) increases binding of monocytes, but not neutrophils, to the endothelium [3]. We have shown that MM-LDL may be produced by phospholipase or iron-induced oxidation of native LDL [4,5] and that cultures of human aortic endothelial cells plus smooth muscle cells can also modify native LDL to form MM-LDL [6]. When monocytes are incubated with such cocultures that have been incubated with LDL they transmigrate across the endothelium [6]. This paper will describe in more detail the molecules induced by MM-LDL that may contribute to monocyte binding and transmigration in vivo and will describe the mechanisms by which the formation and action of MM-LDL are regulated.

Results

MM-LDL regulation of molecules associated with monocyte binding and transmigration

Monocyte transmigration in flowing blood is regulated by at least three types of molecules: (A) molecules that cause rolling, (B) molecules that activate monocytes and (C) endothelial adhesion molecules to which these activated monocytes bind [7]. We have shown that the concentration of molecules associated with the binding and activation process is increased by MM-LDL; this increase is mediated by an accumulation of mRNA, which results in increased levels of protein (Table 1). After a 4-h treatment of human aortic endothelial cells (HAEC) with MM-LDL, the level of mRNA for the binding molecule P-selectin is increased 2- to 3-fold; the levels of mRNA for the activator molecules MCP-1 and GRO protein are increased 25- to 30-fold, and the level of MCSF is increased 3- to 6-fold. Protein levels of these molecules are increased 3- to 20-fold (Table 1). The levels of P-selectin on the cell surface are not increased enough by MM-LDL alone to cause monocyte binding. However, treatment of the cells exposed to minimally oxidized LDL with histamine or with highly oxidized LDL results in a 2- to

Table 1. Increase in levels of mRNA and protein by MM-LDL

Molecule	mRNA	Protein
MCP-1	24-fold	20-fold
MCSF	4-fold	10-fold
GRO/KC	30-fold	20-fold
P-selectin	2-fold	2.5-fold

Magnitude of increases in mRNA and protein for monocyte chemotactic protein 1 (MCP-1), monocyte colony stimulating factor (MCSF), GRO proteins (GRO/KC) and P-selectin produced by a 4-h treatment of human aortic endothelial cells with 100 µg/ml of MM-LDL. Data are the average from four separate studies.

3-fold increase in surface expression of P-selectin. After treatment with MM-LDL the activator molecules MCSF and MCP-1 are released into the medium whereas the GRO protein remains primarily associated with the cell surface [8]. Although we have not yet identified the adhesion molecule increased by MM-LDL, we have published some initial characterization of the molecule and have shown that it is neither ELAM-1, VCAM-1 nor ICAM-1 [9].

Second-messenger pathways for the action of MM-LDL

In published studies we have shown that a major second messenger for the action of MM-LDL is cAMP [5]. We have found that all the changes induced by MM-LDL are also induced by dibutyryl cAMP and cholera toxin. Furthermore the effects of MM-LDL can be inhibited 60% by H8, an inhibitor of protein kinase A. The levels of cAMP in the cell are regulated by two types of G proteins, Gs and Gi. We have recently found that MM-LDL has effects on both of these G proteins. We have found that MM-LDL, but not native LDL, added to membrane preparations from HAEC at a concentration of 100 µg/ml causes a 40% GTP-dependent increase in the levels of cAMP, indicating a regulatory effect of MM-LDL on Gs. In addition we have shown that MM-LDL-treated cells show a complete inhibition of receptor-mediated Gi activity. Thus MM-LDL regulates cAMP by regulating both Gs and Gi.

MM-LDL components responsible for its action

We have previously shown that a component responsible for the action of MM-LDL in inducing monocyte binding is present in the phospholipid fraction of MM-LDL [3]. Recent examination and fractionation of the phospholipid moiety of MM-LDL resulted in the isolation of two peaks that induced monocyte binding and inhibited LPS-induced neutrophil binding, a characteristic function of MM-LDL [10]. These peaks represented a small fraction of the total phospholipid. Treatment of coculture-modified LDL with albumin resulted in loss of activity in the postalbumin LDL. HPLC showed the major phospholipid isolated from this albumin to be similar to that produced by enzymatic modification of LDL, and again represented a small fraction of the total phospholipid. We are currently attempting to identify these active lipids.

The addition of HDL together with LDL to cocultures prevented the formation of MM-LDL [10]. We have recently found that incubation of MM-LDL with one of the enzymes present in HDL, platelet-activating factor acetyl hydrolase (PAF-AH) can inhibit the activity of MM-LDL by as much as 80%. The HPLC peak containing active lipid is markedly decreased by this treatment, which suggests one mechanism by which HDL might regulate monocyte migration.

Regulation of the formation of MM-LDL

We had previously demonstrated that feeding mice a high-cholesterol diet caused an increase in oxidized lipids and heme oxygenase, indicating the presence of oxidative stress [11]. Recently we have shown that in response to an atherogenic diet, a fatty-streak-resistant strain of mice C3H/HEJ exhibited higher levels of liver apoferritin and lower intracellular concentrations of free iron than did the fatty-streak-susceptible strain C57BL/6J. We also showed that addition of ferrous sulfate to a medium containing 5% fetal bovine serum produced a dose-dependent increase in modification of native LDL by cocultures. Moreover, adding LDL to cocultures results in a 2-fold increase in mRNA for the heavy chain of apoferritin and an approximately 2-fold increase in intracellular free iron. Thus our data suggest that the formation of oxidized lipids can be mediated by increased intracellular as well as extracellular iron.

Discussion

These studies have shown that exposure of endothelial cells to MM-LDL causes an accumulation of specific mRNAs in the cells that may promote monocyte entry into the vessel wall. Some members of our group have shown that in L cells, MM-LDL regulates JE (the mouse homologue of MCP-1) at the level of transcription [12]. The present observations suggest that MM-LDL increases the levels of cAMP in endothelial cells, which leads to the activation of a transcription factor which in turn promotes transcription of a set of molecules regulating monocyte–endothelial interactions. We have previously shown that treatment of endothelial cells with MM-LDL activates NFkB [5]. Many of the proteins induced by MM-LDL, including P-selectin [13], MCP-1 [14], M-CSF [15] and GRO [16] have been shown to have an NFkB element in the promoter region. We therefore hypothesize that there are several ways to inhibit the actions of MM-LDL: (A) prevent the oxidation of LDL by increasing HDL levels or the enzymes associated with HDL; (B) inhibit the receptor by which MM-LDL increases the levels of cAMP in cells; (C) prevent elevations in intracellular levels of free iron.

Acknowledgements

This research was supported by NIH Grant HL30568, M01 RR0865 and a grant from the Tobacco Research Foundation and the Laubisch Fund.

References

1. Ross R. Nature 1993;362:801—809.
2. Badimon JJ, Badimon L, Fuster V. J Clin Invest 1990;85:1234—1241.
3. Berliner JA, Territo MC, Sevanian A, Ramin S, Kim JA, Bamshad B, Esterson M, Fogelman AM. J Clin Invest 1990;85:1260—1266.
4. Rajavashisth TB, Andalibi A, Territo MC, Berliner JA, Navab M, Fogelman AM, Lusis AJ. Nature 1990;344:254—257.
5. Parhami F, Fang ZT, Fogelman AM, Andalibi A, Territo, Berliner JA. J Clin Invest 1993;92:471—478.
6. Navab M, Imes SS, Hama SY, Hough GP, Ross LA, Bork RW, Valente AJ, Berliner JA, Drinkwater DC, Laks H, Fogelman AM. J Clin Invest 1991;88:2039—2046.
7. Butcher EC. Cell 1991;67:1033—1036.
8. Schwartz D, Andalibi A, Chaverri-Almada L, Berliner JA, Kirchgessner T, Fang ZT, Tekamp-Olson P, Lusis AJ, Gallegos C, Fogelman AM, Territo MC. J Clin Invest 1994;94:1968—1973.
9. Kim JA, Territo MC, Wayner E, Carlos TM, Parhami F, Smith CW, Haberland ME, Fogelman AM, Berliner JA. Arterioscler Thromb 1994;14:427—433.

10. Watson AD, Navab M, Hama SY, Sevanian A, Prescott SM, Stafforini DM, McIntyre T, La Du BN, Fogelman AM, Berliner JA. J Clin Invest (in press).
11. Liao F, Andalibi A, DeBeer FC, Fogelman AM, Lusis AJ. J Clin Invest 1993;91:2572–2579.
12. Bork RW, Svenson KL, Mehrabian M, Lusis AJ, Fogelman AM, Edwards PA. Arterioscler Thromb 1992;12:800–806.
13. Pan J, McEver RP. J Biol Chem 1993;268:22600–22608.
14. Ueda A, Okuda K, Ohno S, Shirai A, Igarashi T, Matsunaga K, Fukushima J, Kawamoto S, Ishigatsubo Y, Okuba T. J Immunol 1994;153:2052–2063.
15. Rajavashisth TB, Doan K, Mehta J. Faseb J 1993;7:A341.
16. Anisowicz A, Messineo M, Lee SW, Sager R. J Immunol 1991;147:520–527.

Gene expression of oxidative and antioxidative enzymes in atherosclerotic lesions

Seppo Ylä-Herttuala[1,2], Timo Hiltunen[1], Jukka Luoma[1], Ulla Malo-Ranta[1], Helena Viita[1] and Tapio Nikkari[1]

[1]Department of Biomedical Sciences, University of Tampere, P.O. Box 607, 33101 Tampere; and [2]Department of Clinical Chemistry, Tampere University Hospital, Tampere, Finland

Abstract. LDL oxidation takes place in the arterial wall. Several enzymes with antioxidative activity are actively expressed in normal arteries and in atherosclerotic lesions. These include different isoforms of superoxide dismutases (SOD), glutathione peroxidases (GSHPX) and catalase. In some areas of developing lesions the expression of 15-lipoxygenase (15-LO), inducible nitric oxide synthase (iNOS) and myeloperoxidase, and the production of superoxide anions ($O_2 \cdot^-$) by activated macrophages and other cell types, may shift the balance towards pro-oxidative conditions, rendering LDL susceptible to oxidative modification. Characterization of the expression of oxidative and antioxidative enzymes in developing lesions may lead to improved understanding about the pathogenesis of atherosclerosis.

LDL oxidation

Oxidized (Ox) LDL plays an important role in atherogenesis [1–3]. LDL oxidation takes place in the arterial wall, where several mechanisms may contribute to the formation of Ox-LDL (Fig. 1). These include reactions with 15-LO [4], $O_2 \cdot^-$ [5], hydroxyl radical (OH•) [6], peroxynitrite (ONOO⁻) [7], heme proteins [8], myeloperoxidase [9] and ceruloplasmin [10]. When the antioxidative capacity in a lesion/prelesion area is exceeded by one or a combination of these processes, lipid peroxidation proceeds and leads to the formation of Ox-LDL.

Enzymes with oxidative activity

Recent studies have demonstrated that lesion macrophages and/or other cell types express several enzymes with considerable oxidative potential. These include 15-LO [11], myeloperoxidase [9] and iNOS [12,13] (Table 1). Also, under certain conditions the production of $O_2 \cdot^-$ by NADPH oxidase or by other mechanisms may be involved in LDL oxidation [5]. Data regarding quantitative changes in the expression of these enzymes in early lesions are still sparse. However, on the basis of RT-PCR and in situ hybridization analyses, a clear induction of the 15-LO mRNA level has been found in early atherosclerotic lesions of cholesterol-fed New Zealand White rabbits [Hiltunen et al., unpublished observations, 1994].

Enzymes with antioxidative activity

Lipid-soluble antioxidants provide the first line of defense against LDL oxidation [6]. In addition, several enzymatic defense mechanisms protect LDL against lipid peroxidation. These include SODs, GSHPX and catalase [6]. GSHPX, catalase and all major SOD isoforms (i.e., cytosolic CuZn-SOD, mitochondrial Mn-SOD and secreted extracellular (EC)-SOD) are expressed in atherosclerotic lesions [14–16]. As far as CuZn-SOD and

218

OXIDATION OF LDL

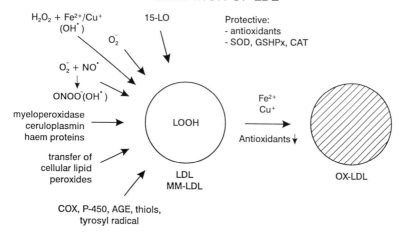

Fig. 1. Mechanisms of LDL oxidation. LDL oxidation takes place in the arterial wall. Several mechanisms may contribute to the formation in LDL of lipid hydroperoxides (LOOH), which play an important role in the early phase of LDL oxidation. In the presence of transition metals and after the depletion of LDL antioxidants, the decomposition of LOOH leads to the formation of fully oxidized LDL. MM-LDL: minimally oxidized LDL; Ox-LDL: fully oxidized LDL; COX = cyclooxygenase; AGE = advanced glycosylation end products; other abbreviations, see text. Reprinted from [3] with permission.

EC-SOD are concerned, no major overall induction in mRNA expression occurs during early atherogenesis, as analyzed by RT-PCR techniques [Hiltunen et al., unpublished observations, 1994]. Thus, as distinct from a clear induction of 15-LO and iNOS expression, it may be the overall conditions in macrophage-rich areas that favor LDL oxidation.

Table 1. Expression of various oxidative and antioxidative enzymes in normal and atherosclerotic human and/or rabbit arteries [3,17]

Enzyme	Normal artery	Fatty streaks	Advanced lesions
15-LO [11]	−	++	+
12-LO[a] [11]	−	−	−
5-LO [11]	−	−	−
iNOS [12,13]	−	++	+
cNOS [18]	+	+	+
Myeloperoxidase [9]	−	+	+
NADPH oxidase [6]	−	+	+
CuZn-SOD [14−16]	+	+	+
EC-SOD [15,16]	+	+	+
GSHPX [14,15]	+	+	+
Catalase [14,15]	+	+	+

[a]Platelet-type 12-LO.
− = no detectable expression; + = moderate expression; + + = strong expression.

Conclusions

The concept of LDL oxidation has provided new insights into the mechanisms by which LDL may exert its atherogenic effects in arteries [1–3]. Although the mechanisms by which LDL is oxidized in the arterial wall remain unknown, it is likely that the local balance between oxidative and antioxidative systems determines the net outcome of the process. Further studies are needed to characterize anatomic, functional and temporal relationships between various oxidative and antioxidative enzymes in atherosclerotic arteries.

Acknowledgements

This study was supported by grants from the Finnish Academy, Sigrid Juselius Foundation and Finnish Heart Foundation.

References

1. Witztum JL, Steinberg D. J Clin Invest 1991;88:1785–1792.
2. Berliner JA, Haberland ME. Curr Opin Lipidol 1993;4:373–381.
3. Ylä-Kerttuala S. Role of lipid and lipoprotein oxidation in the pathogenesis of atherosclerosis. Drugs Today 1994;30(7):(in press).
4. Parthasarathy S, Wieland E, Steinberg D. Proc Natl Acad Sci USA 1989;86:1046–1050.
5. Heinecke LW, Baker L, Rosen H, Chait, A. J Clin Invest 1986;77:757–761.
6. Halliwell B, Gutteridge JMC. edn 2. Oxford: Clarendon Press, 1989.
7. Darley-Usmar VM, Hogg N, O'Learly VJ, Wilson MT, Moncada S. Free Rad Res Comms 1992;17:9–20.
8. Balla G, Jacob HS, Eaton JW, Belcher JD, Vercellotti GM. Arterioscler Thromb 1991;11:1700–1711.
9. Daugherty A, Dunn JL, Rateri DL, Heinecke JW. J Clin Invest 1994;94:437–444.
10. Ehrenwald E, Chisolm GM, Fox PL. J Clin Invest 1994;93:1493–1501.
11. Ylä-Herttuala S, Rosenfeld ME, Parthasarathy S, Glass CK, Sigal E, Witztum JL, Steinberg D. Proc Natl Acad Sci USA 1990;87:6959–6963.
12. Luoma J, Särkioja T, Nikkari T, Ylä-Herttuala S. Atherosclerosis 1994;109:102 (Abstract).
13. Malo-Ranta U, Luoma J, Laukkanen M, Nikkari T, Ylä Herttuala S. Atherosclerosis 1994;109:107 (Abstract).
14. Sharma RC, Crawford DW, Kramsch DM, Sevanian A, Jiao Q. Arterioscler Thromb 1992;12:403–415.
15. Hiltunen T, Luoma J, Ylä-Herttuala S, Nikkari T. Expression of superoxide dismutase in human and rabbit atherosclerotic lesions. XIV Annual European Conference on Vascular Biology, Tampere, 23–27.3.1993 (Abstract) p. 85.
16. Strålin P, Karlsson K, Marklund SL. Extracellular-superoxide dismutase in the vascular wall. XIV Annual European Conference on Vascular Biology, Tampere, 23–27.3.1993 (Abstract) p. 86.
17. Ylä-Herttuala S. Herz 1992;17:270–276.
18. Pollock JS, Nakane M, Butterley LDK, Martinez A, Springall D, Polak JM, Förstermann U, Murad F. Am J Physiol 1993;34:C1379–C1387.

220

Lp(a) oxidation, oxidized sterols and effect of antioxidants

M. Naruszewicz

Regional Center for Atherosclerosis Research, Pomeranian Medical Academy, Powstańców Wielkp. 72, 70–111 Szczecin, Poland

Abstract. By incubation of oxidized Lp(a) with the monocytoid U 937 cell line, we showed that these particles compete more effectively with plasminogen (Pg) binding to cell surface receptors than native Lp(a). Since kringle 4 of apo(a) seemed to be responsible for native Lp(a) binding to the Pg receptor, we concluded that oxidation may have a significant influence on conformational changes in these kringles.

Raised plasma lipid peroxide concentrations have been noted in diabetic subjects. Since circulating monocytes may facilitate removal of oxidized material from the blood as well as from the arterial wall, the oxysterol content of monocytes may represent the increased oxidative stress in the diabetic state. We find a significantly higher content of cholesterol oxides in monocytes from diabetic plasma than from controls.

The antiatherogenic mechanism of β-carotene has not been completely established. We found that β-carotene markedly reduced atherosclerosis in cholesterol-fed guinea pigs. This could be related to: 1) increased HDL-cholesterol levels, and 2) restored activity of the extracellular superoxide dismutase, which has been decreased by the cholesterol diet.

Lp(a) oxidation

There is strong evidence that high levels of lipoprotein (a) [Lp(a)] in plasma represent an independent risk factor for coronary artery disease (CAD) [1]. While this unique lipoprotein class is similar to LDL in many ways, it contains a heavily glycosylated protein, apo(a), which is linked by a disulfide bond to the carboxy-terminal portion of apoB100. The apo(a) structure is strikingly similar to that of plasminogen (Pg), the zymogen of the fibrinolytic plasma protein plasmin. Pg kringle domain 4 is present in many copies in apo(a), contributing to variation in mass [2].

The atherogenic mechanism of Lp(a) is still unknown. However, it could be related to its ready uptake by macrophages, important in atheromata formation, or its inhibition of fibrinolysis at the endothelial cell surface of clots, due to competitive binding to the Pg receptor.

We have shown earlier that Lp(a) particles isolated from human plasma were oxidatively modified when incubated in vitro with human mononuclear cells or Cu^{2+} [3]. This modification, which involved lipid peroxidation measured as thiobarbituric acid-reactive substances (TBARS), caused marked changes in the structure and biological properties of Lp(a). Relative to native Lp(a), oxidized particles showed fewer free amino groups, protein fragmentation, higher negative charge and a high aggregation ability. They were readily taken up and degraded by macrophages in vitro, inducing cholesteryl ester accumulation. When apo(a) was clipped off from oxidized Lp(a) by exposure to dithiothreitol (DTT), the remaining particle was degraded more slowly. This observation implies that the oxidative modification of apo(a) may affect Lp(a) recognition by macrophage scavenger receptors, mediated in part by apo(a) changes, indicated by a stronger negative charge, protein fragmentation and increased immunoreactivity to monoclonal antibody KO7, which also cross-reacted with plasminogen.

223

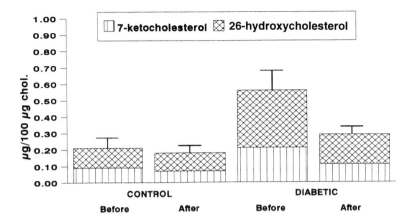

Fig. 1. Cholesterol oxides in monocytes isolated from control and diabetic patients before and after treatment with bezafibrate 600 mg/d for 30 days.

also prevents the oxidation of unsaturated fatty acids in LDL [17]. However, Reaven et al. have shown that enrichment of human LDL in ß-carotene after 6-week dietary supplementation did not reduce LDL susceptibility to oxidation [15]. These discordances among investigations suggest that potentially antiatherogenic properties of ß-carotene could be independent of its influence on LDL oxidation. The present study was undertaken to determine whether β-carotene affects atheromatous lesions and peroxidation indices in the organism.

We investigated the influence of two doses (15 and 30 mg/day) of β-carotene on the extent of aortic lesions in cholesterol-fed guinea pigs. After 12 weeks, the animals were sacrificed and plasma lipids and lipoproteins as well as the activity of antioxidant enzymes (superoxide dismutase-SOD and catalase-CAT) were determined. We found no effect of

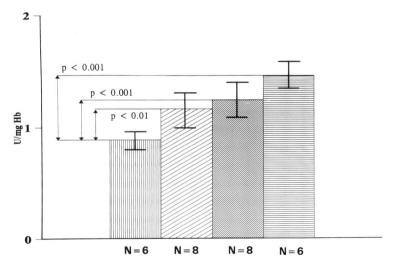

Fig. 2. Effect of β-carotene on activity of superoxide dismutase in cholesterol-fed guinea pigs. Blocks in order: control; cholesterol; cholesterol + 15 mg β-carotene/day; cholesterol + 30 mg β-carotene/day.

224

β-carotene ingestion on the total plasma cholesterol and triglycerides, but significant increases in high density lipoproteins were observed in animals treated with 30 mg of β-carotene per day. Atheromatous lesions of aorta of these animals were significantly fewer than in the cholesterol-only group. No differences in LDL susceptibility to copper-mediated oxidation in vitro were seen between groups. In contrast, β-carotene treatment markedly increased SOD (Fig. 2) and slightly increased CAT, enzymes whose activity had been decreased by the atherogenic diet. These findings show that although β-carotene supplementation does not decrease the susceptibility of LDL to oxidative modification, it may inhibit the progression of atherosclerosis by stimulating the activity of SOD as well as by increasing the level of HDL.

Acknowledgements

This work was supported by grants from Medical Research Council of Canada — UI 0029 and from the State Committee for Scientific Research of Poland PB 0987/S4/93/04. I want to thank Professors Jean Davignon and Światosław Ziemlański for insightful comments and Louise-Marie Giroux, Bogusławie Panczenko-Krasowskiej, Hannie Bukowskiej and Danieli Wirze for their expert technical assistance.

References

1. Scanu AM. Arch Pathol Lab Med 1988;112:1045—1047.
2. Fless GM, Rolih CA, Scanu AM. J Biol Chem 1984;259:11470—11478.
3. Naruszewicz M, Selinger E, Davignon J. Metabolism 1992;41:1—9.
4. Haberland ME, Fless G, Scanu AM et al. J Biol Chem 1992;267:4143—4151.
5. Jürgens G, Ashy A, Esterbauer H. Biochem J 1990;265:605—608.
6. Naruszewicz M, Giroux L-M, Davignon J. Chem Phys Lipids 1994;67/68:167—174.
7. Cushing GL, Gaubatz JW, Nava ML et al. Arteriosclerosis 1989;9:593—603.
8. Rath M, Niendorf A, Reblin T et al. Arteriosclerosis 1989;9:579—592.
9. Simon DI, Schoen FJ, Fless GM et al. Arteriosclerosis 1990;10:812a (abstract).
10. Pepin IM, O'Neil JA, Hoff HF. J Lipid Res 1991;32:317—327.
11. Smith EB, Crosbie L. Atherosclerosis 1991;89:127—136.
12. Naruszewicz M, Mirkiewicz E, Kłosiewicz-Latoszek L. Atherosclerosis 1989;79:261—265.
13. Parthasarathy S, Young SG, Witzum JL et al. J Clin Invest 1986;77:641—644.
14. Naruszewicz M, Selinger E, Dofour R, Davignon J. Metabolism 1992;41:1225—1228.
15. Reaven PD, Khouw A, Beltz WF et al. Arterioscler Thromb 1993;13:590—598.
16. Gaziano JM, Manson JE, Ridker PM et al. Circulation 1990;82(suppl. III):201.
17. Jialal J, Norkus EP, Cristol L, Grundy SM. Biochim Biophys Acta 1991;1086:134—138.

Immunological responses to oxidized LDL

Joseph L. Witztum

Department of Medicine 0682, University of California at San Diego, 9500 Gilman Drive, La Jolla, CA 92093-0682, USA

Abstract. Oxidation of LDL generates neo-epitopes that render it immunogenic. Autoantibodies to malondialdehyde(MDA)-LDL, 4-hydroxynonenal-LDL and Ox-LDL are present in serum of rabbits, mice and man. In man, preliminary studies relate the titer of autoantibodies to the rate of progression of atherosclerosis. ApoE-deficient mice with extensive disease have high titers of autoantibodies. Increasing the titer of autoantibodies to an epitope of Ox-LDL by immunizing WHHL rabbits with homologous MDA-LDL decreased the extent of atherosclerosis. These data are reviewed in the light of increasing evidence that both humoral and cell-mediated immunity may modulate the atherogenic process.

The observation that oxidative modification of LDL would make it immunogenic resulted from the serendipitous observation made some years earlier that the nonenzymatic glycation of LDL rendered it immunogenic. This observation resulted from studies in which LDL and nonenzymatically glycated LDL were injected into human subjects in order to quantify the involvement of the LDL receptor in clearance of the particles. In many persons the die-away curve of glycated LDL was extremely slow and monophasic, consistent with non-receptor-mediated clearance. However, in some diabetic subjects there was very rapid elimination of the tracer, and subsequent studies showed that this was due to the presence of autoantibodies to glycated LDL [1]. Although classical immunological theory suggested that one needs a hapten on a heterologous protein carrier, we showed [2] that even very subtle modifications of autologous LDL such as methylation, ethylation, acetylation or carbamylation were all immunogenic, and gave rise to highly monospecific antisera that recognized the modified lysine residue on the glycated LDL and also on several other similarly modified proteins.

Thus, when we wanted to develop antisera against epitopes of oxidized LDL (Ox-LDL) we reasoned that modifications of the LDL protein would occur and that these would be immunogenic. Since we postulated that breakdown products of lipid peroxidation such as malondialdehyde (MDA) and 4-hydroxynonenal (4-HNE) would bind to lysine residues, we prepared guinea pig LDL that was modified with MDA (MDA-LDL) or with 4-HNE (4-HNE-LDL) and used these to immunize guinea pigs. Similarly, modified mouse LDL was used to generate monoclonal antibodies [3]. We used these reagents to immunostain atherosclerotic lesions of rabbits and man and demonstrated these epitopes in lesions but not in normal arteries [4]. In addition, LDL extracted from atherosclerotic lesions was shown to contain these epitopes, and the serum of man and rabbits to contain such autoantibodies [4]. IgG purified from human subjects could immunostain rabbit atherosclerotic lesions in a manner similar to that of the induced antibodies, and preabsorption with MDA-LDL, for example, could greatly reduce that immunostaining.

In order to determine whether the presence of these antibodies related to the extent of atherosclerosis (or LDL oxidation) occurring in the artery wall, we measured the autoantibody titer to MDA-LDL, in collaboration with Salonen and colleagues [5]. Baseline measurement of carotid atherosclerosis was performed by ultrasound in a large group of asymptomatic middle-aged Finnish men, and a cohort of these were examined again 2 years later. In a nested case-control study we determined the titer of 30 men who had shown the greatest progression of carotid atherosclerosis during this interval, and as controls used 30 individuals who had the least degree of progression. The antibody titer was significantly higher in men with progression, and when a multivariate logistic regression analysis of various risk factors for carotid atherosclerosis was performed only the antibody titer to MDA-LDL and smoking were found to be independent risk factors.

Since that time other reports have documented a relationship between autoantibody titer and various indices of atherosclerotic disease. The fact that the antibody titer correlated with the rate of progression but not with baseline intima-media thickness suggests that it was a marker for the *rate of lesion formation* as related to LDL oxidation. It will require many more epidemiological studies to determine whether autoantibody titer has clinical utility as a marker for extent of lesion formation or of disease activity, but the mere presence of such autoantibodies provides yet another piece of evidence that oxidation of LDL occurs in vivo.

In rabbit lesions large amounts of immunoglobulins occur colocalized with epitopes of oxidized LDL, as well as with complement. When we purified IgG from rabbit atherosclerotic lesions by elution and G-protein chromatography and then tested it in a solid-phase RIA, we documented a high titer of antibody to MDA-LDL and to Ox-LDL but not to native LDL. Furthermore, by preparing specific immunoadsorbents that bound IgG from the lesion and examining the bound material by SDS-PAGE, we demonstrated epitopes of Ox-LDL in the immune complexes. Thus at least a part of the IgG in lesions has specificity for Ox-LDL and is present in immune complexes with it [6].

That the immune system plays an important part of atherogenesis is increasingly apparent [7]. Not only are large numbers of immunocompetent cells present in the lesions, but many of them are activated, as evidenced by expression of CD-25 and class II MHC antigens. In addition, large amounts of immunoglobulin and immunoglobulin–antigen are present and terminal C5b-9 complement complexes are also found. However, there is as yet little information regarding the role these immunological processes actually play. In order to determine if a high titer of autoantibody to an epitope of oxidized LDL could influence the atherogenic process, Palinski et al. [8] isolated LDL from WHHL rabbits, modified it with MDA and used it to immunize a series of 6-month-old WHHL rabbits. Control rabbits were immunized with saline and others with KHL. The rationale for the latter group was that the immune response would be stimulated, but that the antibodies formed would not react with any endogenous epitope. In all case the initial immunization was done with complete Freund's adjuvant, and subsequent immunizations with incomplete adjuvant.

In response to the immunizations a high titer (> 100,000) of antibodies to MDA-LDL was generated in all the immunized rabbits. The control rabbits had no change in antibody titer to MDA-LDL, although at baseline their titers were higher than those of freshly weaned WHHL rabbits. A rise in titer of both IgG and IgA antibodies occurred, but the titer of IgM antibodies did not change. Competition studies showed that the specificity of the antibodies to MDA-LDL was similar to that of the endogenous autoantibodies seen in nonimmunized animals. At the end of the 6-month immunization period, the animals were sacrificed and the extent of atherosclerosis was determined. The extent of atherosclerosis was significantly lower in the total aorta and in the thoracic and abdominal aortas examined individually. The extent of atherosclerosis in the saline-immunized animals was similar to that of the KLH-immunized animals.

The finding that this immunization reduced the extent of atherosclerosis was somewhat surprising. What are potential mechanisms by which immunization could be protective? First, it is possible that the high autoantibody titer promoted rapid clearance from the plasma of minimally modified LDL. Although we had not previously thought that significant modification of LDL occurs in plasma, it is conceivable that mild degrees of oxidation sufficient to cause changes in the protein structure constantly occur, and that such particles might bind circulating immunoglobulins and be removed by Fc receptor-mediated mechanisms in the liver and spleen. Indeed, we have previously documented that LDL glycated to a very slight degree underwent just such enhanced removal when injected into rabbits previously immunized against glycated LDL [9]. The faster removal of such modified LDL from plasma would prevent their entry into the artery, where they would otherwise be more primed for further oxidative modification.

A second possible mechanism could be a faster uptake of modified LDL by macrophages in the intima. We have previously shown [10] that when aggregates of LDL are coated with specific antibodies the uptake into macrophages by the Fc pathway is greatly enhanced. Since oxidation of LDL leads to aggregation, and since autoantibodies are present, such complexes almost certainly exist in vivo and would promote more rapid macrophage uptake. Other laboratories have suggested many ways in which products of minimally modified LDL may be atherogenic, and indeed extracellular oxidized LDL may be more atherogenic than the same materials sequestered within a macrophage.

A third potential mechanism by which immunization may be protective is by stimulation of cell-mediated immunity [8], which much evidence suggests may influence atherogenesis. Oxidized LDL is chemotactic for T-cells and monocytes, and Ox-LDL may activate these cells either directly or via interaction with other cells. Recently, Hansson and colleagues have reported that many CD4+ T-cells specifically respond to Ox-LDL in an HLA-DR-dependent manner that requires the presence of antigen-presenting cells. They previously reported that elimination of T-cells by a monoclonal antibody led to an increase in carotid lesions in rats, and Fyfe, Qiao and Lusis have recently reported that class I MHC-deficient mice have more lesions when fed an atherogenic diet. Thus, it is certainly possible that both humoral and cell-mediated immunity might have a protective role at some stage(s) of the atherosclerotic process.

If we are to study the role of the immune system in detail, it would be helpful to have an animal model in which various components of the immune system were deleted. Many such models exist for mice, and there are also now several excellent murine models of atherosclerosis such as apoE-deficient mice, and LDL-receptor-knockout mice on a Western diet. We have recently found that apoE-deficient mice contain oxidation-specific epitopes in their lesions. Furthermore, there is extensive deposition of IgG and IgM in the lesions, and examination of their sera revealed an extraordinarily high titer of autoantibody to epitopes of MDA-LDL: > 65,000 in 10 of 12 mice studied. They also have elevated titers to other epitopes such as 4-HNE-LDL and copper Ox-LDL itself. The availability of mice with specific defects of both humoral and cell-mediated immunity should allow us to understand the effect of these components on atherogenesis.

Just as with other inflammatory processes, the immune response may play a beneficial role initially, but have adverse consequences later. It is worth noting that many modified proteins and lipids occur in the atherosclerotic lesion and undoubtedly many of these could also be targets of an immune response. Our studies add to the growing body of evidence of a potentially important role for the immune response in atherogenesis. We believe that it is an important area of study, and much remains to be learned.

228

Acknowledgements

The author thanks his many colleagues who have contributed significantly to these studies, and in particular Dr W. Palinski, with whom many of them have been performed.

References

1. Witztum JL, Steinbrecher UP, Fisher M, Kesaniemi A. Proc Natl Acad Sci USA 1983;80:2757–2761.
2. Steinbrecher UP, Fisher M, Witztum JL, Curtiss LK. J Lipid Res 1984;25:1109–1116.
3. Palinski W, Ylä-Herttuala S, Rosenfeld ME, Butler S, Socher SA, Parthasarathy S, Curtiss LK, Witztum JL. Arteriosclerosis 1990;10:325–335.
4. Palinski W, Rosenfeld ME, Ylä-Herttuala S, Gurtner CC, Socher SA, Butler S, Parthasarathy S, Carew TE, Steinberg D, Witztum JL. Proc Natl Acad Sci USA 1989;86:1372–1376.
5. Salonen JT, Ylä-Herttuala S, Yamamoto R, Butler S, Korpela H, Salonen R, Nyyssönen K, Palinski W, Witztum JL. Lancet 1992;339:883–887.
6. Ylä-Herttuala S, Palinski W, Butler S, Picard S, Steinberg D, Witztum JL. Arterioscler Thromb 1994;14:32–40.
7. Libby P, Hansson GK. Lab Invest 1991;64:5–15.
8. Palinski W, Miller E, Witztum JL. Proc Natl Acad Sci USA 1994; (in press).
9. Wiklund O, Witztum JL, Carew TE, Pittman RC, Elam RL, Steinberg D. J Lipid Res 1987;28:1098–1109.
10. Khoo JC, Miller E, Pio F, Steinberg D, Witztum JL. Arterioscler Thromb 1992;12:1258–1266.

Atherosclerosis X.
F.P. Woodford, J. Davignon and A. Sniderman, editors.

LDL oxidation and atherogenesis - studies in nonhuman primates

Alan Chait, Mary Chang, Masakiyo Sasahara, Elaine Raines and Russell Ross
University of Washington, Seattle, Washington, USA

The oxidation of low density lipoprotein (LDL) is believed to play an important role in atherogenesis. If this is correct, antioxidants that inhibit LDL oxidation should inhibit the atherosclerotic process. Several lines of evidence that encompass basic science, epidemiology, animal investigation and limited clinical studies support this hypothesis. Perhaps the strongest evidence is derived from animal studies, in which direct evaluation of the arterial wall is possible. Several different antioxidants (e.g., probucol, butylated hydroxytoluene, vitamin E and diphenylene diamine) have been shown to reduce the extent of atherosclerosis in hypercholesterolemic rabbits, supporting the hypothesis that atherogenesis involves an oxidative process. However, the plasma lipoprotein profile of rabbits differs considerably from that of humans. Therefore, evaluation of the effect of antioxidants on atherosclerosis in nonhuman primates is important, since it tests the role of antioxidants in a species that is similar to humans in lipoprotein particle distribution.

To investigate whether inhibition of LDL oxidation would alter atherogenesis in the nonhuman primate, we administered probucol, a potent antioxidant, to *Macaca nemestrina* fed a high-fat, high-cholesterol diet [1]. After 14 weeks on the hypercholesterolemic diet, probucol was administered daily to half of the 16 animals until sacrifice at 11 months. Histological comparison of lesions at similar sites in control animals showed that aortic lesions in the probucol-treated animals appeared less mature, and had increased accumulation of lipid within smooth muscle cells in contrast to lipid-filled macrophages in the cores of lesions in control animals. Comparison of all control and probucol-treated monkeys demonstrated that intimal lesion areas in the thoracic aortas of the probucol-treated monkeys were smaller by 43% (p < 0.0001), but no significant difference in lesion area was found in the abdominal aortas or in the iliac arteries. To evaluate the antioxidant effect of probucol, the resistance of plasma LDL to ex vivo oxidation was evaluated. Probucol significantly increased the resistance of LDL to oxidative modification, as shown by an increase in the lag time for conjugated diene formation. Evaluation of all 16 animals showed that lesion size was inversely related to oxidation resistance of LDL for all anatomic sites (Fig. 1). The inverse relationship between intimal lesion size and resistance of LDL to oxidation supports a role for lipoprotein oxidation in the development and progression of lesions of atherosclerosis in this species.

To investigate whether cellular and molecular differences were associated with the lower lesion size in the probucol-treated hypercholesterolemic monkeys, detailed quantitative immunocytochemical evaluation of lesions was performed in a subset of the animals [2]. There was no difference between the groups in the extent of immunoreactivity with antibodies generated against either LDL or oxidized LDL. Lesions at all aortic sites in the probucol-treated animals had a 35−80% reduction in the percentage of cells in cell-cycle traverse, as indicated by immunostaining for proliferating cell nuclear antigen

Address for correspondence: Alan Chait, MD, Department of Medicine RG-26, University of Washington, Seattle, WA 98195, USA.

230

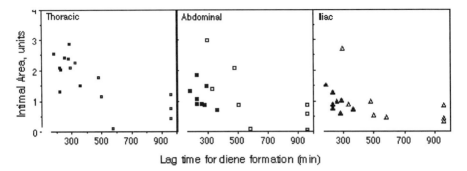

Fig. 1. Relationship between intimal area and lag time for LDL oxidation in control (closed symbols) and procubol-treated (open symbols) monkeys.

(% PCNA (+)). In both groups, macrophages and smooth muscle cells were PCNA (+), but the majority (>60%) of PCNA (+) cells were macrophages. No difference in % PCNA (+) cells was seen in the iliac arteries, where the most advanced lesions were present at the time of initiation of probucol treatment. Since probucol was started after the monkeys had been on the diet for 3.5 months, more advanced fibro-fatty lesions were already present in the iliac arteries, while no lesions or early fatty streaks were present in the thoracic and upper abdominal aorta [3,4]. Analysis of lesions after an additional 7.5 months of hypercholesterolemia demonstrated the greatest reduction in intimal areas and most statistically significant differences in the thoracic aorta. Thus, a potential role for probucol in the treatment of atherosclerosis may be to prevent or decrease the inflammatory response, and thus, early lesion formation and progression. However, it may not alter the cellular characteristics of more advanced lesions of atherosclerosis.

In summary, this study provides evidence for the role of lipoprotein oxidation in atherogenesis in another species, the nonhuman primate. It also suggests that atherogenesis can be inhibited by treatment with probucol, possibly by inhibition of cellular proliferation. Whether probucol's ability to modulate cytokine and growth-factor production, inhibit cellular proliferation and decrease lesion size are directly related to its potency as an antioxidant is not yet known. Therefore, it is not possible to conclusively ascribe probucol's antiatherogenic effects to its antioxidant properties. Since vitamin E also has been shown to reduce carotid atherosclerosis in monkeys, inhibition of oxidative processes may indeed be important in atherogenesis in nonhuman primates and, therefore, also in humans. Additional studies using other antioxidants will be required to confirm this possibility.

References

1. Sasahara M, Raines EW, Chait A, Carew TE, Steinberg D, Wahl P, Ross R. J Clin Invest 1994;94:155—164.
2. Chang MY, Sasahara M, Raines EW, Chait A, Ross R. Circulation 1993;88(suppl 1):3031.
3. Faggiotto A, Ross R, Harker L. Arteriosclerosis 1984;4:323—340.
4. Faggiotto A, Ross R. Arteriosclerosis 1984;4:342—356.

Atherosclerosis X.
F.P. Woodford, J. Davignon and A. Sniderman, editors.

Transcriptional regulation of the lipoprotein lipase gene

Catherine L. Morin and Robert H. Eckel

University of Colorado Health Sciences Center, Colorado, USA

Abstract. Regulation of LPL gene transcription is evident in adipose tissue during differentiation and after tumor necrosis factor-α (TNF-α) treatment. In both conditions, two sets of two unrelated regulatory elements in the LPL promoter appear important for activation of LPL gene transcription. In the differentiated state basal LPL gene expression seems driven largely by the interaction of two transcription factors, OCT-1 and NF-Y, with the LPL promoter. This association is lost with TNF-α treatment. Although several potential regulatory elements have been identified in the LPL promoter, their functional role in vivo remains unproved.

Lipoprotein lipase (LPL) is found predominantly in adipose tissue and muscle including heart and skeletal muscle, and tissue-specific regulation of the enzyme is thought to contribute to whole-body fuel balance [1]. LPL is responsible for the hydrolysis of triglyceride-rich lipoprotein triglycerides, which allows uptake of the resultant lipolysis products by cells. Although it is often stated that many metabolic and nutritional regulators of LPL work at least in part by altering LPL gene transcription, this has rarely been demonstrated. This conclusion has often been based on changes in steady-state LPL mRNA levels, not on direct measurements of LPL gene transcription. There are only a few instances wherein a transcription factor or the requisite consensus sequence on the LPL promoter has been elucidated.

Instances wherein transcriptional regulation contributes to changes in LPL activity include adipose tissue differentiation and the effect of TNF-α on adipose tissue LPL (ATLPL). Adipocyte differentiation, a process which involves several steps, is a clear example of LPL transcriptional regulation. LPL is considered an 'early' gene, because its expression increases early in the differentiation process, and increase in LPL gene expression rapidly follows growth arrest after confluence [2]. Studies performed using the human LPL promoter identified two *cis*-acting elements, LP-α (−702 to −666) and LP-B (−468 to −430), which appear to play a role in the activation of ATLPL during differentiation [3]. These sequences are similar to consensus sequences known to bind the transcription factors HNF-3 and fork head. However, interestingly, these sequences are not present in the murine LPL promoter (Fig. 1).

Another transcription factor implicated in the induction of LPL gene transcription during differentiation is c-fos. After treatment of 0b1771 cells with the c-fos antisense oligonucleotide *sof*, c-fos protein synthesis and the differentiation-dependent increase in LPL mRNA were abolished [4]. Typically, c-fos is a component of the heterodimer AP-1, a transcription factor which appears to be important in the regulation of many adipocyte genes including fatty acid binding protein (FABP). However, the human LPL promoter has no such consensus sequence and the AP-1 consensus sequence in the murine promoter has never been shown to be functionally active, which leaves uncertainty as to whether c-fos has any effect. Many adipocyte genes, including stearoyl-CoA desaturase 1 and FABP, are turned on in the differentiation process through the action of CCAAT-enhancer binding protein (C/EBP), a factor which typically binds to the CCAAT box [5]. This does not appear to be true for LPL. This may be because LPL is expressed early in the

A) Human LPL gene

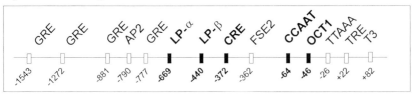

B) Murine LPL gene

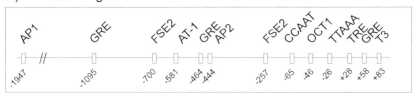

Fig. 1. Cis-acting elements within the LPL promoter are portrayed for the (A) human, and (B) murine promoters. Sequences shown in solid bars with bold labels are regions of the LPL promoter which are important either to basal transcription and/or to transcriptional regulation during adipocyte differentiation or the inhibition of LPL gene transcription in adipocytes by TNF-α.

differentiation process and the C/EBP-regulated genes are induced later. Moreover, C/EBP does not bind to or elicit expression of the LPL gene [3].

Because nutritional and most of the hormonal regulators of LPL, including insulin, thyroid hormone and glucocorticoids, are thought to act posttranscriptionally, the emphasis of work done on LPL gene transcription has focused on transcription factors needed for basal expression. In short, two proteins which bind to the proximal LPL promoter are responsible for most of the basal transcription [6,7]. The first is an octamer-binding protein. Previato originally showed [6], the importance of the octamer-binding sequence (−46 to −39) in basal LPL gene expression by demonstrating that deletions in this area decreased reporter gene expression by 75–80%. Antibodies to the POU domain of octamer proteins also blocked protein:DNA interactions at the octamer consensus sequence. Using electrophoretic mobility shift assays, Currie and Eckel confirmed the importance of this sequence in addition to 5′ and 3′ AT-rich flanking sequences [8]. Currie and Eckel further identified the binding of NF-Y to the LPL CCAAT box (−65 to −61). However, at present, a supershift of OCT-1 and NF-Y:LPL DNA complexes has been accomplished only with antibodies to NF-Y, not OCT-1.

Interestingly, both the octameric sequence and CCAAT box are involved in the ability of TNF-α to decrease LPL gene transcription. TNF-α, originally called cachectin, is a well-known inhibitor of ATLPL, in part by inhibiting LPL gene transcription [9]. Through transfection analysis the region of the LPL promoter necessary to confer the TNF-α effect was located downstream of −180, the area which contains both the CCAAT box and octamer sequence [10]. Electrophoretic mobility-shift assays further suggested the involvement of these *cis*-acting elements (Fig. 2). Using oligonucleotides for the consensus sequences of OCT-1 and NF-Y, we found that specific OCT-1 and NF-Y:LPL DNA interactions were eliminated by TNF-α treatment. Preincubation of the OCT-1 oligonucleotide successfully eliminated one protein:DNA interaction on the LPL promoter

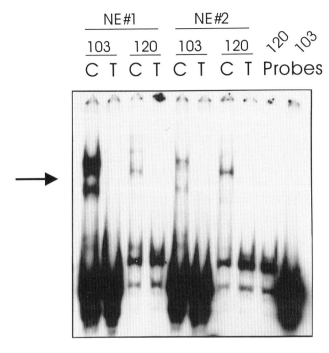

Fig. 2. Electrophoretic mobility-shift analysis of the proximal murine LPL promoter. Nuclear factors from two sets of differentiated 3T3-L1 cells (NE1 and NE2) previously treated with (T) or without (C) 10 ng/ml of TNF-α were compared for their ability to form sequence-specific DNA: protein complexes with oligomers derived from the LPL promoter. Probe 103 (–59 to +44) and probe 120 (–180 to –60) were gel-purified and radiolabeled with α-^{32}P dATP and dCTP. 30-min binding reactions were run on a 3% (60:1) polyacrylamide gel for 1.5 h. Gels were dried and exposed to film.

probe containing the octamer-binding site while other oligonucleotides did not. Preincubation of the NF-Y oligonucleotide was also able to compete away a band on the LPL promoter probe containing the CCAAT box while other oligonucleotides were ineffective. Overall, these experiments suggest that TNF-α can modify the binding of OCT-1 and NF-Y to the LPL promoter, thus reducing LPL gene transcription. Further work has revealed that OCT-1 is probably posttranscriptionally modified by TNF-α, as OCT-1 mRNA and protein are not altered by TNF-α treatment (unpublished data). Although TNF-α frequently works by increasing the activity of the transcription factor NFκB, and indeed TNF-α does increase NFκB in differentiated 3T3-L1 cells [10], there is at present no evidence that this factor can directly alter LPL gene transcription.

Cyclic AMP has also been proposed as a regulator of LPL gene expression [11,12]. A partial cAMP-responsive element is located in the human LPL promoter at –372 to –367. Stimulators of cAMP such as isobutylmethylxanthine are needed for adipocyte differentiation and hence increase LPL. However, in differentiated adipocytes, in vitro work has suggested that cAMP downregulates several adipocyte genes, including LPL [11]. Indeed, at high concentrations (10^{-5} M), isoproterenol (a β-adrenergic agonist) decreases ATLPL gene transcription [12]. Conversely, in brown fat, β-agonists increase LPL mRNA. It remains unclear, however, whether this effect occurs at the level of LPL gene transcription [13]. Thus the role of cAMP on LPL expression is far from clear.

Notably, the cAMP-responsive consensus sequence is conspicuously missing from the murine LPL promoter.

Before the results of these studies on LPL gene transcription are generalized, it is important to consider species and tissue differences further. Undoubtedly LPL is regulated in a tissue-specific manner and as such, physiologic regulators may have differing effects on LPL [1]. For example, although LPL gene regulation in macrophages appears to be differentiation-dependent [14], TNF-α will not decrease macrophage LPL [15]. In addition, despite only 65% homology between the murine and human LPL promoters, there are currently no known functional differences in the in vivo regulation of the lipase gene [7]. This could be because in differentiated tissues, most of the regulation is post-transcriptional. Moreover, in the proximal promoter (first 100 bp), where the control of basal transcription appears to predominate, there is 85% homology between the two species. These differences have been summarized in Fig. 1. An additional example of tissue-specific LPL transcriptional regulation is the extinction of liver LPL gene expression. LPL mRNA is expressed in neonatal liver cells, but during maturation a second transcription factor is produced which binds to an NF-1-like site on the LPL promoter, resulting in decreased transcription [16].

In summary, although much LPL regulation in vivo is posttranscriptional, there are two major exceptions: adipogenesis and the effect of TNF-α on ATLPL. In adipogenesis c-fos may play an important role, whereas in mature adipocytes OCT-1 and NF-Y are responsible for most of the basal promoter activity. Several in vivo regulators of LPL may also work by changing LPL gene transcription, allowing for more long-term regulation, while posttranscriptional mechanisms may serve the need for more rapid regulation of the enzyme activity better [17]. The distinction between the effects of inherent regulators on transcription versus posttranscriptional events is difficult to ascertain in vivo. The use of transgenic animals with variable portions of the LPL promoter offers a unique opportunity to explore more fully the role of regulators at both the transcriptional and posttranscriptional levels.

Acknowledgements

Unpublished work by C.L. Morin was supported by a USDA National Research Initiative Competitive Grants program award #92-37200-7522. This work was also supported in part by a grant from the National Institutes of Health (NIDDK) Grant DK26356. We also thank Isabel Schlaepfer for her technical assistance.

References

1. Eckel RH. N Engl J Med 1989;320:1060–1068.
2. Amri E, Dani C, Doglio A, Grimaldi P, Ailhaud G. Biochem Biophys Res Comm 1986;137:903–910.
3. Enerbäck S, Ohlsson BG, Samuelsson L, Bjursell G. Mol Cell Biol 1992;12:4622–4633.
4. Barcellini-Couget S, Pradines-Figueres A, Roux P, Dani C, Ailhaud G. Endocrinology 1993;132:53–60.
5. Christy RJ, Yang VW, Ntambi JM, Geiman DE, Landschulz WH, Friedman AD, Nakabeppu Y, Kelly TJ Lane MD. Genes Dev 1989;3:1323–1335.
6. Previato L, Parrot CL, Santamarina-Fojo S, Brewer HB Jr. J Biol Chem 1991;266:18958–18963.
7. Hua X, Enerbäck S, Hudson J, Youkhana K, Gimble JM. Gene 1991;107:247–258.
8. Currie RA, Eckel RH. Arch Biochem Biophys 1992;298:630–639.
9. Zechner R, Newman TC, Sherry B, Cerami A, Breslow J. Mol Cell Biol 1988;8:2394–2401
10. Morin CL, Schlaepfer IR, Eckel RH. Circulation 1993 (abstract).
11. Antras J, Lasnier F, Pairault J. Mol Cell Endocrinol 1991;82:183–190; and 1993;132:53–60.
12. Raynolds MV, Awald PD, Gordon DF, Gutierrez-Hartmann A, Rule DC, Wood WM, Eckel RH. Mol Endocrinol 1990;4:1416–1422.

13. Carneheim C, Nedergaard J, Cannon B. Am J Physiol 1988;254:E155–E161.
14. Goldberg DI, Khoo JC. Biochem Biophys Res Comm 1987;142:1–6.
15. White JR, Chait A, Klebanoff SJ, Deeb S, Brunzell JD. J Lipid Res 1988;29:1379–1385.
16. Schoonjans K, Staels B, Devos P, Szpirer J, Szpirer C, Deeb S, Verhoeven G, Auwerx J. FEBS Lett 1993; 329:89–95.
17. Olivecrona T, Liu G, Hultin M, Bengtsson-Olivecrona G. Biochem Soc Trans 1993;21:509–513.

Posttranscriptional regulation of lipoprotein lipase

David L. Severson and Rogayah Carroll

Faculty of Medicine, The University of Calgary, Calgary, AB T2N 4N1, Canada

Abstract. Lipoprotein lipase (LPL) is a glycoprotein that is synthesized in tissue parenchymal cells, and then secreted for translocation to the surface of the vascular endothelium. Potential mechanisms for the posttranscriptional regulation of LPL include alterations in (i) rates of synthesis; (ii) N-linked glycosylation (cotranslational) and processing of oligosaccharide chains by glucosidases in the endoplasmic reticulum (ER); (iii) oligomerization to the active homodimer; (iv) intracellular degradation (ER and/or lysosomes); (v) transfer to the plasma membrane for secretion and translocation to the vascular endothelium; (vi) exchange of endothelium-bound LPL with circulating LPL.

Lipoprotein lipase (LPL) is synthesized in parenchymal cells and is then secreted and translocated to binding sites on the luminal surface of vascular endothelial cells in a number of tissues [1]. The endothelium-bound (functional) enzyme catalyzes the hydrolysis of the triacylglycerol component of circulating lipoproteins; the fatty acid product is then available for tissue (parenchymal cell) utilization as appropriate (esterification or oxidation).

Synthesis, processing and secretion of LPL from parenchymal cells

LPL is synthesized in the rough endoplasmic reticulum (ER) as a 50—55 kDa polypeptide. LPL is a glycoprotein (8—12% carbohydrate), with either two or three oligosaccharide chains. N-linked glycosylation is a cotranslational event, which is followed by processing of the oligosaccharide chains in both ER and Golgi [1].

N-linked glycosylation of LPL is required for catalytic activity, based on results from experiments using tunicamycin to inhibit assembly of the dolichol-linked oligosaccharide that is transferred to the nascent protein [2—4], and on results from site-directed mutagenesis of Asn-43 in human LPL cDNA constructs [5]. Using glycoprotein-processing enzyme inhibitors, a number of investigations have recently shown that acquisition of catalytic activity by glycosylated LPL requires trimming of terminal glucose residues in the oligosaccharide chains by glucosidases in the ER [6—9]. The action of glucosidases must produce a conformational change that results in dimerization and activation of LPL in the ER [10,11]. These results with ER glucosidase inhibitors [6—9] are consistent with observations that LPL retained in the ER by incubation at low temperature, or LPL expressed from an LPL cDNA construct with an ER retention (KDEL) signal, is catalytically active [6].

N-linked glycosylation of LPL is responsible not only for catalytic activity but also for secretion. Thus, inactive nonglycosylated LPL [2,3,5] or inactive glycosylated LPL from cells treated with glucosidase inhibitors [6,9] is not released into the incubation medium. However, after activation (dimerization), further processing of oligosaccharide chains in LPL from high-mannose (ER) to complex forms by processing enzymes in the Golgi apparatus is not required for secretion of the enzyme from cells [4,6,7,9,12]. Processing to complex forms may, however, influence intracellular turnover [9]. The intracellular transfer of LPL through the Golgi to the cell surface can also be disrupted by agents such as brefeldin A [6] and monensin [4]. LPL is secreted from cells constitutively, and can be displaced into the medium from cell-surface binding sites by heparin [1]. The processes responsible for translocation of secreted LPL to functional binding sites on vascular endothelial cells are not well defined.

Posttranscriptional regulation of LPL in the heart

A number of instances where LPL is regulated by posttranscriptional mechanisms have been identified [1,13]. For example, in the heart, LPL is subject to posttranscriptional regulation during development, fasting and diabetes.

Development

Tavanger et al. [14] observed that changes in LPL activity and mass can be dissociated from LPL mRNA levels in the heart at two developmental periods. At the end of gestation and during the 1st 12 h of life, LPL activity and protein mass increase, but LPL mRNA levels remain constant. Conversely, in adult animals, LPL activity and protein decline even though LPL mRNA levels do not change [14].

Fasting

The reciprocal effects of fasting in adipose tissue and heart where LPL activity is reduced and increased, respectively, represents an interesting example of tissue-specific mechanisms for regulation of LPL activity [1]. As a result, fatty acid utilization is targeted according to the metabolic demands of individual tissues; the fasting-induced rise in cardiac LPL activity is important in supplying fatty acids for oxidation and energy production under conditions of caloric deprivation. The increase in LPL activity in fasted hearts is associated with an increase in LPL mass [15], with no change in LPL mRNA [15,16] or in rates of LPL synthesis [15,17] and turnover [17].

Diabetes

The induction of an acute and severe model of insulin-deficient diabetes results in decreased myocardial LPL activity, measured in perfused hearts (functional, endothelium-bound enzyme) and isolated cardiomyocytes (precursor of functional enzyme) [1]. This reduction in cardiac LPL activity is not accompanied by any change in LPL mRNA content (Fig. 1); in contrast, β-actin mRNA levels are reduced in the diabetic heart, as reported in other studies [18].

Sites and mechanisms for posttranscriptional regulation of LPL

Some possible cellular sites and potential mechanisms for the posttranscriptional regulation of LPL are shown in Fig. 2. Parallel changes in LPL activity and mass (with no change in enzyme specific activity) could be due to alterations in the balance between rates of synthesis (translation of LPL mRNA) and degradation. Altered rates of LPL synthesis can be specific or reflect generalized effects on protein synthesis [19]. LPL degradation (ER and/or lysosomes) is a potentially important site of LPL regulation. As much as 80% of newly synthesized LPL is degraded in adipocytes under basal conditions [1]; the turnover of cardiac LPL determined from pulse-chase experiments is much slower [7,17]. The fasting-induced increase in cardiac LPL activity and mass, however, is not accompanied by changes in LPL synthesis or turnover [15,17]. Liu and Olivecrona [17] have suggested,

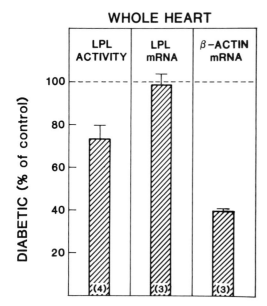

Fig. 1. The activity of LPL and the content of LPL mRNA and β-actin mRNA were measured in whole-heart homogenates from control and diabetic (100 mg/kg streptozotocin; 3–5 days duration) rat hearts. LPL mRNA was quantitated by slot-blot hybridization with an 872-base-pair cDNA clone against rat LPL mRNA (Dr R. Eckel, University of Colorado). Results for diabetic hearts are expressed as the percentage of control hearts (mean ± SE for the number of hearts given in parentheses).

therefore, that the selective increase in functional LPL in fasted hearts is the result of endothelial uptake of circulating LPL which is elevated by fasting. Changes in the dynamic equilibrium that determines LPL content at the vascular endothelium may also be responsible for the selective reduction in functional LPL activity in perfused hearts from mildly diabetic rats, because LPL activity in diabetic cardiomyocytes is unchanged (L. Liu and D.L. Severson, unpublished observations).

An alteration in LPL activity with no change in protein mass (so that enzyme specific activity changes) could be due to mechanisms involving glycosylation and subsequent oligomerization (dimerization) in the ER. Missense mutations in exon 5 of the human LPL gene result in an inactive, monomeric protein [20], indicating that assembly or stability of the active homodimer is inhibited. Defects in the oligosaccharide-processing pathway may be responsible for the observation that inactive, high-mannose LPL is retained in the ER in tissues from the combined lipase-deficient (cld/cld) mouse [1]. The fasting-induced fall in adipose tissue LPL activity may be due to the redistribution of LPL from a secretory pathway into an intracellular degradative pathway; the compensatory increase in synthesis of the inactive, high-mannose LPL precursor is responsible for the observation that total LPL mass (active and inactive) remains constant [15].

Clearly, more research on posttranscriptional mechanisms for LPL regulation is required. Can the ER glucosidases responsible for LPL activation be regulated by hormonal, nutritional or developmental mechanisms? What are the essential requirements for oligomerization to the active homodimer? What determines the fate of cellular LPL (degradation or secretion)? Can the complement of LPL-binding sites on the surface of parenchymal cells and vascular endothelial cells be regulated? How is release of LPL

PARENCHYMAL CELL

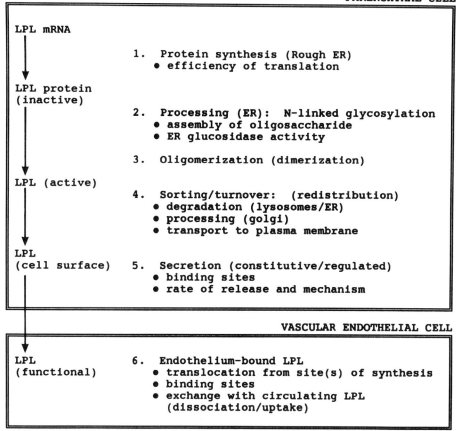

LPL mRNA

1. Protein synthesis (Rough ER)
   - efficiency of translation

LPL protein
(inactive)

2. Processing (ER): N-linked glycosylation
   - assembly of oligosaccharide
   - ER glucosidase activity

3. Oligomerization (dimerization)

LPL (active)

4. Sorting/turnover: (redistribution)
   - degradation (lysosomes/ER)
   - processing (golgi)
   - transport to plasma membrane

LPL
(cell surface)

5. Secretion (constitutive/regulated)
   - binding sites
   - rate of release and mechanism

VASCULAR ENDOTHELIAL CELL

LPL
(functional)

6. Endothelium-bound LPL
   - translocation from site(s) of synthesis
   - binding sites
   - exchange with circulating LPL
     (dissociation/uptake)

Fig. 2. Possible cellular sites and potential mechanisms for the posttranscriptional regulation of LPL.

from the parenchymal cell and translocation to the endothelium controlled? And finally, how important is uptake of circulating LPL as a determinant of functional, endothelium-bound enzyme activity, since this process is entirely independent of LPL regulation in tissue parenchymal cells?

References

1. Braun JEA, Severson DL. Biochem J 1992;287:337–347.
2. Olivecrona T, Chernick SS, Bengtsson-Olivecrona G, Garrison M, Scow RO. J Biol Chem 1987;262: 10748–10759.
3. Friedman G, Chajek-Shaul T, Etienne J, Stein O, Stein Y. Biochim Biophys Acta 1988;960:455–457.
4. Masuno H, Schultz CJ, Park J-W, Blanchette-Mackie EJ, Mateo C, Scow RO. Biochem J 1991;277: 801–809.
5. Semenkovich CF, Luo C-C, Nakanishi MK, Chen S-H, Smith LC, Chan L. J Biol Chem 1990;265: 5429–5433.
6. Ben-Zeev O, Doolittle MH, Davis RC, Elovson J, Schotz MC. J Biol Chem 1992;267:6219–6227.
7. Carroll R, Ben-Zeev O, Doolittle MH, Severson DL. Biochem J 1992;285:693–696.
8. Masuno H, Blanchette-Mackie EJ, Schultz CJ, Spaeth AE, Scow RO, Okuda H. J Lipid Res 1992;33: 1343–1349.

9. Simsolo RB, Ong JM, Kern PA. J Lipid Res 1992;33:1777—1784.
10. Liu G, Bengtsson-Olivecrona G, Olivecrona T. Biochem J 1993;292:277—282.
11. Masuno H, Okuda H. Biochim Biophys Acta 1994;1212:125—128.
12. Semb H, Olivecrona T. J Biol Chem 1989;264:4195—4200.
13. Enerbäck S, Gimble JM. Biochim Biophys Acta 1993;1169:107—125.
14. Tavangar K, Murata Y, Patel S, Kalinyak JE, Pedersen ME, Goers JF, Hoffman AR, Kraemer FB. Am J Physiol 1992;262:E330—E337.
15. Doolittle MH, Ben-Zeev O, Elovson J, Martin D, Kirchgessner TG. J Biol Chem 1990;265:4570—4577.
16. Enerbäck S, Semb H, Tavernier J, Bjursell G, Olivecrona T. Gene 1988;64:97—106.
17. Liu G, Olivecrona T. Am J Physiol 1992;263:H438—H446.
18. Camps M, Castelló A, Muñoz P, Monfar M, Testar X, Palacin M, Zorzano A. Biochem J 1992;282: 765—772.
19. Fried SK, Turkenkopf IJ, Goldberg IJ, Doolittle MH, Kirchgessner TG, Schotz MC, Johnson PR, Greenwood MRC. Am J Physiol 1991;261:E653—E660.
20. Hata A, Ridinger DN, Sutherland SD, Emi M, Kwong LK, Shuhua J, Lubbers A, Guy-Grand B, Basdevant A, Iverius P-H, Wilson DE, Lalouel J-M. J Biol Chem 1992;267:20132—20139.

Regulation of liver lipoprotein lipase gene expression

Johan Auwerx, Kristina Schoonjans and Bart Staels

Laboratoire de Biologie des Régulations chez les Eucaryotes (LBRE), Département d'Athérosclérose, Institut Pasteur, 1 Rue Calmette, 59019 Lille, France

Abstract. Lipoprotein lipase (LPL) is normally absent from adult liver. In neonatal liver, however, LPL mRNA and activity can readily be detected. LPL expression appears to be a characteristic of neonatal or undifferentiated hepatocytes, since its expression can be re-induced in hepatocytes during liver regeneration or after prolonged culture of primary hepatocytes concomitant with a reappearance of other fetal traits. Our studies have shown that this extinction process is mediated by a *cis*-acting element localized between −591 and −288 from the transcription initiation site. A novel nuclear protein, termed RF-2, only present in nuclear extracts obtained from adult liver, might be the *trans*-acting factor or extinguisher involved in this extinction process. Both tumor necrosis factor and peroxisomal proliferators such as fibrate hypolipidemic drugs can reinduce LPL expression in adult liver. For fibrates this reinduction is most probably mediated by the peroxisome proliferator activated receptor (PPAR) interacting with a PPRE in the LPL regulatory region. It is tempting to speculate that fibrates and TNF alter the differentiation characteristics of the hepatocytes.

Lipoprotein lipase (LPL) is a glycoprotein enzyme which is produced in several cells and tissues. LPL belongs to a large lipase gene family which includes hepatic lipase and pancreatic lipase. After secretion, LPL becomes anchored to the luminal surface of capillary endothelial cells. There it hydrolyzes triglycerides in triglyceride-rich lipoproteins, generating free fatty acids which can serve either as a direct energy source or can be stored. Through this action LPL plays a pivotal role both in energy and in lipoprotein metabolism. LPL's role in the removal of triglyceride-rich lipoproteins from the circulation and their subsequent hepatic uptake cannot, however, be wholly ascribed to the remodeling of triglyceride-rich lipoproteins. In fact, LPL could act as a ligand or bridging factor implicated in the retention of lipoprotein particles on the cell surface and hence facilitating their binding and uptake via cell surface receptors. Finally, LPL might also be implicated in the control of lipoprotein production since it has been shown that the net secretion rate of apoB-containing particles is reduced by enhanced re-uptake of nascent lipoproteins, a mechanism facilitated after modification of the newly secreted lipoproteins by the action of LPL.

In this paper we summarize our recent studies regarding the regulation of LPL expression in the liver. For more extensive discussions relating to other aspects of LPL, we refer to some recently published reviews [1–4].

Liver LPL production is associated with a partially differentiated state and is extinguished during development

LPL is synthesized in several differentiated tissues, such as skeletal and heart muscle, macrophages, adipose tissue and the lactating mammary gland. Interestingly, LPL synthesis appears to be induced during development and differentiation of these various tissues. In rats, for example, adipose tissue and heart LPL activity both increase during development. Compared to the basal situation, LPL production is also enhanced in lactating mammary gland (which corresponds to a more differentiated state). Similarly, in monocytes which do not express LPL mRNA or activity, an induction of LPL mRNA is detected upon their differentiation into macrophages [5]. The liver forms a notable exception to the rule that LPL expression is induced during development and differentiation. In this organ LPL activity and mRNA are present at birth at levels comparable to adipose tissue LPL mRNA levels, but LPL mRNA and activity gradually disappears upon development in a fashion reminiscent of the decrease in α-fetoprotein mRNA [6–9]. Further studies are necessary to determine whether LPL mRNA and activity are also present in neonatal human liver.

The expression of LPL mRNA in the neonatal liver and its disappearance during development suggested to us that the expression of LPL mRNA might be a characteristic of relatively undifferentiated or neonatal hepatocytes. Therefore we analyzed the effects of partial two-thirds hepatectomy on liver LPL expression. This procedure induces a transient proliferation of the remaining hepatocytes, resulting in partial liver regeneration, and is associated with a reinduction of several neonatal characteristics. Concomitantly with the reappearance of these fetal traits LPL mRNA was transiently reinduced during the liver regeneration that followed partial hepatectomy (maximal levels 24 h after partial hepatectomy) (Peinado and Auwerx, unpublished data). Furthermore, LPL gene expression could be re-induced in primary cultures of adult rat hepatocytes using specific culture conditions [10] favoring their transition to a fetal phenotype (Staels and Auwerx, unpublished data). It is interesting to note that α-fetoprotein expression is also transiently re-induced during liver regeneration and reappears after prolonged culture of primary hepatocytes.

Next, the expression of LPL was analyzed in various hepatoma cell lines that exhibit different stages of differentiation. Differentiated hepatoma cell lines that exhibit adult characteristics, such as the human cell lines Hep G2 and Hep 3B or rat Fa32 hepatoma cells, do not express LPL mRNA, whereas the fetal hepatoma cell lines mouse BWTG3 or rat McA RH 7777 express substantial amounts of LPL mRNA [11,12]. The production of LPL by hepatoma cell lines expressing fetal traits is consistent with hepatocytes being the source of LPL in the neonatal liver, and thus such cell lines are useful in vitro model systems to study the control of liver LPL gene expression. These data, together with the data obtained using partial hepatectomy and primary hepatocyte culture models, strongly support the notion that LPL production is a fetal hepatocyte trait. LPL would thus belong to a class of hepatic proteins which, like α-fetoprotein, are expressed during fetal hepatic tissue differentiation and are repressed once full tissue maturation is reached.

The extinction of liver LPL production is mediated by a *trans*-acting extinguisher protein

Although we have previously shown that the production of LPL in neonatal rat liver can be modified in vivo by treatment with either glucocorticoid or thyroid hormone [8], several observations suggest that factors other than these hormones are involved in the neonatal extinction process. First, prolonged hypothyroidism in the adult rat did not restore liver LPL production (Staels and Auwerx, unpublished data). Second, glucocorticoid hormone did not influence LPL production in BWTG3 cells [12]. Finally, data obtained from studies of cell hybrids derived from the fusion of LPL-producing mouse hepatoma cell line, BWTG3, with non-LPL-producing rat cells argued strongly against hormonal factors being the sole cause of extinction [11]. In fact, LPL expression is extinguished not only in hybrids formed between cells of different histiotypes (BWTG3 hepatoma cells x fibroblasts) but also in hybrids formed between cells of the same lineage but at different developmental stages (BWTG3 hepatoma cells × adult rat hepatocytes). This situation contrasts with that of the α-fetoprotein gene, which is not extinguished in BWTG3 × hepatocyte hybrids [13]. It has been shown previously by similar somatic cell and microcell hybrid studies that the tissue-specific extinction of several genes implicates specific *trans*-acting factors interacting with specific loci in *cis* (14). Examples of such tissue-specific extinction include the genes for α-fetoprotein, tyrosine aminotransferase, the T-cell antigen receptor, and albumin (see [11] for references). The LPL gene is therefore another example of a gene regulated by extinguisher factors produced by non-LPL-expressing cells, such as adult hepatocytes.

Potential candidates for the extinguisher protein

Using these culture models, we explored the existence of *cis*-acting regulatory sequences within the 5′ upstream region of the LPL gene that could respond to the *trans*-acting extinguisher. Nested deletions of the 5′-LPL regulatory sequences were cloned in front of the reporter gene CAT, and transiently transfected into Hep G2 and BWTG3 cells. The deletion of a region between −852 and −230 (relative to the major transcription initiation site described by Deeb and Peng, 1989 [15]) resulted in the appearance of CAT expression in several non-LPL-expressing cells such as Hep G2 or Hela cells. However, deletion of this sequence did not affect the expression of 5′-LPL-CAT constructs in the LPL-expressing fetal BWTG3 cells. Transfection with constructs containing more defined deletions identified the region important for extinction as being between −591 and −288, indicating that hepatic LPL extinction could occur by interaction of extinguisher proteins with specific DNA motifs in the promotor-enhancer region of its gene. By homology searches three potentially important regulatory elements in the region between −591 and −288 were identified: a potential GRE (at −468/−455), an NF-1 like site (at −514/−487), and a HNF-3 binding site (at −440/−430) (reviewed in [11]). The absence of a footprint on the HNF-3 site using adult liver nuclear extracts made it highly unlikely that the liver-enriched factor, HNF-3, was implicated in the regulation of LPL extinction. Although the presence of a bona fide GRE could be demonstrated by EMSA, its functional significance in liver cells was unclear. In fact LPL gene expression in BWTG3 cells was not affected by glucocorticoid hormones, despite the presence of a functional glucocorticoid receptor [12]. Furthermore, cotransfection of a glucocorticoid receptor expression vector with the LPL-CAT reporter constructs did not alter CAT expression in LPL-expressing BWTG3 hepatoma cells. Using liver nuclear extracts from either neonatal or adult animals, we showed that the NF-1 like site, which showed strong sequence homology to a typical CCAAT box [16], was in fact the only site protected [11]. It is interesting to note that the extent of protection was consistently greater when liver extracts of adult animals were used rather than extracts from neonatal animals. Upon incubation of a double-stranded oligonucleotide encompassing the sequence protected by DNase I footprinting analysis with liver nuclear extracts of neonatal animals in EMSA, a specific protein–DNA complex was identified, which we termed RF-1. In contrast, when liver nuclear extracts from adult animals were used a second complex of slower mobility (termed RF-2) could be visualized in addition to the complex present in neonatal animals [11]. This suggests that the additional factor RF-2, which binds to the LPL-NF-1 site and is present in adult animals only, might be a *trans*-acting factor or extinguisher implicated in the extinction or negative regulation of LPL gene expression. At present the factors binding to this site in neonatal as well as in adult animals are being characterized in more detail in the laboratory.

Re-induction of liver LPL by fibrates and tumor necrosis factor

More recently, two new and apparently unrelated factors, i.e., tumor necrosis factor and fibrates, have been shown to influence liver LPL production. However, the fact that both factors affect cell proliferation and differentiation might provide the link. Tumor necrosis factor was shown to specifically decrease adipose tissue LPL production through inhibition of LPL gene transcription (reviewed in [1,3]), an effect potentially mediated by the anti-adipogenic and dedifferentiating properties of TNF on adipose tissue [17]. Since TNF inhibits the expression of several adipogenic genes, the ultimate effect is a loss of morphologically differentiated adipose tissue and the occurrence of cachexia [17]. In the liver of the adult rat, TNF administration has an opposite effect: a sharp induction of LPL mRNA levels. This shows once more the important tissue-specific differences in the regulation of LPL expression [18]. Recent data from our laboratory extended these observations on the effect of TNF on liver LPL. In transgenic mice with a T-cell targeted overexpression of human tumor necrosis factor a strong expression of liver LPL mRNA was observed, contrasting with the absence of LPL mRNA in livers of their non-transgenic littermates (Staels, Prydz, Auwerx, unpublished results). Whether this re-induction of liver LPL can be explained by the regression of the liver to a more undifferentiated state awaits further study.

Our recent data using fibrates might support the hypothesis that liver differentiation might be involved in the regulation of LPL transcription [9]. Fibrates are potent hypolipidemic drugs which induce peroxisomal proliferation, and upon prolonged administration to rodents can induce proliferation of liver cells, resulting in hepatoma formation [19,20]. Fibrates can furthermore enhance the proliferative capacity of cultured hepatocytes and prevent apoptosis [21,22]. In fact, in adult rats or mice fibric acid derivatives induced a reappearance of LPL transcription and mRNA in the liver [9]. This effect was specific for the liver, since LPL expression did not change in adipose tissue or muscle. Furthermore, fibrate administration could delay the extinction process in neonatal animals [9]. The effects of fibrates on LPL mRNA levels in both neonatal and adult animals occurred through an induction of the transcription of the LPL gene.

Interestingly, it has recently been shown that the effects of fibrates and other peroxisome proliferators on gene expression is mediated via nuclear hormone receptors, termed peroxisome proliferator activated receptors or PPARs (reviewed in [20]). Indeed, the transcriptional activity of these receptors is activated in the presence of peroxisome proliferators such as fibrates, or in the presence of various fatty acids. These activated PPARs then induce the expression of target genes containing a peroxisome proliferator response element (PPRE). Preliminary studies in our laboratory suggest that the effects of fibrates on liver LPL expression are also mediated via interaction of an activated PPAR with a PPRE present in the 5'URS of the LPL gene. In fact a sequence motif in the LPL regulatory region showed a strong homology to a bona fide PPRE and was shown to bind PPAR/RXR heterodimers with high affinity (Schoonjans et al., unpublished data).

It is possible that the common denominator for all conditions in which LPL is expressed in the liver is a relatively undifferentiated state. Therefore, we suggest that the neonatal state, fibrate administration, and TNF administration are accompanied by an increased proliferative capacity of the hepatocytes and a more undifferentiated state. It is not clear whether the hepatic re-induction of LPL by fibrates also occurs in humans, but it is interesting to note that treatment with fibrates augments LPL activity in postheparin plasma [23].

Conclusions

Our data demonstrate that the liver is not only responsible for the degradation and clearance of LPL protein, but can also produce LPL itself. LPL mRNA and activity are readily detectable in neonatal liver, but become extinguished during development, which suggests that LPL production in the liver is associated with a relatively undifferentiated state of the hepatocytes. A novel nuclear factor possibly responsible for this extinction process is currently being characterized in our laboratory. LPL is furthermore re-induced in adult liver by the administration of TNF or fibrates. The effect of fibrates might be mediated by the nuclear receptor PPAR.

Acknowledgements

We appreciate the collaborations and discussions with Drs C. and J. Szpirer, S. Deeb, H. Prydz, J.-C. Fruchart, A. Mahfoudi, T. and G. Olivecrona, J. Brunzell, J. Peinado, M. Llobera, M. Reina, and S. Vilaro during various parts of this work. The technical assistance of D. Cayet, A. Tbaikhi, D. Quincey, L. Troonbeeckx and J. Rosseels are acknowledged. The work reported here has been supported by grants from the CNRS, Association pour la Recherche sur le Cancer (ARC), ARCOL, FGWO, Fondation pour la Recherche Medicale (FRM), Laboratoires Fournier, and the North Atlantic Treaty Organization (NATO).

References

1. Auwerx J et al. Crit Rev Clin Lab Sciences 1992;29:243–268.
2. Lalouel JM et al. Curr Opin Lipid 1992;3:86–95.
3. Enerback S, Gimble JM. Biochim Biophys Acta 1993;1169:107–125.
4. Santamarina-Fojo S, Dugi KA. Curr Opin Lipid 1994;5:117–125.
5. Auwerx J et al. Biochemistry 1988;27:2651–2655.
6. Llobera M et al. Biochem Biophys Res Commun 1979;91:272–277.
7. Burgaya F et al. Biochem J 1989;259:159–166.
8. Peinado J et al. Biochim Biophys Acta 1992;1131:281–286.
9. Staels B, Auwerx J. Development 1992;115:1035–1043.
10. Sirica AE et al. Proc Natl Acad Sci USA 1979;76:283–287.
11. Schoonjans K et al. FEBS Lett 1993;329:89–95.
12. Peinado-Onsurbe J et al. Biochemistry 1992;31:10121–10128.
13. Szpirer J et al. Exp Cell Res 1983;146:224–229.
14. Killary AM, Fournier REK. Cell 1984;38:523–534.
15. Deeb S, Peng R. Biochemistry 1989;28:4131–4135.
16. Dorn A et al. Cell 1987;50:863–872.
17. Torti FM et al. Science 1985;229:867–869.
18. Enerback S et al. Gene 1988;64:97–106.
19. Green S. Biochem Pharmacol 1992;43:393–401.
20. Auwerx J. Hormone Res 1993;38:269–277.
21. Bayly AC et al. J Cell Biol 1994;125:197–203.
22. Bars RGC, Elcombe CR. In: Ciliberto G, Cortese R, Schibler G, Schutz G (eds) Gene Expression During Liver Differentiation and Disease, 1992;IRBM:218.
23. Goldberg AP et al. N Engl J Med 1979;301:1073–1076.

246

Lipoprotein lipase binding to endothelial cells: specific protein–protein and protein–glycosaminoglycan interactions

Ira J. Goldberg[1], Pillarisetti Sivaram[1], Sungshin Y. Choi[1], Narayanan Parthasarathy[2] and William D. Wagner[2]

[1]Department of Medicine, Columbia University, 630 W. 168th Street, New York, NY 10032; and [2]Department of Comparative Medicine, Bowman Gray School of Medicine, Winston-Salem, NC 27157, USA

Abstract. The movement of lipoprotein lipase (LPL) from its site of synthesis in adipocytes and myocytes to its site of physiologic action on the luminal surface of endothelial cells might require a specialized system of transport. A basic biochemical understanding of this transport pathway requires delineation of the various cellular and cell-surface LPL-binding proteins. LPL binds to cell-surface heparan sulfate proteoglycans (HSPG). The specificity of this interaction appears to involve a highly sulfated decasaccharide. LPL also associates with nonproteoglycan proteins, including one found on the endothelial surface that has homology to the amino-terminal region of apolipoprotein B (apoB). Thus, a system analogous to that for growth factors and requiring two molecular interactions may have evolved to allow LPL to associate with endothelial surfaces.

Posttranslational regulation of LPL: potential involvement of the LPL transport pathway

LPL is best known for its physiological actions whereby it hydrolyzes triglyceride circulating in lipoproteins. This allows the catabolism of dietary and endogenous triglycerides and provides for the uptake of calories by muscles and adipose tissue. In addition, in vitro studies by our laboratory and others have demonstrated that LPL can form a molecule bridge between apoB-containing lipoproteins and cell-surface or matrix proteoglycans. This increases lipoprotein retention by the subendothelial matrix and uptake by cultured cells. LPL also increases LDL retention in isolated microvessels [1] and this may be a proatherogenic agent.

Although LPL is a member of the lipase gene family, it has several unique metabolic characteristics that make its biology of special interest. LPL is primarily synthesized and secreted from adipocytes and myocytes. Unlike most secretory proteins, however, LPL appears to reside transiently on the surface of its cell of origin. Studies of cultured adipocytes and immunohistological studies of adipose tissues show that LPL accumulates on the cells and is releasable by heparin. Some of this LPL is probably internalized and degraded by the LPL-synthesizing cells; this is one mechanism of posttranslational LPL regulation. The physiologically active LPL must be released from the cell surface and transferred from the adipocyte to endothelial cells. Then it transverses the endothelium from its abluminal to its luminal surface. During this transit there is potential for LPL, an unstable dimeric protein, to denature.

We have postulated that some of the changes in LPL activity that occur in adipose tissue result from modulation of the LPL transport pathway. When animals or humans are fasted hormone-sensitive lipase is activated, adipocyte fatty acids are released, and the concentration of free fatty acids in the interstitial space is increased. The possible effects of such an increase in free fatty acids on LPL transport were studied using monolayers of cultured endothelial cells [2]. High molar concentrations of oleic acid prevented the movement of LPL across the monolayer. If similar events occur in vivo, fasting would decrease the amount of active LPL present on the endothelial lumen without altering LPL transcription.

LPL interaction with endothelial surface proteoglycans

From the cell biological perspective, LPL interaction with endothelial cells has characteristics that are not similar to other protein–cell associations. Cell-surface LPL is internalized by endothelial cells but it is not degraded in the cell [3]. This may be because these cells do not express the LDL receptor-related protein (LRP) [4] that can bind, internalize and degrade LPL in other cells [5]. Unlike usual receptor–ligand interactions, LPL binding to endothelial cells is increased by acid pH [3]. Moreover, it should be noted that LPL movement across endothelial cells is against the flow of interstitial fluid. Thus a specific system, allowing transcytosis without intracellular degradation, might be operative.

The plasma contains a number of heparin-binding molecules, many of which circulate at concentrations that are orders of magnitude greater than that of LPL. Thus, if LPL binding to endothelial cells involved a nonspecific protein–glycosaminoglycan interaction LPL would be rapidly displaced from the cells. Because LPL is localized to capillary luminal surfaces, allowing for selective tissue triglyceride hydrolysis, LPL endothelial binding must have specific elements that insure its binding.

At least three different classes of HSPG are synthesized by endothelial cells. These include 1) perlecan, a large > 400 kDa basement membrane protein; 2) syndecans, a family of smaller transmembrane proteins; and 3) glipicans, phosphoinositol-anchored proteins [6]. To study the LPL-binding HSPG on the apical surface of cultured bovine aortic endothelial cells, cell surfaces were iodinated or the HSPG were sulfate-labeled. A 220-kDa transmembrane HSPG, which appears to be a member of the syndecan family, was isolated using LPL-Sepharose chromatography [7].

The specificity of most protein proteoglycan interactions resides in the oligosaccharide sequence of the heparan sulfate glycosaminoglycan. Using LPL-affinity chromatography, LPL-binding oligosaccharides were isolated from cultured bovine aortic endothelial HSPG. Endothelial heparan sulfate chains were deacetylated by hydrinolysis, cleaved with nitrous acid and reduced with $NaBH_4$. The resulting N-sulfated glucosamine-rich oligosaccharides were chromatographed on LPL-Sepharose. Over 95% of the HSPG did not bind to the column. An octasaccharide eluted with O.4 M NaCl and a decasaccharide eluted with 1.5 M NaCl. The higher affinity decasaccharide was treated with nitrous acid at low pH. Disaccharide analysis revealed that it contained five repeating disaccharide units of iduronic acid (2-SO_4-glucosamine NSO_4(6- SO_4). This sequence is distinctly different from that which binds to antithrombin and contains a 6-SO_4 that is not required for basic FGF binding to HSPG. A three-dimensional model of this oligosaccharide was constructed and reported [8].

LPL interaction with non-HSPG endothelial proteins

Aside from HSPG, many heparin-binding molecules have additional nonproteoglycan binding proteins. This is true for most growth factors, clotting proteins and apolipo-proteins. Thus, LPL could, like these other proteins, have both HSPG and non-HSPG-binding proteins. Alternatively, like antithrombin, it might interact solely with HSPG.

To further characterize the LPL binding molecules on endothelial cells, we developed a ligand blotting technique. Bovine aortic endothelial cells contained a protein of approximately 116 kDa that both reacted with LPL on ligand blots and bound to LPL-

Sepharose [9]. This protein was originally termed heparin releasable protein-116 (hrp-116) because it dissociated from cells after heparin treatment. Heparin treatment also decreased LPL binding to the endothelial cells. Using heparin-affinity chromatography, the protein was isolated from cell extracts, and amino acid sequence data were obtained [10]. Several peptides were homologous to the amino-terminal region of apolipoprotein. For this reason this LPL-binding protein is now denoted NTAB, N-terminal region of apoB.

LPL interaction with apoB

Does LPL have a protein–protein interaction with apoB? The association of LPL with apoB-containing lipoproteins in human postheparin plasma has been known [11]. In addition LDL is more effectively anchored to cells or matrix than either HDL [12,13] or lipid emulsions [14]. To assess whether the protein portion of LDL was responsible for these observations, LPL–LDL association was studied and compared to LPL association with HDL and lipid emulsion particles (S.Y. Choi, unpublished). Using ligand blotting, LPL was shown to bind to apoB and fragments of the amino-terminal region of apoB, but not to albumin, apoA-I or apoE. The interaction of LPL with apoB-containing lipoproteins was also studied using microtiter plate assays. LPL association with LDL was much greater than with HDL. LPL binding to LDL was not altered by delipidation of the bound LDL and was poorly competed with by lipid emulsion particles. Monoclonal antibodies against the amino-terminal regions of apoB inhibited the LPL–LDL association. Thus, the amino-terminal region of apoB might facilitate LPL association with apoB-containing lipoproteins.

Does NTAB participate in LPL binding to endothelial cells? To study the role of NTAB in LPL binding to endothelial cells, we treated cultured bovine endothelial cells with monoclonal anti-B antibodies. LPL binding to the cells was decreased approximately 60% [10]. When the cells were first treated with heparin, which should remove cell-surface NTAB, the residual binding to the cells was not altered by the antibodies. Thus, we hypothesized that LPL association with endothelial cells requires two interactions to provide specificity and increase the affinity of the LPL association with the endothelial-cell luminal surface.

Conclusions and speculations

LPL resides and works in a very turbulent environment on the luminal surface of endothelial cells. To survive the constant stresses of competing heparin-binding molecules and vascular flow, several molecular interactions must have evolved. One of these is binding to specific heparin-like, oligosaccharide sequences. Additional cell-surface LPL-binding molecules like NTAB might further strengthen this association. Moreover, endothelial cells lack the LPL-degradative pathway via LRP. This might permit these cells to internalize, transport, and recycle LPL without significant amounts of intracellular degradation. Although the molecules that link LPL to the luminal endothelial surface might also play a role in dissociating LPL from adipocytes and affecting their endothelial cell transcytosis, this remains to be proven.

The enzymatic and bridging functions of LPL require its interaction with lipoproteins. The homology of the amino-terminal region of apoB with the endothelial cell-derived LPL-binding protein was an unexpected observation. Both apoB48 and apoB100 contain an approximately 100-kDa globular, cysteine-rich amino-terminal region. This apoB region, which has no known functions, appears to associate directly with LPL.

Because active LPL is dimeric, each LPL molecule should have two NTAB-binding regions. One could hypothesize that NTAB facilitates the interaction of LPL with NTAB on endothelial cells and at the same time LPL could also associate with circulating apoB-containing lipoproteins. Whether such a physiochemical interaction of apoB and LPL is of physiologic importance is currently under investigation.

Acknowledgements

These studies have been facilitated by a series of collaborations and discussions with a number of investigators including Drs A. Attie, L. Curtiss, R. Deckelbaum, I. Edwards, H. Ginsberg, B. Mulloy, J. Rutledge, A. Sasaki, U. Saxena, and S. Sturley. Financial support included grants HL45095 (IJG and WDW), HL21006 SCOR (IJG), HL45848 (WDW) and a grant from the Council for Tobacco Research, USA (IJG).

References

1. Rutledge JC, Goldberg IJ. J Lipid Res 1994;35:1152–1160.
2. Saxena U, Klein MG, Goldberg IJ. Proc Natl Acad Sci USA 1991;88:2254–2258.
3. Saxena U, Klein MG, Goldberg IJ. J Biol Chem 1990;265:12880–12886.
4. Moestrup SK, Glieman J, Pallesen G. Cell Tiss Res 1992;269:375–382.
5. Beisiegel U, Weber W, Bengtsson-Olivecrona G. Proc Natl Acad Sci USA. 1991;88:8342–8346.
6. Lindahl U, Lidholt K, Spillmann D, Kjellen L. Thromb Res 1994;75:1–32.
7. Saxena U, Klein MG, Goldberg IJ. J Biol Chem 1991;266:17516–17521.
8. Parthasarathy N, Goldberg IJ, Sivaram P, Mulloy B, Wagner WD. J Biol Chem (in press).
9. Sivaram P, Klein MG, Goldberg IJ. J Biol Chem 1992;267:16517–16522.
10. Sivaram P, Choi SY, Curtiss LK, Goldberg IJ. J Biol Chem 1994;269:9409–9412.
11. Goldberg IJ, Kandel JJ, Blum GB, Ginsberg HN. J Clin Invest 1986;78:1523–1528.
12. Saxena U, Klein MG, Vanni TM, Goldberg IJ. J Clin Invest 1992;89:373–380.
13. Eisenberg S, Sehayek E, Olivecrona T, Vlodavsky I. J Clin Invest 1992;90:2013–2021.
14. Rumsey S, Obunike JC, Arad Y, Deckelbaum R, Goldberg IJ. J Clin Invest 1992;90:1504–1512.

Transport of lipoprotein lipase in plasma and lipoprotein metabolism

Gunilla Olivecrona, Magnus Hultin, Roger Savonen, Nina Skottova, Aivar Lookene, Yesim Tugrul and Thomas Olivecrona

Department of Medical Biochemistry and Biophysics, Umeå University, Umeå, Sweden

Abstract. There is a low, but significant, amount of active lipoprotein lipase (LPL) in plasma. This level is increased after fat infusions or lipid-rich meals. Most of the LPL in plasma is catalytically inactive. Heparin infusion in humans increases active LPL by several hundred-fold, but inactive LPL by only about 3-fold. When rats were given a bolus injection of a fat emulsion, plasma LPL increased gradually to a maximum at 6–8 min. During this time more than half the triglycerides were cleared. Therefore, the increase in LPL cannot be ascribed to binding to the emulsion particles as such, but is somehow linked to metabolism of the particles.

It has been suggested that LPL can mediate binding of chylomicrons and chylomicron remnants by the liver. To explore this, we perfused doubly-labeled chylomicrons through rat livers in the absence or presence of active or catalytically inactive LPL. Active LPL increased both lipolysis and particle removal in a dose-dependent manner. The same could be accomplished by a bacterial lipase showing that lipolysis, as such, enhanced hepatic uptake. After inhibition by active-site reagents, LPL still caused increased removal of chylomicrons. This suggests that the LPL protein itself enhances binding of chylomicrons in the liver.

Transport of LPL

Lipoprotein lipase (LPL) is synthesized in parenchymal cells in several extrahepatic tissues. After intracellular processing the enzyme is transferred to binding sites at the vascular side of endothelial cells in nearby capillaries and larger vessels [1]. There the enzyme is believed to be anchored via interaction with membrane-associated proteoglycans. Other, more specific, interactions may also be involved [2]. There is a low, but significant, amount of LPL in the circulating blood. Three roles have been suggested for this lipase:

1. The major catabolic route for endothelial LPL is probably transport to and degradation in the liver [3];
2. Transport of LPL in blood results in redistribution of the lipase between tissues, and transfer to sites where the lipase is not locally synthesized [4]; and
3. LPL associated with lipoproteins may target them for binding to cell-surface proteoglycans [5] and/or to specific receptors [6,7].

In the following we will focus on the third function.

LPL in blood

Heparin releases LPL from its endothelial binding sites into blood. This results in a several hundred-fold increase of the lipase activity. The amount of LPL in postheparin plasma is believed to reflect the amount of LPL that was exposed at the vascular

---

Address for correspondence: Gunilla Olivecrona, Department of Medical Biochemistry and Biophysics, Umeå University, S-901 87 Umeå, Sweden. Tel.: +46-90-165234. Fax: +46-90-167840.

endothelium, but does not correlate with the amount of LPL in basal plasma [8]. This suggests that LPL in basal plasma is not in equilibrium with endothelial LPL, but reflects a continuous flux of lipase molecules from sites of synthesis in peripheral tissues to sites for degradation in the liver [3]. This process is apparently influenced by factors other than the amount of lipase present at the endothelium.

Active and inactive forms of LPL in human plasma

The specific activity of LPL in plasma is low, which suggests that most of the lipase molecules have no catalytic activity [9]. That there should be inactive forms of the enzyme is not surprising. Active dimeric LPL has a built-in mechanism to self-destruct through dissociation into inactive monomers [10]. This may be an important aspect of the turnover of endothelial LPL.

Peterson et al. [11] exploited the specificity of two monoclonal antibodies to develop an ELISA technique that could differentiate between active, dimeric LPL and inactive, monomeric forms of the enzyme. By heparin-agarose chromatography they showed that the inactive form of LPL has lower affinity for heparin, and demonstrated that both inactive and active LPL are present in human postheparin plasma. Figure 1 shows an example of such a separation of plasma LPL from a normal individual. In postheparin plasma peaks of lipase activity and mass coincided at around 0.9 M NaCl in the gradient. There was also an earlier peak of inactive lipase that eluted around 0.5 M NaCl. In preheparin plasma only the early, inactive peak was seen. The mass of active lipase in preheparin plasma, corresponding to 1–3 mU/ml, is usually below the limit of detection in the immunoassay. In this experiment the ratio between the active LPL mass and

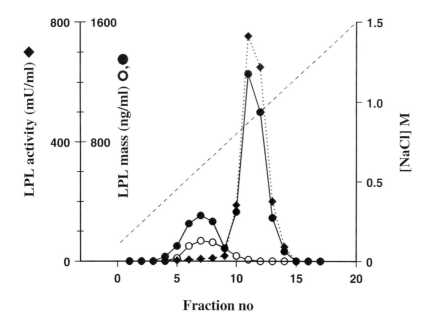

Fig. 1. Separation of active and inactive forms of LPL in plasma by chromatography on heparin-Sepharose. Ten ml of plasma was loaded on a small column of heparin-agarose and eluted by a gradient of NaCl. LPL mass was determined by an ELISA [9]. O LPL mass in preheparin plasma, ● LPL mass in plasma obtained 10 min after i.v. injection of 100 IU heparin/kg body weight, ◆ LPL activity in postheparin plasma.

inactive LPL mass in postheparin plasma was 3.6. Though the lipase activity in plasma increased 325-fold after heparin infusion the inactive LPL mass increased only 2-fold. It follows that whereas most of the lipase that circulates in plasma is inactive, most of the lipase that is released by heparin from binding sites on the vessel walls is active. In analysis of postheparin plasma from six individuals, the ratio between the active peak and the inactive peak was 2.9 ± 0.5. The inactive LPL peak increased 3.0 ± 0.4-fold after heparin infusion.

Increase in active LPL in plasma after lipid meals and after intravenous lipid infusions

Several studies have shown that LPL activity in plasma rises after fat meals [8,12] or after fat infusion [13—15]. The readiest explanation is that the emulsion droplets/chylomicrons bind the lipase, and thereby shift the equilibrium between endothelial binding sites and the circulating blood. There is, however, no consistent relation between the rise of plasma triglycerides and LPL during fat infusion [13,15] or postprandially [8]. It has been suggested that fatty acids rather than the lipoproteins themselves cause the increased release of lipase [8,13].

To further explore the mechanism by which LPL increases in plasma, some of us have studied the effects of a bolus injection of fat emulsion to rats [15]. Plasma LPL activity gradually rose 5-fold to a maximum at 6—8 min. During the same time the concentration of injected triglycerides decreased by half. Hence, the time-course for plasma LPL activity was quite different from that for plasma triglycerides. The disappearance of injected ^{125}I-labeled bovine LPL from the circulation was retarded by the emulsion. This effect was more marked 30 min than 3 min after injection of the emulsion, despite the much lower plasma triglyceride concentration at the later time. These data suggest that release of LPL into plasma is not solely due to binding of the lipase to the emulsion particles as such, but involves metabolism of the particles.

It is still not clear what the mechanism is for the postprandial increase of LPL, but it appears likely that most of the additional LPL is bound to chylomicron remnants. In studies by Karpe et al., LPL activity increased postprandially about 1 mU/ml [8], whereas apoB48 increased about 20 μg/ml [16]. If the increase of LPL was on chylomicron remnants, there would be a lipase molecule on each thousand remnants.

Role of LPL for chylomicron clearance by the perfused rat liver

LPL bound to chylomicron remnants has been suggested to act as a signal for rapid uptake of remnant lipoproteins in the liver [17]. It is known that LPL can mediate binding of lipoproteins to cell surfaces and to components of the extracellular matrix [5]. Furthermore, LPL can mediate binding of lipoproteins to the LDL receptor-related protein, LRP [6,7]. This requires the dimeric (active) form of LPL, since the sites for interaction with lipoproteins and with LRP partly overlap [7]. Binding of lipoproteins to proteoglycans can be mediated also by the monomeric form of LPL [5].

To investigate whether LPL could have a role in the uptake of remnant lipoproteins by the liver we perfused rat livers with chylomicrons doubly labeled in vivo with ^{3}H-retinyl esters and with ^{14}C-triglycerides (Skottova et al., in manuscript). The clearance of chylomicrons from the perfusate was slow without added LPL. Only small amounts of labeled free fatty acids appeared in the perfusate, showing that lipolysis was also slow. When LPL was added, lipolysis increased in a dose-dependent manner. The removal rate for retinyl esters increased dramatically, indicating that remnant particles were taken up by the liver. To test if this effect could be accomplished by any triglyceride lipase with activity against lipoproteins we used a bacterial lipase (*P. fluorescens*). This increased both lipolysis and particle clearance similarly to LPL. Thus, lipolysis as such is an important factor in remnant clearance.

To discriminate between effects of lipolysis and direct effects of the LPL protein for binding of lipoproteins by the liver we used LPL treated with active-site inhibitors. Equimolar amounts of tetrahydrolipstatin inhibited the lipase by more than 95% [18]. However, the conditions used during perfusion allowed rapid reactivation of the lipase, probably by catalytic turnover of the inhibitor. The partially inactivated LPL was more active in stimulating uptake of retinyl esters than was the bacterial lipase when they were compared at similar degrees of lipolysis. This suggested that there might be an additional effect of the LPL protein. With the nonreversible inhibitor hexadecylsulfonylfluoride (HDS) we could show increased clearance of chylomicron particles without concomitant lipolysis. Thus, in this system aimed to mimic the in vivo situation, the LPL protein, as such, enhanced binding of lipoproteins to the liver. This occurred even though the liver contained a full supply of hepatic lipase. Since little lipolysis occurred in the absence of LPL (or bacterial lipase), it must be concluded that hepatic lipase at its physiological site does not efficiently catch the lipoproteins on its own. Our data support a targeting function of LPL traveling with the lipoprotein particles, or already present in the liver.

Acknowledgements

Our studies are supported by grants from the Swedish Medical Research Council (B13X-727), the Bank of Sweden Tercentenary Fund and the Swedish Margarine Industry Fund for Research in Nutrition.

References

1. Olivecrona T, Olivecrona G. In: Schettler G, Habenicht AJR (eds) Principles and treatment of lipoprotein disorders. Berlin: Springer, 1994;175–205.
2. Stins MF, Sivaram P, Sasaki A, Goldberg IJ. J Lipid Res 1993; 34:1853–1861.
3. Vilaró S, Llobera M, Bengtsson-Olivecrona G, Olivecrona T. Am J Physiol 1988;254:G711–G722.
4. Camps L, Reina M, Llobera M, Vilaró S, Olivecrona T. Am J Physiol 1990;258:C673–C681.
5. Eisenberg S, Sehayek E, Olivecrona T, Vlodavsky I. J Clin Invest 1992;90:2013–2021.
6. Beisiegel U, Weber W, Bengtsson-Olivecrona G. Proc Natl Acad Sci USA 1991;88:8342–8346.
7. Nykjær A, Bengtsson-Olivecrona G, Lookene A, Moestrup SK, Petersen CM, Weber W, Beisiegel U, Gliemann J. J Biol Chem 1993;268:15048–15055.
8. Karpe F, Olivecrona T, Walldius G, Hamsten A. J Lipid Res 1992;33:975–984.
9. Vilella E, Joven J, Fernandéz M, Vilaró S, Brunzell JD, Olivecrona T, Bengtsson-Olivecrona G. J Lipid Res 1993;34:1555–1563.
10. Osborne JC Jr, Bengtsson-Olivecrona G, Lee NS, Olivecrona T. Biochemistry 1985;24:5606–5611.
11. Peterson J, Fujimoto WY, Brunzell JD. J Lipid Res 1992;33:1165–1170.
12. Olivecrona T, Hopferwieser T, Patsch JR, Bengtsson-Olivecrona G. In: Windler E, Greten H (eds) Hepatic endocytosis of lipids and proteins. Munich: Zuckschwert Verlag, 1992;288–291.
13. Peterson J, Bihain BE, Bengtsson-Olivecrona G, Deckelbaum RJ, Carpentier YA, Olivecrona T. Proc Natl Acad Sci USA 1990;87:909–913.
14. Nordenström J, Neeser G, Olivecrona T, Wahren J. Eur J Clin Invest 1991;21:580–585.
15. Hultin M, Bengtsson-Olivecrona G, Olivecrona T. Biochim Biophys Acta 1992;1125:97–103.
16. Karpe F, Steiner G, Uffelman K, Olivecrona T, Hamsten A. Atherosclerosis 1994;106:83–97.
17. Felts JM, Itakura H, Crane RT. Biochem Biophys Res Commun 1975;66:1467–1475.
18. Lookene A, Skottova N, Olivecrona G. Eur J Biochem 1994;222:395–403.

Lipoprotein lipase gene haplotypes and dyslipoproteinemias: study of a French-Canadian cohort

Pierre Julien[1], Chandrashekhar J. Savanurmath[2], Suresh P. Halappanavar[2], M.R. Ven Murthy[2], Georges Lévesque[2], François Cadelis[1], Claude Gagné[1] and Paul J. Lupien[1]

[1]Lipid Research Centre, Laval University Medical Centre and [2]Molecular Biology Laboratory on Human Diseases, Department of Biochemistry, Laval University, Canada

Abstract. Three missense mutations in the lipoprotein lipase (LPL) gene have been reported among French-Canadians as causes of primary LPL deficiency. Heterozygotes are characterized by decreased plasma postheparin LPL activity resulting in increased triglyceride levels, larger VLDL particles, denser LDL particles and lower HDL-cholesterol. These abnormal lipoprotein profiles result from impaired clearance of plasma triglycerides due to catalytically defective LPL enzyme. In the present report, we compare the haplotypes of LPL genes of French-Canadians harboring the three known mutations with those of LPL-deficient patients with unknown LPL mutations or with lipemic patients with unknown etiologies. These findings indicate that partial LPL deficiency could be an important component of dyslipidemia in the Québec population.

Lipoprotein lipase (LPL) is a homodimeric protein synthesized by parenchymal cells and transported to its functionally active site, the luminal surface of endothelial cells, where it is anchored by heparan sulfate to membrane glycoproteins [1]. LPL hydrolyzes plasma triglycerides transported by chylomicrons and VLDL. During the catabolism of triglyceride-rich lipoproteins, HDL particles appear to acquire lipid and apoproteins and transform them into more buoyant forms of HDL [2]. LPL also provides fatty acids to the peripheral tissues and affects the maturation of all lipoproteins.

Mutations of the LPL gene

The gene that codes for the LPL protein has been sequenced and a number of mutations affecting the LPL enzymatic activity have been described [3]. Recently, three missense mutations of the LPL gene have been identified in the French-Canadian patients of Québec which result in complete inactivation of the LPL enzyme [4]. Mutations 188 (M-188) and 207 (M-207) are the most frequent and account for 23 and 70% respectively of the mutant alleles. A third mutation, M-250, is also found among French-Canadians, but in much smaller numbers.

Dyslipoproteinemia in homozygotes

There is a relatively high prevalence of familial LPL deficiency in the French-Canadian population of Québec [5]. Clinical manifestations leading to the diagnosis of familial LPL deficiency are characterized by the presence of fasting chylomicrons (plasma triglycerides > 10 mmol/l) and abdominal pain, with pancreatitis as a major complication in the affected patients [6]. They may also manifest splenomegaly, hepatomegaly, lipemia

Address for correspondence: Pierre Julien, Lipid Research Centre, Laval University Medical Centre, 2705 Boulevard Laurier, Ste-Foy, QC, Canada G1V 4G2.

retinalis and eruptive xanthomas. An increase in erythrocyte membrane fluidity has also been reported in these patients and has been attributed to changes in membrane cholesterol and phospholipids in response to abnormal plasma lipoprotein composition [7]. Susceptibility to in vitro hemolysis is often observed in these patients and is presumably mediated by abnormally elevated levels of plasma lysophosphatidylcholine [8].

Several studies emphasize the importance of LPL in the building of fat tissue reserves. However, adiposity is observed to be within the normal range in the LPL-deficient patients, which indicates that normal adiposity can be maintained in the absence of tissue and plasma LPL activity [9]. It has been proposed that fat-tissue homeostasis may be accomplished by hepatic lipase activity or by efficient uptake of plasma free fatty acids in LPL deficiency [10].

Dyslipoproteinemia in heterozygotes

On the basis of the number of homozygote patients referred to the Lipid Clinics from different regions of the Province of Québec, we have estimated the minimum number of heterozygote carriers to be in the order of 45,000. The heterozygote state results in significantly reduced postheparin plasma LPL activity (40% average reduction) as well as in an atherogenic lipoprotein profile characterized by moderately increased plasma triglyceride levels (2.4 ± 0.2 mmol/l, mean ± SEM, n = 50), larger VLDL particles (triglyceride- and cholesterol-rich particles), denser LDL particles and cholesterol-poor HDL particles [4,11]. The dyslipoproteinemia appears to be more pronounced in male than in female heterozygotes and may constitute a sex-dependent form of familial dys-lipoproteinemia associated with a catalytically defective LPL protein.

Lipemia of unknown etiology

We have identified a group of lipemic patients who had no family history of LPL deficiency. Some of them (approximately 13%) were found to be heterozygous for one of the LPL gene mutations [4] and the rest had no mutations identified so far in the LPL gene or other genes involved in lipid metabolism. All the patients in this group showed variable deficiencies in plasma LPL activity and hypertriglyceridemia (triglycerides > 10 mmol/l) several times higher than that observed in heterozygotes containing an LPL gene mutation. Thus, they exhibited a type of lipemia very different from those usually present in simple mutations of the LPL gene, which suggests possible actions of other gene defects on the expression and function of LPL.

LPL gene haplotypes

The study of DNA polymorphisms has demonstrated polymorphic restriction sites in the LPL gene. The HindIII (+/+) genotype has been strongly associated with primary hypertriglyceridemia and lower levels of HDL-cholesterol in Caucasians [12]. Utilizing HindIII and PvuII polymorphisms, we have surveyed different groups of LPL-deficient and other lipemic French-Canadian patients (Table 1). M-188, which appears to be an ancient mutation [13] common to populations of different ancestries (European and East Indian), is associated with the same haplotype H1 (HindIII positive, PvuII negative) in all these races (Table 1). M-207, which so far seems to be specific to the French-Canadian population, is associated with haplotype H2 (HindIII positive and PvuII positive) in all patients. M-250, which has been found in Dutch, French as well as Italian ancestries [4, 14], is also associated in French-Canadians, specifically with haplotype H2.

Table 1. Haplotypes of LPL gene associated with lipemia caused by mutations in the LPL gene or by other undetermined etiologies

Haplotype[a]	Normal allele		Alleles in lipemia due to:							
			LPL gene mutation						unknown etiology	
			M-188		M-207		M-250		unidentified		
	n	%	n	%	n	%	n	%	n	%	n	%
H1	12	32	8	100	0	0	0	0	8	62	14	50
H2	21	55	0	0	11	100	5	100	3	23	12	43
H3	5	13	0	0	0	0	0	0	2	15	2	7
Total	38		8		11		5		13		28	

[a]H1: HindIII+ and PvuII–; H2: HindIII+ and PvuII+; H3: HindIII– and PvuII–. A plus sign denotes the presence of the restriction site, and a minus sign denotes its absence.

It is of interest to note (Table 1) that each of the three mutant alleles in the Québec population are associated with a specific haplotype: M-188 with haplotype 1 and the other two (M-207 and M-250) with haplotype 2, conforming to the hypothesis of a unique origin for each of these mutations. In fact, genealogical reconstruction of 30 families carrying the M-207 has allowed us to identify 16 founders all of whom migrated to Québec in the early 17th century from France, especially from Perche [5]. M-207 is distributed mainly in the eastern part of the Québec Province, while M-188 is found mainly in the western areas [15,16] (Table 2), in agreement with the phenomenon of demographic radiation from focal points where the founders settled originally. The 13 alleles with unidentified mutations did not correspond to a single haplotype, but were distributed among all three haplotypes H1, H2 and H3 in different proportions. Assuming that the unidentified mutations also arose from unique events, this would suggest that there may be at least three additional mutations underlying LPL deficiency in the French-Canadian patients. Among clinically identified homozygote patients, 13 alleles carried an as yet unidentified mutation. These alleles with unknown mutations were associated with H1, H2 and H3 haplotypes.

The great majority of LPL alleles (93%) in lipemics of unknown etiology belong to either haplotype H1 or H2, similar to the known mutant LPL alleles in the French-Canadian population (M-188, M-207 and M-250). The HindIII positive polymorphic site is common to both H1 and H2 haplotypes, which supports the previously described association between LPL gene polymorphisms and hypertriglyceridemia as well as a possible multifactorial control of plasma triglyceridemia [12].

Table 2. Estimation of the heterozygote carrier rate for LPL gene mutations in the province of Québec [6]

Administrative region	Estimated carrier rate
02 Saguenay Lac-St-Jean[a]	1/48
03 Québec (Charlevoix)[a]	1/116
04 Mauricie[b]	1/107
Eastern Québec[a]	1/88
Western Québec[b]	1/220
Whole Québec	1/143

[a]Founding region for mutation M-207; [b]Founding region for mutation M-188.

Conclusion

Our studies on the combined effect of abdominal fat accumulation and reduction in postheparin plasma LPL activity indicate that severe hypertriglyceridemia and elevated fasting insulinemia are strongly associated with waist circumference over the 50th percentile in the heterozygous state, a dyslipidemia more pronounced in male than in female patients [17]. These findings also show that increase in adiposity and reduction in plasma LPL activity have additive deleterious effects on plasma triglyceride levels. Hypertriglyceridemia in heterozygote patients is also associated with smaller and denser LDL and with reduced HDL-cholesterol to produce a lipoprotein profile that is known to increase coronary risk factor. All of these observations, together with the results presented here, support the idea that other genetic and/or environmental factors may interact in the phenotypic expression of the normal and also of the mutant LPL gene.

Acknowledgements

Supported by grants from the Heart and Stroke Foundation of Québec and Parke Davis Canada.

References

1. Brunzell JD. In: Scriver CR, Beaudet AL, Sly WS, Valle D (eds) The Metabolic Basis of Inherited Disease. New York: McGraw-Hill, 1989;1165–1180.
2. Santamarina-Fojo S, Dugi KA. Curr Opin Lipidol 1994;5(2):117–125.
3. Lalouel JM, Wilson DE, Iverius PH. Curr Opin Lipidol 1992;3(2):86–95.
4. Julien P, Gagné C, Murthy MRV, Cantin B, Cadelis F, Moorjani S, Lupien PJ. Can J Cardiol 1994;10 (suppl B):54B–60B.
5. Dionne C, Gagné C, Julien P, Murthy MRV, Roederer G, Davignon J, Lambert M, Chitayat D, Ma R, Henderson H, Lupien PJ, Hayden MR, De Braekeleer M. Hum Biology 1993;65(1):29–39.
6. Gagné C, Brun LD, julien P, Moorjani S, Lupien PJ. Can Med Assoc J 1989;140:405–411.
7. Cantin B, Brun LD, Gagné C, Murthy MRV, Lupien PJ, Julien P. Biochim Biophys Acta 1992;1139:25–31.
8. Cantin B, Boudriau S, Bertrand M, Brun LD, Gagné C, Rogers PA, Murthy MRV, Lupien PJ, Julien P. Hemolysis in primary lipoprotein lipase deficiency. Metabolism 1994 (in press).
9. Peeva E, Brun LD, Murthy MRV, Després JP, Normand T, Gagné C, Lupien PJ, Julien P. Int J Obesity 1992;16:737–744.
10. Cantin B, Brun LD, Gagné C, Murthy MRV, Lupien PJ, Julien P. Atherosclerosis 1994;109:68 (abstract).
11. Julien P, Gagné C, Murthy MRV, Moorjani S, Brunzell JD, Hayden MR, Lupien PJ. Circulation 1992;86 (suppl 4):I–419.
12. Ahn YI, Kamboh MI, Hamman RF, Cole SA, Ferrell RE. J Lipid Res 1993;34:421–428.
13. Ma Y, Henderson HE, Murthy MRV, Roederer G, Monsalve MV, Clarke LA, Normand T, Julien P, Gagné C, Lambert M, Davignon J, Lupien PJ, Brunzell JD, Hayden MR. N Engl J Med 1991;324(25):1761–1766.
14. Ma Y, Ilson BI, Bijvoet S, Henderson HE, Cramb E, Roederer G, Murthy MRV, Julien P, Bakker HD, Kastelein JJP, Brunzell JD, Hayden MR. Genomics 1992;13:649–653.
15. Normand T, Bergeron J, Fernandez-Margallo T, Bharucha A, Murhty MRV, Julien P, Gagné C, Dionne C, De Braekeleer M, Mo R, Hayden MR, Lupien PJ. Hum Genet 1992;89:671–675.
16. Bergeron J, Normand T, Bharucha A, Murhty MRV, Julien P, Gagné C, Dionne C, De Braekeleer M, Brun D, Hayden MR, Lupien PJ. Clin Genet 1992;41:206–210.
17. Julien P, Vohl MC, Lévesque G, Després JP, Murthy MRV, Gagné C, Gaudet D, Brun LD, Cadelis F, Moorjani S, Lupien PJ. American Diabetes Association, Boston, August 1994.

Trans fatty acids and lipoproteins

M.B. Katan[1], R.P. Mensink[2], A. van Tol[3] and P.L. Zock[1]

[1]Department of Human Nutrition, Agricultural University, Bomenweg 2, 6703 HD Wageningen; [2]Department of Human Biology, University of Limburg, P.O. Box 611, 6200 MD Maastricht; and [3]Department of Biochemistry, Erasmus University, Rotterdam, The Netherlands

Abstract. *Trans* fatty acids arise through biohydrogenation in the rumen of cows and sheep or catalytic hydrogenation in industrial hardening of oils. The effects of *trans*-monounsaturates on lipoproteins in man are opposite to those of their *cis*-isomer, oleic acid: *trans* fatty acids raise LDL and Lp(a) and lower HDL, all in a dose-dependent fashion. *Trans* fatty acids raised serum cholesteryl ester transfer (CETP) activity in 52/55 volunteers (mean change 18%, $p < 0.02$) and lowered the ratio of cholesteryl esters to triglycerides in HDL. Lecithin:cholesterol acyl transferase (LCAT) was unchanged. The effects of *trans* fatty acids on HDL and LDL may be mediated through cholesterol ester transfer protein.

Properties and consumption of isomeric fatty acids

Isomeric fatty acids are unsaturated fatty acids in which one or more of the double bonds have an unusual spatial geometry, namely *trans* instead of *cis*, or an unusual position along the length of the molecule, or both. In foods, geometric and positional isomers almost invariably occur together. As it is analytically easier to distinguish *trans* from *cis* isomers than one positional isomer from another, food analyses usually report *trans* fatty acids only rather than total isomeric fatty acids. Wherever this paper discusses effects of dietary *trans* fatty acids the positional *cis* isomers are implicitly included.

Typical intakes of *trans* fatty acids range from almost zero in the traditional Japanese diet to 10–15 g/day in The Netherlands; in most industrialized Western countries mean intakes are some 5–10 g/day.

Small amounts of *trans* fatty acids are continuously formed in the rumen of cows and sheep. *Trans* fatty acids arise here as intermediates in the hydrogenation (saturation) of dietary unsaturated fatty acids by the hydrogen produced during bacterial fermentation. As a result the fat in butter, cheese, and milk contains some 2–8% by weight of *trans* fatty acids, most of the remainder being saturated. Much higher proportions of *trans* fatty acids are formed during the industrial hydrogenation of vegetable oils. Such partially hydrogenated vegetable oils have a particular melting range, stability and mouth feel that makes them suitable for incorporation into a wide range of foods, including baked goods and hard margarines. It should be stressed that only particular types of margarines are high in *trans*, namely brick- or stick-type hard margarines made from partially hydrogenated oils. In contrast, typical levels of *trans* in soft margarines are some 3% of total fatty acids in The Netherlands and 11% in North America. Several brands of soft tub margarines sold in Europe and Canada have *trans* levels of 1% or less, and are also low in saturated fatty acids [1,2].

Address for correspondence: Martijn B. Katan, Department of Human Nutrition, Agricultural University, Bomenweg 2, 6703 HD Wageningen, The Netherlands. E-mail: martijn.katan@et3.voed.wau.nl. Tel.: +31-8370-82646 or +31-8370-82589. Fax: +31-8370-83342.

Effects on serum HDL and LDL concentrations in man

The toxicology of partially hydrogenated vegetable oils has been extensively investigated, and no untoward effects have been detected [3]. However, attention was drawn to *trans* fatty acids when a study in human volunteers [4] showed that *trans* monounsaturated fatty acids, produced through hydrogenation of oleic-acid-rich sunflower oil, lowered HDL- and elevated LDL-cholesterol levels compared with the natural *cis* isomer, oleic acid. A number of studies have appeared since which have largely confirmed these initial findings [5–7]. Figure 1 [8] shows the effects of monounsaturated *trans* fatty acids relative to their *cis* isomer oleic acid across five trials. We adjusted for differences in other fatty acids between the *trans*-enriched diets and the reference diets using regression coefficients from a recent meta-analysis [9]. Figure 1 suggests that the effect of *trans* fatty acids on HDL increases with the amount consumed. Although more experiments would be needed to define the shape of the dose–response curve more precisely, a linear relation appears satisfactory, and there is no evidence for a threshold below which *trans* fatty acids do not affect HDL-cholesterol levels. According to this small meta-analysis, every additional percent of dietary energy as *trans* fatty acids results in a decrease in HDL-cholesterol of 0.013 mmol/l or 0.50 mg/dl ($R^2 = 0.88$, p = 0.0019) and an increase in LDL-cholesterol of 0.040 mmol/l or 1.55 mg/dl ($R^2 = 0.86$, p = 0.0028). This effect on LDL is similar to that of saturated fatty acids [9].

Thus, monounsaturated *trans* fatty acids with a chain length of 18 carbon atoms lower HDL-cholesterol and raise LDL-cholesterol as compared with their *cis* isomer oleic acid, and the effect is proportional to the amount consumed, without evidence for a threshold.

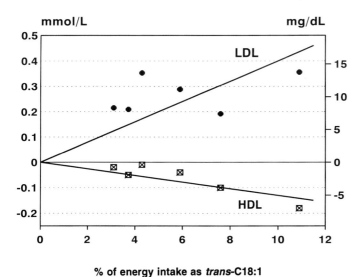

Fig. 1. Effects of monounsaturated *trans trans*-C18:1 on lipoprotein cholesterol levels relative to oleic acid (*cis*-C18:1). Data are derived from six dietary comparisons between *trans* monounsaturates and *cis* unsaturated fatty acids [5–7]. Differences between diets in fatty acids other than *trans* and *cis* monounsaturates were adjusted for by using regression coefficients from a meta-analysis of 27 controlled trials [9]. The regression lines were forced through the origin because a zero change in intake will produce a zero change in lipoprotein levels. Regression coefficients per % contribution of *trans* fatty acids to total daily energy intake are 0.040 mmol/l per en% for LDL ($R^2 = 0.86$, p = 0.0028) and –0.013 mmol/l per en% ($R^2 = 0.88$, p = 0.0019) for HDL-cholesterol.

Effects on lipoprotein(a)

Serum lipoprotein(a) (Lp(a)) is a strong and independent risk factor for coronary heart disease. We therefore examined the effect of *trans* fatty acids on serum Lp(a) levels in controlled trials.

In our first experiment [4] 10% of energy as the cholesterol-raising saturated fatty acids (lauric, myristic, and palmitic acid) was replaced by oleic acid or by *trans*-monounsaturated fatty acids. Each of the 59 participants received each diet for 3 weeks in random order. The median level of Lp(a) was 26 mg/l on the saturated-fat diet; it increased to 32 mg/l ($p < 0.001$) on the oleic-acid diet and to 45 mg/l ($p < 0.001$) on the *trans*-fatty-acid diet [10]. The second experiment [11] involved 56 subjects, who all received 8% of energy from the saturated fatty acid stearic acid, from linoleic acid, or from *trans*-monounsaturates, for 3 weeks each. Median Lp(a) levels were 69 mg/l on both the stearic-acid and linoleic-acid diet, and rose to 85 mg/l ($p < 0.01$) on the *trans*-fatty-acid diet [10].

Our data thus agree with the finding of Nestel et al. [5] in that *trans* fatty acids appear to raise Lp(a), even though the effect is quite small relative to genetically determined differences in Lp(a) levels. The effect of *trans* on Lp(a) is relevant for our understanding of lipoprotein metabolism: both saturates and *trans* fatty acids raise LDL levels in plasma, but *trans* fatty acids raise Lp(a), while saturates, if anything, tend to lower it [10]. This suggests that dietary effects on LDL and on Lp(a) follow different pathways.

Effects on cholesterol ester transfer protein (CETP)

Human plasma contains a protein which transfers cholesteryl esters from HDL to lipoproteins of lower density. We hypothesized that CETP could play a role in the effect of *trans* fatty acids on HDL and LDL levels. We therefore measured the serum activity levels of CETP (using excess exogenous substrate assays) in sera from our second study on *trans* fatty acids (van Tol et al., submitted). The CETP activities measured after the stearate diet and the linoleate diet were identical, despite the higher VLDL + LDL cholesterol levels seen after the stearate diet. The *trans*-diet was accompanied by an 18% increase in CETP activity if all subjects were analyzed together. The increase in CETP activity after the *trans*-diet was seen in 52 out of 55 individuals; one individual showed no effect and two showed a decrease in activity.

The increase in CETP activity coincided with a low cholesteryl esters/triglycerides ratio in HDL. This was to be expected because CETP removes cholesteryl esters from HDL and replaces them with triglycerides. The average molar ratio (±SD) was 6.15 ± 1.83 on the *trans*-diet vs. 6.97 ± 2.19 on the linoleate diet and 6.71 ± 2.25 on the stearate diet ($p < 0.02$).

It was previously reported that high concentrations of elaidic acid (*trans* C18:1 n-9), added in vitro, may increase the transfer of cholesteryl esters from HDL to LDL [11]. Therefore, *trans* fatty acids could act by increasing the serum levels of CETP, as suggested by our data, or by increasing the efficiency of the transfer process, as found in the in vitro experiments. Recently, Abbey and Nestel [12] reported increased CETP activity after substitution of *trans*-elaidic acid for *cis*-oleic acid in the diet. A significant increase was detected only if CETP activity was assayed employing endogenous lipoproteins, but absent if CETP activity was assayed in lipoprotein-deficient plasma. The CETP activity assay used in our present experiments is independent of endogenous lipoproteins and correlates very well with CETP mass. It is therefore possible that dietary *trans* fatty acids increase the transfer of cholesteryl esters by increasing CETP mass as well as by changing the structure of plasma lipoproteins, resulting in their acting as better substrates for CETP action.

Diminished levels of plasma CETP activity are often associated with a low-risk lipoprotein profile, while increased CETP levels are found in patients with various forms of hyperlipidemia. Also, intravenous injection of CETP into rats or introduction of CETP into mice by transgenesis results in a rise in LDL- and a fall in HDL-cholesterol. These changes are similar to those seen in humans consuming high *trans* fatty acid diets. Experiments with mice and monkeys fed atherogenic diets revealed close correlations between atherosclerosis development, LDL-cholesterol concentrations and plasma CETP levels. Our present data thus support the notion that the fall in HDL and increase in LDL on *trans* fatty acids are due to increased CETP activity, and that these lipoprotein changes may contribute to atherogenesis.

Policy implications

Trans fatty acids raise LDL and lower HDL, and if these changes are due to increased activity of CETP then both the rise in LDL and the fall in HDL might promote atherosclerosis. However, it would be erroneous to conclude that dietary fats high in *trans* fatty acids should now be replaced by fats high in saturates and cholesterol. The role of saturated fat and cholesterol in coronary heart disease has been abundantly documented. Also, intakes of saturated fatty acids far exceed intakes of *trans*. It is therefore preferable to count *trans* fatty acids in with the saturates, and aim for a reduction of the sum of the two. This implies replacement of hard fats by oils and margarines low in both *trans* and saturated fatty acids. Such margarines are widely available in Europe and Canada [1]. Their use will make it possible to reduce *trans* intake without reverting to products high in saturated fatty acids and cholesterol.

References

1. Katan MB. J Am Diet Assoc 1994; (in press).
2. Postmus E, deMan L, deMan JM. Can I Food Sci Tech J 1989;22:481—486.
3. Senti FR (ed) Health aspects of dietary *trans* fatty acids. Bethesda, MD: Federation of American Societies for Experimental Biology, 1988.
4. Mensink RP, Katan MB. N Engl J Med 1990;323:439—445.
5. Nestel PJ, Noakes M, Belling GB, McArthur R, Clifton PM, Janus ED, Abbey M. J Lipid Res 1992;33: 1029—1036.
6. Judd JT, Clevidence BA, Muesing RA, Wittes J, Sunkin ME, Podczasy JJ. Am J Clin Nutr 1994;59:861—868.
7. Lichtenstein AH, Ausman LM, Carrasco W, Jenner JL, Ordovas JM, Schaefer EJ. Arterioscler Thromb 1993;13:154—161.
8. Zock PL, Mensink RP, Katan MB. Am J Clin Nutr 1994 (in press).
9. Mensink RP, Katan MB. Arterioscler Thromb 1992;12:911—919.
10. Mensink RP, Zock PL, Katan MB, Hornstra G. J Lipid Res 1992;33:1493—1501.
11. Zock PL, Katan MB. J Lipid Res 1992;33:399—410.
12. Abbey M, Nestel PJ. Atherosclerosis 1994;106:99—107.

Effects of monounsaturated fatty acids on lipoprotein metabolism

B. Jacotot[1], R. Sola[2], C. Motta[3], N. Nicolaiew[1] and J.L. Richard[1]

[1]Unité INSERM 391 and Service de Médecine Interne V, Hôpital Henri Mondor, 94010-Créteil, France; [2]Facultat de Medicina, 43201-Reus, Spain; and [3]Laboratoire de Biochimie, Hôtel-Dieu, 63000-Clermont-Ferrand, France

Abstract. Increased consumption of monounsaturated fatty acids (MUFA) is associated with a low incidence of cardiovascular diseases, but the mechanism of that relation is unclear. We investigated the role of dietary fats on HDL physicochemical characteristics and whether these fats could affect the cholesterol efflux and the intracellular cholesterol in cultured fibroblasts. The HDL_3 obtained from subjects fed the MUFA diet (compared with saturated or polyunsaturated fats diet) induced the highest free-cholesterol efflux, coupled with a reduced content of intracellular cholesterol and a higher LDL-receptor activity of the cells. These variations of cholesterol efflux and the subsequent modulation of cellular cholesterol metabolism appear to be the consequence of modifications of HDL_3 physicochemical parameters, particularly of HDL_3 phospholipid fatty acid composition, fluidity and size.

To demonstrate the effect of dietary fats on the capacity of HDL_3 to remove cellular free cholesterol, we used an in vitro model of $[^3H]$-free cholesterol efflux from cultured fibroblasts to HDL_3. The ability of HDL isolated after different dietary fats to promote free-cholesterol efflux was correlated with the HDL composition, and particularly with the chain length of HDL-phospholipid fatty acids [1]. Variation of HDL-phospholipid fatty acids could be responsible for changes in fluidity of lipoproteins [2], and also in other structural characteristics of these particles such as HDL size. In the present work, we determined whether changes in these physicochemical characteristics of HDL_3 (overall composition, phospholipid fatty-acid composition, fluidity and size) induced by dietary fats could modulate cholesterol homeostasis in human fibroblasts, with particular emphasis on the relative effects of HDL_3 on free-cholesterol efflux, intracellular degradation of LDL and cellular cholesterol content.

Methods

Subjects were 12 healthy women, who adhered strictly to the dietary instructions, with a mean age of 39 (±1) year. Their plasma cholesterol and triglyceride levels were normal, and the body weight, initially in normal range, remained unchanged throughout the study. Four 7-week periods of diet, differing according to their composition of fats, were given successively: 1) saturated fatty acids (SFA); 2) monounsaturated fatty acids (MUFA); 3) n-6 polyunsaturated fatty acids (PUFA n-6); and 4) n-3 polyunsaturated fatty acids (PUFA n-3). The daily intake of fatty acids and polyunsaturated/saturated (P/S) ratio of the four diets are indicated in Table 1.

HDL_3 was isolated by ultracentrifugation (d = 1.120–1.210 g/ml), and its content of cholesterol (free and esterified), triglycerides, phospholipids, and fatty acid composition

Address for correspondence: B. Jacotot, Unité INSERM 391 and Service de Médecine Interne V, Hôpital Henri Mondor, 94010-Créteil, France.

Table 1. Daily intake of fatty acids and P/S ratio of the tested diets

	PUFA	MUFA	SFA	P/S
SFA diet:				0.2
g/day	8.2	23.5	35.3	
%	3.5	10.5	16	
PUFA n-6 diet:				2.4
g/day	32.8	20.5	13.7	
%	14.7	9.2	6.1	
MUFA diet:				0.6
g/day	9.7	42.7	14.6	
%	4.3	19.2	6.5	
PUFA n-3 diet:				1.6
g/day	20.3	34.1	12.6	
%	9.1	15.3	5.6	

For each diet, the daily intake is indicated in g/day per person, and in percentage of the total alimentary energy (%). PUFA = polyunsaturated fatty acids; MUFA = monounsaturated fatty acids; SFA = saturated fatty acids.

of phospholipids was studied [3]. HDL$_3$ fluorescence polarization was used for evaluation of particle fluidity according to Dachet, Motta et al [4], and HDL$_3$ size was determined by gradient gel electrophoresis according to Nichols et al. [5].

Cultured human fibroblasts were used for the determination of [^{3}H]-free-cholesterol efflux and LDL-receptor activity and for measurement of cellular cholesterol content [3].

Results

The overall composition and the phospholipid fatty acid composition of HDL$_3$ was different after the four diets. The HDL isolated after MUFA diet was the richest in cholesteryl esters and triglycerides. In HDL$_3$ phospholipids, the percentage of saturated fatty acids was the highest after SFA diet. The PUFA n-6 diet increased most markedly the proportion of polyunsaturated fatty acids. The percentage of monounsaturated fatty acids was the highest after MUFA and PUFA n-3 diets.

The MUFA diet presented the lowest values of HDL fluorescence anisotropy (Table 2). These values increased nonsignificantly after the PUFA n-6 diet, but significantly after the SFA and PUFA n-3 diets. HDL$_3$ fluorescence anisotropy was negatively correlated with HDL$_3$ phospholipid linoleic/linolenic acid ratio (r = –0.415, p < 0.01), and positively correlated with HDL$_3$ size (r = 0.389, p < 0.01).

The particle diameter of HDL$_3$ was lowest after MUFA, intermediate after SFA and PUFA n-6, and highest on PUFA n-3 (Table 2). For all diets, the HDL$_3$ size was negatively correlated with HDL$_3$ cholesteryl ester content (r = 0.499, p < 0.001).

The HDL$_3$ obtained from the subjects given the MUFA diet induced on fibroblasts the highest [^{3}H]-free-cholesterol efflux (34.5%) coupled with an increased [^{125}I]LDL receptor activity and a reduced content of intracellular cholesterol (Table 2). In contrast, the HDL$_3$ obtained from SFA diet produced the lowest values of cholesterol efflux and LDL-receptor activity, and elevated intracellular cholesterol content. Whereas the HDL$_3$ obtained after PUFA n-6 diet produced intermediate results between the two previous diets, the HDL$_3$ obtained after PUFA n-3 diet produced low values of cholesterol efflux (similar to those of SFA diet). In all the diets, we observed that the free-cholesterol efflux and the LDL-receptor activity varied in the same way, but the intracellular cholesterol

Table 2. Physical characteristics of HDL$_3$ and effects of these particles on cholesterol efflux, LDL degradation and cellular cholesterol content of cultured fibroblasts

Diet	HDL size[a]	Fluorescence anisotropy[b]	Cholesterol efflux[c]	LDL degradation[d]	Cell cholesterol content[e]
SFA	8.98 ± 0.02	0.198 ± 0.001	15.9 ± 1.2	7.8 ± 3.1	48.7 ± 9.8
PUFA n-6	9.09 ± 0.08	0.191 ± 0.001[h]	25.7 ± 2.4[g]	30.0 ± 5.6[g]	15.2 ± 0.8[g]
MUFA	8.71 ± 0.08[f,i]	0.186 ± 0.001[h,j]	34.5 ± 1.5[g,j]	35.1 ± 3.7[g]	26.1 ± 2.5[g]
PUFA n-3	9.00 ± 0.09[k]	0.207 ± 0.002[h,j,k]	11.8 ± 1.7[j,k]	6.5 ± 2.7[j,k]	50.1 ± 5.3[j,k]

[a]HDL$_3$ size in nm; results are expressed as mean ± SE.
[b]HDL fluorescence anisotropy (r) at 37°C, with diphenyl-hexatriene probe (mean ± SE).
[c][^{3}H]cholesterol efflux from cultured fibroblasts in the presence of HDL$_3$; results are expressed in % of the radioactivity of the medium, compared with the total radioactivity (medium + intracellular).
[d][^{125}I]-LDL degradation by cultured fibroblasts in the presence of HDL$_3$, expressed in μg of [^{125}I]-LDL per mg of cell protein per 4 h (mean ± SE).
[e]Intracellular cholesterol content of cultured skin fibroblasts in the presence of HDL$_3$, expressed as μg of free cholesterol per mg of cell protein (mean ± SE).
Significant differences: [f]from SFA at $p < 0.05$; [g]from SFA at $p < 0.01$; [h]from SFA at $p < 0.001$; [i]from PUFA n-6 at $p < 0.05$; [j]from PUFA n-6 at $p < 0.01$; [k]from MUFA at $p < 0.01$.

content changed inversely. The increased intracellular cholesterol was due to high levels of free cholesterol.

The HDL$_3$ fluorescence anisotropy was the most important determinant of free-cholesterol efflux ($R_2 = 0.34$, $p < 0.001$), which was also positively correlated with HDL$_3$ phospholipid linoleic/linolenic acid ratio ($R_2 = 0.12$, $p < 0.02$) and to the cholesteryl ester content ($R_2 = 0.28$, $p < 0.001$). Finally, HDL$_3$ size was negatively related to free-cholesterol efflux ($R_2 = -0.17$, $p < 0.01$).

Discussion

The HDL$_3$ obtained from the subjects who were fed a MUFA diet induced the highest free-cholesterol efflux from cultured fibroblasts, coupled with a reduced content of intracellular cholesterol and a high LDL-receptor activity. Apparently, in response to the variation in capacity of HDL$_3$ to remove cholesterol from cells there exists a change of both the LDL-receptor activity and the intracellular cholesterol content. Thus, HDL$_3$ obtained after SFA or PUFA n-3 diets, which produced the lowest free-cholesterol efflux, presented the lowest LDL-receptor activity and the highest cholesterol content. These two last phenomena could be explained by the fact that these cells contain most of their cholesterol in the free form, which has an inhibiting effect on the biosynthesis of LDL receptor. If these results can be transposed in vivo they lead to the hypothesis that HDL$_3$ from the MUFA diet might increase LDL-receptor activity in tissues by stimulating the efflux of cholesterol, resulting in a more rapid turnover of plasma LDL and perhaps avoiding the accumulation of these lipoproteins in the macrophages, and consequently foam-cell formation. This study confirms the relation between HDL$_3$ capacity to remove cholesterol from cells and its fluidity [2]. Fluidity is an important determinant of the HDL$_3$ capacity to accept cholesterol from cells. Thus, an increase of the lipoprotein fluidity enables the reception of more cholesterol, a well-known stiffening substance [6]. However, an excess of fluidity might lead to perturbations in the lipoprotein functions, as has been observed for cell functions when there is an excess of membrane cell fluidity [7]. There may be a specific degree of HDL fluidity favoring an optimal capacity to remove cellular cholesterol and therefore avoid its accumulation.

The two diets rich in PUFA had opposite effects on HDL_3 fluidity. HDL_3 isolated after PUFA n-6 induced intermediate results in comparison to diets rich in MUFA or SFA, while the HDL_3 obtained after PUFA n-3 were less fluid than those after SFA. The linoleic/linolenic acid ratio is very different in the two PUFA diets (353.0 and 2.9 for the n-6 and n-3 diets, respectively). A lower ratio is likely to induce more rigid lipoproteins. Conversely, an increase of this ratio might produce more fluid HDL_3, though this effect could be modulated by the oleic acid content of HDL_3 phospholipids, another well-known determinant of lipoprotein fluidity [2].

For all diets, a negative correlation was found between HDL_3 size and free-cholesterol efflux, which suggests that smaller particles induce high cholesterol efflux. Moreover, HDL_3 size was negatively correlated with the HDL_3 fluorescence anisotropy, showing that the smallest HDL_3 are the most fluid. Thus, these HDL_3 may have an adequate cholesterol diffusion coefficient and surface area, resulting in a more effective particle for removing cholesterol from cells [8].

In conclusion, this study indicates that HDL_3 physical characteristics, which are influenced by dietary fats, could be determinants of cholesterol efflux. Our results suggest that the relationship between HDL_3 size and free cholesterol efflux are mediated by other covariates, such as HDL_3 fluidity or its cholesteryl ester content. These data also give a new mechanism by which dietary fats exert their effect on the antiatherogenic role of HDL.

Acknowledgements

This work was supported by grants from the European Union and the CETIOM-ONIDOL.

References

1. Esteva O, Baudet MF, Lasserre M, Jacotot. Biochim Biophys Acta 1986;875:174–182.
2. Solà R, Baudet MF, Motta C, Maillé M, Boisnier C, Jacotot B. Biochim Biophys Acta 1990;1043:43–51.
3. Solà R, Motta C, Maille M, Bargallo MT, Boisnier C, Richard JL, Jacotot B. Arterioscler Thromb 1993;13:958–966.
4. Dachet C, Motta C, Neufcour D, Jacotot B. In: Malmendier C, Alaupovic P (eds) Adv Exper Med Biol 243. New York: Plenum Press, 1988;179–184.
5. Nichols AV, Blanche PJ, Gong EL. In: Lewis LA (ed) Handbook of Electrophoresis III. Boca Raton, Florida: CRC Press, 1983;29–47.
6. Shinitzki M. Biochim Biophys Acta 1984;738:251–261.
7. Shinitzki M. Physiology of Membrane Fluidity. CRC Press, 1984.
8. Rothblat GH, Phillips MC. J Biol Chem 1982;257:4775–4782.

Dietary cholesterol, plasma lipoproteins and cholesterol metabolism

Paul John Nestel

CSIRO Division of Human Nutrition, Adelaide, Australia

The relationship between dietary cholesterol and coronary heart disease (CHD) is still not entirely clear. To the extent that eating cholesterol affects plasma lipoprotein concentrations, its influence on CHD is important but indirect. Yet at least one major prospective study has led to the conclusion that dietary cholesterol is independently correlated with future CHD [1] by mechanisms that do not seemingly operate through lipoproteins. In one recent study in subjects with coronary artery disease, the progression of disease was directly correlated with several nutrients, including dietary cholesterol on univariate analysis, which weakened when saturated fat consumption was taken into account [2].

Nevertheless, the most likely link is through change in the atherogenic profile of the lipoproteins. Because the effect of dietary cholesterol in this respect is less than that of saturated fatty acids, public health messages have placed less emphasis on reducing dietary cholesterol.

In Western populations it is difficult to show a clear relationship between mean cholesterol intake and the average plasma cholesterol level, largely because other dietary factors confound the issue. However, in the NHANES II (National Health and Nutrition Examination Survey), among 8,679 Americans, dietary cholesterol was an independent positive predictor of serum cholesterol ($p < 0.04$) [3].

In general, advice to eat less cholesterol is a good example of the possible inappropriateness of targeting an entire population. The variability among individuals in their response to dietary cholesterol is a classic example of genetic influence on nutritional income.

Whereas much has been written about individual variability, it is likely that the serum cholesterol response to dietary cholesterol is almost normally distributed among metabolically normal subjects. This allows identification of both hyporesponders and hyperresponders. Some of this variability can be explained on the basis of cholesterol regulation and on the effectiveness of metabolic compensation in the face of increased cholesterol absorption. To this extent the variability is likely to reflect many genetic points of regulation, justifying the term "polygenic hypercholesterolemia". Findings from metabolic studies with up to one-third of subjects showing a degree of hyperresponsiveness reflect the approximate prevalence of polygenic hypercholesterolemia in the wider population. The genetic contribution to the population variance in the response to dietary cholesterol has been estimated as at least 50%, considerably greater than that for saturated fat. Two extremes are worth commenting on. The Tarahumara Indians of Mexico were reported as showing massive percentage rises in plasma cholesterol [4] whereas New Guinea Highlanders responded minimally to increased intakes of 1 g daily [5].

The lesser influence of dietary cholesterol than of fat was underlined by Keys when

Address for correspondence: Dr P.J. Nestel, CSIRO Division of Human Nutrition, P.O. Box 10041, Gouger Street, Adelaide, SA 5000, Australia. Tel.: +61-8-224-1865. Fax: +61-8-303-8899.

he showed that the change in plasma cholesterol was related only to the square root of the amount of cholesterol eaten.

One important consequence of the square-root relationship is that the effect of a change in intake is less when the total intake is high than when it is low. A recent meta-analysis by Hopkins [6], based on 27 published studies that had utilized controlled diets, has increased the confidence with which the effects of cholesterol intake can be said to influence the plasma cholesterol concentration. The relationship was found to be hyperbolic and dependent partly on baseline cholesterol intakes. Thus the relative rise in plasma cholesterol diminished as cholesterol intake rose and progressively lessened as baseline cholesterol intake rose. Increasing consumption from virtually zero to 500 mg (the approximate US average) increased plasma cholesterol by 12–15%: a substantial change. By contrast, when one or two eggs (200–500 mg) are added to about 500 mg, the change may be so small as to be lost in the variability inherent in such measurements. The failure of many studies to show an average increase in plasma cholesterol has been due to the faulty design of adding cholesterol to an already high intake. Further failures in experimental design are brought about by biological variability in plasma cholesterol and laboratory error. Keys and Parlin [7] had also stressed the variability in an individual's plasma cholesterol, as much as 20 mg/dl (0.5 mmol/l) in free-living subjects. The reproducibility of "responsiveness" has been tested by several workers. We have recently carried out a study in which 15 subjects were tested 6 months apart and given identical high-fat, high-cholesterol supplements. Their responses correlated significantly (r = 0.63, p < 0.01). Further, using a 5% increase in cholesterol as a definition of dietary sensitivity, 70% of the subjects retained their original category [8].

A further possible explanation of some discordant results is the failure to appreciate the interaction between dietary cholesterol and the proportions of saturated and poly-unsaturated fatty acids. Schonfeld et al. [9] have reported significantly lower effects on the serum cholesterol than might have been expected from the Keys equation, as the dietary P/S ratio was increased. We, on the other hand, have found that the degree of saturation of dietary fatty acids did not affect the response to dietary cholesterol [10]. As in our study, neither McNamara et al. [11] nor Brown et al. [12] could find that saturated fatty acids increased the sensitivity to dietary cholesterol. This was also the conclusion reached by Hopkins from a wide survey of available studies [6]. On the other hand, dietary fish oil appears to reduce cholesterol absorption [13].

The rise in the plasma cholesterol due to increased cholesterol consumption reflects changes mostly in LDL, but HDL-cholesterol often increases also. The nature and composition of the LDL remain largely unchanged, indicating that it is the number of LDL particles that rises, reflected in the increase in apoB. The significance of the rise in HDL-cholesterol and mostly also in apoA-I, has been recognized more recently. We have shown that even when total HDL-cholesterol does not change (in people apparently unresponsive to dietary cholesterol), HDL_2-cholesterol does change [10], increasing in size by becoming enriched in cholesterol. We raised the possibility then and confirmed it subsequently that HDL may be the preferred carrier of excess dietary cholesterol, especially in people whose total cholesterol rises minimally.

We have shown that the distribution of cholesterol between LDL and HDL when additional dietary cholesterol is being transported differs among individuals, giving a healthier profile involving mainly HDL or a less desirable profile in which the LDL rise predominates [8]. In general, the "hyperresponsive" hypercholesterolemic subjects show a rise in LDL-cholesterol, whereas normocholesterolemic and relatively unresponsive subjects partition more cholesterol within HDL. Women show a lesser rise in LDL whereas men show a lesser rise in HDL. Older men and hypercholesterolemic people shunt more dietary cholesterol into LDL [14].

When 56 hypercholesterolemic and normocholesterolemic men and women were given approximately 700 mg/day of egg yolk cholesterol in a double-blind, cross-over study there was a 0.23 mmol/l rise in plasma cholesterol after 4 weeks, a 0.19 mmol/l rise in LDL-cholesterol and a 0.07 mmol/l rise in HDL-cholesterol [8]. Normocholesterolemic individuals experienced small, nonsignificant rises in total, LDL- and HDL-cholesterol, respectively and the hypercholesterolemic subjects showed above-average rises.

Since our study also showed a close correlation between responsiveness to dietary saturated fat and to dietary cholesterol, in subsequent studies we compared diets either rich in or poor in both fat and cholesterol. In over 100 men and women we showed several important independent determinants of the nature of the lipoprotein response to changes in the diet including cholesterol (Clifton, Noakes and Nestel, unpublished).

We confirmed our earlier findings of preferential utilization of either HDL_2 or LDL in transporting excess plasma cholesterol. In women only HDL_2-cholesterol concentration rose, whereas rises in LDL-cholesterol occurred in both men and women, more so in the former. The LDL response was significantly and independently related to the baseline LDL level, to age in men, and to the apoE phenotype (rising from the E_2 through to the E_4 phenotype). The rise in HDL_2-cholesterol was significantly influenced by the baseline HDL_2 level and also by the waist:hip ratio (inversely: centrally obese people showed lesser HDL_2 responses). The baseline HDL_2-cholesterol concentration was in turn inversely related to both the fasting insulin level and to the activity of hepatic triglyceride lipase.

Less attention has been paid to the effects of dietary cholesterol on VLDL. Nestel et al. [15] compared the effects of increasing cholesterol consumption from 200–1700 mg. Although the plasma total cholesterol did not change significantly within VLDL, apoE/apoC ratio rose and VLDL became enriched with cholesteryl ester and became smaller. These changed characteristics led to the VLDL becoming bindable to heparin-sepharose, a feature of apoE enrichment and exposure of apoB regions which bind to heparin. The concentration of IDL also rose and led to a further experiment which showed that IDL apoB production was stimulated by a cholesterol-rich diet [16].

Thus, even in the absence of a rise in plasma total cholesterol, the lipoprotein profile may become atherogenic.

The mechanisms responsible for the increase in plasma cholesterol with cholesterol consumption are multiple and complex. Put most simply, there is evidence for both increased hepatic secretion and diminished clearance of lipoproteins. Nestel and Billington [16] showed that IDL production and secretion was raised, suggesting that these particles may have been preferentially secreted from the liver. Packard et al. [17] have also reported increased production of LDL (which are largely derived from IDL), and that the removal of LDL by the LDL-receptor route was impaired. Consistent with this are observations of reduced in vitro uptake of LDL by mononuclear cells of subjects having high cholesterol intakes [18].

The increased formation of IDL and of LDL could be a consequence of the failure of their immediate precursors (e.g., small VLDL) to be cleared by the liver. Feedback inhibition of cholesterol synthesis, measured by sterol balance techniques, has been reported among subjects who show little rise in plasma cholesterol estimated at between three-quarters [19] and two-thirds [11] of Caucasians in an Australian and an American study respectively. The New Guinea Highlanders showed quite marked reductions in cholesterol synthesis [5]. By contrast, Jones et al. [20], who measured the initial rate of cholesterol synthesis within the rapidly turning over pool, using deuterium incorporation into sterol, were unable to show feedback inhibition at cholesterol intakes of 200 mg or so. Increased sterol re-excretion in feces occurs with increased cholesterol consumption but is inadequate to maintain homeostasis. Hopkins in his review [6] concludes that the liver is more efficient at maintaining normal cellular cholesterol concentration in the face of depletion than with overload. Increased fractional absorption of cholesterol is emerging as a factor in diet-induced hypercholesterolemia [21], resembling experimental animal models. This increase in cholesterol absorption efficiency has been reported to be greatest in people with the apoE$_4$ phenotype and to be inversely related to the fractional catabolic (removal) rate of LDL [21]. Increased bile acid synthesis has been difficult to demonstrate in healthy people eating even very large amounts of egg cholesterol; synthesis may even be depressed in people with gallstones [22].

Dietary cholesterol does not appear to influence the clearance of dietary fat, which may reflect the clearance of chylomicron remnants by receptors other than the LDL receptor [23]; this is not surprising since chylomicron removal is generally regarded as occurring normally even in LDL receptor-deficient heterozygotes. Interestingly, transfer of cholesteryl ester among plasma lipoproteins is influenced, rising (as measured by CETP mass) with high cholesterol intakes [23].

References

1. Shekelle RB, Shrock AM, Paul O et al. N Engl J Med 1981;304:65—70.
2. Watts GF, Jackson P, Mandalia S et al. Am J Cardiol 1994;73:328—332.
3. Gartside PS, Glueck CJ. J Am Coll Nutr 1993;12:676—684.
4. Connor W, Cerqueira M, Connor S et al. Am J Clin Nutr 1978;31:1131—1142.
5. Whyte M, Nestel P, MacGregor A. Eur J Clin Invest 1977;7:53—60.
6. Hopkins PN. Am J Clin Nutr 1992;55:1060—1070.
7. Keys A, Parlin RW. Am J Clin Nutr 1965;17:174—178.
8. Clifton PM, Kestin M, Abbey M et al. Arteriosclerosis 1990;10:394—401.
9. Schonfeld G, Patsch W, Rudel LL et al. J Clin Invest 1982;69:1072—1080.
10. Kestin M, Clifton PM, Rouse IL et al. Am J Clin Nutr 1989;50:528—532.
11. McNamara DJ, Kolb R, Parker TS et al. J Clin Invest 1987;79:1729—1739.
12. Brown SA, Morrisett J, Patsch JR et al. J Lipid Res 1991;32:1281—1289.
13. Nestel PJ. Am J Clin Nutr 1986;43:752—757.
14. Clifton PM, Nestel PJ. Arterioscler Thromb 1992;12:955—962.
15. Nestel P, Tada N, Billington T et al. Metabolism 1982;31:398—405.
16. Nestel PJ, Billington T. Metabolism 1983;32:320—322.
17. Packard CJ, McKinney L, Carr K et al. J Clin Invest 1983;72:34—51.
18. Mistry F, Miller NE, Laker M. J Clin Invest 19981;67:493—502.
19. Nestel PJ, Poyser A. Metab Clin Exp 1976;25:1591—1599.
20. Jones PJH, Lichtenstein AH, Schaefer EJ. J Lipid Res 1994;35:1093—1101.
21. Miettinen TA, Kesaniemi YA. Am J Clin Nutr 1989;49:629—635.
22. Kern F. J Clin Invest 1994;93:1186—1194.
23. Ginsberg HN, Karmally W, Siddiqui M et al. Arterioscler Thromb 1994;14:576—586.

Genetic factors in lipoprotein responsiveness to diet in humans

J.M. Ordovas, J. Lopez-Miranda, P. Mata, A.H. Lichtenstein, B. Clevidence and E.J. Schaefer

Lipid Metabolism Laboratory, Jean Mayer USDA Human Nutrition Research Center on Aging at Tufts University, Boston, MA 02111, USA

Abstract. Dietary recommendations to optimize plasma lipid and lipoprotein profiles and reduce the risk of coronary heart disease (CHD) are to reduce the total fat, saturated fat, and cholesterol content of the diet. The extent of the response to changes in the amount or type of dietary fat and cholesterol has been shown to vary between individuals. It has been suggested that the serum lipoprotein response to dietary manipulation has a strong genetic component. Such genetic variability may have a significant impact on the success of public health policies and individual therapeutic interventions. Genetic polymorphisms at the apoA-I, apoA-IV and apoE gene loci appear to affect the level of LDL-cholesterol responsiveness to diet.

It has long been known that in both animals and humans a considerable degree of variability exists with regard to changes in plasma lipoprotein, specifically low density lipoprotein (LDL)-cholesterol levels, and alterations in dietary fatty acids and cholesterol. Such variability has assumed increasing importance as LDL-cholesterol has been identified as a major target of intervention for coronary heart disease risk reduction. Jacobs et al. [1] have documented that 9% of subjects were hypo-responders and 9% of subjects were hyper-responders, based on the < 50% or >150% of predicted response with the Keys equation [2] in well-defined metabolic studies assessing effects of dietary fatty acids and cholesterol on total cholesterol levels. Katan et al. [3] documented a similar variation with regard to response to dietary cholesterol for LDL-cholesterol. These investigators clearly showed a striking variability, ranging from marked hypo- to marked hyper-responsiveness. In our own data we have documented in 43 middle-aged and elderly men and women who had normal or elevated LDL-cholesterol levels a striking variability in response ranging from +1 to –40% LDL-cholesterol lowering in subjects studied on an NCEP step 2 diet, as compared to an average American diet.

It can be assumed that at least some of this variability in response is due to mutations at specific gene loci. Potential candidate gene loci include apoE, apoA-IV, apoA-I, apoB, LDL receptor, lipoprotein lipase, 7 α-hydroxylase, and microsomal transfer protein. In these gene loci there is currently evidence that apoE isoforms [4—8], apoA-IV isoforms [9,10], and the mutation within the apoA-I gene promoter at –78 [11] can all affect dietary responsiveness in LDL-cholesterol to changes in dietary fatty acids and/or cholesterol. These data will be reviewed.

ApoE isoforms

Early studies by Utermann et al. [12] documented the existence of apoE isoforms. The

---

Address for correspondence: Dr Ernst J. Schaefer, Lipid Metabolism Laboratory, Jean Mayer USDA Human Research Center on Aging at Tufts University, 711 Washington Street, Boston, MA 02111, USA.

genetics at the apoE locus was clarified by Zannis et al. [13], and the individual mutations causing the apoE isoforms were elucidated by Rall et al. [14]. Moreover, the apoE2 homozygous state has been associated with dysbetalipoproteinemia, as has familial apoE deficiency [15]. In addition, the apoE*4 allele has been associated with elevated levels of LDL-cholesterol in various population studies [16]. The common allele for apoE, known as apoE*3, has cysteine at residue 112 and arginine at residue 158. The allele frequency in the Framingham Offspring Study was 0.79, consistent with many other previous studies. ApoE*4, a variant allele in which arginine is present instead of cysteine at residue 112 and arginine is present at 158, has an allele frequency of 0.13 in the Framingham Offspring Study, and has been associated with elevated levels of LDL-cholesterol in most population studies. Finally, the apoE*2 variant allele, in which cysteine is present at residues 112 and 158, has an allele frequency in the Framingham Offspring Study of 0.08, and has been associated with lower levels of LDL-cholesterol. It had been suggested that the apoE alleles might account for as much as 14% of the variability in cholesterol levels. In our own recent studies in over 2,000 men and women participating in the Framingham Offspring Study, utilizing previously published equations by Boerwinkle et al. [17,18], only 1% of the LDL-cholesterol variability in men could be accounted for by the apoE alleles, and 0.5% in premenopausal women, but 5% in postmenopausal women [19]. It should be noted that, for data in both men and women, the apoE*2 allele appears to have a somewhat greater effect on LDL-cholesterol lowering than the apoE*4 allele has on raising it. Cross-cultural studies indicate that the apoE alleles have greater effects in populations such as Finland which consume diets higher in total fat, saturated fat, and cholesterol than populations such as Japan, known to consume diets significantly lower in total fat, saturated fat, and cholesterol [16].

Various dietary studies have been designed to address the issue of whether the apoE alleles have an effect on LDL-cholesterol and total-cholesterol response to diets which contain a variable amount of saturated fat, other fatty acids, and cholesterol. An initial study by Miettinen et al. in 1988 [4] documented that the apoE alleles did have a significant effect in predicting LDL-cholesterol response to dietary modification. This was also true for the studies by Tikkanen et al. in 1990 [5], Manttari et al. in 1991 [6], a second study by Miettinen et al. in 1992 [7], and our own recent studies in 1994 [8]. In contrast, studies by Boerwinkle et al. [20], Savolainen et al. [21], Cobb et al. [22], and Martin et al. [23] reported no significant effects of the apoE alleles on dietary LDL-cholesterol response. We have carried out a meta-analysis on 612 subjects participating in all these studies, and this clearly indicates that apoE alleles do have an effect on dietary LDL-cholesterol response when all data are taken into account. The data are consistent with the concept that subjects that carry the apoE*4 allele, especially men, are more responsive to dietary modification with regard to LDL-cholesterol changes than are subjects who do not carry this allele [8].

In our own studies in collaboration with Drs. Clevidence and Judd in Beltsville at the USDA Nutrition Research Center, and Dr Denkle at the University of Texas Southwestern in Dallas, we documented that apoE alleles did have an effect [8]. For example, in 86 male subjects consuming diets meeting NCEP step 1 criteria versus the average American diet, the mean reduction in LDL-cholesterol was 15%. This lowering was 23% in subjects carrying the apoE*4 allele, and 14 and 16% in subjects carrying the apoE*3 allele alone or the subjects carrying both the apoE*2 and the apoE*3 allele. In females the mean reduction in LDL-cholesterol in response to this diet was less, at 8% (47 females) with reductions of 11, 7, and 11% being observed for the different apoE*3/*4, apoE*3/*3 and apoE*2/*3 groups, respectively. None of these differences was statistically significant.

These data are consistent with the concept that male subjects who carry the apoE*4 allele are more responsive to dietary saturated fat and cholesterol restriction than male subjects not carrying this allele.

The question that arises is, how could these apoE alleles affect this response to diet? It is known that dietary saturated fat and cholesterol restriction lowers LDL-cholesterol at least in part by enhanced LDL clearance and increased LDL receptor activity. It is also known that apoE4 has a somewhat higher affinity for triglyceride-rich particles than apoE3, and for this reason it appears that apoE4 may result in somewhat more rapid uptake of such particles by the liver, resulting in excess lipid deposition in the liver and resultant downregulation of the LDL receptor. Presumably this is the mechanism causing the modest LDL-cholesterol elevation that is observed in population studies in subjects carrying the E*4 allele. Therefore, such subjects would be predicted to be more responsive to dietary modification which causes an upregulation of the LDL receptor. In addition to lipoprotein clearance, subjects with different apoE phenotypes have been reported in some studies to have variable efficiencies of intestinal cholesterol absorption [7]. It should be noted here that we have recently investigated the effect of apoE alleles on LDL lowering in response to HMG-CoA reductase inhibitors, as have other investigators. Our own data are consistent with those of Carmena et al. [24] which indicate that the opposite is true with regard to responsiveness to HMG-CoA reductase inhibitors where subjects carrying the apoE*4 allele are less responsive to HMG-CoA reductase inhibitors than other subjects, while subjects carrying the apoE*2 allele appear to be slightly more responsive [25].

ApoA-IV gene locus

A number of mutations have been reported within the apoA-IV gene sequence. The most common mutation is a substitution of glutamine for histidine at residue 360. The allele frequency for this mutation is approximately 0.05 to 0.12 in Caucasians, and it appears to be less common in other races; in some population studies in Caucasians the apoA-IV*2 allele has been associated with higher levels of HDL-cholesterol and/or lower levels of triglycerides, but this association has not been observed in other studies. In our own dietary studies [9], again in collaboration with other investigators at the USDA facility in Beltsville and the University of Texas Southwestern, we have documented that subjects with the apoA-IV*1/*2 phenotype are less responsive to these diets in terms of LDL-cholesterol lowering than subjects who are homozygous for the apoA-IV*1 phenotype. In these studies, in 93 men the mean LDL-cholesterol reduction was 13%, with subjects with the apoA-IV*1/*1 phenotype having a 16% reduction in male subjects with the apoA-IV*1/*2 phenotype having a 17% reduction. In contrast, in 60 women both types of subjects had the same 7% reduction in LDL-cholesterol. These data are consistent with the concept that male subjects with the apoA-IV*1/*2 phenotype are less responsive in terms of LDL lowering to diets meeting NCEP step 1 criteria [9]. In addition, recently McCombs et al. [10] examined the effects of the apoA-IV alleles on changes in lipoproteins in response to cholesterol feeding. They measured plasma lipids and lipoproteins before and after cholesterol feeding, in which the baseline diet contained approximately 200 mg of cholesterol and the intervention diet contained approximately 1,100 mg of cholesterol per day, which was achieved by the addition of four egg yolks per day. In these studies, subjects carrying the apoA-IV*1/*2 allele (n = 11) were documented to have only a 1 mg/dl increase in LDL-cholesterol, while other subjects (n = 12) were documented to have a 19 mg/dl increase in LDL-cholesterol with cholesterol feeding. These data suggest that apoA-IV is an important genetic locus for predicting response to dietary cholesterol. Potential mechanisms could include effects on cholesterol absorption; however, this remains to be determined.

ApoA-I gene locus

A common mutation has been reported in the promoter region for the apoA-I gene, and represents an A for G substitution at 78 base pairs upstream from the apoA-I gene-transcription start site. This allele has been associated with elevated HDL-cholesterol levels, as well as with decreased promoter activity in vitro and with abnormalities in apoA-I production. In our studies in 50 young men [11], subjects were fed a low-fat diet for 25 days, followed by a diet rich in monounsaturated fatty acids which comprised more than 50% of the fat in a 40% fat diet. Subjects were on this higher-fat diet for 28 days, and lipoproteins were measured at the end of each diet phase. Subjects with the GG genotype had a mean 1 mg/dl reduction in LDL-cholesterol, while subjects with the GA genotype had a 10 mg/dl increase in LDL-cholesterol, indicating greater responsiveness in the GA subjects than in the more common GG genotype. These data suggest that this mutation also allows one to predict response to diets altered in fatty acid content. How this mutation precisely affects LDL-cholesterol response is not known.

Conclusions

In the future, these initial studies need to be verified by more investigations in this area, in which all of these mutations are examined and in which BMI and initial LDL-cholesterol as well as age are also controlled for. Moreover, in the future, additional mutations will presumably be identified which also predict variability in LDL-cholesterol response to dietary modification.

In summary, our data indicate that, as in animal studies, humans exhibit a high degree of variability in LDL-cholesterol response to dietary fat and cholesterol modification. Moreover, apoE isoform, apoA-IV isoforms, and the apoA-I gene-promoter mutation all appear to affect the degree of LDL-cholesterol responsiveness to diet.

Acknowledgements

Supported by NIH grant HL 39326 from the National Institutes of Health, and contract 53-3K06-5-10 from the USDA Department of Agriculture Research Service. Dr Lopez-Miranda and Dr Mata were supported by Fellowships from the Spanish Ministries of Health, and Agriculture, Madrid, Spain.

References

1. Jacobs DR, Anderson JT, Hannan P, Keys A, Blackburn H. Arteriosclerosis 1983;3:349–356.
2. Keys A, Anderson JT, Grande F. Metabolism 1965;14:747–758.
3. Katan MB, Beynen AC, de Vries JH, Nobels A. Am J Epidemiol 1986;123:221–234.
4. Miettinen TA, Gylling H, Vanhanen H. Lancet 1988;2:1261.
5. Tikkanen MJ, Huttunen JK, Enholm C, Pietinen P. Arteriosclerosis 1990;10:285–288.
6. Manttari M, Kosninen P, Enholm C, Huttunen JK, Manninen V. Metabolism 1991;40:217–221.
7. Miettinen TA, Gylling H, Vanhanen H, Ollus A. Arterioscler Thromb 1992;12:1044–1052.
8. Lopez-Miranda J, Ordovas JM, Mata P, Lichtenstein AH, Clevidence B, Judd JT, Schaefer EJ. Effect of apolipoprotein E phenotype on diet induced plasma low density lipoprotein cholesterol lowering. J Lipid Res 1994 (in press).
9. Mata P, Ordovas JM, Lopez-Miranda J, Lichtenstein AH, Clevidence B, Judd JT, Schaefer EJ. Arterioscler Thromb 1994;14:884–891.
10. McCombs RJ, Marcadis DE, Ellis J, Weinberg RB. N Engl J Med 1994;331:706–710.

11. Lopez-Miranda J, Ordovas JM, Espino A, Marin C, Salas J, Lopez-Segura F, Perez-Jimenez F. Lancet 1994;343:1246–1249.
12. Utermann G, Hees M, Steinmetz A. Nature 1977;269:604–607.
13. Zannis VI, Breslow JL. Biochemistry 1981;20:1033–1041.
14. Rall SC Jr, Weisgraber KH, Innerarity TL, Mahley RW. Proc Natl Acad Sci USA 1982;79:4696–4700.
15. Schaefer EJ, Gregg RE, Ghiselli G. J Clin Invest 1986;78:1206–1219.
16. Davignon J, Gregg RE, Sing CF. Arteriosclerosis 1988;8:1–21.
17. Boerwinkle E, Sing CF. Am J Hum Genet 1986;39:137–144.
18. Boerwinkle E, Visvikis S, Welsh D, Steinmetz J, Hanash SM, Sing CF. Am J Med Genet 1987;27:567–582.
19. Schaefer EJ, Lamon-Fava S, Johnson S, Ordovas JM, Schaefer MM, Castelli WP, Wilson PWF. Arterioscler Thromb 1994;14:1105–1113.
20. Boerwinkle E, Brown SA, Rohrbach K, Gotto AM Jr, Patsch W. Am J Hum Genet 1991;49:1145–1154.
21. Savolainen MJ, Rantala M, Kervinen K, Jarvi L, Suvanto K, Rantala T, Kesaniemi YA. Atherosclerosis 1991;86:145–152.
22. Cobb MM, Teitlebaum H, Risch N, Jekel J, Ostfeld A. Circulation 1992;86:849–857.
23. Martin LJ, Connelly PW, Nancoo D, Wood N, Zhang ZJ, Maguire G, Quinet E, Tall AR, Marcel YL, McPherson R. J Lipid Res 1993;34:437–446.
24. Carmena R, Roederer G, Mailloux H, Lussier-Cacan S, Davignon J. Metabolism 1993;42:895–901.
25. Ordovas JM, Lopez-Miranda J, Perez-Jimenez F, Rodriguez C, Park J-S, Cole T, Schaefer EJ. Effect of apolipoprotein E and A-IV phenotypes on the low density lipoprotein response to HMG-CoA reductase inhibitor therapy. Atherosclerosis (in press).

Dietary fatty acids and cholesterol: effects on the plasma lipids and lipoproteins

William E. Connor and Sonja L. Connor

The Division of Endocrinology, Diabetes and Clinical Nutrition, Department of Medicine, Oregon Health Sciences University, Portland, OR 97201-3098, USA

Abstract. Dietary saturated fatty acids and cholesterol decrease the LDL-receptor activity in the liver. This impairs LDL removal from the plasma and hence increases plasma LDL concentration. The capacity of a food or diet to affect the plasma LDL concentration can be denoted by a single number, the cholesterol saturated fat index (CSI). Fruits, grains, beans and vegetables are devoid of cholesterol and extremely low in saturated fat, so their CSIs are almost zero, whereas eggs, butter, cheese and fatty meat are just the opposite with CSIs of 10–25. Their consumption elevates plasma LDL concentrations.

The very long-chain polyunsaturated ω-3 fatty acids from fish and fish oil have an especially potent hypotriglyceridemic effect. These fatty acids (EPA and DHA) depress the synthesis of triglyceride-rich lipoproteins, especially VLDL, and improve the clearance of chylomicrons and VLDL from the blood.

A diet low in saturated fat and cholesterol but high in the ω-3 fatty acids would have maximal plasma lipid–lipoprotein lowering effects for both LDL and VLDL in order to prevent coronary heart disease.

Early in this century, de Langen was the first to raise the serum cholesterol levels by feeding foods rich in cholesterol and saturated fat [1]. He fed the Dutch diet (butter, cheese, eggs and meat) to Javanese seamen accustomed to a diet of rice, fruit, fish and vegetables. Then followed hundreds of studies over the next 70 years which indicated that dietary cholesterol and saturated fat are the paramount factors to raise the plasma cholesterol and LDL levels.

This paper will focus upon those two most important pathogenic factors, cholesterol and saturated fat, and upon their combined effect to elevate the plasma low density lipoprotein (LDL) levels. Frequently, these two factors are found together in foods of animal origin although there are exceptions. It is both convenient and educational to generate a single number to indicate the capacity of a given food, recipe or menu to influence the plasma LDL levels from their contents of cholesterol and saturated fat. This number is termed the cholesterol saturated fat index (CSI). A final topic for review is the beneficial effects which result from the group of ω-3 fatty acids derived from fish and fish oil.

Dietary cholesterol and LDL levels

After absorption, dietary cholesterol enters the body via the chylomicron pathway and is removed from the plasma by the liver as a component of chylomicron remnants. Only about 40% of ingested cholesterol is absorbed; the remaining 60% is excreted in the stool.

Address for correspondence: William E. Connor, MD, Department of Medicine, L-465, The Oregon Health Sciences University, Portland, OR 97201-3098, USA. Tel.: +1-503-494-2001. Fax: +1-503-494-6986.

Since the feedback inhibition of cholesterol biosynthesis in humans is only partial even with a large dietary cholesterol intake, dietary cholesterol adds to the amount of cholesterol synthesized by the body [2]. The sterol nucleus cannot be broken down like fat, protein and carbohydrate. As a consequence, cholesterol must be either excreted or stored. Cholesterol is excreted in the bile and, ultimately, in the stool. It is excreted intact or as bile acids synthesized in the liver. Because there is efficient reabsorption of both bile acids and cholesterol, the enterohepatic circulation returns much of what is excreted into the bile back into the body.

After dietary cholesterol is removed by the liver as a component of the chylomicron remnant, it enters the hepatic pool of cholesterol. The quantity of cholesterol in the liver profoundly affects the catabolism of LDL. This effect is mediated through the LDL receptor [3]. In particular, an increase in hepatic cell cholesterol, usually not compensated for by a reduction in cholesterol biosynthesis, will decrease the synthesis of messenger RNA for the LDL receptor which decreases the LDL-receptor activity and, subsequently, causes an increase in the level of LDL-cholesterol in the plasma [4]. Conversely, a drastic decrease in dietary cholesterol will increase the LDL-receptor activity in the liver, enhance LDL removal, and, hence, will lower plasma LDL-cholesterol levels.

Twenty-six separate metabolic experiments over the past 30 years and involving 196 human subjects and patients have shown profound effects of dietary cholesterol upon plasma total and LDL-cholesterol levels [5,6]. These data document the importance of dietary factors in hyperlipidemia associated with any phenotype or genotype. At one extreme are the Tarahumara Indians, who have an average plasma cholesterol level of 120 mg/dl. They consume a low-cholesterol, low-fat diet and respond to an increase in dietary cholesterol with a 20% increase in the plasma cholesterol and a 24% increase in LDL-cholesterol concentrations [7]. This is similar to an increase of 17% in the mean plasma cholesterol that occurred when 1,000 mg dietary cholesterol was added to a cholesterol-free diet in 32 subjects (11 normal and seven with type IIa mild, five with IIa severe, and nine with type IV hyperlipidemia) (Fig. 1). LDL-cholesterol increased very significantly in all groups, again showing indirectly the effects of dietary cholesterol upon the LDL receptor.

Large changes in the amounts of dietary cholesterol will not necessarily increase the plasma cholesterol if dietary cholesterol intake is already substantial. For example, an increase in dietary cholesterol from 475 to 950 mg per day will not elevate the plasma cholesterol level. This phenomenon is restudied from time to time and mistakenly interpreted as showing that dietary cholesterol has no effect on the plasma total and LDL-cholesterol levels. These dietary cholesterol-feeding studies have been exhaustively reviewed for those who wish to explore the subject more fully [6,8].

The effect of gradually increasing amounts of dietary cholesterol upon the plasma cholesterol level is shown in Fig. 2. These findings are supported by both animal and human experiments. In the context of a cholesterol-free diet, the amount of dietary cholesterol necessary to produce a measurable increase in plasma cholesterol is termed 'the threshold amount'. As the dietary cholesterol is increased, the plasma cholesterol level increases and then ultimately plateaus. The amount of dietary cholesterol at this inflection point is termed the *ceiling* amount. Increasing the dietary cholesterol further does not lead to higher levels of plasma cholesterol, even though phenomenally large amounts may be fed. Each animal or human being probably has its own unique threshold and ceiling amount. Generally speaking, the average threshold amount for human beings is about 100 mg/day. The average ceiling is in the neighborhood of 300–400 mg/day. Thus, a baseline dietary cholesterol intake of 500 mg/day from two eggs would, for most

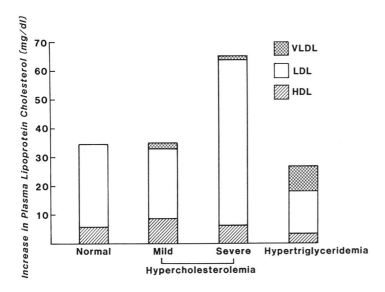

Fig. 1. Effects of a 1,000-mg/day cholesterol diet on the plasma lipoproteins of 25 subjects who comprised a heterogeneous group (normals, moderate and severe hypercholesterolemics and hypertriglyceridemics). The preceding control diet was cholesterol-free. Both dietary periods were 4 weeks in length.

individuals, exceed the ceiling. The addition of two more egg yolks for a total of 1,000 mg/day, however, would not then further increase the plasma cholesterol concentration. Beginning with a low cholesterol diet less than 100 mg/day and adding the equivalent of

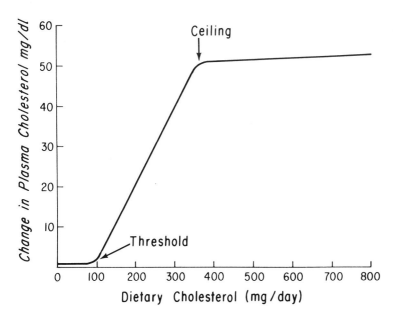

Fig. 2. Effects on the plasma cholesterol level of gradually increasing the amount of dietary cholesterol in human subjects whose background diet is very low in cholesterol. See the text for discussion of the threshold and ceiling concepts.

two egg yolks, or 500 mg, would produce a striking change in plasma cholesterol concentration. This change can be as much as 60 mg/dl [9].

Recent surveys indicate that the average American dietary cholesterol intake is about 400 mg/day for women and 500 mg/day for men [10]. Decreasing these amounts of dietary cholesterol to 100 mg/day, the objective of the therapeutic and preventive diets as will be amplified subsequently, would have a profound plasma cholesterol-lowering effect. Operationally, one would be on the descending limb of the curve illustrated in Fig. 2.

Effects of dietary fats on the plasma lipids and lipoproteins

Both the amount and kind of fat in the diet affect plasma lipid concentrations. The total amount of dietary fat is important in that the formation of chylomicrons in the intestinal mucosa and their subsequent circulation in the blood is directly proportional to the amount of fat which has been consumed in the diet. A fatty meal will result in the production of large numbers of chylomicrons and will impart the characteristic lactescent appearance to postprandial plasma 3–5 h after eating. A typical American diet with 110 g of fat produces 110 g of chylomicron triglyceride per day. 'Remnant' production from chylomicrons is proportional to the number of chylomicrons synthesized. Chylomicron remnants resulting from the action of lipoprotein lipase are cholesterol-rich and are atherogenic particles [11]. Postprandial lipemia is, of course, intense after the usual Western diet and may be present for many hours before being cleared. Not only is this lipemia (the composite of chylomicrons and remnants) atherogenic but it may also promote thrombosis [11]. Postprandial lipemia is lessened by physical activity and by a diet low in fat and/or a diet containing ω-3 fatty acids from fish [12,13]. Postprandial lipemia is intensified and is prolonged in patients with fasting hypertriglyceridemia whose clearance mechanisms are already impaired, e.g., patients with type IV and type V hypertriglyceridemia. There is even impaired chylomicron clearance in patients with familial combined hyperlipidemia whose fasting triglyceride values are elevated [14].

Saturated fatty acids

The chemical structure of different fats will have different effects on plasma cholesterol levels. Fats may be divided into three major classes on the basis of the degree of saturation of its fatty acids. Long-chain, saturated fatty acids have no double bonds, are not essential nutrients, and are readily synthesized in the body from acetate. However, saturated fatty acids in the diet have a powerful hypercholesterolemic effect, increase the concentrations of LDL and are also thrombogenic. All animal fats are highly saturated (30% or more of the fat is saturated) and contain little polyunsaturated fatty acid, in contrast to the fats of fish and shellfish, which are highly polyunsaturated. The molecular basis for the effects of dietary saturated fat on the plasma cholesterol level is now well understood. It rests upon its influence on the LDL-receptor activity of liver cells as described by Brown and Goldstein [3,15]. Dietary saturated fat suppresses messenger RNA synthesis for the LDL receptor which decreases hepatic LDL-receptor activity, decreases the removal of LDL from the blood and thus increases the concentration of LDL-cholesterol in the blood [16,17]. Dietary cholesterol augments the effect of saturated fat by further suppressing hepatic LDL-receptor activity and raising the plasma LDL-cholesterol level. Conversely, a decrease in dietary cholesterol and saturated fat increases the LDL-receptor activity of the liver cells, enhances the hepatic pickup of LDL cholesterol and lowers the concentration of LDL-cholesterol in the blood [16]. Some saturated fats, such as coconut oil, also increase the synthesis of cholesterol and LDL in the liver. Metabolic studies suggest that one can expect an average plasma cholesterol decrease of 20% by maximally decreasing dietary cholesterol and saturated fat.

Besides natural sources of saturated fats, the hydrogenation of liquid vegetable oils can saturate some of the unsaturated fatty acids. Large quantities of highly hydrogenated fat should be avoided to keep the total saturated fat low. Monounsaturated *trans* fatty acids, isomers of the *cis* oleic acid, are important byproducts of the hydrogenation process. It must be appreciated that *trans* fatty acids are also present in butterfat and in beef, for example. The hydrogenation process occurs through bacterial action in the rumen of the cow. *Trans* fatty acids are oxidized for energy as are other fatty acids. In a recent study in which large amounts of *trans* fatty acids were consumed (10% kcal), the plasma LDL-cholesterol level was significantly increased [18]. However, the average *trans* fatty acid intake in the United States is only about 2.5% kcal [19]. This *trans* fatty acid intake is cut in half when a patient reduces fat intake from 40 to 20% kcal. Further, if the patient uses small amounts of liquid vegetable oil and select margarines that have been only lightly hydrogenated (those in which a liquid vegetable oil is listed as the first fat ingredient), the *trans* fatty acid intake will be less than 1% kcal. The softer a margarine is at room temperature the less hydrogenated it is. Peanut butter is so lightly hydrogenated that its fatty acid composition is little affected by this process. The daily use of small quantities of the lightly hydrogenated soft margarines does not constitute a problem in the treatment of hyperlipidemia.

Attention has been called to the fact that some saturated fats do not seem to cause hypercholesterolemia. Medium-chain triglycerides (C8 and C10 saturated fatty acids) are water-soluble and are handled metabolically more like carbohydrate than fat. They are transported to the liver via the portal vein blood rather than as chylomicrons. These fatty acids do not elevate the plasma cholesterol concentration.

Dietary stearic acid, an 18-carbon saturated fatty acid, also has a limited effect upon the plasma cholesterol concentration. Excessive stearic acid from the diet is converted into oleic acid, a monounsaturated fatty acid, by the desaturase enzyme in the liver. Feeding animals large quantities of stearic acid, such as cocoa butter which contains a considerable percentage of its total fatty acids as stearic acid (33%), does not result in the deposition of stearic acid in the adipose tissue, as would occur with mono- and polyunsaturated fat feeding [20]. This again is because of the action of the desaturase enzyme. Instead oleic acid is deposited. The practical importance of these observations about stearic acid is limited because it is present in foods that also contain appreciable amounts of the other saturated fatty acids (palmitic, myristic, lauric) that cause hypercholesterolemia. One of these, palmitic acid, is the most common saturated fat found in our food supply. Palmitic acid has 16 carbons and is intensely hypercholesterolemic. Myristic acid and lauric acid with 14 and 12 carbons, respectively, are also very hypercholesterolemic. It is these fatty acids present in saturated dietary fats that cause their untoward effects. Amounts of stearic acid in the American diet are not great compared with palmitic acid. Also the equations developed for the prediction of plasma cholesterol change have been based upon the changes produced by a given fat including its concentration of stearic acid. Thus, all of the information which has accumulated about the hypercholesterolemic and atherogenic properties of beef fat, butterfat, lard, palm oil, cocoa butter and coconut oil remains completely valid.

The cholesterol saturated fat index (CSI) of foods

As already indicated, the major plasma cholesterol-elevating effects of a given food reside in its cholesterol and saturated fat content. To help understand the contribution of these two factors in a single food item and to compare one food with another, we have computed a cholesterol saturated fat index (CSI) for selected foods [21]. The formulae for the CSI is: CSI = (1.01 × g saturated fat) + (0.05 × mg cholesterol), where the amounts of saturated fat and cholesterol in a given amount of a food item are entered into this equation. The higher the CSI of a food, the greater the hypercholesterolemic and atherogenic effect. This cholesterol saturated fat index is a representation of how much a given food will decrease the activity of the LDL receptor and, hence, will raise the level of LDL cholesterol in plasma.

In this context it is particularly instructive to compare the CSI of fish vs. that of moderately fat beef, both being 85-g portions. An 85-g portion of cooked fish contains 51 mg of cholesterol and 0.14 g of saturated fat. This contrasts to 80 mg cholesterol and 11.3 g of saturated fat in 85 g of 30% fat beef. The CSI for the fish is 3 and for the beef 15, 5 times more. The caloric value of these two portions also differs greatly (71 for fish and 323 kcal for beef). The CSI of cooked chicken and turkey (without the skin) is also lower than that of beef and other red meats. The total fat content is considerably lower. The saturated fat in an 85-g serving is 1.6 g and the cholesterol is 71 mg. The CSI of poultry is 5. Figure 3 lists the CSI for 3 oz of various foods. Shellfish have low CSIs because their saturated fat content is extremely low even though their cholesterol or total sterol content is 2.5–3 times that of fish, poultry or red meat. Shellfish have an average CSI of 4 per 3 oz. This means that, when cholesterol and saturated fat are both taken into account shellfish, like poultry, is a better choice than even the leanest red meats. Shellfish are divided into two groups: higher-CSI shellfish (shrimp, crab and lobster) and lower-CSI shellfish (oysters, clams and scallops). Both contain ω-3 fatty acids and have a low fat content. Because of these differences, higher-CSI shellfish should be more restricted in the daily diet than are the lower-CSI shellfish, i.e., 3 oz vs. 6 oz per day. The lower-CSI shellfish contain sterols (e.g., brassicasterol) that are more similar to plant sterols than cholesterol and are poorly absorbed by humans. Salmon also has a low CSI and is preferred to meat. We have now calculated the CSI for a thousand foods and incorporated this concept in a book along with low-fat, low-cholesterol recipes [21,22].

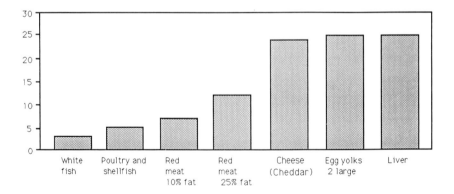

Fig. 3. The cholesterol saturated fat index (CSI) of 3 oz of fish, poultry, shellfish, meat, cheese, egg yolk, and liver. The CSI for poultry is the average CSI for cooked light and dark chicken without skin. The CSI for shellfish is the average CSI of cooked crab, lobster, shrimp, clams, oysters and scallops. The CSI for cheese is the average CSI of cheddar, Swiss and processed cheese.

Polyunsaturated fatty acids

The third class of fatty acids are vital constituents of cellular membranes and serve as prostaglandin precursors. Because they cannot be synthesized by the body and are obtainable only from the diet, they are 'essential' fatty acids [23]. The two classes of polyunsaturated fatty acids are the ω-6 and ω-3 fatty acids. Omega-6 and ω-3 fatty acids are not interconvertible. The most common examples of ω-6 fatty acids are arachidonic acid, 20 carbons in length with four double bonds (20:4), and its dietary precursor, linoleic acid (18:2). Linoleic acid is found in many foods, and especially in vegetable seed oils, whereas there is little arachidonic acid in the diet. Linoleic acid is converted to arachidonic acid in the liver. Since the basic structure of ω-6 fatty acids cannot be synthesized by the body, 2—3% of the total energy in the diet must consist of linoleic acid to meet the metabolic requirements of the body for the ω-6 structure.

Omega-3 fatty acids differ from ω-6 fatty acids in the position of the first double bond. Counting from the methyl end of the molecule, this double bond is at the third rather than the sixth carbon as for the ω-6 fatty acids. Omega-3 fatty acids are also 'essential'. They constitute important membrane components of all organs, but especially the brain, retina and sperm. The dietary sources of ω-3 fatty acids are plant foods, some, but not all, vegetable oils, and leafy vegetables. Fish and shellfish are especially rich in ω-3 fatty acids. Linolenic acid, C18:3, is obtained from vegetable products. Eicosapentaenoic acid (EPA), C20:5, and docosahexaenoic acid (DHA), C22:6, are derived from fish, shellfish and phytoplankton (the plants of the ocean). These fatty acids are highly concentrated in fish oils. Once either the ω-3 or ω-6 structure comes into the body as the 18-carbon linoleic or linolenic acid, the body can synthesize the longer-chain and more highly polyunsaturated ω-6 or ω-3 fatty acids (20 and 22 carbons), but the synthesis is rate-limited. A safe intake of ω-3 fatty acids would be 0.4 to 0.6% of total calories.

EPA and DHA are present in the diet in two forms: as triglyceride in the adipose tissue of fish, usually present between muscle fibers, and as membrane phospholipids of the muscle of fish. These highly polyunsaturated fatty acids occupy the middle position of the glycerol skeleton for both triglycerides and phospholipids. In either of these dietary forms, EPA and DHA are efficiently absorbed from the intestinal tract [24]. After absorption, EPA and DHA readily associate with membranes and are found in the four plasma lipid classes: triglycerides, free fatty acids, cholesteryl esters and phospholipids. Ultimately, they are stored in the adipose tissue and, in experimental animals, we have found they even reach the brain and the retina.

There are distinctly different functions in the body for ω-3 and ω-6 fatty acids [7]. Both serve as substrate for the formation of different prostaglandins and leukotrienes and are abundant in phospholipid membranes. Both ω-3 and ω-6 fatty acids are concentrated in nervous tissue. Omega-3 fatty acids are rich in the retina, brain, spermatozoa, the gonads, and many other organs. Omega-6 fatty acids are concentrated in the different plasma lipid classes (cholesteryl esters, phospholipids, etc.) and, in addition, play a role in lipid transport.

Polyunsaturated fatty acids in large amounts, either the ω-6 or ω-3 structure, reduce plasma total and LDL-cholesterol concentrations in normal and hypercholesterolemic individuals [5]. The situation is somewhat different in hypertriglyceridemic individuals or in those with combined hyperlipidemia. Only the ω-3 fatty acids from fish and fish oil have a decided hypotriglyceridemic effect. VLDL, in particular, is decreased by the ω-3 fatty acids [25]. Isotopic studies have shown that the hypotriglyceridemic effect of ω-3 fatty acids occurs as a result of the depression of triglyceride, VLDL and apoprotein B synthesis in the liver and also of the accelerated catabolism of VLDL from the plasma [26]. In some patients with type IV hypertriglyceridemia and in some patients with combined hyperlipidemia, there have been reports of an increase in LDL as the plasma triglyceride falls after fish-oil administration. This increase in LDL also occurs when gemfibrozil is given to these patients. In the severely hypertriglyceridemic type V patients, however, large doses of fish oil (10–15 g/day) produce a dramatic clearing of chylomicronemia and lower both triglyceride and cholesterol concentrations. Fish oil also promotes the clearing of chylomicrons after the administration of a fatty meal. This would be of particular benefit in the type V patient in whom there is great difficulty in clearing chylomicrons. Most experiments have not shown plasma triglyceride lowering from the ω-6 vegetable oils.

In the early days of dietary therapy for hyperlipidemia, it was suggested that large amounts of a vegetable oil such as corn oil could be used to treat hypercholesterolemia. However, its high content of the ω-6 fatty acid, linoleic acid, was probably not beneficial. It promoted obesity, gallstone formation and, more importantly, may have been carcinogenic, as suggested by animal studies. In current diets for the treatment of hyperlipidemia, ω-6 polyunsaturated fatty acids are not increased from the current amount in the American diet, which averages about 6–8% of the total calories. When saturated and monounsaturated fatty acids are decreased, they should not be replaced by equivalent amounts of polyunsaturated fatty acids from liquid vegetable oil or margarines or shortenings.

Omega-3 fatty acids from fish have important effects whether or not the diet is high in saturated fat. In either instance, ω-3 fatty acids produced lowering of the levels of plasma cholesterol, triglyceride and especially VLDL (about 50%) [27]. With the low-saturated-fat diet, there was an additional action: further plasma cholesterol lowering occurred as LDL declined 25%. Thus, an ideal diet would be low in saturated fat and high in ω-3 fatty acids.

It is not known exactly how much the intake of ω-3 fatty acids should be increased to achieve optimum effects. One study from The Netherlands indicated that men who included fish in their diet twice a week had fewer deaths from heart disease. A similar protective effect from eating fish occurred in Japan. In a prospective trial in Wales, the prescription of two fish meals per week led to both a reduction in total mortality and in coronary events [28]. Even very-low-fat seafood contains an appreciable amount of ω-3 fatty acids, up to 40% or more of total fatty acids. Eating a total of 12 ounces of a variety of fish and shellfish each week would provide 3–5 grams of ω-3 fatty acids as well as protein, vitamins and minerals. The fish could be fresh, frozen or canned without affecting the quantity of ω-3 fatty acids. The patient with hyperlipidemia can expect to have only beneficial effects from following this dietary advice, especially if the fish replaces meat in the diet, meat being a major source of saturated fat. Also to be considered are the antithrombotic actions of fish oil mediated through the inhibition of the thromboxane-A2 in platelets [7] and the enhanced clearance of chylomicrons [12,28,29]. Other effects of fish oil include inhibition of platelet-derived growth factor, alteration of certain functions of leukocytes, reduction of blood viscosity, and greater fibrinolysis as well as inhibition of intimal hyperplasia in vein grafts used for arterial bypass [30]. Fish oil serves as a therapeutic agent in certain hyperlipidemic states, especially the chylomicronemia of type V hyperlipidemia. Thus, fish oils have discrete effects not only upon the plasma lipids and lipoproteins but also upon the atherosclerotic and thrombotic process.

Acknowledgements

Supported by research grants from the National Heart Lung and Blood Institute (HL25,687), the Clinical Nutrition Research Unite (DK40,566) from the National Institute of Diabetes, Digestive and Kidney Diseases and the Clinical Research Center Program (RR334) of the Division of Research Resources of the National Institutes of Health.

References

1. de Langen C. Geneeskd Tijdschr Ned-Indië 1922;62:1–4.
2. Connor WE, Connor SL. In: Havel RJ (ed) Lipid Disorders, 66th edn. Med Clin North Am, 1982;485–518.
3. Brown MS, Goldstein JL. J Clin Invest 1983;72:743–747.
4. Sorci-Thomas M, Wilson MD, Johnson FL, Williams DL, Rudel LL. J Biol Chem 1989;264:9039.
5. Connor WE, Connor SL. In: Stollerman H (ed) Advances in Internal Medicine, 35th edn. Chicago: Year Book, 1989;139–172.
6. Hopkins PN. Am J Clin Nutr 1992;55:1060–1070.
7. Goodnight SH Jr, Harris WS, Connor WE, Illingworth DR. Arteriosclerosis 1982;2:87–113.
8. Roberts SL, McMurry M, Connor WE. Am J Clin Nutr 1981;34:2092–2099.
9. Connor WE, Connor SL. In: Connor WE, Bristow JD (eds) Coronary Heart Disease: Prevention, Complications, and Treatment. Philadelphia: Lippincott, 1985;43–64.
10. Gordon T, Fisher M, Ernst M et al. Atherosclerosis 1982;2:502.
11. Zilversmit DB. Circulation 1979;60:473–485.
12. Harris WS, Connor WE, Alam N, Illingworth DR. J Lipid Res 1988;29:1451–1460.
13. Weintraub M, Rosen Y, Otto R, Eisenberg S, Breslow J. Circulation 1989;79:1007–1014.
14. Cabezas M, de Bruin TWA, Jansen H, Kock LAW, Kortlandt W, Erkelens DW. Arterioscler Thromb 1993; 13:804–814.
15. Brown MS, Goldstein JL. Science 1986;232:34–47.
16. Spady DK, Dietschy JM. J Clin Invest 1988;81:300–309.
17. Fox JC, McGill Jr, Carey KD, Getz GS. J Biol Chem 1987;262:7014.
18. Mensink RP, Katan MB. N Engl J Med 1990;323:439–445.
19. Willett W, Stampfer M, Manson J, Colditz G, Speizer F, Rosner B, Sampson L, Hennekens C. Lancet 1993; 341:581.
20. Lin DS, Connor WE, Spenler CW. Am J Clin Nutr 1993;58:174–179.
21. Connor SL, Artaud-Wild SM, Classick-Kohn CJ, Gustafson JR, Flavell DP, Hatcher LF, Connor WE. Lancet 1986;1:1229–1232.
22. Connor SL, Connor WE. The New American Diet System. New York: Simon & Schuster, 1991;1–574.
23. Neuringer M, Connor WE. Nutr Rev 1986;44:285–294.
24. Nordoy A, Barstad L, Connor WE, Hatcher L. Am J Clin Nutr 1991;99:1185–1190.
25. Phillipson BE, Rothrock DW, Connor WE, Harris WS, Illingworth DR. N Engl J Med 1985;312:1210–1216.
26. Harris WS, Connor WE, Illingworth DR, Rothrock DW, Foster DM. J Lipid Res 1990;31:1549–1558.
27. Nordoy A, Hatcher LF, Ullmann D, Connor WE. Am J Clin Nutr 1993;57:634–639.
28. Burr ML, Gilbert JF, Holliday RM, Elwood PC, Fehly AM, Rogers S, Sweetnam PM, Deadman NM. Lancet 1989;2:756–761.
29. Weintraub MS, Zechner R, Brown, Eisenberg S, Breslow JL. J Clin Invest 1988;82:1884–1893.
30. Connor WE. In: Kritchevsky D, Carroll KK (eds) Nutrition and Disease Update: Heart Disease. Champaign: American Oil Chemists' Society, 1994;7–42.

284

Atherosclerosis X.
F.P. Woodford, J. Davignon and A. Sniderman, editors.

Dietary approach to treatment of the atherogenic dyslipidemia syndrome

Scott M. Grundy

Center for Human Nutrition, Departments of Internal Medicine, Biochemistry and Clinical Nutrition, University of Texas Southwestern Medical Center at Dallas, 5323 Harry Hines Boulevard, Dallas, TX 75235-9052, USA

Abstract. The atherogenic dyslipidemia syndrome is a condition characterized by (a) borderline-high cholesterol levels, (b) elevated triglycerides, (c) small, dense LDL particles, and (d) low HDL-cholesterol levels. These abnormalities frequently occur together in patients with premature coronary disease; this justifies calling their combination a "syndrome". Despite their frequent common association, the etiology of this syndrome appears to be diverse or multifactorial. The first line of therapy for the atherogenic dyslipidemia syndrome is dietary management. Three dietary changes appear to be necessary for effective therapy. These include (a) weight reduction, (b) carbohydrate restriction, and (c) increased monounsaturated fatty acids. The accumulated data on dietary therapy suggests that this combination will produce the best response in all the components of this syndrome.

The major atherogenic lipoprotein is low density lipoprotein (LDL). Evidence of many types indicates that high levels of LDL are a major risk factor for coronary heart disease (CHD). This evidence includes epidemiological data, genetic forms of hyper-cholesterolemia, clinical-trial results, and findings in laboratory animals and model systems [1]. The mechanisms whereby high serum cholesterol levels induce atherosclerosis are not entirely elucidated, but a general understanding of these mechanisms appears to be in place. Because of the strong evidence linking high levels of LDL to atherogenesis, the United States National Cholesterol Education Program (US NCEP) has designated LDL as the primary target of cholesterol therapy in both primary and secondary prevention of CHD [1]. Particular attention should be given to LDL-cholesterol in the so-called 'high-risk' range i.e., at levels ≥ 160 mg/dl.

Although the US NCEP designated a high LDL-cholesterol as the primary target of therapy, it also recognized that other lipoprotein abnormalities participate in the atherosclerotic process. Two of these lipoprotein are very low density lipoprotein (VLDL) and high density lipoprotein (HDL). High levels of VLDL, like those of LDL, appear to be directly atherogenic, whereas high concentrations of HDL impart a degree of protection against the development of CHD. It must be noted, however, that levels of VLDL and HDL are not entirely independent, but are inversely correlated with one another. Moreover, other lipoprotein abnormalities frequently accompany high VLDL and low HDL levels. These are aberrations in the size and composition of LDL particles (called LDL polydispersity) and a mildly elevated (borderline-high) LDL-cholesterol (130–159 mg/dl). Since these abnormalities commonly occur together in one individual, they can be called a "syndrome"; and to distinguish this syndrome from definitely high levels of LDL-cholesterol (hypercholesterolemia), the multiple lipoprotein abnormalities will be named "dyslipidemia". And finally, since this lipoprotein pattern is commonly accompanied by premature CHD, it will be designated the "atherogenic dyslipidemia syndrome." The essential ingredients of this syndrome include: (a) borderline-high cholesterol levels, (b) elevated triglycerides, (c) small, dense LDL particles, and (d) low HDL-cholesterol levels. In this paper, we will examine the relation between the atherogenic dyslipidemia syndrome and CHD risk, its etiology, and the dietary approach to its management.

Relation of the atherogenic dyslipidemia syndrome to coronary heart disease risk

Borderline-high cholesterol levels

In this syndrome, borderline-high levels of cholesterol are the foundation of its atherogenic potential. In populations in whom total (and LDL) cholesterol are very low, atherosclerosis develops too slowly to have a major clinical impact [2]. This is true even when the other components of the dyslipidemia syndrome are present. Whether the other components merely accentuate the atherogenicity of LDL, or in the absence of higher LDL levels they are simply not potent enough to produce advanced atherosclerosis, is unclear. Regardless, for clinically significant coronary atherosclerosis to develop, cholesterol levels must be at least moderately elevated. For present purposes, this degree of elevation will be defined as borderline high, i.e., total cholesterol in the range of 200 to 239 mg/dl. The US NCEP [1] has defined a total cholesterol of below 200 mg/dl as "desirable". Although total cholesterol levels with the range of 160 to 200 mg/dl produce some increase in risk for CHD, the increment in risk is modest. Certainly when total cholesterol levels in the range of 160 to 200 mg/dl are accompanied by other components of the atherogenic syndrome, premature CHD can occur, but the increment is less than when total cholesterol concentrations are in the range of 200 to 239 mg/dl. When cholesterol levels are in this range, risk for CHD increases about 1% for every 1 mg/dl increase in cholesterol levels [1].

Elevated VLDL

The VLDL are major triglyceride-carrying lipoproteins in fasting serum. For this reason, the triglyceride level reflects concentrations of VLDL particles. Perhaps a better indicator of CHD risk than triglyceride levels would be VLDL-cholesterol concentrations, but this parameter is difficult to measure. Several lines of information strongly suggest that high serum concentrations of triglycerides and VLDL particles are atherogenic. This information comes from epidemiological studies [3], animal studies [4] and model systems [5]. Moreover, limited clinical-trial data [6,7] suggest that lowering of VLDL levels will reduce the risk for CHD.

The mechanisms whereby high VLDL levels enhance CHD risk appear to be 2-fold. First, some types of VLDL particles probably are directly atherogenic. This is especially so for small, cholesterol-enriched VLDL called VLDL remnants. But second, the hypertriglyceridemia that accompanies increased levels of VLDL particles may induce changes in other systems that enhance CHD risk. For example, high triglyceride concentrations give rise to small, dense LDL particles and they reduce HDL levels, both of which appear to promote atherogenesis. Moreover, elevated triglycerides may induce a procoagulant state by producing a variety of alterations in the clotting systems [8—19]; the latter changes may increase the likelihood of coronary thrombosis, and hence, myocardial infarction.

Small, dense LDL particles

The presence of abnormalities in LDL-particle size and composition is being increasingly recognized as a component of atherogenic dyslipidemia. Epidemiological studies [20] support this connection. Particularly implicated are abnormally small and dense LDL particles. At least two mechanisms can be visualized whereby small, dense LDL may foster atherogenesis. One of these relates to the observation that rates of filtration of lipoproteins into the arterial wall depend on the size of particles. Hence, the smaller the size of LDL particles, the greater should be their rate of penetration into the intima of the artery [4]. This heightened influx rate of lipoproteins ought to accelerate atherogenesis. Another reason whereby small LDL have increased atherogenicity may be their greater propensity for oxidation, compared to larger ones [21]. If the oxidation of LDL is a key step in atherogenesis, a heightened susceptibility of small LDL to oxidation could help to explain why these particles appear to raise the risk for CHD out of proportion to other types of LDL.

High density lipoproteins

The fourth member of this syndrome is a low level of HDL-cholesterol. The US NCEP defined a low HDL-cholesterol as a level below 35 mg/dl. Epidemiologic observations manifest a strong inverse correlation between HDL-cholesterol concentrations and risk for CHD [22,23]. A portion of this correlation may be understood as an explicit action of HDL to retard the growth of atherosclerotic lesions. Even so, we do not know the precise component of the HDL fraction that is accountable for an antiatherogenic action. Some investigators propose as active agent the HDL subfraction called HDL_2 [24]. Others suggest that a subfraction of the HDL apolipoproteins, (apo) A-I (without apoA-II), is the responsible agent [25]. Regardless, most workers agree that the HDL-cholesterol level correlates with the active subfraction, even if it is not the true antiatherogenic factor.

Moreover, the HDL-cholesterol level may provide a more accurate indicator of CHD risk than would measurement of the specific antiatherogenic factor in HDL. This is because the HDL-cholesterol level often is inversely correlated with other atherogenic lipoproteins (e.g., VLDL remnants and LDL). Thus, HDL-cholesterol levels may indicate the presence of an antiatherogenic HDL subfraction and inversely correlate with the level of other atherogenic lipoproteins. In this double way, the HDL-cholesterol level becomes a strong marker for CHD risk.

Other indicators of risk accompanying the dyslipidemia syndrome

In recent years much interest has centered on the measurements of apolipoproteins as predictors of CHD risk. Two apolipoproteins of particular interest are apolipoprotein B (apoB) and apoA-I. ApoB is the principal apolipoprotein of VLDL and LDL, and it is considered an "atherogenic" apolipoprotein. Several studies [26–28] suggest that apoB levels provide a strong indicator of CHD risk. In contrast, apoA-I levels, like HDL-cholesterol levels, are inversely correlated with risk [29]. The concept has emerged that some patients have elevated concentrations of apoB (as well as decreased apoA-I levels) even in the presence of normal lipid levels. In general, however, such abnormalities are highly linked to the various components of the atherogenic dyslipidemia syndrome (borderline-high cholesterol, increased VLDL-cholesterol, small LDL particles, and low HDL-cholesterol levels). Thus, abnormal levels of apoB and apoA-I may indicate the presence of atherogenic dyslipidemia, but they do not necessarily provide a better indicator of risk accompanying this condition than do measurements of the primary factors.

Indeed, a better marker of risk may be the "cholesterol ratio", i.e., the ratio of total cholesterol to HDL-cholesterol. Investigators of the Framingham Heart Study [22] have long claimed that the total/HDL-cholesterol ratio is the single best lipid determinant of CHD risk. In fact, in the presence of a borderline-high cholesterol level, a high total/HDL-cholesterol ratio almost certainly reveals the presence of atherogenic dyslipidemia. In other words, a high total/HDL ratio will be highly correlated with increased cholesterol, VLDL-cholesterol, and low HDL levels.

Etiology of atherogenic dyslipidemia

Borderline-high-risk LDL-cholesterol

A level of LDL-cholesterol in the borderline-high risk range usually is the result of two defects: a reduced activity of LDL receptors and an overproduction of apoB-containing lipoproteins [30]. A reduced activity of LDL receptors typically is due to (a) an increased dietary intake of cholesterol and cholesterol-raising fatty acids (certain saturated fatty acids and *trans* fatty acids) and (b) the aging process [31]. Baseline LDL-cholesterol levels in humans are about 90 mg/dl, and a relatively high intake of cholesterol-raising fatty acids and cholesterol will raise the levels to about 115 mg/dl. This is a typical LDL-cholesterol concentration in a 20-year-old American adult. Over the next 20–30 years there is a progressive rise of LDL levels that is unrelated to diet; this rise adds another 15 mg/dl to LDL levels. Thus the diet and aging process will bring the LDL-cholesterol level to about 130 mg/dl. Finally, another 15 mg/dl, on the average, is added by increasing body weight with aging. Extra body weight appears to exert its effect on LDL levels by increasing hepatic secretion of apoB-containing lipoproteins [31].

Elevated VLDL

There are three major causes of an increased VLDL level: (a) increased hepatic secretion of VLDL particles, (b) defective lipolysis of VLDL triglycerides, and (c) slow processing of VLDL remnants [32]. Increased hepatic secretion of VLDL particles is due to obesity in most patients. Those with abdominal obesity may be especially vulnerable. Genetic factors may be responsible for high secretion rates for VLDL in some patients, but no defective genes causing high VLDL-input rates have been identified. Defective lipolysis of VLDL triglycerides can be the consequence either of mutations in the lipoprotein lipase (LPL) gene or of reduced expression of this gene. Finally, little is known about regulation of VLDL-remnant processing. Familial dysbetalipoproteinemia, which is due to an abnormal gene for apoE, is a good example of defective remnant processing, but other causes are less well understood; although they are less dramatic than apoE defects, they may be more common and hence clinically more important.

Small, dense LDL particles

These abnormal LDL particles are commonly present in patients who have elevated serum triglycerides [33,34]. A circulating protein, cholesterol ester transfer protein (CETP), is thought to promote exchange of triglycerides and cholesteryl ester between lipoproteins. Seemingly, when triglyceride levels are high, this exchange reaction is accelerated, and LDL-cholesteryl esters are replaced by triglycerides. This reduces the cholesterol content of LDL, but the triglyceride content is increased. However, the triglycerides undergo rapid hydrolysis by hepatic triglyceride lipase (HTGL), and hence the total amount of lipid in the lipoprotein core is reduced. This decreases the size of the LDL particle. Whether this is the only mechanism for the generation of small, dense LDL particles is not known. It has been claimed that some patients have the abnormal particles on a genetic basis [35], but even so, the mechanism could be mediated through a genetic increase in circulating triglycerides.

Low HDL-cholesterol

A low level of HDL-cholesterol can occur by the same mechanism as that for formation of small, dense LDL. In the presence of hypertriglyceridemia, the exchange of triglycerides for cholesteryl ester in the core of HDL particles is augmented, and after hydrolysis of the resulting HDL triglycerides, the HDL particles likewise become small and dense. These small, dense HDL particles are designated HDL_3, and they are to be distinguished from larger, less dense HDL, called HDL_2. The small, dense HDL are seemingly not associated with protection against CHD, at least in epidemiological studies.

Another factor that theoretically could contribute to a reduction of HDL-cholesterol levels is an increase in CETP. Patients with a genetic deficiency in CETP have markedly elevated HDL-cholesterol levels [36]. Recently, we have presented preliminary evidence that the opposite holds, that is, when CETP levels are high, HDL-cholesterol levels tend to be low [37]. This effect appears to be independent of triglyceride levels. Causes of elevated CETP activities are not known at present.

Abnormalities in lipolytic enzymes — LPL and HTGL — have also been associated with low HDL-cholesterol concentrations. These abnormalities include a reduced activity of LPL and an increased activity of HTGL [38]. A high activity of HTGL is apparently the more important cause of a low level of HDL-cholesterol [38]. However, when the ratio of LPL to HTGL is low, due to changes in activities of both enzymes, HDL-cholesterol levels are particularly reduced.

A final basis for a low HDL level is decreased secretion of apoA-I. This apolipoprotein is secreted by both the liver and gut, although the major portion comes from the liver. Secretion rates of apoA-I appear to vary considerably among individuals, and people at the lower end of the spectrum of apoA-I secretion will have lower HDL levels than those at the higher end [39]. A few genetic defects in apoA-I metabolism have been identified that lower HDL-cholesterol levels, but these are rare, and they do not contribute significantly to low secretion rates of apoA-I in the general population. Thus, the reasons for variability in apoA-I secretion rates across the whole population remain to be determined, but this variability clearly contributes to differences in HDL levels.

These considerations make it clear that elevations of serum triglycerides are not the only basis for low HDL levels. Other factors — increased CETP, reduced LPL, increased HTGL, and low apoA-I secretion — can contribute to atherogenic dyslipidemia independently of the triglyceride level. Abnormalities in these other factors may have a genetic basis, but other influences, such as hormonal, may also be at play.

Dietary management of atherogenic dyslipidemia

Changes in diet composition

Reduction in cholesterol-raising fatty acids and cholesterol. Two major dietary factors that contribute to borderline-high cholesterol levels are the cholesterol-raising fatty acids and dietary cholesterol [40]. The former include certain saturated fatty acids, i.e., palmitic acid, myristic acid, and lauric acid, and the unsaturated, *trans* fatty acids. An effort should be made to reduce the intake of these various fatty acids. This can be achieved by decreasing intakes of animal fats, tropical oils, and hydrogenated vegetable oils, as well as products containing these fats and oils. A reduction in dietary cholesterol will produce a further decrease in serum cholesterol levels.

If a significant reduction in intakes of cholesterol-raising fatty acids is achieved, the question can be asked as to what is an appropriate replacement. If a patient is overweight, the offending fatty acids need not be replaced or fully replaced. Their removal from the diet will reduce total caloric intake and will lead to weight reduction, which cause an improvement in the overall lipoprotein pattern. On the other hand, various amounts of caloric replacement may be required if a desirable body weight has been achieved. Two possible substitutions for cholesterol-raising fatty acids can be considered: (a) carbohydrates, (b) unsaturated oils. Each possibility can be discussed briefly.

Carbohydrates. Most authorities recommend replacement of saturated fatty acids with carbohydrates for the purpose of CHD risk reduction. This recommendation is based mainly on the epidemiological observation that populations which consume high-carbohydrate, low-fat diets have relatively low rates of CHD. However, many of these populations have high-energy expenditures that help to overcome some of the potential adverse effects of high-carbohydrate diets. For example, in sedentary and relatively obese populations, high-carbohydrate diets can further raise triglyceride and lower HDL levels [41]. These effects are particularly unwelcome in patients with atherogenic dyslipidemia in whom elevated triglycerides and low HDL levels already are present. Moreover, high-carbohydrate diets do not appear to be effective for lowering total apoB levels [42,43], and thus do not contribute to control of hyperapoB. Therefore, for patients with atherogenic dyslipidemia, carbohydrates do not appear to be the best replacement for cholesterol-raising fatty acids.

Unsaturated fatty acids. These fatty acids, which come from vegetable oils, seem to be a better substitute for cholesterol-raising fatty acids than carbohydrates. They do not raise triglycerides nor do they lower HDL-cholesterol [41], and they are more effective in reducing apoB levels [44,45]. In our view, the monounsaturated fatty acids are preferable to polyunsaturated fatty acids. The former, in contrast to the latter, do not suppress the immune system [46], promote tumorigenesis in animals [47], enhance the susceptibility of LDL to oxidation [48], or induce some reduction in HDL-cholesterol levels [41]. The major vegetable sources of monounsaturated fatty acids are olive oil and canola oil, but high-oleic forms of sunflower seed oil and safflower oil are also available.

Weight reduction. Probably a more important dietary issue in atherogenic dyslipidemia is the need for weight reduction. As indicated before, obesity contributes to all of the lipoprotein abnormalities of atherogenic dyslipidemia, and unless excess body fat is effectively eliminated, it will be difficult to correct these abnormalities. In many patients, even mild-to-moderate obesity can elicit the lipoprotein defects of atherogenic dyslipidemia. In accord, loss of only moderate amounts of weight can produce a striking improvement in dyslipidemia in some patients. Some general principles about weight reduction should be kept in mind. Weight loss obtained from use of very low calorie diets generally cannot be sustained in the long run. A better approach is use of a moderate reduction in caloric intake combined with behavior modification techniques. Assistance from a therapeutic dietitian is helpful in obtaining a successful outcome for many patients.

Exercise. Another valuable adjunct for weight reduction is regular exercise. Regular exercise helps to burn excess calories and can promote weight loss in this way. Some investigators claim that regular exercise suppresses the appetite, at least in some people, and exercise could promote weight loss by this mechanism as well. Further, it tends to lower triglycerides and raise HDL cholesterol concentrations. These responses probably are independent of weight reduction, and thus exercise may be additive to weight loss in reduction in severity of atherogenic dyslipidemia.

When is drug therapy necessary?

In many patients with the atherogenic dyslipidemia syndrome, dietary therapy and exercise do not fully correct all of the lipoprotein abnormalities. There are two reasons for this failure. First, application of therapy may not be complete. Some patients fail to adopt the recommended dietary changes, particularly weight reduction, or they fail to exercise regularly. Others have genetic abnormalities in lipoprotein metabolism that cannot be corrected by dietary therapy and exercise. In these circumstances, consideration must be given to drug treatment. Unfortunately, the ideal drug for treatment of atherogenic dyslipidemia has not been developed. Nonetheless, in many patients the currently available lipid-lowering drugs can be employed with some success. These drugs can be reviewed briefly.

The most effective agent for reversing the various lipoprotein abnormalities in atherogenic dyslipidemia is nicotinic acid [49]. This agent lowers VLDL and LDL levels, and it raises HDL levels. It is the best agent available for raising HDL-cholesterol concentrations [49]. Unfortunately, nicotinic acid has a variety of side effects, e.g., flushing and itching of the skin, skin rashes, hepatic dysfunction, gastrointestinal distress, glucose intolerance, and hyperuricemia. Because of these side effects, only 50—60% of patients can tolerate nicotinic acid long term [49]. Other drugs that have similar effects on lipoprotein metabolism are the fibric acids. These drugs lower VLDL-triglycerides as well as does nicotinic acid, but they are less effective in lowering LDL or in raising HDL levels [49]. Although fibric acids are much better tolerated than is nicotinic acid, their lack of high efficacy for correcting the lipoprotein abnormalities of the dyslipidemia syndromes limits their usefulness for this type of dyslipidemia.

The HMG-CoA reductase inhibitors (statins) also can be considered for atherogenic dyslipidemia, especially when the total cholesterol level is relatively high. These agents effectively lower LDL and VLDL levels, but they produce only modest increases in HDL concentrations [49,50]. The argument can rightly be made that cholesterol lowering takes priority in treatment of dyslipidemias, and if only a single drug can be employed, the statins should be the first choice. This is a logical argument, but if statins are employed, it must be recognized that hypertriglyceridemia and low HDL levels will not be fully corrected, and thus CHD risk will not be reduced to baseline levels.

Finally, for those patients in whom single-drug therapy is not sufficient to normalize lipoprotein levels, consideration can be given to combined drug therapy. Several combinations are available: nicotinic acid + fibric acid; nicotinic acid + statin; and fibric acid + statin. All of these combinations have been tested and proven to be efficacious. However, the side effects accompanying each drug are compounded by their use together, and this fact limits the usefulness of drug combination. A particular problem is the combination of fibric acid + statin in which severe myopathy, myoglobinuria, and acute renal failure may occur. Still, in certain patients who have severe dyslipidemia, combined drug therapy may be warranted, even though careful monitoring for side effects is necessary.

References

1. Expert Panel on Detection Evaluation, and Treatment of High Blood Cholesterol in Adults. National Cholesterol Education Program: second report of the expert panel on detection, evaluation, and treatment of high blood cholesterol in adults (Adult Treatment Panel II). Circulation 1994;89:1329—1445.

2. Grundy SM et al. Eur Heart J 1990;11:462–471.
3. Austin MA. Arterioscler Thromb 1991;11:2–14.
4. Stender S, Zilversmit DB. Arteriosclerosis 1981;1:28–49.
5. Gianturco SH, Bradley WA. Semin Thromb Hemostas 1988;14:165–169.
6. Manninen V et al. Circulation 1992;85:37–45.
7. Carlson LA, Rosenhamer G. Acta Med Scand 1988;223:405–418.
8. Miller GJ. Br J Haematol 1985;59:249–258.
9. Miller GJ. Atherosclerosis 1986;60:269–277.
10. de Sousa JC et al. J Clin Pathol 1988;41:940–944.
11. Mitropoulos KA. Semin Thromb Hemostas 1988;14:246–252.
12. Marckmann P et al. Atherosclerosis 1990;80:227–233.
13. Skartlien AH et al. Arteriosclerosis 1989;9:798–801.
14. Hamsten A et al. N Engl J Med 1985;313:1557–1563.
15. Crutchley DJ et al. Arteriosclerosis 1989;9:934–939.
16. Sundell IB et al. Atherosclerosis 1989;80:9–16.
17. Simpson BCR et al. Lancet 1983;780.
18. Barrowcliffe TW et al. Thromb Haemost 1984;52:7–10.
19. Fox MH et al. J Thorac Cardiovasc Surg 1987;93:56–61.
20. Austin MA et al. Circulation 1990;82:495–506.
21. de Graaf J et al. Arterioscler Thromb 1991;11:298–306.
22. Castelli WP et al. J Am Med Assoc 1986;256:2835–2838.
23. Goldbourt U, Yaari S. Arteriosclerosis 1990;10:512–519.
24. Anderson DW et al. Atherosclerosis 1978;29:161–179.
25. Parra HJ et al. Arterioscler Thromb 1992;12:701–707.
26. Sniderman et al. Proc Natl Acad Sci USA 1980;77:604–608.
27. Sniderman et al. Ann Intern Med 1982;97:833–839.
28. Brunzell JD et al. Arteriosclerosis 1984;4:79–83.
29. Kottke BA et al. Mayo Clin Proc 1986;61:313–320.
30. Vega GL et al. Circulation 1991;84:118–128.
31. Grundy SM. Arterioscler Thromb 1991;11:1619–1635.
32. Grundy SM, Vega GL. Semin Thromb Hemostas 1988;14:149–164.
33. Vega GL, Grundy SM. Arteriosclerosis 1986;6:395–406.
34. Richards EG et al. Am J Cardiol 1989;63:1214–1220.
35. Nishina PM et al. Proc Natl Acad Sci USA 1992;89:708–712.
36. Inazu A et al. N Engl J Med 1990;323:1234–1238.
37. Tato F et al. Clin Res 1994;42:198A
38. Blades B et al. Arterioscler Thromb 1993;13:1227–1235.
39. Gylling H et al. J Lipid Res 1992;33:1527–1539.
40. Grundy SM, Denke MA. J Lipid Res 1990;31:1149–1172.
41. Abate N et al. Atherosclerosis 1993;104:159–171.
42. Dreon DM et al. FASEB J 1994;8:121–126.
43. Ginsberg HN et al. Arterioscler Thromb 1994;14:892–901.
44. Vega GL et al. J Lipid Res 1982;23:811–822.
45. Grundy SM et al. J Am Med Assoc 1986;256:2351–2355.
46. Weyman C et al. Lancet 1975;2:33–34.
47. Reddy BS. Prog Clin Biol Res 1986;222:295–309.
48. Parthasarathy S et al. Proc Natl Acad Sci USA 1990;87:3894–3898.
49. Vega GL, Grundy SM. Arch Intern Med 1994;154:73–82.
50. Vega GL, Grundy SM. J Am Med Assoc 1989;262:3148–3153.

Nutritional determinants of atherosclerosis progression in man: the STARS trial

G.F. Watts[1], B. Lewis[2], P. Jackson[3], E.S. Lewis[2] and V. Burke[1]

[1]University Department of Medicine, University of Western Australia, Perth, Australia; [2]Department of Metabolic Disorders, University of London, London; and [3]Department of Dietetics, St Thomas' Hospital, London, UK

Abstract. The St Thomas' Atherosclerosis Regression Study is a controlled dietary trial designed as a test of the lipid hypothesis of atherogenesis. Relationships between nutrient intakes and progression of coronary atherosclerosis were studied for 39 months in men with coronary artery disease. Progression was defined as reduction in coronary diameter (MW), assessed by serial quantitative angiography. Progression was directly and significantly related to fat intake ($r = 0.55$), saturated fat intake ($r = 0.44$), and energy intake. Saturated-fat intake and plasma LDL-cholesterol were independent predictors of atherosclerosis progression; stearic-acid intake was associated with LDL-independent progression.

Introduction and review

First suggested by numerous feeding experiments in laboratory animals [1—3], the role of nutrition in human atherosclerosis was later evaluated in epidemiological studies of two types. Ecological surveys revealed a strong direct relation between intake of saturated fat and 10-year mortality rates from coronary heart disease (CHD) in different populations ($r = 0.84$) in the Seven Country Study [4], and a similar relation between saturated fat intake and the extent of coronary atherosclerosis as determined in 23,000 autopsies ($r = 0.67$) [5]. Food balance data have also found saturated fat to be related to CHD mortality among countries [6]; in univariate analysis a number of nutrients were so correlated, but bivariate analysis restricted the association to a dietary lipid score that suggested positive associations with saturated fat and cholesterol intakes and a negative association with polyunsaturated fat.

Longitudinal studies in single populations, the second type of study, provide a more rigorous test of the lipid hypothesis, and many have shown similar but weaker associations. Relationships with disease rates are attenuated by the small variance of diet between individuals within a population relative to the variance within individuals over time, coupled with the considerable measurement error in estimating nutrient intake. In one such study CHD incidence was found to be lower in men whose diets were in the upper tertile for the ratio of polyunsaturated fatty acids to saturated fatty acids than in those in the lower tertile [7]. Generally similar conclusions have been drawn from studies based on analysis of adipose tissue and plasma phospholipid fatty acids [8—10], pointing to an inverse relation between polyunsaturated fatty acid percentages and CHD.

In the 19-year Western Electric Study [11] two dietary assessments were made a year apart; low CHD mortality was predicted by a dietary score reflecting low intake of cholesterol and a low ratio of saturated to polyunsaturated fat. Later data from this study revealed the intake of cholesterol to be most significantly and independently predictive of CHD deaths, saturated-fat intake escaping formal statistical significance [12]. The predictive power of dietary cholesterol was also evident in other studies [13,14]. Another long-term study on men of Irish origin showed that those who developed CHD had, at entry, a lower score for foods of vegetable origin, slightly lower fiber intake, slightly higher cholesterol intake, and higher scores indicating saturated-fat and cholesterol intake (directly) and polyunsaturated-fat intake (inversely) [15]. Intake of foods of animal origin were directly related to CHD- and total-mortality rate in a study on Seventh-Day Adventists [16].

Observational studies have not yielded entirely consistent results. No relation between intake of saturated fat and CHD rates was demonstrable in the Zutphen Study [17], and polyunsaturated fat intake was unrelated in an Israeli study [18]. Fish consumption was inversely related to CHD mortality in the Zutphen Study [14] and in other investigations, but contrary findings have also been reported [19].

Using CHD event rates as the primary endpoint, several controlled clinical trials of serum cholesterol lowering by diet have been performed. A recent meta-analysis included eight such trials [20]; CHD event rates in the combined data were decreased by treatment, despite modest cholesterol lowering and relatively short duration. To these studies may be added two not conforming to the inclusion criteria [21,22]; CHD incidence was reduced in both.

Other controlled trials have employed serial coronary angiography to assess the effect of interventions on progression of coronary artery disease. The high degree of consistency of such trials in obtaining favorable outcomes has two possible explanations: the graded nature of the endpoint (contrasting with the counting of clinical events) provides great statistical power for a given sample size, and the consequently smaller size of such trials permits closer supervision and probably better compliance with treatment [23]. The Leiden Study [24] employed a vegetarian diet with a very high ratio of polyunsaturated fat to saturated fat; there was no control group, but favorable changes in coronary angiograms correlated with a fall in the ratio of serum cholesterol to HDL-cholesterol. The Lifestyle Heart Study [25] used five interventions, including a very low intake of total fat, and there was marked weight loss; the treatment group showed favorable change in coronary stenoses. The Heidelberg trial, employing an exercise regime and a lipid-lowering diet, observed angiographic improvement [26]; in the SCRIP trial too, these interventions plus lipid-lowering and antihypertensive drugs reduced progression and increased regression [27].

Of the angiographic trials so far reported, only the St Thomas' Atherosclerosis Regression Study (STARS) has employed a lipid-lowering diet as a unifactorial intervention in a randomized controlled trial [28]. Repeated dietary assessments during the trial provided estimates of average nutrient intake in the 39 month period between initial and final quantitative coronary angiograms. We report the relation between this analysis of ambient nutrient intake and progression or regression of coronary artery disease. Because some participants were consuming their habitual diet and some a therapeutic diet, nutrient intake varied widely.

Subjects and Methods

Men undergoing clinically necessary coronary angiography were eligible for entry if coronary artery disease was present but did not require revascularization, if serum cholesterol levels were > 6.0 mmol/l (232 mg/dl), and if age was <66 years. Ninety men were randomly assigned to receive usual cardiological care, including antismoking counseling and antihypertensive treatment as indicated (group UC), or usual care plus a lipid-lowering diet (group D), or usual care, diet, and cholestyramine (DC). The present report concerns the 50 patients in groups D and UC who completed the study.

The diet employed in group D (Diet C in [29]) has been employed extensively in clinical practice. It utilizes the additive effects of fat modification and soluble fiber in lowering serum cholesterol levels. Observed nutrient intakes in groups D and UC respectively were: energy 2,050 ± 43.7 and 2,175 ± 42.9 kcal/day (means ± SEM), fat 27 ± 1.3 and 39 ± 1.5% energy, saturated fat 9.2 ± 0.57 and 18.4 ± 1.3% energy, polyunsaturated fat 7.5 ± 0.48 and 5.0 ± 0.37% energy, monounsaturated fat 9.2 ± 0.70 and 17 ± 1.1% energy, cholesterol 105 ± 7.1 and 157 ± 10.3 mg per 1,000 kcal, and fiber 28 ± 2.3 and 18 ± 1.3 g/day. Use of soluble fiber was recommended at an intake equivalent to 3.6 g polygalacturonate per 1,000 kcal. Observed nutrient intake was close to the prescribed diet, indicating that compliance was on average good. This was borne out in group D by completion of an average of four 4-day weighed food records during the trial [31].

Dietary assessment was based on the dietary history method [30], performed by the same dietitian throughout the trial. It comprised an interview to record consumption of a wide variety of foods, a 3-day food record, and a cross-check food frequency list. Computerized food composition data, based on data from [32], were used to estimate nutrient intake. Validation was performed by comparing these estimates in group D with those obtained from the multiple weighed food records, by relating energy intake estimated from them to calculated energy balance based on a multiple of basal metabolic rate [33], and by comparing observed reduction in plasma cholesterol in group D with that predicted by Keys' equation [34].

Serial quantitative coronary angiography was carried out with appropriate blinding, using carefully reproduced conditions. Up to 10 proximal coronary segments were analyzed, three selected adjacent frames being digitized at high resolution. After computerized edge detection of arterial segments and catheter, the minimum absolute width of each segment (MW) was calculated in mm, using catheter diameter as reference [35]. Disease progression and regression were defined on the basis of the imprecision of measurement of change in diameter (1.5 SD), based on the variability of repeated analyses of arterial segments.

Results and Discussion

Macronutrients (Table 1)

In the usual-care group 46% of patients showed overall progression of coronary artery disease and 46% showed overall regression; in the diet group 15% showed progression and 38% showed regression (p < 0.02 for trend). Intakes of several nutrients throughout the trial were correlated with angiographic outcome. Saturated-fat intake was strongly inversely related to change in MW (r = –0.44, p = 0.001); thus progression (decreased absolute diameter of stenoses) was associated with greater intake of saturated fat. Dietary cholesterol was related to change in MW (r = –0.27, p = 0.05). These nutrients reflected intake of meat and dairy fats.

Fatty acids (Table 1)

Significant associations with change in MW were not found for intakes of polyunsaturated fat or for P:S ratio despite considerable diversity of intake, nor for total or soluble fibre, protein, carbohydrate or alcohol. Monounsaturated fat intake was inversely related to change in MW (r = –0.33, p = 0.016), i.e., there was no indication of a protective effect; in the British diet meat and dairy fats are significant sources of oleic acid, hence the inverse relation may reflect greater animal fat consumption in those showing progression. The association between intake of saturated fat and progression of coronary artery disease during a 3-year period is concordant with most of the epidemiological studies cited, and

Table 1. Relation between in-trial nutrient intake per day and change in minimum coronary diameter. The STARS Trial. A negative sign indicates a direct relation between nutrient intake and progression of coronary atherosclerosis

	% Variance explained	Regression coefficient (SE)	p
Macronutrients			
energy, kcal	21.7	−0.001 (0.0002)	0.001
fat, g	29.7	−0.01 (0.002)	< 0.001
saturated fat, g	19.5	−0.01 (0.003)	0.001
monounsaturated fat, g	11.4	−0.01 (0.004)	0.016
polyunsaturated fat, g	0.6	−0.006 (0.011)	0.592
cholesterol, mg	7.3	−0.001 (0.001)	0.058
fiber, g	0.7	0.003 (0.006)	0.561
Fatty acids[a]			
14:0	5.7	−0.004 (0.003)	0.221
16:0	13.2	−0.002 (0.0008)	0.026
18:0	17.0	−0.005 (0.001)	0.009
18:1	10.0	−0.001 (0.0007)	0.066
18:1 *trans* (elaidic)	18.0	−0.014 (0.004)	0.001
18:2	11.8	−0.002 (0.0009)	0.039
18:3 n3	9.1	−1.575 (0.8881)	0.083
20:5	2.4	−0.011 (0.042)	0.791
22:6	2.3	0.003 (0.026)	0.898

[a]Adjusted for age, smoking, serum cholesterol, blood pressure, weight and treatment group.

with some dietary clinical trials [20–22]. In the placebo group of the CLAS trial, total fat intake (using 24-h recall) was directly related to visually-assessed progression of coronary disease [36]. Carbohydrate and protein were inversely related; saturated and unsaturated fats shared this direct relation with progression, by contrast with the inverse relation suggested by the Leiden Intervention Trial [24].

In STARS slightly lower energy intake in group D than in group UC was accompanied by a small weight loss (2.0 kg in group D, 0.3 kg in group UC over 3 years). More overweight patients in group D (45%) reduced to a Body Mass Index of <25 than in UC (19%). In the 14-month Lifestyle Heart Trial [25] the favorable outcome was associated with pronounced weight loss.

When multiple regression analysis was employed, the coefficient for saturated fat was independently significant (-0.010 ± 0.004, $p = 0.03$) as was the coefficient for mean LDL-cholesterol concentration during the trial (-0.209 ± 0.014, $p = 0.006$). These associations remained significant after adjustment for age, mean in-trial body weight, smoking, blood pressure, and treatment group assignment.

Hence intake of saturated fat and also LDL-cholesterol level were independently associated with progression of disease. Together these variables "explained" a substantial proportion of the change in MW, R^2 43%, $p < 0.001$. Although the significance of the regression coefficient for the relation between LDL-cholesterol level and progression was greater than that for saturated fat, the effect of saturated fat was not fully explained by its role in elevating plasma LDL-cholesterol. Analogously the association between dietary cholesterol and CHD mortality in a prospective epidemiological study was not fully accounted for by their mutual association with serum cholesterol concentration [12]. The 'additional' effect of saturated fat on progression in STARS may be related to its recognized influence on platelet function [37], coagulation factor VIIc [38], or LDL oxidation [39]. Stearic acid, intake of which 'explained' 17% of variance in change in MW, increases factor VIIc activity [40] but has little effect on serum cholesterol.

The component of the relation between dietary fat and progression that was independent of the effects of this nutrient on plasma cholesterol level was further investigated by adjusting the association for cholesterol level and for age, smoking, weight, blood pressure, and treatment group assignment. In this multiple linear regression analysis, stearic acid intake proved to be the strongest independent predictor ($r < 0.02$).

Conclusion

Over a wide range of intakes, consumption of total fat, saturated fatty acids, the *trans* fatty acid elaidic acid, and dietary energy were predictive of progression of coronary artery disease. No protective effect of unsaturated fatty acids was demonstrable. The relation between saturated fat intake and progression was not fully attributable to its effect in increasing plasma LDL-cholesterol, intake of stearic acid contributing independently to the association.

References

1. Clarkson TB, Lehner ND, Bullock BC, Lofland HB, Wagner WD. Primates Med 1976;9:90—144.
2. Armstrong ML, Warner ED, Connor WE. Circ Res 1970;27:59—67.
3. Anitschow N, Chalatow S. Zentralbl Algemeine Path 1913;24:1—9.
4. Keys A (ed) Seven Countries: a Multivariate Analysis of Death and Coronary Heart Disease. Cambridge, Mass: Harvard University Press, 1980.
5. McGill NC (ed) Geographic Pathology of Atherosclerosis. Baltimore: Williams and Wilkins, 1968.
6. Liu K, Stamler J, Trevisan M, Moss D. Arteriosclerosis 1982;2:221—227.
7. Morris JN, Marr JW, Clayton DG. Br Med J 1977;ii:1301.
8. Simpson NCR, Barker K, Cassels E, Mann JI. Br Med J 1982;285:683—684.
9. Miettinen TA, Naukkarinen V, Nuttunen JK, Mattila S, Kumlin T. Br Med J 1982;285:993—995.
10. Wood DA, Riemersma R, Butler S, Thomson M, Macintyre C, Elton RA, Oliver MF. Lancet 1987;1: 177—183.
11. Shekelle RB, Shryock AM, Paul O, Lepper M, Stamler J, Liu S, Raynor WJ Jr. N Engl J Med 1981;304: 65—70.
12. Stamler J, Shekelle RB. Arch Pathol Lab Med 1988;112:1032—1040.
13. McGee DL, Reed DM, Yano K, Kagan A. Am J Epidemiol 1984;119:667—676.
14. Kromhout D, Bosschieter EB, de Lezenne Coulander C. N Engl J Med 1985;312:1205—1209.
15. Kushi LH, Lew RA, Stare F, Ellison CR, El Lozy M, Bourke G, Daly L, Graham I, Hickey N, Mulcahy R, Kevaney J. N Engl J Med 1985;312:811—818.
16. Phillips RL, Lemon FR, Beeson WL. Am J Clin Nutr 1978;31:191—198.
17. Kromhout D, de Louzenne Coulander C. Am J Epidemiol 1984;119:733—741.
18. Medalie JH, Kahn HA, Riss E, Goldbourt U. J Chron Dis 1973;26:325—349.
19. Vollset SE, Neuch I, Bjelke E. N Engl J Med 1985;313:820—821.
20. Law MR, Wald NJ, Thompson SG. Br Med J 1994;308:357—372.
21. Turpeinen O, Karvonen MJ, Pekkarinen M, Miettinen M, Elosuo R, Paavilainen E. Int J Epidemiol 1979; 8:99—118.
22. Njerrmann I, Velve Byre K, Nolme I, Leren P. Lancet 1981;2:1303—1310.
23. Lewis B. In: Catapano AL, Gotto AM Jr, Smith LC, Paoletti R (eds) Drugs Affecting Lipid Metabolism. Dordrecht: Kluwer Academic Publishers, 1993;241—249.
24. Arntzenius AC, Kromhout D, Barth JD, Reiber JNC, Bruschke AVG, Buis B, van Gent CM, Strikwerde S, Van der Velde EA. N Engl J Med 1985;312:805—811.
25. Ornish D, Brown SE, Scherwitz LW, Billings JH, Armstrong WT, Ports TA, McLanakan SM, Kirkeeide RL, Brand RJ, Gould KL. Lancet 1990;336:129—133.
26. Schuler G, Nambrect R, Schlierf G, Niebauer J, Nauer K, Neumann J, Noberg E, Drinkman A, Bacher F, Grunze M, Kubler W. Circulation 1992;86:1—11.

27. Quinn TG, Alderman E, McMillan A, Naskell W, SCRIP Investigators. Circulation 1992;86:(suppl 1)1–62.

28. Watts GF, Lewis B, Brunt JNH, Lewis ES, Coltart DJ, Smith LDR, Mann JI, Swan AV. Lancet 1992;339: 563–569.

29. Lewis B, Nammett F, Katan MB, Kay RM, Merkx I, Nobels A, Miller NE, Swan AV. Lancet 1981;2:1310–1313.

30. Burke BS. J Am Diet Assoc 1947;23:1041–1046.

31. Bingham SA, Nelson M. In: Margetts BM, Nelson H (eds) Design Concepts in Nutritional Epidemiology. Oxford: OUP, 1991;153–191.

32. Paul AA, Southgate DAT. McCance and Widdowson's The Composition of Foods. 4th ed. London: HMSO, 1988.

33. Black AE, Goldberg GR, Jebb SA, Livingston MBE, Cole TJ, Prentice AM. Eur J Clin Nutr 1991;45: 583–599.

34. Keys A, Anderson JT, Grande F. Lancet 1957;2:959–966.

35. Brunt JNH, Watts GF, Smith LDR, Coltart DJ, Lewis B. Med Eng Physics 1994 (in press).

36. Blankenhorn DH, Johnson RL, Mack WJ, el Zen HA, Vailas LI. J Am Med Ass 1990;263:1646–1652.

37. Hornstra G, Lewis B, Chait A, Turpeinen O, Karvonen MJ, Vergroesen AJ. Lancet 1973;1:1155–1157.

38. Miller GJ, Cruikshank JK, Ellis LI, Thompson RL, Wilkes NC, Stirling Y, Mitropoulos KA, Allison JV, Foz TE, Walker AD. Atherosclerosis 1989;78:19–24.

39. Parathasarathy S, Kheo JC, Miller E, Barnett J, Witztum JL, Steinberg D. Proc Nat Acad Sci USA 1990;87:3894–3898.

40. Mitropoulos K, Miller GJ, Martin JC, Reeves BEA, Cooper J. Arterioscler Thromb 1994;14:214–222.

298

Investigations of the effects of synthetic saponins on cholesterol absorption and serum cholesterol levels

C.A. Dujovne[1], W.S. Harris[1], R.A. Gelfand[2], L.A. Morehouse[2], P.A. McCarthy[2], C.E. Chandler[2], M.P. DeNinno[2], H.J. Harwood Jr.[2], F.A. Newton[2] and C.L. Shear[2]

[1]Lipid and Arteriosclerosis Prevention Clinic, University of Kansas Medical Center, 1348 K.U. Medical Center, 3901 Rainbow Blvd., Kansas City, KS 66160-7374; and [2]Central Research Division, Pfizer Inc., Eastern Point Road, Groton, CT 06340, USA

Abstract. Natural saponins present in a large variety of plants and legumes have physical chemical properties that result, after their oral administration, in an inhibition of intestinal absorption of sterols in animals and humans. A synthetically produced saponin — tiqueside (β-tigogenin cellobioside, CP-88,818) — has been shown to be a safe and effective agent when used to lower serum cholesterol levels in animals and humans. Other synthetic saponins with augmented therapeutic potency are being developed and tested at the present time. One example, CP-148,623, is the subject of several scientific presentations at this meeting.

What are saponins?

Saponins are a structurally diverse group of naturally occurring compounds found mainly in plants [1,2]. Alfalfa sprouts and some types of beans and peas contain the largest concentration of saponins. Chemically, the saponins consist of a steroid or triterpene group (the aglycone) linked to one or more sugar molecules. The molecules are thus amphipathic, giving saponins their characteristic surface activity to which their name refers. This surface activity, and the unique structure of the hydrophilic triterpene or steroid aglycones, has been suggested to be largely responsible for the biological activity of saponins [3].

Natural and synthetic saponins have been shown to reduce plasma cholesterol levels in experimental animals [4–6]. In addition, several human studies have examined the effects on plasma lipids of administration of saponin-containing vegetables. In six of the nine published studies [3], the plasma cholesterol level was reduced by 16 to 24% from baseline, but little effect was seen in the other three studies.

How do saponins affect lipoprotein metabolism?

The best known, well documented, pharmacological effect of the hypocholesterolemic saponins is an inhibition of intestinal cholesterol absorption [1,7]. However, the actual molecular mechanism mediating this effect remains unclear. Since most saponins are very poorly absorbed intact, proposed mechanisms invoke nonsystemic actions in the intestinal lumen. Some saponins, such as digitonin or tomatine, are thought to inhibit cholesterol absorption via the formation of nonabsorbable saponin–cholesterol complexes; indeed, some saponins readily precipitate cholesterol from a micellar solution in vitro. Other saponins also appear to inhibit absorption of bile acids as well as cholesterol, and it has been suggested that these saponins cause the formation of large mixed micelles from which cholesterol, bile acids, and perhaps other micellar constituents are less readily absorbed. Still other mechanisms have been postulated, but because of the lack of definitive in vivo data, the molecular mechanism of action of saponins must be considered still largely undefined.

Safety of saponins

Saponins are found in many different plant species, including beans, peas, oats, garlic and yams [1]. Many, if not most, naturally occurring saponins are poorly absorbed and have been associated with a low order of toxicity when administered orally. For example, no significant toxic effects have been found in rats fed alfalfa saponins at 1% of the diet for up to 6 months [8]. Similarly, the triterpenoid saponins from *Quillaja* (widely used as a food-additive foaming agent) are nontoxic when fed to rats or mice at 1.5% of diet over prolonged periods [9].

Some saponins do possess hemolytic activity and other potentially toxic effects. These effects are highly specific not only to the compound, but to the route of administration [1]. With oral administration of poorly bioavailable saponins, one would expect the gastrointestinal tract to be the major target of any potential toxic effects. No controlled long-term studies in humans have been reported.

A host of other biologic actions have been reported or postulated, including an anti-platelet effect, prevention of liver injury in a rat model, and in vitro anticarcinogenic activity [1]. Again, the ultimate clinical relevance of such potential systemic effects of these very poorly bioavailable compounds is unclear.

The synthetic saponins

Purified, chemically modified or synthetic saponins could potentially have greater capacity to inhibit cholesterol absorption than natural saponins contained in foodstuffs [4]. Encouraged by experiments with alfalfa saponins showing hypocholesterolemic and anti-atherogenic effects, Malinow et al. [5] prepared synthetic glucoside and cellobioside derivatives of several steroidal compounds similar to those found in digitonin. Testing of several of these synthetic saponins indicated that β-tigogenin cellobioside, subsequently termed tiqueside (structure shown in Fig. 1), was the most effective hypocholesterolemic agent among them.

Studies performed at Pfizer Central Research [6] demonstrated that tiqueside inhibits cholesterol absorption, and as a result lowers plasma cholesterol, in a variety of animal species fed either cholesterol-containing or cholesterol-free diets (Table 1). Figure 2 shows the dose-dependent inhibition of cholesterol absorption by tiqueside in the hamster. Unlike its effect to inhibit absorption of cholesterol, tiqueside did not alter intestinal bile acid metabolism.

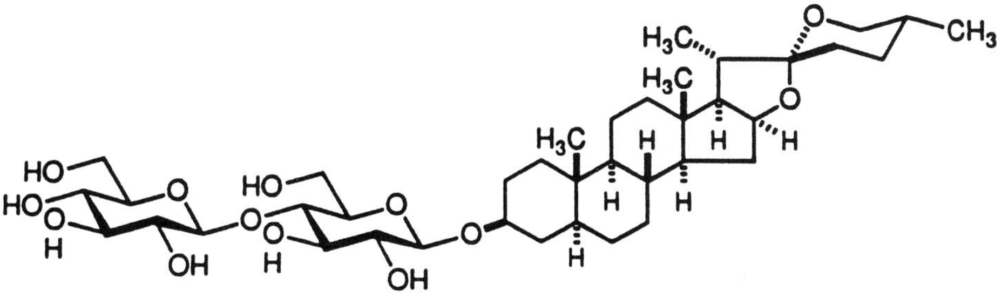

Fig. 1. Structure of β-tigogenin cellobioside, MW = 741.

Table 1. Decrease in serum cholesterol after treatment with CP-88,818 in various species

Species	Dietary cholesterol (%)	Dose (mg/kg)	Duration of treatment (weeks)	Decrease in cholesterol (%)
Rat	0.1	50	2	23
Hamster	0.2	150	2	22
	0.2	200	2	20
Rabbit	0.4	63	3	20
	0.4	125	3	45
	0.4	375	3	86
Sea quail	0.5	20	1	53
	0.5	50	1	64
	0.5	100	1	75
Dog	0.01	250	2	18
	0.01	500	2	24
	0.01	1000	2	30
	0.01	2000	2	41
Rhesus monkey	0.1	24	3	9
	0.1	49	3	19
	0.1	98	3	36

Monkey data are derived from [5].

Effects of tiqueside in humans

Our group at the University of Kansas Medical Center has conducted two small, exploratory clinical studies of the effects of tiqueside administration for 2–3 weeks in healthy volunteers and in hypercholesterolemic patients.

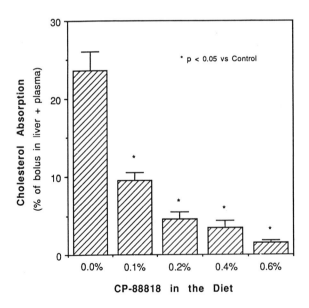

Fig. 2. Dose-dependent inhibition by dietary CP-88-818 (tiqueside) of cholesterol absorption in chow-fed hamsters.

One study involved 15 patients with primary hypercholesterolemia, with an entry LDL-cholesterol level of >160 mg/dl after 4 weeks off all lipid-lowering medications. The study design was multiple-crossover, double-blind, and placebo-controlled. All patients received tiqueside at each of three doses (1, 2 and 3 g/day, given BID with meals) during three separate 2-week treatment periods. The treatment periods were separated from one another by 3-week placebo washout periods. Patients were randomized to one of two treatment sequences. Figure 3 shows that for both treatment sequences, within each tiqueside treatment period mean LDL-cholesterol (bold line) declined, with a rise occurring during each intervening 3-week placebo washout period. Treatment was very well tolerated, with no significant adverse effects. When the data were summarized based on the change in plasma LDL-cholesterol that occurred within each treatment period, clear

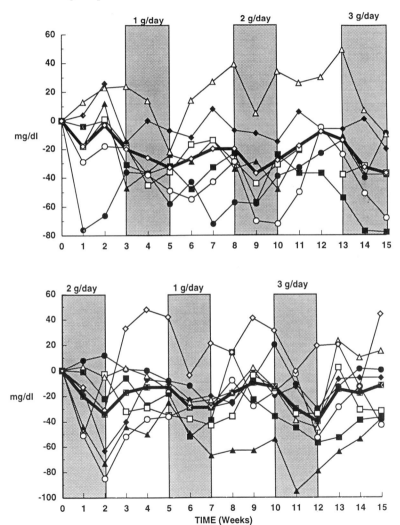

Fig. 3. Change from baseline in LDL-cholesterol in 15 hypercholesterolemic patients receiving tiqueside at each of three different doses (shaded areas), alternating with placebo, according to either of two treatment sequences (top and bottom panels). Mean LDL change is shown by the bold line.

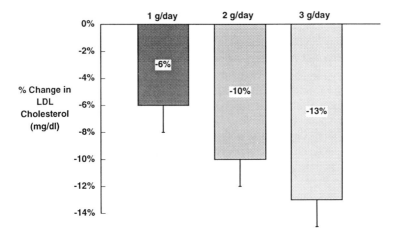

Fig. 4. Mean 2-week change in LDL-cholesterol during crossover treatment with three different doses of tiqueside.

evidence of a dose–response relationship was obtained, as shown in Fig. 4. LDL-cholesterol lowering after 2 weeks of treatment at 3 g/day averaged 13%. These results were considered encouraging, and support dose-dependent LDL-lowering efficacy of tiqueside within the 1–3 g/day range. It must be emphasized, however, that the exploratory design of this small study involved a limited dose range and very short duration of treatment.

In a second study we examined the effects of tiqueside on intestinal cholesterol

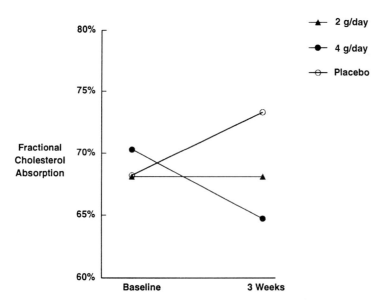

Fig. 5. Fractional cholesterol absorption measured before and after 3 weeks of treatment with tiqueside or placebo, given with a cholesterol-restricted diet. The increase seen in the placebo group probably reflects adaptation to a low-cholesterol diet.

metabolism. Twenty-four healthy male volunteers, with entry plasma total cholesterol >180 mg/dl, were divided into three treatment groups. Two active treatment groups of nine subjects each received either 2 or 4 g/day of tiqueside, while a third group of six subjects received placebo as controls. Unlike the previous study, in this study tiqueside was given as a single daily dose with breakfast. Treatment lasted 3 weeks, and was preceded by a 1-week baseline, diet lead-in period. An NCEP Step-1 diet was consumed throughout the 4-week study period.

Before we discuss the results, a number of caveats should be mentioned. First, because of the very short duration of the diet lead-in period, subjects were not in steady state at the start of the treatment period, and a progressive fall in plasma cholesterol in the diet-alone, placebo group acted to minimize the apparent treatment effect. Second, the once-daily administration regimen is likely to underestimate the effect achievable with divided daily dosing. These caveats notwithstanding, the study results shed important light on the effect of tiqueside on lipid physiology in man.

Figure 5 shows each group's mean fractional cholesterol absorption (measured by the continuous feeding, dual-isotope method) at baseline and after 3 weeks of experimental treatment. Fractional cholesterol absorption rose in the placebo group, did not change in the 2 g/day tiqueside group, and fell in the 4 g/day tiqueside group. The rise in fractional

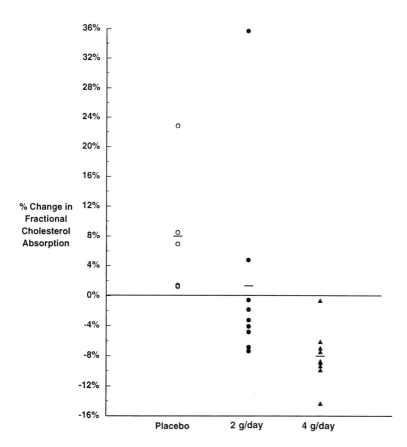

Fig. 6. Individual subject data for groups shown in Fig. 5.

304

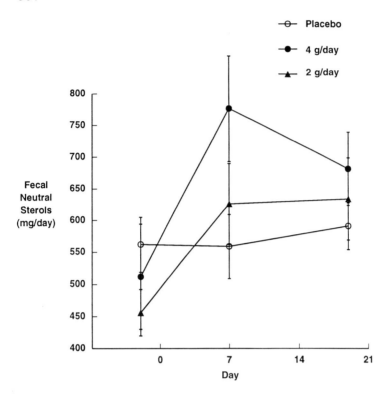

Fig. 7. Increase by tiqueside of fecal neutral sterol excretion in normal volunteers.

absorption observed in the placebo group probably reflects the well-known adaptive response to a cholesterol-restricted diet. Figure 6 shows these individual subjects' 3-week change in fractional cholesterol absorption, and demonstrates a clear dose-dependent inhibition by tiqueside. Consistent with these data based on tracer measurements, total fecal neutral sterol excretion, shown in Fig. 7, rose dose-dependently with tiqueside treatment but was unchanged with placebo. Tiqueside had no effect on fecal bile acid or total fat excretion. Finally, as shown in Fig. 8, the observed reduction in plasma LDL-cholesterol tended to correlate with the observed increase in fecal neutral sterol excretion. This correlation achieved only borderline statistical significance, probably because of the design limitations mentioned earlier. Nevertheless, taken together, these data strongly support the conclusion that tiqueside inhibits cholesterol absorption in humans, and as a consequence reduces circulating LDL-cholesterol levels. The magnitude of cholesterol lowering ultimately achievable clinically with this therapeutic approach was not defined by these small studies. However, interim analysis of a subsequently performed, larger (180 patients), longer-term (8-week) treatment study showed LDL-cholesterol lowering on the order of 20% at a dose of 4 g/day.

Development of new synthetic saponins

A search for other synthetic saponins with greater potential therapeutic efficacy has led to the discovery of CP-148,623. Experimental findings with CP-148,623 are presented by poster at this meeting, as follows. McCarthy et al. [10] describe the structure–activity

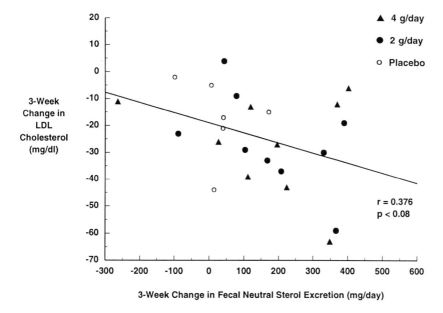

Fig. 8. Relationship of change in plasma LDL-cholesterol to change in fecal neutral sterol excretion after 3 weeks of treatment with tiqueside or placebo in 24 healthy male volunteers.

relationships of a number of synthetic saponins, and have demonstrated that CP-148,623 is more potent than any previously described synthetic saponin. Bangerter et al. [11] show that like tiqueside, CP-148,623 inhibits cholesterol absorption, increases fecal neutral sterol excretion, and prevents diet-induced hypercholesterolemia in hamsters, mice and rabbits. Zaccaro et al. [12] provide evidence that CP-148,623 inhibits the intestinal absorption of biliary cholesterol without affecting intestinal absorption of bile acids. Finally, in support of a site of action that is localized within the intestinal lumen, the Pfizer group has also shown [13] that CP-148,623 specifically prevents the entry of cholesterol into the intestinal mucosa.

Summary and Conclusions

Ingestion of saponin glycosides, which are present in over 500 plant genera, significantly influences cholesterol metabolism in animals and humans. This effect is largely dependent on the chemical structure of the saponin. Our results with the first synthetically produced and pharmaceutically developed such compound — tiqueside — show that synthetic saponins may have a promising role as a safe and effective hypocholesterolemic agent in dyslipidemic patients.

References

1. Price KR, Johnson IT, Fenwick GR. CRC Crit Rev Food Sci Nutr 1987:26;27.
2. Malinow MR. Letter to the Editors. Atherosclerosis 1984;50:117–119.
3. Oakenfull D, Sidhu GS. Eur J Clin Nutr 1990; 44:79–88.
4. Coulson CB, Evans RA. Br J Nutr 1960; 14:121–134.
5. Malinow MR, Gardner, LO, Nelson, JT, McGlaughlin P, Upson B, and Aigner-Held R. Steroids 1986;48: 197–211.

6. Harwood HJ, Chandler CE, Pellarin LD, Bangerter FW, Wilkins RW, Long CA, Cosgrove PG, Malinow MR, Marzetta CA, Pettini JL, Savoy YE and Mayne JT. J Lipid Res 1993;34:377–395.
7. Stredonsky ER. Biochim Biophys Acta 1994; 1210:255–287.
8. Malinow MR, McNulty WP, McLaughlin P, Stafford C, Burns AK, Livingston AL, Kohler GO. Food Cosmet Toxicol 1981:19;443.
9. Gaunt IF, Grasso, P, Gangolli SD. Food Cosmet Toxicol 1974:12;641.
10. McCarthy, PA, DeNinno MP, Morehouse LA, Chandler CE, Beyer TA, Bangerter FW, Cosgrove PG, Duplantier K, Etienne JB, Fowler MA, Wilkins RW, Zaccaro LM, Zawistoski MP. Atherosclerosis 1994;109:309 (abstract).
11. Bangerter FW, Zaccaro LM, Wilkins RW, Woody HA, Wilder DW, Sugarman ED, DeNinno MP, McCarthy PA, Wilson TW, Chandler CE, Morehouse LA. Atherosclerosis 1994;109:309 (abstract).
12. Zaccaro LM, Bangerter FW, Wilkins RW, Woody HA, McCarthy PA, DeNinno MP, Morehouse LA, Chandler CE. Atherosclerosis 1994;109:315 (abstract).
13. Bangerter FW, Wilkins RW, Zaccaro LM, McCarthy PA, DeNinno MP, Morehouse LA, Chandler CE, Cray L and Tso P. Atherosclerosis 1994;109:310 (abstract).

Atorvastatin: a step ahead for HMG-CoA reductase inhibitors

Donald M. Black

Parke-Davis Research Division, Ann Arbor, Michigan, USA

Abstract. Atorvastatin, a synthetic, chiral HMGRI, is in clinical evaluation as a potential new drug. Over 350 patients have been studied in six phase II clinical trials for up to 12 weeks. Dose–response studies in Type IIa/IIb and IV patients have been completed. Several large phase III studies are in progress to assess the long-term safety and efficacy of atorvastatin.

Introduction

The treatment of hypercholesterolemia to prevent early morbidity from atherosclerotic disease remains a high priority in medicine. New recommendations of the NCEP-ATP require a significantly greater reduction in LDL-C in patients with several risk factors for coronary heart disease and pre-existing disease. Patients with evidence of cardiovascular disease are encouraged to reduce their LDL-C below 100 mg/dl (2.6 mmol/l). In large part, the impetus for these recommendations comes from the findings of several studies describing the progression of atherosclerotic disease as the natural outcome of hyper-cholesterolemia, and the attenuation or even reversal of disease with lipid-lowering therapy. Most of these studies have demonstrated positive results with an LDL reduction of 35–45%, often in association with an increase in HDL and/or a decrease in serum triglycerides. Currently available therapies will provide LDL-C reductions of up to 40% at the maximum dose of a single agent, although most of the regression trials have used multiple-drug regimens. Atorvastatin, a new HMG-CoA reductase inhibitor, appears to offer even greater efficacy in the reduction of LDL-cholesterol.

Atorvastatin {[R-(R*,R*)]-2-(4-fluorophenyl)-beta, delta-dihydroxy-5-(1-methylethyl)-3-phenyl-4-[(phenylamino)carbonyl]-1H-pyrloe-1-heptanoic acid calcium salt (2:1)} competitively inhibits HMG-CoA, the rate-limiting step in cholesterol synthesis. Studies in animals and human volunteers indicate that atorvastatin may have greater efficacy in reducing LDL-C and serum triglycerides, and that there was no difference in efficacy when dosed once or twice a day, or between evening and morning. The first study in patients with this compound was 981-04, a parallel-arm, placebo-controlled, dose–response study. Eighty-one subjects with LDL-C levels above 4.1 mmol/l (160 mg/dl), after a diet lead-in period of 8 weeks, were randomized to placebo or 2.5, 5, 10, 20, 40 or 80 mg of atorvastatin once daily for 6 weeks. Lipoprotein levels and routine biochemicals were measured every 2 weeks. At the end of 6 weeks, LDL-C reductions for the seven dose groups were +8, −25, −29, −41, −44, −50 and −61%, respectively. Triglycerides were also reduced by 13–32%, in a non-dose-dependent manner, and HDL-C was modestly increased. The drug was well tolerated, with no significant differences from placebo in adverse events. Over 80% of the lipid-altering effect seen at each dose was evident by the 2nd week of therapy.

Address for correspondence: Donald M. Black MD, Parke-Davis Research Division, 2800 Plymouth Road, Ann Arbor, MI 48105, USA. Tel.: +1-313-996-7466. Fax: +1-313-996-4531.

308

Next, we compared several doses of atorvastatin against previously approved HMG-CoA reductase inhibitors (HMG-RIs). 981-07 was an open crossover study designed to compare the short-term (4-week) effects of atorvastatin 5 and 20 mg per day to those of simvastatin 10 mg and pravastatin 20 mg. Ninety-one patients in The Netherlands and Germany entered the trial after an 8-week diet lead-in, and were randomized to one of four arms (atorvastatin 5 or 20 mg, simvastatin 10 mg or pravastatin 20 mg). After 4 weeks the drug was discontinued, and the subjects were off drugs for 4 weeks. The subjects were then placed on a comparative agent, so that every subject on atorvastatin 5 or 20 mg would take either pravastatin or simvastatin in the second period. The 5-mg dose of atorvastatin reduced LDL-C 27%, as compared to 20 mg pravastatin (26%) and 10 mg simvastatin (29%). The 20-mg dose of atorvastatin reduced LDL-C by 45%. Reductions in triglycerides and increases in HDL-C were approximately the same among all treatments. Again, all four drugs were well tolerated. These results corroborated the findings of 981-04. A comparison of the lipid-lowering profile of atorvastatin to the presently available products — lovastatin, simvastatin, pravastatin and fluvastatin — can be derived from the available literature (Fig. 1).

Preclinical data, as well as the results of studies -04 and -07, indicate the possibility that atorvastatin reduces serum triglycerides to an extent that might be clinically significant. To help explore this issue, we initiated 981-38, a parallel-arm, placebo-controlled, dose–response study in patients with hypertriglyceridemia (serum triglycerides > 4.0 mmol/l). Fifty-six Fredrickson Type IIB and Type IV patients were randomized to placebo or 5, 20, or 80 mg atorvastatin a day for 4 weeks, after an 8-week placebo baseline. Most of the patients in this study were hypertriglyceridemic, with LDL-C levels at baseline of less than 3.1 mmol/l. Reductions in total cholesterol, triglycerides and LDL-cholesterol were dose-dependent. LDL-C was reduced by 6, 19, 31 and 43%, while triglycerides were reduced by 6, 25, 31 and 43%, respectively. HDL-C was increased by 5, 8, 12 and 12%, respectively. This is the first report of the use of an HMG-RI alone in this population, so there are no comparative data for other HMG-RIs. Nicotinic acid and fibrates have similar efficacy in reducing serum triglycerides, but often increase LDL-C

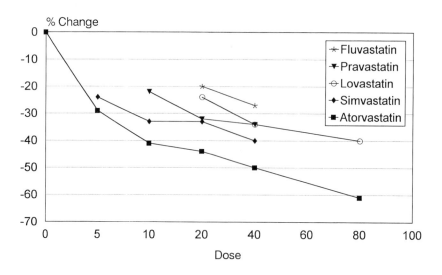

Fig. 1. LDL-C reduction by atorvastatin compared with other HMG-CoA reductase inhibitors.

309

in Type IV patients. These results indicate that atorvastatin may have a greater effect on VLDL-cholesterol than other HMG-RIs, and has led to further research to explore the mechanism of action.

Patients with non-insulin-dependent diabetes mellitus are recognized to have a dyslipidemia due at least in part to the increased production/reduced metabolism of VLDL-cholesterol. Twenty-five subjects with LDL-C >4.1 mmol/l were studied in a parallel-arm study comparing atorvastatin 10 mg to simvastatin 10 mg. After 4 weeks of therapy, LDL-C was reduced in the simvastatin arm by 30%, and in the atorvastatin arm by 39%. Serum triglycerides were reduced by 12 and 22% and HDL-C increased by 4 and 8%, respectively. Parameters associated with stability of diabetic control were also assessed, and indicated that there was little increase in glucose on administration of atorvastatin (+2%), but a considerable increase with simvastatin (+23%). Insulin and hemoglobin A1c were decreased with atorvastatin, and to a lesser degree with simvastatin.

At the other end of the spectrum, 22 patients were identified in South Africa with well-defined LDL-receptor defect. Following a baseline period of 6 weeks, subjects with LDL-C levels > 6.5 mmol/l (average 8.8 mmol/l), were randomized to 40 mg twice a day or 80 mg once a day of atorvastatin for 6 weeks. The drug was tolerated without problems. After treatment, LDL-C in both groups was reduced by 57%, serum triglycerides by 31%, and HDL-C increased by 21%. The effects on LDL-C and triglycerides were expected, and has confirmed the 80-mg response seen in the dose-response study.

Finally, we were interested in comparing the lipid-lowering effects of atorvastatin to a different reference standard, a bile-acid sequestrant, colestipol. This 12-week open-label study was designed to compare the proposed usual starting dose of atorvastatin 10 mg daily to 20 g daily of colestipol. A third arm, combining atorvastatin 10 mg with colestipol 20 g, was included to assess the potential additivity of the lipid effects. One hundred and six patients were randomized to one of the three treatment arms after the 6-week baseline period. After 12 weeks, the change in LDL-C for the colestipol group was –22%, for the atorvastatin group –35%, and for the group on combined colestipol and

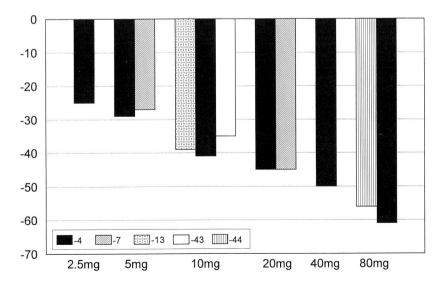

Fig. 2. Mean percentage reduction in LDL-C by atorvastatin in type II patients.

atorvastatin, −45%. Triglycerides were increased in the colestipol group by 18%, but reduced in the atorvastatin and combination groups by 16 and 24%. HDL-C was increased in each of the three groups, by 5, 12 and 13%. Compliance was generally better for the subjects taking atorvastatin, with 90% taking the full prescribed dose, and 70% of the colestipol and 75% of the combination groups taking the full dose. Adverse events were more common on colestipol, with 3 of 44 patients withdrawing from the study because of adverse events on colestipol alone, and only 1 of 41 on atorvastatin alone. None of the combination subjects withdrew because of adverse events. The results of this study indicated that atorvastatin, at the proposed starting dose, had a more beneficial effect on the lipid profile, with fewer adverse effects, than a substantial dose of colestipol.

These six studies represent the use of atorvastatin in 326 patients for 4–12 weeks at doses of 2.5–80 mg a day. The efficacy at the higher doses has not been reported previously with single-agent therapy, and has been corroborated by several small studies (Fig. 2). In the studies completed, there have been no serious attributable adverse events, and no clinically significant increases in muscle enzymes or liver transaminases. Current studies have enrolled 2,700 patients, and patients will be taking 10–80 mg of atorvastatin for up to 1 year. The safety and efficacy of atorvastatin relative to existing therapies will be apparent with the completion of these trials.

©1995 Elsevier Science B.V. All rights reserved.
Atherosclerosis X.
F.P. Woodford, J. Davignon and A. Sniderman, editors.

SCH 48461, a novel inhibitor of cholesterol absorption

Edmund J. Sybertz, Harry R. Davis, Margaret Van Heek, Robert E. Burrier, Brian G. Salisbury, Michael T. Romano, John W. Clader and Duane A. Burnett

Schering Plough Research Institute, 2015 Galloping Hill Rd., Kenilworth, NJ 07033, USA

Abstract. SCH 48461 inhibits cholesterol absorption in rhesus monkeys and other species. The compound prevented the rise in plasma cholesterol and reversed previously established hypercholesterolemia in cholesterol-fed monkeys, with an ED^{50} of 0.12 mg/kg/day. In rats, SCH 48461 prevented the uptake, esterification and secretion of exogenous cholesterol into lymph without affecting the secretion of intestinally synthesized cholesterol into lymph. In vitro, SCH 48461 caused weak inhibition of hepatic microsomal acyl-CoA: cholesterol O-acyltransferase (ACAT) and did not affect enzymatic activity of pancreatic cholesterol esterase. These data suggest that SCH 48461 is a novel inhibitor of the intestinal uptake and absorption of cholesterol.

The liver and intestine are the two major organs regulating whole-body cholesterol homeostasis. In humans, approximately 1,000–1,500 mg of cholesterol is transported through the intestine and about half of this is absorbed [1]. In this paper, we describe SCH 48461, (3R,4S)-1,4-*bis*-(4-methoxyphenyl)-3-(3-phenylpropyl)-2-azetidinone, a potent and specific inhibitor of cholesterol uptake and absorption which reduces plasma cholesterol in cholesterol-fed animals.

Materials and Methods

All animal studies were conducted under approved protocols from an AALAC-accredited institutional animal care and use committee.

Effects on cholesterol absorption and plasma cholesterol in rhesus monkeys

In one study, cholesterol absorption was determined by collecting feces for 7 days from chow-fed and chow-fed SCH 48461-treated rhesus monkeys following an oral dose of ^{14}C-cholesterol and ^{3}H-β-sitosterol [2]. In another study, separate groups of rhesus monkeys were placed on a diet containing 0.25% cholesterol, 15% hydrogenated coconut oil and 7.5% olive oil with or without SCH 48461. Animals were fed once a day for a period of up to 4 weeks. Plasma cholesterol levels were determined weekly on fasting samples. Apoprotein mass and LDL- and HDL-cholesterol were measured at some of the time points [3].

Effects on absorption, synthesis and secretion of cholesterol into lymph in rats

Fasted rats were dosed with vehicle or SCH 48461 (10 mg/kg) 3 h prior to surgery. Rats were anesthetized and the intestine and main mesenteric lymph vessel were cannulated. An emulsion of triolein, phosphatidylcholine, 1 μCi ^{14}C-cholesterol and 10 μCi ^{3}H-mevalonate was placed directly into the duodenum and lymph was collected for 4 h. Lymph cholesterol and cholesteryl esters were separated by thin-layer chromatography and analyzed for radioactivity.

In a separate study, SCH 48461 or vehicle was administered directly into the intestinal cannula of rats in which the lymphatic vessels were left intact. One hour later animals received a solution of monolein, oleate, cholesteryl oleate, 1 µCi cholesteryl ^{14}C-oleate and 2 µCi ^{3}H-cholesteryl oleate via the intestinal catheter. Animals were sacrificed 1.5 h later and plasma was analyzed for ^{14}C and [3]H.

Effects on lipid processing in vitro

In vitro ACAT assays were performed as described previously using rat liver microsomes [4]. Assays to measure the synthesis of cholesteryl esters by bovine pancreatic cholesteryl esterase were performed according to the methods of Kyger et al. [5]. Assays for measurement of the hydrolysis of cholesteryl esters by the same enzyme were performed as described by Camulli et al. [6].

Results

SCH 48461 at 3 mg/kg/day inhibited the absorption of radiolabeled cholesterol by 60% as compared to a control group ($p < 0.05$). SCH 48461 prevented the rise in plasma cholesterol upon cholesterol feeding and rapidly reversed established hypercholesterolemia at 1 mg/kg/day (Fig. 1). The effective dose for causing a 50% inhibition of the rise in plasma cholesterol was 0.12 mg/kg/day. LDL-cholesterol was reduced by 68% at 1 mg/kg/day. HDL-cholesterol was unchanged. ApoB100 levels were reduced 59% whereas levels of apoA1 were unchanged.

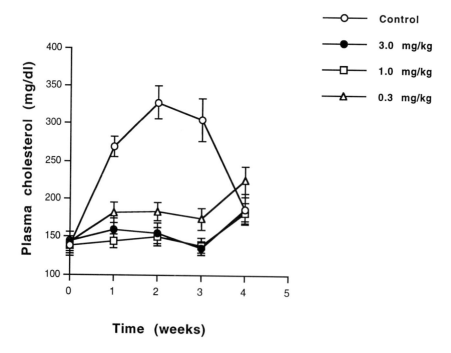

Fig. 1. Effect of SCH 48461 on plasma cholesterol in cholesterol-fed rhesus monkeys. Data are means ± SEM, n = 5 per group. Cholesterol feeding was started on day 0. At week 3, the animals receiving no drug were placed on a diet containing 1 mg/kg/day whereas the other groups were placed on a diet containing no drug. All SCH 48461 groups are different from control from week 1 to 3, $p < 0.05$.

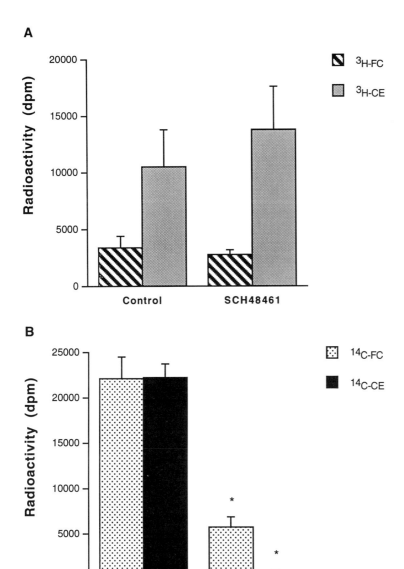

Fig. 2. Effect of SCH 48461 on appearance of radiolabeled cholesterol in the lymph of rats. A: Newly synthesized free cholesterol and cholesteryl ester (from ^{3}H-mevalonate) appearance in lymph. B: Free cholesterol and cholesteryl ester appearance in lymph from exogenous ^{14}C-cholesterol. Data are mean ± SEM, n = 4–7 per group. $^*p < 0.05$ vs. control.

In rats, SCH 48461 did not affect the appearance of newly synthesized free cholesterol or cholesteryl ester into lymph when mevalonate was used as the cholesterol precursor (Fig. 2A). In the same rats (Fig. 2B), the appearance of free and esterified cholesterol from an exogenous source was greatly diminished. The level of radioactivity from cholesteryl ^{14}C-oleate in the plasma was the same in control and treated rats, indicating

314

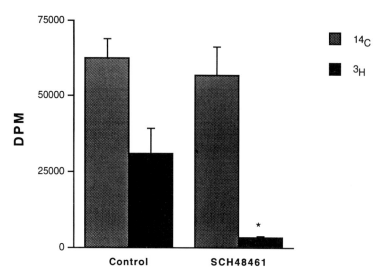

Fig. 3. Effect of SCH 48461 on appearance of [14]C (from cholesteryl ^{14}C-oleate) and [3]H (from ^{3}H-cholesteryl oleate) in plasma. Data are mean ± SEM, n = 5 per group. *p < 0.05 vs. control.

that SCH 48461 did not affect the hydrolysis of cholesteryl ester or the absorption of free fatty acids (Fig. 3). However, the absorption of ^{3}H-cholesterol generated from ^{3}H-cholesteryl oleate was substantially inhibited.

SCH 48461 displayed weak ACAT inhibitory activity when compared to reference standard drugs (IC$_{50}$ = 26 μM). SCH 48461 did not affect the synthetic or hydrolytic activity of pancreatic cholesterol esterase at concentrations as high as 50 μM.

Discussion

The present studies describe the cholesterol absorption-inhibitory and plasma cholesterol-lowering activities of SCH 48461 in rhesus monkeys and its actions in rats. SCH 48461 exerted potent cholesterol-reducing activity in cholesterol-fed monkeys.

SCH 48461 prevented the appearance of free cholesterol and its ester into lymph in the rat. The effect on cholesterol esterification may be a consequence of either weak ACAT inhibitory activity of the compound or reduced delivery of cholesterol to intestinal ACAT. However, SCH 48461 did not affect the appearance of newly synthesized cholesterol in the lymph, which suggests that the main effect is to prevent intestinal uptake of cholesterol and/or its delivery to intracellular processing enzymes.

Pancreatic cholesterol esterase has been implicated in the absorption of cholesterol. The uptake of radiolabel derived from cholesterol ^{14}C-oleate was not impaired by SCH 48461. Moreover, SCH 48461 did not inhibit the enzymatic activity of pancreatic cholesterol esterase in vitro, suggesting that inhibition of pancreatic cholesterol esterase is not the mechanism of action of SCH 48461.

In summary, SCH 48461 is a novel inhibitor of cholesterol absorption which prevents cholesterol and cholesteryl ester from appearing in the lymph and subsequently the plasma. The precise molecular mechanism of action remains to be defined.

References

1. Wilson MD, Rudel LL. J Lipid Res 1994;35:943–953.
2. Bhattacharyya AK, Eggan DA. J Lipid Res 1980;21:518–524.
3. Havel RJ, Eder HA, Bragdon JH. J Clin Invest 1955;34:1345–1353.
4. Burrier RE, Deren S, McGregor DG, Hoos LM, Smith AA, Davis HR. Biochem Pharmacol 1994;47:1545–1551.
5. Kyger EM, Riley DJS, Spilberg CA, Lang LG. Biochemistry 1990;29:3853–3858.
6. Camulli ED, Linke MJ, Brockman HL, Hui DY. Biochim Biophys Acta 1989;1005:177–182.

ACA-147: an inhibitor of ACAT and of the oxidative modification of LDL

Steven J. Adelman, Mar-Lee McKean, Dorothy H. Prozialeck, Donald E. Clark and William F. Fobare

Wyeth-Ayerst Research, C.N. 8000, Princeton, NJ 08543, USA

ACA-147 (5-[[[3,5-*bis*(1,1-dimethylethyl)-4-hydroxyphenyl]amino][[[4-(2,2-di-methylpropyl)phenyl]methyl]hexylamino]methylene]-2,2-di-methyl-1,3-dioxane-4,6-dione), a derivative of Meldrum's acid, was synthesized as an inhibitor of both acyl coenzyme A:cholesterol acyltransferase (ACAT) and of the oxidative modification of LDL. ACAT is an enzyme that has been shown to catalyze the esterification of cholesterol to a variety of fatty acyl CoAs, forming cholesteryl esters [1,2]. The activity of this enzyme is thought to play a role in development of atherosclerosis at three distinct tissue sites: intestine, liver, and cells of the diseased arterial wall such as macrophages. Numerous studies in animal models have demonstrated that ACAT is important for the absorption of dietary cholesterol, leading to the development of hypercholesterolemia [3–6]. Additional studies demonstrate that hepatic ACAT forms cholesteryl esters which are secreted in VLDL [7,8]. Finally, there is strong evidence that ACAT has a direct role in the esterification of cholesterol in cells of the arterial wall, leading to the deposition and accumulation of cholesteryl esters and consequently, formation of atherosclerotic foam cells [9–13]. Therefore, inhibition of ACAT, with all of its purported atherogenic activities, should slow and possibly reverse the development and progression of atherosclerosis directly by effects on arterial foam cells and indirectly by plasma lipid lowering.

A second mechanism reported to participate in atherogenesis is the process of oxidative modification of LDL. Oxidized LDL has been shown to occur in vivo and a number of its properties suggest that it plays a critical role in the development of atherosclerosis, including, through a variety of mechanisms, an induction of extensive cholesteryl ester deposition in atherosclerotic foam cells [14–17]. A number of studies suggest that cells of the arterial wall, including endothelial cells and macrophages, are responsible for the oxidation of LDL leading to its atherogenic activities [14,15,18]. In vitro, exposure of LDL to either Cu^{++} or to cultured cells derived from arterial tissue results in modification of LDL to a lipoprotein which mimics the modified LDL formed in vivo. Probucol (Lorelco®), a commonly prescribed drug used for the treatment of hyperlipidemia, atherosclerosis and coronary heart disease, is thought to exert its antiatherogenic activity, in part, through its ability to inhibit the oxidation of LDL [15].

In the present report, we summarize the effects of ACA-147 on ACAT activity in vitro, as well as its effects on the oxidative modification of LDL. Extending these in vitro observations, we report on the plasma lipid-modulating effects and vascular lesion effects of ACA-147 following oral administration to a wide variety of animal models including the rat, rabbit, dog, quail and cynomolgus monkey.

Results and Discussion

Effects of ACA-147 in in vitro models

ACA-147 was tested in vitro for its effects on ACAT activity and on the oxidative modification of LDL. In the ACAT studies, activity was assessed in rat liver microsomes and estimated in cultured cell lines derived from purported target tissues including the Fu5AH rat hepatoma, the Caco-2 human colon-adenocarcinoma, and the J774 mouse monocyte-macrophage. In these studies, ACA-147 was found to be a potent inhibitor of cholesterol esterification (ACAT). In the cellular assays, selectivity was demonstrated as ACA-147 had no effect on either triglyceride or phospholipid synthesis (Table 1).

The effect of ACA-147 on the oxidative modification of LDL was demonstrated by inhibition of TBARS formation. Hypercholesterolemic rabbit or human LDL were incubated with the compound and exposed to either $CuSO_4$, porcine aortic endothelial cells, CPA-47 bovine aortic endothelial cells or J774 mouse monocyte-macrophages. As shown in Table 2, ACA-147 was similar in potency to probucol in these assays. The inhibitory effects of ACA-147 on LDL modification were confirmed by both conjugated diene formation and changes in LDL electrophoretic mobility.

Effects of ACA-147 in animal models of hypercholesterolemia

In animal models, ACA-147 was found to be effective in reducing intestinal absorption of cholesterol, and to be a potent hypocholesterolemic agent in the presence of dietary-induced hypercholesterolemia. Lesion effects consistent with an antiatherosclerotic agent were also observed.

Inhibition of intestinal cholesterol absorption

In the rat, single oral doses of 1, 2 and 10 mg/kg ACA-147 administered by gavage to

Table 1. Effects of ACA-147 on lipid synthesis in vitro

	Lipid synthesis		
	Cholesteryl ester (IC_{50})[a]	Triglycerides (25 µM)	Phospholipids (25 µM)
Rat liver microsomes	19 nM	—	—
Fu5AH rat hepatoma	0.24 µM	No inhibition	No inhibition
Caco-2 human colon adenocarcinoma	0.24 µM	No inhibition	No inhibition
J774 mouse monocyte-macrophage	0.91 µM	Slight decrease at >5 µM	Slight increase at >5 µM

[a]IC_{50}s were calculated as the concentration which inhibited esterification to radiolabeled oleate by 50%.

Table 2. Effects of ACA-147 on oxidative modification of LDL in vitro

	ACA-147 (IC_{50})[a]	Probucol (IC_{50})[a]
$CuSO_4$-mediated	1.8 µM	0.8 µM
Porcine aortic endothelial cells	0.4 µM	0.2 µM
CPA-47 bovine aortic endothelial cell line	0.34 µM	
	100% at 10 µM	100% at 10 µM
J744 mouse macrophage-like cell line	0.21 µM	0.29 µM

[a]IC_{50}s were calculated as the concentration which reduced TBARS by 50%.

cholesterol-fed animals inhibited the absorption of an oral dose of radiolabeled cholesterol as measured by the appearance of radiolabeled cholesterol in plasma. At both 2 and 10 mg/kg, ACA-147 reduced the C_{max} for plasma radioactivity by 55% and decreased the $AUC_{(0-72\,h)}$ by 46%. ACA-147 at 1 mg/kg reduced the C_{max} by 48% and the $AUC_{(0-72\,h)}$ by 35%. The elimination half-life ($t_{1/2}$) of radiolabeled cholesterol was unchanged by ACA-147, indicating that the overall rate of utilization of circulating plasma cholesterol was unchanged.

Plasma lipid effects

As summarized in Table 3, ACA-147 was found to have potent effects on plasma lipids in a wide variety of species. In Sprague-Dawley rats, oral administration of ACA-147 to male, cholesterol/cholic acid-fed animals produced a dose-dependent inhibition in the development of hypercholesterolemia. ACA-147 completely prevented elevations in plasma total cholesterol (ED_{50} = 0.37 mg/kg, either q.i.d. or b.i.d.) and LDL + VLDL cholesterol (ED_{50} = 0.56 mg/kg) which are induced by the cholesterol-containing diet. A significant elevation in HDL-cholesterol was also observed at doses above 2 mg/kg. Similar activity was demonstrated in animals exposed to the hypercholesterolemic diet for 4 days prior to a single dose of ACA-147.

Orally administered ACA-147 was also found to have potent hypocholesterolemic activity when administered in capsules to male beagle dogs. At doses of 1, 5 and 20 mg/kg/day, postoperatively, ACA-147 prevented by up to 75% the diet-induced hypercholesterolemia in a 3-week study. Cholestyramine, a hypocholesterolemic standard, also reduced the elevation in plasma total cholesterol by up to 50%, but at a dose of 3% of diet (slightly less than 1,000 mg/kg/day). In intervention studies in which ACA-147 (1, 5 or 20 mg/kg/day, postoperatively) was administered to dogs for 2 weeks subsequent to diet-induced elevation of plasma lipids to a stable plateau, plasma total cholesterol was reduced by up to 40% and LDL + VLDL cholesterol by up to 56%.

In cholesterol-fed nonhuman primates (cynomolgus monkeys), oral ACA-147 at 3, 10, 30 or 100 mg/kg/day administered for 8 weeks inhibited the elevation of plasma total cholesterol and LDL + VLDL cholesterol induced by a cholesterol-containing diet. This diet was designed to mimic the average North American human diet, and contained 0.2% cholesterol and 36% fat, 41% of which was saturated fat. There was no dose–response relationship observed at these doses, suggesting that maximal efficacy was achieved at levels down to 3 mg/kg/day. At baseline, total plasma cholesterol levels were 130 mg/dl. After 8 weeks on diet, animals on vehicle alone had plasma total cholesterol levels of 390 mg/dl. On average, ACA-147 administration prevented 75% of the increase above baseline induced by the diet, with plasma total cholesterol of animals of all treated groups averaging 190 mg/dl after 8 weeks of treatment. Thus treated animals had plasma total

Table 3. $ED_{50}s^a$ for reduction of plasma lipids by ACA-147

	Cholesterol			Triglycerides
	Total ED_{50}	LDL + VLDL ED_{50}	HDL	
Rat (prevention and intervention)	0.4 mg/kg	0.5 mg/kg	Elevates	No effect
Dog (prevention and intervention)	1.0 mg/kg	1.0 mg/kg	Elevates	No effect
Monkey (prevention)	<3 mg/kg	<3 mg/kg	Elevates	No effect

$^a ED_{50}s$ were calculated as the dose of compound which gave 50% of the hypocholesterolemic activity.

cholesterol levels approximately 50% lower than vehicle-treated controls. The effect on LDL + VLDL cholesterol was more pronounced, with ACA-147 eliminating approximately 80–90% of the elevation induced by diet, and therefore, treated animals had LDL + VLDL cholesterol levels that averaged 75% lower than controls. ACA-147 also induced a more than 2-fold elevation in HDL-cholesterol. There was no significant effect of the drug on triglyceride levels.

In an intervention study in cynomolgus monkeys, where animals were exposed to the cholesterol-enriched diet for 20 weeks prior to drug administration, ACA-147 was effective over a 24-week treatment period in reducing both plasma total cholesterol and LDL + VLDL cholesterol at doses as low as 3 mg/kg. FPLC analysis demonstrated that approximately 95% of the cholesterol in the LDL + VLDL fraction was in the LDL fraction, and therefore, the primary effect was due to a reduction in LDL-cholesterol.

Aortic atherosclerosis effects
In male rabbits fed a moderately hyperlipidemic diet (0.2% cholesterol, 5% corn oil), ACA-147 admixed in the diet dose-dependently prevented the elevation of plasma total cholesterol and LDL + VLDL cholesterol. After 20 weeks, rabbits fed the hypercholesterolemic diet combined with 0.5% ACA-147 had plasma total cholesterol levels that were 85% lower than controls fed diet without drug; those fed diet combined with 0.1% ACA-147 were 50% lower (Table 4). Similar changes were observed in the LDL + VLDL cholesterol fraction. Probucol (1.0%), a hypocholesterolemic, antiatherosclerotic drug thought to affect lesion development through its antioxidant effects, lowered plasma total cholesterol and LDL + VLDL cholesterol by 30%. As in man, probucol also significantly reduced HDL-cholesterol. In contrast, there was no reduction in HDL by ACA-147, but a significant elevation at the higher dose (0.5%). In this study, a reduction of triglycerides was noted. Additionally, there were no effects of ACA-147 or probucol on fecal lipid excretion (steatorrhea) or on plasma vitamin A levels.

In this same study, ACA-147 substantially decreased the development of aortic atherosclerosis, as defined by percent of aortic surface area stained by Sudan IV. Aortic atherosclerosis was reduced from approximately 60% involvement in cholesterol-fed control animals to < 2.0% in rabbits fed the same cholesterol-containing diet supplemented with ACA-147 at 0.5% (Table 5). Dose dependency was observed as rabbits supplemented with 0.1% ACA-147 had lesions covering 21% of the vessel. Probucol at 1.0% of the diet was also effective in reducing aortic atherosclerosis; only 23% of the vessel was covered. Aortic cholesterol and cholesteryl ester changes were consistent with these observations.

Table 4. Effects of compounds on plasma lipids in cholesterol-fed rabbits

	Probucol	ACA-147	
	1.0%[a]	0.1%[a], p.o.	0.5%[a], p.o.
Plasma total chol.	–34%[b]	–48%[b]	–82%[b]
VLDL + LDL	–33%[b]	–45%[b]	–86%[b]
HDL	–45%[b]	–4%	+32%[b]
Triglycerides	–29%[b]	–19%[b]	–35%[b]
Fecal lipid	No effect	No effect	No effect
Plasma vitamin A	No effect	No effect	No effect

[a]Drug administered as percentage of diet; [b]significantly different from control at $p < 0.05$.

320

Table 5. Percentage area of rabbit aorta covered with atherosclerotic lesion

	Control	Probucol	ACA-147	
		1.0%[a], p.o.	0.1%[a], p.o.	0.5%[a], p.o.
Aortic arch	78%	45%[b]	30%[b]	2%[b]
Thoracic aorta	59%	16%[b]	20%[b]	0.4%[b]
Abdominal aorta	42%	14%[b]	16%[b]	2%[b]
Total aorta	60%	23%[b]	21%[b]	1%[b]

[a]Drug administered as percentage of diet; [b]significantly different from control at $p < 0.05$.

In the final series of studies, ACA-147 administration to male Japanese quail susceptible to experimental atherosclerosis (SEA) inhibited the development of aortic atherosclerosis. In contrast to the lowering of plasma total cholesterol and LDL + VLDL cholesterol demonstrated in the various mammalian species described above, ACA-147 had no statistically significant effect on plasma lipid levels in the quail. Despite this lack of effect on lipid levels, Japanese quail treated with ACA-147 at 34 mg/kg/day had aortic lesions that were approximately 50% that of the vehicle-treated controls.

The results presented here demonstrate the in vitro activities and the lipid-modulating and antiatherosclerotic efficacy of ACA-147 in a wide variety of animal models (rats, dogs, monkeys, rabbits and Japanese quail).

References

1. Spector AA, Mauthur SN, Kaduce TL. Prog Lipid Res 1979;18:31–54.
2. Billheimer JT. Methods Enzymol 1985;111:286–293.
3. Helgerud P, Saarem K, Norum KR. J Lipid Res 1981;22:271–277.
4. Bennett-Clark S, Tercyak AM. J Lipid Res 1984;25:148–159.
5. Heider JG, Pickens CE, Kelly LA. J Lipid Res 1985;24:1127–1134.
6. Largis EE, Wang CH, DeVries VG, Schaffer SA. J Lipid Res 1989;30:681–690.
7. Cianflone K, Yasruel Z, Rodriguez M, Vas D, Sniderman A. J Lipid Res 1990;31:2045–2055.
8. Carr T, Parks J, Rudel L. Arterioscler Thromb 1992;12:1274–1283.
9. St. Clair RW. Ann NY Acad Sci 1976;275:228–237.
10. Brecher PI, Chobanian AV. Circ Res 1974;35:692–701.
11. Hashimoto S, Dayton S, Alfin-Slater RB, Bui PT, Baker N, Wilson L. Circ Res 1974;34:176–183.
12. Brown MS, Ho YK, Goldstein JL. J Biol Chem 1980;255:9344–9352.
13. Bell FP. Exp Mol Pathol 1983;38:336–345.
14. Steinberg D, Parthasarathy S, Carew T, Khoo J, Witztum J. N Engl J Med 1989;320:915–924.
15. Steinberg D, Carew T, Fielding C, Fogelman AM, Mahley RW, Sniderman AD, Zilversmit DB. Circulation 1989;80:719–723.
16. Carew T. Am J Cardiol 1989;64:18G–22G.
17. Steinbrecher U, Zhang H, Lougheed M. Free Radicals Biol Med 1990;9:155–168.
18. Parthasarathy S, Quinn M, Schwenke D, Carew T, Steinberg D. Arteriosclerosis 1989;9:398–404.

CGS 26214, the thyroxine connection revisited

R.E. Steele, J.M. Wasvary, B.N. Dardik, C.D. Schwartzkopf, R. Sharif, K.S. Leonards, C.W. Hu, E.C. Yurachek and Z.F. Stephan

Research Department, Pharmaceuticals Division, Ciba-Geigy Corporation, 556 Morris Avenue, Summit, NJ 07901, USA

Abstract. CGS 26214, a thyromimetic substance devoid of cardiovascular effects in rats and dogs, binds to rat liver nuclear L-T_3 receptors with an IC_{50} of 0.1 nM vs. 0.6 nM for L-T_3, and lowered serum cholesterol in hypercholesterolemic rats at 1 µg/kg vs. 25 µg/kg for L-T_3. In normocholesterolemic dogs and monkeys, CGS 26214 lowered LDL-cholesterol by 59 and 20%, respectively at 1 µg/kg p.o. CGS 26214 decreased Lp(a) by 42% in cynomolgus monkeys at 30 µg/kg p.o., and enhanced postprandial triglyceride clearance in rats. The cardiac-sparing activity is attributed to preferential uptake into hepatocyte nuclei vs. cardiac nuclei of intact cells.

The hypocholesterolemic effect of thyroid hormone (L-T_4, L-T_3) has been well documented in humans and laboratory animals, in which it produces an upregulation of LDL receptors and a marked lowering of LDL-cholesterol [1,2]. However, excessive myocardial activity associated with thyroid hormone and other synthetic thyromimetic agents has limited their use as hypolipidemics. The myocardial activities represent both direct effects on the myocardium and indirect effects associated with the elevations in basal metabolic rate which, by enhancing peripheral tissue oxygen demand, increase the cardiac workload [3]. The high-affinity, low-capacity nuclear receptors for thyroid hormone are believed to be responsible for the initiation of virtually all of the well-documented effects characteristic of thyroid hormone [4]. Thus, if the access of a thyromimetic was largely limited to the liver nuclei (the site of its hypolipidemic effects) and access to the nuclei of cardiac and other tissues was reduced or eliminated, a cardiac-sparing hypolipidemic agent should result. As a preliminary test of this hypothesis we conjugated L-T_3 to cholic acid to produce a liver-targeted compound (CGH 509A). Bile acid conjugation of drugs has previously been used to produce liver-specific drugs [5]. It was noted that while L-T_3 was equally potent at lowering cholesterol in hypercholesterolemic rats and in eliciting cardiovascular (CV) and thyroxine-suppressing effects in normocholesterolemic, euthyroid rats, the cholesterol-lowering effect of CGH 509A was at least 15 and 6 times greater than its CV and thyroxine-suppressing potencies, respectively [6].

CGS 26214 was identified as a cardiac-sparing, lipid-lowering thyromimetic by first identifying its potential thyromimetic activity by means of an in vitro competitive binding assay which uses [^{125}I]L-T_3 and intact rat liver nuclei [6]. The CV properties of CGS 26214 were compared to those of L-T_3 by treating chow-fed, euthyroid rats with various doses of each compound for 7 days, removing and weighing the heart, and measuring in vitro the spontaneous contraction rate of the right atrium and the maximal developed contractile force of the isolated left atrium [6]. In the assay of competitive binding to

Address for correspondence: R.E. Steele, Research Department, Pharmaceuticals Division, Ciba-Geigy Corporation, 556 Morris Avenue, Summit, NJ 07901, USA.

Table 1. Cardiovascular effects of L-T$_3$ and CGS 26214 in rats

	Change from control	
	L-T$_3$ (100 µg/kg)	CGS 26214 (25 mg/kg)
Heart weight (% body weight)	+47%[a]	–3%
Atrial rate (beats/min)	+38%[a]	+2%
Atrial tension	+44%[a]	–3%

[a]$p < 0.05$.

isolated liver nuclei, CGS 26214 was 6 times as potent as L-T$_3$; i.e., the concentration of CGS 26214 which competitively inhibited [^{125}I]L-T$_3$ by 50% (IC$_{50}$) was 0.10 nM, vs. 0.61 nM for L-T$_3$. While L-T$_3$ significantly stimulated heart weight (+47%), atrial rate (+38%), and atrial tension (44%) when given orally at a daily dose of 100 µg/kg, CGS 26214 had no significant effect on any of these parameters at oral doses as high as 25,000 µg/kg (Table 1).

CGS 26214 had no CV effects in the normal rat, but when given to rats made hyper-cholesterolemic by feeding a 1.5% cholesterol, 0.5% cholic acid-modified rat chow diet, CGS 26214 lowered plasma LDL-cholesterol by 35% at a dose of 1 µg/kg and by 50% at 3 µg/kg. A dose 33 times as great was needed for L-T$_3$ to produce similar lipid lowering.

Lipid-lowering and CV studies were also performed in conscious normal chow-fed dogs. Normal chow-fed mixed-breed dogs were fitted with indwelling probes for measuring hemodynamic parameters, and trained to lie on the laboratory table while recordings were made. Recordings were made before and after 7 days of oral treatment with either 100 µg/kg of CGS 26214 or 300 µg/kg L-T$_3$. At these doses L-T$_3$ significantly increased heart rate, cardiac output, force of contraction (dP/dT), and whole body oxygen consumption (Table 2). None of these CV parameters was significantly affected by CGS 26214. CGS 26214 administered daily to normal chow-fed dogs bled before and 7 days after treatment at various doses significantly lowered plasma LDL in a dose-dependent fashion, with 59% reduction at the lowest dose (1 µg/kg) tested.

To determine the mechanism responsible for the dissociation of lipid-lowering from CV effects, we performed cell-free competitive binding studies on rat heart myocyte nuclei isolated nonenzymatically [7]. There was no significant difference between the binding affinity of CGS 26214 for isolated liver nuclei and that for cardiac nuclei to

Table 2. Cardiovascular effects of L-T$_3$ and CGS 26214 in dogs

	Change from baseline	
	L-T$_3$ (300 µg/kg)	CGS 26214 (100 µg/kg)
Heart rate (beats/min)	+53%[a]	+15%
Cardiac output (l/min)	+63%[a]	+19%
Mean arterial pressure (mmHg)	+6%	–5%
dp/dt (mmHg/sec)	+275%[a]	not determined
Whole-body oxygen consumption (ml/min)	+47%[a]	+8%

[a]$p < 0.05$.

Table 3. Competitive binding studies and cellular uptake studies with L-T₃ and CGS 26214

Preparation	IC₅₀ (nM)[a]	
	L-T₃	CGS 26214
Rat liver nuclei	0.61 ± 0.22	0.10 ± 0.02
Rat cardiac myocyte nuclei	0.41 ± 0.10	0.18 ± 0.03[b]
Whole cell nuclear binding HepG2	0.2–0.3	0.1–0.2
Whole cell nuclear binding rat cardiocyte	0.2–0.3	30–40[b]
	Total cellular uptake	
Intact HepG2	62 ± 5	7 ± 2[b]
Intact fetal rat cardiocyte	64 ± 4	14 ± 1[b]

[a]Concentration which inhibited nuclear occupancy by [125I]L-T₃ by 50%.
[b]Difference from L-T₃, $p < 0.05$.

which, as with the liver nuclei, CGS 26214 bound more avidly than L-T₃ (Table 3). Underwood et al. [8] have previously shown that the cardiac-sparing, lipid-lowering thyromimetic SK&F L-94901 bound equally to isolated heart and liver nuclei, but when administered in vivo bound more abundantly to liver nuclei than to cardiac nuclei. Therefore, we incubated CGS 26214 and L-T₃ with [125I]L-T₃ and performed competitive binding studies with intact cells, using human HepG2 cells and fetal rat cardiac myocytes prepared as described by Janero et al. [9]. After the incubation the nuclei were isolated and their [125I]L-T₃ occupancy was determined. As with isolated rat cardiac and rat liver nuclei, L-T₃ bound equally to nuclei from liver and heart (Table 3). However, while CGS 26214 binding to the HepG2 nuclei in intact cells was similar to its binding to isolated rat liver nuclei, its binding to fetal rat myocyte nuclei of intact cells was markedly less than its binding to isolated rat myocyte nuclei (Table 3). These results suggested that the cardiac-sparing property of CGS 26214 was related to impeded access to intact cardiac myocyte nuclei. To determine whether this lack of access was a consequence of a lower uptake of CGS 26214 into rat fetal cardiac cells in culture than into HepG2 cells we incubated [14C]CGS 26214 or [125I]L-T₃ with fetal rat cardiac cells and HepG2 cells and measured the whole cell radioactivity. Less [14C]CGS 26214 than [125I]L-T₃ was taken up by either the HepG2 or fetal rat cardiocyte, and (in contrast to what might be expected) more [14C]CGS 26214 per mg protein was taken up by cardiocytes than by HepG2 cells (Table 3). Thus the greater effect on the hepatocyte than on the cardiocyte is due to differences not in cellular uptake but in cytoplasmic transport to the nuclei.

Normal chow-fed cynomolgus monkeys treated with CGS 26214 orally for 5 days showed a statistically significant reduction (–23%) in their LDL-cholesterol (Table 4). In a subsequent study CGS 26214 (30 µg/kg) was given to chow-fed monkeys for 7 days. Plasma samples were obtained before and after the drug treatment and assayed simultaneously for Lp(a) by ELISA, using an anti-apoA capture antibody and an anti-apoB detecting antibody. CGS 26214 significantly lowered Lp(a) by 43%. This finding is consistent with human studies [10,11] in which thyroid hormone replacement therapy to hypothyroid individuals and inhibition of thyroid hormone secretion in hyperthyroid individuals lowered and increased Lp(a), respectively, as patients became euthyroid.

Both human [12] and rat [13] studies suggest that thyroid hormone promotes the clearance of non-chylomicron triglycerides after a fat load. To determine whether CGS 26214 exerted a similar effect, hypercholesterolemic euthyroid rats maintained for 2 weeks

324

Table 4. Hypolipidemic effects of CGS 26214 (5 days orally) in cynomolgus monkeys

Dose (µg/kg)	Parameter	Before (mg/dl)	After (mg/dl)	Mean % change
1	LDL	95 ± 12^a	74 ± 14	-23^b
30	Lp(a)	$4.5-25^c$	$1.4-12.3$	-43^b

^{a}Mean ± SEM; ^{b}p < 0.05; ^{c}Range.

on a modified rat chow diet containing 1.5% cholesterol and 0.5% cholic acid were treated for 7 days with either vehicle or CGS 26214 (10 µg/kg), after which they were fasted for 18 h and then administered an oral fat load consisting of 320 mg of corn oil and 430 mg of sucrose. Blood was collected at 0, 2, 4, 8 and 24 h after the fat load. Plasma triglycerides returned to preloading values within 4–8 h in the CGS 26214-treated rats whereas this took 24 h in the controls.

These data demonstrate a clear dissociation between the marked lipid lowering by CGS 26214 and its total lack of CV and basal metabolic effects. While the mechanism(s) responsible for this separation of activities is not apparent, it is clearly not attributable to differences between hepatocyte and cardiocyte in the nature of the L-T_3 nuclear receptors or in their cellular uptake. The potent LDL- and Lp(a)-lowering activities of CGS 26214, together with the drug's beneficial effects on postprandial lipid clearance, provide an attractive lipid-lowering profile.

Acknowledgements

We thank Ms C. Laspina for secretarial assistance.

References

1. Thompson GR, Soutar AK, Spengel FA, Jadhav A, Gavigan SJP, Myant, NB. Proc Natl Acad Sci USA 1981;78:2591–2595.
2. Salter AM, Hayashi R, Al-Seeni M, Brown NF, Bruce J, Sorenson O, Atkinson EA, Middleton B, Bleackley RC, Brindley DN. Biochem J 1991;276:825–832.
3. Polikar R, Burger AG, Scherrer U, Nicod P. Circulation 1993;87:1435–1441.
4. Oppenheimer JH, Schwartz HL, Mariash CN, Kinlaw WB, Wong NCW, Freake HC. Endocrinol Rev 1987; 8:288–308.
5. Kramer W, Wess G, Schubert G, Bickel M, Girbig F, Gutjahr U, Kowalewski S, Baringhaus KH, Enhsen A, Glombik H, Mullner S, Neckermann G, Schulz S, Petzinger E. J Biol Chem 1992;267:18598–18604.
6. Stephan ZF, Yurachek EC, Sharif R, Wasvary JM, Steele RE, Howes C. Biochem Pharmacol 1992;43: 1969–1974.
7. Jackowski G, Liew CC. Biochem J 1980;188:363–373.
8. Underwood AH, Emmett JC, Ellis D, Flynn SB, Leeson PD, Benson GM, Novelli R, Pearce NJ, Shah VP. Nature 1986;324:425–429.
9. Janero DR, Burghardt D, Feldman D. J Cell Physiol 1988;137:1–13.
10. de Bruin TWA, van Barlingen H, van Lindesibenius Trip M, van Vuurst de Vries ARR, Akveld MJ, Erkelens DW. J Clin Endocrinol Metab 1993;76:121–126.
11. Engler H, Riesen WF. Clin Chem 1993;39:2466–2469.
12. Abrams JJ, Grundy SM, Ginsberg H. J Lipid Res 1981;22:307–322.
13. Zerbinatti CV, Oliveira HCF, Wechesler S, Quintao ECR. Metabolism 1991;40:1122–1127.

Atherosclerosis X.
F.P. Woodford, J. Davignon and A. Sniderman, editors.

Fibrates and the concept of fraudulent fatty acids

Guido Franceschini and Cesare R. Sirtori
Center E. Grossi Paoletti, Institute of Pharmacological Sciences, University of Milano, via Balzaretti 9, 20133 Milan, Italy

Fatty acids are generally considered as components of energy-supplying foods, but fatty acids also exert pharmacological effects distinct from their caloric contribution to total energy metabolism. Indeed, a number of fatty acid molecules have been proposed for the prevention of diseases and/or for the treatment of specific syndromes. Dietary fatty acids, in particular, may influence the onset and progression of various disease conditions, including atherosclerosis, diabetes and certain types of cancer, by acting at two levels: a) changing the fatty acid composition of membrane phospholipids [1]; and b) directly controlling nuclear events responsible for gene transcription [2]. Thus, a number of cellular functions, including the activity of membrane-bound enzymes and transporters, hormone-binding and signal-transduction mechanisms, may be dependent upon the type of fatty acids in the diet.

A series of synthetic fatty acids have gained an established role in lipid-lowering therapy and atherosclerosis prevention. They are the so-called fibrates or fibric acids, characterized by a common aryloxyisobutyric acid structure, with different substituents on the aromatic ring [3]. Gemfibrozil differs slightly from other fibrates (bezafibrate, ciprofibrate, clofibrate, fenofibrate) in the insertion of three carbons between the isobutyric and the aryloxy moieties. These compounds have well-documented effects on plasma lipids/lipoproteins and hemostatic factors [3]. This pattern of activity is, to some extent, reminiscent of that of n-3 fatty acids, with, however, a more potent and sustained action.

Fibrates, unsaturated fatty acids and other similar compounds: members of the same general family of compounds?

The possibility that different fatty acids, both synthetic and natural, may exert their activities through a common hepatic regulatory pathway has been suggested by the identification of a family of ligand-dependent transcription factors recognizing both fibrates and a number of simpler fatty acids, down to trichloroacetic acid [4]. These factors, named 'peroxisome proliferator-activated receptors' (PPARs), are 'orphan receptors' belonging to the steroid and vitamin nuclear-receptor superfamily [5]. Like other steroid/vitamin receptors, ligand binding to PPAR causes the dissociation of a heat-shock protein (hsp72) from the nascent receptor and converts the receptor into an allosteric form capable of dimerizing with the 9-*cis* retinoic acid receptor (RXR) [6] and of binding to DNA at specific response elements (peroxisome proliferator response elements, PPRE) located at the 5′ end of target genes. The receptor then recruits and stabilizes general transcription factors at target gene promoters and modulates the transcription at the adjacent gene (Fig. 1). Since PPRE sequences have been identified in the 5′ flanking regions of several genes, including those coding for acyl-CoA oxidase, hydratase/dehydrogenase, fatty acid-binding protein and Cyt P450IVA6 [7], fatty acids could modulate the expression of many different genes, thus exerting multiple pleiotropic effects, through PPAR binding and activation. The PPARs are highly expressed in the

326

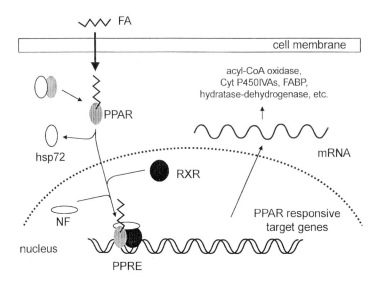

Fig. 1. Hypothetical mechanism by which natural and 'fraudulent' fatty acids (FA) govern gene transcription. PPAR, peroxisome proliferator-activated receptor; hsp72, heat shock protein 72; RXR, retinoid X receptor; NF, nuclear transcription factors; PPRE, peroxisome proliferator response element.

liver, kidney, heart and adipose tissue, very weakly in brain and testis.

The physiological role of PPARs is unknown. The induction of the peroxisomal fatty acid β-oxidation system does, however, indicate a role for the receptor in providing a source of energy via fatty acids. Additional possibilities include the regulation of peroxisomal function or cholesterol metabolism, for example by increasing cholesterol biosynthesis and/or the conversion of cholesterol into bile acids, both occurring mainly in the peroxisomes [8].

The recognition of the PPAR and of the apparently similar ligand properties of fibrates vs. dietary unsaturated fatty acids led to the hypothesis that possibly a wide range of molecules may activate a regulatory pathway in the liver and other tissues, resulting in enhanced fatty acid catabolism. These molecules, tentatively named 'fraudulent fatty acids' [9] in analogy to the 'fraudulent' nucleosides used in cancer therapy, share similar chemical properties. They are characterized by a hydrophobic backbone and by the frequent presence of carboxylic-acid functional groups that can be activated to their CoA esters. In addition to fibrates, a variety of compounds may act as fraudulent fatty acids. Among these are MEDICA 16, a synthetic fatty acid with numerous substituents, indicated as a potential treatment for the polymetabolic syndrome, and thia-substituted fatty acids with powerful triglyceride- and cholesterol-lowering activities [9]. The most widely used fraudulent fatty acids are those derived from fish oil, which share many of the pharmacodynamic properties of fibrates.

Pharmacological properties of fraudulent fatty acids and the mechanism of action of fibrates

The activation of the PPAR by fraudulent fatty acids is followed by a cascade of events now well described in in vitro and in vivo systems. Almost immediately after PPAR activation a dramatic increase in fatty acid metabolism occurs in liver microsomes, through ω-hydroxylation by the Cyt P450IVA system. Both Cyt P450IVA protein and mRNA contents in rat liver increase 10- to 40-fold after induction with fibrates [10]. Cyt P450IVAs exhibit a high preference for hydroxylation at the terminal (ω) methyl group over the internal (ω-n) methylene groups [9]. Proliferation of peroxisomes occurs at approximately the same time in rodent liver, thus leaving some doubts on the exact sequence of events [9]. Figure 2 proposes a scheme suggesting that microsomal activation might be the early event. Following this, enhanced ω-hydroxylation may lead to the formation of peroxidative products, in turn activating peroxisomes in rodents, and mitochondrial enzymes in man. The opposite route, i.e., an early activation of peroxisomes, followed by enhanced microsomal ω-hydroxylation is also a well-founded alternative. Species-specific variability in the biochemical responses may also occur; in certain animal models, the microsomal fatty acid elongation system is affected despite a lack of change in peroxisomal β-oxidation/proliferation [11]. The continuing characterization of the promoter regions of human and animal peroxisomal β-oxidation genes [12] will provide an essential contribution to our understanding of the regulation of these processes by fraudulent fatty acids and in extrapolating their mode of action to humans.

Possible changes of liver peroxisomes in man following the administration of fraudulent fatty acids are controversial [13]. On the other hand, there is clear evidence that 'peroxisomal diseases' do occur. In these conditions, long-chain unsaturated fatty acids are retained in different tissues, leading to neurodegenerative disorders [14]. It is certainly

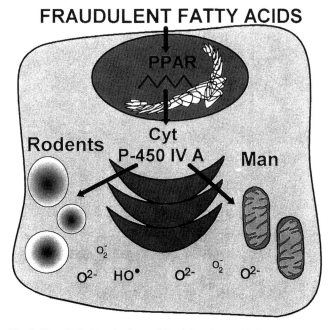

Fig. 2. Hypothetical mechanisms of fraudulent fatty acids in modulating cellular fatty acid metabolism. These molecules interact with PPAR, in turn activating Cyt P450IAs. These cytochromes are directly responsible for the ω-hydroxylation of fatty acids, leading, through as yet unclear mechanisms (formation of peroxidative products?) to enhanced mitochondrial β-oxidation (in man) or peroxisomal β-oxidation (in rodents). Contrasting views explain the mechanism of fraudulent fatty acids by postulating: 1) an initial effect on peroxisomes, followed by the activation of the Cyt P450IVA system; or 2) the direct activation of Cyt P450IVA followed by PPAR recognition of the dicarboxylic acids produced [9].

328

possible that peroxisomal diseases may be secondary to an inefficient activity of PPAR, leading, as a consequence, to a deficient catabolism of very-long-chain fatty acids. Best known and most frequent among peroxisomal diseases is the X-linked adrenoleuko-dystrophy; in this condition, the administration of a mixture of oleic acid (18:1 n-9) and erucic acid (22:1 n-9), widely known as 'Lorenzo's Oil', seemed to lead to some clinical benefit [15].

Most of these findings would point to a predominant mechanism of fraudulent fatty acids in the activation of PPAR, resulting in the stimulation of fatty acid catabolism; through this molecular mechanism, a number of fatty acids, natural or man-made, can exert potentially healthful effects in experimental animals and in man. In the liver, triglyceride synthesis would decrease, with a reduced secretion of very low density lipoproteins (VLDL). In the adipose tissue, the reduction in the cellular content of fatty acids would increase the expression of the lipoprotein lipase (LPL) gene [16], whereas the enhanced uptake of fatty acids would prevent product inhibition of the LPL on the endothelial surface [17]. The final result is an accelerated catabolism of triglyceride-rich lipoproteins (VLDL and chylomicrons) and low plasma triglyceride levels. The concentration of high density lipoproteins (HDL) should increase, either because of the metabolic interrelationship between lipoproteins, or because of a direct effect of fraudulent fatty acids on the expression of apolipoprotein genes or of genes coding for enzymatic determinants of plasma HDL levels (lecithin:cholesterol acyltransferase, cholesteryl ester transfer protein, lipases) [18,19]. Finally, by modulating the recently described fatty acid-activated pathway for low density lipoprotein (LDL) degradation [20], fraudulent fatty acids could lower plasma LDL levels, independent of the classical LDL-receptor pathway.

Indeed, experimental and clinical studies with fibrates and/or n-3 fatty acids have shown a marked triglyceride-lowering effect, consequent on a reduced triglyceride synthesis in the liver and/or to a stimulation of lipase-mediated VLDL chylomicron catabolism [4]. Plasma LDL levels are generally reduced [1,21], except in patients with severe hypertriglyceridemia, by a mechanism independent of HMG-CoA inhibition or LDL-receptor overexpression [21], whereas the concentration of HDL, and in particular of small and dense HDL_3 particles, increases [3]. Other potential consequences, with a less clear relationship with the molecular mechanism suggested above, may be that of reduced fibrinogenemia, decreased platelet aggregability, and activated fibrinolysis [9].

The relatively low ligand specificity of PPAR [4] may allow the recognition of a large number of molecules; at present, probably the major questions are the affinities of the different fraudulent fatty acids for PPAR [5], the relative duration of effects and, most important, the exact nature of the agonist molecule. It is likely that fibrates vs. e.g., n-3 fatty acids, in addition to possessing a higher affinity, may effect more prolonged activation [9], thus leading to a more sustained lipid-lowering activity. New knowledge on the fraudulent fatty acid concept opens up new pathways for the understanding of lipid regulation in man. Activation of the PPAR system might be an ancestral mechanism, allowing the body to dispose of excess fat in different conditions. In addition, fraudulent fatty acids and 9-cis retinoic acid appear to share a signaling pathway that might explain the lipid-modulating effect of vitamin A. Of course, as indicated above, the effects of fraudulent fatty acids on peroxisomal proliferation and/or activation of mitochondrial metabolism might differ among species; in rodents, peroxisomal proliferation may, in special conditions, also be associated with the development of liver tumors [22]. Peroxisomes are essential for the biosynthesis of cholesterol [8] and possibly of other fundamental products of mevalonate metabolism, including prenylated proteins, thus possibly explaining the association between peroxisome proliferation and carcinogenesis.

The understanding of these mechanisms may lead to the design of low-risk molecules with more specific activities on e.g., cholesterol, fibrinogen and the like, and would eliminate the still widely held concept that fibrates are drugs with an 'unclear mode of action'.

References

1. Sirtori CR, Gatti E, Tremoli E, Galli C, Gianfranceschi G, Franceschini G, Colli S, Maderna P, Marangoni F, Perego P, Stragliotto E. Am J Clin Nutr 1992;56:113–122.
2. Clarke SD, Jump DB. Prog Lipid Res 1993;32:139–149.
3. Sirtori CR, Franceschini G. Pharmacol Ther 1988;37:167–191.
4. Gottlicher M, Widmark E, Li Q, Gustafsson J-A. Proc Natl Acad Sci USA 1992;89:4653–4657.
5. Sher T, Yi H-F, McBride OW, Gonzales FJ. Biochemistry 1993;32:5598–5604.
6. Keller H, Dreyer C, Medin J, Mahfoudi A, Ozato K, Wahli W. Proc Natl Acad Sci USA 1993;90:2160–2164.
7. Muerhoff AS, Griffin KJ, Johnson EF. J Biol Chem 1992;267:19051–19053.
8. Biardi L, Sreedhar A, Zokaei A, Vartak NB, Bozeat RL, Shackelford JE, Keller G-A, Krisans SK. J Biol Chem 1994;269:1197–1205.
9. Sirtori CR, Galli C, Franceschini G. Eur J Clin Invest 1993;23:686–689.
10. Sundseth SS, Waxman DJ. J Biol Chem 1992;267:3915–3921.
11. Vázquez M, Alegret M, Adzet T, Merlos M, Laguna JC. Biochem Pharmacol 1993;46:1515–1518.
12. Varanasi U, Chu R, Chu S, Espinosa R, LeBeau MM, Reddy JK. Proc Natl Acad Sci USA 1994;91:3107–3111.
13. Gariot P, Barrat E, Drouin P, Genton JP, Foliguet B, Kolopp M, Debry G. Metabolism 1987;36:203–210.
14. Mose HV, Begin A, Cornblath D. Biochem Cell Biol 1991;69:463–474.
15. Rizzo WB, Leshner RT, Odone A. Neurology 1989;30:1415–1422.
16. Kirkland JL, Hollenberg CH, Kindler S, Roncari DAK. Metabolism 1994;43:144–151.
17. Saxena U, Witte LD, Goldberg IJ. J Biol Chem 1989;264:4349–4355.
18. Hahn SE, Goldberg DM. Biochem Pharmacol 1992;43:625–633.
19. Staels B, van Tol A, Andreu T, Auwerx J. Arterioscl Thromb 1992;12:286–294.
20. Yen FT, Mann CJ, Guermani LM, Hannouche NF, Hubert N, Hornick CA, Bordeau VN, Agnani G, Bihain BE. Biochemistry 1994;33:1172–1180.
21. Franceschini G, Lovati MR, Manzoni C, Michelagnoli S, Pazzucconi F, Gianfranceschi G, Vecchio G, Sirtori CR. Atherosclerosis (in press).
22. Reddy JK, Azarnoff DL, Hignite CE. Nature 1980;283:397–398.

330

Probucol and the PQRST (Probucol Quantitative Regression Swedish Trial): a look back and a look ahead

Göran Walldius[1], Uno Erikson[2], Lott Bergstrand[2], Sven Nilsson[2], Jan Johansson[1,3], Jan Regnström[1], Jan Nilsson[1], Liselotte Schäfer Elinder[1], Karin Hådell[4], Lennart Kaijser[5], Jörgen Mölgaard[6], Claes Lassvik[7], Göran Stenport[8], Ingar Holme[9] and Anders G. Olsson[6]

[1]Department of Internal Medicine, Karolinska Hospital and King Gustaf V Research Institute, Stockholm; [2]Department of Diagnostic Radiology, University Hospital, Uppsala; [3]Centre of General Medicine, North West Health Board, Karolinska Hospital, Stockholm; [4]Department of Dietetics, Karolinska Hospital, Stockholm; [5]Department of Clinical Physiology, Huddinge Hospital, Huddinge; [6]Department of Internal Medicine, Faculty of Health Sciences, Linköping; [7]Department of Clinical Physiology, Faculty of Health Sciences, Linköping; [8]Department of Diagnostic Radiology, Faculty of Health Sciences, Linköping, Sweden; and [9]The Life Insurance Companies Institute for Medical Statistics, Ullevål Hospital, Oslo, Norway

Abstract. Probucol lowers blood cholesterol, reduces xanthomas in hypercholesterolemic patients and prevents development of atherosclerosis in experimental animals. In this trial on 303 hypercholesterolemic patients, probucol plus cholestyramine for 3 years lowered total and LDL-cholesterol but did not reduce or retard femoral-artery atherosclerosis as measured by quantitative arteriography or by several physiologic techniques. However, atherosclerosis did improve in the control group given cholestyramine alone. The lack of effect of probucol may be explained by the reduction of HDL, especially HDL_{2b}, which are thought to be antiatherogenic. Probucol exhibited antioxidant properties measured by cell biological methods but lowered serum β-carotene concentrations. The roles of HDL and antioxidants in the development of atherosclerosis are discussed.

Probucol — a look back

Probucol has been used since the late 1970s in the treatment of different types of hyper-cholesterolemia. Total and LDL (low density lipoprotein)-cholesterol are reduced by about 10—20%. It was soon shown that the drug reduced cutaneous and tendinous xanthomas. In contrast to all other lipid-lowering drugs, probucol decreases HDL (high density lipoprotein)-cholesterol by 20—30% (reviewed in [1]). Interestingly, the regression of xanthomas in man was related to the degree of HDL-cholesterol lowering [2]. These and other results [1] have been taken to indicate that probucol increases reverse cholesterol transport, as one possible mode of action [1,2].

In the early 1980s epidemiological evidence suggested that high levels of HDL-cholesterol were associated with less atherosclerosis [3]. Furthermore, most other lipid-lowering drugs were found to increase HDL-cholesterol [3], which might explain at least in part the beneficial antiatherogenic effects seen in clinical trials, such as the Lipid Research Clinics Coronary Primary Prevention Trial using cholestyramine [4], and in several angiographic trials [5].

It was discovered early on that probucol prolonged the QT interval of the ECG and that this could result in fatal arrhythmias in experimental animals [1]. These findings and the effect of probucol on HDL have been a matter of great concern. In order to evaluate the clinical efficacy of probucol the Probucol Quantitative Regression Swedish Trial (PQRST) was set up. The primary aim was to investigate in hypercholesterolemic individuals whether probucol could retard or even induce regression of atherosclerosis [6]. When PQRST was planned in 1984 little was known about the role of lipid oxidation in atherosclerosis and the possibility of using antioxidants in the treatment of this disease [7]. Thus, PQRST was designed as a cholesterol-lowering and not as an antioxidant trial. The final results were published in November 1994 [8].

PQRST — major design features

The primary endpoint of PQRST was the change in lumen volume, assumed to reflect change in atheroma volume of the femoral artery. It was quantified by computerized evaluation of angiograms obtained before and after 1, 2 and 3 years of treatment with probucol [8]. Femoral arteriography was chosen for ethical reasons and a method was developed [9]. Males and females below 71 years of age were evaluated with respect to inclusion and exclusion criteria [6,8], including total cholesterol >6.88 mmol/l, triglycerides < 4 mmol/l, and a stable clinical condition with respect to coronary and peripheral circulations. All patients were given a moderate lipid-lowering diet and were monitored repeatedly by dietitians throughout the trial. Patients showing signs of atherosclerosis evaluated by pulse plethysmography continued with the diet for 3 months and then cholestyramine 8−16 g/day for 2 months. Those tolerating cholestyramine and responding by at least 8% cholesterol lowering were then given probucol 0.5 mg b.i.d. in addition to cholestyramine for another 2 months. Those responding by a further 8% cholesterol lowering were eligible for the first femoral arteriography to explore for visible atherosclerosis in any of the femoral arteries [6,8]. Eligible patients were then randomized to either probucol 0.5 g b.i.d. or to placebo, while all patients continued with diet and cholestyramine for 3 years. By this procedure all patients were guaranteed a basic lipid-lowering treatment which was judged ethical in the light of results from the LRC-CPPT trial [4]. In order to correlate possible changes in atherosclerosis of the femoral artery with other signs of atherosclerosis we used edge roughness, minimal and maximal width of the femoral artery and visual scoring of an aorto-femoral arteriogram as secondary endpoints [6,8]. Furthermore, bicycle exercise, treadmill tests and pulse plethysmography were performed annually and also used as secondary endpoints [6,8].

Results from PQRST — an overview

Of the 1,496 patients recruited, 303 were randomized to the 3-year double-blind trial. The compliance rate to cholestyramine was about 80% and to probucol about 90%. After 3 years the probucol-treated individuals had 17% lower serum cholesterol, 12% lower LDL-cholesterol, 24% lower total HDL and 34% lower HDL_2-cholesterol than the controls; $p < 0.001$ for all differences.

There was no significant difference in lumen volume change between the probucol and placebo group evaluated by the formal statistical testing procedure. Furthermore, there was no difference between the treatment groups in changes in arterial edge roughness or arterial diameters. Neither were there any differences in the scoring of atherosclerosis in the aortic, pelvic, femoral and popliteal branches. There was no difference in the development of ST-segment depressions on exercise tests or any difference between the treatment groups in ankle/arm blood pressure measured as secondary endpoints. By using a paired within-group statistical test it could be shown that in the control group, the lumen volume increased ($p < 0.001$) and roughness decreased ($p < 0.005$) [8]. In the probucol group there were no such changes over time. Furthermore, there were no differences in clinical events, major side-effects or laboratory tests between the treatment groups.

PQRST — some recent results

After the start of the trial [10] new research had indicated that probucol affected HDL particle size [1] and that probucol possessed antioxidant effects that prevented athero-sclerosis in experimental animals [1,7]. By applying gradient gel electrophoresis we found that probucol lowered the HDL_{2b} concentration by 69% ([10], Johansson et al., in preparation). Cell biology techniques were also used in substudies performed during the prerandomization phase [10] and also during the trial. These analyses showed that probucol markedly reduced the oxidizability of LDL as assessed by a decreased generation of thio-barbituric acid reactive substances (TBARS) and decreased degradation by macrophages of LDL exposed to oxidative stress by Cu^{2+}. The antioxidative effect of probucol remained unchanged throughout the 3-year trial period.

Lipid-soluble vitamins, especially vitamin E and β-carotene, are diet-derived antioxidants. We therefore measured these and other lipid-soluble vitamins during the prerandomization phase [10] as well as during the trial. We found that the probucol-treated patients had a 14% lower serum concentration of vitamin E than controls, subsequent to cholesterol and triglyceride lowering. The 30–50% drop in serum carotenoids in the probucol group was larger than could be explained by the reduction of lipids alone (Schäfer Elinder et al., in preparation).

Discussion

The results from PQRST show that addition of probucol to a lipid-lowering diet and cholestyramine does not reduce or retard atherosclerosis in the femoral artery relative to diet and cholestyramine without probucol. Furthermore, similar results were obtained for all other angiographic and clinical physiologic measurements used as secondary endpoints [8]. Thus, all results from PQRST conclusively point to the lack of antiatherogenic effects of probucol.

One cause for the lack of effect may be the considerable reduction of HDL-cholesterol, especially HDL_2-cholesterol. The largest reduction was found for HDL_{2b} particles, which are thought to be the most antiatherogenic [10]. It should be emphasized that PQRST was not originally planned to study the antioxidant effects of probucol. Nevertheless, results from our add-on studies showed that probucol manifested antioxidant effects not only in the test period for 2 months [10] but also during the 3-year trial phase. Whether or not the displacement of carotenoid substances by probucol from lipoproteins is of any clinical importance remains to be shown.

By applying within-group statistical testing methods [8] we found that those given only diet and cholestyramine benefited from treatment since their femoral lumen volume increased and roughness decreased. These results must be interpreted with some caution since results using arteriographic methods may reflect not only changes of atheroma volume but also changes in vascular dimensions. Compensatory enlargement of the artery with age and/or effects of the treatment on endothelial release of nitric oxide [11] may affect vascular architecture and dynamics. The positive results in the control group could therefore have other explanations. However, whatever is the true change in atherosclerosis, probucol did not favor any of these pathophysiological mechanisms [8]. Furthermore, since we have not studied the effects of probucol on the development of atherosclerosis in other arterial beds like the coronary arteries there is still a possibility that probucol might exert more favorable changes there. In fact, lipid-lowering treatments are known to affect femoral less than coronary atherosclerosis [5].

Probucol — a look ahead

Probucol still has a role in advanced hypercholesterolemia in patients with xanthomas since xanthomas can regress irrespective of or perhaps because of reduction of HDL-cholesterol [2]. The role of HDL in the regression of cutaneous xanthoma vs. the regression of atherosclerosis needs to be studied in more detail. In new trials using probucol, if it is ethically acceptable placebo should be used instead of a basic lipid-lowering treatment in order to simplify interpretation of the results. However, in future probucol will probably be used mainly in combination with other drugs in order to neutralize its presumably negative effects on HDL-cholesterol.

New derivatives of probucol are being developed and will hopefully not lower HDL-cholesterol. Thus, future studies using antioxidant drugs or dietary antioxidants may improve our understanding of atherogenesis. It remains to be shown if antioxidants have a role in primary prevention, presumably by reducing foam-cell generation and early lesion development. New trials are also needed to find out if antioxidants are of value also in secondary prevention of atherosclerosis.

There was one unexpected and in fact so far the only positive result for probucol in PQRST: we found that the QT interval of the ECG was much prolonged throughout the 3-year treatment (Walldius et al., submitted). Despite or perhaps because of these effects various types of arrhythmias were significantly reduced. Whether or not these results indicate anti- rather than arrhythmogenic effects of probucol remains to be elucidated.

Acknowledgements

The work of Inger Malmaeus and the staff at Sema Group InfoData AB, Stockholm, in analyzing all the data is gratefully appreciated. Supported by grants from Marion Merrell Dow Research Laboratories, Cincinnati, Ohio and Kansas City, Missouri, USA and the Swedish Medical Research Council (19X-204, 4494 and 19X-06962) the Swedish Heart-Lung Foundation, the Knut and Alice Wallenberg Foundation, the Torsten and Ragnar Söderberg Foundation, King Gustaf V 80th Birthday Foundation, The Karolinska Institute Foundation, Professor Nanna Svartz' Foundation, the Foundation for Old Servants, the Albert and Gerda Svensson Foundation, Loo and Hans Ostermans Foundation and the Swedish Society for Medical Sciences. Supported also by other funds administered by Universities in Linköping and Uppsala, Sweden.

References

1. Buckley MMT, Goa KL, Price AH, Brogden RN. Drugs 1989;37:762–800.
2. Yamamoto A, Matsuzawa Y, Yokoyama S, Funahashi T, Yamamura T, Kishino B. Am J Cardiol 1986;57:29H–35H.
3. Miller NE. In: Carlson LA (ed) Disorders of HDL. Proceedings of the International Symposium held at the Karolinska Hospital, Stockholm, 7–8 June 1990. London: Smith-Gordon, 1990:1–6.
4. Lipid Research Clinics Program. J Am Med Assoc 1984;251:351–364.
5. Blankenhorn DH. Curr Opin Lipid 1991;2:234–238.
6. Walldius G, Carlson LA, Erikson U, Olsson AG, Johansson J, Mölgaard J, Nilsson S, Stenport G, Kaijser L, Lassvik C, Holme I. Am J Cardiol 1988;62:37B–43B.
7. Steinberg D, Parthasarathy S, Carew TE, Khoo JC, Witztum JL. N Engl J Med 1989;320:915–924.
8. Walldius G, Erikson U, Olsson AG, Bergstrand L, Hådell K, Johansson J, Kaijser L, Lassvik C, Mölgaard J, Nilsson S, Schäfer Elinder L, Stenport G, Holme I. Am J Cardiol 1994;74:875–883.
9. Erikson U, Helmius G, Hemmingsson A, Ruhn G, Olsson AG. Acta Radiol 1988;29:303–309.
10. Walldius G, Regnström J, Nilsson J, Johansson L, Schäfer-Elinder L, Moelgaard J, Hådell K, Olsson AG, Carlson LA. Am J Cardiol 1993;73:15B–19B.
11. Moncada S, Martin JF, Higgs A. Eur J Clin Invest 1993;23:385–398.

Fibrinogen, fibrin and lipoproteins

Elspeth B. Smith

Department of Clinical Biochemistry, University of Aberdeen, Foresterhill, Aberdeen, AB9 2ZD, UK

Abstract. Fibrinogen and lipoproteins cross normal endothelium by vesicular transport. Within the intima a variable proportion of fibrinogen is converted to cross-linked fibrin; fibrin may also be deposited on the luminal surface, and associated with intimal edema. In the edematous gelatinous lesions there is increased fibrin, fibrinogen and fragment X, and fibrin degeneration products derived from cross-linked fibrin. Thrombin binds to fibrin, and α-thrombin is present in lesions. Both FDP and thrombin stimulate proliferation of smooth muscle cells. In intimal extracts, fibrinogen and apoprotein-B (apoB) concentrations are correlated, and apoB and apo(a) concentrations show similar relations to their plasma levels. However, digestion of pre-extracted intima with plasmin or elution with ε-aminocaproic acid releases disproportionate amounts of apo(a). Fibrin appears both to stimulate growth and to contribute to lipid accumulation of lesions by sequestration of Lp(a).

Epidemiological studies have clearly demonstrated that raised plasma fibrinogen is an independent risk factor for ischemic heart disease, re-infarction, and restenosis after bypass grafting and angioplasty. It is also increasingly clear that fibrin deposition plays a significant role in development of atherosclerotic lesions. Its atherogenic activity appears to be multifactorial: deposition on the endothelial surface is associated with intimal edema; smooth muscle cells (SMC) migrate along the fibrin strands, proliferate and deposit collagen; fibrin is a source of fibrin degradation products (FDP) which are both chemoattractive to leukocytes and stimulate SMC proliferation; fibrinogen binds thrombin which is then protected from inactivation by antithrombin III (AT-III) and stimulates SMC proliferation; fibrinogen preferentially binds Lp(a), and so may contribute to lipid accumulation in lesions [1].

Fibrin/fibrinogen-related antigens (FRA) in intima

Soluble fraction

Intimal samples were scissor-minced with 2% EDTA (to prevent clotting) and extracted with buffer containing EDTA and protease inhibitors, and the extracts were analyzed by rocket immunoelectrophoresis, gradient SDS-PAGE and immunoblotting. Most samples contain fibrinogen (Table 1), but whereas in plasma about 70% is fibrinogen I (Mr 340 kDa) with fibrinogens II and III (300 and 280 kDa) accounting for only 25 and 4% of the clottable fibrinogen [2], in intima some samples contained no fibrinogen I, and on average it comprised only 40% of total fibrinogen. All samples contained fragment X, derived from fibrinogen, but further degradation of fibrinogen seems to be limited [3]. In gelatinous lesions and mural thrombi two fragments characteristically derived from cross-linked fibrin, D-dimer-E (DY) and D-dimer (DD), were equally abundant (Table 1). In all but two juvenile fatty streaks the abundant E-fragments failed to react with monoclonal antibodies to fibrinopeptide A, which suggests that they were derived from fibrin, not fibrinogen.

Table 1. Fibrin and soluble fibrin/fibrinogen-related antigens (FRA) in intima

Intimal sample	Concentration (μg/100 mg wet tissue)							
	Fibrinogen	Fragment X	Fibrin	DY	DD	Y	D	ES
Normal (n = 7)	59	32	80	17	21	13	13	30
Gelatinous (n = 15)	112	42	1000	31	29	10	16	36
Thrombus[a] (n = 7)	42	15	b	35	29	13	13	52

[a]Mural thrombi; [b]86% fibrin.

Insoluble fibrin

After exhaustive extraction the residual tissue was incubated with plasmin, and the FDP released was measured by rocket immunoelectrophoresis to give an estimate of the amount of insoluble fibrin. Small amounts of fibrin were found in all normal intimas, but based on the ratio of DY + DD/D-monomer it was poorly cross-linked. By contrast, in gelatinous lesions the fibrin content was 10 times higher (Table 1) and showed the same degree of cross-linking as thrombi. In normal intima the amounts of fibrin and FDP are about the same, which suggests that deposition and lysis are in equilibrium. In gelatinous lesions there is only a small increase in FDP but a 10-fold increase in fibrin (Table 1); apparently, rate of fibrin deposition greatly exceeds its rate of removal.

Histologically, fibrin can be seen at all levels in gelatinous lesions; surface fibrin may be partially or almost entirely covered with endothelium, and SMC and collagen lie along fibrin strands within the lesion. Since deposition of surface fibrin seems to promote intimal edema, leading to increased fibrinogen in the expanded interstitial space, the extent to which the increased fibrin represents incorporation of mural deposits or formation within the intima is not clear. However, Haust [4] demonstrated fibre formation within the plasma insudate, and our recent finding that free α-thrombin is present (see below) suggests that both processes are involved.

Mitogenic activity of FRA

Plasmin digests of clots formed from plasma or purified fibrin stimulate DNA synthesis and angiogenesis in an in vivo model, the chick chorioallantoic membrane (CAM). Intimal extracts also stimulate DNA synthesis, with maximum activity in extracts of gelatinous and early fibrous lesions, in which SMC are presumably proliferating [1,5]. Passing the extracts through anti-(whole serum) affinity columns (which should also remove PDGF) had little effect on activity, but passage through antifibrinogen affinity columns removed most of the activity. Recent studies using antifragment D or antifragment E affinity columns indicate that the mitogenic activity mainly resides in fibrin-derived fragment E. Plasmin digests of fibrinogen and commercial fibrinogen-derived fragment E do not stimulate mitogenesis, but the latter is activated on incubation with thrombin [5]. Fragment E lacking FRA is a consistently abundant constituent of the plaque environment (Table 1).

Prothrombin-related antigens (PtRA) in intima

If fibrinogen is converted to fibrin within the lesion, active α-thrombin must be present. By rocket immunoelectrophoresis we found a concentration of total PtRA in intima that was greater than expected from the relative molecular weight and plasma concentration of prothrombin. However, there were 3 moles of AT-III per mole of PtRA, which suggests that any thrombin would be inactivated. Surprisingly, work in progress using

SDS-PAGE and immunoblotting shows a band migrating with α-thrombin in all intimal samples (Table 2). The expected covalent thrombin/AT-III complex was detected in only two of 16 samples, but a band of 160 kDa in which thrombin/AT-III/vitronectin co-migrated was invariably present (Smith and Crosbie, unpublished). Thus free thrombin is present in lesions where it may recruit more fibrin and independently stimulate SMC proliferation.

Low density lipoproteins in intima

Intimal interstitial fluid contains apparently free LDL in high concentration [6]. In addition, variable amounts may be retained in the intima in the form of complexes, although the nature of the complexes is controversial. In our studies on fibrin we found that incubation of washed intima with plasmin released an apoprotein-B (apoB)-containing lipoprotein in addition to FDP. Elucidation of the structure of lipoprotein(a) suggested that this fibrin-bound fraction might be Lp(a) binding to fibrin through its plasminogen-like kringles.

Incubation of washed intima with plasmin released an apo(a)-containing lipoprotein; it was also effectively eluted by a lysine analogue, ε-aminocaproic acid (ε-aca), which elutes plasminogen from fibrin [7]. As a nonspecific protease, plasmin might degrade apo-proteins, but as ε-aca is a serine protease inhibitor, its use allows further examination of the lipoproteins with less risk of artifacts. In recent studies we have examined the relation between apo(a) and -B as well as the influence of apo(a) isotype on fibrin binding.

LDL and Lp(a) concentrations in serum and intima

Blood samples sent for routine clinical biochemistry were available for some subjects coming to autopsy, and this allowed direct comparison between serum and intimal levels. In buffer extracts (containing aprotinin) of intima the ratios of LDL and Lp(a) were not significantly different from serum (Table 3). In striking contrast, LDL in the ε-aca eluate was only about 25% of that in the buffer extract, whereas significantly more Lp(a) was eluted by ε-aca than by buffer. Similar mechanisms seem to control the uptake of LDL and Lp(a) into intima, but Lp(a) binds much more strongly to fibrin.

Linkage of apo(a) and apoB in intima

In most studies of Lp(a) the samples are reduced, and the disulfide bond between apo(a) and apoB is therefore cleaved. However, it is clearly important to know whether the large Lp(a) molecule remains intact, particularly when bound to fibrin. Serum and intimal samples from two patients with high serum Lp(a) (48 and 66 mg/100 ml) were analyzed, nonreduced, for LDL and Lp(a) on the same gel. In the sera, 67 and 70% of apo(a) co-

Table 2. Prothrombin-related antigens (PtRA) in intima

Intimal sample	Concentration (μg/100 mg)[a]			Molar ratio
	Total PtRA	Prothrombin	α-Thrombin	PtRA/AT-III
Normal (n = 5)	43	9	8	0.3
Gelatinous (n = 15)	72	14	13	0.4
Thrombus (n = 7)	111	22	20	0.6

[a]Dry weight.

Table 3. Relative concentrations of LDL and Lp(a) in serum and intimal extracts

	Patients serum (mg/100 ml)	Intima (µg/100 mg wet wt)		Eluate (% of extract)
		Buffer extract	ε-aca eluate	
LDL (n = 8)	334	279	–	–
Lp(a) (n = 8)	23	25	–	–
LDL (n = 14)	–	345	93	27
Lp(a) (n = 14)	–	41	54	132

migrated with apoB in high molecular mass bands of 700–1,500 kDa, but there were no corresponding bands in the intimal samples. In a total of nine intimal samples from different patients no high molecular weight apoB/apo(a) bands were detected in either buffer extracts or ε-aca eluates. By contrast, in a large mural thrombus the same high-Mr bands were present as in the serum, indicating that cleavage does not occur during the extraction process.

Lp(a) isoforms and fibrin binding

Serum and intimal apo(a) isoform patterns were compared in reduced samples from 10 subjects. The sera exhibited 2–4 isoforms of varying intensity, and in most intimal extracts the same isoforms were present but with a different distribution. The proportion of the largest isoforms was significantly reduced. However, the isoform patterns in buffer extracts and ε-aca eluates of intima were virtually identical; affinity for fibrin does not appear to depend on apo(a) isoform.

Conclusions

Our studies over several years add increasing support to the idea that fibrin deposition plays a significant part in growth and development of fibrous plaques. A new dimension is added by the finding that α-thrombin is present in lesions, and this links lesion growth with recent studies on restenosis [8,9]. The preferential binding of apo(a) within lesions, probably to fibrin, is confirmed in our recent studies. However, the apo(a)–apoB link appears to have been severed, so the Lp(a) is no longer intact, and its role in atherogenesis requires further investigation.

Acknowledgements

The author's work was supported by the British Heart Foundation; the following colleagues collaborated: S. Carey, S. Cochran, L. Crosbie, G.A. Keen, E.M. Staples, C. Stirk, W.D. Thomson.

References

1.   Smith EB, Thompson WD. Thromb Res 1994;73:1–19.
2.   Holm B, Nilsen DWT, Kierulf P, Godal HC. Thromb Res 1985;37:165–176.
3.   Smith EB, Keen GA, Grant A, Stirk C. Arteriosclerosis 1990;10:263–275.
4.   Haust MD. Hum Pathol 1971;1:1–29.
5.   Stirk C, Kochhar A, Smith EB, Thompson WD. Atherosclerosis 1993;103:159–169.
6.   Smith EB, Ashall C. Biochim Biophys Acta 1983;754:249–257.
7.   Smith EB, Crosbie L. Atherosclerosis 1991;89:127–136.
8.   Sarembock IJ, Gertz SD et al. Circulation 1991;84:232–243.
9.   Schwartz SM. J Clin Invest 1993;91:4.

Elastase and cell extracellular matrix interactions in the pathogenesis of intimal proliferation

Marlene Rabinovitch

Division of Cardiovascular Research, Hospital for Sick Children, University of Toronto, Toronto, Canada

Abstract. Endogenous vascular elastase (EVE), a 20-kDa serine proteinase related to adipsin, is expressed in response to pulmonary hypertension-producing stimuli and is directly related to development and progression of vascular disease. Serum or endothelial factors induce EVE via tyrosine kinase intracellular signalling. An EVE is associated with accelerated neointimal formation in coronary arteries after experimental cardiac transplantation, and is probably induced by cytokines as part of an immune/inflammatory response involved in upregulation of fibronectin production. Fibronectin stimulates migration into the subendothelium of smooth muscle cells and inflammatory cells. Cytokine blockade with TNF-α soluble receptor or CS-1 (fibronectin) peptides which bind VLA-4 integrins on lymphocytes reduces by >50% the number of vessels with lesions of neointimal formation and their severity.

Elastase and vascular pathobiology

In an effort to discover the underlying mechanisms causing vascular changes leading to pulmonary hypertension in children with congenital heart defects, we applied ultrastructural analysis to lung biopsy tissue obtained for routine diagnostic purposes. We found that there were indeed structural abnormalities in the endothelial cells of pulmonary arteries, but we also uncovered rather striking changes in the subendothelium [1]. The internal elastic lamina appeared to be fragmented, which suggested that an enzyme, having as one of its proteolytic properties the ability to degrade elastin, might be stimulating the remodeling process (Fig. 1). Increased production of proteolytic enzymes has been associated with tissue remodeling in development and in wound healing. Thus, we proposed that induction of elastolytic activity in the vessel wall might stimulate release of growth factors from the matrix, resulting in smooth muscle cell proliferation and hypertrophy and connective tissue protein synthesis. We further reasoned that continued stimulation of elastolytic activity might further alter smooth muscle cell/extracellular matrix interactions, thereby inducing the production of a new constellation of genes which would change the cell to a migratory phenotype. Migration and proliferation of smooth muscle cells, in association with increased production of connective tissue proteins, would lead to neointimal formation which would become progressively more occlusive (Fig. 2).

To investigate this hypothesis, we measured elastase activity in pulmonary arteries from experimental animals in which pulmonary hypertension was induced by exposure to chronic hypoxia or following injection of the toxin, monocrotaline. In both cases an early rise in elastase activity was observed. In adult rats injected with monocrotaline, which causes progressive and malignant disease, a second rise in elastase activity was also observed, with progression of the disease and the development of early neointimal formation (Fig. 3) [2]. In pulmonary hypertension produced by hypoxia, which is

---

Address for correspondence: Marlene Rabinovitch, M.D., Director, Cardiovascular Research, Hospital for Sick Children, 555 University Ave., Toronto, Ontario, Canada M5G 1X8. Tel.: 416-813-5918; fax: 416-813-7480.

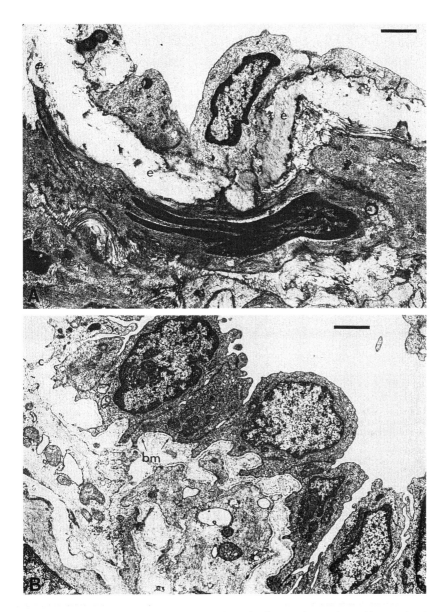

Fig. 1. A: A section of a pulmonary artery 92 μm in diameter in a patient with normal pulmonary artery pressure shows an intact internal elastic lamina(e). B: In a section from a pulmonary artery 108 μm in diameter in a patient with increased pulmonary blood flow and pressure, microfibrillar material is present in the subendothelial layer but there is no true internal elastic lamina. The endothelial and smooth muscle cells are separated by only a thick basement membrane (bm). Bar = 1 μm in both. (From [1], with permission.)

associated with structural changes that are largely reversible upon return of the animals to room air, and in infant rats injected with monocrotaline, which also produces pulmonary hypertension and associated vascular disease that is spontaneously reversible, the second increase in elastase activity does not occur. Subsequent studies showed a cause

340

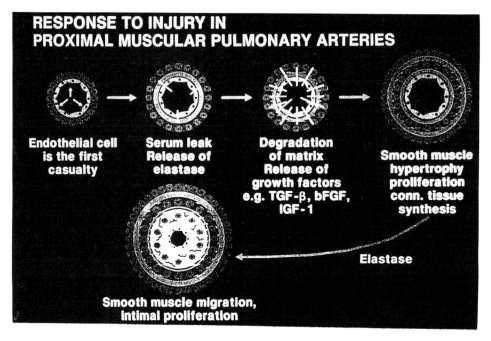

Fig. 2. We have speculated as to how a stimulus, such as the high flow and pressure of a congenital heart defect with a left to right shunt, might induce activity of an elastolytic enzyme and how this might initiate the remodeling process. The process of progressive pulmonary hypertension involves a series of switches in the smooth muscle cell phenotype, i.e., differentiation of muscle from non-muscle precursor cells, smooth muscle cell hypertrophy, and proliferation accounting for medial hypertrophy and smooth muscle cell migration resulting in neointimal formation. We speculate that, in response to a stimulus such as high flow and pressure, the first "casualty" would be the endothelial cell. As a result of structural and functional alterations in endothelial cells, some of the barrier function would be lost, allowing for leak into the subendothelium of a serum factor normally excluded from this region. The serum factor could induce activity of an elastolytic enzyme, as we have shown experimentally. This enzyme released from smooth muscle cells would activate growth factors normally stored in the extracellular matrix in an inactive form, such as basic fibroblast growth factor (bFGF) and transforming growth factor (TGF) β, and might also influence release of insulin-like growth factor (IGF-1). These growth factors are known to induce smooth muscle hypertrophy and proliferation and increases in connective (conn.) tissue protein (e.g., collagen and elastin) synthesis. This would result in hypertrophy of the muscular arteries. Continued elastase activity would cause migration of smooth muscle cells in two ways, first, by removing a physical barrier and also by so changing the cell-extracellular matrix signalling processes such that a new constellation of gene products would be produced, providing the smooth muscle cells with the machinery necessary to switch from the contractile to motile phenotype. Migration of smooth muscle cells and synthesis of extracellular matrix proteins would result in intimal proliferation.

and effect relationship between the induction of elastase activity later found to be serine proteinase in nature and the development and progression of pulmonary hypertension in these experimental models [3,4]. That is, a variety of serine elastase inhibitors either prevented the development of pulmonary hypertension or retarded the progression of pulmonary vascular disease (Fig. 4). Thus, it seemed that this enzyme was important pathophysiologically and further efforts were directed at its characterization.

To identify the elastolytic enzyme, we used a molecular reverse transcriptase (RT)-polymerase chain reaction (PCR) approach. We synthesized degenerate oligonucleotides to conserved regions in serine elastases that shared a similar inhibitor profile to the

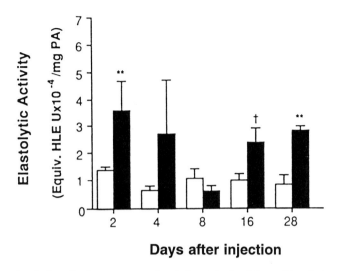

Fig. 3. Central pulmonary artery elastolytic activity in adult rats. Elastolytic activity was observed in all rats and normalized per mg PA. In all control rats, the amount of elastolytic activity remained low throughout the experiment (open bars). Monocrotaline-treated rats (closed bars) had greater elastolytic activity than control rats at 2 and 28 days after injection (**p < 0.05, a trend was observed at 16 days, †p < 0.06). (From [2], with permission.)

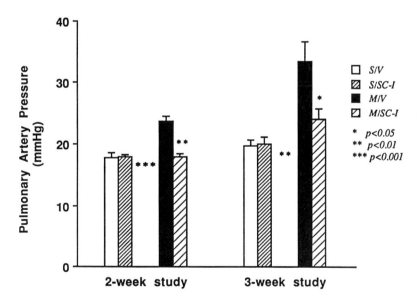

Fig. 4. Mean pulmonary artery pressures. S, saline; V, vehicle; SC-I, SC-37698 (elastase inhibitor) (2 mg/day in 2-wk study and 3 mg/day in 3-wk study); M, monocrotaline. Two-week study: S/V (n = 6), M/V (n = 7), M/SC-I (n = 6). Three-week study: S/V (n = 3), S/SC-I (n = 3), M/V (n = 6), M/SC-I (n = 6). Values are means ± SE. (From [4], with permission). In the 2-week study, the elastase inhibitor was given for 2 weeks elastase. In the 3-week study the elastase inhibitor was given for the last 2 of a 3-week experimental period after injection of the toxin monocrotaline.

endogenous vascular elastase (EVE) (i.e., human leukocyte and porcine pancreatic elastases). These degenerate oligonucleotides were used in an RT-PCR reaction with cDNA reverse-transcribed from rat pulmonary artery (poly-A+) mRNA. Through PCR, a 500 base pair product was generated which was radiolabeled and used to screen a cDNA library from rat pulmonary artery. Three overlapping clones were sequenced and found to have striking homology with rat adipsin [5], a serine proteinase that was not known to be elastolytic, but is a homologue of human complement factor D [6]. Nonetheless, an antibody to mouse recombinant adipsin was used in the three-step immunoaffinity purification procedure to isolate elastase activity from the pulmonary artery and to resolve the proteinase as an enzyme of 20 kDa (Fig. 5). Figure 6 shows that the elastolytic enzyme was localized largely to the smooth muscle cells of the arterial wall.

To understand how elastase activity is increased under pathological conditions, we explored the hypothesis that serum factors which might "leak" into the subendothelium when there is endothelial injury and loss of barrier function could induce the release of EVE from vascular smooth muscle cells. We have, in fact, now shown that elastase activity is induced in pulmonary (as well as systemic) artery smooth muscle cells in a dose-dependent fashion starting with fetal bovine serum concentrations as low as 0.1% (Fig. 7). While the nature of the serum factor was not established, it appears to be both heat- and acid-labile. It operates by binding elastin to smooth muscle cell surfaces and inducing tyrosine kinase activity [7]. Most recent work suggests that this serum factor also binds directly to elastin and, in fact, serum-treated elastin can stimulate elastase activity in much the same manner as serum, but in an accelerated fashion. In addition, an endothelial factor which is similar to the serum factor in physical properties can also

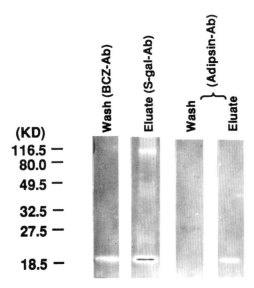

Fig. 5. An elastin substrate gel to resolve the molecular weight of the PA elastase enzyme. A substrate gel with elastin (0.67 mg/ml) impregnated in 10% polyacrylamide shows that in the wash after the BCZ (antielastin binding protein) immunoaffinity column, the eluate after the anti-S-GAL antibody (antibody that recognizes NH$_2$-terminal sequences of elastase) immunoaffinity column, and the eluate after the antiadipsin antibody immunoaffinity column, but not the wash, contain an elastase enzyme (the lytic band at 20 kDa). A band at ~100 kDa in the S-GAL eluate may represent elastase bound to 72-kDa elastin, but it was not seen in the wash and did not bind to the antiadipsin antibody immunoaffinity column. (From [5], with permission.)

343

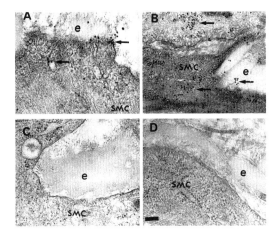

Fig. 6. Representative immunoelectron photomicrographs using an antiadipsin peptide antibody. An antibody was raised in a rabbit to the adipsin sequence: Cys Ala Glu Ser Asn Arg Arg Asp. Goat anti-rabbit antibody was conjugated with 15-nm gold particles and hybridized to the antiadipsin antibody reflecting the antigenic sites (arrows). A: A smooth muscle cell (SMC) from a rat pulmonary artery 28 d after injection of monocrotaline shows adipsin antigenic sites related to the cell surface, secretory vesicles, and in close proximity to elastin (e). B: The antibody is seen more extensively over the SMC and seems to be associated with the Golgi apparatus. C: The antibody has been preabsorbed to an adipsin affinity column and no or only rare antigenic sites were apparent on the tissue. D: The tissue was immunoreacted with normal rabbit serum and there are no positive sites. Magnification 48,600. Bar, 100 nm. (From [5], with permission.)

stimulate smooth muscle cell elastase by a similar mechanism. We have further shown that induction of elastase activity requires new protein synthesis, as well as mRNA transcription (unpublished). Further in vitro work indicates that induction of elastase activity results in the release of basic fibroblast growth factor from the extracellular matrix, thereby further substantiating the way in which activation of an elastolytic enzyme might lead to a complex pathobiologic process.

With this information at hand, we began to investigate whether similar elastases may be involved in the pathobiology of coronary arterial disease. Our laboratory has been specifically interested in the rapidly progressive neointimal formation associated with the coronary arteriopathy that occurs after cardiac transplantation. We have used, as an experimental model, piglets after heterotopic heart transplantation and have shown greater activity of an elastase in the coronary arteries from the donor than the host heart. The increased elastolytic activity was resolved as a 23 kDa protein on an elastin substrate gel. It is inhibited by specific serine proteinase inhibitors such as elafin and is associated, ultrastructurally, with the fragmentation of elastin (Fig. 8). The mechanism of inducing release of this elastase may be similar to that described in pulmonary arteries, but we have evidence that it might also be related to the immune-inflammatory response in the coronary arteries associated with cytokine production. We have further evidence that the induction of elastase in the coronary arteries might stimulate smooth muscle cell migration and transendothelial lymphocyte trafficking by upregulating endothelial and smooth muscle cell production of the matrix glycoprotein, fibronectin.

Critical role of fibronectin in neointimal formation

In an effort to understand the mechanism of smooth muscle cell migration associated with

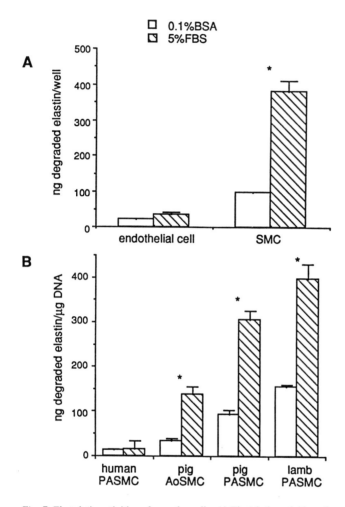

Fig. 7. Elastolytic activities of vascular cells. A) Elastolytic activities of porcine PA endothelial and smooth muscle cell (SMC) with or without FBS. PA endothelial cells had low levels of elastolytic activity under serum-free conditions, and a further increase was not evident following stimulation with 5% FBS. In contrast, porcine PA SMC had higher levels of elastolytic activity under serum-free conditions and showed a greater than twofold increase in activity in response to serum stimulation (*p < 0.01). B) Elastolytic activities in SMC from different sources and species. Adult human PA SMC had low levels of elastolytic activity under serum-free conditions, and no increase in response to serum was evident. In contrast, both Ao and PA SMC from juvenile pigs and fetal lamb PA SMC produced higher levels of elastolytic activity under serum-free conditions than human PA SMC and showed a two- to three-fold increase following serum stimulation (*p < 0.01). Values are mean ± standard error of three separate assays. (From [7], with permission.)

neointimal formation, we studied the ductus arteriosus as a prototype vessel. The ductus, in all species, develops neointimal "cushions" in late gestation; this suggested that ductus arteriosus endothelial and smooth muscle cells were specifically programmed and that these programs might be activated in other vascular cells following pathological stimulation. To elucidate the specific cellular interactions which govern neointimal formation in the ductus arteriosus, we cultured endothelial and smooth muscle cells and

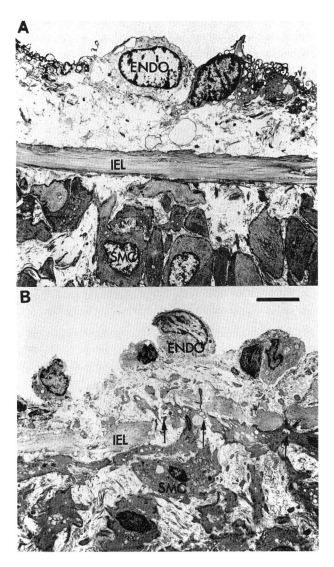

Fig. 8. Representative electron photomicrographs of host (A) and donor (B) coronary artery. No breaks are seen in the IEL of host coronary artery, whereas the IEL of the donor coronary artery is tortuous and a few breaks (arrows) can be seen. ENDO, endothelial cell, SMC, smooth muscle cell. Magnification × 3760; scale bar = 5 μm. (From Oho S and Rabinovitch M. Am J Pathol 1994;145:202–210, with permission.)

compared them to vascular cells from the aorta and pulmonary artery. We have found that, under the stimulation of transforming growth factor-β (TGF-β), ductus endothelial cells produce large amounts of glycosaminoglycans, especially hyaluronans [8,9]. There is increased production of TGF-β by ductus arteriosus endothelial cells. We further showed that an endothelial factor, perhaps also TGF-β, stimulates smooth muscle cell production of glycosaminoglycans, specifically chondroitin sulfate. Chondroitin sulfate removes elastin-binding proteins from ductus smooth muscle cell surfaces and this leads to the impaired assembly of elastin fibers. Moreover, the relative deficiency of elastin-binding proteins in the ductus leads to the production of the truncated 52-kDa tropoelastin [9] which lacks the C-terminal and is likely ineffectively cross-linked [10]. This 52-kDa truncated form of tropoelastin serves as a highly chemotactic fragment which might stimulate smooth muscle cell migration [11]. In addition, we have evidence that elastin peptides probably induce smooth muscle cell migration by upregulating production of fibronectin (unpublished).

Ductus arteriosus smooth muscle cells produce large amounts of cell-associated fibronectin which is responsible for their increased migratory behavior in collagen gels. The phenotype of the migratory ductus smooth muscle cell is also related to increased expression of the receptor for hyaluronan-mediated motility (RHAMM) and this suggests how the ductus smooth muscle cells might migrate upwards into a subendothelium that is enriched in hyaluronan [12] (Figs. 9 and 10). Recent studies in our laboratory have shown that the increased production of TGF-β by ductus endothelial cells, and especially the increased production of fibronectin by smooth muscle cells, may be dependent on a posttranscriptional mechanism of regulation. With respect to fibronectin, this appears to be related to cytoplasmic factors in the ductus smooth muscle cells that bind to an A+U conserved consensus sequence in the 3′ untranslated region of the mRNA.

Fibronectin in the process of neointimal formation in coronary arterial disease

Having established that fibronectin was critical to the process of increased smooth muscle cell migration in the development of neointimal formation in the ductus arteriosus, we next explored whether this glycoprotein was expressed in large amounts in neointima produced in coronary arteries after heterotopic heart transplantation. Using the piglet transplant model described earlier, we showed that the early development of neointimal changes, in donor coronary arteries, included increased expression of MHC Class II antigens on endothelial cell surfaces, interleukin-1β and tumor necrosis factor-α in the endothelium, especially, but also in the subendothelium, and in medial smooth muscle cells to some extent, and increased production of fibronectin [14,15] (Fig. 11). We further elucidated that the increased production of the cytokine interleukin-1β and tumor necrosis factor-α were reciprocally co-inducing the synthesis of fibronectin [16]. With this information in hand, we were able to show that cytokine blockade with the tumor necrosis factor-soluble receptor effectively reduced the incidence and the severity of neointimal formation [15]. On the basis of extensive studies in the literature indicating that fibronectin binds to integrins on lymphocyte surfaces, we investigated whether the increased subendothelial accumulation of fibronectin might serve to traffic T cells into that location whereupon they would, in the activated state, continually express cytokines and growth factors, leading to smooth muscle cell proliferation, hypertrophy, and migration. An in vitro co-culture system was set up in which we documented that the CS-1 peptide, which binds the VLA-4 (α4β1) integrin on T lymphocytes, effectively reduced transendothelial migration of T cells towards smooth muscle cells that were stimulated with IL-1β. RGD peptides also blocked this reaction. This reduced the transendothelial migration of lymphocytes, as did fibronectin antibodies. Further exciting work has shown that the in vivo administration of the CS-1 peptide to rabbits following heterotopic heart transplantation also effectively reduced the incidence and severity of coronary artery neointimal formation.

While we are further investigating the exact mechanism whereby cytokines induce release of fibronectin through elastases, it appears that the induction and the molecular

347

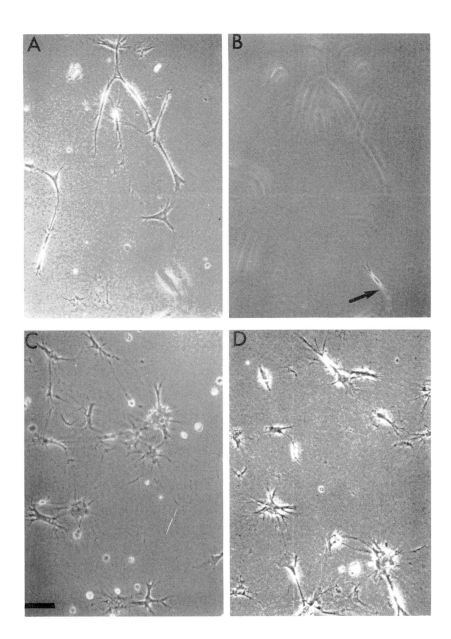

Fig. 9. DA and Ao smooth muscle cells on collagen (2 mg/ml) gels. A: DA smooth muscle cells 2 days following seeding onto the surface of collagen gels. The cells exhibit a spindle-like elongated morphology and the majority of cells are visible on the surface of the gels. B: The arrow indicates the outline of a cell which has migrated below the surface of the gel. By focusing into the gel at a depth of 250 μm this cell comes clearly into focus. C: Ao cells, 2 days following seeding onto the surface of the gel, exhibit a flattened, stellate morphology. D: In the presence of antibodies against fibronectin (1:100) DA smooth muscle cells also display a more flattened, stellate appearance (Bar = 200 μm). (From [13], with permission.)

348

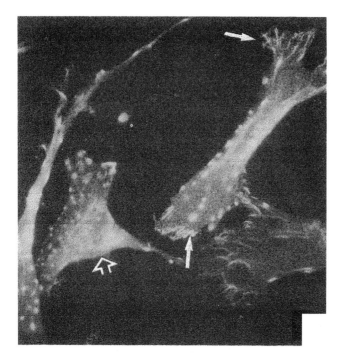

Fig. 10. Immunofluorescent staining of receptor for hyaluronan-mediated mobility of RHAMM on PA smooth muscle cells on glass coverslips using a 1:40 dilution of polyclonal antibodies to HABP and visualized by RITC goat anti-rabbit IgG. Positive staining for RHAMM was prominent in lamellipodia and leading edges as indicated by the closed arrows. (From [13], with permission.)

mechanism whereby cytokines induce production of fibronectin involves transcriptional and post-transcriptional regulatory mechanisms.

Future directions

Future directions will therefore be aimed at targeting EVE(s) by understanding the molecular mechanisms which regulate its induction and its production at the transcriptional and posttranscriptional levels. The factors that induce its release will be elucidated, as will the way in which it, in turn, induces the release and activation of growth factors stored in the extracellular matrix. Further work related to the induction of changes in smooth muscle cell phenotype by elastase revolve around understanding how enzymatic degradation of the matrix leads to the upregulation of fibronectin and the receptor for hyaluronan-mediated motility. This, again, provides a novel therapeutic target whereby inhibition of vascular smooth muscle cell migration will reduce neointimal formation in systemic and pulmonary arteries. Particularly relevant to the inflammatory mechanisms in vascular pathobiology is the way in which fibronectin serves to traffic T cells into the subendothelium. Since fibronectin-binding integrins ($\alpha 4\beta 1$ and $\alpha 5\beta 1$) are present on monocytes, targeting of monocytes into the subendothelium in atherogenesis might also be related to the induction of fibronectin. Thus, it appears that fibronectin provides a dual highway which induces smooth muscle cell migration into the subendothelium and transendothelial migration of lymphocytes and inflammatory cells (lymphocytes and monocytes) from the circulation. Once trafficked into the subendothelium, cytokines,

Post Cardiac Transplant Coronary Arteriopathy

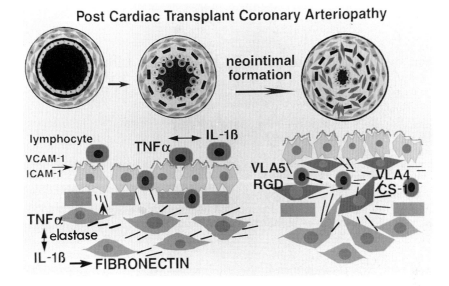

Fig. 11. This schema summarizes our findings related to the pathobiology of postcardiac transplant coronary arteriopathy related to our studies in piglets and rabbits. The activated endothelium displays increased expression of adhesion molecules VCAM-1 and ICAM-1 in addition to MHC class II molecules. The T cell (lymphocytes) adhere and then in the activated state release cytokines IL-1β and TNF-α. These cytokines are then induced in endothelial and smooth muscle cells. Their increased expression in these vascular cell results in the upregulated production of the extracellular matrix glycoprotein, fibronectin. Increased fibronectin in the subendothelium is associated with vascular smooth muscle cell migration as well as transendothelial migration of lymphocytes. There they bind to fibronectin through interactions between RGD and CS-1 peptides and integrins VLA-5 and VLA-4, respectively. This serves to further perpetuate the process which culminates in neointimal formation owing to smooth muscle cell proliferation, migration and increased production of extracellular matrix protein.

especially interleukin-1β and tumor necrosis factor-α, are released and this causes further upregulation of smooth muscle cell proliferation and migration.

References

1. Rabinovitch M et al. Lab Invest 1986;55:632—653.
2. Todorovich-Hunter L et al. Am Rev Respir Dis 1992;146:213—223.
3. Maruyama K et al. Am J Physiol 1991;261:H1716—H1726.
4. Ye C, Rabinovitch M. Am J Physiol 1991;261:H1255—H1267.
5. Zhu L et al. The endogenous vascular elastase which governs development and progression of monocrotaline-induced pulmonary hypertension in rats is a novel enzyme related to the serine proteinase adipsin. J Clin Invest (in press).
6. White RT et al. J Biol Chem 1992;267:9210—9213.
7. Kobayashi J et al. J Cell Physiol 1994;160:121—131.
8. Boudreau N, Rabinovitch M. Lab Invest 1991;64:187—199.
9. Boudreau N et al. Lab Invest 1992;67:350—359.
10. Hinek A, Rabinovitch M. J Biol Chem 1993;268:1405—1413.
11. Hinek A et al. J Clin Invest 1991;88:2083—2094.
12. Hinek A et al. Exp Cell Res 1992;203:344—353.
13. Boudreau N et al. Dev Biol 1991;143:235—247.
14. Clausell N et al. Am J Pathol 1993;142:1772—1786.
15. Clausell N et al. Circulation 1994;89:2768—2779.
16. Molossi S et al. Reciprocal induction of tumor necrosis factor-α and interleukin-1β activity mediates fibronectin synthesis in coronary artery smooth muscle cells. J Cell Physiol (in press).

350

Regulation of proteoglycan synthesis by vascular cells

Thomas N. Wight[1], Elke Schönherr[2], Hannu Järveläinen[3], Michael Kinsella[1], Stephen Evanko[1] and Joan Lemire[1]

[1]*Department of Pathology, University of Washington;* [2]*Institute of Arteriosclerosis, University of Münster, Münster, Germany; and* [3]*University of Turku, Turku, Finland*

Proteoglycans (PGs) are a diverse group of macromolecules which bear one or more linear glycosaminoglycan (GAG) chains usually attached via O-glycosidic linkages to serine residues along a core protein [1]. These macromolecules are located throughout the extracellular matrix of vascular tissue and associated with the surface of vascular cells [2]. The size of the core proteins of the different PGs found in vascular tissue varies considerably as do the number, length and composition of the GAG chains. These variations create enormous structural heterogeneity in these macromolecules which no doubt contributes to differences in their biological functions. A list of some of the PGs present in vascular tissue and synthesized by vascular cells is presented in Table 1.

Proteoglycans are enriched in the arterial intima and accumulate as this layer thickens during the early phases of atherosclerotic disease [3–6]. This accumulation is thought to predispose the hyperplastic intima to additional complications such as lipid accumulation due to the ability of PGs to interact with lipoproteins to form insoluble complexes [7–10]. In addition, PGs accumulate in different vascular lesions characterized by tissue expansion, as is frequently observed in restenosis after balloon angioplasty and in arteriovenous fistulas [11,12]. Since PGs and associated molecules such as hyaluronan (HA) modulate cellular adhesion, proliferation and migration [13], their presence in the vascular intima may in part regulate vascular-cell adhesion, proliferation, and migration which are key events in the genesis of the atherosclerotic plaque [14].

A principal PG present in vascular tissue and synthesized by arterial smooth muscle cells is a large interstitial chondroitin sulfate PG (CSPG) that interacts with HA to form multimolecular aggregates within the vascular extracellular matrix (ECM). Biochemical, immunochemical and cloning studies indicate that this PG is similar, if not identical, to

Table 1. Vascular proteoglycans

Chondroitin sulfate PG
    versican/PGM
Heparan sulfate PG
    perlecan
    syndecan(s)
Dermatan sulfate PGs
    decorin
    biglycan
Keratan sulfate PG
    lumican

Address for correspondence: Thomas N. Wight PhD, Department of Pathology, SM-30, University of Washington, Seattle, WA 98195, USA.

the major mesenchymal CSPG named versican and/or proteoglycan mesenchyme (PGM) [15]. For example, monkey arterial smooth muscle cells (ASMCs) synthesize and secrete a large CSPG (M_r~1.2 × 10^6) which stains on Western blots with antibodies to human versican/PGM [15]. This molecule interacts with HA with high affinity [16] and is co-localized with HA in the vascular intima.

Although it is well documented that PGs and HA are enriched in the arterial intima and change in composition and concentration as vascular lesions develop, little is known as to what factors regulate the synthesis of these important vascular constituents. Growth factors and cytokines play critical roles in vascular biology and are major effectors that regulate ASMC activity following arterial injury and in vascular disease [14,17]. Genes for platelet-derived growth factor (PDGF) and transforming growth factor (TGF-β1) are upregulated after arterial injury [17] and increased expression of TGF-β1 has been observed in the fibroproliferative zone in human restenotic lesions [18]. Areas of the vasculature enriched in growth factors such as TGF-β1 consistently exhibit striking accumulations of PGs [5]. Thus, a fundamental question in vascular biology is whether growth factors known to affect ASMC proliferation and migration also regulate the synthesis of PGs and HA by these same cells.

We have found that PDGF and TGF-β1, while having opposing effects on ASMC proliferation, both stimulate the synthesis of versican/PGM [19] (Fig. 1). Recent experiments also demonstrate increased versican/PGM expression in arteries 2 weeks after balloon catheter injury [20]. On the other hand, the two growth factors have different effects on the levels of mRNA transcripts for the small dermatan sulfate (DS)-containing PGs (decorin and biglycan) that are synthesized by these cells [21]. PDGF does not affect steady-state levels of mRNA for decorin and biglycan following 24-h stimulation while TGF-β1 upregulates biglycan mRNA levels but has no effect on mRNA levels for decorin (Fig. 2). While both PDGF and TGF-β1 upregulate versican/PGM gene expression in cultured ASMC, interleukin-1 (IL-1) has a dampening effect on versican/PGM expression

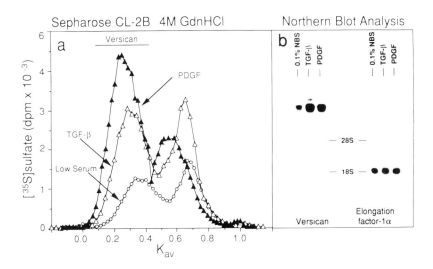

Fig. 1. Growth factors affect versican/PGM expression. A: Molecular sieve (sepharose CL-2B) profile of labeled PGs synthesized by ASMC treated with PDGF or TGF-β1. B: Northern analysis of RNA probed for human versican/PGM. Note that both treatments increase the amount of versican/PGM RNA and PG synthesized by ASMC.

352

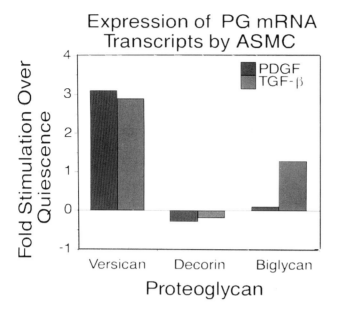

Fig. 2. Relative changes in the amount of mRNA transcripts for versican/PGM, biglycan and decorin induced by a 24-h treatment of cultured ASMC by TGF-β1 and PDGF.

induced by PDGF [22]. These results indicate that versican/PGM core protein synthesis by cultured ASMC is regulated by specific growth factors which are not involved in the regulation of other vascular PGs.

In addition to affecting mRNA transcripts levels for two major ASMC genes, PDGF and TGF-β1 also differentially affect GAG synthesis by these cells. For example, both growth factors cause elongation of the GAG chains attached to three different PG core proteins (i.e., versican, biglycan and decorin), thus increasing overall size of these PGs [19,21]. However, only PDGF and not TGF-β1 induces an enrichment in the chondroitin-6-sulfate to chondroitin-4-sulfate ratio in chains isolated from versican/PGM (Fig. 3),

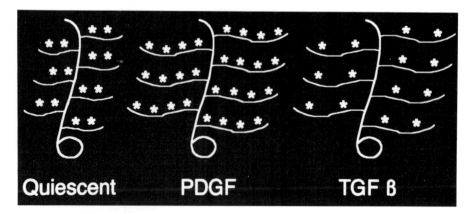

Fig. 3. Model depicting changes in the CS chains of versican/PGM induced by growth factors *chondroitin-6-sulfate.

indicating that chain composition may be related to growth state of the cells. These results suggest that PDGF is capable of regulating PG synthesis through transcriptional/ translational as well as posttranslational mechanisms. The importance of the PDGF receptor in the regulation of versican/PGM synthesis by ASMC is further emphasized by studies which demonstrate that inhibition of tyrosine kinase activity of the PDGF receptor by genistein blocks PDGF-induced synthesis of versican/PGM (Schönherr, Kinsella and Wight, unpublished observations).

Although the significance of these quantitative and qualitative changes in the synthesis of versican/PGM by ASMC induced by PDGF and TGF-β1 is not well understood, these changes have some bearing on the ability of these molecules to bind and trap lipoproteins in the arterial intima. For example, CSPG–lipoprotein complexes have been isolated from atherosclerotic lesions [7], and specific regions within the apolipoprotein (apo) moiety of the lipoproteins interact with CS chains isolated from vascular tissue [9,10]. Chondroitin sulfate has been co-localized with apoB in atherosclerotic lesions [23], and recent experiments demonstrate co-localization of apoE-containing lipoprotein with biglycan [24]. CSPG complexes are avidly taken up by macrophages and contribute to foam-cell formation during atherogenesis [25,26]. Altered GAG chain structure induced by TGF-β1 and PDGF may exhibit different affinities for lipoproteins. For example, CSPGs isolated from proliferating ASMC bind with greater affinity to LDL than those isolated from quiescent ASMC [27]. Length and molecular weight of CS chains have been positively correlated with their ability to complex to low density lipoproteins [28−30]. In addition, predominance of the C-6-S form of the CS chain has been shown to promote lipid interaction and the acceleration of oxidation of LDL [31].

Since versican/PGM from ASMC interacts with HA, and HA is also present in developing vascular lesions, a question of importance is whether HA synthesis is regulated by mechanisms that regulate versican/PGM synthesis by ASMC. Both PDGF and TGF-β1 stimulate HA synthesis by ASMC and this stimulation increases the HA-rich pericellular matrix that surrounds ASMC (Evanko and Wight, unpublished observations). These results suggest that the synthesis of versican/PGM and a versican/PGM-binding glycos-aminoglycan are co-regulated, whether or not the interaction between these two ECM molecules influences the extent of matrix that surrounds ASMC.

In summary, it is clear that the synthesis of specific families of PGs by ASMC is under the control of a specific set of cytokines and growth factors. This regulation involves both core protein synthesis and the GAG synthetic machinery. It is postulated that these structural changes induced in PGs and associated molecules influence the biological activity of these molecules. Identification of the mechanisms that regulate the expression of these molecules offers the potential for targeted therapeutic intervention of vascular lesion development.

Acknowledgements

The authors gratefully acknowledge the assistance of Drs Erkki Ruoslahti, Richard Le Baron of the La Jolla Cancer Research Center and Dr Larry Fisher from National Institute of Dental Research, NIH for providing probes and antibodies used in this study. The work was supported by a grant from the National Heart, Lung, and Blood Institute, NIH, # 18645. Special thanks to Ms Barbara Kovacich for the typing of this manuscript.

References

1. Wight TN, Heinegard D, Hascall VC. In: Hay ED (ed) Cell Biology of the Extracellular Matrix. New York: Plenum Press, 1991;45−78.

2. Wight TN. Arteriosclerosis 1989;9:1−20.
3. Richardson MI, Ihnatowycz I, Moore S. Lab Invest 1980;43:509−516.
4. Stary HC. Eur Heart J 1990;11(suppl E):3−19.
5. Merrilees MJ, Beaumont B. J Vasc Res 1993;30:293−302.
6. Nievelstein PFEM, Fogelman AM, Mottino G, Frank JS. Arteriosclerosis 1991;11:1795−1805.
7. Radhakrishnamurthy B, Srinivasan SR, Vijayagopal P, Berenson GS. Eur Heart J 1990;11:148−157.
8. Wagner WD. Ann NY Acad Sci 1985;454:52−68.
9. Camejo G. Adv Lipid Res 1982;19:1−53.
10. Camejo G, Hurt-Camejo E, Olsson U, Bondjers G. Curr Opin Lipid 1993;4:385−391.
11. Reissen R, Isner JM, Blessing E, Loushin C, Nikol S, Wight TN. Am J Pathol 1994;144:962−974.
12. Swedburg SH, Brown BG, Wight TN, Gordon D, Nichols SC. Circulation 1989;80:1726−1736.
13. Wight TN, Kinsella MG, Qwarnström EE. Curr Opin Cell Biol 1992;4:793−801.
14. Ross R. Nature 1993;362:801−809.
15. Yao LY, Moody E, Schönherr E, Wight TN, Sandell LJ. Matrix 1994;14:213−225.
16. Iwata M, Wight TN, Carlson S. J Biol Chem 1993;268:15061−15069.
17. Miano JM Vlasic N, Tota RR, Stemerman MB. Arterioscler Thromb 1993;13:211−219.
18. Nikol S, Isner JM, Pickering JG, Kearney M, LeClerc G, Weir L. J Clin Invest 1992;90:1582−1592.
19. Schönherr E, Järveläinen HT, Sandell LJ Wight TN. J Biol Chem 1991;266:17640−17647.
20. Nikkari ST, Järveläinen HT, Wight TN, Ferguson M, Clowes AW. Am J Pathol 1994;144:1348−1356.
21. Schönherr E. Järveläinen HT, Kinsella MG, Sandell LJ, Wight TN. Arterioscler Thromb 1993;13:1026−1036.
22. Qwarnström E, Järveläinen HT, Kinsella MG, Sandell LJ, Page R, Wight TN. Biochem J 1993;294:613−620.
23. Galis Z S, Alavi MZ, Moore S. Am J Pathol 1993;142:1432−1438.
24. O'Brien K, Alper CE, Ferguson M, Wight T, Chait A. Am Heart Assoc Meeting 1994 (abstract).
25. Vijayagopal P, Srinivasan SR, Radhakrishnamurthy B, Berenson GS. Biochem J 1993;289:837−844.
26. Vijayagopal P, Srinivasan SR, Xu J-H, Dalferes ER, Radhakrishnamurthy B, Berenson GS. J Clin Invest 1993;91:1011−1018.
27. Camejo G, Fager G, Rosengren B, Hurt-Camejo E, Bondjers G. J Biol Chem 1993;268:14131−14137.
28. Alves CS, Mourão PAS. Atherosclerosis 1988;73:113−124.
29. Cardoso LEM, Mourão PAS. Arterioscler Thromb 1994;14:115−124.
30. Hermann M, Gmeiner B. Arterioscler Thromb 1992;12:1503−1506.
31. Hurt-Camejo E, Camejo G, Rosengren B, Lopez F, Ahlstrom C, Fager G, Bondjers G. Arterioscler Thromb 1992;12:569−583.

Interactions of von Willebrand factor with the vessel wall

D. Baruch, C. Denis and D. Meyer

INSERM U. 143, Hopital de Bicetre, Paris, France

Abstract. Von Willebrand factor (vWF) is a mediator of platelet adhesion to the subendothelium. Using endothelial extracellular matrices (ECM), an in vitro model for the subendothelium, we demonstrated the involvement of subendothelial vWF in platelet adhesion. We also investigated the interaction of vWF with ECM and using purified proteolytic fragments of vWF, we localized the binding domain for ECM on a fragment extending from residues 449 to 728. This fragment, which also contains a binding site for platelets, is able to promote platelet adhesion to the ECM to the same extent as intact vWF. We also characterized the nature of the interactions of vWF with type VI collagen, a potential ligand of vWF in the ECM.

The multimeric protein von Willebrand factor (vWF) is evidently essential for platelet adhesion to the vascular subendothelium under high shear rate conditions, since patients with a quantitative deficiency of vWF have a normal platelet adhesion at low shear rates but a decreased adhesion at high shear rates. Two distinct platelet glycoprotein (GP) complexes can interact with vWF: GPIb-IX mediates the initial platelet contact with the subendothelium and GPIIb-IIIa is mostly involved in platelet spreading and aggregate formation, although it also participates in platelet adhesion. Circulating plasma vWF does not bind to resting, nonactivated platelets, and several mechanisms have been shown to promote vWF interactions with platelets [1]. The antibiotic ristocetin or the venom protein botrocetin are modulators that induce in vitro the binding of soluble vWF to GPIb, through specific sequences located within a region of vWF, extending between amino acids (aa) 474 and 716, the so-called A1 domain, that contains a large disulfide loop between Cys 509 and 695 (Fig. 1). Mutations of patients with the type IIB phenotype (IIB vWD), which is characterized by an increased vWF binding to platelet GPIb, were all identified within the A1 domain. The in vivo counterpart of this modulation is not fully established. A current hypothesis is that the binding of circulating plasma vWF to the subendothelium induces a conformational change of vWF that allows its interactions with platelets [2]. Immobilization of vWF on a plastic surface also favors its interaction with the platelet GPIb in the absence of other agonist [3]. Shear rate may be considered as a modulator of platelet aggregation that changes the specificity of GPIIb/IIIa for its soluble ligand, either fibrinogen at low shear, or vWF at high shear [3].

vWF is synthesized by endothelial cells and deposited in the subendothelium, which contains a variety of potential vWF ligands, like fibrillar type I and III collagens. Our aim is to understand the importance of vWF associated to the subendothelium. To this end, we have studied the interactions of vWF with the extra-cellular matrices (ECM) of endothelial cells, as a model for vascular subendothelium. This paper will focus on the following aspects: 1) role of vWF associated to the ECM in platelet adhesion at high shear rate; 2) localization of the ECM-binding domain of vWF; 3) function of the ECM-binding domain of vWF in platelet adhesion; and 4) identification of the vWF ligand in the ECM.

Address for correspondence: Dr D. Baruch, INSERM U. 143, Hopital de Bicetre, 94275 Bicetre Cedex, France.

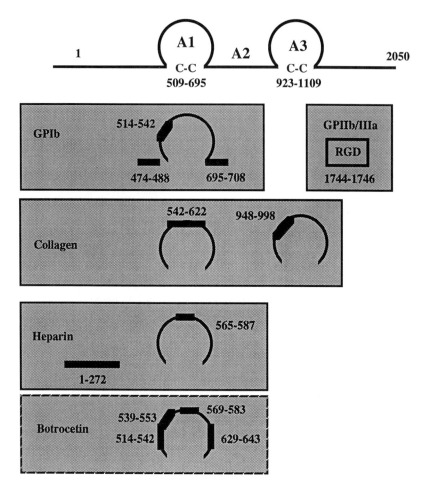

Fig. 1. Schematic representation of the von Willebrand Factor subunit, indicating the position of the disulfide loops, in the A1 domain between Cys 509 and 695, and in the A3 domain between Cys 923 and 1,109, as well as the position of the binding domains to platelet GPIb, GPIIb/IIIa, collagen, heparin and botrocetin.

Role of vWF associated to the ECM in platelet adhesion

In an attempt to clarify the role of ECM-associated vWF in platelet adhesion, we have devised a model of ECM-coated coverslips or microtiter plates that allows comparative studies of vWF binding and of platelet adhesion to either endothelial ECM which contains vWF, or to fibroblastic ECM which is devoid of it. Platelet adhesion was studied in flow conditions by means of the parallel-plate perfusion chamber [2]. We have shown that platelet adhesion to the endothelial ECM is shear rate-dependent as it is increased 3-fold between 100 s^{-1} and 1,600 s^{-1}. In contrast, varying the shear rate from 100 s^{-1} to 2,600 s^{-1} does not significantly alter the adhesion values on fibroblastic ECM. This indicates that endogenous vWF of the endothelial ECM is able to support platelet adhesion [4]. The binding of purified vWF to both types of ECM was assessed in static conditions, and the interaction of vWF with ECM was found to be specific, saturable and of an ionic nature

[4]. Therefore, we investigated whether purified plasmatic vWF, when bound to a fibroblastic ECM, could mimic the function of endogenous vWF of the endothelial ECM as a mediator of platelet adhesion at a high shear rate. We found that platelet adhesion to fibroblastic ECM preincubated with vWF was significantly enhanced, compared to preincubation with an albumin control. Interestingly, the effect of immobilization of vWF onto the fibroblastic ECM produced an increase in platelet adhesion, both in the presence and in the absence of circulating plasma vWF. In contrast, no further enhancement of platelet adhesion was observed when endothelial ECM was preincubated with vWF, and adhesion to endothelial ECM appeared maximal, even in the absence of exogenous vWF. This indicates that endogenous vWF of endothelial ECM is probably present in sufficient amounts or that it is structurally different from plasmatic vWF, so that it can support platelet adhesion at high shear rate. Indeed, we found that vWF deposited in endothelial ECM contains a higher multimeric organization than plasmatic vWF. Thus, these data suggest that endothelial ECM contains the most active form of vWF, whereas plasmatic vWF plays a complementary role when ECM-associated vWF is functionally or quantitatively impaired [4].

Localization of the ECM-binding domain of vWF

Limited proteolytic degradation of vWF to dimeric or monomeric fragments has allowed the identification of different binding domains involved in its functions [1]. The GPIb binding site has been identified on three peptides (aa 474–488, 514–542 and 695–708). The GPIIb/IIIa binding site is located on the C-terminal part and contains an RGD sequence (aa 1,744–1,746) common to several adhesive proteins. Two distinct domains interacting with type I and type III collagen have been described, one between aa 542 and 622 and a second domain between aa 948 and 998. Two binding domains for heparin have also been described, between aa 1 and 272 and between aa 565 and 587. Binding to botrocetin involves four sequences located in the A1 domain: aa 514–542, aa 539–553, aa 569–583 and aa 629–643 (Fig. 1). To assess in more detail the localization of the vWF binding site to the endothelial ECM, we used purified proteolytic fragments of vWF as competitors of the binding of ^{125}I-vWF to the ECM. We compared two complementary fragments: SpII (dimeric, aa 1,366–2,050) and SpIII (dimeric, aa 1–1,365) and found that the vWF domain interacting with the ECM was localized on SpIII [5]. No interaction was obtained in the presence of SpII, in contrast to previously reported data [6]. Three fragments (P34, aa 1–272; T116, aa 449–728; SpI, aa 911–1,365), with sequences overlapping the SpIII fragment, were compared for their ability to inhibit ^{125}I-vWF binding to ECM. We were able to localize a domain responsible for the interaction of vWF with the ECM on the T116 fragment. This fragment was isolated following trypsin cleavage and heparin-Sepharose chromatography; it had an apparent molecular mass of 116 kDa in nonreducing conditions and appeared as a doublet of 52/48 kDa in reducing conditions. The T116 fragment also contains binding domains for GPIb, heparin, type I or III collagen, sulfatides and botrocetin [1]. However, the reduced and alkylated 52/48 kDa fragment has distinct binding properties towards these substrates. Interestingly, we found that the reduced and alkylated 52/48 kDa fragment inhibited ^{125}I-vWF binding either to the ECM or to botrocetin in the same way, requiring a 10-fold higher concentration than the unreduced T116. In contrast, different effects have been reported for the interaction of the 52/48 kDa fragment with fibrillar collagen or with heparin.

Function of the ECM-binding domain of vWF in platelet adhesion

We have demonstrated that when purified plasmatic vWF is bound to the fibroblastic ECM, it can support platelet adhesion to the same extent as endogenous vWF of the endothelial ECM. The aim of the present study was to compare the functional properties of T116 and SpII, since each of these fragments contains a platelet-binding site and has been claimed to contain an ECM-binding site [5,6]. In order to have a sensitive method to detect the effect of vWF on platelet adhesion, we performed subsequent perfusion experiments at a shear rate of $1,600$ s^{-1}. We found that, when bound to fibroblastic ECM, intact vWF, SpIII, and T116 enhanced platelet adhesion to ~40%, as compared with 14.5% on the albumin control. In contrast, adhesion to fibroblastic ECM was not enhanced upon its preincubation with SpII. In addition, when endothelial ECM were preincubated with any of these fragments, no change of adhesion was observed, underlining the essential role of endogenous vWF. These results also indicate that the multimeric structure of vWF is not necessary and that the dimeric T116 is sufficient for platelet adhesion to the subendothelium [7]. Our finding that the T116 fragment can substitute for intact multimerized vWF and support platelet adhesion to the ECM leads to an interesting consideration. Since the early observations of Sakariassen, it has been suggested that a conformational change of vWF is the first step of platelet adhesion [2]. Our data suggest that vWF binding to ECM through the T116 region, also containing the binding sites to the modulator botrocetin, may involve a change of conformation of vWF that allows its interaction with the platelet GPIb. In addition, this region on the vWF subunit appears to contain all the reported mutations in patients with type IIB vWD, characterized by an increased affinity of vWF for GPIb. Investigation of the ability of vWF from these patients or recombinant mutated vWF to bind to the ECM could help elucidate the molecular mechanisms of their abnormal interaction with platelets.

Identification of the vWF ligand in the ECM

The identification of the subendothelium components that bind to vWF is still a matter of debate. Among the components known to bind the T116 fragment, the most likely candidates were fibrillar collagens and glycosaminoglycans. Studies in purified systems have shown that vWF binds to fibrillar collagens types I and III through two distinct binding sites located on the T116 and SpI fragments [1]. Experiments with purified fragments, monoclonal antibodies and a recombinant vWF deleted in the region of the T116 fragment have established that these fragments act independently of each other; however, when both sites are present, they appear to interact. Interestingly, studies with a monoclonal antibody that blocks vWF binding to type I or III collagen via the SpI domain, but not its interaction with the ECM, suggested that no binding to ECM could occur through the SpI fragment, and that fibrillar collagens were not involved as a vWF ligand in the ECM [6]. In agreement with this finding, enzymatic treatment of endothelial ECM with collagenase did not modify vWF distribution [8]. A vWF-binding protein was identified in urea extracts of the subendothelium as type VI collagen, a glycoprotein with a short triple-helical core and large globular domains, that is resistant to the effect of bacterial collagenase [9].

We have identified in endothelial ECM the presence of heparan sulfate, fibrillar type I and type III collagen, all compounds that might be relevant for their interaction with vWF. In addition, we have also shown the presence of nonfibrillar type VI collagen in endothelial ECM, thus confirming the findings of Rand et al. on vascular subendothelium [9]. We then examined whether the present work could help us identify one or more of these compounds as a potential vWF ligand in the ECM.

To follow up the notion that vWF may bind to collagen VI of the ECM, we obtained bovine skin type VI collagen purified in nondenaturing conditions, that retained an intact microfibrillar organization [10]. On the basis of competition studies of ^{125}I-vWF binding to type VI collagen by SpIII subfragments, our results suggest that two vWF fragments, T116 and SpI, are involved in the binding to purified type VI collagen. As the same proteolytic fragments of vWF that bind to type III collagen are also found to bind to type VI collagen, it is tempting to speculate that vWF binds to the fibrillar part of type VI collagen. However, the physiological importance of vWF binding to type VI collagen appears questionable, since we showed that platelet adhesion to purified type VI collagen was not increased at a high shear rate (unpublished observations).

Finally, we have identified the presence in endothelial ECM of heparan sulfate, a negatively charged polysaccharide with a composition very close to that of heparin. We have thus examined the importance of vWF binding to heparin. Heparin binding to vWF and to T116 was clearly shown to be electrostatic in nature, but no data are yet available on heparan sulfate binding to vWF. However, we found two arguments against a role of heparan sulfate as a vWF ligand in the ECM: first, neither heparin nor heparan sulfate was able to inhibit vWF binding to ECM. Second, heparinase treatment of ECM was not associated with a modification of vWF binding. It remains to be determined whether proteoglycans isolated from endothelial ECM or subendothelium are able to bind vWF.

In conclusion, we believe that the identification of the T116 fragment as the vWF domain that binds to the subendothelium helps us understand the mechanism involved in the regulation of platelet adhesion, the first step of primary hemostasis. The difficulties that we met in our attempt to identify a unique component of the ECM as a ligand specific for vWF indicate that the interaction with the ECM, rather than a unique ligand, may involve a network of several components that bind to vWF by an electrostatic mechanism.

References

1. Meyer D, Girma JP. Thromb Haemostas 1993;70:99–104.
2. Sakariassen KS, Aarts PAMM, de Groot PG, Houdijk WPM, Sixma JJ. J Lab Clin Med 1983;102:522–535.
3. Ruggeri ZM. Thromb Haemostas 1993;70:119–123.
4. Baruch D, Denis C, Marteaux C, Schoevaert D, Coulombel L, Meyer D. Blood 1991;77:519–527.
5. Denis C, Baruch D, Kielty CM, Ajzenberg N, Christophe O, Meyer D. Arterioscler Thromb 1993;13:398–406.
6. de Groot PG, Ottenhof-Rovers M, van Mourik JA, Sixma JJ. J Clin Invest 1988;82:65–73.
7. Denis C, Baruch D, Christophe O, Ajzenberg N, Girma JP, Meyer D. Thromb Haemostas 1991;65:798.
8. Wagner DD, Urban-Pickering M, Marder VJ. Proc Natl Acad Sci USA 1984;81:471–475.
9. Rand JH, Patel ND, Schwartz E, Zhou SL, Potter BJ. J Clin Invest 1991;88:253–259.
10. Kielty CM, Cummings C, Whittaker SP, Shuttleworth CA, Grant ME. J Cell Science 1991;99:797–807.

Specific features of lipid deposits associated with arterial collagen and elastin

John R. Guyton and Keith F. Klemp

Departments of Medicine and Pathology, Duke University Medical Center, Durham, North Carolina, USA

Abstract. The patterns of extracellular lipid deposits and their relations to matrix components in human atherosclerosis have been delineated by special ultrastructural techniques. Prominent localization to elastic fibers characterizes early lipid deposits, especially oily droplets comprising cholesteryl ester. Vesicular lipids are found mostly in the "open" space between matrix fibers, but may also appear in clustered masses adjacent to elastin or as isolated vesicles within collagen bundles. In the core of advanced lesions, matrix components are attenuated, and dense lipid deposits assume two contrasting patterns: (a) multilamellar vesicles associated with cholesterol crystals, and (b) small cholesteryl ester droplets.

With aging and with atherosclerosis, human arterial intima accumulates lipid in both cellular and extracellular locations. Much of the extracellular lipid appears derived from intimal lipoproteins via pathway(s) that do not involve foam-cell death. Instead, aggregation and fusion of lipoproteins and their interaction with extracellular matrix are postulated mechanisms of lipid accumulation [1].

Although knowledge about extracellular lipid deposition remains sketchy, existing evidence points toward elastic fibers as favored sites for early lipid deposition and toward proteoglycans as molecular aggregates that may bind lipoproteins containing apoB. Smith found [2] that the age-related development of perifibrous lipid adjacent to elastic fibers in the deep intima was associated with accumulation of intimal cholesteryl ester. Morphometric quantitation of perifibrous lipid visualized by electron microscopy in this laboratory confirmed that these deposits begin at about age 20 and then increase with age [3]. An interaction between intimal lipoproteins and elastin was suggested by Kramsch and Hollander [4]. Subsequent study showed that isolated normal human aortic elastin binds radioiodinated LDL with an apparent affinity constant averaging 3×10^{-8} M [5].

A number of investigators have demonstrated binding of LDL to glycosaminoglycans and, more recently, proteoglycans [6,7]. Peptides apparently derived from elastin were demonstrated among proteoglycan–lipoprotein complexes isolated from human aortic intima by Srinivasan et al. [8].

Approximately a decade ago, this laboratory developed and began to utilize new tissue-processing techniques for electron microscopy which greatly improved the recognition and characterization of extracellular lipid deposits [9]. In this paper we characterize recurring forms of lipid deposits in specimens from human aorta, including normal intima, fatty streaks, fibrolipid lesions, and fibrous plaques.

Address for correspondence: John R. Guyton MD, Department of Medicine, Box 3510, Duke University Medical Center, Durham, NC 27710, USA. Tel.: +1-919-684-3319. Fax: +1-919-681-7775.

Methods

Specimens of human aortic intima, processed by the osmium–tannic acid–paraphenyl-enediamine (OTAP) procedure and embedded in epoxy resin, were selected from tissue blocks previously utilized in a combined biochemical-ultrastructural study of lesion development [1]. Three specimens each from normal intima, fatty streaks, fibrolipid lesions, and fibrous plaques were included. Normal intima and fatty streaks with substantial deep extracellular lipid deposits were chosen for this study. Fibrolipid lesions were defined as lipid-bearing lesions distinctly raised from the luminal surface, covering no more than 16 mm² of surface. These lesions can be considered early fibrous plaques. The shoulder regions of fibrolipid lesions and fibrous plaques were examined. Thin sections were obtained at the level of the first complete elastic lamina in the intima. After locating the elastic membrane at low magnification, four micrographs were obtained at a print magnification of 12,500 at the four corners of the electron microscopic grid square.

For morphometry, a transparent grid marking 2,762 points was placed on each micrograph. When the intersections of grid lines fell on an extracellular lipid deposit, the point was counted as belonging to an oily droplet rather than a lipid vesicle and was further characterized as lipid adjacent to elastin, fibrillar collagen, open reticular space (filled by sparse proteoglycans) or basement membrane.

Results of morphometry

The results (Fig. 1) show the association between elastic fibers and lipid droplets at all four stages of lesion development. Only in more advanced lesions were extracellular lipid droplets found in substantial quantity away from elastic fibers. Lipid vesicles were sparse in normal intima and fatty streaks. In the raised lesions, substantial accumulation of lipid vesicles was demonstrated in the deep intima. Most of these vesicles appeared in the open reticular space. However, appreciable quantities of vesicles were also found associated with both collagen and elastin. Only the fibril-forming, interstitial collagen developed lipid deposits. Basement membranes, which also have a collagenous component, remained remarkably free of lipid.

Matrix components demonstrated a degree of specificity for the type of lipid deposit. Most of the lipid associated with elastic fibers was of the oily droplet form, which largely corresponds to cholesteryl ester. Most of the lipid found among collagen fibrils and in the

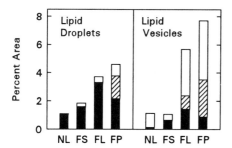

Fig. 1. Bar graph showing the relationship between extracellular lipid deposits and matrix elements at four stages of atherosclerosis development. Area fractions were obtained from 48 micrographs obtained from normal intima (NI), fatty streaks (FS), fibrolipid lesions (FL), and fibrous plaques (FP). Distributions of oily lipid droplets and lipid vesicles are represented as follows: within or adjacent to elastic fibers — solid; within or adjacent to fibrillar collagen — diagonal; in open space between matrix fibers — open.

362

open spaces was of the vesicular type, composed principally of phospholipid and free cholesterol. However, in advanced lesions, substantial amounts of droplet lipid appeared within the collagen bundles.

Specimens examined in this survey were too few to allow statistical analysis, but were representative of large numbers of specimens examined in our laboratory over the past 11 years [1,3,10–12].

Ultrastructural categories of lipid deposits

Figures 2–4 illustrate the relationship between lipid deposits and extracellular matrix. In the interior core of human fibrous plaques, two contrasting types of lipid deposits have

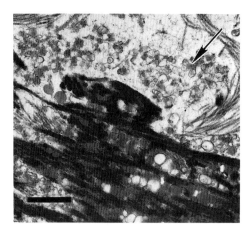

Fig. 2. Electron micrograph from human aortic fibrous plaque demonstrating lipid, mostly oily droplets comprised of cholesteryl ester interspersed with elastic fibers and an accumulation of mostly vesicular lipid (arrow) adjacent to the elastic fibers. In this instance the vesicular lipid appeared to be associated with microfibrils, but such an association was not always evident. Bar = 1 μm.

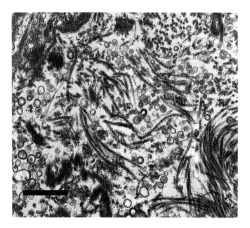

Fig. 3. Electron micrograph from human aortic fibrous plaque showing scattered lipid vesicles associated with collagen fibrils and occupying the open space between tissue matrix elements. Bar = 1 μm.

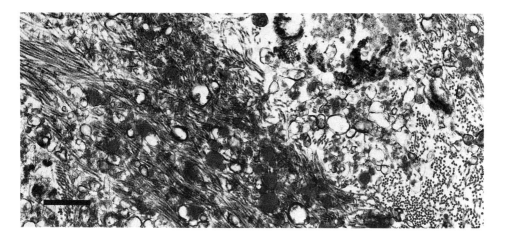

Fig. 4. Electron micrograph of advanced lipid deposition in a human aortic fibrous plaque, demonstrating oily lipid droplets within a bundle of collagen fibrils (center) and mostly vesicular lipid in open spaces (upper right and lower left). Bar = 1 μm.

been found (see micrographs in [1]). The first and slightly more common type is dense vesicular deposits with cholesterol crystals. The same kind of lipid deposition can be found in early fibrolipid lesions and even in flat lesions with the gross appearance of fatty streaks [12]. In contrast to the vesicular deposits are dense deposits of small cholesteryl ester droplets. In a recent study, we found that the fatty acyl groups of the cholesteryl esters in these deposits have a pattern similar to the cholesteryl esters in plasma lipoproteins. This fact suggests that the small cholesteryl ester droplets are derived from relatively direct extracellular processes [1,2].

Hypothetical mechanisms of lipid deposition

The purpose of descriptive research is not so much to form conclusions as it is to shape the hypotheses to be tested in experimental systems. Since lipoprotein aggregation and fusion seems likely to be involved in extracellular oily droplet formation, a pertinent question is whether some component of elastic fibers may promote this process. The hydrophobicity of elastin itself makes it a strong candidate. However, many of the droplets appear at sites where fibrillin, the major component of microfibrils, may be exposed. Finally, there may be a unique proteoglycan associated with elastic fibers. Micrographs by Volker et al. [13] suggest this possibility.

The origin of vesicular lipid is enigmatic, but it may be extraordinarily important, since vesicular deposits arise simultaneously with accumulation of free cholesterol just at the time of transition from fatty streak to fibrous plaque [12]. Hydrolysis of cholesteryl ester is almost certainly involved; hypotheses for the origin of vesicular lipid should answer where and how cholesteryl ester hydrolysis takes place. This is possibly a function of macrophages (via uptake of lipoprotein cholesteryl ester and egress of free cholesterol in some form), smooth muscle cells, an extracellular enzyme, or perhaps even lipoprotein oxidation.

References

1. Guyton JR, Klemp KF. Arterioscler Thromb 1994;14:1305—1314.
2. Smith EB. Adv Lipid Res 1974;12:1—49.
3. Guyton JR, Bocan TM, Schifani TA. Arteriosclerosis 1985;5:644—652.
4. Kramsch DM, Hollander W. J Clin Invest 1973;52:236—247.
5. Podet EJ, Shaffer DR, Gianturco SH, Bradley WA, Yang CY, Guyton JR. Arterioscler Thromb 1991;11:116—122.
6. Wagner WD, Edwards IJ, St Clair RW, Barakat H. Atherosclerosis 1989;75:49—59.
7. Camejo G, H-Camejo E, Olsson U, Bondjers G. Curr Opin Lipid 1993;4:385—391.
8. Srinivasan SR, Yost C, Radhakrishnamurthy B, Dalferes ER Jr, Berenson GS. Atherosclerosis 1981;38:137—147.
9. Guyton JR, Klemp KF. J Histochem Cytochem 1988;36:1319—1328.
10. Bocan TM, Schifani TA, Guyton JR. Am J Pathol 1986;123:413—424.
11. Guyton JR, Klemp KF. Am J Pathol 1989;134:705—717.
12. Guyton JR, Klemp KF. Am J Pathol 1993;143:1444—1457.
13. Volker W, Schmidt A, Buddecke E. Atherosclerosis 1989;77:117—130.

Atherosclerosis X.
F.P. Woodford, J. Davignon and A. Sniderman, editors.

Interaction of low density lipoprotein with proteoglycans: molecular basis and consequences

Germán Camejo[1,2], Eva Hurt-Camejo[1], Urban Olsson[1], Birgitta Rosengren[1] and Göran Bondjers[1]

[1]*Wallenberg Laboratory for Cardiovascular Research, Göteborg University, Göteborg, Sweden;* [2]*Astra Hässle Preclinical Research Laboratories, Mölndal, Sweden*

Abstract. Association of low density lipoproteins (LDL) with intima proteoglycans (PG) is mediated by the surface distribution of positively charged segments of the apoB100. The reversible association with PG and glycosaminoglycans (GAG) induces structural alterations of the LDL particle that increase its uptake by macrophages. In addition, the structural changes accelerate proteolytic and oxidative modifications of LDL. These phenomena, which help to control deposition of apolipoprotein B in the healthy intima, may contribute to atherogenesis if they saturate the tissue capacity to process products of LDL accumulation.

The association of lipoproteins with extracellular proteoglycans (PG) was recognized as an atherogenic mechanism more than 45 years ago [1]. In the intervening years was established the ionic nature of the interaction and that it is modulated by structural features of the apoB100 molecule (for review see [2]). In the extracellular intima of a progressing lesion different types of associations exist between low density lipoproteins (LDL) and PG. We can therefore extract soluble complexes of apoB-lipoproteins with PG from human and rabbit lesions as well as insoluble large aggregates at different stages of modification [3,4]. We studied reversible associations because they may provide insights into the initial phases of LDL immobilization.

Effects of proteoglycans on LDL structure

Aggregates of human LDL with chondroitin sulfate-rich PG of the human arterial intima (versican) are formed at low ionic strength and low Ca^{++}. They are dissociated into molecularly dispersed particles if the NaCl concentration is raised [5]. Low-angle X-ray diffraction and differential scanning calorimetry suggest that after association with versican and dissociation the organization of the lipid and protein moieties of LDL is disrupted. This also causes increased exposure of arginine- and lysine-rich segments on the particle surface [6]. Irreversible aggregates of LDL with arterial PG, with fusion of the lipoprotein particles, are obtained from arterial lesions or can be prepared in vitro by use of high Ca^{++} [4,7].

Molecular basis of the association of apoB100 and proteoglycans

The first approach used to identify segments of apoB100 that bind to GAG was to obtain fragments of apoB100, to establish which of them bind to GAG (mostly to heparin), and finally to sequence them (for a comprehensive review see [8]). We used a strategy that became available once the sequence of apoB100 was known [9]. Segments of apoB100 with a high probability of residing in the particle surface and with an excess of positive charges (Arg, Lys) were identified and chemically synthesized, as well as other regions that do not share such properties. Frontal elution affinity chromatography and competition experiments suggest that a minimum of three noncontiguous segments may be responsible for the association of LDL with the CS-rich arterial versican [10,11]. These segments are: 3147–3157 (SVKAQYKKNKHRH), 3359–3377 (**RLTRKRGLKLATALSLSNK**) and 2106–2121 (**RQVSHAKEKLTALTKK**). The bold letters indicate the positively charged aminoacyl residues; **R** = Arg and **K** = Lys. The helical representation of segments 3147–3157 and 3359–3377 suggests that one side of the region will contain most of the positive charges and the other side an excess of hydrophobic residues. The distribution of positive charges in the apoB100 segments fits reasonably well with the distribution of negative charges suggested by models of an octasaccharide of chondroitin-6-SO$_4$ (C6S) [11]. Olsson, at our laboratory, synthesized a modified apoB segment 3359–3367 in which the positive region was flanked by hydrophobic tails (VVWRLTRKRGLKVVV). This allowed the peptide to be bound to liposomes, LDL and VLDL. The liposomes acquired C6S-binding capacity and the LDL and VLDL markedly increased their affinity for C6S [12].

The apoB100 segments 3147–3157 and 3359–3367 are separated linearly by 202 residues. However, apoB100 appears to have a loop in this region forced by a disulfide bridge between cysteine, residues 3167 and 3297 [9]. The two positive patches 3147–3157 and 3359–3367 could therefore be much closer than their linear separation indicates. To explore the effect of bringing these positive segments together Olsson synthesized a heterodimer where the above segments were separated by a flexible joint of three glycines. The heterodimer showed a much higher affinity for C6S than the individual segments. This suggests that in a large apoB100-containing particle, like VLDL with low affinity for PG and GAG, the positive segments may be separated but that in a smaller one like LDL, with high affinity, they may come together. This model could explain the increase in affinity for C6S observed with diminished triglyceride content (size) of VLDL subfractions [12] and the inverse relationship between size of LDL subfractions and affinity for arterial versican that Hurt-Camejo et al. characterized [13]. In addition we found that small, dense LDL particles have higher affinity for versican. Furthermore, after being associated and dissociated from the PG the small LDL is taken up more efficiently by human macrophages than the less dense, large LDL. The increase in affinity for PG with decreasing size of LDL subfractions was related to a decreased surface area accessible to the apoB100, a situation that could bring closer originally distant segments of apoB100 or increase their exposure to the aqueous milieu. We and others found that LDL with high affinity for arterial proteoglycans is more often found in subjects with signs and symptoms of cardiovascular disease [2]. It should be interesting to explore whether the above correlation is caused by the high prevalence of small, dense LDL in subjects with cardiovascular disease.

Three properties of the PG appear to control their association with apoB-containing lipoproteins: nature of the GAG chains, degree of sulfation of the disaccharide subunits and length of the chains [8]. The C6S-rich versican is the most abundant PG in the extracellular arterial intima. Decorin, a dermatan PG, appears mainly to be a crosslinker of collagen fibers of the intima, whereas heparan PG are mostly associated with the endothelial cells, both at the luminal cell membrane and at the abluminal side forming part of the basement membrane. Versican can form large aggregates with hyaluronic acid and the monomers can contain several GAG chains with different length and proportion of C6S, C4S and dermatan. Wagner et al. found that atherosclerotic lesions contain CS-PG with longer CS chains. In a recent interesting study Mourao et al. [14] showed that the susceptibility to atherosclerosis of human arteries correlates with the in vitro affinity of their CS-GAG for LDL and that the chains of GAG with high LDL affinity were longer than those of low affinity. We found that human arterial smooth muscle cells (HASMC) synthesize versican with longer CS-GAG chains when they are proliferating than when quiescent. Furthermore, both the proteoglycan and GAG of the proliferating cells showed 2–3 times higher affinity for LDL at physiological ionic conditions than the PG and GAG of resting cells [15]. This suggests that at sites of cell proliferation in the intima an extracellular matrix with high affinity for LDL may well exist.

Consequences of the association of LDL with intima proteoglycans

It is not difficult to imagine that increased residence time may provide extended opportunities for hydrolytic (enzymatic) and oxidative modifications of the LDL in the intima. We have discussed how the reversible association with GAG and PG increases the rate of proteolytic fragmentation of apoB100 in LDL. Attack by secretory phospholipase A_2 could explain the enrichment in sphingomyelin observed in apoB-containing particles isolated from lesions. The two products of the reaction, polyunsaturated fatty acids and lysolecithin, will be taken up immediately by the 20–40 mM albumin present in the extracellular milieu. In vitro evidence suggests that binding to PG may increase the susceptibility to Cu^{++} and cell-mediated oxidation, a phenomenon possibly associated with a proteoglycan-induced increased affinity of LDL for Cu^{++} [16].

The alterations in LDL structure induced by the reversible association with intima proteoglycans cause a 2- to 4-fold increase in its binding, uptake and degradation by human monocyte-derived macrophages (HMDM). In 24-h incubations of HMDM with PG-treated LDL, the cells develop lipid vacuoles by a combination of LDL internalization and by increasing the endogenous synthesis of phospholipids, cholesteryl esters and triglycerides. Competition experiments indicate that the pathway followed for LDL internalization uses the apoB,E receptor, not the scavenger receptor. It is unlikely that phagocytosis is involved because in our conditions LDL remains monodisperse. The augmented uptake of LDL was not accompanied by downregulation of the endogenous cholesterol synthesis. Vijayagopal et al. [7] found that HMDM take up PG-LDL aggregates obtained from lesions or formed in vitro at high Ca^{++} via pathways different from the apoB,E receptor. These complexes also caused foam-cell formation. This suggests that HMDM interact with PG-LDL irreversible complexes otherwise than with LDL that has been modified by a reversible association with PG. The two types of LDL may exist in the intima. As discussed above, reversible association of LDL with arterial PG and GAG potentiates its oxidation by Cu^{++}, HMDM and human arterial smooth muscle cells. The rapidly oxidized LDL, depending on the extent of modification, was taken up by macrophages by pathways different from those of the apoB,E and scavenger receptor [16].

Conclusions

It is possible to envision several ways in which the association of apoB100 lipoproteins with PG in the intima may increase their potential atherogenicity by a self-sustained sequence of events. However, in healthy regions of the artery, the interactions constitute part of processes that control the potentially damaging accumulation of the lipoproteins. It is possible that only when the mechanism is saturated by excess lipoprotein entry or accretion of extracellular matrix, as during cell proliferation, do these processes become part of an atherogenic cycle.

368

Acknowledgements

This research was supported by grants from the Swedish Medical Research Council, The Swedish Heart and Lung Foundation and Astra Hässle AB.

References

1. Faber M. Arch Pathol 1949;48:342–350.
2. Camejo G, Hurt-Camejo E, Olsson U, Bondjers G. Curr Opin Lipid 1993;4:385–391.
3. Srinivasan SR, Dolan P, Radhakrishnamurthy B, Pargaonkar PS, Berenson GS. Biochim Biophys Acta 1975;388:58–70.
4. Camejo G, Hurt E, Romano M. Biomed Biochim Acta 1985;44:389–401.
5. Hurt E, Bondjers G, Camejo G. J Lipid Res 1990;31:443–454.
6. Camejo G, Hurt E, Wiklund O, Rosengren B, López F, Bondjers G. Biochim Biophys Acta 1991;1096:253–261.
7. Vijayagopal P. Biochem J 1994;301:675–681.
8. Jackson RL, Busch SJ, Cardin AD. Physiol Rev 1991;71:481–539.
9. Chan L. J Biol Chem 1992;267:25621–25624.
10. Camejo G, Olofsson S-O, López F, Carlsson P, Bondjers G. Arteriosclerosis 1988;8:368–377.
11. Olsson U, Camejo G, Olofsson S-O, Bondjers G. Biochim Biophys Acta 1991;1097:37–44.
12. Olsson U, Camejo G, Bondjers G. Biochemistry 1993;32(7):1858–1865.
13. Hurt-Camejo E, Camejo G, Rosengren B, López F, Wiklund O, Bondjers G. J Lipid Res 1990;31:1387–1398.
14. Cardoso LE, Mourao PA. Arterioscler Thromb 1994;14:115–124.
15. Camejo G, Fager G, Rosengren B, Hurt CE, Bondjers G. J Biol Chem 1993;268(19):14131–14137.
16. Hurt-Camejo E, Camejo G, Rosengren B et al. Arterioscler Thromb 1992;12:569–583.

Atherosclerosis X.
F.P. Woodford, J. Davignon and A. Sniderman, editors.

Vessel wall matrix: an overview

Sean Moore and Misbahuddin Z. Alavi
Department of Pathology, McGill University, 3775 University St., Montreal, Canada H3A 2B4

This workshop has reviewed some of the features of the vessel wall matrix and alterations of it that play significant parts in the genesis and evolution of the atherosclerotic plaque. In a larger perspective it has focused our attention on the changes in the vessel wall that are important in the atherosclerotic process. Sometimes we are inclined to overlook the part played by the vessel wall in atherogenesis. We were reminded of this 60 years ago by Lyman Duff who observed "there is every reason to believe that local injury to the walls of arteries is an essential factor and the primary event in the development of atherosclerosis in man". He also opined that in the lipid-rich arterial lesions, following cholesterol supplementation of the diets of animals, "swelling of the subendothelial ground substance appears always to be the forerunner, and it seems entirely probable therefore that a similar swelling of the intima precedes the earliest deposition of fatty substances". He regarded this experimental model as a form of arterial wall injury, supported by the observation that such diets caused necrosis of aortic, medial smooth muscle cells (SMC). This observation, although confirmed by other investigators, has received scant attention as have the deleterious effects on animals fed large amounts of cholesterol. These include lipid deposition in the monocytes or macrophages of the reticulo-endothelial system, including the Kupffer cells of the liver and the mesangial cells of the renal glomeruli. Hemolytic anemia and eventually cirrhosis of the liver occur.

These early, astute observations by Duff provide a text for considering the role of the matrix in atherogenesis. Moreover, they lend credence to the theory of atherosclerosis as a response to injury. Injury to the endothelium, of almost any type, results in the development of lesions which mimic the human disease. We and others have shown that such lesions accumulate lipid in the thickened neointima, covered by regenerated endothelium [1]. This occurs in the absence of dietary lipid supplements. This fact bears repeating because it still continues to be asserted that atherosclerosis cannot be induced experimentally in the absence of the feeding of cholesterol or saturated fats. Accordingly, I would like to review the evidence that damage to the endothelium alone can reproduce all the kinds of lesions observed in spontaneously occurring human atherosclerosis. While these observations are from our work in the field, they are corroborated by the observations of others. Also, it is of interest to link these observations with those concerning alterations in the vessel matrix that are of importance in atherogenesis.

Our interest in this arose because of a fortuitous observation made when attempting to cause hypertension in rabbits by embolizing the kidneys with aggregates of platelets. The plastic catheters which carried the magnesium–aluminum source of platelet emboli were placed in the aortas of rabbits by way of a femoral artery. In the rabbits after sacrifice it was noticed that raised, yellow lesions were present where the catheter appeared to impinge on the aortic wall. These lesions were similar to the raised lesions of human atherosclerosis and were covered by platelet–fibrin thrombus, beneath which a lipid pool, enclosed by SMC, was present. In the surface thrombus macrophages were seen. Cholesterol clefts in the lipid pool were prominent. Some lesions also showed calcification and ossification. As well as the raised lesions, transient fatty streaks were observed [2]. The lesions induced by catheter placement regressed when the catheter was removed. Exposure of the animals to antiplatelet serum markedly inhibited or prevented the development of the raised lesions. As lesions regressed and lipid was apparently removed, the interstitial content of proteoglycans of large particle size as identified on electron microscopy by ruthenium red staining decreased. This was an indication that lipid accumulation might be related to the presence of proteoglycans in the lesions. Using a Boyden chamber we found that material released from platelets, later shown by Grotendorst to be platelet-derived growth factor, stimulated SMC migration through carbonate filters. This migration only occurred if the filters were coated with gelatin, another indication of the importance of the matrix for cell movement.

In an experiment designed to cause more selective vessel-wall injury, confined to the endothelial layer, a balloon catheter was employed. This caused intimal thickening, composed entirely of SMC. In the areas where lipid accumulated, regrowth of endothelium was observed. In the uncovered areas, morphological evidence of lipid was much less or absent and, if present, was confined to the deep layers of the neointima. A morphometric study showed numerous large-granule proteoglycans in the matrix of the white areas (covered by regenerated endothelium) and very few in the blue areas (remaining uncovered by endothelium). These images are considered to represent either dermatan or chondroitin sulfate-rich proteoglycans [3].

These morphological observations led us to examine more closely the synthesis and accumulation of glycosaminoglycans in atherosclerosis induced by endothelial injury. It was found that synthesis by the neointimal SMCs was increased. The synthesis in the white areas exceeded that in the blue areas. However, GAG was retained in the white areas and quickly lost into the medium from the blue areas in an organ culture system. This led to the concept of the reverse-barrier function of the endothelium, since presumably lipoprotein–proteoglycan (LP-PG) complexes were formed in both areas but equilibrated with the blood stream in the blue areas lacking an endothelial cover. It was further shown that PG from neointima, developed in response to endothelial injury, bound lipoprotein more avidly than proteoglycan recovered from uninjured aortic intima-medial tissue. The binding to very low density lipoprotein (VLDL) was greater than that to low density lipoprotein (LDL), and dietary cholesterol supplementation increased the binding still further [4].

Binding was greater to the proteoglycan-rich aortic tissue extract described by Camejo and since chondroitin sulfate was the chief component of that material we decided to examine the spatial relationships between apolipoprotein (apo)B and chondroitin sulfate in the injured aorta compared to the normal aorta [5]. We had previously shown, using protein-A gold-labeled endogenous rabbit apoB, that it accumulated throughout the injury-derived neointima covered by regenerated endothelium. It was also abundantly present in the normal intima, as had been shown many years ago by Elspeth Smith. In the normal, uninjured endothelium gold-labeled particles were observed in coated pits as well as elsewhere in the membrane, which suggests uptake by receptor-mediated and receptor-independent mechanisms. Using gold immunoconjugates of two different sizes, one on each face of the same grid, viewed on electron microscopy, apoB and chondroitin sulfate colocalization was observed in the neointima in the extracellular space. It was also present on the membrane of SMCs and within the cells. This indicated that LP-PG complexes formed in the extracellular space were taken up and internalized by the SMCs.

This interaction of LP-PG complexes with cultured SMCs was explored. The binding, internalization and degradation of LP and LP-PG complexes by SMC were assayed [6].

Lipoprotein in the LP-PG complexes extracted from normal (uninjured) aortic tissue were bound, internalized and degraded more than LP alone, and LP-PG complexes from injured aorta more than those from normal aorta. Excess unlabeled lipoprotein inhibited all three functions. Cytochalasin also inhibited. However, polyinosinic acid, an inhibitor of the scavenger receptor, had only a small effect. These findings indicate that uptake and degradation are mediated mainly by phagocytosis and by a mechanism or mechanisms which can be inhibited by the presence of excess lipoprotein. This may involve the apoB/E receptor and possibly another receptor mechanism.

These studies of the metabolism of lipoprotein in the neointima of injury-induced atherosclerosis, as they relate to proteoglycans, has another feature, which is of importance in understanding the influence of the various lipoprotein particles on the development of atherosclerosis. This is, that there is no virtually no interaction of high density lipoprotein (HDL) with PG [4]. Thus HDL is not trapped in the neointima and is free to mobilize cholesterol from the arterial wall and to inhibit the binding of other lipoproteins with PG. The many epidemiological studies showing the favorable effects of an increased HDL to LDL ratio are congruent with this observation.

In a study of the reactivity of PG isolated from human aortas with LDL from control subjects compared with LDL-B from subjects with hyperapobetalipoproteinemia, equal reactivity in terms of precipitable complexes was found [7]. This may mean that small-particle LDLs which can more readily traverse the endothelium are equally reactive with arterial wall PG, suggesting a mechanism for increased accumulation of LP in subjects with hyperapobetalipoproteinemia. In previous studies it was shown that permeability of the intima to lipoprotein was increased by injury. Subjects with hyperapobetalipoproteinemia have been shown to be at increased risk for clinical events related to atherosclerosis, even though many have normal blood cholesterol levels. Similar considerations apply to the small-particle LDL associated with hyperinsulinemia.

There are many factors in diabetes mellitus which might facilitate the development of atherosclerosis. We have recently examined changes in glycosaminoglycan content in the aortic intima of human subjects from Type II diabetics and nondiabetics. We found a decrease in the ratio of heparan sulfate to dermatan sulfate, which was greatest in atheromatous plaques from diabetics, followed by plaques from nondiabetics and least from nonlesion areas from diabetics [8]. A similar difference has been observed in Chinese subjects from districts with high and low prevalence of atherosclerosis.

These findings in human atherosclerosis and human atherosclerosis with diabetes differ considerably in terms of GAG content of the PG from those of injury-induced atherosclerosis. Tom Wight has recently shown some differences in PG type between the recurrent lesions after angioplasty and atheromas sampled by atherectomy [9]. Reports by a number of authors have shown that endothelial cells stimulate proliferating SMCs to produce PG, mainly of the chondroitin sulfate-rich variety and that the chain length of these molecules is increased, resulting in larger, isomeric, chondroitin sulfate PGs [10].

It is possible that in the early response to injury or whatever stimulus, presumably signaled by modified or stimulated endothelial cells, causes SMC migration and proliferation, chondroitin sulfate is the main product of SMC synthesis. Later, perhaps, dermatan sulfate may be the chief product.

We have also learned about binding of LP to collagen and elastin, possibly representing a later stage of atherogenesis. In older lesions of atherosclerosis it has been observed that PG content decreases [11]. It is thus feasible to envisage a sequence of matrix changes, all associated with and facilitating lipid deposition, with later uptake by the SMCs, and later still by macrophages in relation to the central lipid core, resulting

372

from cell disintegration.

Apart from binding of lipoprotein causing its retention in the thickened intima, there are many other changes in the matrix regulating the migration, proliferation and adhesion of cells as well as synthesis of agents affecting these processes. Aspects of these have been discussed by the papers of Marlene Rabinovitch (pp 338–349) and Tom Wight (pp 350–354). Elspeth Smith has emphasized (pp 334–347) the importance of fibrinogen and fibrin split products and has related these to a likely early lesion, the gelatinous or edematous plaque. Her paper (pp 334–337) and that of Dominique Baruch (pp 355–359) again emphasize the importance of thrombosis at all stages of the process. The importance of the structural proteins of the matrix in the binding and retention of lipoprotein has been discussed by John Guyton (pp 360–364) and German Camejo (pp 365–368).

All of these observations support a concept of atherogenesis as a response to injury or, if not injury, some mechanism altering the function of endothelial cells, leading to the formation of a neointima. In the intercellular spaces of the neointima, trapping of lipoprotein occurs and one can visualize a sequence of attachment first to fibrin, then to chondroitin sulfate-rich PG, later to PG containing a preponderance of dermatan sulfate, then to collagen and elastica. The ability of SMCs to take up PG-LP complexes has been established. The interaction of complexes of LP with the other structural proteins remains to be explored. Many of the signalling interactions involved in cell proliferation, migration, and matrix production have yet to be elucidated. Further understanding of these processes should enable more rational approaches to modifying or controlling atherogenesis.

References

1. Moore S, Belbeck LW, Richardson M, Taylor W. Lab Invest 1982;47:37–42.
2. Moore S. Lab Invest 1973;29:478–487.
3. Richardson M, Ihnatowycz IO, Moore S. Lab Invest 1980;43:509–516.
4. Alavi MZ, Galis Z, Li Z, Moore S. Clin Invest Med 1991;14:419–431.
5. Galis Z, Alavi MZ, Moore S. Am J Pathol 1993;142:1432–1438.
6. Ismail NAE, Alavi MZ, Moore S. Atherosclerosis 1994;105:79–87.
7. Wasty F, Alavi MZ, Li Z, Cianflone K, Sniderman AD, Moore S. Can J Cardiol 1992;8:605–610.
8. Wasty F, Alavi MZ, Moore S. Diabetologia 1993;36:316–322.
9. Reissen R, Isner JM, Blessing E, Loushin C, Nikol S, Wight TN. Am J Pathol 1994:144:962–974.
10. Vijayagopal P, Ciolino HP, Berenson GS. Biochim Biophys Acta 1992;1135:129–140.
11. Stevens RL, Colombo M, Gonzaless JJ, Hollander W, Schmid K. J Clin Invest 1976;58:470–481.

After quantitative trait locus mapping: isolation of novel genes controlling plasma cholesterol levels in mice and in humans

C.H. Warden and A.J. Lusis

Departments of Medicine and Microbiology and Molecular Genetics, University of California at Los Angeles, Los Angeles, California, USA

Abstract. Systematic detection of genes that control plasma cholesterol levels has been made practical by the discovery of rapid and inexpensive methods for the generation of systematic linkage maps in mouse crosses or in human families. This review focuses on the use of quantitative trait locus (QTL) mapping for the systematic identification of genes that control serum cholesterol levels. QTL mapping uses systematic linkage maps to identify genes that control serum cholesterol levels, or any other indicator of complex disease, without any need for biochemical or physiological understanding of the basis of the disease. Loci identified by systematic linkage maps can then be used to guide studies directed at isolating individual disease-causing genes.

Known mutations affecting plasma cholesterol may account for approximately 10% of population variance, thus novel genes affecting serum cholesterol levels remain to be identified ([1] and Lusis AJ, unpublished calculations).

Quantitative trait locus mapping in mice

Many genes causing complex diseases have been identified by examination of single candidate genes; however, these approaches cannot systematically identify all of the genes causing complex diseases. Quantitative trait locus (QTL) mapping is a general method that does not require any previous knowledge about the underlying physiology of the disease being studied and that can systematically identify loci underlying complex diseases. QTL mapping in mice involves four basic steps: make a F2 intercross or backcross, phenotype and genotype the progeny, and then use statistical methods to find loci that underlie the traits of interest [2].

The principles of QTL mapping can be summarized with a mouse backcross constructed by crossing (C57BL/6J × *M. spretus*) with C57BL/6J. We have measured plasma total cholesterol levels in the backcross mice. Linkage of 148 genes with plasma total cholesterol levels has been tested by LOD score analysis with the MAPMAKER/QTL program that revealed peak LOD scores of 5.6 and 5.8 on mouse chromosomes 6 and 7, respectively [3]. The 90% confidence interval for these QTLs spans 10–20 centimorgans and thus includes many genes. However, these QTLs identify novel loci, since neither QTL contains any candidate genes previously suggested to control plasma cholesterol levels.

Address for correspondence: Craig Warden PhD, Department of Medicine, Division of Cardiology, UCLA, Los Angeles, CA 90024-1679, USA. Tel.: +1-310-206-0133. Fax: +1-310-794-7345. E-mail: warden@biovx1.biology.ucla.edu

QTL mapping can be applied to humans

The principles of human QTL mapping have been previously discussed [4]. Problems with the analysis of complex diseases in humans can include: genetic heterogeneity, incomplete penetrance, and synthetic traits resulting from gene interactions. It is possible to estimate the numbers of families and markers needed to detect the underlying genes, provided one makes several assumptions, primarily about the number of underlying genes. As an approximation, these estimates suggest that complex diseases caused by four or five major genes can be analyzed by looking at 50–100 families with three or more affected sibs, using genetic linkage maps including 300–500 highly informative markers. More complex traits would require more families and more markers.

Since systematic linkage mapping will require hundreds of thousands of genotyping reactions, the success of this approach depends on the speed and quality of genotyping methods. Methods for rapid genotyping using simple sequence-length polymorphism PCR markers that can be scored on automated DNA-sequencing machines with fluorescently labeled primers have been published recently [5]. It was reported that one person could generate 3,000 genotypes per day using the fluorescent genotyping method. This is a pace that will facilitate systematic linkage mapping studies in humans. One of the major problems facing human QTL mapping is that identification of the specific genes underlying disease may be much more difficult than QTL mapping. One approach to isolating genes underlying human QTLs would be to study homologous loci in mouse models and to then use the tools of mouse genetics to isolate the underlying gene. Congenic mouse strains constitute one available tool that may speed the studies of complex traits.

Congenic mouse strains

Congenic mouse strains provide a rich resource for the rapid identification of genes causing complex diseases. A congenic mouse strain is genetically identical to a background strain, except for a small chromosomal region derived from a donor strain. A congenic strain is created by a regimen of crossing and selection that places a gene from donor genetic sources onto a standard inbred-strain background [6,7]. Thus, comparison of phenotypes in background strains with those in congenic strains allows study of the effects of single genes derived from the donor strain, isolated from the effects of other donor strain genes [8]. If the donor DNA of a congenic strain and a QTL include the same genetic locus, and if the congenic differs from the background strain for a quantitative trait, this will provide strong confirming evidence supporting the QTL. Studies of congenic strains are also useful because they can be used to investigate the biochemistry and physiology of single loci underlying plasma cholesterol levels, whether or not the underlying genes are known. Congenic strains can be crossed to background strains to produce F2 mice; since one gene may now control cholesterol levels, these F2s can be used as tools for positional cloning. For instance, typing the F2s for serum cholesterol and genotyping for markers that fall in the donor strain chromosomal regions could be used to identify genetic markers showing no recombination with cholesterol levels.

Congenic mouse strains have been useful in the study of atherosclerosis. The *Ath-1* gene for atherosclerosis susceptibility has been located on distal mouse chromosome 1, near the apolipoprotein A-II (*Apoa2*) gene locus [9]. C57BL/6J mice are susceptible to fatty-streak development on a high-fat diet, while BALB/cJ mice do not develop fatty streaks while on the same diet. The B6.C.H-25^c congenic strain uses C57BL/6J as the background strain with BALB/cJ as the donor strain for the *H-25* minor histocompatibility locus. The *Apoa2* gene of B6.C.H-25^c is also derived from the resistant BALB/cJ. The congenic mice were susceptible to development of atherosclerosis when placed on the high-fat diet and thus the *Apoa2* gene cannot be *Ath-1* [8].

Since human families must be used as we find them, some means other than congenics must be found to narrow the span of human QTLs prior to initiating positional cloning projects.

Isolating genes underlying human QTLs

While systematic linkage maps of family members may detect novel loci controlling plasma cholesterol levels, family data are very inefficient at distinguishing between small recombination fractions, such as 0.5 vs. 5% [10]. This means that other methods must be used to isolate the specific genes that control plasma cholesterol levels. Linkage disequilibrium mapping is one such method. Linkage disequilibrium refers to the existence of nonrandom (nonequilibrium) associations between polymorphisms in the population. As an illustration, suppose alleles "A" and "a" are present in a population with frequencies of 0.5 and 0.5, as are linked alleles "B" and "b". At equilibrium, one would predict frequencies of 0.25 for "AB", "Ab", "aB", and "ab". For example, extreme linkage disequilibrium would be frequencies of 0.5 for genotypes "AB" and "ab", with genotypes "Ab" and "aB" having frequencies of 0. Linkage disequilibrium is useful for refined genetic mapping because it is only apparent over relatively short genetic distances, approximately 0.1 centimorgans. The basic approach to detecting linkage disequilibrium is to saturate the relevant locus with polymorphic markers and to look for ones that have population associations with the disease locus [10]. This approach was very helpful in the search for the Huntington disease gene [11]. However, maximum-likelihood estimates of gene location by measurement of linkage disequilibrium may not provide precise information on map position [12]. Thus, other methods must be used to isolate disease causing genes in the less than 1 centimorgan intervals identified by linkage disequilibrium mapping.

One approach to identify genes controlling plasma cholesterol levels would be to use high-resolution expression maps of cDNA clones [13]. Thousands of random cDNA clones have been isolated and partially sequenced over the last few years [14,15]. Once these cDNA clones are mapped, the resulting expression maps can be used as tools for the positional cloning of genes. Already, chromosomal locations have been determined for 320 genes isolated from a random cDNA library [16]. Integration of expression maps with linkage disequilibrium mapping may speed localization of disease causing genes, by providing a pre-existing list of candidate genes, eliminating the need to isolate expressed genes from the locus identified by linkage disequilibrium mapping. Searches of expression maps for candidate genes may be speeded even more if polished sequences, homology searches, and tissue-specific and developmental expression have been determined for the expressed sequences.

Conclusions

Our work with mice strongly suggests that systematic linkage maps can identify novel genes controlling plasma cholesterol levels. One of the biggest advantages of the systematic linkage approach is that one can narrow the list of candidate genes to those that are present in the QTLs. Identified loci can focus attention on candidate genes included in the locus. This can produce many candidates, since mouse chromosomal linkage maps include several thousand genes. The roles of candidate genes in disease can then be tested by construction of transgenic or knock-out mice and by association and linkage studies using the homologous human loci [17,18]. Loci identified in mouse models can also be used to guide the choice of congenic mouse strains for further studies.

Prospects for the identification of novel human loci causing atherosclerosis by systematic linkage mapping seem good. Nevertheless, several problems remain. Isolation of the specific underlying genes may be even more difficult than QTL mapping, requiring linkage disequilibrium mapping, expression maps, and high-throughput methods for testing dozens to hundreds of candidate genes. Furthermore, QTL mapping will probably not identify all of the genes causing atherosclerosis, because of the problems of gene interactions, high-frequency susceptibility genes, or genes with small effects [4].

Acknowledgements

Supported by DK45066 (JSF).

References

1. Breslow JL. Circulation 1993;87(suppl III):16–21.
2. Lander ES, Botstein D. Genetics 1989;121:185–199.
3. Warden CH, Fisler JS, Pace MJ, Svenson KL, Lusis AJ. J Clin Invest 1993;92:773–779.
4. Lander ES, Botstein D. Cold Spring Harbor Symposia on Quantitative Biology 1986;LI:49–62.
5. Reed PW, Davies JL, Copeman JB, Bennett ST, Palmer SM, Pritchard LE, Gough SCL, Kawaguchi Y, Cordell HJ, Balfour KM, Jenkins SC, Powell EE, Vignal A, Todd JA. Nature Genet 1994;7:390–395.
6. Graff RJ, Snell GD. Transplantation 1968;6:598–617.
7. Bailey DW. Immunogenetics 1975;2:249–256.
8. Mehrabian M, Qiao J-H, Hyman R, Ruddle D, Laughton C, Lusis AJ. Arterioscler Thromb 1993;13:1–10.
9. Paigen B, Mitchell D, Reue K, Morrow A, Lusis AJ, LeBoeuf RC. Proc Natl Acad Sci USA 1987;84: 3763–3767.
10. Bodmer WF. Cold Spring Harbor Symposia on Quantitative Biology 1986;51:1–13.
11. Pritchard C, Cox DR, Myers RM. Am J Hum Genet 1991;49:1–6.
12. Hill WG, Weir BS. Am J Hum Genet 1994;54:705–714.
13. Southern EM. Curr Opin Genet Dev 1992;2:412–416.
14. Okubo K, Hori N, Matoba R, Niiyama T, Fukushima A, Kojima Y, Matsubara K. Nature Genet 1992;2: 173–179.
15. Adams MD, Soares MB, Kerlavage AR, Fields C, Venter JC. Nature Genet 1993;4:373–380.
16. Polymeropoulos MH, Xiao H, Sikela JM, Adams M, Venter JC, Merril CR. Nature Genet 1993;4:381–386.
17. Warden CH, Daluiski A, Lusis AJ. In: Lusis AJ, Rotter JI, Sparkes RS (eds) Monographs in Human Genetics: Molecular Genetics of Coronary Artery Disease. Basel: Karger, 1992;419–441.
18. Friedman JM, Leibel RL, Bahary N. Mamm Genome 1991;1:130–144.

Expression of human apolipoprotein B in transgenic mice

Stephen G. Young[1,2], Sally P.A. McCormick[1,2], Deborah Purcell-Huynh[1,2], MacRae F. Linton[1,2,3] and Robert V. Farese Jr[1,2]

[1]Gladstone Institute of Cardiovascular Disease; [2]Cardiovascular Research Institute, Department of Medicine, University of California at San Francisco, San Francisco, CA 94141-9100; [3]Present address: Vanderbilt University Medical Center, Division of Endocrinology, Medical Center North AA4206, Nashville, TN 37232-2250, USA

Abstract. We used a 79.5-kb fragment of human genomic DNA from a P1 bacteriophage to generate transgenic mice expressing human apolipoprotein (apo)B48 and apoB100. The human apoB transgene was expressed at high levels in the liver but was not expressed in the intestine. The chow-fed females had human apoB levels of ~50–60 mg/dl, nearly as high as those in normolipidemic humans. When the transgenic animals were fed a high-fat diet, the human apoB levels increased by 30–40%, chiefly as a result of higher levels of human apoB48. After 18 weeks on a high-fat diet, the transgenic animals developed extensive aortic atherosclerotic disease.

Development of human apoB transgenic mice

In order to study apoB structure and function, apoB synthesis and secretion, and the role of apoB in atherogenesis, a number of different laboratories have tried to express human apoB in cultured cells and in transgenic mice. Blackhart and co-workers [1] were the first to develop a minigene expression vector for human apoB100. They used this vector to transfect cultured rat hepatoma cells and were able to detect low levels of human apoB in the medium from transfected cells [1]. Unfortunately, their minigene expression vector, even when it was modified to contain appropriate liver-specific promoters, did not prove useful for the expression of human apoB in transgenic mice [2]. Despite extensive efforts with a variety of minigene expression vectors, only a single human apoB transgenic line was developed, and the human apoB levels in the plasma of those mice were barely detectable by a sensitive radioimmunoassay [3].

In 1993, our group undertook a different approach to the development of human apoB transgenic mice. Rather than using a minigene expression vector, we obtained a P1 bacteriophage clone, p158, that spanned the entire human apoB gene (Fig. 1) and used the entire 79.5-kb insert from this clone to generate transgenic mice [2,4]. In addition to containing all 29 exons of the human apoB gene, the insert contained 19 kb of 5′ flanking sequences and 17.5 kb of 3′ flanking sequences. From a single preparation of p158 DNA, we obtained 16 founder transgenic animals that expressed a wide range of human apoB100 levels in their plasma [4]. The animals with the highest expression levels had human plasma apoB levels of ~50 mg/dl, nearly as high as those in normolipidemic humans. We have also used P1 bacteriophage DNA to obtain high levels of human apoB expression in cultured rat hepatoma cells [5]. Our techniques for preparing and purifying P1 DNA for microinjection into murine zygotes and transfection into cultured cells have been published in a recent review [5].

Address for correspondence: Stephen G. Young, Gladstone Institute of Cardiovascular Disease, P.O. Box 419100, San Francisco, CA 94141-9100, USA. Tel.: +1-415- 826-7500. Fax: +1-415-285-5632.

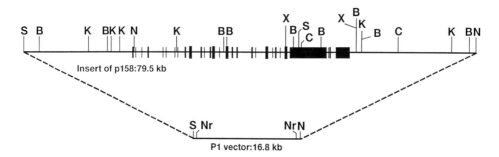

Fig. 1. Restriction map of p158. The insert of p158 is 79.5 kb in length. S, *Sal*I; B, *Bam*HI; K, *Kpn*I; X, *Xho*I; C, *Cla*I; N, *Not*I; Nr, *Nru*I. Reproduced with permission [4].

Tissue sites of transgene expression

Apolipoprotein B is normally expressed in high levels in the intestine and liver [6]; high levels of apoB expression have also been observed in fetal membranes [7]. Because the fragment that we used to generate the transgenic mice contained substantial lengths of 5′ and 3′ flanking sequences, we were hopeful that the transgene would contain all of the tissue-specific elements required for proper expression in both the liver and the intestine. To study the sites of human apoB expression in the transgenic animals, we isolated RNA from a variety of tissues from several transgenic lines and performed RNA slot blots. The results showed several unexpected findings (Fig. 2): first, although there were high levels

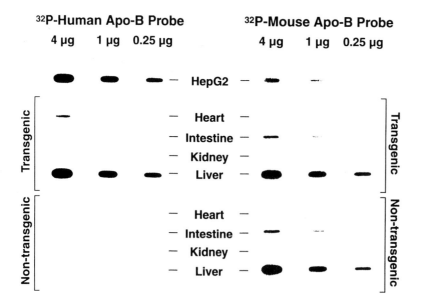

Fig. 2. RNA slot-blot analysis of human and mouse apoB expression. The left side shows a slot-blot probed with a ^{32}P-labeled human apoB cDNA probe; the right side shows an identical blot probed with a ^{32}P-labeled mouse apoB cDNA probe. The endogenous mouse apoB gene is expressed in both the liver and the intestine. The human apoB transgene is largely expressed in the liver, with small amounts of expression in the heart. No intestinal expression could be detected. Reproduced with permission [5].

of the human apoB mRNA in the liver, we observed no expression in the intestine. Second, human apoB transgene expression was detectable in the heart. In control studies in nontransgenic mice, we observed the expected pattern of expression: high levels of murine apoB in both liver and intestine, and no apoB expression in the heart. On the basis of these data, we have generated the tentative hypothesis that the P1 bacteriophage clone lacks the DNA sequences that confer intestinal expression in adult animals. We believe that understanding the DNA sequence elements that govern the intestinal expression of apoB is important and deserves further investigation.

Effects of transgene expression on the plasma lipoproteins

Although we obtained many different lines of human apoB transgenic mice, most of our studies have involved one high-expressing transgenic line (#1102) [4]. Our initial Southern blot experiments suggested that the genomic DNA of the transgenic founder of this line contained approximately 10 copies of the transgene. With transgenic line 1102, chow-fed female hemizygotes have human apoB100 levels of ~60 mg/dl; male animals consistently have lower apoB100 levels, averaging ~40 mg/dl (unpublished observations). We have found that immunoassays that measure total human apoB (apoB100 and apoB48) yield significantly higher values than the assay that measures only apoB100. This result is not surprising, because there is a substantial amount of human apoB48 in the plasma of the transgenic animals. On random blood samples taken during the light cycle, the ratio of apoB100 to apoB48 in chow-fed female transgenics is ~5:1; after a 14-h fast, the ratio is closer to 15:1. Preliminary studies of the lipoproteins of mice that are homozygous for the transgene suggest that the plasma levels of apoB in homozygous animals are twice those of hemizygotes. We have not yet established accurate and reproducible assays for mouse apoB in our laboratory. However, we have used a murine apoB-specific antiserum to probe Western blots of agarose gels, and have found no apparent difference between the amount of mouse apoB in transgenic and nontransgenic animals [4].

The total plasma cholesterol levels in the female transgenic mice are approximately 140 mg/dl, which is 30–50 mg/dl higher than those of the nontransgenic animals [4]. The higher levels in the transgenic mice can be explained by a marked increase in the amount of cholesterol in LDL-sized particles. A large LDL-cholesterol peak can be easily demonstrated by chromatographic separation of mouse plasma on a sepharose column (Fig. 3) or by discontinuous density gradient ultracentrifugation [4]. Male mice have LDL-cholesterol peaks 30–40% lower than those of female mice, a finding that is consistent with the lower levels of human apoB in the plasma of male mice (unpublished observations). The plasma of the human apoB transgenic animals shows a marked increase in the amount of β-migrating lipoproteins on lipid-stained agarose gels (Fig. 4).

The LDL in the transgenic mice has at least one major compositional difference compared with LDL in human plasma: it is enriched in triglycerides [4]. Initially, we proposed the possibility that the high levels of triglycerides in the LDL of the transgenic mice might be due to the fact that mice lack cholesterol ester transfer protein (CETP). However, transgenic mice expressing high levels of both human apoB and human CETP also have triglyceride-rich LDL (David Grass, Stephen G. Young, unpublished observations). An alternative possibility is that the triglyceride-rich LDL may represent nascent hepatic lipoproteins [4].

Both male and female human apoB transgenic mice have approximately 10% lower HDL-cholesterol levels than nontransgenic mice [8]. Although the metabolism of HDL and that of the apoB-containing lipoproteins are known to be highly interrelated [6], the

380

A.   B.

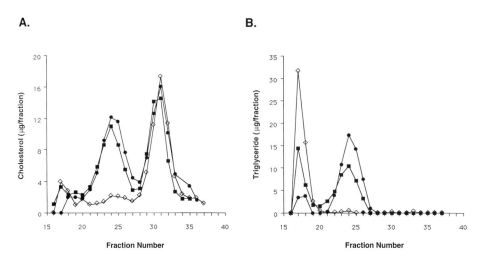

Fig. 3. Superose 6 chromatography studies demonstrating the distribution of (A) cholesterol and (B) triglyceride in plasma of transgenic and nontransgenic mice. Plasma samples (50–100 μl) from individual mice were chromatographed on a Superose 6 10/50 column. Cholesterol and triglyceride levels were measured by a colorimetric method. Fractions 16–20 contain VLDL-sized lipoproteins; fractions 22–27, LDL-sized lipoproteins; fractions 28–34, HDL-sized lipoproteins. Reproduced with permission [4].

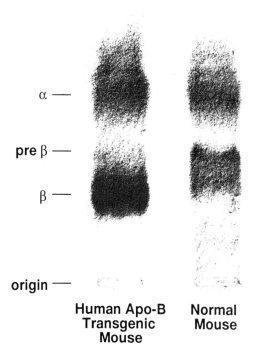

Fig. 4. Agarose gel electrophoresis of the plasma from a human apoB transgenic mouse and a nontransgenic control mouse. The gel was stained for neutral lipids with Fat Red 7B. Reproduced with permission [2].

mechanism for the slightly lower HDL-cholesterol levels in the human apoB transgenic mice is not known.

On a diet rich in fat (15%) and cholesterol (1.25%), the cholesterol levels in the transgenic mice increase by ~160 mg/dl, to ~300 mg/dl; in contrast, cholesterol levels in the nontransgenic animals increase by ~130, to ~230 mg/dl. The total apoB levels increase by ~40% on the high-fat diet, but the apoB100 levels are unchanged. This finding is because human apoB48 levels increase substantially on the high-fat diet [8].

Atherosclerosis in human apoB transgenic mice

We have performed preliminary studies on the susceptibility of the human apoB transgenic mice to the development of atherosclerotic lesions in the ascending aorta [8]. The lesions in the proximal aorta were quantified with a computerized videomicroscopy system. On a chow diet, neither the transgenic nor the nontransgenic animals developed significant atherosclerotic lesions. On a high-fat diet, the nontransgenic animals developed small lesions in the proximal ascending aorta, and most of these lesions were located within 400 μm of the aortic valve cusps. In contrast, the transgenic animals on the high-fat diet developed massive lesions throughout the proximal 1,200 μm of the aorta. The aortic lesions in the transgenic animals were more than 10 times as large as those in the nontransgenic animals. These studies establish that the overexpression of human apoB in transgenic mice causes severe atherosclerotic lesions, but only on a high-fat diet.

Lipoprotein(a) (Lp(a)) transgenic mice

Transgenic mice expressing human apo(a) had been previously developed and characterized by the laboratories of Drs Robert Hammer and Helen Hobbs [9]. The apo(a) circulates free of the lipoproteins in the apo(a) transgenic mice, because mouse apoB100 lacks the ability to bind to apo(a). Thus, the apo(a) transgenic mice have no bona fide Lp(a) in the circulation. Following the initial characterization of the human apoB transgenic mice, we sought to develop transgenic mice expressing Lp(a) [4]. By crossing the human apoB mice with the apo(a) mice, we generated mice that expressed both transgenes [4]. In these mice, all of the apo(a) was covalently bound to human apoB as Lp(a) particles. The Lp(a) could be easily distinguished from the free apo(a) because it migrated at a substantially higher position on SDS-polyacrylamide gels [4]. Interestingly, Western blots indicated that the amount of apo(a) in the plasma of the Lp(a) transgenic mice was approximately twice the amount found in the apo(a) transgenic animals [4]. These data suggest strongly that the metabolism of apo(a) is altered when it is covalently bound to apoB. Callow et al. [10] have also recently reported Lp(a) in the plasma of apo(a)/human apoB transgenic mice.

Our laboratory has also been interested in determining the structural features that are important for the disulfide cross-linking of apo(a) to human apoB100. There have been suggestions that apoB100 cysteine residue-3734 is involved in this interaction [11], but the data cannot be regarded as definitive. To identify the sequences within human apoB100 that are important for this interaction, we expressed human apoB90 (4,084 amino acids in length) in rat hepatoma cells [5] and in transgenic mice [12]. The apoB90 construct was generated by interrupting exon 29 of the full-length human apoB clone, p158, with a transposon [12]. In in vitro incubation experiments, apoB90 completely lacked the capacity to bind to apo(a). Similarly, double-transgenic mice expressing both human apoB90 and apo(a) had little or no Lp(a) in the plasma, as judged by both a sandwich radioimmunoassay and Western blots of SDS-polyacrylamide gels (Fig. 5).

382

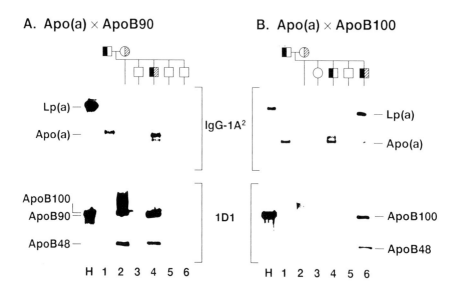

Fig. 5. Panel A shows Western blots demonstrating the absence of Lp(a) in the plasma of a mouse expressing both human apoB90 and apo(a). Plasma (1 μl) from an apo(a) transgenic male (lane 1), an apoB90 transgenic female (lane 2), and the four offspring of one litter (lanes 3–6) were electrophoresed on a 4% SDS-polyacrylamide gel under nonreducing conditions; the separated proteins were transferred to nitrocellulose membrane for immunoblotting with the apo(a)-specific monoclonal antibody, IgG-1A². As a control for the migration of Lp(a), we used 1.0 μl of human plasma (H). In parallel, each of the samples was reduced with 2-mercaptoethanol and electrophoresed on a 4% SDS-polyacrylamide gel for a Western blot with the human apoB-specific monoclonal antibody, 1D1. Panel B shows identical Western blots demonstrating the presence of Lp(a) in the plasma of a mouse expressing both human apoB100 and apo(a) transgenes. ■□, hemizygous for the apo(a) transgene; ▨, hemizygous for the apoB transgene. Reproduced with permission [12].

These studies demonstrate that the carboxyl-terminal 10% of the apoB100 sequence is important for the formation of Lp(a), presumably because it contains the cysteine residue involved in the disulfide bond or because it contains the sequences that are required for the high-affinity interaction between the two molecules. The experiments with human apoB90 obviously provide only preliminary clues regarding the structural features of apoB100 that are necessary for its interaction with apo(a). In the future, newer molecular techniques should make it possible to generate subtle mutations in the full-length human apoB gene construct, and this should permit a more systematic study of important structural domains of the apoB molecule.

Summary

We have used a fragment of genomic DNA spanning the entire human apoB gene to generate human apoB transgenic mice. We expect that these mice will be useful for studying the role of apoB in atherogenesis and metabolism. We have already generated transgenic mice expressing a truncated form of human apoB, and we expect that expression of other mutant apoB proteins will be useful for understanding various aspects of apoB structure and function.

Acknowledgements

We thank L. Hymowitz for preparing the manuscript, L. DeSimone for editorial assistance, and L. Jach for graphics. This work was supported by NIH grant 41633.

References

1. Blackhart BD, Yao Z, McCarthy BJ. J Biol Chem 1990;265:8358—8360.
2. Young SG, Farese RV Jr, Pierotti VR, Taylor S, Grass DS, Linton MF. Curr Opin Lipidol 1994;5:94—101.
3. Chiesa G, Johnson DF, Yao Z, Innerarity TL, Mahley RW, Young SG, Hammer RH, Hobbs HH. J Biol Chem 1993;268:23747—23750.
4. Linton MF, Farese RV Jr, Chiesa G, Grass DS, Chin P, Hammer RE, Hobbs HH, Young SG. J Clin Invest 1993;92:3029—3037.
5. McCormick SPA, Linton MF, Young SG. Genet Anal Tech Appl (in press).
6. Young SG. Circulation 1990;82:1574—1594.
7. Demmer LA, Levin MS, Elovson J, Reuben MA, Lusis AJ, Gordon JI. Proc Natl Acad Sci USA 1986;83: 8102—8106.
8. Purcell-Huynh DA, Farese RV Jr, Flynn LM, Pierotti V, Newland DL, Fein H, Linton MF, Sanan DA, Young SG. Circulation (in press).
9. Chiesa G, Hobbs HH, Koschinsky ML, Lawn RM, Maika SD, Hammer RE. J Biol Chem 1992;267:24369—24374.
10. Callow MJ, Stoltzfus LJ, Lawn RM, Rubin EM. Proc Natl Acad Sci USA 1994;91:2130—2134.
11. Coleman RD, Kim TW, Gotto AM Jr, Yang C-Y. Biochim Biophys Acta 1990;1037:129—132.
12. McCormick SPA, Linton MF, Taylor S, Curtiss LK, Young SG. J Biol Chem (in press).

Macrophage apoE, cholesterol metabolism, and atherosclerosis

Jonathan D. Smith, Claire Grigaux, Edmund H. Wong and Eric Shmookler

The Rockefeller University, 1230 York Avenue, New York, NY 10021, USA

Abstract. The developmental regulation of apolipoprotein (apo)E mRNA in cultured human peripheral blood monocytes and murine bone marrow monocyte-macrophages was investigated. ApoE mRNA induction was blocked by inhibitors of protein kinase C. Human apoE transgenes with various 5′ and 3′ flanking regions have failed to define the DNA regions that control macrophage apoE expression in transgenic mice. To study the role apoE plays in macrophage cholesterol metabolism, we stably transfected the murine macrophage cell line RAW264 with a SV40 promoter-driven human apoE expression vector. After cholesterol loading, only the apoE-expressing cells released free cholesterol into serum-free medium, and only in the presence of cAMP analogues. In a study of the role of monocyte-derived macrophages in atherosclerosis, apoE-deficient mice, which spontaneously develop atherosclerosis, were mated with monocyte-depleted osteopetrotic (op) mice, deficient in the cytokine M-CSF. The double mutant mice had nearly 3-fold higher plasma cholesterol levels yet less atherosclerosis in the proximal aorta than apoE-deficient controls.

Although plasma apolipoprotein (apo)E is derived primarily from liver [1], apoE is synthesized in many nonhepatic tissues including brain, skin, steroidogenic organs, and spleen [2]. Freshly isolated human peripheral blood monocytes do not express apoE mRNA, but after these cells have been cultured for several days apoE mRNA is induced [3]. A similar finding has been reported for murine bone-marrow monocytes which, when cultured for 1 week in the presence of L-cell conditioned medium as a source of macrophage-colony stimulating factor (MCSF), differentiate into macrophages and initiate apoE synthesis [4]. We have found that inhibitors of protein kinase C block the induction of apoE mRNA in these systems. Cholesterol loading of cultured macrophages induces apoE synthesis, which leads to the hypothesis that apoE may be involved in cholesterol efflux from these cells; however, apoE secretion is constitutive while cholesterol efflux depends on the presence of cholesterol acceptors such as HDL [5]. We have re-examined this hypothesis by stably transfecting RAW264 murine macrophages with a human apoE expression vector. In the absence of cholesterol acceptors, we observe cholesterol efflux only from the apoE-secreting cells and only in the presence of a cAMP analogue. Therefore, under certain conditions, apoE may play a role in cholesterol efflux from macrophages.

Current theories of atherosclerosis state that monocyte-macrophage-derived foam cells in early fatty streak lesions precede the development of advanced fibrous plaques. To prove that monocyte-derived macrophages are primarily responsible for the development of arterial foam cells in the hyperlipidemic state, we have bred hyperlipidemic apoE-deficient mice [6] with osteopetrotic (op) mice, which lack MCSF and have greatly reduced levels of circulating monocytes [7,8]. Although the double mutant mice had 2- to 3-fold higher levels of plasma cholesterol they had smaller areas of atherosclerosis lesion than apoE-deficient controls.

Results and Discussion

To probe the mechanism of apoE induction during macrophage differentiation, we cultured both human peripheral blood monocytes and mouse bone-marrow monocytes with or without inhibitors of protein kinase C. ApoE mRNA was not detected in freshly isolated human monocytes, but was found after culturing for 5 days. However, this induction was blocked if the protein kinase C inhibitor H7 was present during the 5 days in culture (Fig. 1A). Similarly, apoE mRNA was not detected in murine bone-marrow cells cultured for 3 days, but was found after culturing for 6 days with L-cell conditioned medium, as a source of MCSF. ApoE mRNA levels were decreased by treatment with 150 nM of the protein kinase C inhibitor calphostin-C, and either higher doses of calphostin C or the inhibitor H7 completely abolished the induction of apoE mRNA (Fig. 1B). These results imply that protein kinase C is involved in the signal transduction pathway leading to apoE mRNA induction during terminal differentiation of monocyte to macrophage.

Using both tissue culture and transgenic mice as assay systems, we have previously defined a 154-bp element, 14 kb 3′ of the human apoE gene that is necessary for hepatic expression of the human apoE gene [9]. None of the apoE-transgenic mice containing 5 kb of 5′ flanking sequence or various 3′ flanking regions have shown expression in peritoneal or bone-marrow-derived macrophages. Thus the DNA element specifying macrophage expression of apoE has not been determined and may be at a distance from the promoter.

In order to probe if macrophage apoE plays a role in cellular cholesterol metabolism, we stably transfected the RAW264 murine macrophage cell line with a human apoE expression vector by cotransfection with a selectable neomycin-resistance plasmid. RAW264 cells did not express endogenous murine apoE mRNA. We selected neomycin-resistant clonal populations and screened for the expression of human apoE by both RNase protection and immunohistochemical assays. Human apoE-expressing (apoE$^+$) and nonexpressing (apoE$^-$) lines were established and compared. Cells were loaded with cholesterol and labeled by overnight incubation with AcLDL preincubated with [^{3}H]cholesterol, and subsequently chased for 24 h in serum-free medium containing 0.2% BSA. Only the apoE$^+$ cells, and only in the presence of 0.1 mM 8-Br-cAMP, secreted a substantial portion of the [^{3}H]cholesterol into the medium (Fig. 2A). Thin-layer chromatography of the secreted radioactivity confirmed that it was >96% free cholesterol. To prove that this indicated a substantial efflux of cholesterol mass, the amounts of cellular free and esterified cholesterol, as well as free cholesterol released into the medium, were determined by gas–liquid chromatography. Cholesterol-loaded apoE$^+$ cells released only 1% of their total cellular cholesterol when chased in serum-free medium for

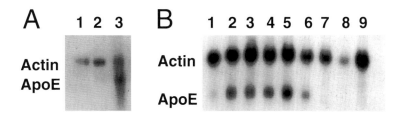

Fig. 1. Inhibition of developmental induction of apoE mRNA by protein kinase C inhibitors. Northern blots of total RNA hybridized with human (A) or mouse (B) apoE and actin riboprobes. A. Human blood monocytes were plated and RNA was prepared after 1 day (lane 1) or 5 days (lanes 2 and 3) in culture. Cells in lane 2 received 25 μM H7 after 1 day in culture. B. RNA from mouse bone-marrow monocytes after 3 days (lane 1) or 6 days (lanes 2–9) in culture. Cells in lanes 4–8 were treated with calphostin C at 5, 50, 150, 500, and 100 nM, respectively. Cells in lane 9 were treated with 25 μM H7.

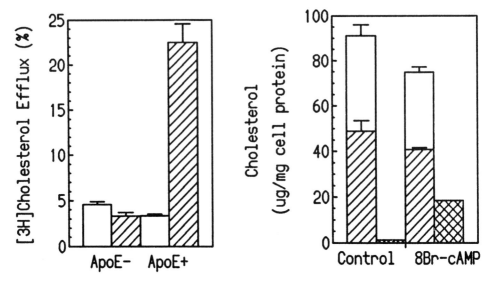

Fig. 2. Effect of 8-Br-cAMP on cholesterol efflux in stably transfected apoE⁺ RAW cells. A: ApoE⁻ and apoE⁺ cells were loaded with cholesterol and labeled with 50 μg/ml AcLDL and 0.33 μCi/ml [³H]cholesterol. Cells were chased for 24 h in serum-free medium in the absence (open bars) or presence (hatched bars) of 0.1 mM 8-Br-cAMP. Cholesterol efflux was calculated as % of total cellular plus medium radioactivity recovered in the medium (n = 3, mean ± SD). B: ApoE⁺ cells were cholesterol-loaded and chased for 24 h in the absence or presence of 0.1 mM 8-Br-cAMP. Cellular free cholesterol (hatched bars), esterified cholesterol (open bars) and medium free cholesterol (cross-hatched bars) were determined by gas–liquid chromatography and normalized to cellular protein content (n = 3, mean ± SD).

24 h, while the addition of 8-Br-cAMP during the chase led to an almost 20% release of the total cholesterol mass (Fig. 2B). Thus apoE appears to promote cholesterol efflux from this cultured macrophage cell line if a cAMP analogue is present. It is not known if macrophage apoE serves a similar function in vivo.

ApoE-deficient mice, created by homologous recombination in embryonic stem cells, are hypercholesterolemic and spontaneously develop atherosclerosis on a low-fat chow diet [6]. We have bred these mice with op mice, which have a reduced number of tissue macrophages, severe deficiencies in osteoclasts and circulating monocytes, and skeletal deformities including the lack of incisors [8,10]. After weaning, mice were maintained on a low-fat powdered diet (4.5% fat by weight) until 16 weeks of age, at which time body weights and plasma cholesterol levels were measured and the mice were sacrificed for a quantitative assay of atherosclerosis in the proximal aorta. We compared three groups: 1) op0/E0, homozygous double mutant, referring to 0 wild-type alleles at both loci; 2) op1/E0, heterozygous for the op mutation on the apoE-deficient background; and 3) op2/E0, wild type at the op locus on the apoE-deficient background. All matings were done with op1/E0 parents so that littermates comprising the three groups could be compared. The op0/E0 mice were smaller, weighing about 75% the weight of mice heterozygous or wild-type at the op locus (Table 1). The mean plasma cholesterol level of op0/E0 mice was 1,372 mg/dl, almost 3 times as high as the mean cholesterol level of the op2/E0 mice, which was 498 mg/dl. There was also a gene dosage effect, such that mean cholesterol levels were ranked, starting with the highest, op0/E0 > op1/E0 > op2/E0, with the differences between each group being statistically significant (Table 1).

Table 1. Weights and cholesterol values in op/E0 mice

Genotype	Weight (g)	Total cholesterol (mg/dl)
op2/E0 (n = 16)	27.4 ± 3.5	498 ± 135
op1/E0 (n = 16)	29.0 ± 2.2	658 ± 255[a]
op0/E0 (n = 14)	21.4 ± 4.8[b]	1372 ± 478[b]

Values are mean ± SD. [a]p < 0.04 compared to op2/E0; [b]p < 0.0005 compared to both op2/E0 and op1/E0.

For the quantitative atherosclerosis assay, the hearts were perfused in situ, removed with the attached proximal aorta, fixed in 10% buffered formalin, gelatin, embedded, cryosectioned, and stained with Oil red O and fast green, as previously described [6]. Figure 3 shows the preliminary data from an ongoing study of total lesion area for individual animals in the three groups. There is a large inter-animal variation within each group in this assay. The mean lesion areas for the op0/E0, op1/E0, and op2/E0 mice were 14,873, 34,188, and 46,345 μm^2, respectively. Although the mean difference between the op0/E0 and the op2/E0 is large, the difference is only marginally significant (p = 0.056) because of the large variation within groups and small sample size. Another way to look at these data is to determine the % of mice with lesion areas < 10,000 μm^2; these were 67, 33, and 17% for the op0/E0, op1/E0, and op2/E0 mice, respectively. Thus, we observe a strong trend towards decreased atherosclerosis lesion area in the proximal aorta of op0/E0 mice, despite their almost 3-fold higher plasma cholesterol. These studies reinforce the concept that monocyte-derived macrophages play a very important role in athero-genesis. The op0/E0 mice with their highly elevated plasma cholesterol levels and fewer monocytes develop less atherosclerosis than their op1/E0 and op2/E0 littermates.

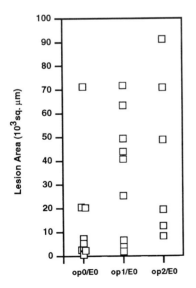

Fig. 3. Atherosclerosis in op/E0 mice. Atherosclerosis lesion area in the proximal aortas was measured from 16-week-old mice with 0, 1, or 2 wild-type alleles at the op locus on the apoE-deficient background.

388

Acknowledgements

This research was supported by a Grant-In-Aid from the American Heart Association. This work was done during the tenure of an Established Investigatorship of the American Heart Association to J.D.S.

References

1. Kraft HG, Menzel HJ, Hoppichler F, Vogel W, Utermann G. J Clin Invest 1989;83:137–142.
2. Mahley RW. Science 1988;240:622–630.
3. Zannis VS, Cole FS, Jackson CL, Kurnit DM, Karathanasis SK. Biochemistry 1985;24:4450–4455.
4. Werb Z, Chin JR. J Cell Biol 1983;97:1113–1118.
5. Basu SK, Goldstein JL, Brown MS. Science 1983;219:871–873.
6. Plump AS, Smith JD, Hayek T, Aalto-Setala K, Walsh A, Verstuyft JG, Rubin EM, Breslow JL. Cell 1992;71:343–353.
7. Wiktor-Jedrzejczak W, Bartocci A, Ferrante AW, Ahned-Ansari A, Sell KW, Pollard JW, Stanley ER. Proc Natl Acad Sci USA 1990;87:4828–4832.
8. Naito M, Hayashi S, Yoshida H, Nishikawa S, Shultz LD, Takashi K. Am J Pathol 1991;139:657–667.
9. Shachter NS, Zhu Y, Walsh A, Breslow J, Smith JD. J Lipid Res 1993;34:1699–1707.
10. Wiktor-Jedrzejczak W, Ahmed A, Szczylik C, Skelly R. J Exp Med 1982;156:1516–1527.

Analysis of the *Apoe* and *Apoc1* genes by targeted mutagenesis in mice

Janine H. van Ree[1,2], Walther J.A.A. van den Broek[3], Marion J.J. Gijbels[2], Bé Wieringa[3], Rune R. Frants[1], Louis M. Havekes[2] and Marten H. Hofker[1]

[1]*MGC-Department of Human Genetics, Leiden University, Leiden;* [2]*TNO-PG, Gaubius Laboratory, Leiden; and* [3]*Department of Cell Biology and Histology, Nijmegen University, Nijmegen, The Netherlands*

Abstract. Recently, the mouse has emerged as an important animal model for the analysis of lipoprotein metabolism and atherosclerosis. The availability of inbred mouse strains and reliable transgenic technology has enabled extremely powerful genetic studies to be done. Additional genes can be introduced in the mouse by conventional transgenic technology to study overexpression, ectopic expression, or expression of mutated genes. In addition, gene targeting via homologous recombination in embryonic stem cells has made it possible to study a wide range of genetic alterations in the endogenous gene, including gene disruptions and the introduction of specific mutations. We have generated mice that overexpress the dominantly mutated APOE3-Leiden gene and mice lacking apolipoprotein e (*Apoe*) or *Apoc1* expression. Mice lacking apoE show high plasma cholesterol levels and develop xanthomatous lesions and are therefore a useful model to study the pathology of familial dysbetalipoproteinemia (FD). Mice lacking apoC1 have provided in vivo evidence that apoC1 plays a role in remnant metabolism.

In our laboratory, the structure of the *Apoe-c1-c2* gene cluster has been investigated both in man [1] and mice [2]. In both species, the gene clusters are remarkably similar in organization (Fig. 1), and map to conserved linkage groups on either human chromosome 19 or mouse chromosome 7. The human locus has expanded, as evidenced by a duplication that yielded the APOC1' pseudogene. Detailed analysis of the mouse gene cluster has led to the discovery of an additional conserved gene located between *Apoc1* and *Apoc2*. This gene has been named *Apoc2* Linked Gene (*Acl*) [3] and is likely to be present in humans as well. The three apolipoproteins of human and mouse share about 70% of sequence homology. Despite differences in lipoprotein metabolism, the high degree of genetic similarity has allowed the generation of extremely useful transgenic animal models.

Apoe has been the primary subject of our transgenic experiments, because of the protein's key role as a ligand for receptor-mediated clearance of lipoprotein remnants. In humans, defective apoE results in the accumulation of VLDL remnants, leading to FD, which is accompanied by premature atherosclerosis. Due to differences in genetic and environmental background, the expression of FD is highly variable in families [4]. Good animal (mouse) models are essential to obtain a better insight into the factors that modulate the expression of FD. Mice overexpressing APOE3-Leiden proved to be a suitable model for FD, since these mice respond dramatically to high-fat diets by accumulating VLDL and developing atherosclerosis [5,6]. We have examined the

Address for correspondence: Marten H. Hofker PhD, MGC-Department of Human Genetics, Sylvius Laboratories, P.O.Box 9503, 2300 RA Leiden, The Netherlands. Tel.: +31-71-276099. Fax: +31-71-276075. E-Mail: Hofker@Ruly46.LeidenUniv.nl.

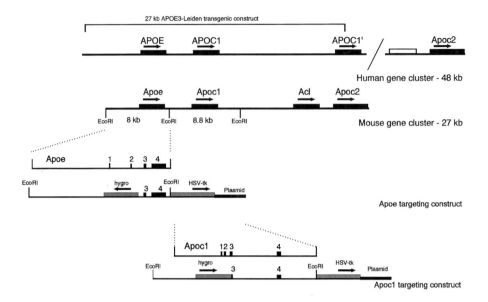

Fig. 1. The human and mouse APOE-C1-C2 gene clusters are schematically represented; genes are solid boxes, and arrows indicate the direction of transcription. The top bar indicates the human APOE3-Leiden transgenic construct. The mouse *Apoe* and *Apoc1* genes are presented in more detail; small solid boxes are the exons. Targeting constructs are shown below the diagrams of both genes. Striped boxes indicate the hygromycin resistance gene and the Herpes simplex thymidine kinase gene (HSV-TK).

pathology of mice lacking apoE and compared it with the effect of overexpression of APOE3-Leiden.

In contrast to apoE and apoC2, insight into the in vivo function of apoC1 is inadequate because of the absence of detectable mutations in human populations. Since apoE and apoC1 might interact in lipoprotein metabolism, an inactivating mutation in the mouse gene has been generated in an attempt to understand the in vivo function of apoC1 better.

Apoe knock-out mice

The mouse *Apoe* gene is 2.7 kb in size, and is encoded by a 1,045 bp mRNA, which is defined by 4 exons [7]. To disrupt the mouse *Apoe* gene, we derived a targeting vector from an 8-kb EcoRI fragment. A hygromycin gene replaced exon 1 and 2, thereby preventing initiation of the transcription and translation of the *Apoe* gene. As a consequence, mice homozygous for this mutation mice completely lack the *Apoe* mRNA and protein, and have a disturbed remnant clearance, similar to the phenotype previously observed by others [8–10]. The accumulation of lipoproteins renders these mice highly susceptible to the development of atherosclerosis [11]. In addition, under relatively mild dietary conditions (Table 1), complete absence of apoE leads to the formation of massive xanthomatous lesions throughout the body [12]. Figure 2 shows the skin near the musculus carnosus of a control mouse, and the same region in an apoE-deficient mouse. In the latter mouse, abundant cholesterol deposits are present. Interestingly, transgenic APOE3-Leiden mice develop an equally profound hyperlipidemia when fed a severe high-fat diet (Table 1). Although this diet causes atherosclerosis in these mice, no signs of xanthomatous lesions have been found. Hence, in the absence of apoE the tissue

Table 1. Serum cholesterol levels and pathology in *apoE*-deficient and APOE3-Leiden mice

Genotype	N	Diet	TC	Pathology	
				Atherosclerosis	Xanthomas
Control	9	HFC 0.5%	4.7	absent	absent
APOE3L	3	HFC 0.5%	60	present	absent
Apoe–/–	5	HFC 0.5%	117	present	present
Apoe–/–	4	HFC	37	present	present

Apoe–/– = homozygous for the *Apoe*-null allele. APOE3L = APOE3-Leiden mice. N = number of animals analyzed. Diets used: HFC = sucrose-based diet containing 0.25% cholesterol and 15% saturated fat (moderate high-fat diet); HFC 0.5% = similar to the HFC diet, but containing 1% cholesterol and 0.5% cholate (severe high-fat diet). Diets are essentially to Nishina et al. [14]. TC = total serum cholesterol.

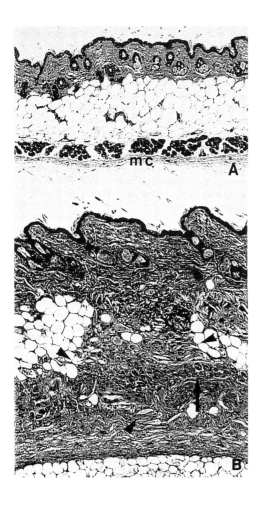

Fig. 2. Panel A shows the skin (× 58) of a control mouse, mc = musculus carnosus. Panel B shows the same section (× 58) in an apoE-deficient mouse. Arrowheads indicate an early xanthomatous lesion in the skin, starting near the musculus carnosus (arrow).

distribution of cholesterol is greatly disturbed. An explanation for this difference could be that, in contrast to *Apoe* knock-out mice, APOE3-Leiden mice still carry a normal mouse *Apoe* gene.

Apoc1 knock-out mice

The mouse *Apoc1* gene is 3.3 kb in size. The 409-bp mRNA is encoded by 4 exons [11]. A replacement-type vector was based on an 8.8-kb *Eco*RI fragment containing *Apoc1*, which was designed to delete exons 1, 2 and a part of exon 3 (van Ree et al., submitted, Fig. 1). Mice homozygous for the *Apoc1*-null allele lack detectable levels of *Apoc1* mRNA in the liver. Heterozygotes have a reduced *Apoc1* mRNA level. Antibodies specific for mouse apoC1 do not detect any apoC1 protein in homozygous mice. In the absence of apoC1, these mice are healthy and do not exhibit overt abnormalities. For each genotype, 9–10 mice were given three different diets for 3 weeks, i.e., normal chow, a moderate high-fat diet and a severe high-fat diet (see above). The serum lipid levels are shown in Table 2. Complete absence of apoC1 leads to a small increase of serum triglyceride levels in mice kept on both chow and the moderate high-fat diet. A more pronounced phenotype was observed in mice kept on the severe high-fat diet. The cholesterol values of apoC1-deficient mice are twice as high as those found in the controls (Table 2). Lipoprotein fractions were analyzed by fast protein liquid chromatography (FPLC) of the pooled serum (van Ree et al., submitted). The accumulation of triglycerides observed in mice fed the moderate high-fat diet occurred predominantly in the VLDL/LDL-sized fractions. In addition, the distribution of cholesterol shifted from the HDL fraction to the VLDL/LDL fraction. The increase of cholesterol found after feeding of the severe high-fat diet is due to the accumulation of VLDL/LDL-sized particles. These data are consistent with a role of apoC1 in remnant metabolism.

However, given the complete disruption of the *Apoc1* gene, the phenotype remains rather subtle, and becomes prominent only after the administration of a severe high-fat diet. Therefore, it is possible that apoC1 shares functions with other apolipoproteins. It would be interesting to test this hypothesis by breeding these *Apoc1* knock-out mice with mice deficient for other apolipoproteins. If certain functions are shared between different lipoproteins, the combination of two knockout mutations in one mouse should unmask

Table 2. Serum cholesterol and triglyceride levels in *apoC1*-deficient mice

Apoc1⁻ genotype	N	Diet	Serum lipids (mean ± SD)	
			TC	TG
+/+	10	chow	3.0 ± 0.6	0.2 ± 0.1
+/–	10	chow	3.0 ± 0.4	0.4 ± 0.1
–/–	10	chow	2.4 ± 0.3	0.4 ± 0.1
+/+	10	HFC	3.9 ± 1.0	0.6 ± 0.4
+/–	10	HFC	3.9 ± 0.6	0.7 ± 0.3
–/–	9	HFC	4.0 ± 0.5	1.1 ± 0.4
+/+	10	HFC 0.5%	5.1 ± 1.6	ND
+/–	10	HFC 0.5%	6.7 ± 1.8	ND
–/–	9	HFC 0.5%	10.7 ± 3.3	ND

SD = standard deviation; N = number of animals analyzed. Chow diet = regular breeder chow; TC = total cholesterol; TG = triglycerides. +/+ = *Apoc1* alleles unaffected; +/– = heterozygous for the *Apoc1*-null allele; –/– = homozygous for the *Apoc1*-null allele; ND = not detectable.

these functional redundancies. Moreover, phenotype rescue can explain why the phenotype of *Apoc1* knock-out mice does not mirror the effect of overexpression. The latter mice become hypertriglyceridemic [13]. It is likely that both types of mice, knockouts and conventional transgenics, will be required to unravel in vivo the function of apoC1.

Acknowledgements

The authors would like to thank Dr K. Willems van Dijk for critically reviewing the manuscript.

References

1. Smit M, Van der Kooij-Meijs E, Frants RR, Havekes LM, Klasen EC. Hum Genet 1988;78:90–93.
2. Hoffer MJV, Hofker MH, Van Eck MM, Havekes LM, Frants RR. Genomics 1993;15:62–67.
3. Van Eck MM, Hoffer MJV, Havekes LM, Frants RR, Hofker MH. Genomics 1994;21:110–115.
4. De Knijff P, Van den Maagdenberg AMJM, Stalenhoef AFH, Gevers Leuven JA, Demacker PNM, Kuyt LP, Frants RR, Havekes LM. J Clin Invest 1991;88:643–655.
5. Van den Maagdenberg AMJM, Hofker MH, Krimpenfort PJA, De Bruijn I, Van Vlijmen B, Van der Boom H, Havekes LM, Frants RR. J Biol Chem 1993;268:10540–10545.
6. Van Vlijmen BJM, Van den Maagdenberg AMJM, Gijbels MJJ, Van der Boom H, HogenEsch H, Frants RR, Hofker MH, Havekes LM. J Clin Invest 1994;93:1403–1410.
7. Horiuchi K, Tajima S, Menju M, Yamamoto A. J Biochem 1989;106:98–103.
8. Zhang SH, Reddick RL, Piedrahita JA, Maeda N. Science 1992;258:468–471.
9. Plump AS, Smith JD, Hayek T, Aalto-Setälä K, Walsh A, Rubin EM, Breslow J. Cell 1992;71:343–353.
10. van Ree JH, van den Broek WJAA, Dahlmans VEH, Groot PEH, Vidgeon-Hart M, Frants RR, Havekes LM, Hofker MH. Diet-induced hypercholesterolemia and atherosclerosis in heterozygous apolipoprotein E-deficient mice. Atherosclerosis 1994 (in press).
11. Hoffer MJV, Van Eck MM, Havekes LM, Hofker MH, Frants RR. Genomics 1993;18:37–42.
12. van Ree JH, Gijbels MJJ, van den Broek WJAA, Hofker MH, Havekes LM. Atypical xanthomatosis in apolipoprotein E-deficient mice after cholesterol feeding. Atherosclerosis 1994 (in press).
13. Simonet WS, Bucay N, Pitas RE, Lauer SJ, Taylor JM. J Biol Chem 1991;266:8651–8654.
14. Nishina PM, Verstuyft J, Paigen B. J Lipid Res 1990;31:859–869.

Cloning and expression of ACAT gene

T.Y. Chang

Department of Biochemistry, Dartmouth Medical School, Hanover, NH 03755, USA

Acyl-coenzyme A:cholesterol acyltransferase (ACAT) is an intracellular enzyme that catalyzes the conjugation of long-chain fatty acids and cholesterol to form cholesterol esters. ACAT is believed to play important roles in lipoprotein assembly, in dietary cholesterol absorption and in cholesterol homeostasis. In hepatocytes, ACAT is believed to compete for a regulatory pool of intracellular cholesterol generated from either exogenously delivered cholesterol or endogenously synthesized cholesterol. Under pathological conditions, accumulation of ACAT reaction products as foamy lipid droplets in the cytoplasm of macrophages and smooth muscle cells is a characteristic feature of early lesions of atherosclerotic plaques.

ACAT is an integral membrane protein located in the endoplasmic reticulum (ER). The ACAT protein has been solubilized and reconstituted in lipid vesicles from various cultured cells and tissues. However, this protein exists only in minute quantities and little progress has been made to significantly purify the protein in an active form from crude cell homogenates. Recently, our laboratory reported the cloning of human ACAT cDNA K1 by a somatic cell genetic and molecular biological approach [1]. This gene has been localized to human chromosome 1 q 25 [2]. Upon transfecting the coding region of cDNA K1 into ACAT-deficient mutant CHO cells, the ACAT activity has been expressed in these cells. Heat inactivation studies indicated that the expressed ACAT activities were of human origin. This result, along with protein-sequence homology analysis, indicated that the open reading frame (ORF) of cDNA K1 encodes a polypeptide essential for ACAT catalysis. Whether this predicted polypeptide alone is sufficient to constitute the ACAT holoenzyme or whether it is one of the catalytic subunits of ACAT protein cannot be determined by these data.

With the aim of determining if cDNA K1 alone is sufficient to produce ACAT activity, we now report the expression of this cDNA in insect Sf9 cells, which were derived from ovarian tissue of the fall army worm *Spodoptera frugiperda*. This cell line does not contain detectable ACAT-like activity. Recently, a baculovirus expression vector system has been employed to express a number of integral membrane proteins in functionally active forms. We have found that, after Sf9 cells had been infected with recombinant virus containing the coding region of cDNA K1, significant ACAT activity was produced. The emergence of ACAT activities coincided with the appearance of two new polypeptides, sized at 56 and 50 kDa by SDS-PAGE. We have validated the use of a specific antipeptide antibody in recognizing these two polypeptides in Western blot analysis, and characterized the enzymatic properties of the ACAT activity expressed.

References

1.   Chang CCY, Huh HY, Cadigan KM, Chang TY. J Biol Chem 1993;268:20747−20755.
2.   Chang CCY, Noll W, Nutile-McMenemy N, Lindsay EA, Baldini A, Chang W, Chang TY. Somat Cell Mol Genet 1994;20:71−74.

Apolipoprotein B mRNA editing protein: dimeric structure, chromosomal localization of its gene and potential utility as a therapeutic agent

Lawrence Chan[1], Paul P. Lau[1], BaBie Teng[1] and Antonio Baldini[2]

[1]Departments of Cell Biology and Medicine; and [2]Department of Molecular and Human Genetics, Baylor College of Medicine, One Baylor Plaza, Houston, TX 77030, USA

Abstract. We recently cloned a human apolipoprotein (apo)B mRNA editing protein gene and localized it to chromosome band 12p13.1–p13.2 by in situ hybridization. The 28-kDa editing protein undergoes spontaneous homodimerization. Dimerization does not require glycosylation and is not mediated by disulfide bridge formation. Expression of the editing protein cDNA in HepG2 cells results in editing of the intracellular apoB mRNA. We also found that adenovirus-mediated transfer of the editing protein in the mouse liver in vivo results in the production of apoB48 in place of apoB100 and the virtual elimination of LDL. Further experimentation on the treatment of hypercholesterolemia by somatic gene transfer of the editing protein gene is warranted.

Apolipoprotein B (apoB) exists in two forms, apoB100 and apoB48 [1]. ApoB100 is synthesized by the liver and secreted in association with very low density lipoproteins (VLDL). It is an obligatory structural component of VLDL, intermediate density lipoproteins (IDL), low density lipoproteins (LDL) and lipoprotein(a). ApoB48 is synthesized by the small intestine as an essential component of chylomicron. It is tightly associated with chylomicron and chylomicron remnants and is essential for efficient fat absorption from the small intestine. ApoB100 contains 4,536 amino acid residues and apoB48 2,152 residues.

ApoB48 mRNA is produced from apoB100 mRNA by a process known as apoB mRNA editing ([2,3], reviewed in [4]), which consists in a CU conversion involving the first base of the codon CAA encoding glutamine-2153 in apoB100 mRNA to UAA, a stop codon at the same position in apoB48 mRNA. ApoB mRNA editing is mediated by a multicomponent enzyme complex containing a catalytic subunit called an apoB mRNA editing protein and other protein(s) which have not been characterized.

The cDNA for a rat apoB mRNA editing protein was cloned by Teng et al. [5]. The cDNA for the corresponding human editing protein was recently cloned by Hadjiagapiou et al. [6] and Lau et al. [7]. The mRNA for the human editing protein is detected exclusively in the small intestine. The tissue distribution of the editing protein mRNA indicates that the presence or absence of this protein determines whether a specific tissue has apoB mRNA editing activity. This is an important observation because the editing activity requires the participation of other protein(s) which seem to occur in numerous tissues including those that do not synthesize apoB.

The genomic sequences of the human apoB mRNA editing protein were cloned by Lau et al. [7]. Two λ phage clones from an EMBL 3 human genomic library and two P1 clones from a P1 human genomic library were identified and characterized. Three of these clones were used as hybridization probes for fluorescence in situ hybridization to metaphase chromosomes. *Alu* PCR was performed on the P1 clones; the PCR product was labeled by nick-translation using biotin-14-dATP. Hybridization to standard chromosome spreads from a male donor was performed [8]. Biotin-labeled DNA was detected using

396

fluorescein isothiocyanate-conjugated avidin DCS. At least 10 metaphases were analyzed per experiment. Hybridization signals from the two P1 clones and one λ phage clone were observed in 90—95% of chromosome 12s and were located in the interval 12—13.1—p13.2 (Fig. 1). No hybridization was observed in other chromosomes.

Lau et al. [7] showed that the human apoB mRNA editing protein undergoes spontaneous dimerization. The mechanism of dimerization is unclear. There are eight cysteine residues in the human editing protein (Fig. 2). However, intermolecular disulfide linkage mediated by one or more of these cysteine residues has been excluded as a mechanism because reduction of the newly synthesized editing enzyme by incubating it in the presence of the reducing agent dithiothreitol failed to disrupt the dimer. There is a leucine zipper-like sequence motif spanning residues 173—216 of the editing protein (Fig. 2). This region encompasses two overlapping heptad leucine-rich repeats. The first heptad repeat (residues 173—189) contains three leucines in a span of 17 amino acids flanked by proline residues. The second heptad repeat (residues 182—216) contains five repeat units with two proline residues immediately after the first repeat. Classical leucine zippers are thought to mediate dimer formation through interacting amphipathic α-helices,

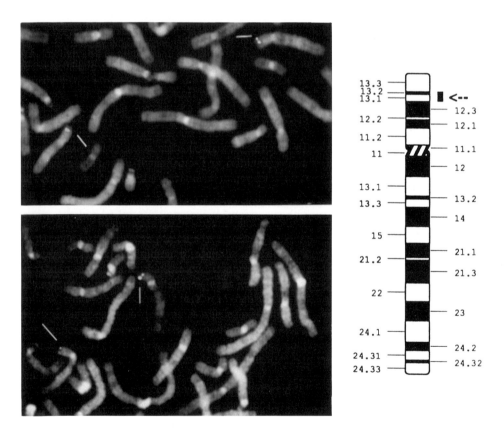

Fig. 1. Fluorescence in situ hybridization of apoB mRNA editing protein P1 genomic clones. A (left). Examples of hybridization experiments using a P1 clone containing the human editing protein gene as hybridization probe. Two partial metaphase spreads; the two chromosome 12s carrying the hybridization signal are indicated by bars. B (right). Ideogram of chromosome 12. The bar indicates the interval within which the hybridization signal from the genomic clones for the apoB mRNA editing protein has been observed.

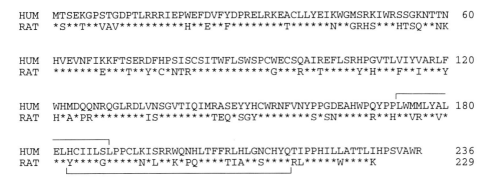

```
HUM  MTSEKGPSTGDPTLRRRIEPWEFDVFYDPRELRKEACLLYEIKWGMSRKIWRSSGKNTTN 60
RAT  *S**T**VAV**********H**E**F*********T******N**GRHS***HTSQ**NK

HUM  HVEVNFIKKFTSERDFHPSISCSITWFLSWSPCWECSQAIREFLSRHPGVTLVIYVARLF 120
RAT  *******E***T**Y*C*NTR***********G***R**T*****Y*H***F**I***Y

HUM  WHMDQQNRQGLRDLVNSGVTIQIMRASEYYHCWRNFVNYPPGDEAHWPQYPPLWMMLYAL 180
RAT  H*A*PR********IS********TEQ*SGY********S*SN****R**H**VR**V*

HUM  ELHCIILSLPPCLKISRRWQNHLTFFRLHLGNCHYQTIPPHILLATTLIHPSVAWR    236
RAT  **Y****G*****N*L**K*PQ****TIA**S****RL****W****K            229
```

Fig. 2. Aminoacid sequence of human apoB mRNA editing protein and alignment with the rat editing protein. The sequences are displayed in single-letter amino acid codes. The human editing protein sequence is from Lau et al. [7] and the rat sequence from Teng et al. [5]. The human sequence contains 236 amino acid residues and is seven residues longer than the rat sequence. Identical residues are indicated by stars. The two overlapping leucine-rich heptad repeats are indicated by braces above and below each sequence. The first leucine-rich domain is flanked by proline dipeptides. The second domain is interrupted by a proline dipeptide after the first repeat. In this domain, after the proline dipeptide there are still three uninterrupted leucine-rich motifs in which the leucine residue in the first repeat is substituted by a serine residue in the human sequence.

forming coiled coil proteins [9]. Inspection of the human and rat editing protein sequences reveals that there is potential for the leucine zipper-like region to form two long coiled coils separated by a proline-proline dipeptide (Fig. 2). Similar coiled coils serve as dimerization interfaces in both structural and nonstructural proteins. The coiled coils are static structures in structural proteins, but they mediate dynamic conformational change in many nonstructural regulatory proteins. It is tempting to speculate that dimerization in the apoB mRNA editing protein is mediated by the leucine zipper-like sequences and dimerization may play a key role in regulating the interaction of the editing protein with other accessory proteins in the editing complex thereby controlling enzyme catalysis. Like the cytidine deaminase from *Escherichia coli* [10], the homodimeric form of the apoB mRNA editing protein is almost certainly the catalytically active form of the protein. Additional studies are needed to define the potential role of the leucine zipper-like region in dimerization and in the interaction of the editing protein with other components of the editing complex.

The existence of a multicomponent editosome involved in apoB mRNA editing was first postulated by Smith et al. [11]. The demonstration that the cloned editing protein requires accessory proteins before it catalyzes the sequence-specific deamination of apoB mRNA in vitro provides definitive support for the editosome hypothesis. Interestingly, extracts from numerous tissues are competent in complementing the editing protein in editing apoB mRNA in vitro. Expression of the human and rat editing proteins in HepG2 cells results in the editing of the endogenous apoB mRNA [7,12]. We have taken advantage of this observation and tested the potential utility of the editing protein in gene therapy.

ApoB100 is a major determinant of plasma LDL and lipoprotein(a), two of the most atherogenic lipoproteins. If we can substantially lower the production of apoB100, the level of LDL and lipoprotein(a) will also fall. In fact, many pharmaceutical companies are actively screening for compounds that downregulate the transcription of the apoB or the apo(a) (an essential component of lipoprotein(a)) gene. To date, there has been little success in this endeavor. This is not surprising because the transcription of both the apoB and the apo(a) genes appears to be constitutive and relatively resistant to experimental manipulations. With the discovery of apoB mRNA editing and the cloning of an editing enzyme, we believe that we have a potentially powerful therapeutic tool in our hand. If we can convert a constant amount of apoB mRNA from the unedited (apoB100) form to its edited (apoB48) form, apoB48 will be produced in place of apoB100 leading to a lowering of plasma apoB100-containing lipoproteins, which include LDL and lipoprotein(a). All this can be accomplished by the successful transfer and expression of the editing protein gene to the liver, the main site of apoB100 production.

On the basis of this premise, we have initiated experiments on the adenovirus-mediated transfer of the rat apoB mRNA editing enzyme in mice. We have selected adenovirus as the gene-transfer vehicle because it has been shown to mediate the efficient in vivo transfer of therapeutic genes to the liver in different animal models [13–15]. Furthermore, different laboratories have initiated efforts to modify the existing adenoviral vectors to make them much more versatile, and to enable them to allow the long-term expression of therapeutic genes at the target tissue [16]. Our preliminary experiments indicate that within 2 weeks of intravenous administration in normal mice of an adenovirus vector containing a rat apoB mRNA editing protein cDNA, there is high-level expression of the editing protein in the liver, apoB100 synthesis is almost completely inhibited and circulating plasma LDL is essentially eliminated in these animals.

Since the discovery of apoB mRNA editing, much effort has been directed to the elucidation of the molecular mechanism involved in the editing process. The cloning of the editing protein gene represents an important step in this direction. It also opens up the possibility of somatic gene therapy for hyperlipidemia involving apoB100-containing lipoproteins.

Acknowledgements

We thank Ms Sally Tobola for expert secretarial assistance. The work performed in this chapter in the authors' laboratories was supported by grants from the National Institutes of Health (HL27341 for a Specialized Center of Research in Arteriosclerosis at Baylor College of Medicine to L.C., and HG00210 for a Human Genome Center to A.B.).

References

1. Chan L. J Biol Chem 1992;267:25621–25624.
2. Powell LM, Wallis SC, Pease RJ, Edwards, YH, Knott TJ, Scott J. Cell 1987;50:831–840.
3. Chen SH, Habib G, Yang C-Y, Gu ZW, Lee GR, Weng S-a, Silberman SR, Cai S-J, Deslypere JP, Rosseneu M, Gotto AM Jr, Li W-H, Chan L. Science 1987;238:363–366.
4. Chan L. BioEssays 1993;15:33–41.
5. Teng BB, Burant CF, Davidson NO. Science 1993;264:1816–1819.
6. Hadjiagapiou C, Giannoni F, Funahashi T, Skarosi SF, Davidson NO. Nucl Acids Res 1994;22:1874–1879.
7. Lau PP, Zhu H-J, Baldini A, Charnsangavej C, Chan L. Proc Natl Acad Sci USA 1994;91:8522–8526.
8. Baldini A, Ross MT, Nizetic D, Vatcheva R, Lindsay EA, Lehrach H, Siniscalco M. Genomics 1992; 14:181–184.
9. O'Shea EK, Rutkowski R, Kim PS. Science 1989;243:538–542.
10. Betts L, Xiang S, Short SA, Wolfenden R, Carter CW Jr. J Mol Biol 1994;235:635–656.
11. Smith HC, Kuo S-R, Backus JW, Harris SG, Sparks CE, Sparks JD. Proc Natl Acad Sci USA 1991;88: 1489–1493.
12. Gionnoni F, Bonen DK, Funahashi T, Hadjiagapiou C, Burant CF, Davidson NO. J Biol Chem 1994;269: 5932–5936.

13. Ishibashi S, Brown MS, Goldstein JL, Gerard RD, Hammer RE, Herz J. J Clin Invest 1993;92:883–893.
14. Kozarsky KF, McKinley DR, Austin LL, Raper SE, Stratford-Perricaudet LD, Wilson JM. J Biol Chem 1994;269:13695–13702.
15. Kay MA, Landen CN, Rothernberg, SR, Taylor LA, Leland F, Wiehle S, Fang B, Bellinger D, Finegold M, Thompson AR, Read M, Brinkhous KM, Woo SLC. Proc Natl Acad Sci USA 1994;91:2353–2357.
16. Engelhardt JF, Ye X, Doranz B, Wilson JM. Proc Natl Acad Sci USA 1994;91:6196–6200.

Role of the hormone response elements (HRE) and the apoCIII enhancer in the transcription regulation of genes involved in lipid transport

Vassilis Zannis[1], Christos Cladaras[1†] and Iannis Talianidis[2]

[1]*Section of Molecular Genetics, Boston University Medical Center, Boston, Massachusetts, USA; and* [2]*University of Crete Medical School and Institute of Molecular Biology and Biotechnology of Crete, Greece*
[†]*Deceased.*

Systematic analysis of five apolipoprotein promoters resulted in the identification of 37 regulatory elements [1—6]. Four elements were also identified in the proximal apoE promoter [7,8] and several elements in the distal 3' and 5' regulatory regions of apoB [9,10]. Careful examination of the activities that have been identified indicates that several previously described factors participate in the transcriptional regulation of the apolipoprotein genes [6]. This includes the liver-enriched factors C/EBP, HNF-1, HNF-3, HNF-4 [11—14] as well as ubiquitous factors such as NF1, NFY, SP1, GABP/Ets-1 [15—18]. The binding sites of these factors on the apolipoprotein promoters are shown in Table 1. Elements which did not correspond to the binding sites of previously described factors were used either as ligands for purification of new transcription factors or as probes for the isolation of potentially new factors from expression cDNA libraries. A summary of the factors purified is shown in Table 2. Although Table 1 indicates that several previously described transcription factors may recognize different apolipoprotein promoters, the arrangement of the factors within each promoter is unique. This unique arrangement of the regulatory elements and the factors bound to them (referred to as *promoter context*) may allow the formation of a unique, stereospecific DNA protein complex which results in the transcriptional activation of the corresponding gene.

Analysis of the promoter strength by transcription assays using wild-type and mutated promoter CAT constructs showed that despite the apparent complexity of the apolipoprotein promoters, only a few regulatory elements and the corresponding factors may be essential for optimal transcription in cell culture.

Transcriptional activation of the apoA-I, apoCIII, apoA-IV gene complex: role of the apoCIII enhancer and the nuclear receptors

The apoCIII gene is closely linked to the human apoA-I and apoA-IV genes [19]. Expression of segments of the apoA-I:CIII:A-IV gene cluster indicated that hepatic transcription requires only 5' regulatory elements in the apoA-I and apoCIII genes, whereas the intestinal transcription of the apoA-I and apoA-IV gene requires elements localized in the intergenic sequence between apoCIII and apoA-I genes extending 1.4 kb upstream of the apoCIII gene [20—22]. As shown in Table 1, a common feature of several apolipoprotein promoters is that they contain a hormone response element (HRE) which binds the orphan receptors HNF-4, ARP-1, EAR-2 and EAR-3. The HRE is also

Address for correspondence: Vassilis Zannis, Section of Molecular Genetics, Boston University Medical Center, 700 Albany Street, Boston, MA 02118-2394, USA.

Table 1. Binding sites for C/EBP, nuclear receptors, CIII-B1, HNF-1 and HNF-3 in apolipoprotein promoters

Human gene	Elements (binding sites)	Human gene	Elements (binding sites)	Human gene	Elements (binding sites)
	C/EBP		*Nucl. recpt.*		*HNF-1*
ApoA-I	(AIC)	ApoA-I	(AIB)	ApoA-II	(AIIN)
	(AIC)		(AID)		(AIIH)
ApoA-II	(AIIAB)	ApoA-II	(AIIJ)	ApoB	(E)
	(AIIC)		(BAI)		
	(AIID)		(Reducer		*HNF-3*
	(AIIF)		element)	ApoB	(BC)
	(AIIG)	ApoCIII	(CIIIB)		
	(AIIL)		*CIII-BI*		
ApoB	(BA2)	ApoA-II	(AIIAB)		
	(BA3)		(AIIK)		
ApoCIII	(CIIIC)		(AIIL)		
	(CIIID)	ApoCIII	(CIIIB)		

recognized by homodimers of *cis*-retinoic acid receptor RXR and heterodimers of RXR with trans-retinoic acid receptor RAR and thyroid hormone receptor THR [6,23–29].

Transactivation of the human apoCIII gene by HNF-4 and repression by EAR-2, EAR-3 and ARP-1

The regulatory element B of apoCIII binds within overlapping sites I and II the orphan receptors (HNP-4, ARP-1, EAR-2, EAR-3) as well as a heat-stable activity which we have purified and designated CIIIB1 (Table 2). The hormone receptors bind to site I and CIIIB1 binds to site II. Recent experiments in our laboratory also showed that site I is also recognized by the newly described transcription factor SREBP-1 (Kan, Pissios and Zannis, unpublished). It has been shown that this factor binds to the sterol-response elements of the LDL-receptor and is regulated by sterols [30–33].

Table 2. Purification of factors bound to apolipoprotein promoters

Factor (Element bound)	M_r kDa (Heat stability)
NF-BA1 (HNF-4-related) (A of apoB; B of apoCIII; D of apoA-I; J of apoA-II)	60 (stable)
CIII B1 (new factor) (B of apoCIII; A,B,K,L of apoA-II)	41 (stable)
CIII C1 (new factor) (C,D of apoCIII; D of apoA-II)	100 (labile)
BCB 1,2,3 (HNF-3-related) (B,C of apoB)	— (labile)
Heat-stable proteins (HS) NF-BA2, NF-BA3 (C/EBP-related) (Heat-stable proteins (HS); A,B,C,E of apoB; C of apoA-I; C,D of apoA-II; C,D of apoCIII)	— (stable)
AII D2 (GABP-Ets-1-related) D of apoA-II	54,57,63 (labile)

Cotransfection experiments using CAT constructs under the control of wild-type and mutated apoCIII promoter regions and HNF-4 expression plasmids showed that HNF-4 activated the apoCIII transcription 7- to 8-fold whereas ARP-1, EAR-2, EAR-3 inhibited transcription to less than 10% of control [6,29]. Cotransfection with increasing concentrations of HNF-4 could reverse the ARP-1-mediated activation of transcription. The HNF-4-dependent transactivation was severely affected by mutations which diminished the binding of HNF-4 to the hormone-receptor binding site (site II) but not by mutations which affected the binding of CIIIB1 to its cognate sequence (site I). The proximal regulatory elements of apoCIII were not sufficient for HNF-4-mediated transactivation [29]. Optimal transactivation required the presence of the distal regulatory elements [29] and was severely affected by mutations in the upstream regulatory elements H and G [34]. DNA-binding and competition assays showed that the regulatory element H forms three DNA protein complexes (Fig. 1). Competition experiments performed with oligonucleotides corresponding to the distal regulatory elements of the apoCIII as well as with oligonucleotides containing the binding site of the transcription factor SP1 showed

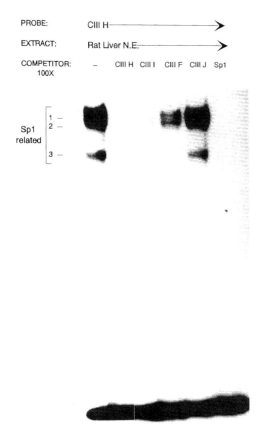

Fig. 1A,B. Panel A. DNA-binding gel electrophoresis and competition assay using the upstream apoCIII regulatory elements H (–705 to –690) as probe and rat liver nuclear extracts. Competitor oligonucleotides were added in all except the first lane at 100-fold molar excess relative to the ^{32}P-labeled oligonucleotides. The oligonucleotides used are indicated by abbreviations at the top of the figure.

that all three complexes bound to the oligonucleotide CIII H were competed with completely by oligonucleotides CIII H, CIII I and SP1. Oligonucleotide CIII F competed out the formation of complex 3 and partially that of complex 1 and 2, whereas oligonucleotide CIII J did not compete out any of the complexes (Fig. 1). Analysis of nuclear extracts from different tissues and cells showed that the activity which binds to the regulatory element H is ubiquitous. These findings suggested that the factors which bind to the regulatory elements H, I and F of apoCIII may be related to SP1 [34].

Figure 2 shows putative paths of transcriptional activation or repression of the human apoCIII gene. Strong activation requires the binding of positive regulators in the upstream regulatory elements as well as binding of HNF-4 or other positive activator(s) to the hormone-receptor binding site (site II). If element B is occupied by CIIIB1 (site I), the transcriptional activation is lower. Finally, if the hormone-receptor binding site (site II) is occupied by negative regulators, ARP-1, EAR-2, EAR-3, the transcription is repressed. Repression of transcription may also occur if negative regulator(s) bind to the distal regulatory elements. Experiments are in progress to determine the role of SREBP-1 on the regulation of transcription of the human apoCIII gene. The observation that SREBP binds to the HRE (site I) of the apoCIII promoter raises an exciting possibility of coordinated regulation of the LDL-receptor and apolipoprotein genes by sterol.

Role of apoCIII enhancer and of nuclear receptors on the transcriptional activation of the apoA-IV gene

The apoA-IV gene displays a tissue-specific expression in primates, with the intestine being the major and the liver the minor site of apoA-IV mRNA synthesis [35]. Previous

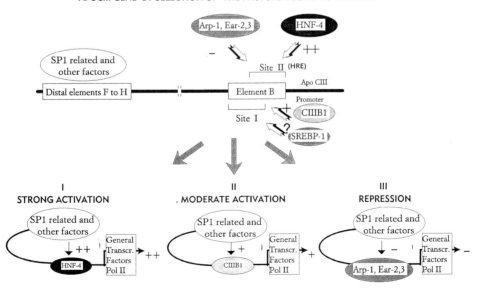

Fig. 2. A schematic representation showing potential interactions of the factors which bind to the distal and proximal regulatory sites of apoCIII. The putative interaction depicted leads either to strong or moderate activation or to repression of transcription of the apoCIII gene.

studies have shown that only a large DNA segment extending up to $-7,700$ nucleotide position from the transcriptional start site was able to drive apoA-IV transcription in transgenic mice [21]. This construct contained the apoCIII promoter region which is located approximately at a $-6,000$ bp distance [2,19].

To investigate the mechanism controlling apoA-IV transcription we have analyzed its promoter region by in vitro DNA binding and competition assays and transient transfection experiments.

DNase I footprinting analysis of the proximal apoA-IV promoter with rat-liver nuclear extract showed the presence of four protected regions: AIVA (-32 to -22), AIVB (-84 to -42), AIVC (-148 to -120), and AIVD (-274 to -250) [3]. DNA binding, competition, and methylation interference assays showed that element AIVC is a hormone-response element which binds the orphan receptors HNF-4, ARP-1, and EAR-3 with similar affinity ($Kd = 4-7$ nM) (Table 1). Antibodies raised against HNF-4 which recognize only HNF-4, and COUP-TF which recognizes ARP-1 and EAR-3 but not HNF-4, supershifted part of the complex formed on the AIVC site [3]. A substantial amount of unaltered activity remained when both antibodies were included in the binding reaction, which indicates that besides these hormone-receptors other nuclear factors can also recognize this element [3]. Methylation interference of nuclear protein binding to the AIVC oligonucleotide probe indicated that HNF-4, ARP-1 and EAR-3 recognize highly overlapping parts of the AIVC regulatory region [3]. Transient transfection assays showed that the proximal apoA-IV promoter region -700 to $+10$ had very low activity in cells of hepatic (HepG2) or intestinal (CaCo-2) origin. As shown in Fig. 3, the promoter activity was increased 10- and 9-fold in HepG2 and CaCo-2 cells when the apoCIII promoter (-65 to -890) was linked to it in tandem or the reverse orientation. Deletion analysis of the apoCIII promoter in the 5' and the 3' direction localized the optimal enhancer activity within the -890 to -500 apoCIII promoter sequence (Fig. 3, lines 3 and 4). This sequence contains the distal regulatory elements F to J of the apoCIII gene [2]. The enhancer activity was practically abolished by terminal 5' deletion of elements J and I, and was reduced to 16 and 32% of control in HepG2 and CaCo-2 respectively by 3' deletions of elements F and G (Fig. 3; compare line 4 with lines 6 and 7). Combinations of one or two elements of the apoCIII enhancer with the proximal apoA-IV promoter had no effect on the apoA-IV promoter strength (Fig. 3; compare line 4 with lines 8 and 9). This finding indicated that one or more proteins bound to the proximal apoA-IV HRE and the entire protein complex which assembles on the apoCIII enhancer is required for optimal enhancement of transcription. Mutagenesis of the HRE of the proximal apoA-IV promoter which abolished hormone-receptor binding reduced the enhancer activity to 21 and 29% in HepG2 and CaCo-2 cells respectively (Fig. 3; compare line 4 with line 5), indicating the importance of the factors bound to the HRE for transactivation.

The HNF-4-mediated transactivation of the apoA-IV gene can be explained by synergistic interactions between HNF-4 bound to the HRE and Sp1 and other factors bound to the apoCIII enhancer

Cotransfection experiments showed that HNF-4 transactivated chimeric constructs containing three intact AIVC sites in front of the heterologous thymidine-kinase minimal promoter, while ARP-1 and EAR-3 repressed this activation. Increasing amounts of HNF-4 alleviated ARP-I- or EAR-3-mediated repression, which suggests that the observed opposing effect is a result of direct competition of these factors for the same recognition site [3]. HNF-4 also transactivated the fused intact apoCIII enhancer/apoA-IV promoter

THE DISTAL APOCIII REGULATORY ELEMENTS F TO J OF THE APO CIII PROMOTER ACT AS AN ENHANCER IN APOA-IV TRANSCRIPTION

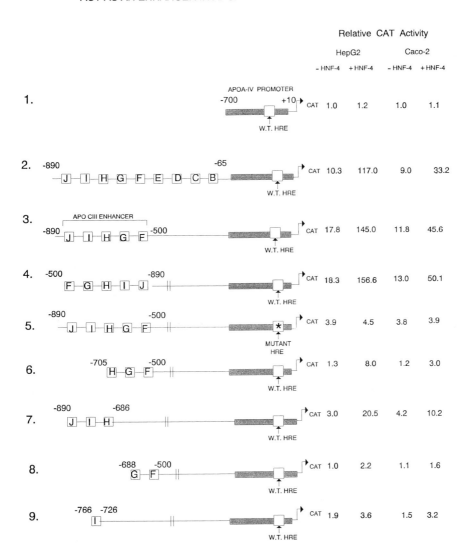

Fig. 3. Localization of the elements of the distal apoCIII enhancer and proximal apoA-IV promoter required for the transcriptional activation of the apoA-IV gene. HepG2 and CaCo-2 cells were transfected with 2 μg of reporter plasmids shown on the left side in the presence (+) or absence (–) of 2 μg of an HNF-4-expression vector. The numbers represent mean values of normalized CAT activities with less than 10% standard deviation, from five independent experiments with at least two different plasmid preparations. The data are presented relative to the activity obtained with AIV-CAT.

CAT construct approximately 150- and 50-fold respectively in HepG2 and CaCo-2 cells (Fig. 3, lines 3 and 4). Truncated apoCIII-enhancer regions lacking the 5′ elements J and I were insufficient to support the HNF-4-dependent transactivation (Fig. 3, line 6).

Similarly, the truncated apoCIII-enhancer region lacking the 3′ elements G and F caused a relatively small HNF-4-dependent transactivation (20 and 10% in HepG2 and CaCo-2 respectively) (Fig. 3, line 7). Combination of one or two elements of the apoCIII enhancer with the proximal apoA-IV promoter had practically no effect on the HNF-4-dependent transactivation (Fig. 3, lines 8 and 9). The HNF-4-dependent transactivation of the apoCIII enhancer/apoA-IV promoter CAT construct was also abolished by mutations which eliminated the binding of HNF-4 to its cognate site on element AIVC (Fig. 3, line 5). In general there was a correlation between the effect of the apoCIII mutations on the strength of the proximal apoA-IV promoter and the HNF-4-dependent transactivation of the promoter (Fig. 3, lines 1–9). The findings suggest that the enhancer effect is mediated by synergistic interactions between Sp1-related factors and other activities that bind to the apoCIII enhancer, and HNF-4 or other nuclear receptors that bind to the proximal regulatory element C of the apoA-IV promoter which is a HRE. This synergism can be deduced from the findings of Fig. 3, lines 1, 4 and 5. Thus Fig. 3 indicates that promoter construct 1, which contains an intact HRE, and construct of line 5, which contains an intact apoCIII enhancer but a mutated HRE, were transactivated 1.2- and 4.5-fold respectively by HNF-4 (the sum of transactivation being 5.7). In contrast, the construct of line 4, which contains both an intact apoCIII enhancer and an intact HRE, was transactivated 157-fold. This provides an increase in transactivation by a factor of 27.5 (157:5.7 = 27.5). The findings of Fig. 3, lines 1, 4 and 5 also suggest synergistic interactions between the factors bound to the HRE and the factors bound to the apoCIII enhancer in HepG2 and CaCo-2 cells in the absence of HNF-4. In this case, however, there is an increase in the transactivation in HepG2 and CaCo-2 cells by a factor of approximately 4 and 3 respectively as opposed to factors of 27.5 and 10 respectively observed in the presence of HNF-4. This can be explained by the fact that the element AIVC in hepatic cells, in addition to HNF-4, may bind other nuclear receptors which may have lower activation potential than HNF-4. Cotransfection of these cells with HNF-4 results in a very large increase in the concentration of HNF-4 in the nuclei of the transfected cells. The excess of HNF-4 may displace the other factors from the HRE site, and this in turn may lead to increased synergistic transactivation of the apoA-N gene. Similar effects of synergism of SP1 and nuclear receptors were deduced from the analysis of constructs containing the adenovirus major late promoter, an HRE site and the apoCIII enhancer [3] as well as constructs containing the apoCIII enhancer in the context of the apoCIII or apoA-I promoter.

Conclusions and future directions

The transcription of eukaryotic genes is a complex biological event involving numerous proteins including RNA polymerase II, the proteins of the basal transcription initiation complex and a variety of promoter- and enhancer-specific transcription factors, and requiring an ATP-dependent activation step [36]. Numerous studies have established that there exists a precise array of regulatory elements in each promoter/enhancer which are occupied by transcription factors. It has been proposed that this promoter/enhancer-specific arrangement of factors permits the formation of stereospecific DNA–protein complexes [37]. These complexes may directly or indirectly interact with the basal transcription system, leading to transcriptional activation of the target gene (Fig. 4).

Transcription factors participate in the final step(s) of signal transduction pathways, leading to transcriptional activation or repression of specific genes. New insights into gene regulation will require a better understanding of a) the three-dimensional interactions of

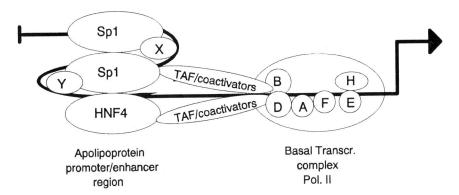

Fig. 4. Schematic representation showing the putative interactions of the proteins bound to the apoCIII enhancer/apoA-IV promoter with the proteins of the basal transcription complex. The figure implies DNA binding caused by transcription factors, and the presence of TAFs/coactivators which link the transcription factors with the proteins of the basal transcription complex.

the regulatory proteins within the specific promoter/enhancer complex; b) the potential activation or repression of the function of a transcription factor by dimerization and/or interaction with ligands; c) the direct or indirect interaction of the transcription factors via their activation domains with the components of the basal transcription systems; d) the intra- or extracellular stimuli which initiate the signal transduction pathway that leads to transcriptional activation or repression. Understanding the mechanism of transcriptional regulation may allow us in the long run to switch the apolipoprotein genes on and off selectively. As indicated, upregulation of the apoA-I gene and/or downregulation of apoB, apoA-II and apoCIII genes may have beneficial effects in protecting humans from hyperlipidemia and atherosclerosis.

Acknowledgements

This manuscript is dedicated to the memory of our close associate and friend Christos Cladaras, who died on August 10, 1994. This work was supported by grants from the National Institutes of Health (HL-33952), and a grant from the EEC (BIOT-CT93-0473). We would like to thank Maria Laccotripe, Effie Tzameli and Anne Plunkett for excellent technical assistance, and Dr Savvas Makrides for carefully reading the manuscript.

References

1. Papazafiri P, Ogami K, Ramji DP, Nicosia A, Monaci P, Cladaras C, Zannis VI. J Biol Chem 1991;266: 5790–5797.
2. Ogami K, Hadzopoulou-Cladaras M, Cladaras C, Zannis VI. J Biol Chem 1990;265:9808–9815.
3. Ktistaki E, Lacorte JM, Katrakili N, Zannis VI, Talianidis I. Nucl Acids Res 1994 (in press).
4. Kardassis D, Zannis VI, Cladaras C. J Biol Chem 1992;267:2622–2632.
5. Chambaz J, Cardot P, Pastier D, Zannis VI, Cladaras C. J Biol Chem 1991;266:11676–11685.
6. Zannis VI, Kardassis D, Cardot P, Hadzopoulou-Cladaras M, Zanni EE, Cladaras C. Curr Opin Lipidol 1992;3:96–113.
7. Smith JD, Melian A, Leff T, Breslow JL. J Biol Chem 1988;263:8300–8308.
8. Chang DJ, Paik YK, Leren TP, Walker DW, Howlett GJ, Taylor JM. J Biol Chem 1990;265:9496–9504.
9. Paulweber G, Brooks AR, Nagy BP, Levy-Wilson B. J Biol Chem 1991;266:24161–24168.
10. Paulweber B, Sandhofer F, Levy-Wilson B. Mol Cell Biol 1993;13:1534–1546.
11. Sladek FM, Zhong W, Lai E, Darnell JE Jr. Genes Dev 1990;2353–2365.

12. Frain M, Swart G, Monaci P, Nicosia A, Stampfli S, Franck R, Cortese R. Cell 1989;59:145–157.
13. Costa RH et al. Mol Cell Biol 1989;9:1415–1425.
14. Landschulz WH, Johnson PF, Adashi E, Graves BJ, McKnight SL. Genes Dev 1988;2:786–800.
15. Jones KA, Kadonaga JT, Rosenfeld PJ, Kelly TJ, Tjian R. Cell 1987;48:79–89.
16. Hooft van Huijsduijnen R, Li XY, Black D, Matthes H, Benoist C, Mathis D. EMBO J 1990;9:3119–3127.
17. Briggs MR, Kadonaga JT, Bell SP, Tjian R. Science 1986;234:47–52.
18. Lamarco KL, Thompson CC, Byers BP, Walton EM, McKnight S. Science 1991;253:789–792.
19. Karathanasis SK. Proc Natl Acad Sci USA 1985;82:6374–6378.
20. Walsh A, Ito Y, Breslow JL. J Biol Chem 1989;264:6488–6494.
21. Walsh A, Azrolan N, Wang K, Marcigliano A, O'Connel A, Breslow JL. J Lipid Res 1993;34:617–623.
22. Lauer SJ, Simonet WS, Bucay N, de Silva HV, Taylor JM. Circulation 1991;84:1390.
23. Miyajima N, Kadowaki Y, Fukushige S, Shimizu S, Semba K, Yamanashi Y, Matsubara K, Toyoshima K, Yamamoto T. Nucl Acids Res 1988;16:11057–11074.
24. Ladias JA, Karathanasis SK. Science 1991;251:561–565.
25. Rottman JN, Widom RL, Nadal-Ginard B, Mahdavi V, Karathanasis SK. Mol Cell Biol 1991;11:3814–3820.
26. Mietus-Snyder M, Sladek FM, Ginsburg GS, Kuo CF, Ladias JAA, Darnell JE Jr, Karathanasis SK. Mol Cell Biol 1992;12:1708–1718.
27. Ladias JAA, Hadzopoulou-Cladaras M, Cheng J, Zannis VI, Cladaras C. Circulation 1993;88:464.
28. Tzameli E, Cladaras C, Zannis VI. Circulation 1993;88:422.
29. Ladias JAA, Hadzopoulou-Cladaras M, Kardassis D, Cardot P, Cheng J, Zannis VI, Cladaras C. J Biol Chem 1992;267:15849–15860.
30. Briggs MR, Yokoyama C, Wang X, Brown MS, Goldstein J. J Biol Chem 1993;68:14490–14496.
31. Wang X, Briggs MR, Hua X, Yokoyama C, Goldstein JL, Brown MS. J Biol Chem 1993;268:14497–14504.
32. Yokoyama C, Wang X, Briggs MR, Admon A, Wu J, Hua X, Goldstein JL, Brown MS. Cell 1993;75:187–197.
33. Wang X, Sato R, Brown MS, Hua X, Goldstein JL. Cell 1994;77:53–62.
34. Ktistaki E, Lacorte JM, Katrakili N, Zannis V, Talianidis I. Circulation 1994 (in press).
35. Karathanasis SK, Yunis I, Zannis VI. Biochemistry 1986;25:3962–3970.
36. Gill G, Paccal E, Tseng Z, Tjian R. Proc Nat Acad Sci USA 1994;91:192–196.
37. Tjian R, Maniatis T. Cell 1994;77:5–8.

Regulation of hepatic secretion of lipoproteins

Henry N. Ginsberg[1] and Joseph L. Dixon[2]
[1]Columbia University, New York, New York; and [2]University of Missouri, Columbia, Missouri, USA

Regulation of the assembly and secretion of apoprotein B (apoB)-containing lipoproteins (LPs) has become an active area of investigation as it is recognized that overproduction of apoB-containing LPs may be responsible for hyperlipidemia in a large percentage of patients [1—5]. ApoB-containing lipoproteins must be secreted to meet the challenge posed to the liver by the delivery of dietary cholesterol and triglyceride, and plasma fatty acid. Although the liver makes a range of apolipoproteins, including apoA-I, apoC-II, apoC-III and apoE, it is apoB that is necessary for the secretion of the lipoproteins that carry the bulk of lipid from the liver to the peripheral tissues.

ApoB100 is a large hydrophobic protein of 4,536 amino acids and a molecular weight of approximately 520 kDa that is synthesized in the liver [6—9]. The endoplasmic reticulum is the site of initial assembly of apoB100 with core lipids; maturation of the nascent lipoprotein occurs in the Golgi apparatus of hepatocytes prior to secretion [10]. ApoB mRNA level has been found not to change in many situations where apoB secretion from cultured liver cells is altered over a wide range, and so it appears that apoB secretion is not typically regulated at the transcriptional or mRNA level. Pullinger et al. [11] found that the level of apoB mRNA in HepG2 cells was refractory to treatment with oleate or insulin, although the former stimulated and the latter inhibited secretion of apoB. Similar discordant effects of oleate on apoB message and secretion were obtained by Moberly et al. [12]. Dashti et al. [13] also showed that apoB mRNA levels were unaffected by oleate or insulin treatment. These observations on the refractory nature of apoB mRNA levels in HepG2 cells are in agreement with several studies of the effects of diet on the levels of apoB mRNA in nonhuman primates [14,15] and rabbits [16].

The studies described above do not, however, rule out some transcriptional regulation of apoB secretion. Cebus monkeys fed diets containing coconut oil and cholesterol for 3 years or longer had hepatic levels of apoB mRNA that were 87% higher than those of animals fed corn oil without cholesterol [17]. Dashti [18] reported an increase in apoB mRNA after treating HepG2 cells with 25-hydroxycholesterol. The addition of free cholesterol to HepG2 cells did not, in the same study, alter apoB mRNA. We showed that incubation of HepG2 cells with VLDL was associated with modest increases in apoB mRNA levels and apoB synthesis [19]. These reports, together with the study by Theriault et al. [20] demonstrating that thyroid hormone increased mRNA levels in HepG2 cells, suggest that transcriptional regulation of apoB secretion does occur.

Despite the studies described above, available evidence suggests that the physiologically significant regulation of apoB secretion occurs posttranslationally. The first indication that this is so came in the studies of Borchardt et al. [21], who reported that only 36 and 60% of newly synthesized apoB100 and apoB48, respectively, were secreted by primary rat hepatocytes in culture. These results indicated that a large percentage of both forms of nascent apoB was being degraded intracellularly. Bostrom et al. [22] noted that the inclusion of oleate in the medium of HepG2 cells increased the proportion of the intracellular pool of apoB that was secreted. Sato et al. [23] and Furakawa et al. [24] demonstrated that apoB in HepG2 cells was degraded in the ER, indicating that posttranslational regulation is involved in modulating apoB secretion in these cells. Furthermore, Dixon et al. [25] observed that the extent of intracellular apoB degradation could be modulated by treatment of the cells with oleate, such that in the presence of oleate, apoB degradation was decreased and its secretion increased. Whereas oleate protected apoB, treatment of cultured rat hepatocytes with 10 nM insulin has been shown by Sparks and Sparks [26] to stimulate the intracellular degradation of newly synthesized apoB100. Wang et al. [27] reported that the ω-3 fatty acids EPA and DHA increased intracellular degradation of apoB in primary cultures of rat hepatocytes.

The basis for posttranslational regulation appears to be the prolonged association of newly synthesized apoB with the ER membrane. Thus, although secretory proteins are typically synthesized in association with the cytosolic surface of the rough endoplasmic reticulum (RER) and then directed to the lumen of the RER by rapid translocation through the membrane [28], this does not seem to be the case for apoB. Although this proposal is not accepted by all investigators [29], there are now numerous reports indicating that apoB becomes associated with the ER membrane, either cotranslationally or very early in the posttranslational period. Studies by Olofsson and his colleagues [22,30,31] indicated that most of the newly synthesized apoB isolated in the ER of HepG2 cells was membrane-associated, and that once apoB was transferred to the ER lumen it was quickly secreted from the cell. Bamberger and Lane [32] confirmed that apoB was located in the ER membrane: they found that approximately 40% of apoB remained in the membrane fraction after alkaline treatment of both heavy and light ER isolated from chick hepatocytes. Davis et al. [33] reported that apoB was not only associated with the ER membrane, but was, in fact, located on the outer surface of the ER membrane. Dixon et al. [34,35], using immunoelectron microscopy, observed that 96% of a gold-labeled antibody to chick apoB was clearly associated with the membrane of isolated RER vesicles. Furthermore, apoB could not be dislodged from the ER membrane by treatment at pH 9.1 (which causes the formation of small pores in the membrane), but could be almost completely removed from the membrane upon carbonate (pH 11) treatment. These data indicate that although apoB is tightly associated with the ER membrane, it is not an integral membrane protein in the classical sense.

Most recently, we have observed proteinase K sensitivity of apoB in permeabilized HepG2 cells. Indeed, a significant proportion of newly synthesized apoB is sensitive to exogenous proteases for as long as 1 h in this cell system. These latest studies provided further support for the hypothesis that apoB domains are exposed on the cytosolic surface of the ER for significant periods of time after completion of translation. The molecular basis of the prolonged association of nascent apoB with the ER membrane has not been defined clearly. Chuck and Lingappa have suggested that structural information present within the extremely long apoB peptide chain provides the signal for a "pause" during apoB translocation [36,37].

The synthesis of triglyceride, cholesterol or cholesteryl ester have been proposed as regulators of apoB secretion in various model systems. It is possible that the availability of these lipids influence the posttranslational metabolism of apoB, and therefore its secretion rate. At present, numerous studies suggest that triglyceride availability is the major factor in the posttranslational regulation of apoB secretion. Furthermore, stimulation of triglyceride synthesis appears to be the mechanism for the well-established stimulation of apoB secretion by fatty acids [38]. The role of triglyceride synthesis in regulating apoB secretion was also studied by Arbeeny et al. [39] using primary hamster hepatocyte cultures. When the cells were treated with TOFA (5-(tetradecyloxy)-2-furancarboxylic acid), an inhibitor of actyl CoA carboxylase, the synthesis of fatty acids and triglyceride and the secretion of triglyceride were inhibited 98, 76, and 90%, respectively. TOFA also inhibited apoB secretion (50%) and cholesteryl ester synthesis (38%). Our group has observed similar effects with Triacsin D, a competitive inhibitor of fatty acyl synthetase, in HepG2 cells. In the presence of triacsin D, synthesis of triglyceride and secretion of apoB are reduced in parallel. In addition, low levels of triacsin D can abolish the stimulation of apoB secretion by oleate.

There have also been reports that the availability of cholesterol or cholesteryl esters may be important in regulating hepatic apoB secretion [4,40–43]. Because of the sensitivity of cells to the cholesterol content of membranes, the free cholesterol pool in the cell is usually maintained at a precise level. Thus it is likely that if effects of cholesterol on apoB secretion are important, they occur through changes in the cell content of cholesteryl esters. The fact that the enzyme which esterifies cholesterol with fatty acid, acyl-CoA:cholesterol acyltransferase (ACAT), is located predominantly in the RER of rat liver [44–46], adds strength to the idea that cholesteryl esters may be important. Cianflone and Sniderman [42] concluded that the stimulation in the rate of apoB secretion with exogenous free fatty acid occurred through effects on triglyceride synthesis or cholesteryl ester synthesis. They observed that when either lovastatin or the ACAT inhibitor 58-035 was added to oleate-stimulated cells, both the accumulation of apoB in medium and the synthesis of cholesteryl ester decreased, whereas the synthesis of triglyceride remained relatively unchanged [42]. However, in extensive studies, Wu et al. [47] were not able to reproduce those findings. In fact, these authors demonstrated that triglyceride and not cholesteryl ester content was critical for the secretion of apoB-containing LPs from HepG2 cells. Thus, triacsin D, which inhibits both triglyceride synthesis and apoB secretion, does not affect cholesteryl ester synthesis. Uncertainty about the role of cholesterol or cholesteryl ester synthesis or availability in the regulation of apoB secretion also come from studies on the effects of inhibitors of HMG-CoA reductase on apoB production in cells not stimulated with fatty acids. Rather than inhibiting apoB secretion, inhibitors of HMG-CoA reductase either stimulated or had no effect on apoB secretion in rat hepatocytes [48] or HepG2 cells [23], respectively. Finally, in studies with VLDL, Wu et al. [19] demonstrated that increases in cellular triglyceride but not cholesteryl ester content was associated with increases in apoB secretion.

Availability of newly synthesized triglyceride appears to facilitate the translocation of newly synthesized apoB across the ER membrane. Thus, although the cysteine-protease inhibitor, ALLN, can prevent the rapid degradation of nascent apoB, it does not accelerate apoB secretion; only after the addition of oleate can we observe rapid secretion of an enlarged, protected pool of nascent apoB [49]. It is likely that in the absence of protease inhibitors, newly synthesized triglyceride can also accelerate the translocation of apoB across the ER membrane, allowing formation of the nascent lipoprotein in the ER lumen, and thus avoiding degradation. The recent observations that microsomal transfer protein (MTP) appears to play an essential role in the assembly and secretion of apoB-containing lipoproteins suggests that MTP is the link between newly synthesized triglyceride and translocation of apoB [50–52].

Availability of one or more lipid class is not only important in the posttranslational regulation of apoB secretion, but also in determining what type of lipoprotein is secreted. Thrift et al. [53] demonstrated that HepG2 cells, when grown under serum-free conditions, secrete a majority of their apoB in LP particles having a buoyant density in the LDL range, as only 1% of the protein found in the d < 1.063 g/ml fraction floated in the d < 1.006 range. These particles were also observed to be similar in size to LDL (25 nm) [54]. However, Ellsworth et al. observed that when HepG2 were incubated with 0.8 mM oleate, secreted apoB and triglyceride were both redistributed from the LDL to the VLDL density range [55]. In contrast to the heterogeneous particles secreted by HepG2 cells, the characteristic apoB-containing LP particle secreted by rat liver [56] and rat hepatocytes in culture [57] is VLDL. However, there are conditions under which smaller particles are secreted by rat liver. In both nephrosis [58] and cholestasis [59], rat liver secretes a more heterogeneous mixture of apoB-containing particles, including those which float in the IDL and LDL fractions. In cultured rat hepatocytes, too, it appears that the density of the nascent apoB-containing LP secreted is dependent upon the dietary regimen of the donor rat and/or the culture conditions employed. Belle-Quint and Forte [60] showed that hepatocytes obtained from fasted rats secreted lower amounts of triglyceride and VLDL than controls, whereas hepatocytes from sucrose-fed rats secreted 10 times more VLDL than fasted rats. In VLDL and LDL isolated from the medium of control rat hepatocytes after short-term incubations (<6.5 h), 56% of the total LP mass was found in VLDL, 20% in LDL, and 24% in HDL [60]. Patsch et al. [61] also reported a similar distribution for rat hepatocytes cultured on a fibronectin matrix for 16 h, with 43% of apoB in VLDL, 27% in LDL, and 29% in HDL (determined by chromatography on Sepharose 6B). However, when Belle-Quint and Forte [60] cultured rat hepatocytes for longer periods (17 and 48 h), the VLDL fraction contained only approximately 20% of the total LP mass, possibly because of a lower rate of triglyceride synthesis due to lower availability of precursor substrates, or because the hepatocytes were becoming dedifferentiated [62,63].

In summary, the assembly and secretion of apoB-LPs in hepatocytes is complex, and appears to be modulated by a variety of factors. In particular, posttranslational degradation of nascent apoB which is associated with the ER membrane plays a major role in determining how much apoB is secreted. The availability of core lipids, particularly triglyceride, seems to play a major role in both targeting apoB for secretion and in determining the density of the secreted lipoproteins.

References

1. Janus ED, Nicoll A, Wootton R, Turner PR et al. Eur J Clin Invest 1980;10:149−159.
2. Sigurdsson G, Nicoll A, Lewis B. Eur J Clin Invest 1976;6:167−177.
3. Teng B, Sniderman AD, Soutar AK, Thompson GR. J Clin Invest 1986;77:663−672.
4. Arad Y, Ramakrishnan R, Ginsberg HN. J Lipid Res 1990;31:567−582.
5. Vega GL, Denke MA, Grundy SM. Circulation 1991;84:118−128.
6. Cladaras C, Hadzopoulou-Cladaras M, Nolte RT, Atkinson D et al. EMBO J 1986;5:3495−3507.
7. Knott TJ, Pease RJ, Powell LM, Wallis SC et al. Nature 1986;323:734−738.
8. Yang C, Kim TW, Weng S, Lee B et al. Proc Natl Acad Sci USA 1990;87:5523−5527.
9. Lawson SW, Grant K, Higuchi A, Hospattankar K et al. Proc Natl Acad Sci USA 1986;83:8142−8146.
10. Olofsson SO, Bjursell G, Bostrom K, Carlsson P et al. Atherosclerosis 1987;68:1−17.
11. Pullinger CR, North JD, Teng B-B, Rifici VA et al. J Lipid Res 1989;30:1065−1076.
12. Moberly JB, Cole TG, Alpers DH, Schonfeld G. Biochim Biophys Acta 1990;1042:70−80.
13. Dashti N, Williams DL, Alaupovic P. J Lipid Res 1989;30:1365−1373.
14. Sorci-Thomas M, Wilson MD, Johnson FL, Williams DL et al. J Biol Chem 1989;264:9039−9045.
15. Kushwaha RS, McMahan CA, Mott GE, Carey KD et al. J Lipid Res 1991;32:1929−1940.
16. Kroon PA, DeMartino JA, Thompson GM, Chao Y-S. Proc Natl Acad Sci USA 1986;83:5071−5075.
17. Hennessy LK, Osada J, Ordovas JM, Nicolosi RJ et al. J Lipid Res 1992;33:351−360.
18. Dashti N. J Biol Chem 1992;267:7160−7169.
19. Wu X, Sakata N, Dixon JL, Ginsberg HN. J Lipid Res 1994;35:1200−1210.
20. Theriault A, Ogbonna G, Adeli K. Biochem Biophys Res Commun 1992;186:617−623.
21. Borchardt RA, Davis RA. J Biol Chem 1987;262:16394−16402.
22. Bostrom K, Borén J, Wettesten M, Sjöberg A et al. J Biol Chem 1988;263:4434−4442.
23. Sato R, Imanaka T, Takatsuki A, Takano T. J Biol Chem 1990;265:11880−11884.
24. Furukawa S, Sakata N, Ginsberg HN, Dixon JL. J Biol Chem 1992;267:22630−22638.

25. Dixon JL, Furukawa S, Ginsberg HN. J Biol Chem 1991;266:5080–5086.
26. Sparks JD, Sparks CE. J Biol Chem 1990;265:8854–8862.
27. Wang H, Chen C, Fisher EA. J Clin Invest 1993;91:1380–1389.
28. Palade G. Science 1975;189:347–358.
29. Pease RJ, Harrison GB, Scott J. Nature 1991;353:448–450.
30. Bostrom K, Wettesten M, Borén J, Bondjers G et al. J Biol Chem 1986;261(29):13800–13806.
31. Borén J, Wettesten M, Sjöberg A, Thorlin T et al. J Biol Chem 1990;265:10556–10564.
32. Bamberger MJ, Lane MD. J Biol Chem 1988;263:11868–11878.
33. Davis RA, Diuz SM, Leighton JK, Brengase VA. J Biol Chem 1990;284:8970–8977.
34. Dixon JL, Battini R, Ferrari S, Redman CM et al. Biochim Biophys Acta 1989;1009:47–53.
35. Dixon JL, Chattapadhyay R, Huima T, Redman CM et al. J Cell Biol 1992;117:1161–1169.
36. Chuck SL, Lingappa VR. Cell 1992;68:9–21.
37. Chuck SL, Yao Z, Blackhart BD, McCarthy BJ et al. Nature 1990;346:382–385.
38. Dixon JL, Ginsberg HN. J Lipid Res 1993;34:167–179.
39. Arbeeny CM, Meyers DS, Bergquist KE, Gregg RE. J Lipid Res 1992;33:843–851.
40. Ginsberg HN, La N-A, Short MP, Ramakrishnan R et al. J Clin Invest 1987;80:1692–1697.
41. Khan B, Wilcox HG, Heimberg M. Biochem J 1989;258:807–816.
42. Cianflone KM, Yasruel Z, Rodriguez MA, Vas D et al. J Lipid Res 1990;31:2045–2055.
43. Fuki IV, Preobrazhensky SN, Mishavin AY, Bushmakina NG et al. Biochim Biophys Acta 1989;1001:235–238.
44. Hashimoto S, Fogelman AM. J Biol Chem 1980;255:8678–8684.
45. Balasubramaniam S, Venkatesan S, Mitropoulos KA, Peters TJ. Biochem J 1978;174:863–872.
46. Spector AA, Mathur SN, Kaduce TL. Prog Lipid Res 1979;18:31–53.
47. Wu K, Sakata N, Lui E, Ginsberg HN. J Biol Chem 1994;269:12375–12382.
48. Ribeiro A, Mangeney M, Loriette C, Thomas G et al. Biochim Biophys Acta 1991;1086:279–286.
49. Sakata N, Wu K, Dixon JL, Ginsberg HN. J Biol Chem 1993;268:22967–22970.
50. Wetterau JR, Aggerbeck LP, Bouma ME, Eisenberg C et al. Science 1992;258:999–1001.
51. Sharp D, Blinderman L, Combs KA, Kienzle B et al. Nature 1993;365:65–69.
52. Shoulders CC, Brett DJ, Bayliss JD, Narcisi TM et al. Hum Mol Genet 1993;2:2109–2116.
53. Thrift RN, Forte TM, Cahoon BE, Shore VG. J Lipid Res 1986;27:236–250.
54. McCall MR, Nichols AV, Blanche FJ, Shore VC et al. J Lipid Res 1989;30:1579–1589.
55. Ellsworth JF, Erickson SF, Cooper AD. J Lipid Res 1986;27:858–874.
56. Hamilton RL. In: Glaumann Jr H, Peters T, Redman C (eds) Plasma Protein Secretion by the Liver. London and New York: Academic Press, 1983;357–374.
57. Davis RA, Engelhorn SC, Fangburn SH, Weinstein DB et al. J Biol Chem 1979;254:2010–2016.
58. Marsh JB, Sparks CE. J Clin Invest 1979;64:1229–1237.
59. Felker TE, Hamilton RL, Havel RJ. Proc Natl Acad Sci USA 1978;75:3459–3463.
60. Bell-Quint J, Forte J. Biochim Biophys Acta 1981;663:83–98.
61. Fatsch W, Franz S, Schonfeld G. J Clin Invest 1983;71:1161–1174.
62. Jefferson DM, Clayton DF, Darnell J, Reid LM. Mol Cell Biol 1984;4:1929–1934.
63. Clayton DF, Harrelson AL, Darnell J. Mol Cell Biol 1985;5:2623–2632.

Nascent VLDL assembly occurs in two steps in the endoplasmic reticulum (ER) of hepatocytes

R.L. Hamilton, S.K. Erickson and R.J. Havel

Cardiovascular Research Institute and Departments of Anatomy and Medicine, UCSF School of Medicine, San Francisco, CA 94143-0130, USA

Abstract. A novel method was developed which recovers large amounts of rough endoplasmic reticulum (RER) from rat liver. Separation of RER membranes from contents revealed small (~150–250 Å) HDL/LDL-like particles enriched in apolipoprotein B (apoB) and containing small amounts of core lipids. ApoB-deficient particles of Golgi nascent VLDL size and core lipid composition were also isolated from RER contents. These findings are consistent with a two-step model of apoB core lipidation in the ER in VLDL assembly. The first step is the core lipidation of RER-bound apoB by microsomal triglyceride-transfer protein, which is required to dissociate apoB from the membrane. A larger (VLDL size) TG-rich but apoB-deficient particle is formed by unknown mechanisms in the smooth ER. The second step is the coalescence between one apoB-rich small particle with one apoB-deficient large TG-rich particle forming one nascent VLDL.

Expression of message for apolipoprotein B (apoB mRNA) by specific cell types is strong indirect evidence that those cells secrete triglyceride-rich particles into extracellular fluids for lipid transport to distant cells for nutrition. Only two specific types of epithelial cells express substantive amounts of apoB mRNA in adult mammalian tissues: hepatocytes and absorptive enterocytes, which secrete nascent VLDL and nascent chylomicrons respectively. Chylomicron assembly and secretion provides an efficient mechanism for transport of dietary long-chain fatty acids, cholesterol and fat-soluble vitamins. Hepatocytes secrete VLDL, providing a mechanism for exporting excess long-chain fatty acids and cholesterol that the liver takes up from blood or synthesizes. VLDL also serve the function of generating LDL particles that deliver cholesterol to extrahepatic tissues in addition to liver.

Although there is only one known apoB gene, there are two variants of apoB mRNA-translating proteins of widely different molecular weights (apoB48 ~ 264 kDa and apoB100 ~ 550 kDa) due to a unique editing event. In most adult mammals studied, intestinal apoB mRNA is edited at high levels whereas editing of apoB mRNA is virtually absent in adult livers from human, monkey, pig, cow, sheep and cat [1] such that virtually all hepatocytic VLDL contain apoB100. However, in some other species (dog, horse, rat and mouse) hepatic apoB mRNA editing [1] probably results in plasma VLDL particles that contain either one mole of apoB48 or one mole of B100.

The genetic disease abetalipoproteinemia (abeta) is characterized by the virtual absence of all plasma lipoproteins containing apoB, in which chylomicrons and VLDL are not secreted, although apoB mRNA is expressed in intestine and liver, and apoB of appropriate molecular weight is synthesized [2]. The genetic defect in this disorder is the apparent absence of a protein heterodimer called microsomal triglyceride-transfer protein (MTP), which comprises protein disulfide isomerase (PDI) and a protein of about 88 kDa [3]. MTP stimulates the transfer of phospholipids between liposomes, as well as the triglycerides (TG) and cholesteryl esters (CE) that form the core (nonpolar lipids) of plasma lipoproteins. Because this heterodimer was discovered in hepatic microsomes and is unique among cellular transfer proteins in its capacity to stimulate nonpolar lipid transfer between liposomes, it was originally hypothesized to be a participant in VLDL assembly [4]. Convincing experiments have recently showed the apparent absence of the 88-kDa subunit of MTP in intestinal biopsies from several abeta subjects [5]. The question now is: how does the absence of MTP explain abetalipoproteinemia in which apoB and its message are present in fatty enterocytes?

One possible explanation may be provided by the two-step model of apoB core lipidation in the endoplasmic reticulum of enterocytes and hepatocytes [6]. In 1976 we reported that antibodies to rat apoB (from rat LDL and rat VLDL) that were cross-linked to horseradish peroxidase failed to immunostain lipid-rich particles of VLDL size in the lumen of the smooth endoplasmic reticulum (SER) of rat hepatocytes. By contrast, Golgi nascent VLDL within vesicles and putative remnants in the space of Disse stained intensely for apoB, as did long stretches of RER cisternae in which no particles of VLDL size were evident [7]. This suggested the hypothesis that apoB is added to TG-rich particles formed in the SER when these particles reach the junctional region that joins the SER and RER compartments. This concept is compatible with a hypothesis developed from studies on Hep G2 cells that secrete apoB in small particles, namely that these transformed cells lack a "second stage" of VLDL assembly present in normal liver cells whereby nascent apoB-containing particles acquire additional lipid to form large VLDL, 400–600 Å in diameter [8]. We subsequently interpreted the concept of two-staged VLDL assembly to be two steps in the core lipidation of apoB [9], because there are probably many steps in the complicated processes by which nascent VLDL assembly occurs. Our new research began with the goal of determining the nature of apoB in the contents of the lumen of the RER [7]. We believed that standard techniques of isolating microsomal membrane fractions were inadequate for our purpose, which was to obtain RER contents in adequate amounts for chemical characterization. Because classical RER fractions require day-long ultracentrifugal runs, yield relatively small amounts of material, and represent vesicles which may have lost contents following shear-induced rupture and resealing, we looked for a rapid nonultracentrifugal method. Schenkman and Scinti described a nonultracentrifugal method of isolating rat liver ribosomal-rich membranes by calcium precipitation which was, in addition, also quite rapid [10]. We modified their method to finally achieve a highly purified RER fraction from rat liver in 2–3 h. This cell fraction almost exclusively contains elongated strips of ribosomal-rich membranes. It is highly enriched in ER markers such as glucose-6-phosphatase, acylCoA:cholesterol acyltransferase (ACAT) and diacylglycerol acyltransferase (DGAT) activity. It has low levels of markers for plasma membranes, endosomes, mitochondria, and Golgi membranes.

We found that small amounts of proteins of appropriate molecular mass for apoB100 and apoB48 were released from the RER fraction by two techniques: treatment with sodium carbonate (pH 11.3) and rupture in the French pressure cell. These proteins, which sedimented to the bottom of ultracentrifuge tubes together with serum albumin, a well-known secretory protein of hepatocytes, were identified by Western blotting with rat apoB antisera. We found that the bulk of the apoB remained firmly bound to the RER membranes. When the apoB- and albumin-containing fraction was layered under a stacked sucrose gradient and ultracentrifuged overnight in a swinging bucket rotor, two pearly bands were found near the top of the gradient separated by a clear zone of about 1–2 mm. In negative stains, electron photomicrographs of these two bands showed round, lipoprotein-like particles (150–250 Å diameter) characterized by a small electron-lucent core. The topmost band contained many particles with an electron-lucent core close to 100 Å diameter whereas the second band contained particles in which the lucent core was smaller and more difficult to measure. Chemical analyses showed that both fractions contained more TG than CE and that the less dense particles were more enriched in these nonpolar lipids. By Western blotting, both bands were found to be enriched in apoB, particularly apoB48. The question follows: do these apoB-rich small particles of HDL/LDL size and density from the lumen of the RER fraction represent artifacts generated by the procedures used to release content proteins or do they represent early physiologic stages in the normal process of VLDL assembly? If the latter is correct, conditions may occur in nature in which small apoB-rich particles are secreted by hepatocytes and by enterocytes as well. This appears to be a plausible explanation for the transformed human liver HepG2 cells and human intestinal CaCo$_2$ cells, both of which secrete most apoB in particles of HDL/LDL size and density, rather than VLDL or chylomicrons [11,12]. Moreover, when rat livers are perfused without added FFA for 5—6 h, perfusate apoB accumulates in HDL fractions [13] and this fraction is more than doubled when cholestatic livers are perfused under the same conditions [14]. Finally, HDL particles containing apoB have been obtained from rat intestinal cell fractions [15], which suggests that the processes of VLDL assembly by hepatocytes and chylomicron assembly by enterocytes share a common mechanism for core lipidation of apoB.

After release of protein contents from our RER fraction by both methods, and an overnight centrifugation at ~100,000 xg to sediment proteins, a turbid layer, similar to that of plasma VLDL, is always present at the top of the tube. Electron microscopy of negative stains of this fraction showed that it comprised electron-lucent particles, largely of 400—600 Å diameter. By Western blotting, only small amounts of apoB48 were evident. Concentrating this VLDL-like fraction by ultracentrifugation removed most apoB, but also appeared to cause coalescence of some of the apoB-deficient particles. Incubation with anti-apoB IgG followed by centrifugation sedimented a portion of the particles away from those that lacked apoB, although both fractions resembled plasma VLDL in size and negative staining properties. Preliminary analyses have shown that the proportions of cholesteryl esters and triglycerides in these apoB-deficient VLDL-like particles are similar to those of Golgi nascent VLDL.

These studies support the two-step model for core lipidation of apoB. A number of studies have established that apoB becomes firmly bound to the membrane of the RER before it is either degraded by proteolysis, or is released into the lumen [16]. We propose that the first step of core lipidation of apoB in the RER requires MTP to release apoB from its membrane-binding site. When MTP is absent or structurally defective, the first step cannot occur as is the case in abeta. The second step depends on the formation of a larger TG-rich microemulsion particle within the lumen of the SER, which occurs by unknown processes in the absence of apoB. This SER capacity is most highly developed in enterocytes and is induced by fat absorption. Little of this SER capacity is found in the rat yolk-sac endoderm, which assembles and secretes TG-rich particles that are mostly of LDL size and density [17]. The second step of apoB core lipidation in the assembly of hepatocytic VLDL or enterocytic chylomicrons depends upon the coalescence of one apoB-rich particle formed in the RER with one TG-rich apoB-deficient particle formed in the SER. Because apoB-rich small particles from the RER appear to be secreted whereas the apoB-deficient TG-rich particles are not, apoB must contain information permitting TG-rich particles to enter the secretory pathway. Another function of apoB may be to stabilize large TG-rich particles in the circulating blood.

Possible functional advantages of the second step of the two-step model are illustrated in Fig. 1. ApoB message is constitutively expressed, and strong evidence supports the concept that proteolytic degradation of RER-bound apoB is important in regulating apoB

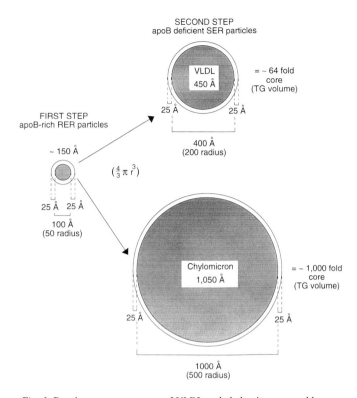

Fig. 1. Putative two-step process of VLDL and chylomicron assembly.

secretion [16]. The first step may protect apoB from degradation by dissociating it from the RER membrane in the formation of the small apoB-rich particle containing some core lipids. The core of the small apoB-rich particle is about 100 Å diameter but the thickness of the surface monolayer of phospholipid is constant (about 20–25 Å) in microemulsion particles [8]. Thus, the coalescence of the small apoB-rich particle in the hepatocyte with an apoB-deficient particle of average VLDL size of ~450 Å would result in little change in diameter, but the ratio of TG to apoB would be increased 64-fold (Fig. 1). In the absorptive enterocytes of the small intestine where fat availability varies greatly, the second step would increase the TG load for each mole of apoB 1,000-fold in the formation of an average-size chylomicron as shown in Fig. 1. Thus, an important question for future research is to investigate the mechanisms of forming TG-rich microemulsion particles in the absence of apoB within the SER.

Acknowledgements

The authors' research is supported by Arteriosclerosis SCOR HL-14237, and the Department of Veterans Affairs.

References

1. Greeve J, Altkemper I, Dieterich J-H, Greten H, Windler E. J Lipid Res 1993;34:1367–1383.
2. Kane JP, Havel RJ. In: Scriver CR, Beaudet AL, Sly WS, Valle D (eds) The Metabolic Basis of Inherited Disease. New York: McGraw-Hill, 1994:1853–1886.

418

3. Wetterau JR, Combs KA, Spinner SN, Joiner BJ. J Biol Chem 1990;265:9800–9807.
4. Wetterau JR, Zilversmit DB. Chem Phys Lipids 1985;38:202–222.
5. Wetterau JR, Aggerbeck LP, Bouma M-E et al. Science 1992;258:999–1001.
6. Hamilton RL. Trends Cardiovasc Med 1994;4:131–139.
7. Alexander CA, Hamilton RL, Havel RJ. J Cell Biol 1976;69:241–263.
8. Spring DJ, Chen-Liu LW, Chatterton JE, Elovson J, Schumaker VN. J Biol Chem 1992;267:14839–14845.
9. Hamilton RL, Havel RJ. Hepatology 1993;18:460–463.
10. Schenkman JB, Scinti DL. Methods Enzymol 1978;52:83–89.
11. Thrift RN, Forte TM, Cahoon BE, Shore VG. J Lipid Res 1986;27:236–250.
12 Hughes TE, Sasak WU, Ordovas JM, Forte TM, Lamon-Fava S, Schafer EJ. J Biol Chem 1987;262:3762–3767.
13. Fainaru M, Felker TE, Hamilton RL, Havel RJ. Metabolism 1977;26:999–1004.
14. Felker TE, Hamilton RL, Vigne J-L, Havel RJ. Gastroenterology 1982;83:652–663.
15. Magun AM, Brasitus TA, Glickman RM. J Clin Invest 1985;75:209–218.
16. Thrift RN, Drisko J, Dueland S, Trawick JD, Davis RA. Proc Natl Acad Sci USA 1992;89:9161–9165.
17. Plonné D, Winkler L, Franke H, Dargel R. Biochim Biophys Acta 1992;1127:174–185.

Endosomal and extra-endosomal intracellular trafficking of lipoproteins

Stefan Jäckle, Franz Rinninger, Ulrike Beisiegel, Andreas Block, Oluf Braren, Walter Tauscher, Michael Biermer, Heiner Greten and Eberhard Windler
Medizinische Kernklinik und Poliklinik, Universitäts-Krankenhaus Eppendorf, Martinistr. 52, D-20246 Hamburg, Germany

Abstract. LDL, chylomicron remnants and HDL-particles are taken up first into a compartment where receptors and ligands are uncoupled and are subsequently transferred to the prelysosomal compartment of multivesicular bodies. These endosomal fractions are characterized by high concentrations of annexin VI, which has recently been identified as the main constituent of hepatocytic endosomes. Small chylomicron remnants bind predominantly to the LDL receptor, by which they are taken up into endosomes. However, large chylomicron remnants bind initially to hepatic lipase and require further processing before the remnant particle is internalized by an endocytic receptor. HDL particles are transported into endosomes and are finally subjected to lysosomal degradation, while HDL-cholesteryl esters accumulate in a nonendosomal, nonlysosomal compartment.

The terminal catabolism of most plasma lipoproteins occurs chiefly in the liver by means of receptor-mediated endocytosis [1]. In research on the hepatic endocytosis of lipoproteins we have isolated three morphologically distinct endosomal fractions from rat liver [2,3]. Ligands and receptors, which are internalized via receptor-mediated endocytosis, accumulate first in a "compartment of uncoupling of receptor and ligand" (CURL) and later in multivesicular bodies (MVB), the immediate prelysosomal compartment [2,4]. The receptor recycling compartment (RRC), which is derived from the membranous appendages of the vesicular endosomes (CURL, MVB), is enriched in various recycling receptors and in transferrin, which escape lysosomal degradation and recycle back to the cell surface. The RRC fraction is depleted of receptors and ligands such as apolipoprotein B (apoB)-containing lipoproteins, epidermal growth factor (EGF) and the EGF receptor, which are subjected to lysosomal degradation [4].

The most prominent membrane protein of these endosomes is one of 68 kDa, as revealed by silver and Coomassie brilliant blue staining of SDS gel electrophoretograms. This protein dominates profiles obtained from purified membranes of CURL, MVB, and RRC, but is greatly reduced or undetectable in those obtained from plasma membranes and lysosomes. Six tryptic fragments of the endosomal 68-kDa protein share 91 and 96% identity with corresponding sequences of human and mouse annexin VI, respectively. Using immunoblotting we detected high concentrations of annexin VI with an apparent molecular weight of 68 kDa in endosomal membranes. Annexin VI was also detected in Golgi membranes, but the concentration there was substantially lower than that of the three endosomal fractions, for which annexin VI may serve as a characteristic marker protein. Incubation of intact endosomes with pronase leads to a complete degradation of annexin VI without any detectable disintegration of proteins on the luminal surface of endosomal membranes. Evidently, annexin VI is confined to the cytoplasmic leaflet of the membrane of endosomes. It appears to get attached to early endosomes and leaves them before they are transformed to secondary lysosomes. Annexin may therefore serve as an anchor for the cytoskeleton and may be important in endosomal intracellular trafficking [5].

Chylomicron remnants are rapidly taken up by the liver and have been shown to be internalized by hepatocytes, yet the endocytosis-mediating receptor is unidentified. Two hepatocytic receptors which follow the classical endosomal pathway are known to bind apoE and thus would be able to bind chylomicron remnants: the low density lipoprotein (LDL) receptor and the LDL receptor-related protein (LRP). In earlier research, we obtained evidence that in the rat, endocytosis of a major fraction of chylomicron remnants is mediated by the LDL receptor in vivo [6]. This is in line with many observations in vitro showing that chylomicron remnants bind to the LDL receptor, their uptake being mediated by the LDL receptor in different cell lines [1]. However, humans, rabbits, and mice lacking functional LDL receptors do not accumulate chylomicron remnants in their plasma. In the rat, hepatic uptake and endocytosis of chylomicron remnants could be inhibited by the receptor-associated protein (RAP), a negative regulator of LRP function [7]. Recently, Willnow and co-workers showed that inactivation of LRP by RAP was associated with a marked accumulation of chylomicron remnants in mice lacking the LDL receptor and to a lesser degree in normal mice; this suggests that both the LDL receptor and LRP are involved in remnant clearance [8]. The endocytosis of chylomicron remnants is delayed after hepatic uptake from the blood of normal rats, which suggests that extracellular processing of chylomicron remnants by the liver precedes receptor-mediated endocytosis [3]. No such delay was observed in estradiol-treated rats, whose LDL receptors had been induced several-fold [9]. Shafi and co-workers showed that hepatic lipase participates in the initial uptake and processing of chylomicron remnants in isolated, perfused rat livers [10]. In a current study, uptake and internalization of small chylomicron remnants from glucose-fed rats and large chylomicron remnants from fat-fed rats were measured and provided interesting insights into the extracellular processing and endocytosis of chylomicron remnants in the fasting and postabsorptive state. Plasma clearance and liver uptake of large chylomicron remnants occur more rapidly than those of small chylomicron remnants. However, the internalization of large chylomicron remnants into endosomes of estradiol-treated and untreated rats is substantially slower than the endocytosis of small chylomicron remnants. Extracellular processing of large chylomicron remnants seems to be much more important than that of small chylomicron remnants; the delay in endocytosis of large chylomicron remnants cannot be abolished by stimulation of the LDL receptor. From our findings (see contribution of Windler et al.) we conclude that large chylomicron remnants bind initially to hepatic lipase and require further processing before the remnant particle is internalized by an endocytic receptor. However, small chylomicron remnants bind in estradiol-treated rats exclusively and in normal rats predominantly to the LDL receptor, by which they are taken up into endosomes.

High density lipoproteins (HDL) are believed to play an important role in the transport of excess cholesterol from extrahepatic tissues to the liver for re-utilization or excretion into bile, referred to as reverse cholesterol transport. The liver takes up cholesteryl esters of HDL at a greater fractional rate than apoA-I. Three different mechanisms for the hepatic uptake and intracellular processing of HDL particles, and of cholesteryl esters selectively taken up from HDL, have been proposed in reverse cholesterol transport [11]: a) binding of HDL particles to the cell surface without internalization, yet selective delivery of cholesteryl esters to the cell, b) internalization of HDL particles and retroendocytosis after unloading of cholesteryl esters within the cell, or c) internalization and lysosomal degradation of HDL particles plus selective uptake of cholesteryl esters from surface-bound noninternalized HDL. The trafficking of apoE-deficient HDL particles and their component cholesteryl esters in rat hepatocytes were studied. Human HDL$_3$, labeled with two nondegradable, intracellularly trapped tracers in their apoA-I and their cholesteryl esters, were injected into rats, and five subcellular fractions were isolated from the liver after various times. In endosomes and lysosomes the two labels were recovered at a ratio near unity, indicating that HDL are endocytosed as particles, transported to early and late endosomes and finally subjected to lysosomal degradation. However, no significant amounts of label were found in receptor-recycling endosomes. Thus, we found no evidence for the proposition that HDL may recycle to the plasma after intracellularly unloading cholesterol. In contrast to the endocytic organelles, label of HDL-associated cholesteryl esters in the whole liver exceeded 2- to 3-fold the label of HDL-associated apoA-I, which is compatible with selective separate uptake of HDL-cholesteryl esters in addition to uptake of whole HDL particles. The excess cholesteryl esters accumulated in a nonendosomal fraction, whose major proteins clearly differed from the integral proteins of endosomes. These data thus indicate two distinct intracellular routes of hepatocytic HDL trafficking in vivo [11].

Acknowledgements

This work was supported by the Deutsche Forschungsgemeinschaft, Sonderforschungsbereich 232. For excellent technical assistance we thank Birgit Biermann, Anke Grigoleit, Walter Tauscher, Christine Voss, and Wilfried Weber.

References

1. Havel RJ, Hamilton RL. Hepatology 1988;8:1689—1704.
2. Belcher JD, Hamilton RL, Brady SE, Hornick CA, Jäckle S, Schneider WJ, Havel RJ. Proc Natl Acad Sci USA 1987;84:6785—6789.
3. Jäckle S, Runquist E, Brady S, Hamilton RL, Havel RJ. J Lipid Res 1991;32:485—498.
4. Jäckle S, Runquist E, Miranda-Brady S, Havel RJ. J Biol Chem 1991;266:1396—1402.
5. Jäckle S, Beisiegel U, Rinninger F, Buck F, Grigoleit A, Block A, Gröger I, Greten H, Windler E. J Biol Chem 1994;269:1026—1032.
6. Jäckle S, Rinninger F, Greeve J, Greten H, Windler E. J Lipid Res 1992;33:419—429.
7. Mokuno H, Brady S, Kotite L, Herz J, Havel RJ. J Biol Chem 1994;269:13238—13243.
8. Willnow TE, Sheng Z, Ishibashi S, Herz J. Science 1994;264:1471—1474.
9. Jäckle S, Brady SE, Havel RJ. Proc Natl Acad Sci USA 1989;86:1880—1884.
10. Shafi S, Brady SE, Bensadoun A, Havel RJ. J Lipid Res 1994;35:709—720.
11. Jäckle S, Rinninger F, Lorenzen T, Greten H, Windler E. Hepatology 1993;17:455—465.

Mechanisms regulating hepatic chylomicron remnant uptake and metabolism

E. Windler[1], S. Jäckle[1], J. Greeve[1], W. Daerr[1], F. Rinninger[1], O. Braren[1], C. Pox[1], D. Puchta[1], D. Petkova[2], H. Robenek[3] and H. Greten[1]

[1]*Medizinische Kernklinik und Poliklinik, Universitäts-Krankenhaus Eppendorf, Martinistraße 52, D-20246 Hamburg, Germany;* [2]*Department of Lipid Protein Interactions, Bulgarian Academy of Sciences, Sofia, Bulgaria; and* [3]*Institute for Arteriosclerosis Research, University of Münster, Münster, Germany*

Abstract. Removal of small chylomicron remnants by rat livers closely correlates with the LDL-receptor mRNA modulated by various interventions. In contrast, removal of remnants of large chylomicrons is not appreciably influenced by the activity of the hepatic LDL receptor. Their primary removal depends on a heparinase-sensitive binding site, presumably hepatic lipase. Despite their more rapid removal from plasma, large chylomicron remnants appear in hepatocytic endosomes only after some delay. In contrast to small chylomicron remnants, endocytosis of large chylomicron remnants is apparently a two-step process in which they are first rapidly bound to hepatic lipase, and secondly passed on to an endocytosis-mediating receptor.

Results and Discussion

In the rat, hepatic LDL-receptor mRNA is suppressed by exogenous cholesterol, dietary saturated fatty acids and bile acids and by intravenously injected high doses of β-VLDL. For the determination of LDL-receptor mRNA a quantitative reverse transcription PCR was developed. Insertion of a DNA fragment led to an allelic variant of the LDL-receptor cDNA, which was cloned in plasmid pT3T7 and transcribed by T7-RNA polymerase in vitro. This variant mRNA was amplified together with endogenous mRNA by RT-PCR using ^{32}P-labeled primers to enable quantification.

In vivo and in isolated perfused rat livers, the rate of uptake of the postlipolytic remnants of triglyceride-rich lipoproteins was determined. As a surrogate for VLDL remnants containing apolipoprotein (apo)B100, β-VLDL was tested [1]. Their uptake paralleled the activity of the LDL receptor, as estimated from LDL-receptor mRNA. But the mechanism of uptake of chylomicron remnants containing apoB48 is still not settled. On the one hand they contain apoE, a high-affinity ligand for the LDL receptor, on the other hand a lack of LDL receptors does not result in gross hypertriglyceridemia or apparent remnant accumulation. When remnants from small chylomicrons were tested a clear dependence of the hepatic uptake on the activity of the LDL receptor was observed. This is in line with many observations in vitro in various cell lines showing that chylomicron remnants bind to the LDL receptor and their uptake is mediated by the LDL receptor.

When LDL-receptor mRNA was suppressed to undetectable levels, the rate of uptake of small chylomicron remnants was as low as that of their parent lymph chylomicrons. Since these do not contain apoE and have been shown to have a very slow removal rate compared with remnants, the uptake under these conditions probably reflects nonspecific association in the liver. This would mean that, at least in rodents, the LDL receptor is the single most important binding site mediating endocytosis of small chylomicron remnants in the liver.

However, humans, rabbits, and mice lacking functional LDL receptors do not accumulate chylomicron remnants in their plasma. Thus, under nonphysiological conditions alternative mechanisms have to act as substitutes for the LDL receptor. One likely alternative is the LDL receptor-related protein (LRP). In rats and mice, accumulation of chylomicron remnants has been noted when LRP was inhibited by RAP, a receptor-associated protein which is able to inhibit binding to LRP very effectively [2]. The rate of internalization mediated by LRP, however, appears to be quite slow. RAP also associates with the LDL receptor, but with much lower affinity, and association with additional as yet unidentified receptors has not been excluded with certainty. However, experiments using RAP or observations in animals deficient in the LDL receptor did not distinguish between possible differences of effects on remnants from chylomicrons of various sizes, which are synthesized under different nutritional states.

The observations relating chylomicron remnant uptake to the activity of the LDL receptor hold only for remnants from small chylomicrons as they are formed in the fasting state. When remnants from large chylomicrons, produced under postprandial conditions, were used, results differed greatly. In vivo their half-life in the circulation of rats is shorter than that of small chylomicron remnants, and the rate of uptake in liver perfusions has been shown to be higher. Their uptake is not, however, influenced by modulation of the activity of the LDL receptor. The percentage of uptake during one passage in single-pass liver perfusions is similar to that found for small chylomicron remnants, and downregulation of the LDL-receptor activity did not lower the rate of uptake. Nor did upregulation of the LDL receptor markedly enhance the uptake at lower concentrations. Yet an additional effect of the LDL receptor cannot be excluded under conditions of high concentrations of remnants, when the capacity of the primary binding site of large chylomicron remnants is saturated. Observations compatible with this concept were made in the rat in vivo.

Thus, in contrast to small chylomicron remnants, large chylomicron remnants appear to bind initially to a site that is unregulated, or else differently regulated from the LDL receptor. When livers were flushed with heparin or heparinase prior to studies of uptake, the removal of large chylomicron remnants was greatly retarded, while that of small chylomicron remnants remained unaffected. These interventions eliminate as binding sites the heparan sulfates and substances like hepatic lipase attached to these proteoglycans. Although evidence has been obtained from in vitro studies that triglyceride-rich lipoproteins may bind to heparan sulfates after enrichment in apoE or lipoprotein lipase, there is no evidence that such a mechanism operates in vivo [3]. However, recently it has been demonstrated that hepatic lipase participates in the initial uptake of chylomicron remnants [4]. In isolated perfused rat livers it has been shown that the effect induced by treatment with heparin is due to the elimination of hepatic lipase, since a specific antibody to hepatic lipase had the same effect in abolishing uptake of remnants by the liver. From this it is concluded that large, in contrast to small, chylomicron remnants initially bind to hepatic lipase. This accounts for their fast removal from plasma and the lack of response to modulation of the LDL-receptor activity.

Hepatic lipase is not known to mediate endocytosis. This fits the observation that large chylomicron remnants are internalized much more slowly than small chylomicron remnants. Kinetics of intrahepatocytic trafficking have been determined [5]. Endosomal fractions were isolated 30 min after injection of remnants into rats and the specific activity of the radiolabel of the injected remnants was determined (see pp 419–421). Much less of the dose of large chylomicron remnants was recovered in isolated early hepatic endosomes (the compartment of uncoupling of receptors and ligands and that of recycling

424

receptors), as well as in late endosomes (the multivesicular bodies). Thus, in comparison to small chylomicron remnants, despite their more rapid removal from plasma large chylomicron remnants appear to pass through a delay compartment before being internalized. This fits the view that hepatic lipase, to which large chylomicron remnants apparently bind initially, inefficiently mediates endocytosis.

Endocytosis has probably to be envisioned as a two-step process in which the large chylomicron remnants are first rapidly bound to hepatic lipase. Here, further hydrolysis of the remnants may modulate the particle and possibly unmask apoE to initiate the second step, in which the remnants are passed on to a receptor that is able to mediate endocytosis. This again may be the LDL receptor. Thus, modulation or absence of LDL-receptor activity is not reflected in disappearance from the plasma. Interestingly, it has been shown that upregulation of the LDL receptor by estrogen can partially overcome a delay in remnant removal and enhance the endocytosis [6]. Thus, all speculations on the function of the LDL receptor in the removal of remnants derived from plasma kinetics may be inappropriate. In the case of lack of LDL receptors alternative binding sites may substitute for the initiation of endocytosis. LRP is one alternative, and the asialoglycoprotein receptor may function as an additional endocytosis-mediating binding site [7,8].

The hypothesis of this function for the asialoglycoprotein receptor has been challenged by expressing the receptor in cultured cells. COS-7 cells were transfected with the cDNAs of the two components of the heterodimer human asialoglycoprotein receptor. Only transfected cells bound asialoglycoproteins and their binding capacity for chylomicron remnants increased by up to 50%. Similar results have been obtained using stably transfected cells. Degradation was increased likewise. Although these results may point to a role of the asialoglycoprotein receptor in the hepatic uptake of chylomicron remnants under conditions of impaired LDL-receptor activity, the physiological significance needs to be evaluated and demonstrated in vivo.

The structural differences between large and small chylomicron remnants which determine their different modes of hepatic uptake are currently under investigation. It becomes evident that not merely the size of the particles is significant for their metabolic fate. Other structural determinants seem to be more important and may not only determine the initial mechanism of uptake of intestinal lipoproteins, but are conceivably also decisive for the hepatic catabolism and fate of their constituents [9], and may also apply to structural variants of triglyceride-rich lipoproteins of hepatic origin [10].

Acknowledgements

This research was supported by grants from the Deutsche Forschungsgemeinschaft SFB 232.

References

1. Jäckle S, Rinninger F, Greeve J, Greten H, Windler E. J Lipid Res 1992;33:419–429.
2. Mokuno H, Brady S, Kotite L, Herz J, Havel RJ. J Biol Chem 1994;269:13238–13243.
3. Beisiegel U, Weber W, Bengtsson-Olivecrona G. Proc Natl Sci 1991;88:8342–8346.
4. Shafi S, Brady SE, Bensadoun A, Havel RJ. J Lipid Res 1994;35:709–720.
5. Jäckle S, Runquist E, Brady S, Hamilton RL, Havel RJ. J Lipid Res 1991;32:485–498.
6. Jäckle S, Brady SE, Havel RJ. Proc Natl Acad Sci USA 1989;86:1880–1884.
7. Windler E, Greeve J, Levkov D, Därr W, Greten H. Biochem J 1991;276:79–87.
8. Willnow TE, Sheng Z, Ishibashi S, Herz J. Science 1994;264:1471–1474.
9. Smit JS, Kuipers F, Vonk RJ, Temmermann AM, Jäckle S, Windler E. Hepatology 1993;17:445–454.
10. Greeve J, Altkemper I, Greten H, Windler E. J Lipid Res 1993;34:1367–1383.

Atherosclerosis X.
F.P. Woodford, J. Davignon and A. Sniderman, editors.

425

Chylomicron-remnant uptake by rat liver and biliary secretion of chylomicron cholesterol

Th.J.C. Van Berkel, M.C.M. Van Dijk, G.J. Ziere, M.N. Pieters and J.K. Kruyt

Division of Biopharmaceutics, Leiden-Amsterdam Center for Drug Research, Sylvius Laboratories, University of Leiden, P.O. Box 9503, 2300 RA Leiden, The Netherlands

Abstract. Recognition of chylomicron remnants by the parenchymal liver cells is due to the remnant receptor which in rats is also responsible for β-VLDL uptake. In vivo, the uptake of both ligands can be effectively blocked by lactoferrin, a 76.5-kDa glycoprotein with an amino acid sequence similar to that of the recognition site of apolipoprotein E (apoE). The efficiency of the liver uptake of chylomicron remnants, the conversion of its cholesterol (esters) into bile acids and their secretion into bile determines the fate of intestinally absorbed cholesterol (esters). In rats provided with permanent catheters inserted into the bile duct, the heart and the duodenum, it was determined that 72 h after injection of [3H]-cholesteryl ester-labeled chylomicrons 70% of the injected dose has appeared in bile, mainly as bile acids (>90%). Prior lactoferrin injection reduced the biliary secretion of radioactivity to 58%. It can be concluded that the processing of chylomicron-remnant cholesterol components in the liver and the subsequent excretion in bile is very efficient and the hepatic remnant receptor is essential to achieve this high percentage of removal and thus protect against extrahepatic cholesterol (ester) deposition.

Chylomicrons are produced in the intestinal enterocytes and secreted into the lymph. After drainage of the lymph into the bloodstream, chylomicrons are processed by the action of endothelial cell-bound lipoprotein lipase and high density lipoprotein (HDL) [1]. The resulting chylomicron remnants are rapidly taken up by the liver. Uptake is primarily carried out by the parenchymal cells, while Kupffer and endothelial cells play a minor role [2]. Chylomicron remnants are taken up by the parenchymal cells via the remnant receptor, which in rats is also responsible for the in vivo uptake of β-migrating very low density lipoprotein (β-VLDL) [2,3]. This conclusion is based upon studies which showed that the uptake in vivo of both ligands by parenchymal cells was effectively blocked by lactoferrin, a 76.5-kDa glycoprotein with a similar cluster of arginine residues at the N-terminus to apolipoprotein (apoE). In vitro data also indicated that the two lipoproteins compete for the same high-affinity site on isolated parenchymal cells [2]. The efficiency of intestinal cholesterol absorption, chylomicron (remnant)-mediated transport to the liver and conversion to bile acids is an important feature, as it determines the effect of cholesterol feeding on cholesterol (ester) deposition. To protect the body against extrahepatic (atherosclerotic) accumulation of cholesterol (esters), it is necessary that these lipoproteins are rapidly removed from the blood circulation, coupled with an efficient secretion of the cholesterol components into the bile.

This study was performed to characterize the kinetics of secretion of chylomicron (remnant) cholesterol components into the bile after uptake by liver parenchymal cells. Chylomicrons were labeled with [3H]cholesteryl esters and the kinetics of bile secretion were determined in unrestrained rats provided with permanent catheters inserted into the bile duct, the heart and the duodenum [4]. In addition we analyzed the effect of a temporarily lactoferrin blockade of the liver uptake of chylomicron remnants on the bile secretion of chylomicron-remnant cholesterol components, in order to determine to what extent the efficiency of liver uptake could affect the total proportion of cholesterol (esters) secreted into the bile. The chylomicron (remnant) data were compared with those of β-VLDL in order to determine to what extent the initial recognition determines the final efficiency of bile secretion.

Methods

Bile was collected from unrestrained male Wistar rats (mass 350–450 g), as described previously [4]. Permanent catheters were inserted into the bile duct, the heart and the duodenum, and tunneled subcutaneously to the skull. The bile duct and the duodenum catheters were connected to each other immediately after surgery in order to maintain an intact enterohepatic circulation. The rats were allowed to recover from the operation for 1 week. At 11 am, lipoproteins (50 µg of apolipoprotein/kg body wt, both for chylomicrons and β-VLDL) were administered via the heart catheter. If indicated, rats received a prior injection of 70 mg/kg lactoferrin via the heart catheter. Animals were not anesthetized during the experiments. The bile duct was immediately connected to a fraction collector and bile was collected continuously in 15-min fractions for 3 h, followed by 1-h fractions for the remaining period.

Results

After injection of [3H]cholesteryl ester-labeled chylomicrons into rats, the liver uptake proceeded rapidly up to a maximum of 71.8% of the injected dose, 20 min after injection (Fig. 1A). The serum radioactivity showed the characteristic biphasic decay which is explained by extrahepatic processing of chylomicrons to chylomicron remnants and decreases to 12.6% of the injected dose 30 min after injection (Fig. 1B). The initial extrahepatic processing of chylomicrons is apparently not influenced by lactoferrin. A

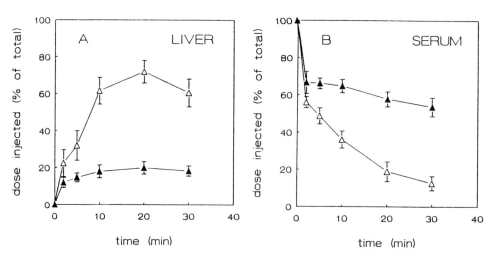

Fig. 1. Effect of lactoferrin on liver uptake and serum decay of [3H]cholesteryl ester-labeled chylomicrons. Labeled chylomicrons (50 µg apolipoprotein/kg body wt) were injected into anesthetized rats. At the times indicated, liver association (A) and serum decay (B) were determined in rats not pretreated (Δ) or rats previously injected with lactoferrin (▲; 70 mg/kg body wt 1 min before injection of radiolabeled chylomicrons). Liver values are corrected for radioactivity present in serum. Values are means ± SEM of four experiments with two different preparations of labeled chylomicrons in four different rats.

prior injection of 70 mg/kg lactoferrin, 1 min before injection of chylomicrons, largely inhibited the liver uptake of chylomicrons (72% inhibition at 20 min after injection; Fig. 1A). Concomitantly, the serum radioactivity remained at much higher levels, indicating that the residence time of chylomicron remnants in the bloodstream was increased (Fig. 1B).

Cellular distribution and processing of chylomicrons

[³H]cholesteryl ester-labeled chylomicrons were injected into rats and 15 min after injection, the different liver cell types were isolated by a low-temperature cell isolation procedure. It appeared that of the total liver-associated radioactivity, 88.2% was associated with the parenchymal cells, 1.4 % with the endothelial cells and 9.5% with the Kupffer cells. Up to 10 min after injection of chylomicrons, the ratio of cholesteryl esters to cholesterol in liver reflected that of chylomicrons (approximately 75% in cholesteryl esters). Between 10 and 60 min after injection, hydrolysis of cholesteryl esters to unesterified cholesterol took place (Fig. 2).

Kinetics of biliary excretion of ³H from chylomicrons and the effect of lactoferrin

After injection of ³H-cholesteryl ester-labeled chylomicrons, radioactivity appeared in bile within the first 15 min. Secretion of radioactivity (plotted as counts collected/15 min) reached a plateau 1 h after injection (Fig. 3A).

Injection of lactoferrin 1 min prior to injection of chylomicrons considerably reduced the secretion of radioactivity in bile. Especially during the first hour after injection, a strong reduction in biliary secretion of radioactivity was noted (Fig. 3A). From 12 to 72 h after injection, biliary secretion of radioactivity was almost identical between control

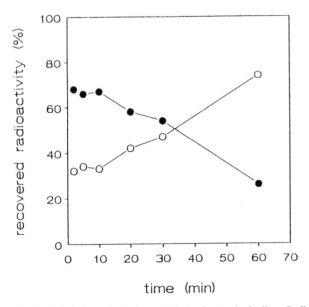

Fig. 2. Hydrolysis of chylomicron cholesteryl esters in the liver. Radiolabeled chylomicrons were injected into anesthetized rats (50 μg apolipoprotein/kg body wt). At the times indicated, liver samples were taken and lipid was extracted, [³H]cholesterol (O) and [³H]cholesteryl ester (●) were separated by TLC and radioactivity was determined.

428

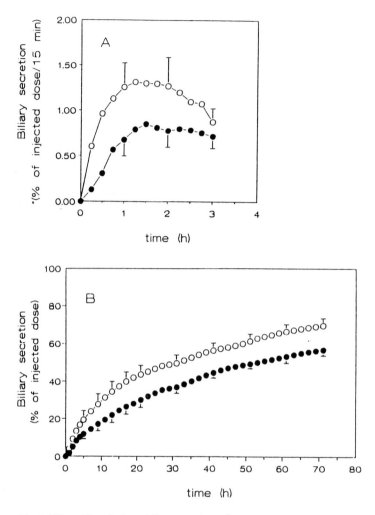

Fig. 3. Effect of lactoferrin on biliary secretion of ^{3}H radioactivity after administration of [3H]cholesteryl ester-labeled chylomicrons. Chylomicrons were injected into rats not pretreated (O) or preinjected with lactoferrin (●). Bile was collected in 15-min fractions during the first 3 h (A) and subsequently in 1-h fractions (B), and fractions were analyzed for radioactivity. Values are means of four experiments ± SEM (two different preparations used for four different rats).

and lactoferrin-preinjected rats (Fig. 3B). Analysis of the bile composition revealed that at all time points in this study, most (>90%) of the radioactivity was present in (water-soluble) bile acids. At 24 and 72 h after injection, accumulation increased to respectively 44 and 70% of the injected dose (Fig. 3B), whereas after lactoferrin the amount recovered at 72 h was only 58% of the injected dose.

Discussion

This study describes the in vivo processing of chylomicron-remnant cholesterol components by rat liver. Cholesterol ester-labeled chylomicrons injected into rats were rapidly taken up from the circulation by liver parenchymal cells. Initially (up to 10 min after injection) the cholesterol/cholesteryl ester ratio reflected that of the injected chylomicrons but subsequently the cholesteryl esters were hydrolyzed, so that 1 h after injection, 75% of the radioactivity is present as free cholesterol which was used for bile acid synthesis and excreted into the bile. At 72 h after injection, the total recovery of chylomicron radioactivity in bile was 70.0%. We used lactoferrin in order to study if inhibition of the liver uptake of chylomicron remnants would influence the efficiency of cholesterol (ester) processing by the liver and thus increase the flux of cholesterol (esters) into the extrahepatic sites. It appears that lactoferrin not only delays the rate of excretion into the bile but also reduces the total amount of radioactivity recovered there, which underlines the importance of efficient hepatic uptake of chylomicron cholesterol (esters) to prevent or minimize extrahepatic deposition of cholesterol.

Acknowledgement

Hille Bakkeren is thanked for surgical assistance.

References

1. Redgrave TG. Int Rev Physiol 1983;28:103–130.
2. Van Dijk MCM, Ziere GJ, Boers W, Linthorst C, Bijsterbosch MK, van Berkel ThJC. Biochem J 1991;279: 863–870.
3. Harkes L, van Duijne A, van Berkel ThJC. Eur J Biochem 1989;180:241–248.
4. Kuipers F, Havinga R, Bosschieter H, Toorop GP, Hindriks FR, Vonk RJ. Gastroenterology 1985;88:403–411.

Cholesterol transport mediated by sterol carrier protein 2 (SCP2)

U. Seedorf[1], P. Brysch[1], T. Engel[1], S. Scheek[1], M. Raabe[1], M. Fobker[1], T. Szyperski[2], K. Wüthrich[2], N. Maeda[3] and G. Assmann[1]

[1]*Institut für Arterioskleroseforschung, Westfälische Wilhelms-Universität, Münster, Germany;* [2]*Swiss Institute of Technology, ETH-Hönggerberg, Zurich, Switzerland; and* [3]*Institute of Pathology, University of North Carolina at Chapel Hill, Chapel Hill, North Carolina, USA*

Abstract. Two sterol carrier proteins, SCP2 and SCPx, are expressed from the same gene via alternative splicing or alternative transcription initiation. The sterol transfer domains of the two proteins consist of a unique plate-like structure. The flat bottom is created by a five-stranded β-sheet, whereas three α-helices make up its rim, creating a hydrophobic cavity. Moreover, we found that SCPx, but not SCP2, functions as a previously undescribed peroxisomal 3-ketoacyl-CoA thiolase (EC 2.3.1.16) with intrinsic sterol- and phospholipid-transfer activities. We currently assume that this multifunctional protein participates in the peroxisomal β-oxidation pathway involved in the oxidative degradation of various fatty acids, xenobiotics, and the cholesterol side-chain. In addition, the protein may facilitate the intraperoxisomal movement of sterols and various other lipids. To evaluate this hypothesis, we started to construct mice lacking the SCP2/SCPx-gene function by introducing a neo®-gene into exon 14 of the gene. The murine SCP2/SCPx-gene is shown to consist of 16 exons spanning almost 100 kb. The coding information of exons 1 to 16 is used to generate SCPx whereas exons 12 to 16 are used to create SCP2. These ongoing studies should therefore provide a mouse strain deficient in SCP2 and SCPx that should provide an ideal model to study the functions of the two sterol carrier proteins in vivo.

According to current concepts, intracellular trafficking of cholesterol and related sterols is not simply mediated by nonspecific diffusion but requires target-specific transport mechanisms. Earlier studies performed in our and other laboratories indicated that the bulk flow of de novo synthesized cholesterol from the endoplasmic reticulum to the plasma membrane is a fast, energy-requiring, vesicular process that proceeds independently of the secretory protein pathway [1]. Specific transport mechanisms have also been suggested for the transfer of cholesterol from the membrane of secondary lysosomes to the endoplasmic reticulum, the intracellular site of cholesterol esterification catalyzed by the enzyme acyl-CoA:cholesterol acyl transferase (ACAT), and the delivery of sterols to mitochondria and peroxisomes [2]. The latter pathways are primarily required for the synthesis of pregnenolone and bile acids. The precise mechanisms involved have not, however, been elucidated.

Sterol transport via a soluble carrier protein is an attractive hypothesis. The protein could harbor signals mediating target specificity and, at the same time, shield the lipophilic transport substrates from the aqueous phase. The most likely known candidate for a sterol carrier is sterol carrier protein 2 (SCP2). SCP2, also known as the nonspecific lipid transfer protein, promotes the exchange of a wide variety of lipids and sterols between membranes in vitro [3]. In addition, the protein activates the enzymatic conversion of 7-DHC to cholesterol by liver microsomes [4]. It also stimulates the ACAT-mediated esterification of intracellular cholesterol [5] and the introduction of the less polar

---

Address for correspondence: Dr Udo Seedorf, Institut für Arterioskleroseforschung, Universität Münster, Domagkstr. 3, 48149 Münster, Germany. Tel.: +49-251-836197. Fax: +49-251-836208.

substrates in bile acid biosynthesis to the membrane-bound enzymes in vitro [6]. Moreover, the protein may be required for the intracellular transfer of cholesterol which is needed for pregnenolone synthesis in adrenals [7] and ovaries [8]. On the other hand, purified SCP2 does not contain any bound lipid [9], and a stable association between SCP2 and phospholipids or cholesterol could not be demonstrated [10]. It was therefore proposed that the protein either binds lipids with low affinity [11] or does not function as a typical binding protein but facilitates lipid exchange between membranes by other means [12]. Moreover, in view of the high degree of specificity which is required for intracellular sterol transport, the structural simplicity of SCP2 deduced from its primary sequence [13] seems to be at least surprising.

To evaluate the hypothesis that SCP2 functions as an intracellular sterol carrier employing methods of current molecular biology, we first cloned and sequenced SCP2-encoding cDNAs from the rat [14], mouse [15], and human (Seedorf, unpublished). These studies indicated that mammalian SCP2 is synthesized as a 143-amino-acid precursor that is processed to the 123-amino-acid mature SCP2. In addition, SCP2-related transcripts encoding larger proteins that are identical at their C-terminal domains with pre-SCP2 are present in the livers of all mammalian species studied. The complete cDNA encoding one of these proteins has an open reading frame of 547 codons, representing an extension of 404 codons at the initiator methionine of pre-SCP2. The open reading frame was predicted to encode a previously undescribed fusion protein containing a 143-amino-acid C-terminal lipid-transfer domain and a 404-amino-acid N-terminal domain with unknown biochemical activity or function. The fact that SCP2 is completely contained within this sequence suggested possible sterol carrier activity, and we assigned the predicted protein the provisional name *sterol carrier protein x* (SCPx) [14].

Most recent work in our laboratory focused on the mouse model. As shown in Fig. 1, SCP2 and SCPx are encoded by a single gene consisting of 16 exons spanning almost 100 kb located on murine chromosome 3 or 4. SCP2 and SCPx transcripts are most probably

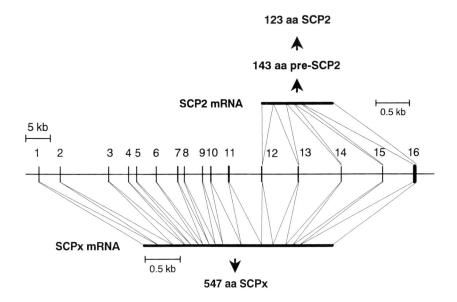

Fig. 1. Structure of the murine SCP2/SCPx-gene and presumed alternative splicing pathways.

432

produced by alternative splicing, but alternative transcription initiation cannot be completely excluded as the underlying mechanism. The coding information of exons 1–16 is used to generate SCPx whereas exons 10–16 are spliced to create the SCP2 transcript. Further transcript heterogeneity results from alternative polyadenylation of the two types of transcripts [15]. In addition, we have isolated and characterized two SCP2-related pseudogenes, SCP2-ps1 and SCP2-ps2, both of which have similar structures lacking introns and are not transcribed ([15]; Seedorf and Raabe, unpublished).

To elucidate possible biological functions of SCPx, we expressed the entire rat SCPx (SCPx-547) and a peptide consisting of the thiolase-like SCPx-specific domain (residues 1 to 383, SCPx-383) in *E. coli*. Subcellular fractionation followed by Western blotting analysis with antibodies against SCPx-383, which did not cross-react with SCP2, revealed that SCPx is primarily localized within peroxisomes [16]. This result was confirmed by immunocytochemistry, which revealed SCPx-383 epitopes within the matrix of organelles containing an electron-dense lattice-like structure, characteristic of peroxisomes. In contrast, relatively little SCP2 was detected in this organelle, which suggests that this protein has wider intracellular localization [16].

Since the sequence of the N-terminal 400 amino acids of SCPx is known to be vaguely related to acetoacetyl-CoA and 3-ketoacyl-CoA thiolases we further investigated whether SCPx-547 has thiolase activity if tested in an in vitro β-oxidation system [16]. As shown in Table 1, SCPx-547 efficiently catalyzes the thiolytic cleavage of a wide variety of 3-oxoacyl-CoA substrates. The highest specific activity was obtained with 3-oxooctanoyl-CoA (V_{max} = 120 U/mg). Acyl chain lengths above or below 8 resulted in a gradual decrease in specific activity. The enzyme is a very poor catalyst of the thiolytic cleavage of acetoacetyl-CoA (specific activity of 2.5 U/mg). The activities obtained with the unsaturated substrate 3-oxooleoyl-CoA (C18:1) and the saturated substrate 3-oxostearoyl-CoA (C18:0) were similar (33.3 and 26.7 U/mg) (Table 1). The essentially parallel straight lines provided by the kinetic analyses shown in Fig. 2 are compatible with a ping-pong reaction mechanism. The apparent K_M values for CoA are 2.9 ± 0.59 and 6.3 ± 1.3 μM ([3-oxooctanoyl-CoA] = 2.5 and 10 μM), which suggests that the enzyme has a high affinity for CoA. The apparent K_M values of 5.4 and 7.9 μM ([CoA] = 150 μM) obtained for 3-oxooctanoyl CoA and 3-oxopalmitoyl-CoA point to a somewhat higher affinity for the medium- than for the long-chain acyl substrate (Fig. 3). The classical Michaelis-Menten kinetic relationship between substrate concentrations and initial velocities found for the medium-chain acyl substrate 3-oxooctanoyl-CoA is altered to a sigmoidal curve for the

Table 1. Specific activities of SCPx-547 determined with various 3-oxoacyl-CoA substrates. For experimental details see [16]

Acyl-CoA substrate	Acyl chain length and no. of double bonds	V_{max} (U/mg)
Acetoacetyl-CoA	C4:0	2.5
3-oxohexanoyl-CoA	C6:0	55.4
3-oxooctanoyl-CoA	C8:0	120
3-oxodecanoyl-CoA	C10:0	48.9
3-oxoundecanoyl-CoA	C11:0	53.3
3-oxomyristoyl-CoA	C14:0	35.3
3-oxopalmitoyl-CoA	C16:0	30.6
3-oxostearoyl-CoA	C18:0	26.7
3-oxooleoyl-CoA	C18:1	33.3

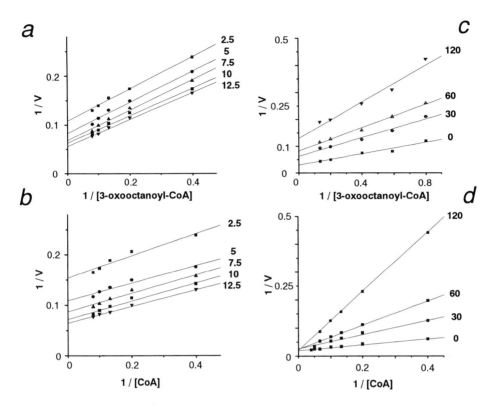

Fig. 2. Kinetic analyses of the SCPx-547 3-oxoacyl-CoA thiolase activity. (a) Lineweaver-Burk plots for 3-oxooctanoyl-CoA obtained with 2.5, 5, 7.5, 10, and 12.5 µM coenzyme A. (b) Lineweaver-Burk plots for coenzyme A obtained with 2.5, 5, 7.5, 10, and 12.5 µM 3-oxooctanoyl-CoA. (c) Lineweaver-Burk plots for 3-oxooctanoyl-CoA obtained in the presence of 0, 30, 60, and 120 µM acetyl-CoA. (d) Lineweaver-Burk plots for coenzyme A obtained in the presence of 0, 30, 60, and 120 µM acetyl-CoA.

long-chain acyl substrate 3-oxopalmitoyl-CoA (Fig. 3). Therefore, efficient thiolytic cleavage of the long-chain acyl substrate is dependent in vitro on relatively high substrate concentrations.

The latter finding discriminates the novel thiolase from the previously described peroxisomal 3-oxoacyl-CoA thiolase that has been reported [17] to exhibit significantly higher affinities for long than for medium acyl chain substrates. Peroxisomal 3-oxoacyl-CoA thiolase was further shown to be regulated by acetyl-CoA-mediated product inhibition. It was suggested that acetyl-CoA binds to the CoA site of the enzyme as a dead-end inhibitor, resulting in strong product inhibition at acetyl-CoA concentrations as low as 30 µM [17]. As shown in Fig. 2c,d, SCPx-547 shows a different behavior. Acetyl-CoA is competitive with respect to CoA (K_I: 20.4 ± 2.0 µM) and noncompetitive with respect to 3-oxooctanoyl-CoA (K_I: 29.0 ± 5.5 µM), which suggests that acetyl-CoA reacts with the enzyme as the first product in the ping-pong mechanism. This result supports a reaction mechanism in which the first partial reaction is the formation of acetyl-CoA and an acyl$_{(n-2)}$-S-enzyme whereas in the second partial reaction the acyl$_{(n-2)}$ moiety is transferred to CoA, resulting in saturated fatty acyl$_{(n-2)}$-CoA and the free enzyme form.

Since SCPx-547 contains the SCP2-identical domain at its C-terminus, we also investi-

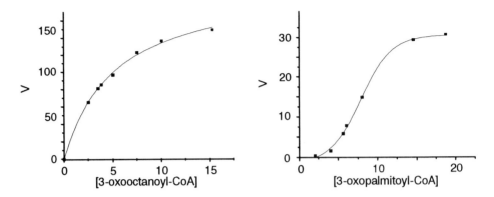

Fig. 3. Relationship between initial velocities and substrate concentrations for 3-oxooctanoyl-CoA (left) and 3-oxopalmitoyl-CoA (right) obtained with SCPx-547.

gated whether the protein has the same ability to stimulate the microsomal conversion of 7-dihydrocholesterol (7-DHC) to cholesterol as SCP2 (known as sterol carrier activity). As shown in Fig. 4a, SCPx-547 stimulates this in vitro reaction, though to a lesser extent than SCP2. To exclude a direct stimulatory effect of SCPx-547 on microsomal sterol Δ^7-reductase, the enzyme catalyzing the reaction, we also measured the transfer of 7-DHC from small unilamellar vesicles to *Bacillus megaterium* protoplasts directly. As shown in Table 2, SCPx-547 transfers 16.3 nmol/(nmol × h) representing 53% of the value for SCP2 (30.6 nmol/(nmol × h)). Moreover, SCPx has almost the same sterol-transfer activity as an artificial fusion protein constructed between glutathione-S-transferase and SCP2 (GST-SCP2), which suggests that the N-terminal thiolase-like domain has no specific influence on the transfer activity of SCPx-547 (Table 2). Another well-documented activity of SCP2 is the transfer of phosphatidylcholine (PC) from donor small

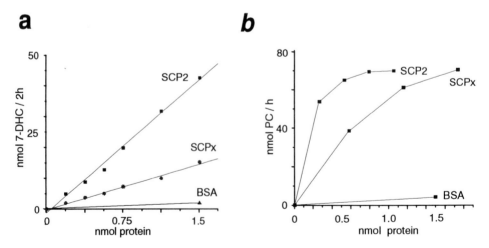

Fig. 4. Sterol-carrier and phosphatidylcholine-transfer activity of SCPx-547. (a) Stimulation of the microsomal conversion of 7-dehydrocholesterol to cholesterol in the presence of increasing concentrations of SCP2, SCPx-547 (SCPx) and BSA, determined as described in [16]. (b) Transfer of phosphatidylcholine from small unilamellar vesicles (donors) to *Bacillus megaterium* protoplasts (acceptors) as described in [16]. BSA: bovine serum albumin.

Table 2. Transfer of 7-dehydrocholesterol from small unilamellar vesicles (donors) to *Bacillus megaterium* protoplasts (acceptors) as described in [16]. BSA: bovine serum albumin, GST: glutathione-S-transferase

	Transfer of 7-dehydrocholesterol (nmol/(nmol proteins × h))
SCP2	30.6
SCPx-547	16.3
GST-SCP2	16.9
BSA	1.3

unilamellar vesicles to *Bacillus megaterium* protoplasts [18]. We deduce from Fig. 4b that SCPx-547 transfers 64 nmol PC/(nmol × h) representing 34% of the molar activity of SCP2 (189 nmol/(nmol × h)).

What is the structural basis of SCP2- and SCPx-mediated sterol and phospholipid transfer? We addressed this question by site-directed mutagenesis of recombinant human SCP2 combined with three-dimensional nuclear magnetic resonance spectroscopy with [^{15}N] human SCP2 [18,19]. Three α-helices comprising the polypeptide segments of residues 9–22, 25–30, and 100–102 were identified by sequential and medium-range nuclear Overhauser effects (NOE). The analysis of long-range backbone–backbone NOEs further revealed a five-stranded β-sheet including the residues 33–41, 47–54, 60–62, 71–76 and 100–102. Figure 5 shows the ribbon drawing of residues 8–76 and 99–103 of the optimized conformer, omitting helix C, since its precise arrangement has not yet been elucidated. SCP2 consists of a very unusual α–β-tertiary fold. No near identity was found

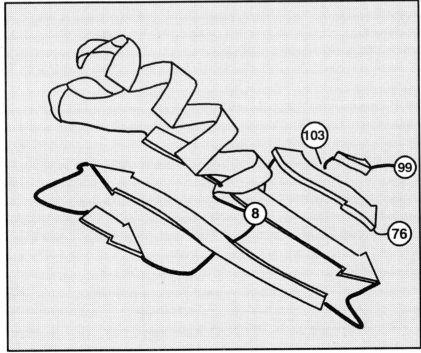

Fig. 5. Three-dimensional polypeptide backbone fold of human SCP2. Ribbon drawing generated with program Molscript of residues 8–76 and 99–103 of the optimal DIANA conformer without helix C. For methodological details see [19].

with any of the protein-folding types which are known to exist. The central feature of the molecular architecture consists of the five β-strands. The first three strands are arranged in an antiparallel fashion, the polypeptide chain then crosses over this sheet in a right-handed sense so that the fourth strand is added parallel to the first one. The fifth strand runs antiparallel to the fourth one, so that the total topology is +1, +1, -3x, -1. The β-sheet forms a flat, nearly oval-shaped, structure which is surrounded by three amphiphatic α-helices. Schematically, the whole structure resembles a plate or dish consisting of a hydrophilic outer part and an essentially hydrophobic inner part. Currently, we believe that the latter part is involved in the interaction between lipids and the protein. This view is clearly supported by the results of our site-directed mutagenesis study. Mutations which interfere with helix A or the integrity of the central β-sheet lead to drastic inactivation of SCP2-mediated sterol and lipid transfer. In contrast, mutations outside this structure or mutations which would have no effect on this structure have almost no effect on SCP2 activity [18].

The in vivo function of the novel peroxisomal 3-oxoacyl-CoA thiolase with intrinsic in vitro sterol carrier and PC transfer activity remains to be elucidated. Since another peroxisomal 3-oxoacyl-CoA thiolase has already been known for more than 10 years, the idea that this enzyme which exists in two closely related isoforms is completely sufficient to catalyze the thiolytic cleavage of all 3-oxoacyl-CoA substrates occurring in peroxisomal β-oxidation in vivo has to be reassessed [20]. We think that the catalytic properties of the novel thiolase imply an important role in peroxisomal β-oxidation. One major function discriminating peroxisomal from mitochondrial β-oxidation is to supply acetyl-CoA for anabolic reactions when the cells are well supplied with energy [21]. It is believed that the rate-limiting step in peroxisomal β-oxidation is the acyl-CoA oxidase reaction [22]. However, because of its high relative affinity for long 3-oxoacyl-CoA substrates, thiolysis of medium-chain substrates by the conventional peroxisomal 3-oxoacyl-CoA thiolase may become inefficient at high levels of long-chain substrates (e.g., postprandially in the liver). Under these circumstances, one possible function of the novel thiolase activity may be to act preferentially on medium-length 3-oxoacyl-CoA substrates, thus preventing their thiolytic cleavage from becoming rate-limiting. Another major function of peroxisomal β-oxidation is the oxidative degradation of xenobiotics and the cholesterol side-chain. So it is also possible that the novel SCP2/3-oxoacyl-CoA thiolase participates in these pathways in vivo.

One approach that can be used in order to investigate this hypothesis is to generate mice lacking the gene function. We applied this approach to SCP2 and SCPx by constructing a gene-targeting vector. An approx. 7-kb EcoRI fragment containing exon 14 of the murine SCP2/3-ketoacyl-CoA thiolase gene and the flanking intron regions was isolated from a genomic λ-clone and subcloned in the vector pBluescript. The continuity of exon 14 was then disrupted by inserting a neo^R-gene and the resulting DNA-fragment was cloned in the vector pPNT (Fig. 6). Subsequently, this vector was used in collaboration with Dr Maeda (UNC at Chapel Hill) to transfect E14TG2a mouse embryonic stem cells. Selection with G418 and gancyclovir led to the isolation of 182 resistant clones. Southern blotting analyses revealed two clones in which homologous recombination had occurred between the vector and the endogenous exon-14 region of the SCP2/SCPx-gene (Fig. 6). These clones were subsequently used to generate chimeric mice which are currently being crossed with C57BL/6-mice in order to identify transmitters and ultimately generate a strain of mice deficient in SCP2 and SCPx. We hope that the phenotypic characterization of these mice will help us to understand the roles of the two sterol carrier proteins in sterol trafficking and sterol metabolism.

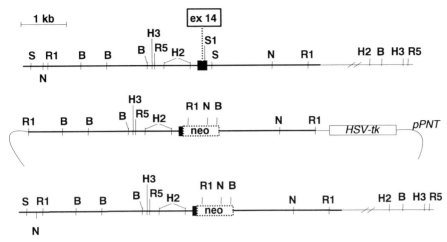

Fig. 6. Restriction nuclease map of the exon-14 region of the murine SCP2/SCPx-gene (top). Structure of the gene replacement vector constructed for disruption of exon 14 (middle). Restriction nuclease map of the exon-14 region as determined after homologous recombination had occurred in clones 20 and 110. S: Spe1, N: Nco1, R1: EcoR1, B: BamH1, H3: Hind3, R5: EcoR5, H2: Hind2, S1: Sal1.

Acknowledgements

This work was supported by the Deutsche Forschungsgemeinschaft (grant Se 459/2-1), the Land Nordrhein Westfalen, and a grant from Bristol Myers Squibb.

References

1. Seedorf U, Fobker M, Assmann G. Circulation 1992;86(suppl):1–549.
2. Liscum L, Dahl NK. J Lipid Res 1992;33:1239–1254.
3. Reinhart MP. Experientia 1990;46:599–611.
4. Noland BJ, Arebalo RE, Hansbury E, Scallen TJ. J Biol Chem 1980;255:4282–4289.
5. Gavey KL, Noland BJ, Scallen TJ. J Biol Chem 1981;256:2993–2999.
6. Seltman H, Diven W, Rizk M, Noland BJ, Chanderbhan R, Scallen TJ, Vahouny GV, Sanghvi A. Biochem J 1985;230:19–24.
7. Chanderbhan R, Noland BJ, Scallen TJ, Vahouny GV. J Biol Chem 1982;257:8928–8934.
8. Chanderbhan R, Tanaka T, Strauss JF, Irwin D, Noland BJ, Scallen TJ, Vahouny GV. Biochem Biophys Res Commun 1983;117:702–709.
9. Chanderbhan R, Noland BJ, Scallen TJ, Vahouny G. J Biol Chem 1982;257:8928–8934.
10. Van Amerongen A, Teerlink T, Van Heusden GPH, Wirtz KWA. Chem Phys Lipid 1985;38:195–204.
11. Schroeder F, Butko P, Nemecz G, Scallen TJ. J Biol Chem 1990;265:151–157.
12. Wirtz KWA, Gadella TWJ Jr. Experientia 1990;46:592–599.
13. Pastuszyn A, Noland BJ, Bazan JF, Fletterick RJ. J Biol Chem 1987;262:13219–13227.
14. Seedorf U, Assmann G. J Biol Chem 1991;266:630–636.
15. Seedorf U, Raabe M, Assmann G. Gene 1993;123:165–172.
16. Seedorf U, Brysch P, Engel T, Schrage K, Assmann G. Sterol carrier protein x is peroxisomal 3-oxoacyl-CoA thiolase with intrinsic sterol carrier and lipid transfer activity. J Biol Chem (in press).
17. Miyazawa S, Furuta S, Osumi T, Hashimoto T, Ui N. J Biochem (Tokyo) 1981;90:511–519.
18. Seedorf U, Scheek S, Engel T, Steif C, Hinz HJ, Assmann G. J Biol Chem 1994;269:2613–2618.
19. Szyperski T, Scheek S, Johansson J, Assmann G, Seedorf U, Wüthrich K. FEBS Lett 1993;335:18–26.
20. Hijikata M, Wen JK, Osumi T, Hashimoto T. J Biol Chem 1990;265:4600–4606.
21. Leighton F, Nicovani S, Soto U, Skorin C, Necochea C. In: Fahimi HD, Sies H (eds) Peroxisomes in Biology and Medicine. Heidelberg: Springer, 1987;177–188.
22. Hryb DJ, Hogg JF. Biochem Biophys Res Commun 1979;87:1200–1206.

F.P. Woodford, J. Davignon and A. Sniderman, editors.

Characterization of Chinese hamster ovary cell lines defective in intracellular cholesterol transport

Neera K. Dahl and Laura Liscum

Tufts University School of Medicine, Department of Physiology, Boston, Massachusetts, USA

Abstract. Our objective is to identify gene products involved in intracellular cholesterol transport and regulation. We have isolated somatic cell mutants that are defective in the intracellular transport of low density lipoprotein (LDL)-derived cholesterol. Complementation analysis between seven independently isolated mutants reveals that at least two genes control LDL-cholesterol signaling and transport. The first mutant class exhibits the same biochemical phenotype as classical Niemann-Pick type C fibroblasts, with impaired LDL-cholesterol transport and signaling commensurate with an accumulation of LDL-cholesterol in lysosomes. The second mutant class expresses a variant phenotype with normal movement of LDL-cholesterol but defective signaling to LDL-sensitive homeostatic responses.

Mammalian cells tightly regulate their cholesterol content and its intracellular disposition. Cholesterol is not uniformly distributed among cell membranes, and activities that modulate cholesterol levels (rates of cholesterol biosynthesis, LDL internalization and cholesterol esterification) are sensitive to the cellular content of free cholesterol. Neither the sensing mechanism nor the mechanism by which cholesterol is compartmentalized within cells is well understood (reviewed in [1] and [2]).

To identify multiple cell components involved in intracellular cholesterol movement and regulation, we have taken a somatic cell genetic approach. We isolated Chinese hamster ovary (CHO) cell mutants that express defective mobilization of LDL-derived cholesterol from lysosomes to the plasma membrane [3]. Biochemical analysis of several allelic mutant lines revealed a phenotype resembling classical Niemann-Pick disease type C (NPC). They exhibit grossly defective LDL stimulation of cholesterol esterification and impaired LDL suppression of 3-hydroxy-3-methylglutaryl coenzyme A reductase, the rate-limiting enzyme for cholesterol synthesis. However, these activities are modulated normally in response to 25-hydroxycholesterol or mevalonate. The LDL-specific regulatory defects are predicated by the inability of the mutants to mobilize LDL-cholesterol from lysosomes.

Results

Complementation analysis was performed between six of our cholesterol transport-defective CHO cells (designated 1-2, 2-2, 3-6, 4-4, 5-1 and 10-3), which were isolated from independently mutagenized pools [4]. The analysis also included CT, a cholesterol-transport mutant isolated in T.Y. Chang's laboratory (Dartmouth University) using a vastly different selection protocol [5]. Complementation required cell lines bearing selectable markers. Wild-type CHO and mutant 4-4 lines resistant to 5 μg/ml thioguanine and 0.4–1

Address for correspondence: Laura Liscum, Tufts University School of Medicine, Department of Physiology, 136 Harrison Avenue, Boston, MA 02111, USA.

mM ouabain were isolated and are designated CHO (HAT^s oua^r) and 4-4 (HAT^s oua^r). Resistance to thioguanine confers sensitivity to medium containing HAT (hypoxanthine, aminopterin, and thymidine).

Somatic cell fusions were performed using polyethylene glycol and hybrids selecting in medium containing HAT and ouabain [4]. Complementation was assayed by examining the ability of LDL to stimulate cholesterol esterification in hybrids. Cholesterol esterification was measured by determining the incorporation of [^{3}H]oleate into cholesteryl [^{3}H]oleate and normalized for [^{3}H]triglyceride synthesis. This was chosen as the complementation test because it is the homeostatic response that is most profoundly defective in the cholesterol transport mutants. Assays of the hybrids formed by fusion of cholesterol-transport defective mutants with LDL-receptor-defective met-18b-2 cells served as a positive control for complementation [6].

The results of five separate experiments are shown in Table 1. When cells were cultured in medium without LDL, the amount of cholesterol esterified was similar in all cell lines, ranging from 4 to 12. 25-Hydroxycholesterol, at 2 mg/ml, stimulated cholesterol esterification in all cell lines and hybrids. The addition of LDL to 40 µg/ml also stimulated cholesterol esterification. Table 1 gives the relative cholesterol esterified in response to LDL. In Experiment 1, LDL stimulated cholesterol esterification to 158 in CHO cells, but did not stimulate cholesterol esterification at all in 2–2 or 4-4 cells or in 4-4/2-2 hybrids. Therefore, there was no complementation between mutants 4-4 and 2-2. Experiments 2 and 3 show complementation between mutants 4-4 and 3-6, but no complementation between mutants 4-4 and either 1–2 or 5–1.

Our finding that mutants 4-4 and 3-6 are in different complementation groups was

Table 1. LDL stimulation of cholesterol esterification

Experiment	Cell line or hybrid	Relative cholesterol esterified
1	CHO	158
	2–2	6
	4-4	4
	4-4/2–2	3
2	CHO	155
	4-4	4
	3-6	30
	4-4/3-6	76
3	4-4/CHO	62
	4-4/1–2	4
	4-4/5–1	4
	4-4/3–6	36
4	CT/CHO	129
	CT/18b–2	82
	CT/4-4	20
	CT/2–2	18
5	CHO	142
	CT	62
	3-6	31
	CT/3-6	118

Cells and hybrids were grown as described [4]. Cells were incubated for 5 h in medium with 40 µg/ml LDL, then pulsed for 3 h with [^{3}H]oleate. The cellular content of cholesteryl [^{3}H]oleate and [^{3}H]triglyceride was determined after extraction and thin-layer chromatography. Relative cholesterol esterification represents the incorporation of [^{3}H]oleate into (cholesteryl [^{3}H]oleate/[^{3}H]triglyceride) × 1,000.

confirmed in our analysis of mutant CT. Experiment 4 shows the expected complementation between CT, a cholesterol-transport mutant, and met-18b-2 cells, which are LDL-receptor defective, but no complementation between CT and either 4-4 or 2–2, indicating that CT, 4-4 and 2–2 are defective in the same gene. Experiment 5 indicates that CT and 3-6 are in different complementation groups.

Because mutant 3-6 is clearly in a different complementation class from the six other mutants tested, we wanted to characterize other aspects of LDL-derived cholesterol transport in 3-6 to determine which aspects are similar to the classic NPC phenotype. Our analysis showed the following: (i) Mutant 3-6 exhibited impaired LDL-mediated regulatory responses (stimulation of cholesterol esterification and suppression of HMG-CoA reductase activity), but normal responses were seen with 25-hydroxycholesterol. (ii) Mutant 3-6 grew poorly when LDL was the sole cholesterol source. Thus in its cholesterol homeostatic responses, mutant 3-6 exhibited the classical NPC phenotype. (iii) The relative rate of movement of LDL-derived cholesterol to the plasma membrane was normal in 3-6 cells. Therefore, while the 2–2 and 4-4 gene defect alters cholesterol egress from lysosomes [3], the 3-6 gene defect appears to affect signaling and not LDL-cholesterol transport to the plasma membrane.

Discussion

Niemann-Pick disease type C is an autosomal recessive lysosomal storage disease characterized by the accumulation of unesterified cholesterol, sphingomyelin, glucosyl-ceramide, and bis(monoacylglycero)phosphate [7]. Variations in expression of the disease are characterized clinically by age of onset and development of symptoms, and biochemically by responsiveness to LDL [8,9].

Biochemically, three subtypes of NPC are found. The classical phenotype shows levels of LDL-stimulation of esterification less than 10% of normal controls and increased lysosomal accumulation of unesterified cholesterol in response to LDL. A variant phenotype shows a slight defect in LDL-stimulation of cholesterol esterification and partial downregulation of cholesterol synthesis [8,9]. LDL-cholesterol is transported normally to the plasma membrane in these cells [9]. A third group appears intermediate [8]. NPC patients with the most severe clinical presentation generally exhibit the classical biochemical phenotype while adult onset patients fall into the variant group [8]. For the majority of patients, biochemical phenotype expression does not correlate well with severity or progression of NPC disease. However, expression of a phenotype seems restricted within families [8], which indicates that a genetic basis exists for the biochemical differences.

Our collection of cholesterol transport-defective CHO cell mutants include many with a biochemical phenotype identical to the classical NPC phenotype. Our hypothesis is that this complementation class expresses defects that directly affect LDL-cholesterol movement, i.e., in a lysosomal membrane protein/lipid required for cholesterol egress, a soluble cholesterol transport molecule, or a factor involved in vesicular trafficking.

Among our collection of mutants are a minority that do not resemble the classical NPC phenotype. Some, such as 3-6, more closely resemble a variant NPC phenotype, which is relatively rare [8]. The defect expressed in this complementation class could reflect the need for a protein to direct the effluxed cholesterol to proper intracellular targets or to relay intracellular regulatory signals.

Acknowledgements

This work was supported by the National Institutes of Health, and the American Heart Association, Bristol-Myers and Parke-Davis. NKD received support from the American Liver Foundation and Berlex Laboratories.

References

1. Liscum L, Dahl NK. J Lipid Res 1992;33:1239—1254.
2. Liscum L, Faust JR. Curr Opin Lipidol 1994;5:221—226.
3. Dahl NK, Reed KL, Daunais MA, Faust JR, Liscum L. J Biol Chem 1992;267:4889—4896.
4. Dahl NK, Daunais MA, Liscum L. J Lipid Res 1994;35(in press).
5. Cadigan KM, Spillane DM, Chang T-Y. J Cell Biol 1990;110:295—308.
6. Faust JR, Krieger M. J Biol Chem 1987;262:1996—2004.
7. Vanier MT, Wenger DA, Comly ME, Rousson R, Brady RO, Pentchev PG. Clin Genetics 1988;33:331—348.
8. Vanier MT, Rodriguez-Lafrasse C, Rousson R, Gazzah N, Juge M-C, Pentchev PG, Revol A, Louisot P. Biochim Biophys Acta 1991;1096:328—337.
9. Argoff CE, Comly ME, Blanchette-Mackie J, Kruth HS, Pye HT, Goldin E, Kaneski C, Vanier MT, Brady RO, Pentchev PG. Biochim Biophys Acta 1991;1096:319—327.

Processing of oxidized LDL in macrophages

Henry F. Hoff, June O'Neil and George Hoppe
Department of Cell Biology, Research Institute, Cleveland Clinic Foundation, 9500 Euclid Ave., Cleveland, OH 44195, USA

Abstract. We investigated whether the poor processing of oxidized (ox-) LDL in macrophages could be due in part to inactivation of lysosomal proteases by oxidized LDL. We found that pretreatment of mouse peritoneal macrophages (MPM) with ox-LDL resulted in less degradation, relative to cells pretreated with LDL or acetyl LDL, of not only subsequently added labeled ox-LDL, but other lipoproteins as well. Extracts of such cells pretreated with ox-LDL also demonstrated a reduction in thiol protease activity at low pH, specifically cathepsin B. When extracts of untreated macrophages or mixtures of cathepsin B and D were incubated with ox-LDL, LDL, or acetyl LDL, only ox-LDL reduced cathepsin B activity. It is suggested that ox-LDL might directly bind to the thiol group at the active site of cathepsin B, thereby inactivating it.

Oxidation of LDL is believed to play a major role in the pathogenesis of atherosclerosis by virtue of its unregulated uptake by tissue macrophages leading to lipid loading (foam cell formation) [1,2]. However, after internalization by macrophages in culture, ox-LDL was shown to be processed less efficiently than acetyl LDL, resulting in the accumulation of undegraded or partially degraded apolipoproteinB (apoB) [1–5], eventually leading to the formation of insoluble lipid–protein complexes called ceroid [6]. It was suggested that this was the result of the inability of lysosomal cathepsins to degrade apoB in ox-LDL following inter- and intramolecular cross-linking in apoB induced by reactive aldehydes such as 4-hydroxynonenal (HNE) formed during the oxidative process [4,5]. However, it is also possible that such deficient proteolysis is the result of direct inactivation of lysosomal cathepsins by ox-LDL. We therefore tested whether ox-LDL was capable of reducing cathepsin activity in extracts of mouse peritoneal macrophages (MPM) incubated with ox-LDL and whether this resulted in a reduced ability of cells pretreated with ox-LDL to degrade subsequently added ox-LDL. We also tested whether ox-LDL could directly inactivate such cathepsins in extracts of untreated macrophages or in mixtures of cathepsins.

Results and Discussion

We first assessed whether preincubation of MPM with LDL that had been extensively oxidized with 10 μM Cu^{++} for 24 h at 20°C led to a reduction in degradation of subsequently added labeled ox-LDL relative to cells pretreated with LDL. As shown in a more detailed communication [7], we found that cells preincubated for 21 h with ox-LDL showed dramatically less degradation of ox-LDL than cells preincubated with LDL (Fig. 1). Since much of the extensively oxidized LDL is aggregated, we also tested whether LDL that was induced to aggregate by vortexing (vx-LDL) had the same ability to induce this inhibition in lipoprotein (LP) degradation in MPM as ox-LDL. However, cells pretreated with vx-LDL showed no difference from cells pretreated with LDL in their ability to degrade ox-LDL. Yet MPM pretreated with ox-LDL showed the same reduced degradation of labeled vx-LDL as was shown for labeled ox-LDL (Fig. 1). Degradation of labeled LDL and to a lesser degree acetyl LDL was also less in MPM

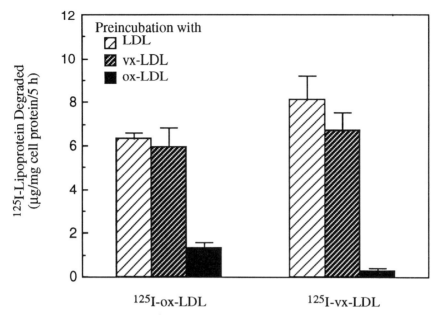

Fig. 1. Preincubation of MPM with ox-LDL leads to inhibition of subsequent LP degradation. MPM were incubated with 50 µg/ml of LDL, vx-LDL or ox-LDL for 21 h at 37°C. Cells were then washed and incubated for 5 h with fresh medium containing 20 µg/ml of ^{125}I-ox-LDL or ^{125}I-vx-LDL. The amount of labeled ligand degraded as iodine-free trichloracetic acid-soluble radioactivity (TCA) in the medium was determined.

preincubated with ox-LDL than in cells pretreated with LDL. That the described reduction in LP degradation was not the result of reduced uptake by MPM rather than degradation: uptake was unaffected by preincubation with ox-LDL. Collectively, these results indicate that if macrophages internalize ox-LDL, they become less able to degrade any subsequently added LP, especially if they are in an aggregated state.

To assess whether this reduced ability to degrade LP by MPM pretreated with ox-LDL was related to a reduction in their lysosomal protease activity, we determined the ability of crude extracts of MPM pretreated with ox-LDL, LDL, or vx-LDL for 21 h to degrade ^{125}I-LDL during a 1.5-h incubation. As seen in Fig. 2a and as shown recently by us [7], total protease activity was reduced by treating MPM with ox-LDL. However, when we determined the ability of thiol proteases in such extracts to degrade labeled LDL by looking only at the dithiothreitol (DTT)-dependent activity (difference between activities in the absence and presence of DTT), we found that the reduction in ability to degrade labeled LDL was even more dramatic than found for total protease activity (Fig. 2a). We also found that the reduction in DTT-dependent activity (ability to degrade ^{125}I-LDL) coincided with the reduction in cathepsin B activity as determined by assessing the hydrolysis of the artificial substrate Na-CBZ-L-lysine *p*-nitrophenyl ester (CLN) [8].

We next asked whether ox-LDL would specifically reduce thiol protease activity such as cathepsin B by directly interacting with the enzyme in crude extracts of untreated MPM at the lysosomal pH of 4.0. When such extracts were incubated with ox-LDL, LDL, vx-LDL or acetyl LDL, only ox-LDL induced a reduction in DTT-dependent thiol protease activity (Fig. 3), even though total protease activity was not reduced. In studies published elsewhere [7] we found that commercial purified cathepsin B, but not cathepsin D, was

444

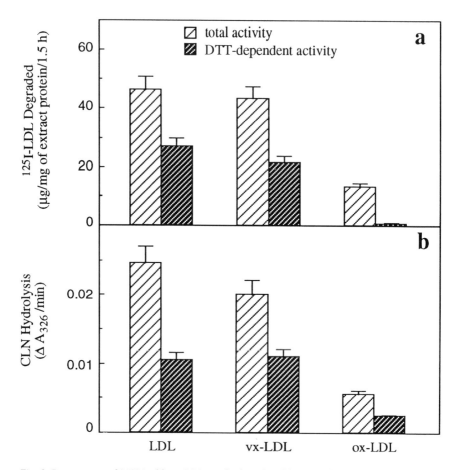

Fig. 2. Pretreatment of MPM with ox-LDL results in reduced lysosomal thiol protease activity. MPM were incubated with medium containing LP under conditions as described in Fig. 1. Cells were washed and cell extracts prepared by freezing-thawing and subsequent sonication. 5 µg of protein from each extract were incubated with 150 µg of ^{125}I-LDL in a final volume of 100 ml of acetate buffer, pH 4.0 for 1.5 h with and without DTT, and the amount of TCA-soluble label was determined (Fig. 2a). 0.1 µg of each extract was mixed with 2×10^{-4} M CLN in a final volume of 500 µl of acetate buffer, pH 4.0 with and without DTT (Fig. 2b). Hydrolysis of CLN was expressed as changes in absorbance at 326 nm/min. DTT-dependent activity represents the difference in activity in the absence and presence of DTT.

inactivated by ox-LDL but not by LDL, vx-LDL or acetyl LDL. When the ability of individual samples of ox-LDL to inactivate cathepsin B was compared, we found a significant negative correlation between enzyme activity remaining after incubation with ox-LDL and the degree of oxidation of the LDL used, as assessed either by their individual conjugated diene contents or specific fluorescence at 360 excitation/430 emission [9] (Fig. 4). Collectively, these studies show that there is a direct link between the reduced degradation of LP in cells pretreated with ox-LDL and a reduction in lysosomal cathepsin B activity. Furthermore, they show that this reduction in enzyme activity can be induced by directly interacting cathepsin B with ox-LDL in vitro.

The mechanism responsible for this inactivation has not yet been elucidated. However,

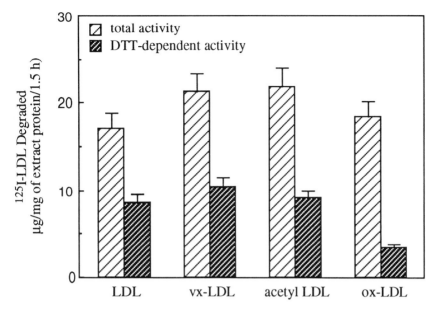

Fig. 3. Direct incubation of extracts from untreated MPM with ox-LDL reduces lysosomal thiol protease activity. Untreated MPM were homogenized to obtain crude extracts which were then incubated directly with LDL, vx-LDL, acetyl LDL, or ox-LDL (1:1 wt:wt) extract protein:LP protein for 5 h in the presence or absence of DTT. The mixture was subsequently incubated with ^{125}I-LDL for 1.5 h and the degradation determined as described for Fig. 2.

certain reactive aldehydes formed during the decomposition of lipid hydroperoxides such as 4-hydroxynonenal (HNE) [9] were shown to form thioether linkages with cysteines in proteins [10]. If this were to occur at the active site of the thiol protease, cathepsin B [8], inactivation of the enzyme would occur. In preliminary studies we have found that ox-LDL forms covalent complexes with other proteins under the conditions at which cathepsin B inactivation takes place, i.e., at pH 4.0, but not at pH 7.4. We propose that

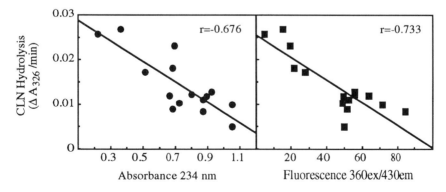

Fig. 4. The ability of individual samples of ox-LDL to inactivate cathepsin B correlates with their degree of oxidation. Separate samples of LDL oxidized for 24 h with 10 μM Cu^{++} were incubated for 1 h with cathepsin B at pH 4.0 and the levels of enzyme activity were determined from the hydrolysis of the artificial substrate, CLN as described for Fig. 2b. The degree of oxidation was determined from the conjugated diene content (absorbance at 234 nm) and fluorescence at 360ex/430em.

446

at low pH, reactive sites on ox-LDL become exposed that can form thioether linkages with the active site of the enzyme. Since in further preliminary studies we could show that HNE-modified LDL mimicked ox-LDL in ability to inactivate cathepsin B and covalently bind to protein at low but not at high pH, it is likely that reactive groups in HNE covalently bound to apoB in ox-LDL become exposed at low pH that are responsible for this binding and enzyme activation. Since excess amount of DTT as well as covalent blockage of thiols on proteins with N-ethylmaleimide inhibited both binding of ox-LDL and of HNE-modified LDL to protein, it is likely that enzyme inactivation is mediated by a thioether linkage between the reactive aldehyde and the active site of the enzyme, as was proposed earlier for other enzymes [10]. Further studies are needed to elucidate the underlying mechanism.

Acknowledgements

This work was supported by NIH Program Project Grant HL29582.

References

1. Witztum JL, Steinberg D. J Clin Invest 1991;88:1785–1792.
2. Steinbrecher UP, Zhang H, Lougheed M. Free Rad Biol Med 1990;9:155–168.
3. Sparrow CP, Parthasarathy S, Steinberg D. J Biol Chem 1989;264:2599–2604.
4. Lougheed M, Zhang H, Steinbrecher UP. J Biol Chem 1991;266:14519–14525.
5. Jessup W, Mander EL, Dean RT. Biochim Biophys Acta 1992;1126:167–177.
6. Ball RY, Bindman JP, Carpenter KLH, Mitchinson MJ. Atherosclerosis 1986;60:173–181.
7. Hoppe G, O'Neil J, Hoff HF. Inactivation of lysosomal proteases by oxidized LDL is partially responsible for its poor degradation by mouse peritoneal macrophages. J Clin Invest 1994 (in press).
8. Bajkowski AS, Frankfater A. Anal Biochem 1975;68:119–127.
9. Esterbauer H, Schaur RG, Zollner H. Free Rad Biol Med 1991;11:81–128.
10. Uchida K, Stadtman ER. Proc Natl Acad Sci USA 1992;89:5611–5615.

Molecular heterogeneity of familial hypercholesterolemia in the Arab communities in Israel

E. Leitersdorf and A. Reshef

Division of Medicine and The Center for Research, Prevention and Treatment of Atherosclerosis, Hadassah University Hospital, 91120 Jerusalem, Israel

Abstract. The Arab population of Israel consists of several well-defined communities. Among them, increased prevalence of familial hypercholesterolemia (FH) has previously been identified in Christian Arabs and Druze. These populations may represent only a minor fraction of the corresponding communities that reside in the region and it may be postulated that some of the mutations identified in Israel originated in the neighboring countries. Convincing evidence for this emerged through the identification of the Lebanese allele at the LDL-receptor gene locus (stop 660) in homozygote FH cases from Lebanon and in Israeli Christian Arabs. Other mutations, including the J.D. mutation which is of Italian-Syrian origin (Y807C) and the Jerusalem mutation (E187K), have recently been identified in Israel. With the identification of a mutation in Moslem Arabs (delta G165) which is reported here for the first time, it is now possible to extend the search for FH cases in the region and determine the relative importance of each of these mutations in the local FH patients.

Familial hypercholesterolemia (FH) is a dominantly inherited disease with an estimated worldwide prevalence of 1 in 500. Heterozygote FH patients may be clinically identified by elevated plasma low density lipoprotein cholesterol (LDL-C) levels, premature ischemic heart disease (IHD) and the presence of tendon xanthomas. Homozygote patients have much higher plasma cholesterol levels and often die in childhood of premature coronary atherosclerosis [1]. In several population groups, the disease is much more common [2–4]. In these populations most of the FH subjects living in the same area have the same LDL-receptor mutation [5–8], presumably as a result of a founder gene effect.

Khachdurian and Uthman [2] observed an increased prevalence of FH in Lebanon. A single mutation in the LDL-receptor gene (a nucleotide substitution that produces a premature termination codon and a truncated receptor) was subsequently found to be responsible for most of the Lebanese homozygote cases. The possible existence of other mutations responsible for elevated LDL-C in this community has also been suggested [5]. This mutation was later identified in the Galilee region of northern Israel in Christian-Arab patients whose origin was traced back to Lebanon. It was evident that more than one mutation exists [9]. In another sect of the Israeli Arab population, the Druze from the Golan Heights in northern Israel, another mutation in the LDL-receptor gene was reported [10]. This mutation is a single base substitution, resulting in a premature termination codon at amino acid 167 in the fourth repeat of the binding domain of the receptor. In both of these Israeli Arab populations because of the high degree of consanguinity, as well as the existence of the populations in a delimited area for an extended period, a significant founder effect with high frequency of the mutant gene reported is to be expected.

Here we report the identification of three LDL-receptor gene mutations in a third sect of the Israeli Arab population, the Muslims. Patients were recruited from the city of Genin and the village of Kara. In this population, as with the Christian and Druze Arabs, consanguineous marriages particularly among first-degree cousins are very common.

Identification of these mutant alleles can therefore simplify further screening, analysis and genetic counseling for hypercholesterolemia in the Muslim Arab sect living in Israel.

Materials and Methods

Recruitment of patients and families and biochemical analysis

Israeli-Arab Muslim patients were recruited through the outpatient clinic of the Center for Research, Prevention and Treatment of Atherosclerosis of the Division of Medicine of the Hadassah University Hospital in Jerusalem. For each patient and family member a fasting blood sample was collected in 0.15% (w/v) EDTA. Plasma total triglycerides, cholesterol, and HDL-C levels were determined using commercially available diagnostic kits (Boehringer Mannheim, Germany). Plasma LDL-C levels were calculated according to the Friedewald-Levy formula [11]. For each index case, a pedigree was constructed and verified through personal interviews with all available family members. Family FH# 375 was recruited from the city of Genin and FH# 373 from village of Kara.

Identification of the LDL-receptor gene mutations

Genomic DNA was extracted from blood leukocytes. Oligonucleotides (Biotechnology, Rehovot Israel) flanking the promoter region and each of the 18 exons of the LDL receptor gene and 0.1 µCi of [α-^{32}P]-dCTP were used for PCR amplification. The PCR product was analyzed using SSCP (single strand conformation polymorphism). In brief, the DNA fragments were denatured and subjected to electrophoresis on a 6% polyacrylamide gel containing 10% glycerol for 16 h at 250 V and for 4 h at 50 W. The fragments were observed by autoradiography on a Kodak XAR-5 film. After identification of an abnormally migrating band in SSCP, the corresponding region was re-amplified. The PCR product was subjected to electrophoresis on a low-gelling SeaPlaque® agarose (FMC, Bio Products, USA). The PCR band was excised and its DNA was purified and directly sequenced using the corresponding oligonucleotide primers and a Sequenase® version 2 kit (United States Biochemicals, La Jolla, California).

Results

The lipid profile of the index case FH 373-9 was: total cholesterol (TC) 547 mg/dl, LDL-C 488 mg/dl, HDL-C 40 mg/dl and triglycerides (TG) 97 mg/dl. The patient had had two myocardial infarctions at the age of 13, followed by a coronary arterial bypass graft (CABG). The lipid profile of index case FH 375-1 during treatment with 40 mg/day of lovastatin was TC 340 mg/dl, LDL-C 301 mg/dl, HDL-C 24 mg/dl and TG 76 mg/dl. The patient had a CABG operation at the age of 18. Both these profiles are compatible with the clinical diagnosis of homozygote FH. Parental consanguinity could not be demonstrated in either family. PCR-SSCP analysis of FH 373-3 and FH 375-1 showed band shifts in exon 17 and in exon 4 of the LDL receptor respectively. The PCR products of these exons were directly sequenced. FH 373-3 was found to be homozygous to an A to G substitution at residue 807 (exon 17), leading to a tyrosine to cysteine transversion. This mutation has previously been described and designated as the Italian-Syrian mutation [12]. In FH 375-1 direct sequencing of exon 4 indicated a G to A change at residue 187, of one allele, that caused glutamine to lysine transversion. This mutation too has been previously described and designated the Jerusalem Moslem mutation [12]. Further sequencing of exon 4 revealed that the other allele carries a second mutation, a deletion of guanine at residue 165, that had not been previously reported and was designated the Genin mutation.

After identifying the three mutations in the Israeli Muslim Arabs, we established PCR-based assays for screening and genetic counseling for FH in this population. To identify the Jerusalem mutation (FH 375, allele A), PCR-PIRA (primer-introduced restriction analysis) [13] was planned. Two oligonucleotides, an upstream SP15A (5'-CCCCAGC-TGTGGGCCTGCCAGAACG-3') which is complementary to a 5' sequence within exon 4, and a downstream oligonucleotide 375MUT (5'-CAGCGCCAGCTGGAGTGGATGC-ACA-3') which is complementary to a 3' sequence in exon 4 (except for the underlined adenosine (A) that has been introduced instead of thymidine (T)) were used for PCR amplification. After this amplification a new NspI (recognition sequence (AG)CATG(TG)) is created exclusively in the mutant gene. To identify the newly discovered Genin mutation (FH 375 allele B), the mutated allele was isolated and purified from a compound heterozygote case that carries also the Jerusalem mutation described above. Two oligonucleotides, an upstream LDLR61C (5'-GCTGGTGTTGGGAGACTTCACACG-3') which is complementary to 3' sequences of intron 3 and a downstream oligonucleotide LDLR51E (5'-TGCATGTTGTTGGAAATCCACTTCG-3') which is complementary to 5' sequences of intron 4 were used for PCR amplification. The PCR product of exon 4 (where both mutations are located) was digested with NspI and subjected to electrophoresis on 4.5% Nusieve agarose. The longer fragment (23 bp longer), which does not carry the Jerusalem mutation and is therefore not digested by NspI, was repetitively purified, re-amplified by PCR, redigested by NspI and extracted from the Nusieve agarose gel. This highly purified allele can now serve as a PCR template for PCR-SSCP analysis of the Moslem mutation. To identify the previously described [12] Italian-Syrian mutation (FH 373-3), PCR-SSCP using FH 373-3 DNA as a positive control was performed as described above.

Discussion

In the present study we have identified three LDL-receptor mutations in FH families of Muslim origin who reside in Israel. Two mutations, the Italian-Syrian (Y807C) and the Jerusalem-Arab (E187K) have been previously described [12]. The third mutation, delta G 165, has not been previously reported. Due to high consanguinity rates in the Muslim Arab population residing in Israel, as well as their remaining in a relatively small region for a long time, a significant founder effect with high frequency of the mutant gene reported is expected. It can therefore be postulated that establishment of detection assays for these mutations will simplify the extended search for new FH cases in this population and enable prenatal diagnosis, as for the "Lebanese mutation" in Christian Arab families living in Israel [14].

The Arab population of Israel consists of several well-defined communities that at least partially reflect the demographic characteristics of the neighboring countries. As the Arab population of Israel may represent only a minor fraction of the corresponding communities that reside in the region, at least some of the mutations identified here may have originated in a neighboring country. Convincing evidence for this emerged from the identification of the "Lebanese allele" at the LDL-receptor gene (stop 660) in several homozygote FH cases from Lebanon and the subsequent proof that this mutant allele is the most important cause of FH in the Christian Arab community in Israel. This is also true for the J.D. mutation of Italian-Syrian origin that has now been identified in Israel. The result of the current investigation will allow extension of the search for additional FH cases in neighboring Arab countries and eventually determine the relative importance of each of these mutations in the local FH population.

450

Acknowledgements

This research was supported by the Endowment Fund for Basic Research in the Life Sciences Dorot, administered by the Israel Academy of Sciences Foundation and Humanities. We thank Liat Triger for excellent technical assistance.

References

1. Goldstein JL, Brown MS. In: Scriver CR, Beaudet AL, Sly WS and Valle D (eds) The Metabolic Basis of Inherited Disease, 6th edn. New York: McGraw-Hill, 1989;1215—1250.
2. Khachadurian AK, Uthman SB. Nutr Metabol 1973;15:132—140.
3. Seftel HC, Baker SG, Jenkins T, Mendelsohn D. Am J Med Genet 1989;34:545—547.
4. Moorjani S, Roy M, Gagne C, Davignon J, Brun D, Toussaint M, Lambert M, Campeau L, Blaichman S, Lupien P. Arteriosclerosis 1989;9:212—216.
5. Lehrman MA, Schneider WJ, Brown MS, Davis CG, Elhammer A, Russell DW, Goldstein JL. J Biol Chem 1987;262:401—410.
6. Hobbs HH, Brown MS Russell DW, Davignon J, Goldstein JL. N Engl J Med 1987;317:734—737.
7. Leitersdorf E, van Der Westhuyzen DR, Coetzee GA, Hobbs HH. J Clin Invest 1989;84:954—961.
8. Leitersdorf E, Tobin EJ, Davignon J, Hobbs HH. J Clin Invest 1990;85:1014—1023.
9. Oppenheim AY, Friedlander Y, Dann EJ, Berkman N, Pressman Schwartz S, Leitersdorf E. Hum Genetics 1991;88:75—84.
10. Landsberger D, Meiner V, Reshef A, Levy Y, van der Westhuyzen DR, Coetzee GA, Leitersdorf E. Am J Hum Genet 1992;50:427—433.
11. Friedewald WT, Levy RI, Fredrickson DS. Clin Chem 1972;18:499—502.
12. Hobbs HH, Brown MS, Goldstein JL. Hum Mutation 1992;1:445—466.
13. Meiner V Marais DA, Reshef A, Björkhem I, Leitersdorf E. Hum Mol Genet 1994;3:193—194.
14. Reshef A, Meiner V, Dann EJ, Granat M, Leitersdorf E. Hum Genetics 1992;89:237—239.

Chicken oocyte growth: novel insights into the LDL-receptor gene family

Hideaki Bujo, Marcela Hermann, Johannes Nimpf and Wolfgang Johann Schneider
Department of Molecular Genetics, Biocenter and University, Vienna, Austria

Abstract. Deposition of the yolk mass components of chicken oocytes, namely very low density lipoprotein (VLDL) and vitellogenin (VTG), is mediated by a 95-kDa plasma membrane protein, termed VLDL/VTG receptor (VLDL/VTGR). Molecular characterization of the VLDL/VTGR revealed that it is a member of the LDLR gene superfamily, and harbors eight complement-type, cysteine-rich ligand-binding repeats at the amino-terminus. Such ligand-binding domain structure is the hallmark of the recently discovered mammalian so-called VLDLRs, whose true physiological function remains to be elucidated. The oocyte receptor's key role in avian reproduction and extremely high evolutionary conservation shed new light on VLDLR function in mammals, which also express the gene in ovaries.

Recent cloning efforts in several laboratories have identified an ever-increasing number of relatives of the mammalian low density lipoprotein receptor (LDLR). Probably the most fascinating aspect of this gene family is that the physiological roles of its members appear to be quite diverse, although they have several common structural elements. These modules comprising the receptors are (i) the so-called "binding repeats", complement-type domains consisting of ~40 residues displaying a triple-disulfide-bond-stabilized negatively charged surface (certain head-to-tail combinations of these repeats are believed to specify ligand interaction); (ii) epidermal growth factor precursor-type repeats, also containing six cysteines each; (iii) modules of ~50 residues with a consensus tetrapeptide, Tyr-Trp-Thr-Asp (YWTD); and (iv), in the cytoplasmic region, signals for receptor internalization via coated pits, containing the consensus tetrapeptide, Asn-Pro-Xaa-Tyr (NPXY). The best characterized binding domain is that of the LDLR, which consists of seven ligand-binding repeats and recognizes apoB and apoE [1]. Both naturally occurring and site-specifically introduced mutations have defined the minimal requirements for recognition of ligands via either of the two apolipoproteins.

Recently, a receptor with a single cluster of eight binding repeats has been added to the list of LDLR gene family members [2]. The hitherto identified preferred ligand of this receptor is very low density lipoprotein (VLDL) rather than LDL, hence its designation VLDLR. The structural basis for preferential recognition of VLDL, in particular the role of the extra aminoterminal ligand-binding repeat relative to the LDLR, has not been investigated.

Our own studies [3–7] on the LDLR gene family of the chicken — particularly in the laying hen — constitute a different approach to cell type-specific receptor expression and function observed in this gene family. The aspects amenable to investigation in the laying hen result from the unique physiological challenges posed by egg-laying, coupled to an otherwise typical network of receptor-mediated systemic transport pathways. Studies in our laboratory to date have revealed that in order to meet these challenges, the laying hen expresses at least four related genes belonging to the LDLR family. One of these specifies a 95-kDa protein that binds VLDL and VTG (the VLDL/VTG receptor), whose absence leads to the failure of oocyte growth and consequently the failure to produce offspring [4].

We have previously isolated and characterized the 95-kDa VLDL/VTGR from growing chicken oocytes in order to obtain partial protein-sequence data and detailed knowledge about its ligand specificity [3,7]. The most surprising findings were (i) the ability of the VLDL/VTGR to bind, in addition to apoB, also apoE [7], a protein not synthesized by chickens, and (ii) its immunological cross-reactivity with mammalian LDLRs [3]. These properties suggested that the 95-kDa protein was a bona-fide LDLR, further strengthened by the fact that the somatic cell-specific 130-kDa receptor was shown to be incapable of interaction with apoE [5]. In order to facilitate the delineation of molecular details underlying the LDLR pathway dichotomy in the laying hen, we now report new information about the abundant oocytic 95-kDa protein. Surprisingly, its ligand-binding domain consists of eight, not seven, ligand-binding repeats, and thus it is the chicken homologue of mammalian VLDL receptors.

Results

Molecular characterization of the chicken oocyte receptor

In order to identify a chicken VLDL/VTGR cDNA by the polymerase chain reaction (PCR), two degenerate oligonucleotides (17-mers) corresponding to tryptic peptide sequences of the purified receptor [7] were designed and synthesized. Using these degenerate oligonucleotides as primers to amplify cDNAs prepared from poly(A$^+$)-RNA of mature chicken ovaries, a ~0.8 kb PCR fragment, C8-1, was obtained, subcloned into a plasmid vector, and further analyzed. The deduced amino acid sequence of C8-1 indicated that it was highly homologous to VLDL and LDL receptors. C8-1 was then used to probe a chicken ovary cDNA library. The screening resulted in the identification of a 3.3-kb cDNA insert, CVR-1, encoding the entire VLDL/VTGR sequence (amino acid sequence shown in Fig. 1).

Sequencing of CVR-1 defined an open reading frame of 2589 bp (coding for 863 amino acids). A single ATG (methionine) codon is present in the 5′ part of the open reading frame, followed by a stretch of hydrophobic amino acid residues that presumably function as a cleavable signal sequence. Moreover, the ATG codon fulfilled the rules for translation initiation, and is therefore likely to represent the translation initiation site. The preferred cleavage site for the signal peptidase, 44 residues downstream, was predicted according to von Heijne. Another hydrophobic region, presumably representing a putative transmembrane domain, is found at amino acid residues 744–765. The putative extracellular domain has a cysteine-rich region (see below) with two potential N-glycosylation sites. The calculated molecular weight of the mature protein is 90,230, in good agreement with the apparent M$_r$ of 95,000 of the purified VLDL/VTGR protein determined by nonreducing SDS-PAGE [7]. The deduced amino acid sequence of CVR-1 contains all known tryptic peptide sequences of the isolated VLDL/VTGR (amino acids 466–474, 502–510 and 775–783; [7]).

Alignment of the amino acid sequence of the chicken VLDL/VTGR with those of the rabbit VLDLR and LDLR (Fig. 1), the human VLDLR and LDLR and other LDLRs (not shown) suggests that the chicken VLDL/VTGR is, in fact, a homolog of the mammalian VLDL receptor. This notion is based on the presence of eight ligand-binding repeats at the amino-terminus (1 to 8 in Fig. 1); the cluster of eight rather than seven such repeats — as present in LDLRs — is the signature of all VLDLRs characterized to date. Furthermore, as in other LDLRs and VLDLRs, the carboxyterminal 3 repeats are separated by a "linker" region from the aminoterminal 4 (in LDLRs) or 5 (in VLDLRs) repeats (Fig. 1). All cysteine residues in the ligand-binding domains of LDLRs, the

453

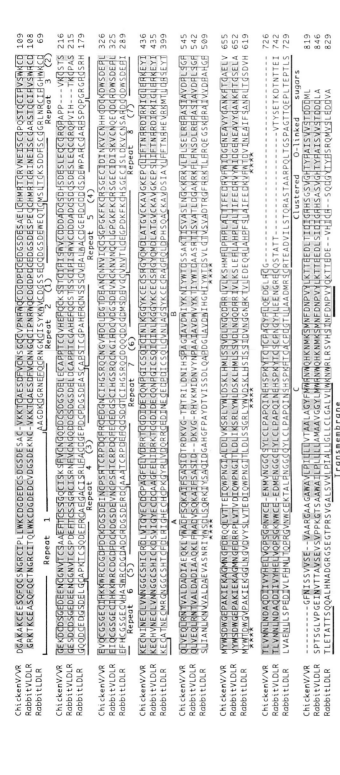

Fig. 1. Comparison of the amino acid sequences of the chicken VLDL/VTG receptor, the rabbit VLDL receptor [2] and the rabbit LDL receptor. The amino acids are numbered from the N-terminus of the putative mature protein of each receptor. Gaps have been introduced to optimize the alignment. Amino acids identical in the chicken VLDL/VTG receptor and the rabbit VLDL receptor and among three receptors including the rabbit LDL receptor are noted by shading with light gray and boxed, respectively. The ~40 amino acid repeats 1~8 (1~7 of the LDL receptor) in the ligand-binding domains, cysteine-rich repeats A, B and C in the EGF precursor homology domains, clustered O-linked sugar regions and transmembrane domains are shown. The YWTD sequences are indicated by asterisks, and the FDNPVY sequence, required for clustering of the LDL receptor in coated pits, is indicated by a heavy underline. V/V receptor, VLDL/VTG receptor.

chicken oocyte receptor, and VLDLRs are in identical positions. The eight repeats are followed by an EGF precursor homology domain (A to C in Fig. 1), a putative trans-membrane region, and a carboxyterminal domain of 54 amino acid residues; all other VLDLRs and LDLRs harbor these domains. Remarkably, despite the evolutionary distance between chicken and rabbit, the amino acid sequences of their VLDLRs show extremely high conservation. Identical residues are present in 93% of the positions in the cyto-plasmic domains, 85% in the EGF precursor homology domains, and 84% in the ligand-binding domains. Even the membrane-spanning domain, generally the least conserved region in the LDLR gene family [8], shows 64% identity. As Fig. 1 shows, the identity between rabbit and chicken eight-repeat receptors is much greater than between LDL and VLDL receptors of the rabbit (this is also true for chicken vs. human; data not shown).

However, in contrast to the rabbit VLDLR, the chicken oocyte VLDL/VTGR lacks a serine- and threonine-rich domain that is likely to carry clustered O-linked carbohydrate groups. When present, the O-linked sugar domains of members of the LDLR gene family are highly variable in length and sequence (e.g., only 20% identity between rabbit VLDLR and LDLR, Fig. 1; and [2] and [8]). In addition, splice variants of the human VLDLR mRNA specifying two putative forms of VLDLR, with or without this domain, have been identified. In the chicken, preliminary PCR-based experiments also suggest the presence of a VLDLR mRNA encoding an O-linked sugar domain-containing receptor different from that in oocytes (H. Bujo, unpublished observations). Five repeats containing a signature tetrapeptide (indicated by asterisks in Fig. 1) between repeats B and C of the EGF precursor homology domain, and the internalization signal (Phe-Asp-Asn-Pro-Val-Tyr) are conserved in the chicken VLDL/VTGR (Fig. 1).

Ligand-binding function of the receptor expressed in COS-7 cells

In order to test whether the expressed protein is capable of binding both VLDL and VTG as demonstrated for the isolated oocyte receptor [7], we performed surface ligand-binding studies on the transfected COS-7 cells. As Fig. 2 shows, the cells expressing the chicken VLDL/VTGR showed saturable, high-affinity binding of both ligands, with maximal amounts of binding 2–3 times that of control-transfected cells. An exact determination of binding parameters for the expressed heterologous receptor is not possible due to saturable ligand binding to endogenous sites (open circles); however, maximum binding of VLDL and VTG to transfected cells were comparable, and the K_d values for both ligands were in the range of 3–5 μg/ml, both in excellent agreement with previous results on isolated oocyte receptor [7].

Discussion

The finding that the chicken oocyte 95-kDa receptor, previously shown to be responsible for the uptake of VLDL and VTG into growing oocytes [3–7], is a homolog of the mammalian so-called VLDL receptor rather than the LDL receptor was somewhat surprising at first. Inasmuch as (i) the chicken LDL receptor, a 130-kDa sterol-regulated protein of somatic cells, does not bind apoE [5], but the oocyte 95-kDa protein does recognize apoE, a hallmark property of LDLRs, and (ii) antibodies against mammalian LDLRs were cross-reactive against the chicken oocyte receptor but not the chicken fibroblast receptor [3,5], we expected the oocyte lipoprotein receptor to be a cell-specific type of LDLR. However, as reported here, this key receptor for oocyte growth is in fact a relative of the mammalian VLDLRs, warranting careful consideration of the possible physiological roles of VLDLRs in mammals and egg-laying species.

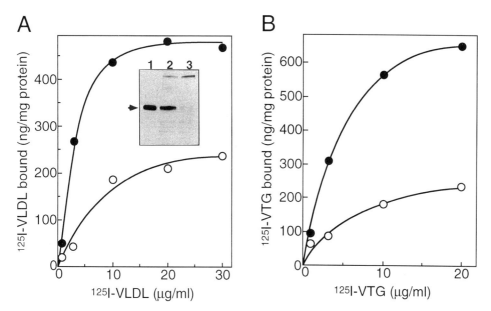

Fig. 2. Functional analysis of VLDL/VTG receptor expressed in COS-7 cells. Surface binding of (A) ^{125}I-VLDL (482 cpm/ng) and (B) ^{125}I-VTG (613 cpm/ng) to monolayers of pCDMCVR-1-transfected (closed circles) and vector-only-transfected (open circles) COS-7 cells. The data are the average of duplicate determinations and represent high-affinity binding, which is the difference between binding in the absence and presence of excess unlabeled ligand (1 mg/ml VLDL, panel A; and 750 µg/ml VTG, panel B). The insert in panel A shows the results of immunoblotting with an antireceptor carboxyterminal IgG; lane 1, 1 µg oocyte membrane protein; lanes 2 and 3, 60 µg protein of pCDMCVR-1 transfected or control COS-7 cells, respectively.

One of the remarkable aspects of VLDLRs is that their degree of conservation of common domains, as indicated by amino acid identity, is greater than that among LDLRs. LDLRs of rabbit and man show identities of 75%, but rabbit and human VLDLRs are 97% identical; the identities between the eight-repeat receptors from chicken and rabbit as well as from chicken and man are 84%. This conservation, together with the fact that naturally occurring mutations in the VLDLR gene have not been reported to date, may point to great importance of the receptors with eight ligand-binding repeats. Our finding that the receptor critical to the most important biological function, i.e., reproduction of the species *Gallus gallus* is such a protein, supports this hypothesis.

The finding of multiple ligand binding to single LDLR family members requires further structural refinement of the receptor molecules and their ligands in order to gain understanding of the molecular basis for their interaction. In comparing LDLRs with VLDLRs, the contribution of the eighth binding repeat, and also of the conserved acidic tetrapeptide Glu-Asp-Glu-Glu in the third repeat of VLDLRs, will be of particular interest. Studies to address these questions are now under way. These investigations are hoped to be feasible in the case of receptors containing single clusters of binding repeats, in contrast to the complex situation in LRP, which contains four clusters of 2–11 binding repeats each (31 to 35 in total, depending on species). In such receptors, ligand specificity may be defined by the overall conformation of more than one cluster of repeats. In addition, the exact range of physiological ligands of LRP is not known. Current evidence suggests that LRP is a multifunctional receptor in vivo, responsible for the systemic

456

clearance of spent, biologically inactive and/or unwanted plasma carrier complexes, as well as certain toxins. Indeed, preliminary ligand-binding experiments with the comparatively small chicken oocyte VLDL/VTGR suggest that it may be a superior model system to unravel structure/function relationships of LDLR-gene family members.

Acknowledgements

This work was supported by grant P-9040-MOB (to WJS), and HB held a Lise Meitner Postdoctoral Fellowship of the Austrian Science Foundation. We are grateful to R. Lo and M. Blaschek for excellent technical assistance.

References

1. Russell DW, Brown MS, Goldstein JL. J Biol Chem 1989;264:21682—21688.
2. Takahashi S, Kawarabayasi Y, Nakai T, Sakai J, Yamamoto T. Proc Natl Acad Sci USA 1992;89:9252—9256.
3. George R, Barber DL, Schneider WJ. J Biol Chem 1987;262:16838—16847.
4. Nimpf J, Radosavljevic MJ, Schneider WJ. J Biol Chem 1989;264:1393—1398.
5. Hayashi K, Nimpf J, Schneider WJ. J Biol Chem 1989;264:3131—3139.
6. Stifani S, Barber DL, Aebersold R, Steyrer E, Shen X, Nimpf J, Schneider WJ. J Biol Chem 1991;266:19079—19087.
7. Barber DL, Sanders EJ, Aebersold R, Schneider WJ. J Biol Chem 1991;266:18761—18770.
8. Mehta KD, Chen WJ, Goldstein JL, Brown MS. J Biol Chem 1991;266:10406—10414.

The VLDL receptor and related molecules: role and function

Tokuo Yamamoto and Juro Sakai

Tohoku University Gene Research Center, Sendai 981, Japan

Abstract. The VLDL receptor is specific for apolipoprotein E (apoE)-containing lipoproteins and consists of five functional domains that resemble the LDL receptor. Although structurally the VLDL receptor is closely related to the LDL receptor, the tissue expression and regulation of the two receptors are different. The VLDL receptor is abundant in muscle and fat cells and the expression of the receptor is not downregulated by its ligands, whereas the LDL receptor is most abundant in liver and is downregulated by sterols.

Lipoprotein receptors mediate the uptake of plasma lipid-carrying lipoproteins, thereby playing a key role both in intracellular lipid metabolism and in the clearance of lipoproteins from the plasma. The LDL receptor, consisting of five functional domains, binds lipoproteins that contain apolipoprotein B100 (apoB100) and/or apoE, and carries them into cells [1]. The VLDL receptor, also, consists of five functional domains, resembling the LDL receptor, but binds only apoE-containing lipoproteins: VLDL, IDL and β-VLDL [2,3]. The VLDL receptor is a member of the rapidly expanding LDL-receptor family which includes LDL-receptor-related protein (LRP) [4], gp330 [5] and the LDL-receptor itself. Within this supergene family, the VLDL receptor is the most closely related to the LDL receptor, with respect to domain structure and the binding of apoE lipoproteins. However, the expression and function of the two receptors are different. In this paper, we compare the structure and properties of the VLDL receptor with those of the LDL receptor.

Structure and genomic organization of the VLDL and LDL receptors

The VLDL and LDL receptors [1,6] consist of five functional domains (Fig. 1): (i) an amino-terminal ligand-binding domain consisting of many cysteine-rich repeats; (ii) an EGF (epidermal growth factor) precursor homology domain; (iii) an O-linked sugar domain; (iv) a transmembrane domain; and (v) a cytoplasmic domain with a coated-pit signal, FDNPVY [7]. The only structural difference between the two receptors is the number of cysteine-rich repeats that form the ligand-binding domains (Fig. 1): seven in the LDL receptor [6] and eight in the VLDL receptor [2,8]. Excluding an additional repeat at the N-terminus of the VLDL receptor, 56% of the amino acids within the ligand binding domain of the two human receptors are identical. The amino acids of two functionally important domains, EGF precursor homology and cytoplasmic domains, are also highly conserved: 53 and 48%, respectively (Fig. 1) [8]. This striking similarity of the two receptors suggests that they perform similar functions.

Consistent with the similarity of the functional domains of the two receptors, the genomic organization of the human VLDL receptor gene [8] is almost the same as that of the LDL receptor gene [9], except for an extra exon that encodes the additional repeat at the N-terminus of the VLDL receptor. However, although the structure and organization of the VLDL- and LDL-receptor genes are highly similar, they are located on different chromosomes: the LDL-receptor gene on chromosome 19 [10] and the VLDL-receptor gene on chromosome 9 [8,11]. A most unexpected finding was the extremely high

458

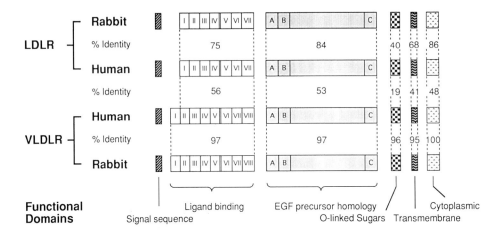

Fig. 1. Comparison of the structures of the VLDL and LDL receptors. Five functional domains in the receptors (VLDLR and LDLR) are shown. The number of identical residues (expressed as a percentage) in a given domain is indicated between adjacent proteins. The cysteine-rich repeats in the ligand-binding domain are assigned roman numerals; those in the EGF precursor homology domain are lettered A to C.

conservation of the amino acids of the entire region of the VLDL receptor among species: approximately 95% of the amino acids in the VLDL receptor are identical in the human, rabbit and mouse receptors [8,12]. In contrast, only 76% of the amino acids are conserved between human and rabbit LDL receptors [13]. Extremely high conservation of the VLDL receptor sequence among species suggests that it plays a crucial role in lipoprotein metabolism.

Expression of the VLDL and LDL receptors

VLDL receptor mRNA is abundant in heart, muscle, adipose tissue and brain [2], whereas that of LDL receptor is expressed in most tissues, including adrenal gland, liver and fibroblasts [13]. Despite the importance of the liver in cholesterol homeostasis in vivo, only trace amounts of VLDL-receptor mRNA are detectable. Transcription of the LDL-receptor gene in mammals is downregulated by cholesterol [14]. This feedback regulation is mediated via SRE-1 (sterol regulatory element-1) found in the promoter regions of genes for the LDL receptor [15] and HMG-CoA synthase [16]. The 5' flanking region of the VLDL-receptor gene contains two copies of SRE-1-like sequences [8]. Despite the conservation of SRE-1-like sequences, the levels of VLDL-receptor mRNA in THP-1 cells were unchanged in the presence of excess LDL or β-VLDL, indicating that the SRE-1-like sequence is inactive in vivo. In addition to the SRE-1-like sequences, the promoter region of the VLDL-receptor gene contains a half-site for interaction with estrogen receptor. To test whether estrogen activates the expression of the VLDL-receptor in vivo, we treated rabbits with estradiol and analyzed the levels of VLDL-receptor mRNA. Pharmacological doses of estradiol enhanced the expression of VLDL mRNA several-fold in rabbit heart, suggesting that estradiol exerts its effects on VLDL-receptor gene expression [17].

Polymorphic triplet repeat

The 5'-untranslated region of the human VLDL-receptor mRNA contains a polymorphic triplet (CGG) repeat sequence. Expansion of a triplet repeat sequence has been implicated as the cause of heritable human diseases including spinal and bulbar muscular atrophy [18], fragile X syndrome [19], myotonic dystrophy [20], and Huntington's disease [21]. In the normal population, the CGG repeat polymorphism displays at least five discrete alleles ranging from four to nine repeat units. Jokinen et al. analyzed the expansion length of the repeats in patients with type III hyperlipidemia, familial hypertriglyceridemia, familial combined hyperlipidemia and type V hyperlipidemia and no expansion was found [22]. However, despite the apparent lack of expansion of the repeat, this unstable triplet sequence is a potential site of possible defects in the VLDL-receptor gene.

Implication of the roles of the VLDL receptor

On the basis of the expression of the VLDL receptor in tissues performing active fatty-acid metabolism, it is proposed that the basic function of the receptor is to provide muscle and fat cells with fatty acids [3]. The uptake of fatty acids into these cells has been believed to be mediated via lipoprotein lipase (LPL) [23]. However, there is no evidence for abnormal energy production or fat deposition in patients lacking LPL. The abundant expression of the VLDL receptor in fat cells may account for the accumulation of fats in adipose tissue in patients lacking LPL.

Acknowledgements

We thank Dr Ian Gleadall for helpful comments on the manuscript. This research was supported in part by research grants from the Ministry of Education, Science and Culture of Japan, the Ono Medical Research Foundation, Takeda Medical Research Foundation and the Mochida Memorial Foundation for Medical and Pharmaceutical Research.

References

1. Brown MS, Goldstein JL. Science 1986;232:34–47.
2. Takahashi S, Kawarabayasi Y, Nakai T, Sakai J, Yamamoto T. Proc Natl Acad Sci USA 1992;89:9252–9256.
3. Yamamoto T, Takahashi S, Sakai J, Kawarabayasi Y. Trends Cardiovasc Med 1993;3:144–148.
4. Herz J, Hamann U, Rogne S, Myklebost O, Gausepohl H, Stanley KK. EMBO J 1988;7:4119–4127.
5. Raychowdhury R, Niles JL, McCluskey RT, Smith JA. Science 1989;244:1163–1165.
6. Yamamoto T, Davis CG, Brown MS, Schneider WJ, Casey ML, Goldstein JL, Russell DW. Cell 1984;39:27–38.
7. Chen W–J, Goldstein JL, Brown MS. J Biol Chem 1990;265:3116–3123.
8. Sakai J, Hoshino A, Takahashi S, Miura Y, Ishii H, Suzuki H, Kawarabayasi Y, Yamamoto T. J Biol Chem 1994;269:2173–2182.
9. Südhof TC, Goldstein JL, Brown MS, Russell DW. Science 1985;228:815–822.
10. Lindgren V, Luskey KL, Russell DW, Francke U. Proc Natl Acad Sci USA 1985;82:8567–8571.
11. Gåfvels ME, Caird M, Britt D, Jackson CL, Patterson D, Strauss III JF. Som Cell Mol Genet 1993;19:557–569.
12. Gåfvels ME, Paavola LG, Boyd CO, Nolan PM, Wittmaack F, Chawla A, Lazar MA, Bucan M, Angelin B, Strauss III JF. Endocrinology 1994;135:385–394.
13. Yamamoto T, Bishop RW, Brown MS, Goldstein JL, Russell DW. Science 1986;232:1230–1237.
14. Goldstein JL, Brown MS. Nature 1990;343:425–430.
15. Smith JR, Osborne TF, Goldstein JL, Brown MS. J Biol Chem 1990;265:2306–2310.
16. Smith JR, Osborne TF, Brown MS, Goldstein JL, Gil G. J Biol Chem 1988;263:18480–18487.
17. Masuzaki H, Jingami H, Yamamoto T, Nakao K. FEBS Lett 1994;347:211–214.
18. La Spada AR, Wilson EM, Lubahn DB, Harding AE, Fischbeck KH. Nature 1991;352:77–79.
19. Fu Y-H, Kuhl DPA, Pizzuti A, Pieretti M, Sutcliffe JS, Richards S, Verkerk AJMH, Holden, JJA, Fenwick RG Jr, Warren ST, Oostra BA, Nelson DL, Caskey CT. Cell 1991;67:1047–1058.

20. Brook JD, McCurrach ME, Harley HG, Buckler AJ, Church D, Aburatani H, Hunter K, Stanton VP, Thirion J-P, Hudson T, Sohn R, Zemelman B, Snell RG, Rundle SA, Crow S, Davies J, Shelbourne P, Buxton J, Jones C, Juvonen V, Johnson K, Harper PS, Shaw DJ, Houseman DE. Cell 1992;68:799—808.
21. The Huntington's Disease Collaborative Research Group. Cell 1993;72:971—983.
22. Jokinen E, Sakai J, Yamamoto T, Hobbs HH. Hum Mol Genet 1994;3:521.
23. Eckel RH. N Engl J Med 1989;320:1060—1068.

Analysis of ligand binding to the low density lipoprotein receptor-related protein (LRP)

Thomas E. Willnow and Joachim Herz

Department of Molecular Genetics, University of Texas, Southwestern Medical Center, Dallas, TX 75235, USA

Abstract. LRP is a large multifunctional receptor implicated in the clearance of a multitude of different ligands including lipoproteins, proteases and protease–inhibitor complexes. To localize individual ligand binding sites on LRP we constructed truncated forms of the receptor that actively endocytose ligands from the extracellular space but are restricted in their ligand recognition profile. Using these minireceptors we were able to map the binding sites for the receptor-associated protein, tissue-type plasminogen activator and tissue-type plasminogen activator–inhibitor-1 complex on LRP.

LRP is a member of the LDL-receptor gene family

LRP [1], a 600-kDa cell-surface receptor, is a member of the LDL-receptor gene family, which also includes the LDL receptor [2], the VLDL receptor [3] and gp330 [4]. Each of these proteins is characterized by cysteine-rich repeats of the complement or ligand-binding type, by epidermal growth factor precursor homologous domains and by a single membrane-spanning segment. Their cytoplasmic domains contain at least one copy of the NPxY motif, which directs internalization of the receptors through coated pits (reviewed in [5]).

All members of the gene family mediate endocytosis of ligands from the plasma or extracellular space in general. Ligand binding to the receptors is calcium-dependent. The LDL receptor, the paradigm of this gene family, binds lipoprotein particles containing apolipoprotein E (apoE) and apoB100. These ligands are bound to the ligand-binding type repeats, which are present in seven copies in the N-terminal part of the receptor. All repeats with the exception of the first one contribute to the ligand-binding sites [6].

LRP contains 31 ligand-binding-type repeats and exhibits a rather complex ligand-binding profile (reviewed in [7]). Ligands binding to LRP include apoE-enriched β-migrating very low density lipoproteins, lipoprotein lipase (LPL) and lactoferrin. Furthermore, LRP has been shown to bind and internalize urokinase-type and tissue-type plasminogen activators (uPA, tPA) and complexes of these proteases with their specific protease inhibitor plasminogen activator inhibitor-1 (PAI-1). In addition, LRP has also been identified as the receptor for α_2-macroglobulin–serine protease complexes.

LRP is composed of individual ligand-binding sites

Cross-competition experiments have been carried out both in vitro and in vivo to map the relative localization of ligand-binding sites on LRP. The results of these studies, summarized in Table 1, have demonstrated that some of the ligands binding to the receptor are able to compete to a variable extent for receptor binding, while others fail to do so. This would argue for the presence of individual binding sites on the receptor, some of which are recognized by more than one ligand. In addition, a 39-kDa receptor-associated protein (RAP) has been shown to bind to multiple sites on LRP and, in doing so, displaces all the other known ligands [13,19]. This led to a proposed role for RAP as

462

Table 1. Competition of ligand binding to LRP in vitro, in cultured cells or in vivo.

Ligand	Competitor		
apoE	α_2M*	±	[8–12]
	Lactoferrin	+	[9,13]
LPL	Lactoferrin	+	[13]
	α_2M*	+	[14]
α_2M*	apoE	±	[8,10–12]
	LPL	±	[12,15]
	Lactoferrin	–	[9,13]
tPA/PAI-1	LPL	–	[13]
	Lactoferrin	–	[13]
	apoE	–	[13]
	α_2M*	–	[13]
	tPA	+	[16,17]
uPA/PAI-1	α_2M*	–	[18]
	tPA	–	[18]
	tPA/PAI-1	+	[18]
	PAI-1	+	[18]

+ = competition; α_2M* = methylamine- or protease-activated α_2-macroglobulin.

a regulator of receptor function. Taken together, these findings suggest that LRP is composed of a complex pattern of individual ligand-binding and regulatory sites.

Identification of binding sites for RAP, tPA/PAI-1 and tPA on LRP

The extracellular portion of LRP can be broken down into four individual regions, I–IV. Each of these regions is composed of a cluster of N-terminal ligand-binding type repeats and one or more domains homologous with epidermal growth factor precursor, thus resembling the structure of the LDL receptor (Fig. 1). We used a PCR-based cloning approach to construct LRP minireceptors containing regions II and IV fused to the membrane anchor and cytoplasmic domain of the receptor (Fig. 1). These minireceptors were overexpressed in the Chinese hamster ovary cell line ldlA7 [20].

In ligand-binding assays performed on membrane extracts of minireceptor-expressing cells, both Region II and IV bind RAP. Region II also binds complexes of tPA and PAI-1. As has been shown for the wild-type receptor, ligand binding to the individual regions is dependent on calcium and can be inhibited by the addition of RAP. Expressed mini-receptors are functional and bind and internalize ligands. This can be demonstrated by an increased rate of degradation of ^{125}I-labeled RAP in cell lines expressing Region II or Region IV (R-II, R-IV) over the parental cell line (ldlA7, Fig. 2). In addition, the cells expressing Region II also exhibit on average a 5-fold higher rate of degradation of ^{125}I-tPA/PAI-1 complex, consistent with the binding of this ligand to Region II on ligand blots. In separate experiments the binding site for free tPA could also be localized to Region II of the receptor. Neither Region II nor Region IV is able to bind methylamine-activated α_2-macroglobulin, as the rate of degradation of this ligand was similar in all three cell lines, reflecting the basal activity of wild-type LRP present in the cells. This suggests that the binding sites for α_2-macroglobulin and tPA or tPA/PAI-1 complexes are different.

Conclusion

The nature of the ligands binding to LRP suggest that this receptor is involved in

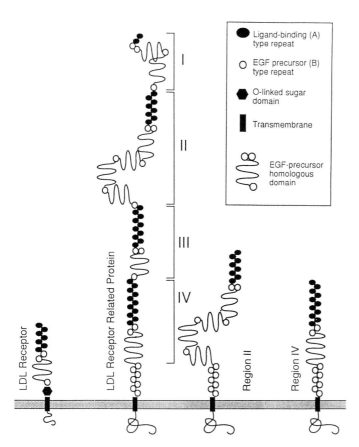

Fig. 1. Structural organization of the LDL receptor and wild-type and truncated LRP. Extension of the individual extracellular regions of LRP (I-IV) are shown. The constructed minireceptor Region II contains the leader peptide and the first seven amino acids of the mature LRP followed by region II (residues 836-2501) and the COOH-terminal membrane anchor and cytoplasmic tail of the receptor (starting at residue 4164). Region IV begins at residue 3316 of wild-type LRP and is also preceded by the leader peptide and the first seven amino acids of the mature LRP. All segments of the minireceptors were generated by PCR from the human cDNA of LRP.

regulation of lipoprotein metabolism as well as fibrinolysis. Disturbances in both of these diverse biological processes contribute to the development of atherosclerotic lesions. To better assess the role of LRP in these processes, it is important to understand the mechanism of interaction of the receptor molecule with a multitude of different ligands and regulators. In this study we have shown that recombinant LRP minireceptors with restricted ligand-binding profiles can be constructed. Using these truncated receptors we were able to map binding sites for RAP, tPA/PAI-1 and free tPA on LRP. Similarly it should be feasible to generate minireceptors that contain only a single binding site for any of the known proteins binding to the receptor.

Acknowledgements

This work was supported in part by National Institutes of Health Grant HL 20948 and a

464

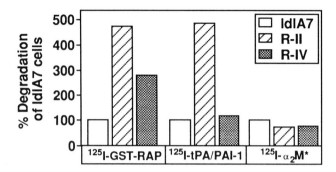

Fig. 2. Degradation of ^{125}I-labeled ligands by transfected and nontransfected cell lines. Chinese hamster ovary cells (ldlA7) were transfected with cDNA constructs for Region II and IV and lines stably expressing the minireceptors were isolated (R-II, R-IV). Subsequently 2.5×10^5 cells/well of cell lines ldlA7, R-II and R-IV were seeded into 12-well plates and grown for 24 h. Replicate monolayers of cells received 1 ml of DMEM containing 0.2% (w/v) bovine serum albumin and either ^{125}I-labeled glutathione-S-transferase–RAP fusion protein (^{125}I-GST-RAP), ^{125}I-tPA/PAI-1 complex or ^{125}I-labeled human α_2-macroglobulin that had been activated with methylamine (^{125}I-α_2M*). After incubation for 7 h (^{125}I-GST-RAP) or 20 h (^{125}I-tPA/PAI-1 and ^{125}I-α_2M*), the amount of ^{125}I-labeled degradation products secreted into the medium was determined. Each value represents the mean of duplicate incubations and is expressed as % amount of degradation products of the nontransfected parental cell line ldlA7, set at 100%.

grant from the Perot Family Foundation. T.E.W is a recipient of a fellowship from the Deutsche Forschungsgemeinschaft. J.H. is supported by the Syntex Scholar Program and the Lucille P. Markey Foundation.

References

1. Herz J, Hamann U, Rogne S, Myklebost O, Gausepohl H, Stanley KK. EMBO J 1988;7:4119–4127.
2. Brown MS, Goldstein JL. Science 1986;232:34–47.
3. Takahashi S, Kawarabayasi Y, Nakai T, Sakai J, Yamamoto T. Proc Natl Acad Sci USA 1992;89:9252–9256.
4. Raychowdhury R, Niles JL, McCluskey RT, Smith JA. Science 1989;244:1163–1166.
5. Brown MS, Herz J, Kowal RC, Goldstein JL. Curr Opin Lipidol 1991;2:65–72.
6. Russell DW, Brown MS, Goldstein JL. J Biol Chem 1989;264:21682–21688.
7. Krieger M, Herz J. Ann Rev Biochem 1994;63:601–637.
8. Hussain MM, Maxfield FR, Más-Oliva J, Tabas I, Ji ZS, Innerarity TL, Mahley RW. J Biol Chem 1991; 266:13936–13940.
9. Huettinger M, Retzek H, Hermann M, Goldenberg H. J Biol Chem 1992;267:18551–18557.
10. van Dijk MCM, Ziere GJ, van Berkel TJC. Eur J Biochem 1992;205:775–784.
11. Choi SY, Cooper AD. J Biol Chem 1993;268:15804–15811.
12. Jaeckle S, Huber C, Moestrup S, Gliemann J, Beisiegel U. J Lipid Res 1993;34:309–315.
13. Willnow TE, Goldstein JL, Orth K, Brown MS, Herz J. J Biol Chem 1992;267:26172–26180.
14. Chappell DA, Fry GL, Waknitz MA, Muhonen LE, Pladet MW, Iverius PH, Strickland DK. J Biol Chem 1993;268:14168–14175.
15. Chappell DA, Fry GL, Waknitz MA, Iverius PH, Williams SE, Strickland DK. J Biol Chem 1992;267: 25764–25767.
16. Orth K, Willnow TE, Herz J, Gething MJ, Sambrook JF. LRP is necessary for the internalization of both tPA/PAI-1 complexes and free tPA. J Biol Chem (in press).
17. Camani C, Bachmann F, Kruithof E. J Biol Chem 1994;269:5770–5775.
18. Nykjaer A, Petersen CM, Moller B, Jensen PA, Moestrup SK et al. J Biol Chem 1992;267:14543–14546.
19. Williams SE, Ashcom JD, Argraves WS, Strickland DK. J Biol Chem 1992;267:9035–9040.
20. Kingsley DM, Krieger M. Proc Natl Acad Sci USA 1984;81:5454–5458.

Characterization and purification of the lipolysis-stimulated receptor

Bernard E. Bihain, Frances T. Yen, Lydie M. Guermani, Armelle A. Troussard, Jamila Khallou, Bernadette Delplanque and Christopher J. Mann
INSERM U391, Université de Rennes, 35043, Rennes, France

The molecular events underlying clearance of chylomicrons (CM) from the circulation have received considerable interest. These large lipoproteins are synthesized by the intestine to transport dietary triglyceride and cholesterol. Once in the circulation, rapid hydrolysis of their triglyceride core by lipoprotein and hepatic lipases leads to formation of CM remnants, which enter the space of Disse in the liver, and are subsequently removed by hepatocytes [1].

One mechanism able to clear CM remnants is the LDL receptor. This receptor binds these particles with high affinity and has been estimated, in normal subjects, to account for half of CM-remnant removal [2,3]. However, subjects with familial hyper-cholesterolemia (FH) who lack functional LDL receptor do not accumulate CM remnants in their circulation [4], which indicates that there are one or more alternative routes for uptake of these particles. Several studies have suggested a role for the LDL receptor-related protein (LRP). This large multifunctional receptor, which is identical to the α_2-macroglobulin (α_2MG) receptor [5], has been shown to clear β-VLDL when the latter is enriched with additional exogenous apoE [6]. The ability of a receptor-associated protein (RAP), which co-purifies with LRP, to induce marked accumulation of CM remnants in LDL receptor-deficient mice has led to the proposal that LRP is a second remnant receptor [7].

However, a third potential mechanism exists for clearance of CM remnants, known as the lipolysis-stimulated receptor (LSR). This receptor is able to bind apoB and apoE lipoproteins with high affinity, but only when activated by the presence of free fatty acids (FFA), the products of lipoprotein-triglyceride hydrolysis. We summarize here the observations that have led to characterization and purification of the LSR.

In vitro characterization of LSR activity

The capacity of FFA to induce binding, internalization and degradation of apoB-containing lipoproteins was initially observed in human FH fibroblasts [8]. The first step of this pathway is the binding of the lipoprotein to a single class of sites on the plasma membrane: under conditions of equilibrium with 1 mM oleate, the apparent K_d for ^{125}I-LDL binding was found to be 12 μg protein/ml. That this binding provides the committed step for lipoprotein clearance was demonstrated by the presence of suramin during incubation of the FH cells with oleate and ^{125}I-LDL: by reversing the ^{125}I-LDL specific binding to the cell surface, both uptake and degradation were inhibited in parallel. Degradation of the lipoproteins occurs within the lysosomal compartment, as evidenced by the dose-dependent inhibition of degradation that occurs with chloroquine, a known inhibitor of lysosomal function [9]. Binding, uptake and degradation all approached saturation at 50 μg/ml ^{125}I-LDL, and levels of oleate as low as 25 μM were sufficient to significantly activate each of the three steps. The species of FFA is an important determinant of the degree of activation of LSR. Short-chain FFAs were shown to be poor activators, while unsaturated FFAs were more efficient than their saturated analogues; the monounsaturates were the most effective. That the effect of FFA is dependent on the hydrophobic chain was shown by similar stimulatory effects achieved with FFA analogues substituted on the carboxylic group with uncharged residues. These data thus indicated that the presence of specific FFA at the cell surface induce LSR to bind, internalize and deliver LDL to lysosomes.

The use of LDL as ligand for such studies was motivated by technical considerations, namely that LDL contain solely apoB, which is a nonexchangeable apoprotein that displays few nonspecific interactions [10]. Nevertheless, the affinity of LSR for CM is many times greater than for LDL (Fig. 1) [11], which is consistent with a role of LSR as receptor of intestinally derived lipoproteins. A similarly strong affinity of the receptor for triolein phosphatidylcholine emulsions supplemented with apoE (Fig. 1) indicates that it is this apoprotein that forms the recognition site on CM. We therefore know that LSR recognizes lipid particles containing solely apoB, both apoB and apoE, or solely apoE, but with preference for the larger apoE-containing particles. Interestingly, while normal VLDL showed an affinity intermediate between CM and LDL, VLDL isolated from a type III hyperlipidemic patient with the apoE2/E2 phenotype were unable to bind to LSR (Fig. 1). The ligand specificity of LSR is thus consistent with its putative function as CM-remnant receptor.

With this perspective of LSR as remnant receptor, we investigated the effect on LSR of lactoferrin, a milk protein that delays the clearance of CM remnants in vivo [12]. Human lactoferrin was able, in a parallel and dose-dependent manner, to completely inhibit LSR-mediated binding, uptake and degradation in FH fibroblasts [11]. By contrast,

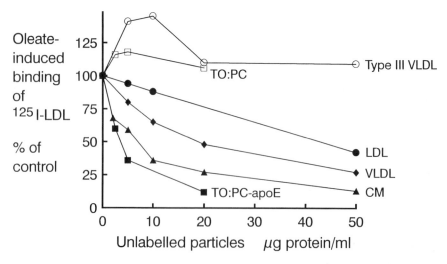

Fig. 1. Curves showing competition of different lipoproteins with ^{125}I-LDL for binding to LSR. FH fibroblasts were incubated at 37°C with 1 mM oleate, 20 µg/ml ^{125}I-LDL, and the indicated concentrations of unlabeled lipoproteins. After cell washing, the amount of ^{125}I-LDL specifically bound to the cell surface was determined by incubation with 10 mM suramin for 60 min at 4°C, and subsequent measurement of radioactivity in the medium. TO:PC = triolein/phosphatidylcholine emulsion. (Reproduced with permission from Biochemistry, 1994;33:1175.)

a related protein, transferrin, which is unable to delay remnant clearance in vivo [12], was unable to block LSR.

While the presence of LSR in human FH fibroblasts shows that it is genetically distinct from the LDL receptor, we questioned whether LSR activity was mediated by LRP. Five different lines of evidence failed, however, to show biochemical identity between LSR and LRP [11]. Firstly, the LRP ligand, activated α_2MG (α_2MG*), does not bind to oleate-activated LSR. Secondly, oleate has no effect on the binding of α_2MG* to LRP. Thirdly, unlike LRP activity, LSR activity is independent of Ca^{2+}. Fourthly, ligand-blotting studies using FH fibroblasts revealed two plasma membrane proteins of 115 and 85 kDa that were able to bind ^{125}I-LDL after exposure to oleate; these proteins are considerably smaller than the 600-kDa LRP. Finally, low concentrations of RAP (5 µg/ml) sufficient to block LRP in FH fibroblasts were unable to inhibit LSR (Fig. 2). It should be noted, however, that elevated concentrations of RAP markedly inhibited LSR activity (Fig. 3). Thus, at sufficiently high concentrations, RAP is capable of inhibiting not only LRP [7] and the LDL receptor [13], but also LSR (Fig. 3).

For LSR to play a role in clearance of CM remnants, it is necessary for the receptor to be expressed by the cells that directly participate in remnant removal. We therefore tested the effect of FFA on lipoprotein uptake by hepatocytes in culture. Primary hepatocytes isolated from both rats and WHHL homozygous rabbits showed oleate-induced LSR activity with kinetic characteristics similar to those observed in human normal and FH fibroblasts.

Because LSR activity appeared only after 24 h of culture of primary hepatocytes, we questioned whether this protein was also expressed in the living animal. To investigate

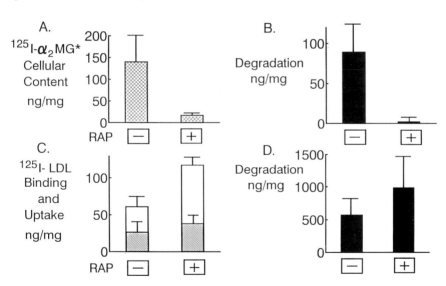

Fig. 2. Effect of low-concentration RAP on activities of LRP (panels A and B) and LSR (panels C and D) in FH fibroblasts. One set of cells was incubated for 90 min at 37°C with 1 µg/ml ^{125}I-α_2MG* in the absence or presence of RAP (5 µg/ml). The cell monolayers were washed, and ^{125}I-α_2MG* cellular content (A) and degradation (B) were measured. A second set of cells was incubated for 90 min at 37°C with 50 µg/ml ^{125}I-LDL and 0.2 mM oleate in the absence or presence of RAP (5 µg/ml). The cells were washed, and ^{125}I-LDL binding (C, hatched bar), uptake (C, open bar) and degradation (D) were measured as previously described [8]. (Reproduced with permission from Biochemistry 1994;33:1176.)

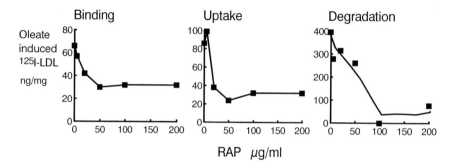

Fig. 3. Effect of high concentrations of RAP on LSR binding, uptake and degradation in FH fibroblasts. Cells were incubated for 2 h at 37°C with 20 μg/ml ^{125}I-LDL, 0.4 mM oleate and the indicated concentrations of RAP. The cells were washed, and ^{125}I-LDL binding (A), uptake (B) and degradation (C) were measured as previously described [8].

this, an assay was developed to measure and observe LSR activity in isolated rat liver membranes under different conditions. Briefly, membranes were first incubated with oleate to activate LSR, washed to remove excess FFA, and then further incubated with ^{125}I-LDL. Bound ^{125}I-LDL was separated from unbound ^{125}I-LDL by centrifugation of the membrane through a cushion of 5% BSA. EDTA (2 mM) was present at all stages to suppress LDL-receptor activity. ^{125}I-LDL binding studies showed saturation of LSR activity at 50 μg ^{125}I-LDL/ml, and with similar kinetic characteristics to that observed in intact cells (Mann et al., unpublished data).

Mechanism of LSR activation in rat liver membranes

Using this assay, LSR was found to be trypsin-sensitive, but not affected by heparinases or chondroitinase. Thus, LSR activity is mediated by a protein and not a proteoglycan. Furthermore, perfusion of intact livers with trypsin prior to membrane preparation, to selectively degrade cell-surface proteins, showed that more than 60% of LSR is on the external surface of the plasma membrane. The inability of trypsin perfusion to suppress LSR activity completely is consistent with a fraction of total cellular LSR residing within the cell. Indeed, membranes from isolated endocytic organelles — multivesicular bodies, compartment of uncoupling of receptor and ligand, and retrosomes — are more than 10-fold higher in LSR activity than total liver membrane [11]. These data are consistent with LSR, expressed on the cell surface, being able to mediate endocytosis.

   Ligand blotting was then performed to identify the rat-liver membrane protein responsible for LSR activity. Under specific conditions, these studies revealed a single 90-kDa protein able to bind ^{125}I-LDL after exposure to oleate (Fig. 4). Other ligand-blot studies showed the presence of an additional band of 180 kDa (not shown). We speculate that this larger protein represents a dimer of the 90-kDa protein. That both the oleate-activation and the lipoprotein-binding steps occurred with LSR separated from lipid and other proteins showed that these two steps result from direct interactions with the LSR protein. Furthermore, the failure of ^{125}I-LDL to recognize LSR incubated with lactoferrin (Fig. 4, lane 3) demonstrates that lactoferrin also acts directly on the receptor.

   From the latter set of data, we speculated that if lactoferrin recognizes only the active form of the receptor, this would indicate that the action of FFA is effected by inducing a conformational change of the LSR. To test this, rat membranes were treated with

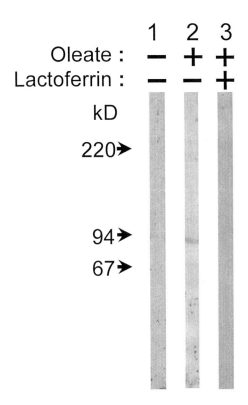

Fig. 4. Ligand blot of LSR from rat liver membrane. Solubilized membrane proteins were separated by SDS-PAGE and transferred to nitrocellulose by the method described previously [11]. After blocking, the nitrocellulose strips were incubated at 37°C for 60 min first in the absence (lane 1) or presence (lanes 2 and 3) of 1 mM oleate, then in the absence (lanes 1 and 2) or presence (lane 3) of 2 mg/ml lactoferrin, and finally with 20 μg/ml ^{125}I-LDL. The radioactivity of ^{125}I-LDL bound to LSR was revealed by exposure to a phosphor screen, and image analysis (PhosphorImager SF, Molecular Dynamics).

lactoferrin (2 mg/ml) before or after the oleate-activating step. While exposure of oleate-activated LSR to lactoferrin blocked ^{125}I-LDL binding, exposure of LSR to lactoferrin prior to oleate activation was unable to induce any inhibition of binding. Lactoferrin thus appears to act as a nonlipoprotein ligand requiring for its binding the conformational shift of LSR.

Further evidence that FFA alter the structure of LSR was provided by the observation that incubation of a solubilized membrane protein preparation with oleate increased the relative affinity of LSR for anion-exchange resin; this occurred without a change in the profile of the total proteins. It is our hypothesis that FFA interacts with a domain on LSR which induces a rearrangement of the folding of the protein, and thereby unmasks a series of negatively charged residues that serves as a binding site for apoB, apoE, or lactoferrin. Whether the FFA per se forms part of the binding site remains to be investigated. Experiments conducted to modulate the exposure of LSR to FFA showed that the conformational change of LSR remains fully reversible while the binding domain is unoccupied. By contrast, the modulatory effect of FFA is lost after formation of the receptor–lipoprotein complex, indicating that occupation of the binding domain with a ligand stabilizes the active conformation of the receptor.

Using anion-exchange chromatography and electrophoretic size separation, a protein of 90 kDa has been purified from rat-liver membranes. Elution of the relevant protein from the gel, incorporation into synthetic phospholipid liposomes, and testing for LSR activity showed that this protein could be induced by oleate to bind ^{125}I-LDL. N-terminal sequence analysis of this isolated protein showed no known homology with currently reported proteins. Experiments are presently under way to gather further information on LSR sequence in order to determine whether this newly characterized protein belongs to the LDL-receptor family.

Conclusion

LSR is a membrane protein that undergoes conformational change upon binding to FFA. This conformational shift allows recognition of specific classes of lipoproteins and of lactoferrin. We propose as a working hypothesis that the products of lipolysis generated in the space of Disse by lipolytic enzymes serve as signal molecules recruiting this receptor, which therefore provides a potential new model for the clearance of chylomicrons.

References

1. Sherill BC, Dietschy DM. J Biol Chem 1978;253:1859—1867.
2. Brown MS, Goldstein JL. Science 1986;232:34—47.
3. Choi SY, Fong LG, Kirven MJ, Cooper AD. J Clin Invest 1991;88:1173—1181.
4. Rubinsztein DC, Cohen JC, Berger GM, Van der Westhuyzen DR, Coetzee GA. J Clin Invest 1990;86: 1306—1312.
5. Strickland DK, Ashcom JD, Williams S, Burgess W, Migliorini H, Argraves WS. J Biol Chem 1990;265: 17401—17404.
6. Kowal RC, Herz J, Goldstein JL, Esser V, Brown MS. Proc Natl Acad Sci USA 1989;86:5810—5814.
7. Willnow TE, Sheng Z, Ishibashi S, Herz J. Science 1994;264:1471—1474.
8. Bihain BE, Yen FT. Biochemistry 1992;31:4628—4636.
9. De Duve C. In: De Reuck AVS, Cameron MP (eds) Lysosomes. Boston: Little, Brown and Co., 1963;1.
10. Elovson J, Jacobs JC, Schumaker VN, Puppione DL. Biochemistry 1985;24:1569—1575.
11. Yen FT, Mann CJ, Guermani LM, Hannouche NF, Hubert N, Hornick CA, Bordeau VN, Agnani G, Bihain BE. Biochemistry 1994;33:1172—1180.
12. Huettinger M, Retzek H, Eder M, Goldenberg H. Clin Biochem 1988;21:87—92.
13. Mokuno H, Brady S, Kotite L, Herz J, Havel RJ. J Biol Chem 1994;269:13238—13243.

Atherosclerosis X.
F.P. Woodford, J. Davignon and A. Sniderman, editors.

Physiological role of macrophage scavenger receptors

M. Honda[1], Y. Wada[2], H. Suzuki[2,3], K. Jishage[3], Y. Kawabe[2,4], T. Shimokawa[2,5], Y. Kurihara[2], H. Kurihara[2], H. Asaoka[5], A. Matsumoto[2,5], H. Itakura[2,5], Y. Yazaki[2], M. Naito[6], T. Mori[7], K. Takahashi[7], H. Nakamura[8], M. Matsushita[1], M. Emi[9], T. Doi[10] and T. Kodama[2]

[1]Departments of Psychiatry and [2]Internal Medicine III, University of Tokyo, Hongo Tokyo 113; [3]CSK Research Park and [4]Chugai Pharmaceutical, Gotenba; [5]National Institute of Nutrition and Health, Tokyo; [6]Department of Pathology, Niigata University, Niigata; [7]Department of Pathology, Kumamoto University, Kumamoto; [8]Protein Engineering Institute, Osaka; [9]Institute for Gerontrogy, Nippon Medical School, Kanagawa; and [10]Department of Pharmaceutical Sciences, University of Osaka, Japan

Both type I and type II macrophage scavenger receptors (MSR) consist of six domains, and each of the protein domains, which are encoded by separate exons, mediate particular cellular functions. Domain 1 (cytoplasmic) mediates rapid internalization and has a novel endocytosis motif. Domain 4 (α-helical coiled coil) is essential for trimer formation. In this domain the histidine interrupting heptad repeats of leucines is essential for acid-dependent ligand dissociation and for recycling of the receptor. Domain 5 (collagen-like) is essential for the binding of both acetyl-LDL and oxidized-LDL. Domain 6 is a type-specific domain, but the function remains obscure. MSR are expressed in macrophage lineage cells in various organs, and this macrophage-specific epitope helps define novel macrophage lineage cell types such as Mato's fluorescent granular perithelial cells in the brain. The wide distribution of MSR along blood vessels suggests that this receptor is essential for maintenance of the vascular system. Both type I and type II receptors are also co-expressed in atherosclerotic lesions. A MSR-deficient mouse strain generated by gene targeting is expected to be of help in the further analysis of physiological role of this receptor and its role in the development of atherosclerosis.

Structure of the MSR

The human MSR gene

We have cloned the 80-kilobase human MSR gene and localized it to band p22 on chromosome 8 near the LPL gene locus, by fluorescent in situ hybridization and genetic linkage analysis using three common restriction fragment length polymorphisms [1]. The human MSR gene consists of 11 exons, and two types of mRNAs are generated by alternative splicing from exon 8 to either exon 9 (type II) or exons 10 and 11 (type I). Figure 1 summarizes the domain structure of the human MSR, whose gene consists of a mosaic of exons that encode the functional domains.

Domain structure of MSR

Domain 1: N-terminal cytoplasmic domain

The N-terminal cytoplasmic domain consists of about 50 amino acid residues [2,3]. Immunoelectron-microscopic studies have revealed that at 4°C, MSR are gathered in the coated pit, but when the temperature is raised to 37°C, MSR are internalized and accumulate in the endosomes of the macrophages [4]. The results of experiments using mutant receptors indicate that residues 12–18, which can form a tight-turn secondary

472

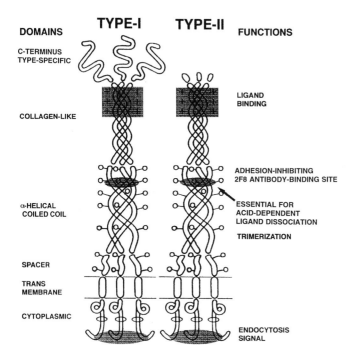

DOMAINS **TYPE-I** **TYPE-II** **FUNCTIONS**

C-TERMINUS
TYPE-SPECIFIC

LIGAND
BINDING

COLLAGEN-LIKE

ADHESION-INHIBITING
2F8 ANTIBODY-BINDING SITE

α-HELICAL
COILED COIL

ESSENTIAL FOR
ACID-DEPENDENT
LIGAND DISSOCIATION

TRIMERIZATION

SPACER

TRANS
MEMBRANE

CYTOPLASMIC

ENDOCYTOSIS
SIGNAL

Fig. 1. Schematic model of the postulated structures for type I and type II scavenger receptors and the functions of each domain.

structure, are essential for the endocytosis of MSR. The EDXDSCSE structure that appears in the MSR cytoplasmic domain is a new type of tight-turn motif which adds to the known tight-turn endocytosis signals such as NPXY and YXRF [5,6].

Domain 2: membrane-spanning domain
The transmembrane domain consists of a stretch of 26 hydrophobic amino acids [2,3].

Domain 3: spacer domain
A 32-amino-acid domain connects the membrane-spanning domain to the long fibrous coiled-coil domain [2,3].

Domain 4: α-helical coiled coil domain
Domain 4 contains as many as 23 7-amino-acid "heptad" repeats. Experiments using C-terminally truncated mutant receptors indicate that an α-helical coiled-coil structure mediates the assembly of the functional trimeric receptor [7].

The presence of histidines at positions 168 and 260, which disrupt the heptad repeats, is another conserved characteristic of this domain. We transformed His168 or His260 into leucine, a hydrophobic amino acid, and measured the ability of the resultant proteins to dissociate their ligands at acidic pH. The 260His→Leu substitution resulted in the loss of acid-dependent ligand-dissociation activity, whereas the 268His→Leu substitution did not affect it. Immunoelectron-microscopic studies show that the 260His→Leu mutant receptors appear in the lysosome compartments with their ligands, 30 min after warming, whereas normal receptors had already dissociated their ligands and appeared in transgolgi and other recycling pathways. These results indicate that His260 is essential for the pH-dependent conformational change of MSR, which leads to dissociation of their ligands at acidic pH [8].

Domain 5: collagen-like domain
Domain 5 consists of 23–24 uninterrupted Gly-X-Y tripeptide repeats that form a collagenous triple helix. Experiments using C-terminus-deleted receptors indicate that the 22 C-terminal amino acids of domain 5, which contains a cluster of basic amino acids, is essential for ligand binding and uptake. Experiments using point mutant receptors indicate that substitution of lysine 337 by alanine abolished acetyl-LDL degradation and binding at 37°C, but did not abolish the 4°C binding. In contrast, substitution of more than two lysines in this region was needed to abolish the oxidized-LDL degradation and 37°C binding [7]. This observation is consistent with reported nonreciprocal cross-competition. The results of direct binding experiments show that the binding activities of certain mutants at 4°C were different at 37°C. On the basis of a computational model of this domain using the coordinates of backbone atoms given by X-ray fiber diffraction for poly (L-prolyl-glycyl-L-proline), we built a structure of this domain, and have named it the "charged collagen" model [7].

Domain 6: C-terminal type-specific domain
By alternative splicing of 3′ exons, two C-terminally different receptor subunits were generated [1,9,10]. The type I C-terminal domain contains six conserved cysteines, consisting of scavenger-receptor cysteine-rich (SRCR) domains. When transfected separately, both type I and type II receptors mediate the scavenger function [2,9]. The expression of type I mRNA and protein increased during differentiation from monocytes to macrophages, which is associated with an increase in receptor activity, whereas type II expression did not change as dramatically [11].

Expression in various organs and atherosclerotic lesions

Tissue distribution and cell-type specificity

Table 1 summarizes the results of immunohistochemical studies of MSR-positive cells. These studies indicate that MSR are expressed in most macrophage lineage cells. Double immunostaining studies show that both type I and type II receptors are co-expressed in the same human macrophages [12]. Adding to the known macrophage lineage cells, MSR were also detected in a particular group of cells surrounding brain microvessels [13]. These cells contain spontaneous fluorescence, and have been named Mato's fluorescent granular perithelial cells (Mato cells). In addition to Mato cells, MSR has been detected in perivascular cells surrounding the microarteries of several organs. Among the various macrophage lineage cells, macrophages with high scavenging activity, such as alveolar macrophages or Kupffer cells in the liver, expressed a high level of MSR protein, but macrophage lineage cells specifically differentiated for antigen presentation, such as dendritic cells, had little receptor protein [12]. Aortic endothelial cells did not express MSR protein [12,15]. Sinusoid endothelial cells of the liver expressed immunoreactive receptor protein, but the immunoreactivity was different from the receptor in macrophages. Against the bovine MSR, two types of monoclonal antibody, IgG-D1 and D2, have been established. IgG-D2, which recognizes domain 4, cannot bind to sinusoidal endothelial cells [12], but IgG-D1, whose epitope is not known, recognizes these cells [14].

Table 1. Distribution of scavenger-receptor-positive cells

Tissues and sites	Cell type
Lymph nodes	
Sinus	Sinus macrophage
Germinal centers	Tingible body macrophage
Paracortical area	Macrophage
Medullary cords	Macrophage
(Interdigitating cells: negative)	
Liver	Kupffer cells
Sinusoid	Endothelial cells[a]
(Hepatocyte, fat-storing cells: negative)	
Spleen	
Red pulp	Macrophage
White pulp	Macrophage
Heart	
Connective tissue	Macrophage
Aorta	
Adventitia	Macrophage
Atherosclerotic lesion	Foam cells
(Smooth muscle cells, endothelial cells: negative)	
Lung	
Alveolar space	Alveolar macrophage
Esophagus	
Submucosa	Macrophage
Stomach	
Lamina propria	Macrophage
Intestine	
Lamina propria	Macrophage
Pancreas	
Connective tissue	Macrophage
(Pancreatic parenchymal cells: negative)	
Kidney	
Connective tissue	Perivascular macrophage
Adrenal	
Interstitial	Macrophage
Skin	
Dermis	Histiocytes
Uterus	
Endometrium	Macrophage
Myometrium	Macrophage
Ovary	Macrophage
Brain	
Cerebrum	Mato's FGP cells
Cerebellum	Mato's FGP cells
Subarachnoid space	Macrophages
Peripheral nerve	Perineurium macrophage

[a] A monoclonal antibody (IgG-D2 anti-bovine macrophage receptor) was unable to recognize this cell type.

Monoclonal antibody against murine MSR can recognize the sinusoidal endothelial cells (I. Fraser, S. Gordon et al., personal communication). These results suggest that sinusoidal endothelial cells express sMSR with a minor structural difference.

Intracellular pathway of scavenger receptor

By the use of gold-labeled acetyl-LDL and immunoelectron microscopy, the intracellular pathway of MSR has been elucidated [4,16]. They bind their ligand at the cell surface, accumulate into coated pits, internalize and dissociate in the endosome, and recycle via the trans-Golgi apparatus. The histidine 260 which interrupts the leucine zipper structure in the α-helical coiled-coil domain is essential for acid-dependent ligand dissociation and recycling of the receptor [8].

Expression in atherosclerotic lesions

Both type I and type II receptor proteins and mRNAs have been detected in the foam cells of atherosclerotic lesions [12,15]. Neither receptor protein nor mRNA has been detected in smooth muscle cells or aortic endothelial cells in human lesions [12,15].

Physiological role of MSR

MSR are expressed in macrophages active in the scavenging of various denatured and modified substrates and in sinusoidal endothelial cells. MSR can bind various negatively charged macromolecules by means of a charged collagen structure, after which it can internalize and recycle. The structure of this receptor is suitable for scavenging various compounds from various tissues and from the blood. The presence of MSR in Mato cells and other perivascular cells surrounding microarteries suggests that MSR is also important for the maintenance of vessel systems.

In 1993, Fraser et al. [17] reported an unexpected function of MSR. They developed a monoclonal antibody 2F8, which can inhibit the cation-independent adhesion of murine macrophages. In macrophages, β2-integrin and the complement type 3 receptor function as cation-dependent adhesion molecules. Using the mutant receptor expressed in CHO cells, we have shown the 2F8-binding site to localize in the α-helical coiled-coil domain (I. Fraser, S. Gordon, M. Honda and T. Kodama, unpublished). This domain is not a ligand-binding domain, but a domain which mediates the acid-dependent ligand dissociation. Cation-independent adhesion and the uptake of various negatively charged macromolecules are two of the most important characteristics of macrophages. The fact that both adhesion and uptake function are mediated by MSR suggests that macrophages may be recruited to lesions where denatured or modified materials accumulate, such as oxidized LDL in atherosclerotic lesions, and MSR then process these substrates using the same receptor. These findings may explain why such a large number of macrophages accumulate in lesions and form fatty streaks.

Scavenger-receptor-deficient mice and future problems

Using gene targeting in ES cells, a mouse strain deficient in MSR has recently been established by Suzuki and colleagues. Homozygote mice with MSR deficiency look normal. The number of peritoneal macrophages obtained from these mice is increased. Macrophages obtained from homozygous mice retained about 25% of the acetyl-LDL degradation activity and 30% of the oxidized-LDL degradation activity. Future investigations with this mouse strain will provide important information on the physiological roles of MSR and the roles they play in the development of atherosclerosis.

476

References

1. Emi M, Asaoka H, Matsumoto A et al. J Biol Chem 1993;268:2120–2125.
2. Kodama T, Freeman M, Rohrer L, Zabrecky J, Matsudaira P, Krieger M. Nature 1990;343:531–535.
3. Matsumoto A, Naito M, Itakura H et al. Proc Natl Acad Sci USA 1990;87:9133–9137.
4. Naito M, Kodama T, Matsumoto Doi T, Takahashi K. Am J Pathol 1991;139:1411–1423.
5. Kurihara Y, Matsumoto A, Itakura H, Kodama T. Curr Opin Lipidol 1991;2:295–300.
6. Wada Y, Doi T, Kodama T et al. Ann NY Acad Sci 1994 (in press).
7. Doi T, Higashino K, Kurihara Y et al. J Biol Chem 1993;268:2126–2133.
8. Doi T, Wada Y, Kodama T et al. J Biol Chem 1994 (in press).
9. Rohrer L, Freeman M, Kodama T, Penman M, Krieger M. Nature 1990;343:570–572.
10. Freeman M, Ashkenas J, Rees DJ et al. Proc Natl Acad Sci USA 1990;87:8810–8814.
11. Geng J, Hanson G, Kodama T. Arterioscler Thromb 1994 (in press).
12. Naito M, Suzuki H, Mori T, Matsumoto A, Kodama T, Takahashi K. Am J Pathol 1992;141:591–599.
13. Mato M, Sakamoto A, Kodama T et al. Proc Natl Acad Sci USA 1994 (in press).
14. Kodama T, Reddy P, Kishimoto C, Krieger M. Proc Natl Acad Sci USA 1988;85:9238–9242.
15. Luoma J, Hiltunen T, Sarkioja T, Moestrup KS, Gliemann J, Kodama T, Nikkari T, Yla-Herttuala S. J Clin Invest 1994;93:2014–2021.
16. Mori T, Naito M, Takahashi K et al. Life Sciences 1994 (in press).
17. Fraser I, Hughes D, Gordon S. Nature 1993;364:343–347.

Atherosclerosis X.
F.P. Woodford, J. Davignon and A. Sniderman, editors.

Characterization of abnormal macrophage metabolism in a normocholesterolemic kindred with xanthoma

Claude Giry, Louise-Marie Giroux, Madeleine Roy, Jean Davignon and Anne Minnich
Clinical Research Institute of Montreal, 110 Pine Ave West, Montreal, Quebec, Canada H2W 1R7

Abstract. We have observed in two siblings (FC, LC) extensive xanthelasma and planar xanthomas in the absence of hyperlipidemia. Monocyte scavenger receptor (SR) expression was markedly higher than normal and rose rapidly during maturation in both patients and controls. In the FC kindred, markedly high monocyte SR mRNA segregated with abnormal cellular phenotype characterized by lipid overaccumulation. Thus, the presence of xanthoma in the absence of hyperlipidemia was associated with precocious expression of the SR mRNA in monocytes. These studies will help to clarify the regulation of SR expression and the role of this receptor in foam-cell formation and atherogenesis.

Monocyte-derived macrophages are implicated in the formation of foam cells in atherosclerotic lesions [1]. These foam cells are characterized by a high content of cellular cholesteryl esters. The human macrophage SR cDNA has recently been cloned [2]. The ligand specificity of this receptor is broad [3] and includes two forms of modified lipoprotein: oxidized LDL, a physiological form, and acetylatedLDL (AcLDL), often used in vitro to assay SR activity. It is known that two forms of the SR, designated as type I and type II, are generated from alternative splicing of the same gene [4]. These forms differ in the carboxyl-terminal region in that the type I receptor contains a 110-amino-acid cysteine-rich carboxyl-terminal domain of unknown function while the 17-amino-acid carboxyl terminus of the type II receptor contains no cysteines. Since both forms take up acetylated and oxidized LDL equally well in transfected cells, the relative physiological significance of the two forms is unknown [5].

In addition to arterial foam-cell formation, it is also believed that the presence of cutaneous xanthomas in hyperlipidemia results from the uptake of plasma LDL, which may be modified as a result of prolonged circulation, by monocyte-macrophages and subsequent foam-cell formation. We have observed in one proband (FC) and her brother (LC) attending our clinic planar xanthomas in the absence of hyperlipidemia or any other detectable etiology. We have therefore hypothesized that this phenotype is related to abnormal activity of the SR. This report, which characterizes SR overexpression in monocytes from these subjects and in their family members, contains data to support this hypothesis.

Results and Discussion

Blood monocyte-macrophages from the original proband FC, in whom planar xanthomas of the face and neck were observed despite normolipidemia, were markedly visually abnormal in that they differentiated rapidly in culture and appeared foam-cell like. SR activity in her macrophages was markedly above normal. Because of her unfortunate death, subsequent studies were performed in her brother LC, in whom a similar phenotype was observed.

In THP-I cells, a human monocytic cell line frequently used to study monocyte

478

maturation, SR activity and message is induced after stimulation of maturation with phorbol ester [6–8]. In monocytes isolated from normal subjects' fresh blood, SR activity and mRNA increased approximately 3- and 100-fold, respectively, during 7 days in culture in the presence of autologous serum (Fig. 1). Thus, as expected, SR expression is induced during human monocyte maturation. In repeated experiments, monocyte SR activity and mRNA were on average 3- and 8.5-fold, in LC than in control subjects (Fig. 1). Thus, the phenotype of xanthomas in the absence of hyperlipidemia is associated with precocious expression of the SR in monocytes, and perhaps with precocious monocyte maturation.

Family study of FC kindred

SR mRNA was measured in several family members. SR mRNA levels in blood monocytes from two of the three brothers examined and from the son of LC were several times higher than controls, although these family members did not display detectable xanthomas. Only one brother (II-8) displayed relatively normal SR mRNA levels. In addition, 3-fold greater expression of SR mRNA in monocytes from sibling II-9 than in those from II-8 was associated with markedly greater SR activity in 2-day-old monocytes, as assessed by uptake of DiI-labeled AcLDL. The difference in SR activity between these two subjects was even more apparent in 7-day-old macrophages.

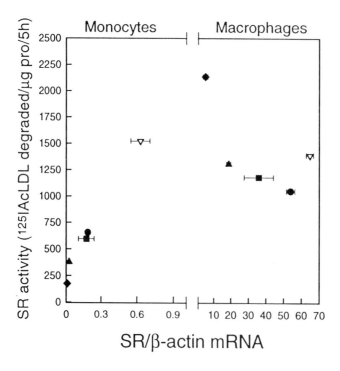

Fig. 1. Scavenger receptor activity and mRNA in monocytes and macrophages from LC vs. controls. SR mRNA was measured by RT-PCR with SR-specific primers [2] and fluorescence quantification of the PCR fragments. For controls, each point represents the mean (error bars indicate standard errors) of triplicate determinations. Closed and open symbols represent controls and LC, respectively. Monocytes, measurements 1 day after monocyte isolation; macrophages, 7 days.

Cellular cholesterol levels in affected and unaffected subjects

Macrophages from LC accumulated more total cholesterol than did those from control subjects, with over 80% as esterified cholesterol. Large cellular lipid accumulation was observed in macrophages from LC by Oil Red O staining and microscopy, in contrast to those from a control subject. Thus, apparent SR overexpression in monocytes from LC is associated with excess accumulation of cellular lipid in cultured macrophages. In siblings, high monocyte SR gene expression was associated with abnormal cellular phenotype, also characterized by lipid accumulation, despite the absence of xanthomas in these subjects. The additional genetic or environmental factor(s) which predispose some but not other members of this kindred to the xanthoma phenotype are not known, but may be related to the extent of SR overexpression.

Expression of SR isoforms

In normal subjects, the rise in SR expression during monocyte maturation into macrophages (7 days in culture) was associated with increases in both the type I and type II SR mRNA. This result contrasts with a previous observation that monocyte maturation was associated with a specific increase in the type I message [9]. Since the two messages share a common promoter but differ with respect to their 3′ sequence, which region is generally believed to mediate mRNA stability, the relative increase in the two isoforms during monocyte maturation may have implications regarding the molecular mechanisms underlying this induction. Preliminary results of SR mRNA quantification after actinomycin treatment of monocytes and macrophages suggests that neither the increase in SR mRNA during maturation nor the overexpression in LC can be ascribed to differences in message stability, so that these phenomena may be transcriptionally mediated.

SR gene expression in the absence of autologous serum

Since human blood monocytes are normally cultured in the presence of autologous serum, it was possible that the apparent overexpression of the SR in monocytes from LC and his family members might be related to some component in their serum. We therefore compared SR gene expression in monocytes from LC and his son and from a control subject cultured in the presence and absence of autologous serum. For this purpose, Nutridoma®, a media supplement shown to support growth and maturation of human monocytes [10], was used. In a control subject, LC, and his son, monocyte SR mRNA was similar in the presence or absence of autologous serum, and was 10- and 4-fold higher in LC and his son, respectively, than in the control. In all three subjects, SR expression rose after maturation into macrophages, to a similar degree (10- to 15-fold) in the presence or absence of autologous serum. This is consistent with the previous observation that Nutridoma® supports monocyte maturation even in the absence of autologous serum [10]. Thus, monocyte SR overexpression in LC does not appear to depend on a serum component.

Summary

We have described a genetic condition characterized by precocious blood monocyte maturation, SR overexpression, and abnormal lipid accumulation, sometimes associated with cutaneous planar xanthoma in the absence of hyperlipidemia. The cellular phenotype appears endogenous to the monocyte and independent of serum components. However, it is not clear whether the apparent SR overexpression in monocytes from members of the

480

kindred is the cause or consequence of precocious monocyte maturation. Although the phenomenon appears to be genetic, whether the SR gene itself or some other gene involved in monocyte maturation is implicated remains to be determined. Experiments to address these questions will undoubtedly elucidate the physiological role of the SR in monocyte maturation and foam cell formation as well as physiological mechanisms for regulation of SR gene expression.

Acknowledgements

We are grateful to Guy Lepage, Department of Gastroenterology and Nutrition, Ste. Justine Hospital for measurements of cellular cholesterol. We thank Dr Ross Milne for measurement of anti-LDL antibody. We thank Ghilaine DeLangavant for measurement of plasma antioxidants, Lucie Boulet for measurement of cellular cholesterol, Francois Pepin and Christian Charbonneau for photography, and Dr Djamel Ramla for assistance with preparation of cells for microscopy. We are grateful to Dr T. Kodama for the gift of the scavenger receptor cDNA. We thank Dr Marek Naruszewicz for helpful discussions during the project. We are deeply indebted to FC and her family for their cooperation in these studies. This work was supported by the Heart Stroke Foundation of Quebec.

References

1. Gerrity RG. Am J Pathol 1981;103:181–200.
2. Matsumoto A, Naito M, Itakura H, Ikemoto S, Hitoshi A, Hayakawa I, Kanamori H, Abutatani H, Takaku F, Wydro R, Housman DE, Kodama T. Proc Natl Acad Sci USA 1990;87:9133–9137.
3. Brown MS, Goldstein JL. Ann Rev Biochem 1983;52:223–261.
4. Emi M, Asaoka H, Matsumoto A, Itakura H, Kurihara Y, Wada Y, Kanamori H, Yazaki Y, Takahashi E, Lepert M, Lalouel J-M, Kodama T, Mukai T. J Biol Chem 1993;268:2120–2125.
5. Freeman M, Ekkel Y, Rohrer L, Penman M, Freedman NJ, Chisolm GM, Krieger M. Proc Natl Acad Sci USA 1991;88:4931–4935.
6. Akeson AL, Schroeder K, Woods C, Schmidt CJ, Jones WD. J Lipid Res 1991;32:1699–1707.
7. Moulton KS, Wu H, Barnett J, Parthasarathy S, Glass CK. Proc Natl Acad Sci USA 1992;89:8102–8106.
8. Kodama T, Freeman M, Rohrer L, Zabrecky J, Matsudaira P, Krieger M. Nature 1990;343:531–535.
9. Geng Y, Kodama T, Hansson GK. Arterioscler Thromb 1994;14:798–806.
10. Banka CL, Black AS, Dyer CA, Curtiss LK. J Lipid Res 1991;32:35–43.

Cholesterol efflux from cells in culture

P.G. Yancey[1], G.H. Rothblat[1], W.S. Davidson[1], E.P.C. Kilsdonk[1], V. Atger[2] and M. de la Llera Moya[1]

[1]Department of Biochemistry, Medical College of Pennsylvania, 2900 Queen Lane, Philadelphia. Pennsylvania, USA; and [2]Hôpital Broussais, Paris, France

Abstract. We examined what properties of acceptors influence cholesterol efflux. The most complex acceptor was human serum. Efflux was correlated with the concentrations of specific lipoproteins, and the order was: total HDL > HDL_3 = LpAI > HDL_2 > LpAI/AII suggesting that many HDL populations contribute to efflux. Lipid-free apolipoprotein A-I (apoA-I) and synthetic peptides containing amphipathic helical segments were the simplest acceptors. With these acceptors there was efflux of both cholesterol and phospholipid from macrophages, which suggests that amphipathic helices are required. This process was dependent on helical length and number, but was independent of amino acid sequence. When apoA-I or peptides were complexed to phospholipid to form discs, the peptide/phospholipid discs were equally or more efficient than apoA-I-containing discs. Our results suggest that efflux does not require interaction of acceptors with specific cell-surface receptors.

The first step in the process of reverse cholesterol transport is the release of cholesterol from cells to acceptor lipoproteins. Both cellular and acceptor factors affect the rate at which cholesterol molecules desorb from the cell plasma membrane and are solubilized by acceptors. We have conducted studies using acceptors of different complexity to gain more insight into what factors affect acceptor efficiency. Human whole serum was used as the most complex acceptor of cholesterol from cells while the simplest acceptors employed were lipid-free apoA-I and synthetic peptides consisting of amphipathic helical segments. Acceptors of intermediate complexity and of a uniform population were formed by complexing either the apoA-I or synthetic peptides to phospholipid to form discs. Release of radiolabeled cholesterol from cells was used as a measure of cholesterol efflux in these studies. In the experiments using discs and lipid-free peptides as acceptors, the release of radiolabeled cholesterol into the medium represents net cholesterol efflux or a decrease in the mass of cholesterol in the cells since these acceptors initially are free of cholesterol and there would be little influx of cholesterol. When whole serum is used as an acceptor, quantitation of radiolabeled cholesterol in the medium would not necessarily reflect a net change in cell cholesterol content since influx of cholesterol would occur from the various lipoproteins present in serum.

Release of cholesterol to whole serum

Mouse L-cells and the rat hepatoma cell line, Fu5AH, were used to test a large number of human serum samples for their ability to promote the efflux of cell cholesterol [1]. The measurement of cholesterol efflux obtained with each sample was correlated with the serum concentrations of different parameters including lipids (i.e., cholesterol, triglycerides), and apolipoproteins (i.e., apoA-I, apoA-II, apoB) and lipoproteins (i.e., HDL_2, HDL_3, LpAI, LpAI/AII). Colleagues from the clinical chemistry laboratory at the Hôpital Broussais in Paris, France kindly provided the human serum samples used in these studies.

All serum samples were obtained from men who had been chosen via a cholesterol screening program conducted at their place of employment.

Statistically significant correlations were observed between cholesterol efflux and levels of serum parameters associated to HDL. The strongest relationship was observed between cholesterol efflux and the serum concentration of total HDL-cholesterol ($r = 0.68$, $p = < 0.0001$, $n = 113$). Similarly, high correlations were obtained when comparing cholesterol efflux with either HDL_2 or HDL_3. The efflux of cell cholesterol was found to be more strongly correlated with serum LpAI levels ($r = 0.57$, $p = < 0.0001$) than with LpAI/AII levels ($r = 0.26$, $p = 0.002$). While there was a strong relationship between cell-cholesterol efflux and serum total HDL-cholesterol concentrations, there were many times in which different samples having the same HDL levels promoted very dissimilar rates of cholesterol release. A large overlap amongst HDL populations is obtained when the different subfractions are quantitated by their content of cholesterol or apoproteins. Thus, when the data are analyzed by partial correlation, LpAI and HDL_3 become the strongest independent serum parameters affecting the release of cholesterol from cells. No correlations were observed between efflux of cell cholesterol and the serum parameters related to the apoB-containing lipoproteins. Therefore, although LDL can accept and exchange cholesterol with cells [2—6], the apoB-containing lipoproteins do not affect the rate of cholesterol efflux from cells.

Release of cellular lipid to lipid-free apoA-I and peptides

We used peptides of defined structure to determine what structural properties of lipid-free apoA-I mediate efflux of cholesterol and phospholipid from mouse peritoneal macrophages and L-cells. ApoA-I and the other exchangeable apolipoproteins contain repetitive α-helical domains which are amphipathic and mediate interaction of the protein with phospholipid [7]. The synthetic peptide 18A consists of 18 amino-acid residues that form one amphipathic helical segment. This helix is similar to the Class A helical segments present in apolipoproteins [7,8]. Peptide 37pA contains two helical segments and is a dimer consisting of two 18A molecules covalently joined by a proline residue [7]. Blocked 18A ($Ac18ANH_2$) is an 18A molecule where the charges at the H-terminal and C-terminal have been neutralized by the addition of an acetyl group and an amide group, respectively. The modification effectively lengthens and stabilizes the helical segments, giving this peptide a higher lipid-binding affinity than 18A [9]. The order of lipid-binding affinity of the peptides is 37pA > $Ac18ANH_2$ > 18A [7,9].

The order of efficiency with which the acceptors promoted cholesterol efflux, as assessed by the molar acceptor concentration (EC_{50}) which promoted half-maximum efflux from mouse macrophages and L-cells, is apoA-I > 37pA > $Ac18AHH_2$ > 18A. On a mass basis, the order of efficiency of the acceptors was similar to when the data were expressed in molar concentrations, except that apoA-I and 37pA were equally effective. The order of efficiency of the acceptors in stimulating phospholipid efflux was similar to that observed for cholesterol efflux. There was saturation of cholesterol efflux when either apoA-I or the peptides were used as acceptors. In contrast, there was saturation only of phospholipid efflux when apoA-I was used as the acceptor. In addition, the amount of phospholipid release from macrophages and L-cells was much higher in the presence of the peptides than when incubated with apoA-I. The EC_{50} values were similar for cholesterol and phospholipid efflux in the presence of apoA-I. However, the EC_{50} values for phospholipid efflux were 2—5 times higher than those for cholesterol efflux when the peptides were used as acceptors.

Release of cholesterol to reconstituted particles

The three Class A helical peptides and apoA-I were complexed to dimyristoyl phosphat-idylcholine (DMPC) to gain more insight into the effects of amphipathic helical structure on the efflux of cholesterol from cells. When the peptides are complexed to DMPC, the discs formed are similar in diameter (11–12 nm) to that of the particles with apoA-I and DMPC, at a phospholipid to protein ratio of 2.5:1 (w:w). When compared at saturating acceptor concentrations (> 200 µg DMPC/ml), the four types of discs were equally efficient in stimulating cell-membrane cholesterol removal. However, at the same phospholipid concentration, protein-free small unilamellar vesicles (SUV) of DMPC were significantly less efficient. The V_{max} for the SUV was 10 times lower than that observed when apolipoprotein/DMPC discs were used as acceptors. We suggest that this difference in V_{max} is due to a reversible interaction of the apolipoproteins or peptides with the plasma membrane that changes the lipid-packing characteristics in such a way as to increase the rate of desorption of free cholesterol from the cell surface. This interaction would require amphipathic α-helical segments but would not be influenced by the length, number, and lipid-binding affinity of the helices.

The abilities of the peptides and apoA-I-containing particles to stimulate the efflux of lysosome-derived free cholesterol were also examined. To achieve this, L-cells were incubated with medium containing reconstituted LDL (rLDL) that contained [^{3}H]-cholesteryl oleate. Efflux of cholesterol from the plasma membrane was examined simultaneously by previously exchange-labeling the cells with [^{14}C]-cholesterol. At low concentrations of acceptor (< 100 µg DMPC/ml), the 18A/DMPC disc was the most effective acceptor of cell membrane cholesterol while the apoA-I-containing discs were the least efficient. The AC-18A-NH$_2$/DMPC and 37pA/DMPC complexes accepted cholesterol with an intermediate efficiency. Qualitatively similar results were observed for the efflux of free cholesterol originating from both the plasma membrane and the lysosome, showing that the peptide- and apoA-I-containing complexes have the same relative ability to remove free cholesterol from the two different cellular pools.

Discussion

The results of the present studies on the efflux of cell cholesterol to the different extracellular acceptors cannot be explained by a single mechanism for the release of cholesterol from cells. Clearly, the desorption of cholesterol from the cell plasma membrane is a fundamental mechanism, and it may be the predominant process governing efflux to acceptors such as small unilamellar vescles that contain no protein [10]. The data in these studies show that when either apoA-I or synthetic peptides are complexed to phospholipid to form discs, the maximal rate of cholesterol efflux from cells is greater than when SUV are used as acceptors. We propose that the efflux of cell cholesterol to acceptors which contain apoproteins is mediated, at least in part, by the interaction of the apoprotein with the plasma membrane. Although the synthetic peptides used in these studies have no sequence homology to apoA-I, peptide/DMPC complexes were equally effective as apoA-I/DMPC discs in enhancing the rate of cholesterol release from cells. Thus, the interaction of apoproteins and peptides with the plasma membrane would not be mediated by a specific cell-surface receptor. It is more likely that the facilitated rate of cholesterol efflux to apoprotein-containing particles is due to a relatively nonspecific interaction of the apoprotein with the plasma membrane. There are two possibilities for such an interaction. First, the apoprotein could remain associated with the lipoprotein and still interact with the cell surface, possibly at specific domains on the plasma membrane

484

[11]. Second, the interaction could involve the apoprotein disassociating from the lipoprotein. Here, the unassociated apoprotein could bind to the cell surface and modify the lipid-packing characteristics of the plasma membrane in such a way as to facilitate the desorption rate of cholesterol molecules [12]. As discussed with the data above, the interaction of the lipid-free apoprotein with the plasma membrane could also stimulate phospholipid efflux, resulting in the formation of nascent particles capable of accepting cell cholesterol. It is probable that all of the proposed mechanisms of cholesterol efflux can take part in the release of cellular cholesterol, and that the relative contribution of each mechanism to overall efflux is dependent on the combination and types of acceptors present in the interstitial fluid at the cell surface.

Acknowledgements

This work was supported by Program Project Grant HL22633 and a Minority Investigator Research Supplement (MIRS) to this grant, NSF Research Planning Grant MCB-9308279 (MM), National Institutes of Health Training Grant HL07443, a predoctoral fellowship to W.S. Davidson from the American Heart Association, Southeastern Pennsylvania Affiliate, a grant from Pfizer, Inc., and NATO Collaboration Research Grant 930317 (VA). We wish to thank Drs G.M. Anantharamaiah and J.P. Segrest for supplying the synthetic peptides used in these studies.

References

1. de la Llera Moya M, Atger V, Paul JL, Fournier N, Moatti N, Giral P, Friday KE, Rothblat GH. Arterioscler Thromb 1994;14:1056–1065.
2. Bates SR, Rothblat GH. Biochim Biophys Acta 1974;360:39–55.
3. Johansson J, Carison LA, Landou C, Hamsten A. Arterioscler Thromb 1991;11:174–182.
4. Lund-Katz S, Hammerschlag B, Phillips MC. Biochemistry 1982;21:2964–2969.
5. Francone OL, Fielding CJ, Fielding PE. J Lipid Res 1990;31:2195–2200.
6. Nakamura R, Ohta T, Ikeda Y, Matsuda I. Arterioscler Thromb 1993;13:1307–1316.
7. Segrest JP, Jones MK, De Loof H, Brouillette CG, Venkatachalapathi YV, Anantharamaiah GM. J Lipid Res 1992;33:141–166.
8. Anantharamaiah GM, Jones JL, Brouilleffe CG, Schmidt CF, Chung SH, Hughes TA, Shown AS, Segrest JP. J Biol Chem 1985;260:10248–10255.
9. Venkatachalapathi YV, Phillips MC, Epand RM, Epand RF, Tytler EM, Segrest JP, Anantharamaiah GM. Proteins 1993;15:349–359.
10. Johnson WJ, Mahlberg FH, Rothblat GH, Phillips MD. Biochim Biophys Acta 1991;1085:273–298.
11. Rothblat GH, Mahlberg FH, Johnson WJ, Phillips MD. J Lipid Res 1992;33:1091–1098.
12. Letizia JY, Phillips MD. Biochemistry 1991;30:866–873.

Atherosclerosis X.
F.P. Woodford, J. Davignon and A. Sniderman, editors.

Role of second messengers in cholesterol efflux

E.L. Bierman, M.A. Deeg, A.J. Mendez, W.S. Garver, B.M. Hokland, J.P. Slotte and J.F. Oram

Division of Metabolism, Department of Medicine, University of Washington, Seattle, Washington, USA

HDL binding to a cell-surface binding site transduces signals that stimulate translocation of excess cholesterol from apparent intracellular pools to the plasma membrane, from where it can desorb onto acceptor particles such as HDL. Recent studies indicated that protein kinase C (PKC) is activated by binding of intact HDL to several cell types [1], preceded by formation of the PKC activator diacylglycerol [2,3], possibly from phosphatidylcholine [4]. HDL-binding sites may be linked to phospholipase C via G proteins, since pertussis toxin, which inactivates G proteins, blocks HDL_3-mediated diacylglycerol formation [3,5]. Inhibition of PKC by chronic phorbol ester treatment or by sphingosine decreases HDL_3-mediated translocation and efflux of intracellular sterol [3]. This signal-transduction pathway is also attenuated if HDL particles are modified by treatment with tetranitromethane or trypsin, which indicates that HDL apolipoproteins rather than lipids are involved.

Specific cellular proteins that are phosphorylated in response to HDL binding have now been identified that may play a role in the HDL-mediated translocation and efflux pathway. HDL stimulation increased phosphorylation of at least two acidic proteins (quantified by phosphor imaging of 2-D gels of total cell phosphorylated proteins after preincubation of cholesterol-loaded fibroblasts with $^{32}P_i$ and then HDL_3) with apparent M_r of 18 (pp18) and 80 kDa (pp80) [6]. The time courses of phosphorylation differed: pp80 increased within 30 s of HDL_3 stimulation, while the increase in pp18 was apparent after 2 min. Phosphorylation of both proteins remained elevated for at least 30 min. Phorbol ester (PMA), but not a cAMP derivative, increased phosphorylation of these proteins, consistent with PKC activation. Based on the M_r and pI, pp80 has the characteristics of MARCKS (myristoylated alanine-rich C kinase substrate), consistent with HDL-mediated protein kinase C activation. However, the identities and function of pp18 and pp80 are as yet unknown. A hypothetical scheme for the HDL-stimulated protein kinase C signalling pathway is depicted in Fig. 1. Additional studies are required to demonstrate a possible link between these and other phosphorylated proteins and translocation of intracellular sterol to the plasma membrane.

Cholesterol efflux may be controlled by other messengers as well. Activation of cAMP-dependent protein kinase also resulted in stimulation of translocation and efflux of intracellular sterols in cholesterol-loaded cells, as evident from studies using cAMP analogues (N^6-cAMP and 8t-cAMP), an adenylyl cyclase activator (forskolin), a phosphodiesterase inhibitor (IBMX), and an inhibitor of cAMP-dependent protein kinase (H8) [7]. However, unlike PKC, cAMP-dependent protein kinase (PKA) was not activated in response to HDL binding, since HDL did not increase cell cAMP levels and inhibition of either adenylyl cyclase or PKA had no effect on sterol efflux promoted by HDL_3. Further, stimulation of PKA by a cAMP analogue did not increase phosphorylation of pp80 and pp18. A hypothetical scheme for the involvement of the cAMP signalling pathway in cholesterol trafficking is depicted in Fig. 2. Although HDL binding to the cell

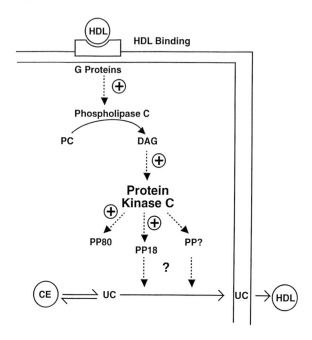

Fig. 1. A hypothetical scheme for the HDL-stimulated protein kinase C signalling pathway.

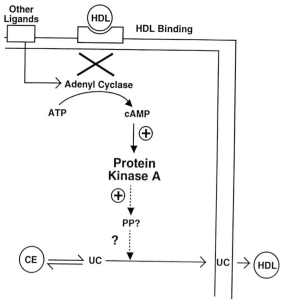

Fig. 2. A hypotheical scheme for the involvement of the cAMP signalling pathway in cholesterol trafficking.

surface does not appear to activate PKA, other ligands that activate adenylyl cyclase could play a role in translocation of intracellular sterol.

In summary, at least two distinct protein kinase signalling pathways modulate movement of intracellular sterols in cholesterol-loaded cells, only one of which, the PKC pathway, appears to be activated by HDL cell-surface binding.

References

1. Mendez AJ, Oram JF, Bierman EL. J Biol Chem 1991;266:10104–10111.
2. Theret N, Delbart C, Aguie G, Fruchart JD, Vassaux G, Ailhaud G. Biochem Biophys Res Commun 1990;173:1361–1368.
3. Mendez AJ, Oram JF, Bierman EL. Trans Assoc Am Physicians 1991;104:48–53.
4. Nazih H, Devred D, Martin-Nizard F, Fruchart JC, Delbart C. Thromb Res 1990;59:913–920.
5. Nazih H, Devred D, Martin-Nizard F, Clavey V, Fruchart JC, Delbart C. Thromb Res 1992;67:559–567.
6. Deeg MA, Garver WS, Bierman EL, Oram JF. Circulation 1993;88:227.
7. Hokland BM, Slotte JP, Bierman EL, Oram JF. J Biol Chem 1993;268:25343–25349.

Structural determinants of apoA-I and apoA-II–receptor interaction

Noel Fidge and Dmitri Sviridov

Baker Medical Research Institute, P.O. Box 348 Prahran, Victoria 3181, Australia

Abstract. The major proteins of circulating high density lipoprotein, AI and AII apoproteins, play many roles in lipid transport. Some recent evidence suggests that apoA-I, through interaction with a previously unrecognized high-affinity site on liver cells, may participate in receptor-linked regulation of other biochemical pathways. Our laboratory has recently identified receptor-binding domains in the C-terminal region of apoA-I, a finding which has been confirmed elsewhere. This receptor-binding site may or may not correspond exactly with other sites involved in cellular cholesterol efflux, which suggests that high-affinity receptor binding and interactions connected with cholesterol efflux may involve different structural properties of apoA-I.

The fate of circulating high density lipoprotein (HDL) is determined in large part by its major constitutive protein moieties, AI and AII apolipoproteins. Although secondary structural features, such as α-helices which provide the amphipathic properties essential for assembly of lipid-protein complexes, are shared in common with other apolipoproteins, apoA-I and apoA-II appear to confer specific roles on the particles on which they reside. Thus lipid-binding domains and enzyme (LCAT) recognition sites have been identified on apoA-I, while more recently specific cellular binding domains that recognize the putative HDL receptor have also been reported to exist on apoA-I [1]. Our laboratory first identified a previously unrecognized high-affinity site for HDL (K_d 3 × 10^{-9} M) on liver plasma membranes, a finding confirmed recently by Barbaras et al. [2], who further showed that this site was specific for free apoA-I as opposed to lipid-associated apoA-I. Taken together, the evidence points to the existence of a physiological receptor for at least one of the HDL apoproteins (AI), further stimulating investigation of the association between structure and function of this HDL apoprotein moiety. In addition, the existence of these high-affinity sites for apoA-I is persuasive evidence for a receptor-mediated regulatory role of apoA-I in cell metabolism that may or may not be related to lipid transport. Indeed, one hypothesis is that the high-affinity sites, possibly through cell-signalling processes, regulate the function of the lower-affinity HDL binding sites.

That apoA-II, as well as apoA-I, is involved in HDL–receptor interactions is suggested by many studies. ApoA-II apparently binds to the same receptor sites as apoA-I since we have shown that both apoproteins bind to two candidate HDL receptors, HB$_1$ and HB$_2$ [3], when subjected to ligand blotting. However, the binding parameters of HDL particles containing exclusively apoA-I differ from apoA-II-containing particles, which show a higher affinity but lower capacity than the apoA-I particles. To accommodate these differences, we formulated a model [4] of interaction that fitted these binding parameters. This model proposes that apoA-II-containing particles occupy four receptors for a single receptor occupied by apoA-I particles, a model subsequently supported when we demonstrated that each monomer of the homodimer apoA-II is capable of binding to HB$_1$ and HB$_2$ [5]. The existence of two molecules of apoA-II on each HDL particle that contains apoA-II is consistent with the predicted model. We further observed a strong homology between the putative receptor-binding domain in the C-terminal region of apoA-I and the C-terminal region in apoA-II, which strengthened the binding relationship between them. Because of its higher affinity apoA-II would, at higher concentrations, compete effectively with apoA-I-rich HDL particles; this antagonistic potential is consistent with the hypothesis that apoA-II-rich HDL particles inhibit cholesterol flux between cells and particles [6], with important consequences for the efficiency of reverse cholesterol transport.

Several apoproteins that include those of AI, AII, E and AIV share common structural features in the form of repeating units and a high level of α-helical content. The amphipathic property arising from this secondary structure is thought to provide the explanation for the unique lipid-binding properties on the one hand, but the water solubility of these proteins on the other. However, evidence reported in this laboratory, and more recently confirmed by others, supports the notion that sequences of specific amino acid residues may influence binding between cell membranes and HDL. In fact, several domains may be involved. Our studies using direct binding assays with fragments of apoA-I suggest that binding domains reside in the C-terminal region [3]. This has been supported by Swaney's laboratory [7], which used protease digestion to produce sequential truncation of apoA-I and subsequently found that a domain spanned by residues 149-219 possesses the capacity to bind to hepatic membrane proteins. Availability of epitope-specific monoclonal antibodies (mAbs) has aided these investigations. We found that mAbs against the C-terminal domain inhibited binding to the receptor, which is consistent with the results obtained in our direct binding studies [8]. Whether or not cellular, or more precisely receptor, recognition of apoA-I is restricted to only one domain requires more investigation and will probably be resolved only when a membrane protein that unconditionally fulfills the criteria of a lipoprotein receptor is cloned and expressed and with which highly specific interactions of the ligand can be observed.

In contrast to these observations, Leblond and Marcel [9] found little difference in the degree of inhibition of HDL–cell interactions using mAbs against apoA-I and concluded that optimal binding involves accessibility of the entire apoA-I molecule, particularly the amphipathic α-helical repeats. Conceivably, none of the experiments with mAbs, which depend on steric hindrance of a site by a bound antibody molecule, has yet provided a definitive answer because none of these antibodies binds to the precise binding domain in question. Antibodies, especially IgG molecules, may also obscure an active site, even though it binds to an unrelated region.

That binding of HDL, mediated by apoproteins and apparently involving specific regions, occurs in vitro is less controversial than is the evidence for a physiological event that is dependent on the specificity of binding. This question has been the subject of much recent attention although the reports so far have mainly addressed studies of cholesterol flux (and its dependence on apoprotein specific determinants) as opposed to other biochemical pathways (such as cellular signalling) which may be stimulated by the binding of an HDL apoprotein. Again, these investigations have involved the use of apoA-I-specific mAbs. Banka et al. [10] used a panel of eight mAbs to test the hypothesis that discrete structural domains of the molecule mediate cholesterol efflux. Only two antibodies inhibited the in vitro flux of ^{14}C-cholesterol to HDL or apoA-I proteoliposomes, their epitopes overlapping and corresponding to either residues 74-105 or 96-111 respectively. This region of apoA-I is highly conserved phylogenetically, is involved in LCAT activation and is highly antigenic. Within this domain, a pair of amphipathic α-helices of 22 amino acid residues is reputed to contain a structural feature which acts as a "hinge". This hinge domain provides mobility and thus may confer functional as well as structural properties on apoA-I which are crucial in lipid–protein interactions. The authors interpreted their findings as evidence that the immobilization of the hinge domain, caused by one of the antibodies, is unfavorable for promoting cholesterol efflux from the plasma membrane of cells.

Other studies implicate the involvement of specific sequences of apoA-I in cholesterol efflux. Fielding's laboratory [11] recently demonstrated that two mAbs which recognize epitopes involving apoA-I residues 137-144 or 113-128 inhibit binding by approximately 36%. Noting that this central region is part of, or at least juxtaposed to, the putative hinge domain, these authors also speculate that this region is active in the efflux of cellular cholesterol. Moreover, they found that the antibodies which inhibited efflux coincidentally recognized apoA-I residing on pre β1-HDL, but not pre β2-HDL particles, which suggests that the active domain for cholesterol efflux is exposed only on specific particles.

Work in our laboratory also provides evidence for the involvement of structural sites on apoA-I in cholesterol efflux. Using a panel of mAbs whose epitopes spanned amino and carboxy termini, and central regions, we observed significant suppression of flux of ^{14}C-cholesterol by one mAb recognizing residues 140–147 and by another mAb of undefined epitope but involving the C-terminus. Anti-apoA-I polyclonal antibodies inhibited cholesterol efflux by 55%, which suggests that more than one region may be implicated in the process. In our experiments, antibodies were preincubated with serum which was added to cell culture medium as a source of cholesterol acceptors. It is conceivable, therefore, that the mAbs which produced a modest but significant (35%) inhibition in cholesterol efflux recognized a structural region that is exposed in only a small population of HDL particles, consistent with the observations of Fielding et al. [11]. Partial inhibition could also be explained by the fact that HDL particles which are preferentially used as acceptors are substituted by other particles, e.g., Lp(a) or LDL present in serum when blocked by antibodies. Of some importance, none of the antibodies used in our studies affected cholesterol efflux from the plasma membrane of HepG2 cells. Only the flux of intracellular cholesterol pools labeled by incubating cells for short periods (1.5 h) with ^{14}C-acetate (to minimize redistribution of isotopic cholesterol) were inhibited by the antibodies.

One interpretation of these data is that the signal for transport of intracellular cholesterol, mediated by apoA-I high-affinity receptors, has been inhibited by antibodies which bind and therefore block the active domain of the ligand. It seems unlikely that most of the ^{14}C-cholesterol used to label cells would have occupied only the cholesterol-rich domains of plasma membranes of the cultured cells which, according to Rothblat and co-workers [12], are more resistant to cholesterol efflux than cholesterol-poor domains.

Conclusions

Evidence is accumulating that protein–protein interactions, presumably resembling ligand–receptor systems, influence the mechanisms by which HDL regulate cellular metabolism. Several apolipoproteins may share common properties in mediating HDL binding or stimulating cholesterol efflux, but there is a consensus that apoA-I is a major influence on these events. Such a view is strengthened by the recent identification of receptor-binding domains that are present on apoA-I [1,3], a finding subsequently confirmed by others [2,7]. It now appears that specific regions of apoA-I are concerned in the process of cholesterol efflux and that these regions may or may not be identical with those principally responsible for determining the binding of HDL to cells. It is clear that we are approaching a phase of fuller understanding of the manner by which apolipoprotein specificity regulates cell metabolism, the attainment of which will allow manipulation of important functions such as reverse cholesterol transport.

References

1. Morrison JR, McPherson GA, Fidge NH. J Biol Chem 1992;267:13205−13209.
2. Barbaras R, Collet X, Chap H, Perret B. Biochemistry 1994;33:2335−2340.
3. Morrison J, Fidge NH, Tozuka M. J Biol Chem 1991;266:18780−18785.
4. Vadiveloo PK, Fidge NH. Biochem J 1992;284:145-151.
5. Vadiveloo PK, Allan CM, Murray BJ, Fidge NH. Biochemistry 1993;32:9480−9485.
6. Barbaras R, Puchois P, Fruchart J-C, Ailhaud G. Biochem Biophys Res Commun 1987;142:63−69.
7. Dalton MB, Swaney JB. J Biol Chem 1993;268:19274−19283.
8. Allan CM, Fidge NH, Morrison JR, Kanellos J. Biochem J 1993;290:449−455.
9. Leblond L, Marcel YL. J Biol Chem 1991;266:6058−6067.
10. Banka CL, Black AS, Curtiss LK. J Biol Chem 1994;269:10288−10297.
11. Fielding PE, Kawano M, Catapano AL, Zoppo A, Marcovina S, Fielding CJ. Biochemistry 1994;33:6981−6985.
12. Rothblat GH, Mahlberg FH, Johnson WJ, Phillips MC. J Lipid Res 1992;33:1091−1097.

ApoA-I- and A-IV-containing particles in reverse cholesterol transport

J.C. Fruchart[1], N. Duverger[2], G. Castro[1] and P. Denèfle[2]

[1]*Serlia & U. 325, Institut Pasteur de Lille, France; and* [2]*Rhône-Poulenc-Rorer, Vitry Sur Seine, France*

High density lipoproteins (HDL) may facilitate reverse transport of cholesterol from peripheral cells to the liver for excretion in the bile [1]. This process involves several steps. Interactions between HDL and HDL binding sites are generally believed to facilitate egress of cholesterol from cells to the plasma lipoproteins [2], and particularly to a small pre-β-migrating HDL [3]. This incorporation of free cholesterol into acceptor lipoproteins, facilitating its esterification by lecithin:cholesterol acyltransferase (LCAT, phosphatidyl-choline-sterol acyltransferase, EC 2.3.1.43) and cholesterol ester transfer protein (CETP), mediates transfer to very-low-density lipoproteins and exchange for TG [4]. Apolipo-protein A-I (apoA-I), apoA-II and apoA-IV represent more than 90% of the total apolipoprotein content of HDL and bind specifically and with high affinity to the surface of several cell types [5,6]. We proposed that apoA-I and apoA-IV play the role of agonists and apoA-II that of antagonist of cholesterol efflux from cells [7]. The purpose of this paper is to review the role of particles containing apoA-I and apoA-IV in reverse cholesterol transport and to demonstrate a connection between cholesterol efflux and atherosclerosis risk.

Role of apoA-I- and apoA-IV-containing lipoprotein particles in reverse cholesterol transport

It is now recognized that HDL contains at least four types of lipoprotein particles defined by their apolipoprotein content: LpA-I, LpA-I:A-II, LpA-I:A-IV and LpA-IV [7,8].

We have reported that human plasma LpA-I, LpA-IV and LpA-I:A-IV promote cholesterol efflux more effectively than LpA-I:A-II from cholesterol-loaded ob1771 cells, a mouse adipocyte cell line [5,6]. LpA-I is highly heterogeneous and includes three different subclasses of different size. All LpA-I subclasses promoted cholesterol efflux from the ob1771 cells but on a molar basis, medium-sized particles were more effective than large particles [9].

LpA-I:A-II were less able to reduce the cholesterol content of some type of cells and blocked the ability of LpA-I in promoting cholesterol efflux [10,11]. In contrast, studies using other cell types have shown LpA-I and LpA-I:A-II to be equally effective in promoting efflux of plasma membrane or lysosomal cholesterol [12–14].

Incubation of cholesterol-preloaded adipose cells with both subpopulations of apoA-IV-containing lipoprotein particles promoted cholesterol efflux from cells, with slightly greater cholesterol efflux promotion by LpA-IV than LpA-I:A-IV [8].

Correlation between in vivo atherogenesis, in vitro cholesterol efflux and formation of lipoproteins with pre-β mobility

A recent study in transgenic mice confirmed the protective role of apoA-I for athero-sclerosis, while the overexpression of human apoA-II in human apoA-I transgenic mice appears to promote aortic fatty-streak development [15].

In order to examine the biochemical mechanisms underlying these in vivo observations, we have tested sera from human A-I transgenic and human apoA-I/apoA-II transgenic mice for participation in cholesterol efflux in vitro. Analysis of cholesterol efflux from Fu5AH cells according to the method described by Moya et al. [16] revealed that the serum from human A-I transgenic mice produced a significantly higher level of cholesterol efflux than serum from human apoA-I/apoA-II transgenic mice [17] (Fig. 1). This study shows for the first time a correlation between in vivo atherogenesis and in vitro cholesterol efflux.

Since pre-β migrating small apoA-I-containing particles have been associated with the early steps in cholesterol efflux in man, we examined by two-dimensional electrophoresis the plasma from the various types of transgenic mice. The control mice contained particles with primarily α mobility. In contrast, the apoA-I-overexpressing animals had close to 30% of the apoA-I particles with pre-β mobility (Fig. 2). We counted five different pre-β particles with molecular weights of approximately 43, 70, 92, 116 and 256 kDa.

In order to evaluate further the extent of protection against atherosclerosis induced by apoA-I overexpression, we have used a rabbit model because advanced human-type lesions can be rapidly obtained in this model.

Rabbits transgenic for human apoA-I were created and compared with controls. Human apoA-I overexpression in the rabbit resulted in a nonatherogenic lipoprotein profile [18] (Fig. 3) and we are now testing the protective role of this overexpression against atherosclerosos induced by a cholesterol-rich diet. Studies of cellular cholesterol efflux with Fu 5AH cells showed a connection between changes in lipoprotein profile, cholesterol efflux and formation of apoA-I-containing pre-β lipoprotein particles [19].

Expression of human apoA-IV in a strain of mice susceptible to atherosclerosis on a high-fat diet is also protective against the development of atherosclerosis (submitted for

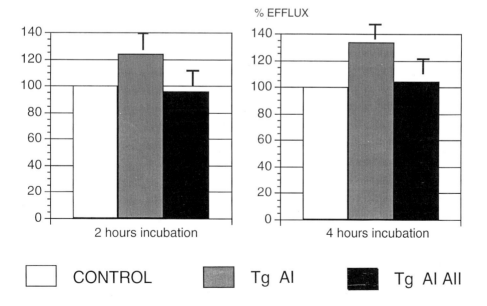

Fig. 1. Human apoA-I and human apoA-I:A-II transgenic (Tg) mice and cholesterol efflux from FU 5AH hepatoma cells.

494

CONTROL MOUSE

TRANSGENIC APO A-I MOUSE

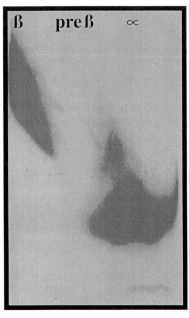

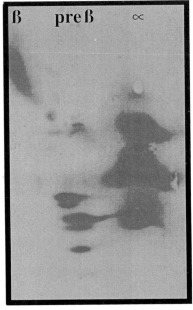

Anti mouse apo A-I immunoblot

Anti human apo A-I and anti mouse apo A-I immunoblot

Fig. 2. Pre-β fraction in transgenic apoA-I mouse.

publication). This protection can be related to the in vitro observation that apoA-IV promotes cholesterol efflux from cholesterol-preloaded cells [5]. This observation is qualitatively similar to that previously reported with human apoA-I overexpression in transgenic mice, but there are at least two important differences between the two studies. First, the quantitative effect of apoA-IV expression appears to have been even greater than that of apoA-I in protecting against atherosclerosis, although more studies will be required. Second, and perhaps more importantly, the effect of the apoA-IV in preventing atherosclerosis occurred despite a relatively modest effect on HDL-cholesterol levels. This is in marked contrast to the apoA-I studies, in which HDL-cholesterol levels were substantially elevated. This suggests that apoA-IV can inhibit atherogenesis without substantially elevating HDL-cholesterol, and provides the first example of atherosclerosis inhibition in an animal model without marked elevation of HDL.

Conclusion

As peripheral cells are unable to degrade cholesterol, a pathway by which intact cholesterol molecules can be removed from the cells is essential for cholesterol homeostasis. We report here that apoA-I and apoA-IV play an important role in reverse cholesterol transport. Both apolipoproteins not only activate LCAT but also promote

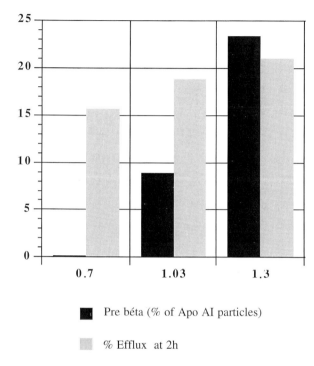

Pre béta (% of Apo AI particles)

% Efflux at 2h

Fig. 3. Correlation in an antiatherogenic role between pre-β fractions, cholesterol efflux and human apoA-I levels in human apoA-I transgenic rabbits. x-axis, plasma apoA-I level (mg/ml) in transgenic rabbit; y-axis, % efflux.

cholesterol efflux from peripheral cells and decrease atherogenesis. The effect of the apoA-IV in preventing atherosclerosis may help to explain the lack of premature coronary artery disease in diseases characterized by very low apoA-I levels, such as Tangier disease and LCAT deficiency, in which apoA-IV levels are normal or elevated. Our results also confirm that apoA-II modulates reverse cholesterol transport. In vitro and in vivo results demonstrate the antagonistic role of apoA-II towards cholesterol efflux and formation of pre-β LpA-I particles. These findings suggest new avenues towards diagnosis and treatment of atherosclerosis.

References

1. Glomset JA. J Lipid Res 1968;9:155–167.
2. Oram JF, Albers JJ, Cheung MC, Bierman EL. J Biol Chem 1981;256:8348.
3. Castro GR, Fielding PE. Biochemistry 1988;27:25–29.
4. Fielding CJ, Fielding PE. Proc Natl Acad Sci USA 1980;77:3327–3330.
5. Steinmetz A, Barbaras R, Ghalim N, Clavey V, Fruchart JC, Ailhaud G. J Biol Chem 1990;265:7859–7863.
6. Barbaras R, Puchois P, Fruchart JC, Pradines-Figueres A, Ailhaud G. Biochem J 1990;269:767–773.
7. Fruchart JC, Ailhaud G, Bard JM. Circulation 1993;87/III:22–27.
8. Duverger N, Ghalim N, Ailhaud G, Steinmetz A, Fruchart JC, Castro G. Arterioscler Thromb 1993;13: 126–132.
9. Duverger N, Rader D, Duchateau P, Fruchart JC, Castro G, Brewer HB. Biochemistry 1993;32:-12372–12379.
10. Fruchart JC, De Geteire C, Delfly B, Castro GR. Atherosclerosis (in press).

11. Barkia A, Puchois P, Ghalim N, Torpier G, Barbaras R, Ailhaud G, Fruchart JC. Atherosclerosis 1991;87:135—146.
12. Johnson WY, Kilsdonk EPC, Van Tol A, Philips MC, Rothblat GH. J Lipid Res 1991;32:1993.
13. Ohta T, Nakamura R, Ikeda Y, Shinshara M, Minjazaki A, Horiuchi S, Matsuda J. Biochim Biophys Acta 1992;1165:119.
14. Oikawa S, Mendez A, Oram JF, Bierman EL, Cheung MC. Biochim Biophys Acta 1993;1165:327.
15. Schultz JR, Verstugft JG, Goug EL, Nichols AV, Rubin EM. Nature 1993;365:761.
16. Moya, Atger V, Paul JL, Fournier, Moatti N, Giral, Friday, Rothblat G. Arterioscler Thromb (in press).
17. Castro GR, Nihoul L, Dengremont C, Tailleux A, Duverger N, Denèfle P, Rubin EM, Fruchart JC. 67th Scientific Sessions of American Heart Association, Dallas, 14—17 November 1994. Circulation (in press).
18. Duverger N, Emmanuel F, Viglietta C, Tailleux A, Benoit P, Attenot F, Cuine S, Fievet C, Laine B, Fruchart JC, Houbebine LM, Denèfle P. 67th Scientific Session of American Heart Association, Dallas, 14—17 November 1994. Circulation (in press).
19. Castro G. Satellite of the Xth International Symposium on Atherosclerosis "The Molecular Basis of HDL Antiatherogenicity", Halifax, 14—16 October 1994.

Atherosclerosis X.
F.P. Woodford, J. Davignon and A. Sniderman, editors.

Release of hepatic lipase from the liver does not affect the uptake of HDL-cholesteryl esters

Arie van Tol, Teus van Gent, Ina Kalkman and Hans Jansen

Department of Biochemistry, Cardiovascular Research Institute (COEUR), Faculty of Medicine and Health Sciences, Erasmus University Rotterdam, Rotterdam, The Netherlands

Abstract. Heparin-releasable hepatic lipase (salt-resistant lipase, HL) may be part of a selective uptake mechanism for HDL-cholesterol and -cholesteryl esters (CE) in the liver, facilitating the uptake of plasma cholesterol for bile acid synthesis and excretion. It is not clear whether the binding of HL to the endothelial liver cells is essential for its physiological function or not. We measured the effects of a shift of HL from liver to plasma, induced by heparin injection, on the plasma turnover and tissue uptake of HDL-CE in rats.

The tissue uptake of HDL-^{3}H-CE (biologically labeled in vivo in the cholesterol moiety) was measured in animals treated with hourly intravenous injections of heparin. Heparin treatment released a substantial part (47–63%) of total HL into the plasma compartment, but did not affect the plasma decay of HDL-^{3}H-CE. Almost half of the label left the plasma compartment in 3 h (with or without heparin treatment), and 25.4 ± 2.9% of the injected dose was taken up in the liver of heparin-treated rats vs. 26.8 ± 1.9% in the liver of control animals. Adipose tissue and skeletal muscle each contained 4–6% of the injected dose with or without heparin treatment.

We conclude that intravenous injection of heparin into rats releases half to two-thirds of the total HL activity. This substantial release of HL from the liver into plasma does not affect hepatic HDL-CE uptake. The high HL activity in rat liver may be in excess of that necessary for optimal HDL-CE metabolism.

In hepatic lipase (HL) deficiency, all endogenous lipoproteins (VLDL, IDL, LDL and HDL) may be elevated, suggesting a multifunctional role of the enzyme [1]. Functions in VLDL-IDL-LDL conversion as well as in HDL metabolism have been proposed [2–4]. Extrahepatic lipoprotein lipase (LPL) and HL are part of the lipase family. Both enzymes are located on endothelial cells and released into the plasma compartment by intravenous heparin injection. It was recently proposed that HL and LPL, in addition to their lipolytic function, may act as ligands in the hepatic uptake of chylomicron remnants, probably via the LDL receptor-related protein (LRP), a multiligand receptor [5–7].

Heparin-releasable (salt-resistant) hepatic lipase may be part of a selective uptake mechanism for HDL-cholesterol [8] and HDL-cholesteryl esters (HDL-CE) in the liver [9], facilitating the uptake of plasma cholesterol for bile acid synthesis and excretion. In agreement with this proposed function, it was shown that HL specifically acts on HDL$_2$-phospholipids [10]. This could induce the transfer of cholesterol and cholesteryl esters from HDL to liver cells and result in conversion of HDL$_2$ into HDL$_3$ [8,11,12].

It is unclear whether the binding of HL to hepatic endothelial cells is essential for its physiological function or not. Appreciable activities of salt-resistant lipase are present in native (preheparin) plasma/serum of several species, in addition to the hepatic activity. Native plasma/serum of man and rat have very low activity levels (<5 mU/ml), while high

Address for correspondence: Dr A. van Tol, Department of Biochemistry, Faculty of Medicine and Health Sciences, Erasmus University Rotterdam, P.O. Box 1738, 3000 DR Rotterdam, The Netherlands.

activities of salt-resistant lipase are found in native plasma/serum of hamsters and mice (>100 mU/ml) [13,14]. In the present experiments we looked for an effect of the location of HL (plasma vs. liver) on HDL metabolism in rats and tested the effect of a shift of HL from liver to plasma, induced by heparin, on the in vivo turnover and tissue uptake of HDL-CE.

Methods

Male Wistar rats were used, weighing 291 ± 9 g (mean ± SD). The animals had free access to food (normal rat chow) and water. Preparation of HDL labeled with ^{3}H-CE, assay of plasma turnover of HDL and tissue uptake of labeled HDL-CE were performed as described [9]. The in vivo tissue uptake of HDL-^{3}H-CE was measured 3 h after intravenous injection in control rats and in heparinized rats. At this time the animals were bled from the abdominal aorta, followed by whole-body perfusion via the left ventricle for 3 min with 90 ml of saline. Blood was removed from most tissues, including the liver. All intravenous injections and the bleeding were performed under light ether anesthesia.

75 IU of heparin were injected intravenously at 0 h, and additional amounts of 75 IU at 1 and 2 h after injection of labeled HDL. Control animals were injected with saline. The activities of HL and LPL in plasma and of HL in liver extracts were measured at 5, 30, 90 and 150 min after the start of the experiments (labeled HDL was injected at t = 0).

Activities of hepatic (salt-resistant) lipase was measured in liver extracts and in serum/plasma as described [15,16]. Both activities were inhibited >90% by antibody to rat HL.

Results and Discussion

Heparin injection induced a substantial shift of HL from the liver to the plasma compartment. In normal rats the plasma activity is very low (<5 mU/ml), while the activities in postheparin plasma ranged from 250 to 450 mU/ml, if measured at the different time points in heparin-treated animals. Heparin was injected at 0, 1 and 2 h. As mentioned above, the lipase activities were measured at 5, 30, 90 and 150 min after the start of the HDL turnover experiments. The activities of HL, measured in livers obtained at the same time points, as well as those in control livers, are shown in Fig. 1. Our data indicate that a substantial amount of HL is circulating in plasma of heparin-treated animals (not shown), but also that the livers of heparin-treated rats are not devoid of HL activity. Figure 1 shows that these livers still contain between 1/3 and 1/2 of the original HL activity. At present the exact location of this remaining part of HL is unknown. Heparin will primarily release HL bound to extracellular sites which are easily accessible. A substantial part of the remaining HL will probably be located intracellularly.

Table 1 shows that the shift of HL activity from liver to plasma induced by heparin injection has no significant effect on the plasma turnover and tissue uptake of HDL-CE. Heparin treatment did not affect the plasma decay of HDL-^{3}H-CE. Almost half of the injected label left the plasma compartment during the 3 h of the in vivo experiment (with or without heparin treatment); 25.4 ± 2.9% of the injected dose was taken up in the liver of heparin-treated rats and 26.8 ± 1.9% in the liver of control animals. Other quantitatively important tissues for the uptake of HDL-^{3}CE were adipose tissue and skeletal muscle, each containing 4–6% of the injected dose with or without heparin treatment.

We conclude that intravenous injection of heparin in rats releases half to two-thirds of the total HL activity from the liver. This substantial release of HL into plasma does not affect hepatic HDL-CE uptake. Our data are not necessarily in conflict with earlier

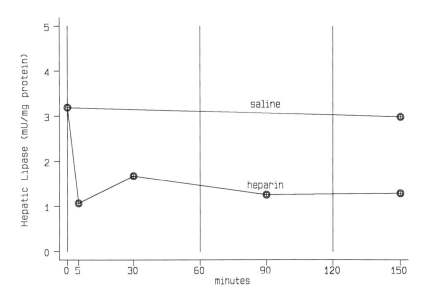

Fig. 1. Hepatic lipase activity levels in livers from heparin-treated and control animals treated with saline. Each point gives the average hepatic activities in six animals. The activities are expressed per mg of total liver protein. The vertical lines indicate the time points (0, 1 and 2 h) of saline or heparin injection.

[2–4,8,9] and recent work [17,18] suggesting a role for HL in HDL metabolism. It is conceivable that the relatively high HL activity in normal rat liver is in excess of that necessary for optimal HDL-CE metabolism. However, a different situation may exist in other species. The present data clearly show that liver/plasma activity ratios for HL of >100 (normal rats) or <1.0 (heparinized rats) are compatible with identical fractional turnovers and hepatic uptake of HDL-CE. Mice and hamsters fed normal chow have liver/plasma activity ratios of about 0.4 and 1.3, respectively [13,14]. Future research is necessary to find out if the distribution of HL between the liver and plasma compartment in these species has an impact on lipoprotein metabolism.

Table 1. Uptake of injected HDL-^{3}H-CE in tissues of heparin-treated rats and control animals

	Heparin-treated	Saline-treated
Plasma	51.8 ± 4.1	53.1 ± 6.3
Lungs	1.2 ± 0.3	1.2 ± 0.3
Liver	25.4 ± 2.9	26.8 ± 1.9
Adrenals	0.1 ± 0.0	0.1 ± 0.1
Adipose tissue	5.9 ± 1.3	4.1 ± 0.7
Testes	0.5 ± 0.2	0.6 ± 0.2
Skeletal muscle	5.7 ± 1.6	5.9 ± 0.6

All values are given as % of the injected dose present in the total tissues at 3 h after injection of labeled HDL (means ± SD, n = 5). No significant differences were present between heparin-treated and saline-treated animals (Mann-Whitney test).

500

References

1. Breckenridge WC. Am Heart J 1987;113:567–573.
2. Jansen H, Van Tol A, Hülsmann WC. Biochem Biophys Res Commun 1980;92:53–59.
3. Rao SN, Cortese C, Miller NE, Levy Y, Lewis B. FEBS Lett 1982;150:255–259.
4. Demant T, Carlson LA, Holmquist L, Karpe F, Nilsson-Ehle P, Packard CJ, Shepherd J. J Lipid Res 1988;29:1603–1611.
5. Kowal RC, Herz J, Goldstein JL, Esser V, Brown MS. Proc Natl Acad Sci USA 1989;86:5810–5814.
6. Beisiegel U, Weber W, Ihrke G, Herz J, Stanley KK. Nature 1989;341:162–164.
7. Shafi S, Brady SE, Bensadoun A, Havel RJ. J Lipid Res 1994;35:709–720.
8. Jansen H, Hülsmann WC. Trends Biochem Soc 1980;5:265–268.
9. Van 't Hooft FM, Van Gent T, Van Tol A. Biochem J 1981;196: 877–885.
10. Groot PHE, Jansen H, Van Tol A. FEBS Lett 1981;129:269–272.
11. Van Tol A, Van Gent T, Jansen H. Biochem Biophys Res Commun 1980;94:101–108.
12. Johnson WJ, Mahlberg FH, Rothblat GH, Phillips MC. Biochim Biophys Acta 1991;1085:273–298.
13. Jansen H, Lammers R, Baggen MGA, Wouters NMH, Birkenhäger JC. Biochim Biophys Acta 1989;1001:44–49.
14. Peterson J, Bengtsson-Olivecrona G, Olivecrona T. Biochim Biophys Acta 1986;878:65–70.
15. Jansen H, Birkenhäger JC. Metabolism 1981;30:428–430.
16. Schoonderwoerd K, Jansen H. Lipids 1989;24:1039–1042.
17. Marques-Vidal P, Azéma C, Collet X, Vieu C, Chap H, Berret B. J Lipid Res 1994;35:373–384.
18. Busch SJ, Barnhart RL, Martin GA, Fitzgerald MC, Yates MT, Mao SJT, Thomas, CE, Jackson RL. J Biol Chem 1994;269:16376–16382.

Towards gene therapy targeting HDL

P.P. Denèfle[1], S. Hughes[2], C. Desurmont[1], E. Vigne[3], L. Bassinet[1], J. Verstuyft[2], M. Perricaudet[3], P. Benoit[1] and E.M. Rubin[2]

[1]*Rhône-Poulenc Rorer SA, Vitry, France;* [2]*Lawrence Berkeley Laboratory, Berkeley, USA; and* [3]*Institut Gustave Roussy, Villejuif, France*

Abstract. To evaluate the feasibility of impeding atherogenesis by somatic gene therapy, we have developed recombinant adenoviral vectors to achieve in vivo overproduction of some of the proteins which participate in HDL metabolism, such as apolipoprotein A-I (apoA-I). Intravenous injection into mice of viral preparations succeeded in producing significant plasma concentrations of human apoA-I which was found associated with the HDL fraction. The expression lasted for several weeks, but was strongly dependent on the type of promoter chosen. In treated apoA-I knockout mice, a several-fold increase in HDL-C was accompanied by the appearance of a characteristic bimodal density distribution of HDL containing human apoA-I. A 3-week regression study on C57Bl/6 mice with predeveloped aortic lesions was undertaken. The Ad-apoA-I treated group experienced a transient increase in HDL-C levels of 80% but the lesion progression was not significantly reduced. These studies demonstrate the ability to raise HDL-C levels by infection of animals with recombinant adenoviruses, but suggest that the duration of expression with the present series of vectors may need to be improved to reduce atherogenesis.

The recent spectacular development of transgenic animal models as a tool to dissect out the individual role of genetic risks factors in the physiopathology of atherosclerosis has raised the possibility of monitoring candidate genes for their potential in somatic gene therapy. However, the central issues concerning the future applications of gene therapies to the treatment of cardiovascular diseases and in particular atherosclerosis are i) a better understanding of the causes of the disease, ii) elucidation of the molecular lesions and the relative phenotypic relevance of particular gene mutations, iii) the choice of vectors for gene transfer into specific organs or cell subtypes, iv) the existence of animal models which can be used to test novel therapeutic strategies and v) development of appropriate strategies to achieve a significant and cost-effective therapeutic goal in human clinical trials.

For the time being, in vivo gene transfer to the whole adult animal can be used as a research tool to study the impact of the overexpression of these genes on the course of atherogenesis and lipid metabolism.

Candidate genes

Much recent evidence indicates that high density lipoproteins (HDL) and their major protein component apolipoprotein A-I (apoA-I) are directly protective against the development of atherosclerosis [1]. A clear-cut demonstration was recently provided with genetically engineered mice overexpressing human apoA-I, in which the onset of atherogenesis is strikingly lower than isogenic inbred mice [2,3]. Overexpression of human apoA-I in rabbits has confirmed those results in our group. ApoA-I therefore

Address for correspondence: Patrice P. Denèfle, Biotechnology Department, Rhône-Poulenc Rorer SA, 13 quai Jules Guesde, 94403, Vitry s/Seine, France.

502

constitutes the most promising gene candidate to evaluate for gene therapy. However, as apoA-I defects account for less than 1—2% of low HDL-C levels in humans, one has to consider other genes involved in HDL metabolism. To that aim, we have also developed new recombinant adenoviral vectors to achieve in vivo overproduction of some of the proteins which participate in HDL metabolism, such as apoA-I, apoE, apoA-IV and LPL.

Compared with commonly used retroviral systems, adenovirus-mediated gene transfer has several advantages in that adenovirus can infect a large variety of cells independently of their growth state, and persistent expression of the foreign gene can be maintained despite a lack of integration of the vector into the host cell genome. Viral stocks of extremely high titer, essential for in vivo infection experiments, can be produced by infection of the human replication permissive 293 cell line with the replication-deficient recombinant virus [4]. The main disadvantage of the adenovirus system is that vectors are replication-deficient, so that replication of infected cells will eventually dilute the population of cells expressing the foreign gene, with corresponding decline in expression. For this reason, the adenovirus system is best suited for targeting gene expression to tissues having a low rate of cell division. Use of recombinant adenovirus has proven highly effective for transduction of hepatocytes in vivo, as demonstrated for expression of ornithine transcarbamylase [5] and the LDL receptor [6] in mouse liver. In addition, studies of the distribution of tissues affected by intravenous administration of adenovirus vectors directing β-galactosidase expression have clearly shown that liver can be transfected with very high efficiency [5,7].

In the present study, we have investigated the suitability of two distinct constitutive viral promoters to drive human apoA-I expression from an adenovirus vector (Fig. 1). The parameters documented are related to the level and duration of expression of human apoA-I in mice treated with these vectors as well as the effect on HDL size of scattered apoA-I production sites.

In order to determine whether adenovirus-mediated gene transfer of the human apolipoprotein A-I to either normal or A-I knockout mice could lead to significant and persistent production of the human protein, we injected by the i.v. route 10^{10} pfu of different recombinant virus preparations containing either the β-galactosidase bacterial gene (fused to a nuclear addressing signal, Ad-βgal) or the apoA-I cDNA placed under the control of two different virus-derived promoters (CMV, Ad-CMV/AI, or LTR-RSV: Ad-RSV/AI). ApoA-I plasma levels were monitored by direct protein ELISA assay using a mixture of monoclonal antibodies. As shown in Fig. 2, the maximum plasma levels of human apoA-I were in the range of 1—5 mg/dl and were obtained 96 or 168 h after

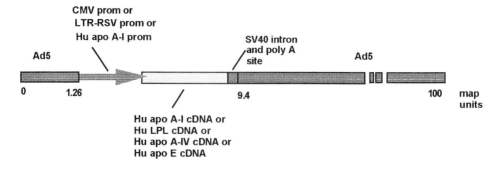

Fig. 1. Map of current recombinant adenovirus vectors (first-generation vectors).

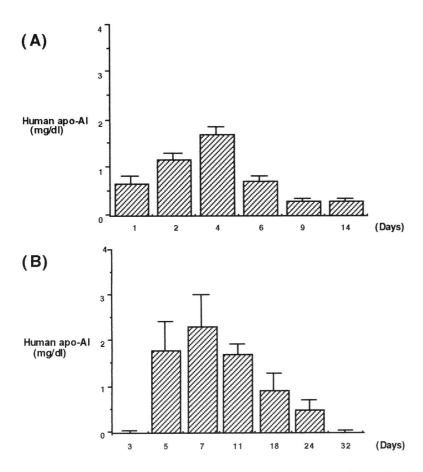

Fig. 2. Concentration of human apoA-I in C57BL/6 mice infected with recombinant adenoviruses. Mice were infected through the tail vein at Day 0 with either 10^{10} pfu Ad-CMV/AI (panel A) or Ad-RSV/AI (panel B). On the days indicated, blood was taken from the mice and plasma human apoA-I levels were determined. Each bar represents the mean and standard deviation for three or more animals.

infection, depending on the type of viral promoter.

Interestingly, CMV-driven production of human apoA-I reached peak levels more quickly than with the RSV-LTR promoter. Significant levels of human apoA-I were found in the plasma of the Ad-RSV/AI-injected mice for at least 4 weeks. The duration of expression was shorter in the case of the CMV construct, for which human apoA-I could be detected in the plasma of infected mice only until day 14. This suggests a possibly important but as yet unravelled control of viral promoters in transgene expression.

Assembly of vector-derived human apoA-I into HDL particles was studied in mice rendered deficient in apoA-I by gene targeting. These mice have extremely low levels of HDL particles which are totally devoid of apoA-I, providing an ideal background for measuring net changes in HDL concentration and particle size distribution. As shown in Fig. 3, HDL-cholesterol levels were elevated 4-fold at 48 h after injection of apoA-I knockout mice with Ad-CMV/AI, coinciding with peak levels of vector-driven human apoA-I expression.

504

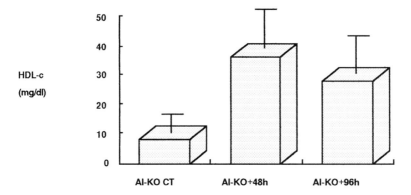

Fig. 3. HDL levels in apoA-I knockout mice infected with adenovirus. Levels presented are from the analysis of 3–4 animals in each group just prior to infection and at the indicated time points thereafter.

Particle-size distribution of HDL in A-I knockout mice treated with the adenoviral vectors was determined by GGE of plasma lipoprotein fractions (d < 1.21). Human apoA-I derived from vector expression was incorporated into HDL particles having a bimodal size distribution similar to that seen in human apoA-I transgenic mice. Blotting with antiserum to human apoA-I confirmed that HDL in Ad-CMVAI-treated mice did contain apoA-I, while HDL produced in the mice treated with vector alone did not.

On finding that vector-driven expression of human apoA-I could produce significant plasma apoA-I concentrations and elevate HDL levels, we designed an initial study to evaluate the ability of these conditions to reduce atherosclerosis in C57Bl/6 mice fed a diet high in fat and cholesterol. Four groups of mice were given the high-fat diet for 14 weeks, at which time one group was sacrificed for size determination of the initial lesions. The remaining three groups were injected with: A) 2×10^{10} pfu Ad-RSV/AI, B) 2×10^{10} pfu Ad vector only, C) vehicle only. These three groups were continued on the high-fat diet for 3 weeks, a period of time which we felt adequately balanced the limited duration of vector-driven apoA-I expression with the time required to detect any changes in lesion size. Mice were sacrificed at the end of this period for quantitation of lesions as well as HDL-C measurement. Mice injected with Ad-RSV/AI experienced a significant (+80%) and transient elevation of HDL-C, coincident with the time course of vector-driven apoA-I expression. However, these changes had little or no effect on the progression of atherosclerosis in these animals: the mean lesion areas were not significantly different. These studies demonstrate the ability to raise HDL-C levels by infection of animals with recombinant adenoviruses, but suggest that the duration of expression with the present series of vectors may need to be improved to alter atherosclerosis susceptibility. The most suitable avenue we are now following is to complete the deletion of some of the remaining adenoviral genes critically involved in the residual viral gene expression, which has been recently confirmed to be involved in cellular response against adenovirus-infected cells in vivo [8].

In addition to apoA-I, we also paid attention to other possible candidate genes such as apoE, LPL, and apoA-IV, for which solid data from transgenic experiment in mice are now available. Nevertheless, what is presented here may well constitute the first step towards somatic gene therapy of atherosclerosis by an HDL apolipoprotein.

Ackowledgements

Dr N. Maeda, of the University of North Carolina, for kindly providing the apoA-I knockout mice used in these studies. Drs J-C. Fruchart, J-F. Mayaux & J-B. Le Pecq for constant support and stimulating discussions all along this work. This project was supported by the Bio/Avenir Program (Rhône-Poulenc SA and Ministère de la Recherche et de l'Industrie), National Institutes of Health Grants to E.R., PPG HL18574, and a grant funded by the National Dairy Promotion and Research Board and administered in cooperation with the National Dairy Council. E.R. is an American Heart Association Established Investigator. Research was conducted both at the Lawrence Berkeley Laboratory (Department of Energy Contract DE-AC0376SF00098), University of California, Berkeley, USA, at the Laboratoire des Virus Oncogènes (Institut Gustave Roussy), Villejuif, France, and at the Biotechnology Department, Centre de Recherche de Vitry-Alfortville, Rhône-Poulenc Rorer SA, Vitry, France.

References

1. Miller NE. Am Heart J 1987;113:589−597.
2. Rubin EM, Krauss RM, Spangler EA, Verstuyft JG, Clift SM. Nature 1991;353:265−267.
3. Pászty C, Maeda N, Verstuyft, J Rubin EM. J Clin Invest 1994;94:899−903.
4. Graham FL, Smiley J, Russel WC, Nairn R. J Gen Virol 1977;36:59−72.
5. Strafford-Perricaudet LD, Levero M, Chasse J, Perricaudet M, Briand P. Hum Gene Ther 1990;1:241−256.
6. Ishibashi S, Brown MS, Goldstein JL, Gerard RD, Hammer RE, Herz J. J Clin Invest 1993;92:883−893.
7. Li QT, Kay MA, Finegold M, Stratford-Perricaudet LD, Woo SLC. Hum Gene Ther 1993;4:403−409.
8. Yang Y, Nunes FA, Berencsi K, Furth EE, Gönczöl E, Wilson JM. Proc Natl Acad Sci USA 1994;91: 4407−4411

Elevated human apolipoprotein A-I and HDL: impact on atherogenesis in apolipoprotein(a) transgenic and apolipoprotein E knockout mice

Mary E. Stevens and Edward M. Rubin

Human Genome Center, Lawrence Berkeley Laboratory, University of California, Berkeley, California, USA

Abstract. Apolipoprotein E (apoE)-deficient mice are hypercholesterolemic and develop diet-independent atherosclerosis, while apo(a) transgenic mice are susceptible to diet-induced atherosclerosis independent of changes in their lipoprotein profile. Studies have demonstrated that overexpression of a human apoAI transgene and associated increases in HDL result in the protection of C57BL/6 mice from diet-induced atherosclerosis. To investigate the effect of elevation of HDL levels in differing proatherogenic genetic milieus, we have introduced the human apoAI transgene into the apoE knockout (KO) background as well as into mice also expressing the apo(a) transgene. In both settings, elevations of human apoAI and HDL were associated with a marked reduction in atherogenesis. The finding of decreased atherosclerosis concomitant with both elevated apo(a) and a lack of apoE suggests that elevations of apoAI and HDL may prove to be a useful approach for treating unrelated causes of heightened atherosclerosis susceptibility.

Introduction

The mouse has been increasingly useful as a model system to study the genetics of atherosclerosis [1,2] because this organism can be manipulated both genetically and environmentally in a manner not possible in humans. Three recently developed strains of engineered animals — apoA-I transgenics [3,4], apo(a) transgenics [5,6], and apoE KO [7,8] mice — have significantly contributed to our ability to address issues relevant to human atherosclerosis previously unavailable. Transgenic mice expressing human apoA-I have been created in the C57BL/6 background [9]. The C57BL/6 strain is an atherosclerosis-susceptible inbred strain which differs from resistant inbred strains (e.g., Balb/c, C3H) in that its HDL concentration decreases when fed an atherogenic diet. The C57BL/6 mice expressing the human apoA-I transgene have been shown in several studies to have higher plasma concentrations of human apoA-I and HDL than nontransgenic C57BL/6 mice and to be resistant to diet-induced atherogenesis [3,10].

ApoE KO mice derived from embryonic stem cells in which the murine apoE gene has been inactivated have provided a new murine model for studying atherosclerosis susceptibility [7,8]. These animals lacking apoE, a critical ligand involved in the removal of nearly all classes of lipoproteins from the plasma, have massive hypercholesterolemia and susceptibility to atherosclerosis. The apoE KO mice develop atherosclerosis independent of a dietary insult and have lesions that mimic many of the features observed in human atheromas.

Mice expressing a human apo(a) transgene provide a second, recently developed, model of heightened atherosclerosis susceptibility [5,6]. Although apo(a) is normally lacking in mice, high plasma levels of human apo(a) in the transgenic animals are

---

Address for correspondence: Edward M. Rubin, Human Genome Center, Lawrence Berkeley Laboratory, University of California, One Cylclotron Road – M/S 74-157, Berkeley CA 94720, USA.

associated with increased diet-induced atherosclerosis. A novel aspect of the apo(a) transgenic animals and their susceptibility to diet-induced atherosclerosis is the lack of differences in the lipoprotein profiles between transgenic atherosclerosis-susceptible animals and the control atherosclerosis-resistant mice. Since both groups of animals have nearly identical lipoprotein profiles, the increased atherosclerosis in the apo(a) transgenic animals is probably related to the atherogenic properties intrinsic to apo(a) itself, independent of its effect on the organism's lipoprotein profile.

A further strength of the mouse system in addressing genetic issues relevant to diseases such as atherosclerosis is the ability to cross-breed animals rapidly and create defined strains with combinations of transgenes or targeted alleles. This provides a practical approach for investigating the interaction of several genetic elements and to examine whether different factors act along similar or distinct metabolic pathways with regard to their effect on a singular phenotype — in this case, atherogenesis. Although it has been known for several decades that HDL concentration and atherosclerotic risk are inversely related [11], the question of whether HDL acts directly as an antiatherogenic factor is still contested. In order to investigate the antiatherogenic properties of HDL in settings beyond that of the relatively HDL-deficient C57BL/6 mouse, we have bred the human apoA-I transgene into the background of mice with increased atherosclerosis susceptibility due either to expression of the apo(a) transgene [12] or to a deficiency of apoE [13]. Lipoproteins and atherogenesis were then assessed in the resulting animals.

Results

ApoA-I transgene corrects apoE deficiency-induced atherosclerosis

To examine if increases in apoA-I and HDL are effective in minimizing apoE deficiency-induced atherosclerosis, we introduced the human apoA-I transgene into the hyper-cholesterolemic apoE KO background [13].

Apolipoproteins and lipoproteins

We first examined apolipoproteins and lipoproteins in apoA-I transgenic, apoE KO, apoA-I transgenic/apoE KO, and control mice (Table 1). As has previously been noted [4,9], animals with high levels of human apoA-I have low levels of endogenous murine apoA-I. The antibody used in detecting human apoA-I shows no cross-reactivity with murine apoA-I, demonstrated by the absence of human apoA-I in the control or the apoE KO mice. Similar elevations of total plasma cholesterol occurred in the apoE KO mice and in the apoE KO animals also expressing the human apoA-I transgene. The apoA-I transgenic/apoE KO animals, however, had a 2- to 3-fold increase in HDL.

The relative concentration and size distribution of the VLDL and LDL particles were similar in the apoE KO and the apoA-I transgenic/apoE KO mice [13]. In addition to increased concentration, HDL from the apoA-I transgenic/apoE KO mice showed a polydispersity of particle sizes, in contrast to the unidispersity of HDL particle size in the apoE KO mice. This polydispersity of HDL size is consistent with previous analyses of HDL in mice expressing human apoA-I transgenes [4,9].

Effects of apoE KO and apoA-I transgene alleles on atherosclerosis

Highly significant differences in the area of fatty streaks in the proximal aorta were observed in the different groups of mice when fed the low-fat mouse chow diet (Fig. 1A). Consistent with prior studies, the C57BL/6 mice did not develop aortic fatty streaks when

508

Table 1A,B. Apoliproteins and lipoproteins (mg/dl) in the different mouse strains

Genotype	(n)	Murine apoE	Murine apoA-I	Human apoA-I	HDL-C	Non-HDL(c)
ApoA-I/E KO	22	0	8 ± 1	82 ± (8)	101 ± 3	465
E KO	34	0	53 ± 3	0	31 ± 2	447

Female mice fed mouse chow diet at 8 weeks of age.

Genotype	(n)	Apo(a)	HDL-C	Non-HDL-C
Apo(a)	32	3.6 ± 0.2	43.6 ± 4.0	127
ApoA-I	23	0	99.7 ± 7.0	79
Apo(a)/apoA-I	22	3.2 ± 0.2	115.2 ± 11.2	82
Control	25	0	53.6 ± 9.2	126

Female mice at 8 weeks of age placed on high-fat, high-cholesterol diet [3] for 16 weeks [12].

fed mouse chow, while the apoE KO mice fed the same chow diet developed large fatty streaks. In contrast to the pronounced atherogenesis observed in all the apoE KO mice, of the 27 apoA-I/apoE KO mice studied, more than 90% of the animals either had no lesions or extremely small lesions (mean lesions <1,000 mm^2/section). In summary, the mean lesion area per section per animal of the apoA-I/apoE KO mice was 6 times lower than that of the apoE KO mice (p < 0.0001). The lesions in the apoE KO mice differed significantly from the small lesions that developed in a limited number of the apoA-I/apoE KO animals. The former had large lesions, with extensive lipid-staining material infiltrating the disrupted media of both the proximal aorta and more distal locations in the aorta. All animals expressing the apoA-I transgene had, at most, small fatty-streak lesions that did not extend into the media.

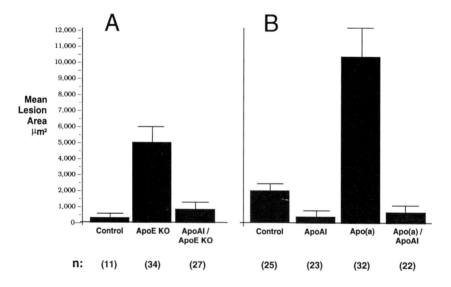

Fig. 1. Atherogenesis as measured by area of aortic fatty-streak lesions. A: Mouse chow diet (4% fat); animal examined at 12 weeks of age; B: After high-fat, high-cholesterol diet [3] for 12 weeks [12].

Human apoA-I prevents atherosclerosis associated with apo(a) in transgenic mice

Elevated levels of apo(a) are associated with increased atherosclerosis risk whereas elevated apoA-I levels are associated with decreased atherosclerosis risk. To examine the interactions of these two important lipid-associated proteins, we have assessed the effect on atherogenesis of human apoA-I and human apo(a) transgenes alone, and in combination [12].

Apolipoprotein and lipoprotein measurements of the apo(a), apoA-I, and apo(a)/apoA-I transgenic mice

Apo(a) levels were similar in all groups of animals expressing the apo(a) transgene, either alone or in combination with the apoA-I transgene (Table 1B). Human apoA-I levels were also similar in animals expressing either the human apoA-I transgene alone or in combination with the apo(a) transgene (data not shown). As was observed in the apoE KO and the C57BL/6 mouse background, high-level expression of the human apoA-I transgene was associated with an 8- to 10-fold decrease in endogenous murine plasma concentrations in both the apoA-I or the apo(a)/apoA-I mice (data not shown). The apoA-I and apo(a)/apoA-I groups had approximately twice the HDL concentrations of those in apo(a) or the nontransgenic control mice. In summary, comparing the four groups of animals — control, apo(a), apoA-I, and apo(a)/apoA-I — only animals expressing the apoA-I transgene showed any alteration of lipoprotein levels, namely an increase in the HDL component.

Atherogenesis studies show that human apoA-I and elevated HDL prevent the atherosclerosis associated with apo(a) in transgenic mice

The area of the oil red O staining regions of the aorta for the four groups of animals — nontransgenic controls, apo(a) transgenics, apoA-I transgenics, and combined apo(a)/apoA-I transgenic animals — following a 6-week exposure to an atherogenic diet are shown in Fig. 1B. By far the greatest degree of atherogenesis was seen in animals expressing the apo(a) transgene alone.

In agreement with prior studies [6], animals that expressed the apo(a) transgene alone had significantly larger lesions than control nontransgenic mice. The mean lesion area of the apo(a) transgenics was approximately 25 times that in mice expressing either the apoA-I transgene alone or both the apo(a) and apoA-I transgenes. Of the 32 apo(a) animals examined, 27 had significant atherosclerotic lesions with mean lesion areas greater than 2,000 mm^2, while of the 22 apo(a)/apoA-I animals examined, only one animal demonstrated an atherosclerotic lesion area greater than 2,000 mm^2. There were no histological differences noted between the apo(a) transgenics and the other groups other than the fact the lesions were larger and more numerous in the apo(a) animals.

Discussion

This study supports earlier results showing increased atherosclerosis susceptibility in mice expressing an apo(a) transgene and mice homozygous for the apoE KO allele. It extends these studies by showing that the presence of the human apoA-I transgene protects animals against atherogenesis in two different genetic settings which are usually associated with increased atherogenesis. Together, the results suggest that elevations of apoA-I and HDL plasma concentrations may serve to counter different causes of heightened atherosclerosis susceptibility.

In earlier studies with apoA-I transgenic mice, it was shown that increasing levels of apoA-I in the atherosclerosis-susceptible C57BL/6 strain, a strain with lower HDL concentrations than resistant inbred strains, resulted in elevated HDL and lower atherosclerosis susceptibility. The present study, in contrast to the studies using relatively HDL-deficient C57BL/6 mice or hypercholesterolemic apoE KO mice, shows that elevation of apoA-I and HDL can prevent atherosclerosis in mice with heightened susceptibility that is not associated with alterations of their lipoprotein profile. These findings support the utility of the mouse in distinguishing the interactions of various pro- and anti-atherogenic factors and suggest that the antiatherogenic role of apoA-I and HDL is effective in countering heightened atherosclerosis susceptibility due to the presence of apo(a) or the absence of apoE in the plasma of mice.

Acknowledgements

This work was supported by National Institutes of Health Grants to: E.M.R. PPG HL18574, R.M.L. PPG48638-01, and A.C.L. NRSA HL08733-02. E.M.R is also funded by a grant from National Dairy Promotion and Research Board and administered in cooperation with the National Dairy Council. E.M.R. is an American Heart Association Established Investigator. Research was conducted at the Lawrence Berkeley Laboratory (Dept. of Energy Contract DE-AC0376SF00098), University of California, Berkeley.

References

1. Ishida BY, Paigen B. In: Lusis Aj, Sparkes SR (eds) Genetic Factors in Atherosclerosis: Approaches and Model Systems. Basel: Karger, 1989;189—222.
2. Breslow JL. Proc Natl Acad Sci USA 1993;90:8314—8318.
3. Rubin EM, Krauss RM, Spangler EA, Verstuyft JG, Clift SM. Nature 1991;353:265—267.
4. Chajek-Shaul T, Hayek T, Walsh A, Breslow JL. Proc Natl Acad Sci USA 1991;88:6731—6735.
5. Chiesa G, Hobbs HH, Koschinsky ML, Lawn RM, Maika SD, Hammer RE. J Biol Chem 1992;267: 24639—24374.
6. Lawn RM, Wade DP, Hammer RE, Chiesa G, Verstuyft JG, Rubin EM. Nature 1992;360:670—672.
7. Plump AS, Smith JD, Hayek T, Aalto-Setala K, Walsh A, Verstuyft JG, Rubin EM, Breslow JL. Cell 1992;71:343—353.
8. Zhang SH, Reddick RL, Piedrahita JA, Maeda N. Science 1992;258:468—471.
9. Rubin EM, Ishida BY, Clift SM, Krauss RM. Proc Natl Acad Sci USA 1991;88:434—438.
10. Schultz JR, Verstuyft JG, Gong EL, Nicholas AV, Rubin EM. Nature 1993;365:761—764.
11. Gofman JW, Lindgren F, Elliott H. Science 1950;11:166—171.
12. Liu AC, Lawn RM, Verstuyft JG, Rubin EM. Human apoliprotein A-I prevents atherosclerosis associated with apoliprotein(a) in transgenic mice. J Lipid Res (in press).
13. Paszty C, Maeda N, Verstuyft J, Rubin EM. Apoliprotein A-I Transgene Corrects Apoliprotein E Deficiency-Induced Atherosclerosis in Mice. J Clin Invest 1994;94:899—903.

Plurimetabolic syndrome or syndrome X: an overview

Gaetano Crepaldi

Department of Internal Medicine, University of Padua, Padua, Italy

During the first annual meeting of the European Association for the Study of Diabetes, in a paper entitled "Essential hyperlipemia, obesity and diabetes" we presented some observations made in our patients. We concluded that there is "a plurimetabolic syndrome including hyperlipemia, obesity and diabetes" and that "the development of ischemic heart disease and, less frequently, of arterial hypertension is often found in these patients" [1].

In this description of the association of clinical and metabolic abnormalities we underlined the heterogeneity of these patients with regard to hypertension. Indeed, only about 50% of the patients with abnormal plasma lipid and glucose concentrations also had elevated blood pressure levels. Our conclusions came exclusively from the clinical observation of the patients affected by an association of metabolic disorders (hyperlipidemia, diabetes or impaired glucose tolerance, obesity, hyperuricemia) and we were far from considering hypertension as a metabolic disease, as it would be now. Since then several authors recognized the frequent association of the above-mentioned diseases, and each author stressed some aspects of this syndrome.

In 1986 W.P. Castelli observed that Framingham data suggested the existence of "a new syndrome, characterized by a high triglyceride level, a normal cholesterol level, and a low HDL level" [2]. Overweight, diabetes mellitus, and often elevated serum uric acid levels were considered part of this syndrome. In 1987 Ferrannini et al. [3] reported an association between impaired insulin-induced extrahepatic carbohydrate utilization and hypertension in lean patients with essential hypertension. These findings suggested a pathogenic link between an impaired insulin sensitivity and the development of hypertension. Such a mechanism has been tentatively associated with the occurrence of hyperinsulinemia, which could in turn determine sodium retention, adrenergic overactivity and vascular abnormalities.

In 1988 R.R. Williams and coworkers in a population study observed a syndrome consisting of hypertension, mixed lipid abnormalities (high triglycerides, high LDL, low HDL-cholesterol) and moderate obesity [4]. In the same year G.R. Reaven revisited the role of insulin resistance in human disease. In his review data were presented to support the hypothesis that resistance to insulin-stimulated glucose uptake, glucose intolerance, hyperinsulinemia, increased VLDL-triglyceride, decreased HDL-cholesterol and hypertension tend to occur in the same patient. This syndrome was called "syndrome X" [5].

All these observations contributed greatly to a better understanding of the vascular risk in many patients and gave important hints to the research into the physiopathological mechanisms linking such different diseases as hypertriglyceridemia, obesity, diabetes, and hypertension.

However, the definition of "syndrome X" appeared slightly puzzling since this term

Address for correspondence: Gaetano Crepaldi, Istituto di Medicina Interna, Patologia Medica I, Policlinico Universitario, Via Giustiniani 2, 35128 Padua, Italy. Tel.: +39-49-8212150. Fax: +39-49-657647.

512

had already been used for years to identify patients with chest pain and normal coronary arteriograms, in whom symptoms are due to myocardial ischemia with reduced coronary perfusion reserve [6].

In our opinion as part of the "syndrome X" or "plurimetabolic syndrome" we must include hypertriglyceridemia and/or low HDL-cholesterol with or without high LDL-cholesterol, insulin resistance or impaired glucose tolerance or type 2 diabetes, hyperuricemia, central obesity and the frequent occurrence of microalbuminuria, polycythemia, respiratory disorders, sodium retention, cardiovascular events and cardiomegaly or organomegaly. The family history of the individuals with these clinical features is also frequently characterized by cardiovascular diseases.

The definition of "syndrome" usually indicate "a group of symptoms and signs of disordered function, related to one another by means of some anatomic, physiologic or biochemical peculiarity. It also embodies a hypothesis concerning the deranged function of an organ, organ system or tissue" [7]. The definition of "syndrome X" as formulated by Reaven and modified by De Fronzo et al. [8] as "insulin resistance syndrome" maintains that impaired insulin sensitivity is the common denominator responsible for the association of obesity, hypertension and insulin resistance with dyslipidemia in all patients. However, in order to gain further insights into the pathogenesis of these clinical disorders it is vital to recognize that the association among these four factors is not obligatory; on the contrary, these individual clinical features can occur independently. In fact, in our original report we pointed out that the association of hypertension with diabetes and hyperlipemia was observed in some but not all patients with the plurimetabolic syndrome [1].

More recently we found an association between hypertension and impaired insulin sensitivity at extrahepatic level in non-insulin-dependent diabetes but not in essential hypertension [9–12]. Familial genetic traits and racial differences have been shown to play a role in determining a heterogeneous association among abnormalities in blood pressure levels and carbohydrate and lipid metabolism [4,13]. Although the reasons accounting for this heterogeneous association do not appear immediately understandable, I believe it is important to consider that the link among hypertension, dyslipidemia and insulin resistance again is not mandatory. All these clinical findings suggest that hyperinsulinemia itself does not lead to hypertension, but that insulin resistance and blood pressure are linked indirectly and through a variety of mechanisms.

The question then arises at to the nature of these hypothetical inherited or acquired mechanisms. Overweight does not appear to be the major determinant of the association between hypertension and insulin resistance, since several reports show a stronger relation between insulin sensitivity and abnormalities in cellular ion handling [14,15]. Results from our laboratory indicate that in non-insulin-dependent diabetes, as already observed in essential hypertension, a constellation of clinical and biochemical abnormalities such as hypertension, extrahepatic rather than hepatic insulin resistance, dyslipidemia, obesity, microalbuminuria and abnormalities in ion handling tend to cluster in the same cohort of patients [9,10,12]. The identification of such cohorts of patients will certainly be useful in gaining further insights into the pathogenesis of these clinical disorders, possibly confirming the hypothesis that a common genetic defect leads to the development of different phenotypic abnormalities.

It is interesting to note that about one out of three hypertriglyceridemic patients turns out to be hypertensive, one out of two has overt diabetes or impaired glucose tolerance, 44% are overweight, and 44% have elevated serum uric acid levels [16]. When these patients have high levels of triglyceride-rich particles in plasma they also have LDL particles that are smaller and denser than normal [17]. Hypertriglyceridemic patients have lower than normal HDL-cholesterol and when they are treated by diet the LDL abnormalities are rather easily normalized while the HDL abnormalities (particularly the absence of HDL$_2$) are not corrected [18]. These observations point to several physico-chemical alterations of the plasma lipoprotein particles in hypertriglyceridemic patients. From a clinical point of view it is important to emphasize that these alterations are associated with an increased risk of cardiovascular diseases [19].

When examining type 2 diabetic patients we should consider that some of these patients might be affected by both type 2 diabetes and a genetic form of hyper-triglyceridemia. We have examined a population of well-controlled type 2 diabetic patients, excluding patients with possible genetic forms of hypertriglyceridemia, and we observed that plasma triglyceride and HDL-cholesterol levels are not significantly different from controls. These diabetic patients had a higher body weight than controls and their lipid values were significantly related to body weight but not to the indices of metabolic control. This observation suggests that insulin resistance is associated with lipoprotein level alterations [20].

We have analyzed lipoprotein levels and the LDL and HDL particle size by gradient gel electrophoresis in type 2 diabetic patients: normotensive and nonmicroalbuminuric, hypertensive nonmicroalbuminuric, and hypertensives with microalbuminuria. Diabetic patients with hypertension and with hypertension and microalbuminuria are characterized by lower HDL (particularly HDL$_{2b}$) cholesterol levels than controls. The LDL particles were smaller in diabetic patients than in controls, particularly in NIDDM patients with hypertension without microalbuminuria and in NIDDM patients with both hypertension and microalbuminuria [21].

Overweight and obesity are associated with hypertriglyceridemia and more often with low HDL-cholesterol levels. These associations seem stronger for the visceral type of obesity rather than for the subcutaneous [22]. Visceral obesity is also more linked to insulin resistance and associated with higher blood pressure. When an oral glucose tolerance test is performed in viscerally obese subjects, both the plasma glucose and insulin levels are higher than in patients with the same body mass index but with a subcutaneous deposition of the body fat [22].

Also, patients with visceral obesity have higher cholesterol, triglyceride and uric acid and lower HDL-cholesterol levels than in patients with subcutaneous obesity. Quite recently some authors observed that subjects with a high waist to hip ratio, independently of body weight, have higher levels of small dense LDL. Our own observations in morbidly obese patients before and after gastroplasty confirm higher amounts of such small dense LDL particles than in controls [23].

In patients with essential hypertension, whole-body glucose utilization was significantly lower in patients with elevated albumin excretion rate than in patients with a normal albumin excretion rate during euglycemic insulin-glucose clamp at ~100 µU/ml plasma insulin. In patients with NIDDM, whole-body glucose utilization (during euglycemic clamp with similar plasma insulin concentrations) was significantly lower in patients with hypertension without altered albumin excretion rate, in patients with altered albumin excretion rate without hypertension, and in patients with hypertension and altered albumin excretion rate, than in controls [9,10,12]. In contrast, diabetic patients with normal blood pressure levels and albumin excretion rate had normal insulin sensitivity [9,10,12]. Insulin release, as assessed by plasma C-peptide response to glucagon challenge, was impaired in all diabetic patients, irrespective of blood pressure and albumin excretion-rate dif-ferences [9,10].

No differences were found in total serum cholesterol concentrations between patients with essential hypertension and controls, whereas HDL-cholesterol was significantly lower in patients with altered albumin excretion rate than in those with normal albumin excretion rate and in controls. Serum triglyceride concentrations were on the contrary higher in hypertensives with high than in hypertensive patients with normal albumin excretion rate and in controls [12,15].

Patients with essential hypertension had an average ultrasound index of left ventricular mass higher than controls. However, despite similar blood pressure levels, patients with microalbuminuria had a more elevated value of left ventricular mass index than hypertensives without microalbuminuria. Diabetic patients with hypertension had a higher ultrasound index of cardiac mass than normotensive diabetic patients and controls. Interestingly, left ventricular mass was also greater than in controls in microalbuminuric diabetic patients, even though their blood pressure levels were normal [15].

With regard to kidney ultrasound imaging, patients with essential hypertension and microalbuminuria had greater renal volume than patients without microalbuminuria. All non-insulin-dependent diabetic patients had elevated values of renal volume. A significant difference between controls and diabetic patients was, however, found only in hypertensive groups and in microalbuminuric normotensive patients [15].

Patients with essential hypertension and microalbuminuria had significantly higher Na^+/Li^+ countertransport activity in red blood cells than controls as well as hypertensive without altered albumin excretion rate. With regard to non-insulin-dependent diabetes a significantly higher value of Na^+/Li^+ countertransport in red blood cells was shown by hypertensive patients and by microalbuminuric patients with and without hypertension, but not by normotensive and normoalbuminuric patients [15]. The LDL size as well as the plasma triglyceride levels were significantly related (LDL size inversely, triglyceride directly) to the Na/Li countertransport activity [24].

In our opinion these results in patients with NIDDM and essential hypertension indicate that: 1) insulin resistance can occur without hypertension, and conversely hypertension is not necessarily linked to insulin resistance, 2) altered albumin excretion rate is associated with insulin resistance, irrespective of blood pressure levels, 3) there is a strong relation between insulin-induced glucose utilization and sodium-lithium counter-transport activity in red blood cells, and 4) a constellation of biochemical and morphological abnormalities, such as dyslipidemias as well as cardiac and renal hyper-trophy, tend to cluster in a cohort of patients characterized by elevated sodium-lithium countertransport activity in red blood cells.

Thus, in patients with essential hypertension and NIDDM elevated blood-pressure levels, altered albumin excretion rate and impaired insulin action are not necessarily associated. Conversely, whenever insulin resistance and microalbuminuria do occur, either together or separately, an abnormality in cell ion handling, namely sodium-lithium countertransport activity in red blood cells, is also found.

A definition of "syndrome X" that maintains that the association of obesity, hypertension, insulin resistance and dyslipidemia necessarily occurs in all patients could be misleading. In fact, if we deem that the link among these abnormalities is mandatory we can fail to recognize the unknown nature of the pathogenetic mechanisms responsible for the development of the constellation of these clinical disorders. Since we do not yet know the pathogenesis of insulin resistance, we should pay more attention, at the moment, to the variety of clinical facets with which hypertension and insulin resistance do occur in vivo.

References

1. Avogaro P, Crepaldi G. Diabetologia 1965;1:137(abstract 53).
2. Castelli WP. Am Heart J 1986;112:432−437.
3. Ferrannini E, Buzzigoli G, Bonadonna E. N Engl J Med 1987;317:350−357.
4. Williams RR, Hunt SC, Hopkins PN et al. J Am Med Assoc 1988;259:3579−3586.
5. Reaven GM. Diabetes 1988;37:1595−1607.
6. Anonimous. Lancet 1987;2:1247−1248.
7. Harrison's Principles of Internal Medicine, In: Braunwald E, Isselbacher KJ, Petersdorf RG et al. (eds) 11th edn. New York: McGraw Hill 1987;3.
8. De Fronzo RA, Ferrannini E. Diabet Care 1991;14:173−194.
9. Nosadini R, Solini A, Velussi M et al. Diabetes 1994;43:491−499.
10. Nosadini R, Manzato E, Solini A et al. Eur J Clin Invest 1994;24:258−266.
11. Doria A, Fioretto P, Avogaro A et al. Am J Physiol 1991;261:E684−E691.
12. Zambon S, Manzato E, Solini A et al. Arterioscler Thromb 1994;14:911−916.
13. Saad MF, Lilloja S, Nyomba BL. N Engl J Med 1991;324:733−739.
14. Nosadini R, Fioretto P, Trevisan R et al. Diabet Care 1991;14:210−219.
15. Nosadini R, Semplicini A, Fioretto P et al. Hypertension 1991;18:191−198.
16. Crepaldi G, Fellin R, Briani G et al. Atherosclerosis 1977;26:593−602.
17. Manzato E, Zambon S, Zambon A et al. Clin Chim Acta 1993;219:57−65.
18. Manzato E, Marin R, Gasparotto A et al. Eur J Clin Invest 1986;16:149−156.
19. Austin MA. Arterioscler Thromb 1991;11:2−14.
20. Manzato E, Zambon A, Lapolla A et al. Diabet Care 1993;16:469−475.
21. Zambon S, Manzato E, Solini A et al. Arterioscler Thromb 1994;14:911−916.
22. Enzi G, Pavan M, Digito M et al. Diab Nutr Metab 1993;6:47−55.
23. Manzato E, Zambon S, Zambon A et al. Int J Obes 1992;16:573−578.
24. Manzato E, Zambon S, Cortella A et al. Acta Diabetologica 1992;29:231−233.

Epidemiology of the plurimetabolic syndrome

Barbara V. Howard

Medlantic Research Institute, Washington DC, USA

Abstract. The plurimetabolic syndrome, often referred to as the insulin resistance syndrome, is a precursor of non-insulin-dependent diabetes mellitus (NIDDM). Dyslipidemia often accompanies this disorder in all populations examined to date. This dyslipidemia, or alterations in lipoprotein composition and metabolism, typically includes increased VLDL, LDL compositional changes, and decreased HDL with concomitant compositional changes. Insulin resistance contributes to the incidence of these abnormalities, the existence of which relates directly to increased risk of cardiovascular disease.

The plurimetabolic, or insulin resistance, syndrome has been defined as the presence of increased insulin concentrations in association with other disorders, including visceral obesity, hyperglycemia, hypertension, dyslipidemia, and sometimes hyperuricemia and renal dysfunction. This syndrome has particular significance because it has been shown to be an antecedent of both non-insulin-dependent diabetes mellitus (NIDDM) and atherosclerosis. Dyslipidemia (high VLDL, low HDL, and altered LDL composition) accompanies this syndrome and may be a major factor in the increased risk for cardiovascular disease.

Insulin and lipoprotein concentrations

A possible relationship between insulin and plasma lipids was suggested as early as the 1960s, soon after techniques for measuring plasma insulin became available. The relationships between insulin and plasma lipids were first noted in metabolic ward studies focusing on individuals with triglyceride disorders. Subsequently, a consistent relationship between insulin and plasma lipids has been established in many population-based studies. These studies (summarized in Table 1) show positive associations between insulin and plasma triglycerides (VLDL), and negative associations between insulin and HDL-cholesterol that remain strong despite gender and ethnic variations and after adjustments for covariates such as age and obesity.

Dyslipidemia and insulin resistance

There appears to be a direct relationship between insulin action and both increased triglycerides and lowered HDL (literature summary in Table 2).

Dyslipidemia in individuals with insulin resistance also appears to include LDL depleted in core cholesteryl ester and relatively enriched in apolipoprotein B (apoB), and with a smaller diameter and a higher average density. In 1993 Selby et al. showed that LDL size and the B subclass pattern were associated with an array of risk factors defining the insulin resistance syndrome [1] and Haffner et al. confirmed the association of LDL

Address for correspondence: Barbara V. Howard, Medlantic Research Institute, 108 Irving Street NW, Washington, DC 20010, USA. Tel.: +1-202-877-6530. Fax: +1-202-877-3209.

Table 1. Summary of population-based studies of links between insulin and lipoproteins (adapted from [4])

Reference	N	Sex	Age range	Race (country)	Lipoprotein	Covariates
Orchard et al. 1983 [5]	323	M/F	3–66	White (USA)	VLDL, LDL HDL (-)	Age, BMI
Howard et al. 1984 [6]	1391	M/F	15–79	American Indian (USA)	VLDL HDL (-)	Age, alcohol, BMI, glucose, smoking
Cambien et al. 1987 [7]	2144	M	43–54	White (France)	VLDL HDL (-)	Age, alcohol, BMI, glucose, smoking
Donahue et al. 1987 [8]	87	M	20–24	White (USA)	HDL (-)	BMI, TG
Haffner et al. 1988 [9]	606	M/F	25–64	Hispanic (USA)	VLDL HDL (-)	BMI, WHR
Burchfield et al. 1990 [10]	856	M/F	20–74	Hispanic (USA)	VLDL HDL (-)	–
McKeigue et al. 1989 [11]		M/F	35–69	East Asian (UK)	VLDL HDL (-)	–
Modan et al. 1988 [12]	542	M/F	38–70	White (Israel)	VLDL, LDL HDL (-)	Age, BMI
Zavaroni et al. 1985 [13]	607	M/F	22–73	White (Italy)	VLDL HDL (-)	Alcohol, glucose, physical activity
Manolio et al. 1990 [14]	4576	M/F	18–30	Black/ White (USA)	VLDL HDL (-)	Age, BMI
Fontbonne et al. 1992 [15]	1686	M	20–60	Black (French Caribbean)/ White	VLDL	Age, alcohol, BMI, BP, glucose, plasma insulin
Howard et al. 1992 [16]	1161	M/F	45–74	Native American (USA)	VLDL, HDL (-)	Age, BMI, waist-hip ratio, plasma glucose, physical activity

Table 2. Summary of studies that establish the associations between plasma lipoproteins and insulin action

Reference	Finding
Abbott et al. 1987 [17]	Insulin-mediated disposal, storage, and oxidation of glucose inversely related to total/VLDL triglyceride and directly related to HDL in Native Americans. Relationship was found to be independent of obesity and fasting insulin, and the relationships of triglyceride and HDL-cholesterol with insulin action were independent of each other
Garg et al. 1988 [18]	Association between lipoproteins and in vivo insulin action among non-diabetic white males
Laakso et al. 1990 [19]	Association, in groups with various degrees of glucose intolerance (normal, impaired, NIDDM), of lower concentrations of HDL and higher total VLDL-triglycerides with increased insulin resistance. Associations were independent of fasting insulin, age, obesity, waist-hip ratio, 2-hour glucose and fatty acid concentrations, and HDL-cholesterol and VLDL triglycerides were independently associated with insulin action.
Godsland et al. 1992 [20]	Association of insulin action with triglycerides and independent association of hepatic insulin throughput with HDL_2-cholesterol. Relationships were independent of age, BMI, and body-fat distribution.

518

size and pattern with a clustering of risk factors of the insulin resistance syndrome [2]. In another 1993 study, by Reaven et al., a negative association between LDL size and insulin action was reported, and insulin-resistant individuals were found to have a higher proportion of LDL subclass pattern B [3].

Mechanisms

The possible mechanisms for the association between insulin resistance and lipoprotein alterations are summarized in Table 3. Although there is disagreement in the literature as to whether hyperinsulinemia is a major determinant of elevated VLDL in insulin-resistant subjects, the insulin-resistant state itself may induce elevated VLDL. The complexity of the mechanisms controlling HDL metabolism and the lack of understanding of many of the key mechanisms regulating HDL impede the examination of possible associations between insulin resistance and HDL. Although low HDL often accompanies elevated VLDL, some studies have demonstrated that the relationship between HDL and insulin/insulin action is independent of VLDL concentrations, which suggests that a more direct connection may exist between insulin resistance and HDL metabolism. With respect to alterations in LDL composition, the literature overwhelmingly demonstrates a strong inverse relationship between VLDL concentrations and LDL size. Although the metabolic mechanisms controlling the size of LDL are not well understood, it is hypothesized that impaired lipase activity in insulin-resistant subjects, or the exchange of triglyceride for cholesteryl ester in the LDL core followed by lipolysis, may result in smaller LDL particles.

Conclusions

Dyslipidemia appears to be an integral part of the insulin resistance syndrome and is associated with hyperinsulinemia in individuals over a wide range of age and ethnic groups. The relevant elements of this dyslipidemia are elevated VLDL, lowered HDL, and the presence of small, dense LDL. These changes are associated with atherogenesis [4]. The lipoprotein alterations in insulin resistance are no longer thought to be caused by elevated insulin concentrations, but to result from the effects of the insulin-resistant state on lipoprotein metabolism. Thus, basic aspects of insulin-resistant muscle, adipose tissue, and/or liver must cause the defective lipoprotein metabolism. A logical unifying hypothesis for the dyslipidemia associated with insulin resistance starts with an increase in free fatty acid flux that probably results from the central obesity that accompanies insulin resistance. It is likely that the insulin-resistant liver, presented with an increased

Table 3. Possible mechanisms for lipoprotein alterations associated with insulin resistance

Alteration	Possible mechanism
Elevations in VLDL	Elevated free fatty acids and glucose flux to liver
	Elevated VLDL-triglyceride production
	Increased VLDL-apoB
	Lowered LPL activity
Decreases in HDL	Impaired lipolysis of triglyceride-rich lipoproteins
	Increased HTGL
	Decreased hepatic production
Small dense LDL	Impaired lipolysis
	Depletion of core cholesteryl ester because of exchange with VLDL triglyceride

flux of free fatty acids and elevated levels of glucose, overproduces VLDL and either produces less HDL or accelerates its clearance [4]. Subsequently, small dense LDL result either from the impaired metabolism of VLDL (insulin-resistant LPL) or through the lipoprotein transfer process in which triglycerides are exchanged for cholesterol in the LDL core. The mechanisms that control VLDL, LDL, and HDL metabolism and how they are altered in the insulin-resistant state are topics for further study. This knowledge will undoubtedly shed light on the etiology of the insulin resistance syndrome and aid in the development of possible strategies for prevention of the associated atherosclerosis.

References

1. Selby JV, Austin MA, Newman B et al. Circulation 1993;88:381–387.
2. Haffner SM, Mykkanen L, Vadez RA et al. Arterioscler Thromb 1993;13:1623–1630.
3. Reaven GM, Chen YDI, Jeppesen J et al. J Clin Invest 1993;92:141–146.
4. Howard BV. Ann NY Acad Sci 1993;683:1–8.
5. Orchard TJ, Becker DJ, Bates M et al. Am J Epidemiol 1983;118:326–337.
6. Howard BV, Knowler WC, Vasquez B et al. Arteriosclerosis 1984;4:462–471.
7. Cambien FJ, Warnet M, Eschwege E et al. Arteriosclerosis 1987;7:197–202.
8. Donahue RP, Orchard TJ, Becker DJ et al. Am J Epidemiol 1987;125:650–657.
9. Haffner SM, Fing D, Hazuda HP et al. Metabolism 1988;37:338–345.
10. Burchfiel CM, Hammon RF. Marshall JA et al. Am J Epidemiol 1990;131:57–70.
11. McKeigue PM, Miller GJ, Marmot MG. J Clin Epidemiol 1989;42:597–609.
12. Modan M, Halkin H, Lusky A et al. Arteriosclerosis 1988;8:227–236.
13. Zavaroni I, Dall'Anglio E, Alpi O et al. Atherosclerosis 1985;55:259–266.
14. Manolio TA, Savage PJ, Burke GL et al. Arteriosclerosis 1990;10:430–436.
15. Fontbonne A, Papoz L, Eschwege E et al. Diabetes 1992;41:1385–1389.
16. Howard BV, Welty TK, Fabsitz RR et al. Diabetes 1992;14:4–11.
17. Abbott WGH, Lillioja S, Young AA et al. Diabetes 1987;36:897–904.
18. Garg AJ, Helderman H, Koffler M et al. Metabolism 1988;37:982–987.
19. Laakso M, Sarlund H, Mykkanen L. Arteriosclerosis 1990;10:223–231.
20. Godsland IF, Crook D, Walton C et al. Arterioscler Thromb 1992;12;9:1030–1035.

The plurimetabolic syndrome and mortality: the diabetes intervention study (DIS)

M. Hanefeld

Department of Metabolic Research, Technical University, Dresden, Germany

Abstract. Non-insulin-dependent diabetes mellitus (NIDDM) leads to a reduction of life expectancy of 1—15 years, depending on age at onset and associated risk factors. DIS is a prospective controlled trial with 1,139 middle-aged newly diagnosed NIDDM patients classified as diet-controlled at entry. Patients were recruited by complete registration in a population survey. Follow-up time was at least 11 years; 197 (19.8%) out of 993 died. Cardiovascular diseases were the major cause of death. In multivariate analysis blood pressure, triglycerides, male sex, age, smoking, hematocrit and fasting blood glucose were independent risk factors for MI. Risk factors for early death were smoking, blood pressure, male sex, triglycerides, age and fasting blood glucose. The plurimetabolic syndrome entails risk for MI and death.

G. Grepaldi in 1965 inaugurated "a plurimetabolic syndrome including hyperlipemia, obesity and diabetes" and stated that "the development of ischemic heart disease and, less frequently, of arterial hypertension is often found in these patients". In 1968 I presented at the Dresden Medical Conference a more comprehensive concept that puts atherosclerosis into the center. In a review [1] in 1981 we defined the metabolic syndrome "as a cluster of obesity, hyper- and dyslipoproteinemia, maturity-onset diabetes (type II), gout and hypertension connected with an increased incidence of atherosclerotic vascular diseases, fatty liver and cholelithiasis that develops on the basis of a genetic susceptibility under conditions of overnutrition and low physical activity". More recent investigations by G. Reaven [2] focused on insulin resistance as the primary defect in the so-called syndrome X. The insulin-resistance/hyperinsulinemia syndrome is considered by many investigators as a common basic defect for non-insulin-dependent diabetes (NIDDM), android obesity, dyslipoproteinemia and hypertension leading to a clustering of these diseases.

The prognosis of NIDDM is still poor. Little has changed since the first reports about an excessive mortality in diabetes in controlled prospective studies by Pell and D'Alonzo in 1970 [3] and Garcia et al. in 1974 [4]. In 1981 Panzram and Zabel-Langhennig [5] reported that the excess mortality in a complete survey of a geographically defined diabetic population with NIDDM ranged from 2.1 to 1.0. It is a consistent finding that, decreasing with age at onset, cardiovascular causes account for the majority of deaths (30—60%). It appears that there exist a commonality of risk factors for coronary heart disease and total mortality in NIDDM. The question is whether the lower life expectancy in NIDDM is not at least related to the quality of metabolic control and a clustering of risk factors. So far, little is known about the impact of the metabolic syndrome on the incidence of myocardial infarction (MI) and mortality. There is consistent evidence that the relative risk for MI in NIDDM is 2—4 times higher than in age-adjusted nondiabetic

Address for correspondence: M. Hanefeld, Department of Metabolic Research, Technical University, 01307 Dresden, Fetscherstr. 74, Germany.

populations [6]. Furthermore there obviously exists a sex paradox that diabetic women exhibit a twice higher odds ratio for MI than diabetic men versus nondiabetic controls. Prospective studies with NIDDM revealed by multivariate analysis high blood pressure, smoking, dyslipoproteinemia, blood glucose and ischemic ECG at baseline as independent risk factors [7]. We therefore analyzed these questions with the patients of the Diabetes Intervention Study (DIS).

Short description of the DIS trial

DIS is a prospective controlled trial with 1139 newly diagnosed NIDDM aged 30–55 years at entry. The patients were classified as diet-controlled after a 6-week screening phase with conventional dietary advice. Important exclusions were clinical manifestations of macroangiopathy (myocardial infarction, stroke, gangrene) and severe life-threatening diseases. Details of the recruitment, study population and design were previously published [8]. The average follow-up time was 12 years, minimum 11 years; 993 (87.2%) completed the study, 197 documented deaths (19.83%) inclusive. Myocardial infarction was defined as: documented death by MI (fatal), clinical MI according to WHO criteria and/or newly detected ECG changes according to Minnesota codes 1.1 or/and 1.2 (silent MI).

The metabolic syndrome was defined as the common prevalence of NIDDM with hypertension (HT, BP160/95 mmHg and/or hypertensives), hypertriglyceridemia (HTG, $\geq$2.3 mmol/l), hypercholesterolemia (HCH, $\geq$6.5 mmol/l) or obesity (BMI, $\geq$25 kg/m^2).

Prevalence of the metabolic syndrome

As shown in Fig. 1, about 70% of the patients at entry exhibit one or several components of the metabolic syndrome when diabetes is first detected. Females show a somewhat

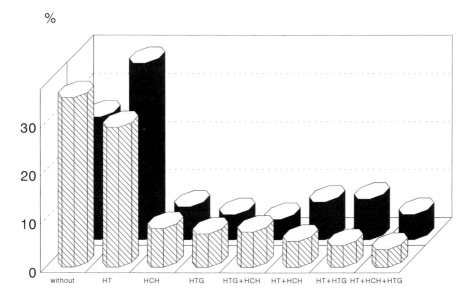

Fig. 1. Frequency of associated risk factors in newly detected NIDDM by sex (DIS, at entry) (▨ men, ■ women).

522

higher prevalence of associated risk factors, in particular with respect to hypertension. Obesity was present in 80.5% of the men and 85.3% of the women. Hyperinsulinemia (>1 SD above the normal range) was associated with a higher level of risk factors and worse glucose control (Fig. 2) at the 5-year follow-up in patients not treated with insulin. At that time 12.6% of the patients exhibited HDL-cholesterol <0.9 mmol/l.

Coronary death and myocardial infarction

As shown in Fig. 3 the classical risk factors for MI also act in NIDDM. In contrast to nondiabetics hypertriglyceridemia is a prominent independent risk factor whereas plasma cholesterol seems to be of less importance. In multivariate analysis for cardiovascular death, diastolic blood pressure, log triglycerides, male sex, age, smoking, systolic blood pressure, hematocrit and fasting blood glucose, in that order, were independent risk factors for cardiovascular death. Low HDL-cholesterol was a significant contributor for MI in patients with hypertension and as a part of the lipid triad (TG >2.3 mmol/l and cholesterol >6.5 mmol/l).

Mortality

Coronary heart disease (25.9%) was the major cause of death, followed by neoplasm (17.8%) and liver cirrhosis (10.2%). In 14.2% no exact diagnosis was obtained. Thus, the frequency of cardiovascular complications could be somewhat higher. This is in the same range as described by Panzram [5] in a 10-year follow-up for diabetics aged 40–59 years. The cumulative survival time classified by sex is shown in Fig. 4. In multivariate analysis smoking, systolic blood pressure, male sex, log triglycerides, age and fasting blood glucose at entry were significant predictors of early death. Our data confirm that even

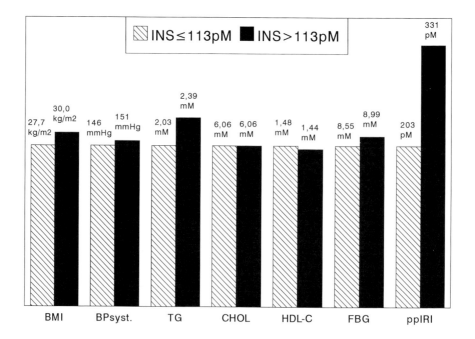

Fig. 2. Impact of hyperinsulinemia on level of risk factors (DIS, 5-year follow-up).

%

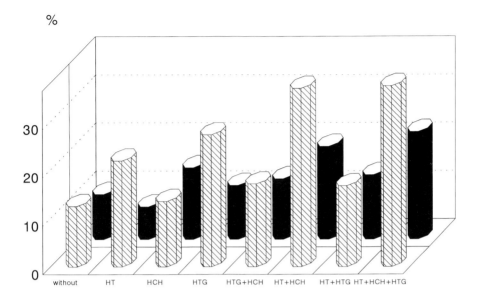

Fig. 3. Incidence of myocardial infarction (M = 92, F = 39) in newly detected NIDDM by sex (DIS, 11+ years follow-up) (▨ men, ■ women).

presumably mild NIDDM exhibits an excessive mortality. It is an impressive finding that the classic risk factors, except cholesterol, also operate for total mortality. Even more important: high blood glucose at the time of diabetes detection is an indicator for early death.

By extrapolation, our data suggest that the metabolic syndrome is a common companion of NIDDM and, if present, it raises the risk of cardiovascular complications and early death.

Cum.prop.survival

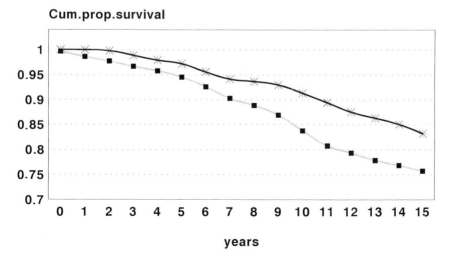

Fig. 4. Survival analysis (■ men, ✳ women in the Diabetes Intervention Study).

524

References

1. Hanefeld M, Leonhardt W. Dtsch Ges Wesen 1981;35:545–551.
2. Reaven GM. Diabetes 1988;37:1595–1607.
3. Pell S, D'Alonzo CA. J Am Med Assoc 1970;214:1833–1840.
4. Garcia MJ, McNamara PM, Gordon T, Kannel WB. Diabetes 1974;23:105–111.
5. Panzram G, Zabel-Langhennig R. Diabetologica 1981;20:587–591.
6. Pyörälä K, Laakso M, Uusitupa M. Diabet Metab Rev 1987;3:463–524.
7. Uusitupa MIJ et al. Diabetologica 1993;36:1175–1184.
8. Hanefeld M et al. Diabet Care 1991;14:308–317.

Atherosclerosis X.
F.P. Woodford, J. Davignon and A. Sniderman, editors.

Clustering of clinical features identifies a subset of non-insulin-dependent diabetic patients who have a predisposition to cardiovascular diseases

Romano Nosadini, Sabina Zambon, Andrea Carraro and Enzo Manzato
Department of Internal Medicine, University Hospital, Padua, Italy

Abstract. Insulin resistance may be a mechanism linking non-insulin-dependent diabetes mellitus (NIDDM) to hypertension and to cardiovascular mortality. Microalbuminuria is also an independent risk factor for cardiovascular mortality and hypertension. Little information is available in the literature on the relationship between microalbuminuria and insulin action. We have compared clinical features of patients with NIDDM who develop cardiovascular diseases with those of NIDDM patients without such complications.

Seventy-three normotensive and normoalbuminuric NIDDM subjects took part in a 6-year follow-up study. They were divided into two groups with insulin-induced whole body glucose utilization below (cohort A, n = 45) and above (cohort B, n = 28) the mean value minus one standard deviation in normal controls. During the follow-up cohort A diabetics more frequently developed hypertension (30 vs. 14%, p < 0.01), microalbuminuria (15 vs. 7%, p < 0.01) and cardiovascular events than did cohort B diabetics. Cohort A NIDDM patients were also characterized by the so-called atherogenic lipoprotein phenotype (small dense low density lipoproteins), which is known to be linked to cardiac ischemic disease in the nondiabetic population. Insulin resistance in extrahepatic tissues and atherogenic lipoprotein phenotype seem to precede the onset of hypertension, microalbuminuria and cardiac ischemic disease of NIDDM patients, independently of diabetic disease itself.

It has been suggested that insulin resistance may be a mechanism linking non-insulin-dependent diabetes mellitus (NIDDM) to hypertension [1]. Evidence supporting this view is provided by the observation that essential hypertension is an insulin-resistant state and that plasma insulin concentrations and blood pressure levels are correlated in lean, hypertensive subjects [2]. Furthermore, obesity and NIDDM, two syndromes primarily characterized by insulin resistance, have a high prevalence of hypertension [3].

Although evidence favoring a link between insulin resistance and hypertension has been provided, numerous studies have reported little or no relation between insulin concentration and blood pressure. This could be accounted for by the possibility that hypertension and insulin resistance are not universally associated in all subjects. In fact, insulin sensitivity is impaired in only 40–50% of the patients with essential hypertension [4]. Moreover, micro- and macroalbuminuria have also been reported to be associated with impaired insulin-induced glucose uptake in essential hypertension [4] and in insulin-dependent diabetes [5]. Furthermore, microalbuminuria is an independent risk factor of cardiovascular mortality in diabetic and nondiabetic subjects. It has been reported that insulin resistance is highly predictive of cardiovascular mortality [6]. The presence of small dense LDL particles (LDL pattern B) was recently identified as a genetic trait

Address for correspondence: Dr Romano Nosadini, Istituto di Medicina Interna, Patologia Medica I, Policlinico Universitario, Via Giustiniani 2, 35128 Padua, Italy. Tel.: +39-49-8212176. Fax: +39-49-657647.

associated with an increased prevalence of cardiovascular disease in the general population [7].

The aim of the present study was to investigate from a prospective point of view the relationships among hypertension, insulin-induced glucose uptake (considered the true clinical hallmark of extrahepatic insulin sensitivity), lipoprotein abnormalities, microalbuminuria and cardiovascular events in NIDDM.

Patients and Methods

Consecutive NIDDM patients who came to our clinic between January 1983 and December 1985 were recruited to take part in the study. Diagnosis of NIDDM was made when fasting plasma glucose was higher than or equal to 7.8 mmol/l on two different occasions. Baseline blood pressure was measured 3 times in both arms after 15 min supine rest. In agreement with the Statement of the Working Group on Hypertension in Diabetes [8], hypertension was considered as BP levels above 145/90 mmHg. Three 24-h urine collections were requested from each patient to evaluate albumin excretion rate. Microalbuminuria was defined as an albumin excretion rate higher than or equal to 15 µg/min in two out of three urine collections.

73 normotensive NIDDM patients who had never been treated with antihypertensive agents and whose albumin excretion rate was lower than or equal to 15 µg/min were directed to come for regular examinations at our outpatients' clinic every 3 months, for a 6-year period from 1985 to 1991. At each examination medical history was collected and HbA1c and blood pressure levels were measured. The diagnosis of arterial hypertension was made when diastolic blood pressure, measured as detailed above, exceeded 90 mmHg on at least three different occasions separated by 2- to 3-week intervals.

Once a year each patient was admitted to the hospital. At that time three 24-h urine collections were made over a 1-week period to determine albumin excretion rate. History of the patients along with their medical records as outpatients or as inpatients were reviewed for evidence of cardiovascular events, including myocardial infarction and cardiac angina (WHO definition and ECG and/or CPK-MB enzyme abnormal value). The patients were divided into two cohorts on the basis of their whole-body glucose uptake during the second-step insulin infusion euglycemic clamp. 45 patients in cohort A had a whole-body glucose utilization rate below and the 28 in cohort B above the mean value minus one SD in the overall normal population in our lab (688 mg/min/1.73 m^2). No difference was found between the two cohorts during the clamp with regard to hepatic glucose output, which was higher in both cohorts than in the controls (cohort A vs. cohort B vs. controls: 200 ± 42 vs. 195 ± 48 vs. 66.4 ± 31 µmol/min per 1.73 m^2, $p < 0.01$ vs. both). Thus both cohort A and B patients were resistant to insulin action at the hepatic level.

Whenever hypertension did occur this was recorded, as well as the patient's albumin excretion rate in the 6 months preceding this event. Adequate antihypertensive therapy was commenced and the patient was excluded from further evaluation. Abnormalities in albumin excretion rate (>20 µg/min during the 24-h collection) were not considered a criterion for exclusion unless associated with hypertension.

If diastolic blood-pressure levels remained below 90 mmHg, the follow-up evaluation of these patients was completed in the 6th year (between January 1989 and December 1991, depending upon when they were first seen at baseline). Data evaluation on whole-body glucose utilization rate, i.e., the selection criterion for the two cohorts, was begun in January 1990. Thus throughout the follow-up period neither patients nor doctors were aware of the patient's classification standing.

Insulin sensitivity was assessed using the euglycemic multiple-step insulin clamp technique [4,9,10]. Glycated hemoglobin A1c (HbA1c) was measured by high pressure liquid chromatography and blood glucose by enzymatic technique. Lipoprotein size was measured by nondenaturing polyacrylamide gradient gel electrophoresis [9,11]. Differences among groups were tested by analysis of variance. If a significant difference was found, differences between individual groups were tested by the Tuckey method.

Results

Gender, age, glycated hemoglobin A1c, fasting plasma glucose, fasting plasma insulin, plasma C-peptide, blood pressure and albumin excretion rate in cohort A were all similar, at baseline, to those in the cohort B patients. Patterns on sulphonylurea treatment (42 vs. 52%, respectively) were likewise similar in the two cohorts. LDL size at follow-up was smaller in cohort A than in cohort B (25.9 vs. 27.1, p < 0.01); diastolic blood pressure and albumin excretion rate were higher in cohort A than in cohort B. More particularly, 15 out of 45 (30%) patients in cohort A had blood pressure above 90 mmHg, whereas only 4 out of 28 patients (14%) in cohort B registered such levels (p < 0.01). Micro-albuminuria was likewise found more frequently in cohort A than cohort B (7 out of 45, 15% vs. 2 out of 28, 7%; p < 0.01). Angina pectoris (3/28 vs. 9/45, p < 0.01), silent angina with resting positive ECG (3/28 vs. 9/45, p < 0.01) and positive exercise ECG (4/28 vs. 11/45, p < 0.01) occurred more frequently in cohort A.

Discussion

The novel finding of the present study is that in NIDDM, insulin resistance in extrahepatic tissues precedes the onset of hypertension, microalbuminuria and cardiac ischemic disease. Furthermore, the cohort of patients with such a clustering of clinical features are characterized by an atherogenic lipid profile (i.e., small dense LDL), which is a pheno-typic marker of predisposition to myocardial infarction in nondiabetic populations. Insulin resistance and small dense LDL seem to identify a subset of NIDDM patients with poorer atherosclerotic prognosis which appears to be independent of the challenge of the diabetic disease itself.

The rate of insulin-induced whole-body glucose utilization in NIDDM patients without hypertension and microalbuminuria was on average similar to that in controls. Recently Laakso et al. [12] observed that in extrahepatic tissues insulin resistance is more pronounced in hypertensive than in normotensive nonobese NIDDM subjects. These authors concluded that since hypertension increases insulin resistance only in nonobese patients with NIDDM, this might mean that the etiology of insulin resistance in nonobese and obese subjects with NIDDM is different when hypertension is present. Our data, in keeping with the observations of Laakso et al. [12] and with our previous reports [9–11], provide further evidence supporting the view that the etiology of insulin resistance is different in normotensive and hypertensive NIDDM patients. In fact, impaired insulin-induced glucose uptake by extrahepatic tissues was a clinical hallmark only in those NIDDM patients characterized by abnormalities in blood pressure and in albumin excretion rate.

An important limitation of previous studies linking insulin resistance and hyperin-sulinemia to other metabolic variables is that they have all been cross-sectional. As a result, insulin resistance could conceivably be a consequence of hypertension, rather than a cause of these disorders.

More recently the San Antonio Heart Study reported 8-year prospective data showing a relation between fasting insulin and the incidence of hypertension and NIDDM in Mexican Americans and non-Hispanic whites [13]. This study, however, is based on the assumption that fasting insulin concentration closely reflects insulin resistance despite the observation that insulin resistance is frequently not associated with hyperinsulinemia after an overnight fast.

Our data demonstrate that lower rates of insulin-induced whole-body glucose utilization (a true physiological index of extrahepatic insulin sensitivity) precedes the development of hypertension and microalbuminuria in NIDDM patients.

Questions have arisen concerning the nature of the link between hypertension, microalbuminuria and extrahepatic — rather than hepatic — insulin resistance. Obesity, however, does not appear to be the major factor determining the association between hypertension and insulin resistance, as the San Antonio Heart Study shows that the association between hyperinsulinemia and hypertension was not attributable to differences in baseline obesity [13].

Our study shows that the risk of atherosclerotic vascular complications is not present in all NIDDM patients but is limited to those patients who present at the same time abnormalities in blood pressure, extrahepatic insulin sensitivity, and lipid metabolism. Therefore it seems unlikely that diabetic disease itself is the only determinant of vascular damage in NIDDM, and it is conceivable that other pathogenetic factors play a major role. LDL alterations alone may be responsible for the eventual vascular damage in the subset of NIDDM patients. Identification of the genetic alterations responsible for such an association of clinical abnormalities would allow not only a better understanding of the pathophysiology of the plurimetabolic syndrome but also a more effective prevention of vascular clinical events.

Acknowledgements

Work in part supported by the Italian National Research Council (CNR) grant no. 880193604, Progetto Finalizzato Invecchiamento.

References

1. Reaven GM, Hoffman BB. Lancet 1981;2:435–437.
2. Ferrannini E, Buzzigoli G, Bonadonna E et al. N Engl J Med 1987;317:350–357.
3. Chiang BN, Perlman LV, Epstein FH. Circulation 1969;39:403–413.
4. Doria A, Fioretto P, Avogaro A et al. Am J Physiol 1991;261:E684–691.
5. Trevisan R, Nosadini R, Fioretto P et al. Kidney Int 1992;41:861–885.
6. De Fronzo R, Ferrannini E. Diabet Care 1991;14:173–194.
7. Austin MA, Breslow JL, Hennekens CH et al. J Am Med Assoc 1988;260:1917–1921.
8. The Working Group on Hypertension in Diabetes. Arch Int Med 1987;147:830–842.
9. Nosadini R, Manzato E, Solini A et al. Eur J Clin Invest 1994;24:258–266.
10. Nosadini R, Solini A, Velussi M et al. Diabetes 1994;43:491–499.
11. Zambon S, Manzato E, Solini A et al. Arterioscler Thromb 1994;14:911–916.
12. Laakso M, Sarlund H, Mykkanen L. Eur J Clin Invest 1989;19:518–526.
13. Haffner S, Valdez R, Hazuda H et al. Diabetes 1992;41:715–722.

Neuroendocrine anomalies

Per Mårin

Departments of Medicine and Heart and Lung Diseases, Sahlgren's Hospital, University of Göteborg, Sweden

Several neuroendocrine anomalies have been described in human and experimental obesity. It is becoming increasingly clear that some of these perturbations are found particularly often in visceral obesity, also called abdominal or central obesity. This condition is the entity of human obesity which is particularly closely statistically associated with cardiovascular disease (CVD), non-insulin-dependent diabetes mellitus (NIDDM) and stroke, as well as the established metabolic risk factors for these diseases, including elevated blood pressure [1]. Visceral distribution of body fat seems to be equally common in this cluster of symptoms and diseases as any of the metabolic components [2], and is therefore probably an integrated part of what has been called the metabolic syndrome, Syndrome X or the insulin resistance syndrome.

It should be emphasized that obesity, defined as an increased mass of total body fat, is not essential for this coupling. In epidemiological studies the waist/hip ratio (WHR) is a risk factor independent of obesity (body mass index, BMI) for CVD, NIDDM and stroke. This is particularly striking in men, where the risk of CVD is most pronounced in the leanest men with an elevated WHR. Furthermore, the association with perturbations of metabolism and blood pressure is equally pronounced at low and high BMIs [3]. In summary, obesity is often found in this syndrome, but is not obligatory. The statistical power of associations is usually more pronounced and independent for the distribution factor (WHR or visceral fat by computerized tomography) than for obesity [2]. This is an important distinction, because as will be seen below, there is now considerable evidence to suggest that neuroendocrine anomalies are the main background factors not only for visceral distribution of body fat, but also for the associated metabolic aberrations. The central origin of these neuroendocrine anomalies may well be related to the same regulatory system as energy balance, providing the possibility of understanding why obesity is often, but not always, part of the syndrome.

Cortisol secretion in obesity has been studied previously [4]. Vague [5] and Krotkiewski [6] were early researchers who started to distinguish abnormalities in this variable in relation to android and gynoid obesities. It should be noticed that visceral obesity has several clinical, anthropometric, and metabolic features in common with Cushing's syndrome. It is therefore not far-fetched to examine cortisol concentrations, secretion and turnover in visceral obesity. Recently, this area has attracted renewed attention, providing results which promise to be highly informative. We were able to show that there is a significant increase of urinary output of free cortisol in relation to the WHR or sagittal, abdominal diameter [7], an anthropometric measurement of visceral distribution of body fat [8]. After stimulation of the adrenals with ACTH, cortisol secretion was elevated in this category of subjects, and physical and mental stress tests also showed elevated cortisol responses in subjects with high WHR. We considered this to indicate

Address for correspondence: Per Mårin, Departments of Medicine and Heart and Lung Diseases, Sahlgren's Hospital, University of Göteborg, S-413 45, Sweden. Tel.: +46-31-603995. Fax: +46-31-820600.

increased sensitivity of the limbic-hypothalamo-pituitary-adrenal (LHPA) axis [7]. The elevated response to mental stress tests has recently been confirmed [9]. In addition, Pasquali and his associates confirmed the sensitivity of the peripheral part of the axis, and have provided another piece of important evidence, namely that the response of ACTH and endorphin to corticotrophin-releasing hormone (CRH) is also elevated in women with a high WHR [10]. Evidence presented recently from the same group shows that a similar sensitivity to arginine vasopressin (AVP) is at hand (Pasquali, personal communication, 1994).

There is thus evidence from several groups that the LHPA axis is hypersensitive in subjects with abdominal body fat distribution. The regulation of this axis is dependent on several factors that promote or inhibit the activity. Increased response to stimulation is provided by increased sensitivity of the CRH receptors in the hypophysis, which is dependent on AVP [11]. However, an increased sensitivity is also found proximal to these receptors in the physical and mental stress tests, which suggests that proximal, central nervous system regulations are involved. I discuss this later.

Inhibitory activity is provided via cortisol binding to glucocorticoid receptors (GR), mainly in the hippocampus region of the brain [12]. These GRs are regulated by cortisol secretion in such a way that elevated cortisol secretion downregulates their activity, and may even cause irreversible damage [12]. There is considerable evidence that this occurs in human conditions with increased cortisol secretion such as Cushing's syndrome [13], depression and alcohol abuse [14]. One would then suspect that an increased LPHA axis activity in the metabolic syndrome may in fact cause a downregulation of the GR secondary to increased cortisol secretion, amplifying the cortisol response due to deficient inhibiting activity of the GRs in the brain.

This abnormality can be tested by dexamethasone inhibition tests, where the hypothalamo-pituitary-adrenal (HPA) axis is inhibited by GR effects on CRH secretion. We have performed such tests with the conventional technique without finding certain abnormalities [7]. This problem requires, however, more refined techniques to allow safe conclusions.

As mentioned above, an increased sensitivity proximal to the hypothalamus is suggested by laboratory stress tests [7,9]. One may therefore seek evidence for a primary lesion at this level. The signal systems in brain are involved in these transmissions, where environmental stress might be involved, and the activity of the GRs seems to be regulated via specific 5-hydroxytryptamine receptors [12]. Serotonergic neurons are also of interest from an other aspect. We have found that depressive and anxiety symptoms are coupled to an elevated WHR with associated metabolic perturbations [15,16] as well as increased carbohydrate appetite (unpublished). The role of serotonin in these phenomena is well established [17]. Taken together, these observations suggest an involvement of serotonergic neurons in the metabolic syndrome.

The results from laboratory stress tests mentioned above suggest that environmental stress factors might be involved in the syndrome, sensitizing the distal regulatory stations of the LPHA axis. Such involvement is suggested by other observations. Starting out from an elevated WHR, corrected statistically for the influence of BMI, we have found in population studies relationships to other signs of putative consequences of stress [15,16]. Persons so affected are often absent from work and they have diseases of a psychosomatic character such as peptic ulcer and stomach bleeding. They use free health-care facilities such as X-ray examination frequently. They are often smokers and consume more alcohol than average. Sleep disturbances are common. In addition, psychiatric complaints are significantly more common, including depression and anxiety treated by medication.

These complaints might have a stressful environment as a common background, based on insufficient coping abilities in susceptible personalities. Personality characteristics were also different [15]. Women with a high WHR had high scores of extroversion and affiliation. As mentioned above, they were more often smokers and used more strong liquor than average. This might be considered to be a type of woman with "sensation-seeking" behavior, which might be considered to expose them to frustration and strain, with frequent stress arousals. Women with an elevated BMI (adjusted for WHR) were quite different, with low scores for achievement, aggression and dominance and high scores in sociability [15]. Thus women with elevated WHR seem to be more prone to react badly to a stressful environment than those with an elevated BMI. Such information is not yet available in men. However, men with elevated WHR had signs of socio-economic handicap: low social class, poor education, lack of qualifications and poorly paid jobs [16]. It might be hypothesized that when such men are exposed to environmental stress they will have difficulties meeting it because of the socio-economic handicaps.

In summary, these observations have led us to suggest that psychosocial and socio-economic factors in relation to susceptible personalities are followed by poor coping with stress, and that this might be a reason for sensitization of the LHPA axis. Several of these observations have recently been confirmed.

Finally, the possibility of several interconnected endocrine disturbances in the metabolic syndrome must be discussed in some detail. First, the increased cortisol secretion in visceral-obese subjects can explain directly several of the disturbances recognized in the metabolic syndrome, i.e. insulin resistance, accumulation of visceral fat and hypertension. An increased cortisol secretion can also explain both the relatively low testosterone levels [18] and the signs of decreased growth hormone activity observed in visceral-obese men [19] by inhibiting the secretion and/or action of these hormones. If an increased cortisol secretion is actually responsible for several of the disturbances described in the metabolic syndrome, the use of drugs with cortisol-antagonistic activity would be expected to reduce these disturbances, especially the insulin resistance. At our laboratory we are currently evaluating the effects of ketoconazol (Fungoral™). We have found that this drug dramatically improves insulin resistance in people with visceral obesity and severe insulin resistance and also acts positively on other parts of the metabolic syndrome. Future studies are needed to evaluate the importance of this novel type of treatment further.

References

1. Björntorp P. Obes Res 1993;1:206–222.
2. Lapidus L, Bengtsson C, Björntorp P. Obes Res 1994;2:372–377.
3. Andersson B, Lapidus L, Bengtsson C, Björkelund C, Björntorp P, Lissner L, Lundberg P-A, Lindstedt G. SHBG concentration and hypertension. Results from the population study of women in Göteborg, Sweden. Abstract, 7th International Congress on Obesity 1994.
4. Björntorp P. Diabet Metab Rev 1988;4:615–622.
5. Vague J, Vague P, Boyer J, Cloix MC. In: Rodriguez et al. (eds) Proceedings of the VII Congress of the International Diabetes Function. Excerpta Medica International Congress Series 1970;23:517–525.
6. Krotkiewski M, Butruk E, Zembrzuska Z. Le Diabète 1966;19:229–233.
7. Mårin P, Darin N, Amemiya T, Andersson B, Jern S, Björntorp P. Metabolism 1992;41:882–886.
8. Kvist H, Chowdhury B, Grangård U, Tylén U, Sjöström L. Am J Clin Nutr 1988;48:1351–1361.
9. Moyer AE, Rodin J, Grilo CM, Cummings N, Larson LM, Rebuffé-Scrive M. Obes Res 1994;2:255– 262.
10. Pasquali R, Cantobelli S, Casimirri F, Capelli M, Bortoluzzi L, Flamia R, Labate A, Barbara L. J Clin Endocrinol Metab 1993;77:341–346.
11. Chrousos G, Gold P. J Am Med Assoc 1992;267:1244–1252.
12. Sapolsky R, Krey L, McEwen B. Endocrinol Rev 1986;7:284–301.

532

13. Schteingart GR, Starkman MN, Gebarski SS, Berent S, Schteingart DE. Biol Psychiatry 1992;32:756–765.
14. von Bardeleben U, Holsboer F. J Neuroendocrinology 1989;1:485–488.
15. Lapidus L, Bengtsson C, Hällström T, Björntorp P. Appetite 1989;12:25–35.
16. Larsson B, Seidell JC, Svärdsudd K, Welin L, Tibblin G, Wilhelmsen L, Björntorp P. Appetite 1989;13: 37–44.
17. Eriksson E, Humble M. In: Pohl R, Gershow W (eds) The Biological Aspects of Psychiatric Treatment. Basel: Karger, 1990;3:66–119.
18. Mårin P, Holmäng S, Jönsson L, Kvist H, Sjöström L, Holm G, Björntorp P. Obes Res 1993;1:245–251.
19. Mårin P, Kvist H, Lindstedt G, Sjöström L, Björntorp P. Int J Obes 1993;17:83–89.

Atherosclerosis X.
F.P. Woodford, J. Davignon and A. Sniderman, editors.

Increased prevalence of e4 allele in patients with the plurimetabolic syndrome

I. Reiber[1], J. Schaper[2], H. Eckardt[2], A. Bimmermann[2] and E. Steinhagen-Thiessen[2]

[1]First Department of Internal Medicine, St. George's Hospital Székesfehérvár, Hungary; and [2]Fettstoffwechselambulanz des UKRV der Freie Universität Berlin, Germany

Abstract. The distribution of apolipoprotein E phenotypes in 402 patients with dyslipidemia of different origin has been investigated. Special attention was focused on patients with metabolic syndrome (n = 86). The prevalences of the most frequent apolipoprotein E phenotypes in the whole study group were as follows: E 3/3, E 4/3 and E 3/2: 45.5, 31.3 and 10.2% respectively. The highest prevalence of E 4/4 and E 4/3 was observed in patients with plurimetabolic syndrome (5.8 and 41.9%). The allele frequencies in this group were: e2: 12.8%, e3: 58.7%*** and e4: 28.5%*** vs. 8.2, 78.2 and 13.6% (*** $p < 0.001$) in a normal German population. A possible association is suggested between apolipoprotein E polymorphism and the plurimetabolic syndrome: a significantly higher prevalence of e4 allele was shown in patients with the syndrome.

In numerous epidemiological investigations it has been shown that there is a close correlation between central obesity, hyperinsulinemia, disturbances of carbohydrate, fat and purine metabolism, and hypertension [1]. This cluster of risk factors (summarized under the heading "plurimetabolic syndrome or syndrome X") is closely related to an increased prevalence of cardiovascular diseases and occurs frequently in certain families. The mechanism of how these metabolic disturbances exercise mutual influence is not yet well defined.

The evidence associating apolipoprotein E (apoE) polymorphism with altered lipid and lipoprotein levels and atherosclerosis has been a source of major interest in recent years. The polymorphic gene for apoE is located on chromosome 19: three common alleles, designated e4, e3 and e2, code for three major apoE isoforms in plasma, respectively designated apoE4, apoE3 and apoE2. The mean serum cholesterol concentration is influenced by the different apoE phenotypes (E4 with high, E2 with low cholesterol level). ApoE polymorphism shows association with some kinds of dyslipoproteinemia (type III; familial hypercholesterolemia) [2].

Our study investigated the distribution of apoE phenotypes in patients with dyslipidemia of different origin, with special attention focused on patients with the plurimetabolic syndrome.

Patients and Methods

The retrospective Berlin Outpatient Clinical Study (BOCS) comprised a total of 402 patients (213 males and 189 females) with dyslipidemia (HLP) from the lipid clinics of Freie Universität Berlin. Hypercholesterolemia (HCH) was defined as serum cholesterol >200 mg/dl (5.2 mmol/l) (n = 173); hypertriglyceridemia (HTG) as serum triglycerides >200 mg/dl (2.3 mmol/l) (n = 12) and combined hyperlipidemia (CHL) as both cholesterol

---

Address for correspondence: Dr Reiber, István I. Belgy, Szent György Kórház, 8000 Székesfehérvár, Seregélyesi u. 3. Hungary.

and triglycerides being supranormal (n = 131). 86 subjects were defined as patients with the plurimetabolic syndrome. They had simultaneously hyperlipidemia, diabetes mellitus type II, increased uric acid level (>420 μmol/l), obesity (body mass index ((BMI) >27 kg/m^2) and hypertension (RR >140/90 mmHg).

Serum was collected from a control group of 1,557 normolipidemic factory employees in connection with an epidemiological study, the Munster "Prospective Cardiovascular Study" (PROCAM) [3]. Blood samples in our study were obtained after a 12-h fast. A plasma sample was used for measurement of total cholesterol, high density lipoprotein (HDL)-cholesterol, triglycerides and apoB. ApoE phenotype was determined by isoelectrofocusing from delipidated very low density lipoprotein. Percentage distributions of apoE phenotypes were statistically analyzed (by Student's t-test) and compared to the data of PROCAM Study by means of the SPSS package of statistical programs.

Results

Plasma lipid and lipoprotein levels and BMI for the six apoE phenotypes are given in Table 1.

Figure 1 shows the prevalence of six apoE phenotypes in the dyslipidemic individuals and in the patients with syndrome X and in the control group. The percentage distributions of different apoE phenotypes in the whole study group (HLP) were as follows: homozygous phenotypes E 3/3, E 4/4 and E 2/2 45.5***, 5*** and 4.2%*** respectively (vs. 62.2, 2.2 and 0.9% in PROCAM, *** p < 0.001), heterozygous phenotypes E 4/3, E 3/2 and E 4/2: 31.3%***, 10.2 and 3.7% respectively (vs. 19.9, 11.7 and 2.9% in PROCAM). In the patients with syndrome X as a group, E 4/3 occurred significantly more frequently (41.9%***) and E 3/3 less frequently (31.4%) than in the normal group (19.9 and 62.2% respectively). The similar trend was found in the other hyperlipidemic individuals (HCH and CHL).

Figure 2 shows the allele frequencies of apoE in the five above-mentioned groups. The frequency of e3 allele is significantly (p < 0.001) lower in the group of patients with syndrome X and in individuals with combined hyperlipidemia than in the group of normal individuals. The frequency of e4 allele is significantly (p < 0.001) higher in the whole dyslipidemic population, in the group of patients with CHL and with syndrome X. The allele frequencies in metabolic group were: e2 12.8, e3 58.7*** and e4 28.5%*** vs. 8.2, 78.2 and 13.6% in the normal German population.

Table 1. Plasma lipid and lipoprotein levels (mg/dl) and BMI (kg/m^2) in apoE phenotypes

	E 4/4	E 4/3	E 4/2	E 3/3	E 3/2	E 2/2
Chol	339.0	325.6	322.0	350.3	258.4	281.2
	(±42.5)	(±184.9)	(±161.6)	(±135.1)	(±92.9)	(±70.2)
TG	720.7	631.6	933.7	1035.7	537.0	557.5
	(±414.6)	(±1077.2)	(±917.5)	(±1616.3)	(±561.1)	(±193.5)
HDL-C	23.3	35.9	23.0	36.4	34.9	39.5
	(±12.0)	(±12.2)	(±4.6)	(±11.6)	(±7.2)	(+13.2)
apoB	210.5	160.6	247.3	185.3	153.0	154.2
	(±88.4)	(±39.4)	(±204.5)	(±67.8)	(±72.5)	(±39.4)
BMI	27.3	30.6	29.0	29.0	31.3	27.2
	(±1.8)	(±3.5)	(±1.0)	(±2.9)	(±3.5)	(±2.8)

Values are given as mean ± SD.

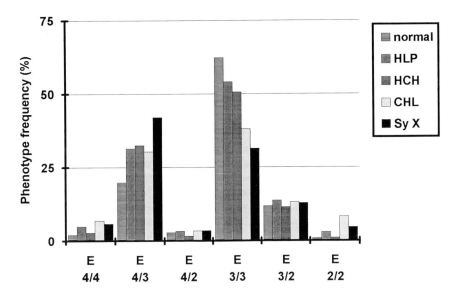

Fig. 1. Prevalence of the six apoE phenotypes in the normal population and in the study groups. HLP, dyslipidemia; HCH, hypercholesterolemia; CHL, combined hyperlipidemia; Sy X, Syndrome X (plurimetabolic syndrome).

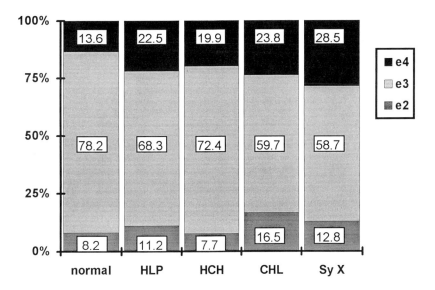

Fig. 2. Allele frequencies of apoE in the normal population and in the study groups.

Discussion

It is well known that the apoE allele exerts a significant effect on plasma lipoprotein concentrations in man. A higher efficiency of enteral cholesterol absorption in subjects with the e4 allele than with e3 or e2, together with the high affinity to apoE4 for lipoproteins of lower density and the faster postprandial fat clearance of E4 individuals, are possible explanations for the elevated plasma and LDL-cholesterol levels seen in carriers of the e4 allele.

In recent years numerous investigations have shown that hyperinsulinemia and insulin resistance are associated with altered concentrations and compositions of lipoproteins [4]. Furthermore there is a close correlation between hyperinsulinemia and hypertension [5].

All the biological processes implicated in the pathogenesis of CHD are likely to have genetic determinants [6]. The gene for apoE is located on chromosome 19 (19q13.2) where it is closely linked to the genes for apoC-I (19q12.2), apoC-II (19q13.2), insulin receptor (19q13.3) and transforming growth factor β-I (19q13.1) and more distantly linked to the gene for the LDL receptor (19p13.3). The major finding of this study was the high prevalence of the e4 allele of apoE in the group of patients with plurimetabolic syndrome compared with subjects without dyslipoproteinemia or with hypercholesterolemia only. Our data suggest that there is an important association between apoE polymorphism and multimetabolic syndrome. Clearly, much more needs to be done to assess the genetic background of this polygenic phenomenon.

References

1. Kaplan NM. Arch Int Med 1989;149:1514–1520.
2. Davignon J et al. Arteriosclerosis 1988;8:1–21.
3. Assmann G et al. Clin Chem 1984;30:641–643.
4. Donahue RP. Endocrinologist 1994;4:112–116.
5. Reaven GM, Hoffmann BB. Lancet 1987;2:435–436.
6. Zebra KE. Curr Opin Lipidiol 1993;4:152–162.

The protective role of the macrophage in atherogenesis: insight from using M-CSF

Robert G. Schaub[1], Lori Hayes Donnelly[1], Thomas S. Parker[2], Steven K. Clinton[3] and Marc B. Garnick[1]

[1]Genetics Institute, Inc., Cambridge, Massachusetts; [2]The Rogosin Institute, New York, NY 10021; and [3]Dana Farber Cancer Institute, Boston MA 02115, USA

Abstract. The pharmacologic administration of recombinant human macrophage colony-stimulating factor (rhM-CSF) decreases plasma cholesterol in normocholesterolemic and hypercholesterolemic animals and also slows progression and enhances regression of atherosclerotic lesions in animal models. Two mechanisms have been postulated to account for these effects. rhM-CSF enhances liver uptake and clearance of serum cholesterol by a mechanism which does not require functional LDL receptors. rhM-CSF may also enhance and stimulate functions related to the catabolism and export of lesion lipids. rhM-CSF increases immunoreactive apolipoprotein E (apoE) within atherosclerotic lesions and increases cholesterol efflux from lipid-laden arteries. Preliminary clinical studies suggest that the hypocholesterolemic effects of rhM-CSF are observed in humans. rhM-CSF may be a useful therapeutic agent for the treatment of severe hyperlipidemia refractory to other treatments or to promote regression of atherosclerotic lesions.

Monocyte-derived macrophages are a major source of lipid-filled foam cells within atherosclerotic lesions [1,2]. Infiltration of monocytes into arteries is one of the earliest events in experimental atherosclerosis and in the pathogenesis of human disease [1,3]. The cascade of signaling events leading to monocyte accumulation may be initiated when oxidatively modified LDL stimulates endothelial cells and induces the expression of the chemokine monocyte chemotactic protein-1 (MCP-1) and VCAM-1 [4,5]. Although macrophage recruitment has classically been interpreted as enhancing lesion development, it is not unreasonable to postulate that these steps are important host responses designed to limit vessel damage to oxidized lipids. However, as the macrophages accumulate lipid, their mobility and metabolic activities are impaired. More monocytes are recruited into the artery while few foam cells migrate out. As lesions become larger and more complex, many of the foam cells die and become the nidus for the necrotic core and cholesterol clefts observed in advanced atherosclerosis. Interventions which can improve the viability, mobility and metabolic activity of macrophages within the vessel wall could be expected to promote lesion regression and reduce lesion progression. For example, lipid-laden macrophages secrete enormous amounts of apolipoprotein E (apoE), an important mediator of reverse cholesterol transport [6,7].

Macrophage colony stimulating factor (M-CSF) is a hematopoietic growth factor that promotes the differentiation, proliferation and activation of cells of the monocyte/macrophage lineage [8,9]. The cloning and expression of recombinant human protein (rhM-CSF) has provided material for experimental studies on atherosclerotic lesion development in

Address for correspondence: Robert G. Schaub PhD, Genetics Institute, Inc., 87 Cambridge Park Drive, Cambridge, MA 02140, USA.

both genetic and diet-induced models of atherosclerosis [10]. The results of these studies have shown that the systemic administration of pharmacologic doses of rhM-CSF has effects on cholesterol clearance and vessel wall biology which reduce progression and enhance regression of atherosclerotic lesions.

rhM-CSF decreases plasma cholesterol

Normocholesterolemic animals

Normocholesterolemic nonhuman primates receiving rhM-CSF by continuous infusion at doses of 25 to 175 µg/kg/day for 14 days had a mean decrease in plasma total cholesterol of 16 ± 8%. Bolus administration of 1 mg/kg/day to nonhuman primates reduced total cholesterol by 43% and LDL-cholesterol by 55% [11].

Infusion of rhM-CSF into normocholesterolemic New Zealand White (NZW) rabbits for 7—14 days reduced total cholesterol from 83 ± 26 mg/dl to 63 ± 23 mg/dl. Studies in normal rabbits infused with ^{125}I-labeled LDL exhibited enhanced clearance of labeled lipid when given rhM-CSF at 100 µg/kg/day (3.75 pools per day vs. 2.07 pools per day) [11].

Hypercholesterolemic animals

More profound effects of rhM-CSF on plasma cholesterol were observed in LDL-receptor-defective Watanabe heritable hyperlipidemic (WHHL) and English half-lop (EHL) rabbit strains. EHL rabbits were treated by intravenous bolus injection with rhM-CSF at doses of 100, 300 or 1,000 µg/kg/day for 7 days. There was a dose-related decrease in serum total cholesterol which was evident by day 3. Nadir was reached by day 5 at 30, 49 and 73% of baseline at 100, 300 and 1,000 µg/kg/day respectively. Most of the decrease in plasma cholesterol was due to a lowering of LDL-cholesterol: 423 ± 81 mg/dl in the control group vs. 246 ± 40, 150 ± 90 and 63 ± 19 mg/dl in the respective treatment groups. A dose-related increase in HDL-cholesterol was observed that seemed to lag behind the fall in plasma LDL-cholesterol by 1—2 days [12]. WHHL rabbits were treated with rhM-CSF at a dose of 100 µg/kg/day by constant intravenous infusion (CIVI) for 14 days. Plasma cholesterol decreased from 606 ± 166 mg/dl to 363 ± 64 mg/dl. The decrease in LDL-cholesterol accounted for almost the entire decline (475 ± 147 mg/dl vs. 292 ± 37 mg/dl). HDL-cholesterol increased over 400% from 6 ± 1 mg/dl to 25 ± 7 mg/dl during treatment. ^{125}I-labeled LDL was cleared more rapidly from the plasma of WHHL rabbits treated with rhM-CSF. Their mean fractional catabolic rate was 1.23 pools per day compared with 0.43 pool per day in untreated WHHL rabbits [11].

rhM-CSF enhances biliary excretion of cholesterol

Bile fistulas were placed into three EHL rabbits to permit collection of bile during rhM-CSF (500 µg/kg/day, CIVI) treatment. Treated rabbits had a 200 mg/dl lower plasma cholesterol than nontreated controls with bile fistulas. Total cholic acid excretion into the bile was increased over 50% (Fig. 1). This increase in cholic acid output over the 3—5 days of rhM-CSF treatment is equivalent to an additional 266 mg of cholesterol excreted. Cholesterol-fed (0.25% cholesterol/4.75% hydrogenated coconut oil/95% rabbit chow) NZW rabbits were treated with rhM-CSF (200 µg/kg/day, CIVI, n = 6) or vehicle (n = 6) using implanted ALZET™ pumps. Plasma cholesterol was decreased by 50% in rhM-CSF-treated animals. Bile was collected on the last day of treatment. The increase in bile salt concentration (625 ± 269 mM vs. 350 ± 162 mM) in the rhM-CSF-treated animals

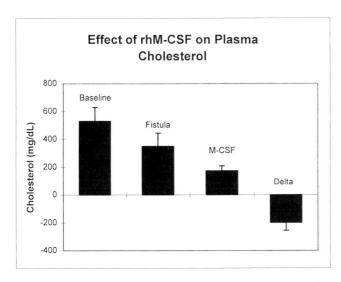

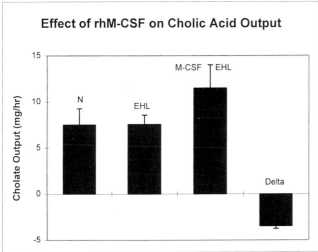

Fig. 1. rhM-CSF administration to EHL rabbits (500 µg/kg CIVI) induced a decrease in plasma cholesterol in excess of that produced by the presence of the bile fistula (upper panel). Baseline cholic acid secretion in bile-fistula WHHL rabbits was similar to normal rabbits (N) (lower panel). rhM-CSF treatment increased bile cholic acid secretion of EHL rabbits (lower panel) in parallel with the decrease in plasma cholesterol. The delta value represents the change in output produced by rhM-CSF treatment.

was consistent with the increased hepatic cholesterol clearance observed in studies of rabbits with a bile fistula.

rhM-CSF promotes reverse cholesterol transport from peripheral tissue

rhM-CSF (128 ng/ml) was found to enhance the uptake and degradation of both ^{125}I-oxidized and ^{125}I-acetyl-LDL in cultured macrophages [13]. rhM-CSF increased the B_{max} for degradation 5-fold for acetyl-LDL and 2-fold for oxidized LDL, but did not change

540

the K_m of degradation significantly [13]. rhM-CSF can also enhance cholesterol efflux from macrophages. Acetyl-LDL pretreated macrophages were incubated in lipoprotein-deficient serum medium for 8 h in the presence or absence of rhM-CSF (128 ng/ml). Cellular cholesterol decreased almost 50% in the treated cells compared to only 10% in the untreated cells [13]. In this same study, the specific radioactivity of plasma cholesterol was measured 1 month after injection of 150 μCi of [³H]cholesterol. rhM-CSF administered at 300 μg/kg/day for 7 days decreased plasma cholesterol by 21% and increased the specific activity of HDL-cholesterol 1.4-fold, which suggests movement of cholesterol from tissue to plasma. During rhM-CSF treatment (100, 300, 1,000 μg/kg/day for 7 days) of EHL rabbits, lipoprotein size was also measured by nondenaturing polyacrylamide gradient gel electrophoresis. HDL particle size was shifted to larger diameters in a dose-dependent manner (Fig. 2). This increased HDL particle size correlated with a decreased plasma cholesterol concentration. The increased HDL size is consistent with increased cholesterol accumulation onto the HDL particle, as occurs with reverse cholesterol transport.

rhM-CSF decreases atherosclerotic lesion formation

To evaluate the effect of rhM-CSF on atherosclerotic lesion formation, we treated WHHL rabbits with rhM-CSF at 100 μg/kg/day for 5 weeks followed by 300 μg/kg/day for an additional 3 weeks by CIVI or vehicle. rhM-CSF treatment significantly decreased plasma cholesterol through weeks 1–4 (p < 0.05). Plasma cholesterol remained lower than controls from weeks 5–8, but due to the increasing concentrations of host anti-rhM-CSF antibody the biological activity of administered rhM-CSF was reduced. Lesion distribution in both the thoracic (47 ± 27% in rhM-CSF vs. 73 ± 16% in control) and abdominal (57

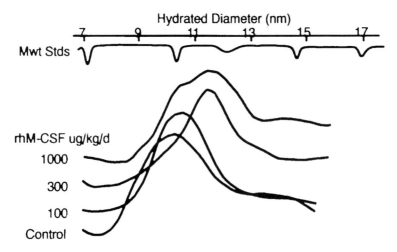

Native Gradient Gel Electrophoresis 4-30% of Rabbit HDL

Hydrated Diameter (nm)

Representative scans from plasma taken after 5-days of rhM-CSF

Fig. 2. HDL particle size was shifted to larger diameters in a dose-dependent manner following rhM-CSF treatment (100, 300, 1,000 μg/kg/day). The increase in HDL particle size correlated with a decrease in plasma cholesterol concentration.

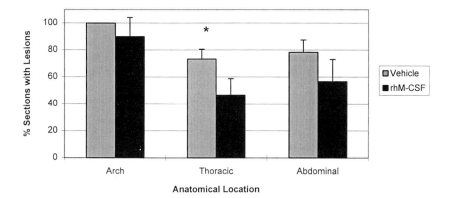

Fig. 3. Mean percent sections with atherosclerotic lesions. The thoracic and abdominal aortas of rhM-CSF treated WHHL rabbits had fewer histologically identified atherosclerotic lesions than vehicle control rabbits in the nonarch thoracic region (p < 0.05) and the abdominal region (ns).

± 17% in rhM-CSF vs. 78 ± 20% in controls) aortas was also decreased (Fig. 3). Total aortic cholesterol content was decreased, although not significantly, in rhM-CSF treated rabbits (2.1 ± 0.8 µg/mg in rhM-CSF vs. 1.6 ± 0.3 µg/mg in controls, p > 0.05) (Fig. 4). However, aortic cholesteryl ester concentrations were significantly lower in the rhM-CSF-treated animals (0.2 ± 0.3 µg/mg) than in controls (1.0 ± 0.1 µg/mg) (p < 0.05). Cholesterol lowering induced by rhM-CSF has also been correlated with decreased foam-cell development in macrophage-rich carrageenan-induced granulomas in WHHL rabbits and with enhanced regression of atherosclerotic lesions in WHHL and cholesterol-fed New Zealand white rabbits [14,15].

Immunoreactive M-CSF and apoE in atherosclerotic lesions of WHHL rabbits is increased by rhM-CSF treatment

Aortic tissues from rhM-CSF treated and control rabbits were examined by immunohisto-chemistry for localization and distribution of immunoreactive M-CSF and apoE. Atheromata of vehicle-treated animals showed both M-CSF and apoE located in medial macrophages closest to the lumen, while deeper regions of lesion exhibited less intense staining. Treatment with rhM-CSF increased the intensity of immunoreactive M-CSF within the medial region of lesions. Lesion apoE staining appeared to be increased after rhM-CSF treatment, especially within the intracellular and extracellular space (Fig. 4).

Discussion

The importance of endogenous cytokines, growth factors and immunomodulators in atherogenesis is now appreciated but not well understood [16]. M-CSF is one of the few cytokines which is found in biologically active concentrations in the plasma of healthy individuals [17]. Over 90% of M-CSF is selectively cleared by the macrophage receptor (c-fms), which suggests an important feedback control mechanism between the cytokine and its target cell population [18]. It is interesting that partially oxidized LDL will both induce the expression of M-CSF in cultured endothelial cells and cause the release of M-CSF into serum following intravenous administration, which suggests a relationship between atherogenic lipids and M-CSF production [19]. M-CSF gene expression and immunoreactive protein has been demonstrated within the endothelium, smooth muscle

542

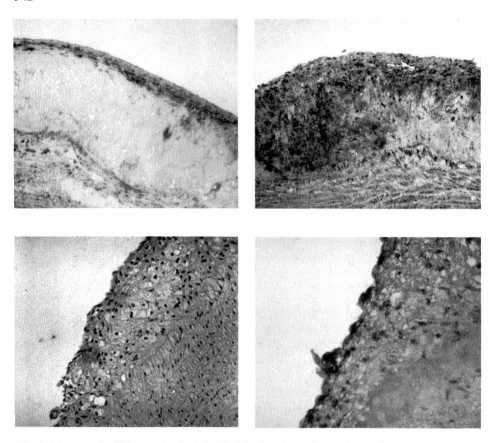

Fig. 4. Atheroma of vehicle-treated animals had both M-CSF (upper left) and apoE (lower left) localized in luminal macrophages (dark grey, black areas). Treatment with rhM-CSF increased the intensity of immunoreactive M-CSF (upper right) within the medial region of lesions. ApoE staining (lower right) increased in the lumen and the medial area in what appeared to be both foam cell-associated and extracellular accumulation.

cells and macrophages associated with atherosclerotic lesions [20,21]. The presence of M-CSF within the arterial lesion has led to speculation that the protein may play a role in promoting atherosclerosis by enhancing monocyte recruitment, proliferation, foam-cell development and the release of monocyte-derived growth factors for smooth muscle cells and pathogenic cytokines [22]. The importance of M-CSF as a maintenance factor for monocyte/macrophages has also led to the speculation that M-CSF may be important in maintaining long-term survival of macrophages within lesions and that necrosis of foam cells in advanced lesions may occur because of a deficiency in local M-CSF production [15,21]. The role of endogenously produced M-CSF by endothelial cells, smooth muscle cells and macrophages within the vessel wall will depend on the forms of M-CSF expressed as well as the balance and coordination of the broader cytokine network.

rhM-CSF injection produces a rapid decline in total plasma cholesterol to levels which have been demonstrated to reduce the rate of progression and promote the regression of atherosclerotic lesions in humans [23]. The correlation of the plasma cholesterol decrease with increased biliary secretion of cholesterol would suggest that much of this decrease is due to excretion by the liver. The fact that this rapid decrease in cholesterol can occur in LDL-receptor-deficient animals suggests a mechanism unrelated to this receptor. LDL-receptor-independent clearance of cholesterol accounts for 40—60% of LDL removal by the liver, depending on species and conditions [24,25]. Recent evidence has indicated that a number of additional receptors and other mechanisms can have a role in cholesterol clearance. Two of these pathways are the apoE-binding protein known as the LDL-receptor-related protein (LRP) and the lipolysis-stimulated receptor [26,27]. Although we have no direct evidence that rhM-CSF enhances expression of these alternative receptors, it has been shown that LRP expression of bone marrow-derived macrophages is increased by M-CSF [28]. rhM-CSF administration may also improve the efficiency of hepatic receptor function. rhM-CSF administration induces the proliferation and activation of the Kupffer cells (hepatic macrophages) within the hepatic sinusoids. M-CSF will also induce synthesis of both apoE and lipoprotein lipase by macrophages [20,29]. Both of these factors are important in coordinating the uptake of lipids by the LRP receptor [6,7,30,31]. Indirect support for this hypothesis is found in the study by Cai et al. in which monocyte-macrophage activation by systemic administration of zymosan to cholesterol-fed rats significantly decreased plasma VLDL and LDL by increased hepatic clearance of lipids [32].

The studies reported here would suggest that pharmacologic doses of M-CSF can significantly reduce the development of atherosclerosis in animal models. The mechanism(s) responsible for this beneficial effect appear to be related to M-CSF's effect on plasma lipids and to M-CSF-induced changes within the atherosclerotic lesion. Taken together, these data suggest a potentially important role for M-CSF in regulating the metabolism and clearance of atherogenic lipids. M-CSF may be the first example of an endogenous factor capable of regulating reverse cholesterol transport.

Acknowledgements

The authors wish to thank Audry Rudd, Joseph Loscalzo, Daniel Levine, Thomas Donnelly, Mark Bree, Thomas Ferranti, Liz Lavigne, Larry Mason, Jamie Erickson, Joanne Donovan, David Bilheimer and John Stoudemire for their assistance and collaboration in the performance of the studies discussed in this manuscript.

References

1. Faggiotto A, Ross R, Harker L. Arteriosclerosis 1984;4:323—340.
2. Gerrity RG. Am J Pathol 1981;103:181—190.
3. Ross R. Am J Pathol 1993;143:987—1002.
4. Navab M, Imes SS, Hama SY, Hough GP, Ross LA, Bork RW, Valente AJ, Berliner JA, Drinkwater DC, Laks H, Fogelman AM. J Clin Invest 1991;88:2039—2046.
5. Cybulski M, Gimbrone M. Science 1991;251:788—791.
6. Yamada N, Inoue M, Harada K, Watanabe Y, Shimano H, Gotoda T, Shimada M, Kohzaki K, Tsukada T, Shiomi M, Watanabe Y, Yazaki Y. J Clin Invest 1992;89:706—711.
7. Rosenfeld ME, Butler S, Ord VA, Lipton BA, Dyer CA, Curtiss LK, Palinski W, Witztum JL. Arterioscler Thromb 1993;13:1382—1389.
8. Metcalf D. J Cell Physiol 1970;76:89—100.
9. Stanley ER, Guilbert LJ, Tushinski RJ, Bartelmez SH. J Cell Biochem 1983;21:151—159
10. Wong GG, Temple AA, Leary AC, Witek-Giannotti JS, Yank Y-C, Ciarletta AB, Chung M, Murtha P, Kriz R, Kaufman RJ, Ferenz CR, Sibley BS, Turner KJ, Hewick RM, Clark SC, Yanai N, Yokota H, Yamada M, Saito M, Motoyoshi K, Takaku F. Science 1987;235:1504—1508.
11. Stoudemire JB, Garnick MB. Blood 1991;77:750—755.
12. Parker TS, Levine DM, Donnelly TM, Stoudemire JB, Garnick MB. Circulation 1990;82(suppl III):III—233.
13. Yamada N, Ishibashi S, Shimano H, Inaba T, Gotoda T, Harada K, Shimada M, Shiomi M, Watanabe Y, Kawakami M, Yazaki Y, Takaku F. Proc Soc Exp Biol Med 1992;200:240—244.

544

14. Inoue I, Inaba T, Moyoyoshi K, Harada K, Shimano H, Kawamura M, Gotoda T, Oka T, Shiomi M, Watanabe Y, Tsukada T, Yazaki Y, Takaku F, Yamada N. Atherosclerosis 1992;93:245–254.
15. Schaub RG, Bree MP, Hayes LL, Rudd MA, Rabbani L, Loscalzo J, Clinton SK. Arterioscler Thromb 1994;14:70–76.
16. Clinton SK, Libby P. Arch Pathol Lab Med 1992;116:1292–1300.
17. Bartocci A, Pollard JW, Stanley ER. J Exp Med 1986;164:956–961.
18. Bartocci A, Mastrogiannis DS, Migliorati G, Stockert RJ, Wolkoff AW, Stanley ER. Proc Natl Acad Sci USA 1987;84:6179–6183.
19. Liao F, Berliner JA, Mehrabian M, Navab M, Demer LL, Lusis AJ, Fogelman AM. J Clin Invest 1991;87:2253–2257.
20. Clinton SK, Underwood R, Hayes L, Sherman ML, Kufe DW, Libby P. Am J Pathol 1992;140:301–316.
21. Rosenfeld ME, Herttuala S, Lipton BA, Ord VA, Witztum JL, Steinberg D. Am J Pathol 1992;140:291–300.
22. Shyy Y-J, Wickham LL, Gagan JP, Hsieh H-J, Hu Y-L, Telian SH, Valente AJ, Sung K-LP, Chien S. J Clin Invest 1993;92:1745–1751.
23. Brown G, Albers JJ, Fisher LD, Schaefer SM, Lin J-T, Kaplan C, Zhao X-Q, Bisson BD, Fitzpatrick VF, Dodge HT. N Engl J Med 1990;323:1289–1298.
24. Meddings JB, Spady DK, Dietschy JM. Am Heart J 1987;113(IIpt2):475–481.
25. Spady DK, Huettinger M, Bilheimer DW, Dietschy JM. J Lipid Res 1987;28:32–41.
26. Beisiegel U, Weber W, Ihrki G, Herz J, Stanley KK. Nature 1989;341:162–164.
27. Yen FT, Mann CJ, Bihain BE. Arterioscler Thromb 1991;11:1410a.
28. Hussaini IM, Srikumar K, Quesenberry PJ, Gonias SL. J Biol Chem 1990;265:19441–19446.
29. Goldman R, Sopher O. Biochim Biophys Acta 1989;1001:120–126.
30. Shimano H, Shimada M, Gotoda T, Herada K, Yamada N. Circulation 1993;88:I–2.
31. Mann A, Meyer N, Weber W, Rinninger F, Greten H, Beisiegel U. Circulation 1993;88:I–321.
32. Cai H-J, He Z-G, Ding Y-N. Biochim Biophys Acta 1988;959:334–342.
33. Shimano H, Yamada N, Ishibashi S, Harada K, Matsumoto A, Mori N, Inaba T, Motoyoshi K, Itakura H, Takaku F. J Biol Chem 1990;265:12869–12875.

Atherosclerosis X.
F.P. Woodford, J. Davignon and A. Sniderman, editors.

Calcium antagonists and atherosclerosis: current status, new directions

Nemat O. Borhani

Internal Medicine, School of Medicine, University of California, Davis and School of Medicine, University of Nevada, Reno, Nevada, P.O. Box 969, Carnelian Bay, CA 96140, USA

Abstract. The process of atherosclerosis begins with a sustained injury to the surface of endothelium. Hypertension causes such an injury. Thus, control of hypertension should, at least in theory, prevent atherosclerosis. Calcium antagonists are new antihypertensive agents with different degrees of potency in their antiatherogenic properties. For example, isradipine, which like nifedipine is a dihydropyridine calcium antagonist, has shown in animal models more pronounced antiatherogenic effects than nifedipine. Clinical trials have been conducted to test the anti-atherogenic effect of calcium antagonists in man, of which one was the Multicenter Isradipine Diuretic Atherosclerosis Study (MIDAS). Results of MIDAS over 36 months showed that isradipine generally had a positive effect (p = 0.02) on progression of extracranial carotid intima-media thickness (IMT), a surrogate for atherosclerosis.

With the advent of noninvasive methods such as B-mode ultrasound, the prevalence of subclinical atherosclerotic disease in the population can be detected. Its magnitude is not trivial. For example, in a study of men and women aged 65 years and above, 37.2% had evidence of subclinical atherosclerotic disease (e.g., common carotid wall thickness in the upper 80th percentile, or carotid artery stenosis of more than 25%) with no history or symptoms of clinical manifestation of atherosclerosis [1]. Obviously, prevention of the progression from subclinical to clinical disease should have a major impact on morbidity and mortality statistics.

Results of recent studies of the cellular and molecular biology of the arterial wall have focused our attention on the pathogenesis of atherosclerosis. They have shown that injury to the surface of the endothelium, caused by hypertension, cigarette smoking, hyper-lipidemia, and diabetes, disrupts vascular integrity, causes endothelial dysfunction, and results in the formation of atherosclerotic lesions [2]. These observations confirm what we have known from numerous epidemiologic studies, that certain risk factors, such as hypertension, are independent predictors of morbidity and mortality. These risk factors are known to cause injury to the surface of endothelium. Thus, an effective strategy for prevention must address the issue of how these factors could be altered in the general population. In this presentation I have chosen hypertension as a model to address this question.

Hypertension and atherosclerosis

The endothelial cells respond to uncontrolled hypertension by making adaptive changes which are characterized by increased migration and proliferation of smooth muscle cells, production of vasoactive substances such as endothelium-derived relaxing factors (EDRF), endothelin, angiotensin converting enzyme (ACE), and platelet-derived growth factor (PDGF). These adaptive changes set the stage for vasoconstrictive response to the vasoactive substances [3]. The risk of clinical manifestations of atherosclerotic diseases, such as acute myocardial infarction, rises with increasing severity of hypertension. Further, hypertension in the presence of other risk factors exerts a synergistic effect on the risk of atherosclerotic disease [4]. Although the reported efficacy of drug treatment of hypertension in reducing morbidity and mortality from stroke has been very impressive and according to expectation, this has not been consistently the case for coronary heart disease [5]. There are several explanations for this paradox. On the one hand, the adverse metabolic effects of antihypertensive drugs used in clinical trials may have blunted the beneficial effect of drug therapy on the incidence of coronary heart disease. On the other hand, the use of clinical events as primary endpoints for these trials may not have been appropriate. The development of alternatives to traditional antihypertensive drugs and the search for a suitable endpoint as a surrogate for clinical events have been the focus of recent research. Considerable progress has been made on both fronts. New classes of antihypertensive agents, such as calcium antagonists, have been developed and studied for their antiatherogenic properties; and B-mode ultrasound has been utilized to test the effect of therapy on the atherosclerotic process whose first result is thickening of the intimamedia.

Calcium antagonists and atherosclerosis

The principal mechanism of action of calcium antagonists is to interfere with calcium uptake by vascular smooth muscle cells, causing vasodilatation. By inhibiting transmembrane calcium-ion flux, these agents produce arterial vasodilation and a reduction in blood pressure [6]. Thus, they are capable of reversing the main hemodynamic abnormality in essential hypertension (i.e., peripheral vasoconstriction and vascular resistance). In addition, calcium antagonists, especially those in the dihydropyridine class, have shown, mostly in animal experiments, a specific antiatherogenic property. A study in cholesterol-fed rabbits first demonstrated [7] the antiatherogenic properties of relatively high doses of nifedipine. Isradipine in smaller doses, similar to those recommended for treatment of hypertension in man (2.5–5.0 mg/kg), inhibited the formation of intimal plaque, which usually develops after balloon injury to the rat carotid artery [8]. Other studies have shown that isradipine reduces, in cholesterol-fed rabbits, the impairment of endothelium-dependent relaxation, and the uptake of cholesterol by the arterial wall [9,10].

Several hypotheses have been postulated to explain the mechanism for the antiatherogenic action of calcium antagonists. Most of these hypotheses deal with the antihypertensive action of these drugs, and postulate that hemodynamically these agents reduce the level of blood pressure and hence the shear stress on the arterial wall. Also, it has been suggested that calcium antagonists repress myoproliferation in response to injury by inhibiting thymidine incorporation into smooth muscle DNA [11]. The antiatherogenic properties of isradipine may lie in its ability to inhibit gene expression for scavenger receptors, leading to a reduction in the formation of foam cells and fatty streaks, and this inhibition of the development of fatty streaks may be due to a reduction in the volume of cellular and noncellular components of the intima [12]. Results from these animal experiments have stimulated clinical trials to test the antiatherogenic properties of calcium antagonists in man, such as INTACT, The Montreal Heart Institute Study, and MIDAS [13–15].

MIDAS was a double-blind, randomized, positive controlled clinical trial. The primary endpoint of the trial was to compare, using B-mode ultrasound, the effect of two drugs (isradipine and a diuretic) on the progression of the mean maximum intima-media thickness (IMT) in carotid artery walls. A total of 883 patients who met all the inclusion

Table 1. Description of MIDAS population characteristics at baseline

Variables	Isradipine	HCTZ[a]	Total
Mean age (yr)	58.2	58.7	58.5
Mean systolic BP (mmHg)	150.6	148.9	149.7
Mean diastolic BP (mmHg)	96.7	96.2	96.5
Mean serum cholesterol (mmol/l)	5.6	5.6	5.6
Mean maximum IMT 12 walls (mm)	1.17	1.17	1.17
Mean maximum IMT 6 near walls (mm)	1.16	1.16	1.16
Mean maximum IMT 6 far walls (mm)	1.18	1.20	1.19
Mean maximum IMT Common carotid (mm)	0.98	0.98	0.98
Mean maximum IMT Bifurcation (mm)	1.45	1.44	1.45

[a]Hydrochlorothiazide. IMT = intima-media thickness.

Table 2. The primary and secondary B-mode endpoints (outcome measures) in MIDAS

Outcome measures	Mean IMT change from baseline to 3 years (mm)		Absolute difference (mm)	p value drug effect
	Isradipine	Hydrochlorothiazide		
Primary endpoint IMT overall	0.121	0.149	−0.028	0.02
Secondary endpoints				
Diseased segment	0.086	0.121	−0.035	0.02
Common carotid	0.064	0.061	0.003	0.07
Bifurcation	0.154	0.208	−0.054	0.01
Far walls of common carotid and bifurcation	0.178	0.200	−0.022	<0.01

criteria, and who gave informed consent, were randomized into the two treatment groups, and were monitored for 3 years. Table 1 presents a summary description of the MIDAS population characteristics at baseline. Both drugs were equally effective antihypertensive agents.

Table 2 presents a summary of the findings on the primary and secondary B-mode endpoint measurements. Overall, the progression of IMT from baseline to the 36th month had slowed more in the isradipine-treated group than in the diuretic group (p = 0.02). This difference between the two drug regimens was observed at the 6-month visit and persisted for the duration of the trial. The beneficial effect of isradipine on the progression of IMT was most pronounced at the bifurcation (p = 0.01), in the far walls of the combined bifurcation and common carotid artery (p < 0.01), and in the diseased segment of the carotid arteries.

Future directions

For the immediate future the focus of attention should be towards identification of a precise molecular mechanism of the antiatherogenic action of calcium antagonists, at first

548

in animal models. Attention should also be directed to the role of other channels, such as the R channel [16] as well as the action of these agents on glycosaminoglycans.

References

1. Kuller LH, Borhani NO et al. Am J Epidemiology 1994;139:1164—1179.
2. Ross R. N Engl J Med 1986;314:488—500.
3. Dzau VJ. J Cardiovasc Pharmacol 1990;15(suppl 5):S59—S69.
4. Borhani, NO. In: Yanowitz FG (ed) Coronary Heart Disease Prevention. New York, Basel, Hong Kong: Marcel Dekker Inc. 1992;251—272.
5. Collins R, Peto R et al. Lancet 1990;335:827—838.
6. Man In't Veld AJ. Am J Med 1989;86(suppl 4A):6—14.
7. Henry PD, Bentley KL. J Clin Invest 1981;68:1366—1369.
8. Handley DA, Van Valen RG et al. Am J Pathol 1986;124:88—93.
9. Habib JB, Bossaller C et al. Circ Res 1986;58:305—309.
10. Weinstein DB, Heider JG. Am J Cardiol 1987;59:163B—172B.
11. Jackson CL, Bush RC et al. Atherosclerosis 1988;69:115—122.
12. Skepper JN, Kappagoda CT. Atherosclerosis 1992;96:17—31.
13. Lichtlen PR, Hugenholtz PG et al. Lancet 1990;335:1109—1113.
14. Waters D, Lesperance J et al. Circulation 1990;82:1940—1953
15. Borhani NO, Miller ST et al. J Cardiovasc Pharmacol 1992;19(suppl 3):S16—S20.
16. Bkaily G, Economos D. Mol Cell Biochem 1992;117:93—106.

Radical therapy of atherosclerosis by apheresis or liver transplantation

G.R. Thompson and A. Sussekov

Lipoprotein Team, MRC Clinical Sciences Centre, Hammersmith Hospital, Royal Postgraduate Medical School, London, UK

Abstract. The commonest indication for radical antiatherosclerotic therapy is severe familial hyper-cholesterolemia (FH) i.e., homozygotes or drug-resistant heterozygotes. Liver transplantation can completely normalize plasma lipoproteins, including Lp(a), in homozygous FH, but necessitates long-term immunosuppression. Extracorporeal cholesterol removal by plasma exchange or LDL apheresis is less effective but safer. It has been shown to increase life-expectancy in homozygotes but offers no advantage over combination drug therapy in most heterozygotes, even those with high Lp(a) levels. Evidence from angiographic trials suggests that the pathogenicity of Lp(a) is diminished if accompanying levels of LDL are kept low. To obtain more direct evidence a pilot study of Lp(a) apheresis was undertaken in four heterozygotes with markedly raised Lp(a) and persistent coronary disease and endothelial dysfunction despite normalized LDL levels. The results were equivocal and whether therapeutic reduction of Lp(a) is advantageous remains unresolved at present.

Radical therapy is used mainly to treat patients with familial hypercholesterolemia (FH) which is unresponsive to conventional lipid-lowering drug therapy. Patients who fall into this category are mainly homozygotes, but heterozygotes with coronary heart disease (CHD) who are refractory to or intolerant of drug therapy are also eligible.

Plasmapheresis and LDL apheresis

As reviewed in 1989 [1] plasmapheresis plays an important role in the management of severe FH. Initially, plasma exchange was used and this has markedly improved the life expectancy of treated homozygotes [2], as shown in Table 1. Plasma exchange is still used in some centers but is becoming obsolete with the introduction of more specific methods of extracorporeal cholesterol removal.

LDL apheresis has largely replaced plasma exchange in the treatment of a raised LDL-cholesterol although double-filtration apheresis provides a compromise between the two types of procedure in cost and specificity. The two most popular techniques for LDL apheresis are the Kaneka twin-column MA01 system, which uses dextran sulfate to adsorb LDL from plasma and the Braun HELP System, which uses heparin to precipitate LDL at low pH.

One of the theoretical advantages of LDL apheresis is that not only LDL but also Lp(a) is removed from plasma. However, data from a regression trial using diet and exercise [3] suggest that Lp(a) loses its adverse influence on CHD if accompanying LDL-cholesterol levels are sufficiently low. This conclusion is supported by the results of the FH Regression Study, which compared LDL apheresis plus simvastatin with colestipol plus simvastatin in patients with heterozygous FH [4]. The reduction in both LDL and

Address for correspondence: Dr G.R. Thompson, Lipoprotein Team, MRC Clinical Sciences Centre, Hammersmith Hospital, Royal Postgraduate Medical School, London W12 0NN, UK.

Table 1. Age now or at death of five pairs of homozygous siblings according to whether or not they were plasmapheresed (updated from [2])

	Male/Female	Age (SD)	Deceased
Untreated	4/1	17.7[a] (3.8)	5/5
Treated	4/1	29.0[a] (2.4)	3/5

[a]$p < 0.001$.

Lp(a) achieved by apheresis plus simvastatin was no more advantageous in arresting progression or inducing regression of coronary disease than the reduction in LDL alone resulting from dual drug therapy.

Lp(a) apheresis

In an attempt to determine whether Lp(a) is pathogenic in the absence of a raised LDL-cholesterol, a small pilot study was undertaken of Lp(a) apheresis in FH heterozygotes with markedly raised Lp(a) levels and evidence of persistent CHD, despite effective reduction of LDL-cholesterol by conventional drug therapy. Immunoadsorption columns (Pocard, Moscow) were used to selectively remove Lp(a) from plasma, as described by Pokrovsky et al. [5]. Combination drug therapy was maintained throughout and progress was monitored by noninvasive indices of arterial endothelial function.

Patients were randomly allocated to receive no additional treatment (controls) or to undergo Lp(a) apheresis at weekly intervals for 6 months. Initially one immunoadsorption column was used per procedure, but to obtain greater reduction of Lp(a) two columns were used sequentially for the second 3 months of the study. No serious side effects were observed but the impact of Lp(a) apheresis on indices of endothelial function was equivocal, as shown in Table 2. Flow- and nitrate-mediated vasodilatation improved but exercise tolerance and von Willebrand factor levels did not change. The main limitation was the inadequate reduction in Lp(a) achieved owing to its rapid rate of rebound.

For the present it seems advisable to reduce LDL-cholesterol but not Lp(a) in those with established CHD. However, in view of the data that elevated levels of Lp(a) adversely affect endothelial function [6], larger studies are needed using Lp(a) apheresis combined with an adjuvant form of drug therapy which slows Lp(a) rebound without

Table 2. Pilot study of Lp(a) apheresis in four men with FH and CHD receiving anion-exchange resin and simvastatin therapy. Mean values are shown

	Control group (n = 2)			Apheresis group (n = 2)		
	Baseline	3 months	6 months	Baseline	3 months	6 months
Lp(a) (mg/dl)	154.5	159.5	168.5	141	92.6[a]	84.4[a]
LDL-C (mmol/l)	3.35	3.15	3.50	3.6	3.9[a]	3.8[a]
FMVD (%)	2	–	2.5	0.5	3.0	6
NMVD (%)	10.3	–	3	15	19.5	24.5
RPP at –1 mm	165	–	156.5	189	220	195
vWF (U/ml)	0.95	–	1.23	0.80	1.57	0.87

FMVD and NMVD = flow-mediated and nitrate-mediated vasodilatation as gauged by change in brachial artery diameter; RPP at –1 mm = rate pressure product at 1 mm ST segment depression using Bruce protocol; vWF = von Willebrand factor. [a]Integrated mean over each 3-month period.

Table 3. Known instances of liver transplantation (Tx) with or without cardiac transplantation in FH homozygotes

Authors	Procedure	Outcome	Adjuvant statin therapy
Statzl et al. (1984)	Double Tx	Died after 5 years	Yes
Shaw et al. (1985)	2 double Tx's	Operative deaths	–
Bilheimer (personal communication)	Double Tx	Operative death	–
Hoeg et al. (1987)	Liver Tx	Alive after 9 years	No
Valdivieso et al. (1988)	Double Tx	Alive after 8.5 years	Yes
Barbir et al. (1992)	Double Tx	Alive after 4 years	No

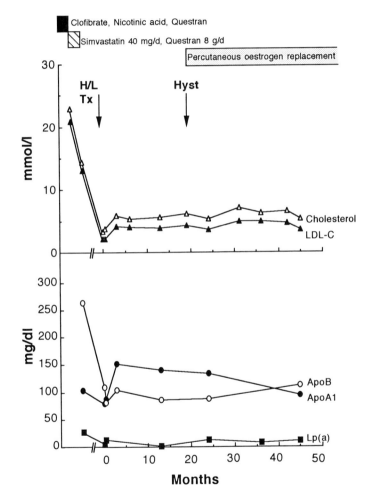

Fig. 1. Total and LDL-cholesterol, apolipoprotein A-I, B and Lp(a) levels in serum before and after combined heart and liver transplantation (H/L Tx) and bilateral oophorectomy/hysterectomy (Hyst).

altering other variables which influence atherosclerosis. Lp(a) apheresis is a valuable research tool but is unlikely to prove useful as a clinical procedure since LDL apheresis removes Lp(a) from plasma just as efficiently as LDL.

552

Liver transplantation

The first combined heart and liver transplantation on an FH homozygote was successfully performed 10 years ago. Subsequent treatment with lovastatin resulted in complete normalization of LDL turnover [7], indicating the dominant role normally played by hepatic LDL receptors in the regulation of plasma LDL levels. This patient subsequently died, as did three others who underwent liver transplantation combined with cardiac transplantation (Table 3). However, the last three cases to be published [8–10], two of them double transplants, have now survived for periods of 9, 8½ and 4 years respectively.

As shown in Fig. 1 the most recently transplanted patient has shown complete normalization of serum lipids and apolipoproteins, including Lp(a). She receives cutaneous estrogen replacements following hysterectomy and bilateral oophorectomy for endometriosis and remains well, apart from slightly impaired renal function attributable to cyclosporin. The necessity for long-term immunosuppression is the main drawback to liver transplantation, which in other respects represents the most definitive therapy currently available for homozygous FH. However, the operation itself is not without risk, especially when combined with cardiac transplantation, and LDL apheresis provides a safer means of improving the prognosis of this fatal disorder.

Acknowledgements

We are grateful to Dr J Deanfield for the measurements of flow- and nitrate-mediated vasodilatation, to Dr M Barbir for providing the data used in Fig. 1, to Clare Neuwirth for skilled assistance, and to Kaneka for loan of a SA-01 apheresis module.

References

1. Thompson GR, Barbir M, Okabayashi K, Trayner I, Larkin S. Arteriosclerosis 1989;9(Suppl I):I-152—I-157.
2. Thompson GR, Miller JP, Breslow JL. Br Med J 1985;291:1671—1673.
3. Marburger C, Hambrecht R, Niebauer J, Schoeppenthau M, Scheffler E, Hauer K, Schuler G, Schlierf G. Am J Cardiol 1994;73:742—746.
4. Thompson GR, on behalf of the FHRS Investigators. JACC 1994;131-A.
5. Pokrovsky SN, Sussekov AV, Afanasieva OI, Adamova IY, Lyakishev AA, Kukharchuk VV. Chem Phys Lipid 1994;67/68:323—330.
6. Sorensen KE, Celermajer DS, Georgakopoulos D., Hatcher G, Betteridge DJ, Deanfield JE. J Clin Invest 1994;93:50—55.
7. East C, Grundy SM, Bilheimer DW. J Am Med Assoc 1986;256:2843—2848.
8. Hoeg JM, Starzl TE, Brewer HB. Am J Cardiol 1987;59:705—707.
9. Valdivielso P, Escolar JL, Cuervas-Mons V, Pulpon LA, Chaparro MAS, Gonzalez-Santos P. Ann Int Med 1988;108:204—206.
10. Barbir M, Khagani A, Kehely A, Tan K-C, Mitchell A, Thompson GR, Yacoub M. Quart J Med 1992;85:807—812.

Gene therapy for dyslipoproteinemia and atherosclerosis

Louis C. Smith[1], James T. Sparrow[1], Stephen Gottschalk[2] and Savio L.C. Woo[2,3]

[1]Department of Medicine, [2]Department of Cell Biology and [3]Howard Hughes Medical Institute, Baylor College of Medicine, One Baylor Plaza, Houston TX 77030, USA

Current treatment of dyslipoproteinemia relies primarily on reduction of plasma cholesterol and/or triglycerides by life-long medications or costly procedures. With technologies for successful gene transfer that give constitutive expression in vivo, therapeutic genes can now be introduced somatically into the proper organs for expression that may provide a long-term cure for these diseases. Efficient expression of genes to control the metabolism of plasma lipoproteins may prove to be an effective treatment for atherosclerosis in man. The initial experimental approaches have relied on recombinant viruses as gene-delivery systems. Novel nonviral DNA delivery systems based on synthetic peptides should provide effective gene transfer and avoid many limitations of viral delivery systems.

The basic science investment of this society in the study of human diseases has yielded an understanding of the molecular pathologies of many inherited metabolic disorders. Unfortunately, for many debilitating hereditary disorders, there are no specific therapies, only complex strategies to minimize the progression and complications of the particular disease. A prime example is familial hypercholesterolemia (FH), which is caused by defects in the receptor which mediates the internalization of low density lipoprotein (LDL) [1]. This disease is associated with severe hypercholesterolemia and premature coronary artery disease, and frequently is resistant to conventional drug therapy.

One alternative for these diseases is somatic gene therapy [2], whereby a functional gene is introduced into the cells where the expression of that gene has been compromised, and the gene product is expressed in amounts sufficient to affect the course of the disease. Thus, rather than treat the disease, the underlying genetic defect would be corrected and thereby prevent, reverse, stabilize or at least slow the progression of the disease, depending upon the nature of the disease and when in the course of the disease treatment is initiated. At present, gene therapy offers the potential of a complete cure for metabolic or cardiovascular disorders in which the mechanism and progress of the disease process is well understood.

Somatic gene therapy can be considered when three conditions are met: (a) The potentially therapeutic gene is cloned. (b) Delivery systems for the transfer of the gene into the appropriate somatic cell targets have been developed. (c) An animal model is available for establishing the relative efficiencies of different methods of gene transfer. Two conceptually different approaches have been examined for the delivery of therapeutic genes. The first, an ex vivo approach, involves the removal of the target cells from the subject, the introduction of therapeutic genes into these cells using retroviral vectors or other transfecting agents, and the return of the transduced cells into the subject by autologous transplantation to reconstitute the missing function or functions. While the ex vivo approach is conceptually straightforward, there are two limiting features. Tissue removal may require a major surgical procedure, and the culturing of the cells is a labor-intensive, expensive procedure. The second approach, the in vivo approach, involves the direct introduction of genetic material into specific tissue sites. Although the in vivo approach is conceptually simple, it requires the ability to direct the injected genetic material, either by injection or using a targeting mechanism, into the proper tissues or organs to be effective.

Recombinant retroviruses

Recombinant retroviruses have many desirable features as vectors for somatic gene therapy, including their broad host cell range, their established safety record, and their ability to stably integrate into the host cell genome. Although the response to ex vivo retroviral hepatic transduction of the LDL receptor was modest in WHHL rabbits [3], these experimental findings provided the necessary background for ex vivo gene therapy directed to the liver of a patient with familial hypercholesterolemia [4], using a recombinant retrovirus containing a normal copy of the human LDL receptor gene. There was no apparent pathology in a liver biopsy sample at 4 months and in situ hybridization showed single cells expressing the gene. The level of serum LDL-cholesterol after gene therapy was 17% lower than the pretreatment baseline. The lowering of LDL-cholesterol was attributed to an acceleration of the receptor-mediated uptake of LDL into the liver. This interpretation has been disputed by Brown et al. [5], who noted that no pre- and post-treatment studies of LDL turnover had been performed. Because the decline in serum LDL-cholesterol could be due either to diminished lipoprotein production or to enhanced activity of the patient's own LDL receptors, no conclusions can be reached about the efficacy of the ex vivo gene transfer procedure performed on this patient. Thus, it is critically important that the criteria described by Brown et al. [5] are met in subsequent studies of gene therapy of lipid disorders in humans.

For treatment of disorders that require only small amounts of the therapeutic gene product to be expressed, retroviral vectors may be useful. The principal limitations of recombinant retroviral vectors are their inability to integrate in nondividing cells and their relatively low transduction efficiency in vivo.

Recombinant adenoviruses

Recombinant adenoviral vectors have the highest transduction efficiency in vivo. They can infect not only lung and other epithelial-derived tissues but also nonproliferating cell types such as hepatocytes. In liver, 100% of all mouse hepatocytes could be transduced following intraportal infusion of recombinant adenoviral vectors [6]. The extremely high transduction efficiencies suggested that recombinant adenoviral vectors would be excellent candidates for the in vivo delivery of therapeutic genes to the liver. In animal models for diseases caused by hepatic deficiencies such as PKU, hemophilia B, and FH, infusion of recombinant adenoviral vectors containing the appropriate therapeutic cDNAs gave normal or supernormal levels of the missing gene products and completely normalized the disease phenotype [7,8]. In vivo administration of a recombinant adenovirus containing the LDL receptor to LDL, receptor knockout mice [9] increased the half-lives for intravenously administered ^{125}I-VLDL and ^{125}I-LDL 30-fold and 2.5-fold, respectively. An estimated 90% of the parenchymal cells in liver expressed the adenovirus-transferred genes as judged by immunofluorescence. Recombinant, replication-defective adenoviruses expressing the LDL receptor infused into the portal vein of WHHL rabbits gave similar results [10,11]. Transgene expression was stable for 7—10 days and diminished to undetectable levels within 3 weeks. Although adenovirus-encoded LDL receptors can acutely reverse the hypercholesterolemic effects of LDL-receptor deficiency, the presence of neutralizing antibodies to the recombinant adenovirus prevent further treatment by a second dose. The issues of viral genome instability and blocking immune response need to be overcome before the promise of this technical approach can be fully realized.

Nonviral DNA delivery systems

This conceptually different approach is based on the premise that an effective nonviral DNA delivery systems can be constructed from the information about how viruses penetrate cells and take control of cellular components for viral replication and maturation. The effectiveness of a virus or of a direct gene-delivery system in vivo depends on the route of administration, uptake by a specific cell type, escape from lysosomal degradation, transit through the cytoplasm, transport through the nuclear membrane, and recognition and utilization by nuclear enzymes and transcription factors for expression. As a pseudo-virus, a synthetic targeted gene delivery system needs at least five components: (a) a DNA sequence with a marker or therapeutic gene; (b) a cationic DNA-binding template that condenses DNA sufficiently for packaging; (c) a ligand that recognizes and binds with high affinity to a cell-surface receptor; (d) a lytic peptide to rupture the endosomes to release the complex directly into the cytoplasm; and (e) at least one nuclear localization sequence to enhance delivery of the DNA to the nucleus. Several different types of synthetic DNA-binding molecules are available, so that receptor ligand, lytic peptide and nuclear localization sequence can be attached to separate templates.

The principal advantage of this approach is its flexibility. By design, the composition of the final complex can be easily modified in response to experimental results in vitro and in vivo. This design flexibility is important since there is little quantitative information about how efficiently the vector is processed through each stage of the complex processes of cellular uptake and transport to the nucleus. The processes that might account for the observed low efficiency of the existing methods of nonviral gene delivery remain to be identified. In addition to sequences for endosome lysis and nuclear uptake, there may be other essential but as yet unidentified functions of viral proteins. The stepwise assembly of DNA complexes using small peptides which are functional equivalents of the much larger, more complex, viral and cellular proteins should also improve our understanding of how viruses invade and replicate.

Two unique features of nonviral DNA delivery systems are the absence of (a) biohazards related to the viral genome as well as the production of the viral vector and (b) limitations on the size of the therapeutic genes that can be inserted in the recombinant viral vector. In principle, if the gene can be cloned into an expression vector, it can be delivered as a synthetic DNA complex. Finally, since these synthetic delivery systems are composed of small peptides which are poorly antigenic, they hold the promise of repeated gene administration, a highly desirable feature which will be important for gene targeting in vivo to endothelial cells, monocytes and other cell types that normally turn over at relatively high rates.

We have used a series of synthetic poly-L-lysine analogs that contain a central cluster of 4–8 lysine residues as the DNA-binding template to condense a CMV-β-galactosidase expression vector to a monodisperse 60-nm particle. Measurements of particle size using laser light-scattering techniques show that the condensed particles are stable for at least a week. These complexes are also stable when incubated with serum or with tissue homogenates under conditions that degrade free DNA.

For nonviral DNA to be effective for gene transfer, there must be a mechanism to lyse the endosome after internalization; otherwise, the endosomal contents will be delivered to the lysosomes or returned to the cell surface. Cationic lipids, pH-sensitive liposomes,

556

chemically inactivated adenoviruses, and synthetic peptides from the hemagglutinin proteins have been used, with limited success, for direct DNA delivery in vitro. In our experiments, we have used several different amphipathic negatively charged peptides as lytic agents. They have been included in a positively charged DNA:polylysine complex that is effective in promoting gene transfer. Using β-galactosidase expression as an index of transduction, the efficiency of delivery varied from 1 to 90% in about 20 different types of cultured cells. Typically, 10–40% of the cells are transduced. Molecular modeling and structure prediction programs suggest that the hydrophobic face of the peptide will orient the peptides to form pores in one side of an endosomal membrane, thereby destabilizing the membrane which then ruptures.

Only a few reports describe in vivo applications of DNA/protein complexes, with limited transduction efficiency of hepatocytes or other target cells [12–15]. The chief limitations are the low transduction efficiencies in vivo and a lack of persistence of the exogenous DNA. Since most metabolic diseases will probably be treated by these vectors only in vivo, significant improvement will be required in several areas before clinical applications can proceed. However, even at their present state of development, it is clear that synthetic DNA delivery systems have several significant advantages over other vector systems and will be important delivery systems in the future.

Perspective

The routine use of gene therapy in the treatment of metabolic and cardiovascular disease lies in the near future. The refinement of existing viral-based methods of gene delivery and the development of novel nonviral delivery systems are occurring at an ever-increasing rate. The molecular biology of tissue-specific expression of exogenous genes is also developing rapidly. One of the first applications of these systems will be in experimental animal systems to test the accuracy of the currently accepted understanding of the relationships of risk factors to cardiovascular disease, inferred in large part from epidemiological studies.

References

1. Goldstein JL, Brown MS. In: Scriver CR, Beaudet AL, Sly WS, Valle D (eds) Metabolic Basis of Inherited Disease. New York: McGraw-Hill, 1989;1215–1250.
2. Morgan RA, Anderson WF. Annu Rev Biochem 1993;62:191–217.
3. Chowdhury JR, Grossman M, Gupta S, Chowdhury NR, Baker JR Jr, Wilson JM. Science 1991;254:1802–1805.
4. Grossman M, Raper SE, Kozarsky K, Stein EA, Engelhardt JF, Muller D, Lupien PJ, Wilson JM. Nature Genetics 1994;6:335–341.
5. Brown MS, Goldstein JL, Havel RJ, Steinberg D. Nature Genetics 1994;7:349–350.
6. Li QT, Kay M, Finegold M, Stratford-Perricaudet L, Woo SLC. Hum Gene Ther 1993;4:403–409.
7. Fang B, Eisensmith RC, Li XHC, Finegold MJ, Shedlovsky A, Dove W, Woo SLC. Gene Ther 1994;1: 247–254.
8. Kay MA, Landen CN, Rothenberg SR, Taylor LI, Leland F, Wiehle S, Fang B, Bellinger D, Finegold M, Thompson AR, Read M, Brinkhous KM, Woo SLC. Proc Natl Acad Sci USA 1993;91:2353–2357.
9. Ishibashi S, Brown MS, Goldstein JL, Gerard RD, Hammer RE, Herz J. J Clin Invest 1993;92:883–893.
10. Kozarsky KF, McKinley DR, Austin LL, Raper SE, Stratford-Perricaudet LD, Wilson JM. J Biol Chem 1994;269:13695–13702.
11. Li J, Fang B, Eisensmith RC, Li XHC, Nasonkin I, Lin-Lee YC, Mims M, Hughes A, Montgomery C, Roberts J, Parker T, Levine D, Woo SLC J Clin Invest 1994;(in press).
12. Wu GY, Wu CH. J Biol Chem 1988;263:14621–14624.
13. Wu CH, Wilson JM, Wu GY. J Biol Chem 1989;264:16985–16987.
14. Wu GY, Wilson JM, Shalaby F, Grossman M, Shafritz DA, Wu CH. J Biol Chem 1991;266:14338–14342.
15. Chowdhury NR, Wu CH, Wu GY, Yerneni PC, Bommineni VR, Chowdhury JR. J Biol Chem 1993;268:11265–11271.

Antioxidant vitamins and cardiovascular disease mortality: experiences from the Alpha-Tocopherol, Beta-Carotene (ATBC) Lung Cancer Prevention Study

Jussi K. Huttunen, Demetrius Albanes, Jarmo Virtamo, Jaason Haapakoski, Olli P. Heinonen, Juni Palmgren, Pirjo Pietinen, Janne Rapola, Matti Rautalahti and Philip Taylor
National Public Health Institute, Helsinki, Finland; and Cancer Prevention Branch, Division of Cancer Prevention and Control, National Cancer Institute, Washington DC, USA

Abstract. The mortality data of the Alpha-Tocopherol, Beta-Carotene Cancer Prevention Trial do not support the hypothesis that supplemental intake of β-carotene or α-tocopherol protects against lung cancer or ischemic heart disease in man. On the contrary, the study has raised the possibility that these substances, when used in pharmacological doses, may have deleterious side-effects. Final conclusions on the benefits or adverse effects of these compounds must, however, await results from other continuing randomized trials.

There is increasing evidence that oxidative and antioxidative factors may play an important role in the development of atherosclerosis [1]. Reactive oxygen molecules and other free radicals have been shown to transform low-density lipoproteins (LDL) into an oxidized form. Oxidized LDL has several actions that could contribute both to the initiation and progression of atherogenesis. If oxidative modification of LDL is an important mechanism in the causation of atherosclerosis, intake of dietary antioxidants might be protective against coronary heart diseases. Indeed, epidemiological studies have suggested that high intake of antioxidant vitamins may prevent coronary heart disease in man [2,3].

Final proof for the beneficial effects of antioxidant vitamins and antioxidant drugs can be obtained only from sufficiently large controlled clinical trials. This report examines the mortality data from the Alpha-Tocopherol Beta-Carotene (ATBC) Cancer Prevention Trial, a controlled, double-blind, primary prevention trial studying the efficacy of long-term supplementation with antioxidant vitamins among male smokers in Finland [4,5].

Participants and Methods

The rationale, methods, participant characteristics and preliminary results of the ATBC Study have been described elsewhere [4,5]. The participants (n = 29,133) were recruited from postal survey respondents (n = 224,377) residing in the study region with a total population of 290,406. To be eligible, the subjects had to smoke five or more cigarettes per day at entry. Potential participants with prior cancer, serious disease limiting the capacity to participate, or use of vitamin E, vitamin A or β-carotene supplements in excess of predefined doses were excluded.

Participants were randomly assigned to one of the four intervention groups of α-tocopherol alone, β-carotene alone, α-tocopherol and β-carotene, or placebo to receive a single capsule daily. Treatment assignments were based on a 2 × 2 factorial design to

Address for correspondence: Dr Jussi Huttunen, National Public Health Institute, Mannerheimintie 166, SF-00300 Helsinki, Finland.

558

allow assessment of two separate factors independently in a single trial. Thus, half of the participants received α-tocopherol while half did not. Similarly, half received β-carotene and half did not. At the end of 5–8 years of intervention (median 6.1 years), 20,072 participants were still active in the trial, and 25,563 were alive.

Identification of incident cancers was primarily via the Finnish Cancer Registry. Deaths were verified via the Central Population Register, and death certificates were checked for the underlying cause of death. The noncancer diagnoses were ascertained through the National Hospital Discharge Register. Endpoints were correlated with trial treatment according to the "intention to treat" principle. Standard survival analysis methodology was used, including plots of Kaplan-Meier survival curves and computation of log rank statistics.

Results

A total of 3,570 deaths occurred during the trial. Total mortality was 2% higher among the participants who received α-tocopherol than those who did not (95% confidence interval, –5 to 9%; p = 0.6). Among the men who received β-carotene, an excess of cumulative total mortality was observed after 5 years, resulting in an 8% difference in total mortality by the end of the study (95% confidence interval, 1–16%; p = 0.02).

The causes of death among subjects who received α-tocopherol or β-carotene and among those who did not are shown in Table 1. The number of deaths from hemorrhagic stroke was higher and the number of ischemic strokes slightly lower among subjects who received α-tocopherol than among those who did not. The difference in mortality from hemorrhagic stroke appeared early during the course of the intervention and persisted throughout the trial. Ischemic heart disease mortality was lower in the groups that received α-tocopherol than in those that did not, but the difference was only 5%.

The excess of total mortality in the groups that received β-carotene was primarily due to higher mortality from lung cancer (+15%) and ischemic heart disease (+11%). The difference in mortality from ischemic heart disease appeared 3 years after the beginning of the intervention, and was most evident among subjects with a history of myocardial infarction at the onset of the study.

Discussion

The results of the Alpha-Tocopherol, Beta-Carotene Cancer Prevention Trial do not support the hypothesis that α-tocopherol or β-carotene supplements protect against cancer

Table 1. Disease-specific causes of death among participants who received α-tocopherol (AT) supplements and those who did not and among participants who received β-carotene (BC) supplements and those who did not[a]

Cause of death	Treatment			
	AT	No AT	BC	No BC
Lung cancer	285	279	302	262
Other cancer	294	258	280	272
Ischemic heart disease	602	637	653	586
Hemorrhagic stroke	66	44	59	51
Ischemic stroke	56	67	68	55
Other cardiovascular disease	129	122	125	126
Injuries and accidents	166	170	172	164
Other causes	200	191	191	200

[a]The cause of death was unknown for four participants.

or cardiovascular diseases. On the contrary, they have raised the possibility that supplements of β-carotene might increase the risk of lung cancer or death from ischemic heart disease and that supplements of α-tocopherol might be associated with excess deaths from hemorrhagic stroke. Caution should, however, be exercised in the interpretation of the data. Lack of protective effect of antioxidant vitamins on lung cancer may have several explanations. The 5—8 years of intervention may have been too short, as the initial stage of carcinogenesis that is potentially sensitive to the effects of antioxidants precedes the symptomatic phase by many years. The dose of β-carotene may have been too high, and a beneficial effect might have been observed if supplements closer to nutritional intakes had been studied. Finally, the effect of antioxidant vitamins may not become apparent in a well-nourished population.

Lack of protective effect of α-tocopherol on coronary heart disease mortality and an excess of ischemic heart disease deaths in the β-carotene groups is a startling observation in view of the wealth of evidence supporting the role of oxidized LDL in the pathogenesis of coronary heart disease. The dose of α-tocopherol (50 mg/day) may, however, have been too low to influence LDL oxidation. Furthermore, even relatively high intakes of β-carotene have failed to influence LDL oxidation in man. On the other hand, in sharp contrast to the present results, preliminary data from another trial suggested that β-carotene protects against cardiovascular events in men with pre-existing disease [6]. Clearly, final conclusions on the role of antioxidant vitamins in prevention of atherosclerotic diseases can be drawn only after the incidence data from this trial and the results from other randomized trials [7—9] become available.

An apparently higher risk of hemorrhagic stroke was observed among the participants who received α-tocopherol than among those who did not. This difference was balanced with an excess of ischemic strokes among participants not receiving this supplement. Although the difference in hemorrhagic strokes was nominally significant, it may have been due to chance in view of the large number of comparisons. A causal effect remains, however, a possibility, as other studies have suggested that α-tocopherol influences platelet function.

Oxidative damage to DNA, proteins, and lipids has been postulated to be a major type of endogenous damage leading to aging. Furthermore, it has been argued that dietary intake of antioxidants might retard the aging process and promote longevity [10]. The results of the ATBC Study are not consonant with this hypothesis. In fact, total mortality was higher among subjects who received β-carotene or α-tocopherol than among those who did not. These results seem to exclude the possibility that supranutritional intakes of these vitamins substantially prolong lifespan in man.

References

1. Witztum JL. Br Heart J 1993;69:512—518.
2. Rimm EB, Stampfer MJ, Ascherio A et al. N Engl J Med 1993;328:1450—1456.
3. Stampfer MJ, Hennekens CH, Manson JE et al. N Engl J Med 1993;328:1444—1449.
4. The Alpha-Tocopherol, Beta-Carotene Cancer Prevention Study Group. N Engl J Med 1994;330:1029—1035.
5. The ATBC Cancer Prevention Study Group. Ann Epidemiol 1994;4:1—10.
6. Gaziano JM, Manson JE, Ridker PM et al. Circulation 1990;82(suppl III)III—201.
7. Omenn GS, Goodman G, Thornquist M. Cancer Res 1994;54(suppl):2038s—2043s.
8. Steering Committee of the Physicians' Health Study Research Group. N Engl J Med 1989;321:129—135.
9. Buring JE, Hennekens CH. J Myocardial Isch 1992;4:27—29.
10. Ames BN, Shigenaga MK, Hagen TM. Proc Natl Acad Sci USA 1993;90:7915—7922.

The Heidelberg regression study

Christian Marburger, Josef Niebauer, Rainer Hambrecht, Klaus Hauer, Michael Schöppenthau, Reinhard Ziegler, Wolfgang Kübler, Gerhard Schuler and Günter Schlierf

Medizinische Universtätsklinik, Bergheimerstr. 58, 69115 Heidelberg, Germany

Abstract. The aim of this randomized intervention trial was to determine the influence of physical exercise and a cholesterol-lowering diet on the progression of coronary artery disease (CAD) in middle-aged men. Patients (n = 113) were recruited after coronary angiography for suspected CAD (56 intervention, 57 control group). In 92 patients a second coronary angiography was performed after 1 year, and the results were correlated with changes in metabolic and hemodynamic data.

Patients in the intervention group showed better results with respect to: 1. lipid values (cholesterol −10 vs. 0% in the control group, LDL-cholesterol −8 vs. +2%, triglycerides −24 vs. −17%); 2. physical work capacity (+23 vs. +6%), myocardial oxygen consumption as estimated from maximal rate-pressure product (+10 vs. −4%), and stress-induced myocardial ischemia detected by myocardial scintigraphy (reversible perfusion defect −10 vs. −2%); and 3. CAD progression (regression in 30 vs. 4% of the patients, no change in 50 vs. 54%, progression in 20 vs. 42%).

Regression of CAD correlated tendentially with lower total and LDL-cholesterol and significantly with the amount of leisure-time physical activity in a subgroup of 62 patients (29 intervention, 33 control group). Lipoprotein(a) and fibrinogen levels showed no correlation with progression of the disease.

In addition to the above, 5-year follow-up data from our pilot study were available for evaluation. Patients of the intervention group (n = 18) still showed a significant lower serum cholesterol and greater physical work capacity after 5 years than the control group. There was also a tendency towards a slower progression of CAD in the intervention group than in the control group (n = 18).

In summary, a cholesterol-lowering diet plus physical exercise showed favorable effects on lipid metabolism, physical work capacity and progression of CAD.

It has been shown that cholesterol lowering is an effective method of secondary prevention in coronary artery disease (CAD) [1]. In the past decade several studies demonstrated regression of coronary atheromatous lesions in coronary angiograms [2]. Most investigators, however, have included patients with overt familial hyperlipidemia or dyslipidemia, and have used lipid-lowering drugs to achieve this goal. Cholesterol-rich, hypercaloric diet and sedentary lifestyle are widespread habits in Western populations and are associated with an increase in serum cholesterol and with the incidence of CAD. Thus, prudent dietary behavior and regular physical activity instead of lipid-lowering drugs should also lower cholesterol levels and possibly favorably alter the natural progressive course of CAD. The Heidelberg Regression Study was designed to test this hypothesis in middle-aged men with CAD. Results have been published previously [3–7,9] and will be summarized here.

Address for correspondence: Christian Marburger MD, Institut für Herzinfarktforschung, Medizinische Universitätsklinik, Bergheimerstr. 58, 69115 Heidelberg, Germany.

Methods

In a pilot study 18 patients were enrolled in a 1-year program with intensive physical exercise and dietary counseling. Changes in lipid profile, in hemodynamic variables, and in coronary angiograms performed after 1 year were compared with changes in 18 control patients (matched-pair design), who had been instructed according to the same guidelines on diet and exercise once, but received "usual care" by their private physician.

In the second, larger study 113 men with CAD were randomly assigned to an "intervention group" (n = 56) or a "control group" (n = 57). Again, intervention consisted of repeated dietary counseling for a low-fat, low-cholesterol diet (fat <20% of energy intake, cholesterol <200 mg, polyunsaturated-to-saturated fatty acid ratio >1) and for regular physical exercise. Patients were lent cycle ergometers for home use of at least 30 min per day, and they were to attend 1-h group training sessions at least twice a week. Familial hypercholesterolemia (LDL >200 mg/dl) was an exclusion criterion and lipid-lowering drugs were not used during the study period.

Every 3 months, serum lipoproteins were determined, and an exercise test was performed. At the beginning and after 1 year quantitative coronary angiography with evaluation by digital image processing and thallium-201 scintigraphy were performed. Dietary compliance was assessed by detailed 24-h protocols in all patients and by measuring fatty acid composition in adipose tissue. Leisure-time physical activity was estimated by a questionnaire in a subgroup of 62 patients. Lipoprotein(a) and fibrinogen were determined in 102 patients and were correlated with progression of CAD. All methods have been described in detail previously [3—6].

After 1 year patients of both trials were asked to proceed with the program. Metabolic follow-up and exercise testing was then performed annually, and repeat coronary angiography was performed again after 5 years [7]. This follow-up of the second study is still in progress.

Results and Discussion

Both studies revealed essentially identical results at 1 year. Therefore, and because of limited space, 1-year results from the larger and randomized trial are presented. Patient characteristics are listed in Table 1. During the study period, metabolic variables improved significantly in the intervention group: body weight decreased by 5%, total cholesterol by 10%, LDL-cholesterol by 8%, and triglycerides by 24%. HDL-cholesterol remained essentially unchanged. In the control group, triglycerides decreased by 17%. All other variables showed no significant changes.

Physical work capacity, maximal rate pressure product, maximal oxygen uptake and reversible myocardial ischemia (assessed by scintigraphy) all improved significantly in the intervention group and showed no changes in the control group. Likewise, coronary morphology changed favorably in the intervention group compared to the control group (Fig. 1) [3]. Patients with overall lesion regression had a tendency towards higher HDL-cholesterol and lower LDL-cholesterol than patients with lesion progression. Surprisingly, there was no correlation between the improvement of hemodynamic variables and changes in coronary lesions. However, there was a strong correlation between regression and the amount of energy expenditure during leisure-time physical activity. Regression occurred only in patients exercising at intensity levels above 1,600 kcal/week [5].

Progression, however, occurred also in some patients with excellent dietary and exercise compliance. The search for predictors of progression in these patients remained unsuccessful. For example, lipoprotein(a) and fibrinogen — risk factors apparently

562

Table 1. Patient characteristics in the larger trial (mean ± SD)

	Intervention	Control
No. of randomized patients	56	57
Age (years)	52.8 ± 5.8	54.2 ± 7.7
Smokers (no. (%))	6 (11)	6 (11)
Previous myocardial infarction (no. (%))	31 (60)	40 (70)
Body mass index (kg/m^2)	26.7 ± 2.5	26.4 ± 2.2
Cholesterol (mg/dl)	234 ± 39	235 ± 40
HDL-cholesterol (mg/dl)	36 ± 9	36 ± 7
LDL-cholesterol (mg/dl)	164 ± 27	164 ± 33
Triglycerides (mg/dl)	175 ± 72	191 ± 110
Resting heart rate (min^{-1})	74 ± 11	76 ± 12
Resting systolic blood pressure (mmHg)	128 ± 19	128 ± 21
Maximal heart rate (bpm)	142 ± 17	151 ± 20
Maximal systolic blood pressure (mmHg)	188 ± 24	190 ± 27
Physical work capacity (Watt)	159 ± 53	163 ± 47
Maximal oxygen uptake (l/min)	1.8 ± 0.4	1.9 ± 0.5
Maximal rate pressure product (×10^3)	26.9 ± 5.0	28.6 ± 6.0
^{201}Tl perfusion defect (°)	44 ± 44	42 ± 37
Gensini score	28.8 ± 16	27.6 ± 19
Left ventricular ejection fraction (%)	57 ± 9	55 ± 8

No significant difference was detected for any variable between groups (Mann-Whitney U-test). Table adapted from Table 1 in [4].

associated with the development of CAD — showed no correlation with disease progression [6].

After 5 years of the pilot study, patients of the intervention group still showed a

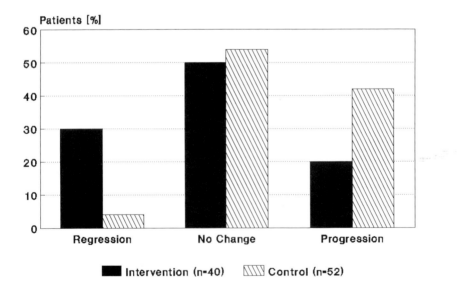

Fig. 1. Changes of relative diameter reduction of coronary lesions quantified by digital image processing after 1 year. In the intervention group progression was seen in eight (20%), no change in 20 (50%) and regression in 12 (30%) patients; in the control group in 22 (42%), 28 (54%), and two (4%) patients, respectively. Groups differed significantly from each other (p < 0.001; Mann-Whitney U-test). Figure adapted from Fig. 3 in [4].

significant reduction of triglycerides and total cholesterol vs. baseline values, whereas body weight and LDL-cholesterol had returned to pre-intervention levels [7]. Myocardial infarctions occurred in four patients (none related to exercise), coronary balloon dilatations (PTCA) were performed in three and coronary bypass operations (CABG) in four patients (in total six patients with events). In the remaining 12 patients significant improvement of the hemodynamic variables lasted throughout the 5 years (Table 2) due to a constant exercise compliance of 64% (68% during year 1). Coronary angiograms (13 patients) revealed lesion progression in eight, no change in three and continued regression in two patients. New lesions had developed in two patients.

In the control group, triglycerides were also markedly lowered after 5 years, but body weight and LDL-cholesterol had significantly risen above baseline levels. In this group, eight patients suffered from myocardial infarctions, three required PTCA, and CABG had to be performed in two (nine patients with events in total). One patient died of cancer. Hemodynamic variables in 12 patients showed no difference as compared to the beginning of the study. Angiograms showed lesion regression in one, no change in one, and progression in 10 patients. New lesions had developed in eight patients.

Between both groups, 5-year results show a significant difference strongly in favor of the intervention, although fading dietary compliance was observed when compared to the first study year. Still, the tendency towards a slower progression of CAD in these patients suggests a continuing positive effect of the intervention program. Adherence to the proposed measures, however, remains a continuous challenge for both patients and their physicians.

Although physical exercise in patients with CAD has been shown to be rather safe during supervised training sessions, there are dangers of acute exercise including ischemia-induced arrhythmia and acute myocardial infarction [8]. In our pilot study, there were no exercise-related events during 5 years of intervention. In the larger trial exercise-related cardiac arrest occurred in two patients, in one of them during a training session. At the

Table 2. Hemodynamics in patients of the pilot study

	Begin (B)	1 year	5 years (5Y)	B vs. 5Y	5Y vs. control
Intervention (n = 12)					
HRmax (min-1)	148 ± 23	153 ± 18	159 ± 15	$p < 0.03$	$p < 0.006$
SBPmax (mmHg)	168 ± 15	177 ± 17	194 ± 14	$p < 0.003$	p = n.s.
RPPmax (×10³)	25 ± 6	27 ± 5	32 ± 4	$p < 0.004$	$p < 0.03$
PWC(Watt)	169 ± 40	208 ± 46	205 ± 50	$p < 0.01$	$p < 0.02$
201Tl PD (°)	41 ± 36	16 ± 13	29 ± 29	p = n.s.	p = n.s.
Control (n = 12)					
HRmax (min-1)	137 ± 18	139 ± 19	132 ± 24	p = n.s.	
SBPmax (mmHg)	182 ± 28	170 ± 22	189 ± 32	p = n.s.	
RPPmax (×10³)	25 ± 6	24 ± 6	26 ± 8	p = n.s.	
PWC(Watt)	165 ± 45	163 ± 43	142 ± 62	p = n.s.	
201Tl PD (°)	32 ± 24	41 ± 44	23 ± 18	p = n.s.	

HR = heart rate; SBP = systolic blood pressure; RPP = rate pressure product; PWC - physical work capacity; 201TI PD = scintigraphic myocardial perfusion defect; AP = angina pectoris during stress test. For explanation of patient numbers see text. Values represent mean ± standard deviation; p was calculated by the Mann-Whitney U-test. Table adapted from Table VII in [7].

time of cardiac arrest the patient happened to undergo Holter monitoring during swimming. Evaluation of the recordings revealed heart rates more than 130% above his recommended training heart rate and severe ST-segment depression that degenerated into ventricular tachyrhythmia. In a subgroup of patients Holter monitoring was obtained during swimming as well as during different forms of exercise. Results revealed that ST-segment depression indicating myocardial ischemia during exercise sessions was almost exclusively seen in patients exceeding their recommended training heart rates (95% of maximal heart rate during symptom-limited exercise testing) [9]. Therefore, patients should be taught to measure and control their training heart rates and should be repeatedly observed concerning their exercise intensities. Holter monitoring has been shown to be helpful in identifying patients at risk. In contrast, medical history, number of affected vessels, or left ventricular ejection fraction were no predictors of cardiac events in our study groups.

In conclusion, the course of CAD can be favorably altered by physical exercise coupled with dietary reduction of atherogenic plasma lipoproteins. Since this was a multifactorial intervention, it is not possible to measure the individual contribution of a single component such as diet or exercise. Still, the correlations between lesion regression and both lowered LDL-cholesterol and leisure-time physical activities suggest that both diet and exercise were effective. Lesion regression can be seen as early as 1 year after change of life style. Also, results of the pilot study show a tendency towards slower progression during intervention after 5 years.

Although diet and exercise have clearly been shown to be effective measures for secondary prevention in our trials, patients' dietary compliance has been fading during the study course. It should be emphasized that adherence to dietary recommendations and physical activities remains a day-to-day challenge for patients and physicians alike.

Acknowledgements

The support of Bundesministerium für Forschung und Technologie and of Verein zur Förderung der Herzinfarktforschung, Heidelberg is gratefully acknowledged.

References

1. Rossouw JE, Lewis B, Rifkind BM. N Engl J Med 1990;323:1112–1119.
2. Brown G, Albers JJ, Fisher LD, Schaefer SM, Lin JT, Kaplan C, Zhao XQ, Bisson BD, Fitzpatrick VF, Dodge HT. N Engl J Med 1990;323:1289–1298.
3. Schuler G, Hambrecht R, Schlierf G, Grunze M, Methfessel S, Hauer K, Kübler W. J Am Cell Cardiol 1992;19:34–42.
4. Schuler G, Hambrecht R, Schlierf G, Niebauer J, Hauer K, Neumann J, Hoberg E, Drinkmann A, Bacher F, Grunze M, Kübler W. Circulation 1992;86:1–11.
5. Hambrecht R, Niebauer J, Marburger C, Grunze M, Kälberer B, Hauer K, Schlierf G, Kübler W, Schuler G. J Am Cell Cardiol 1993;22:468–477.
6. Marburger C, Hambrecht R, Niebauer J, Schoeppenthau M, Scheffler E, Hauer K, Schuler G, Schlierf G. Am J Cardiol 1994;73:742–746.
7. Niebauer J, Hambrecht R, Marburger C, Schlierf G, Kälberer B, Kübler W, Schuler G. J Cardiopulm Rehab (in press).
8. Mittleman MA, Maclure M, Tofler GH, Sherwood JB, Goldberg RJ, Muller JE. N Engl J Med 1993;329:1677–1683.
9. Niebauer J, Hambrecht R, Hauer K, Marburger C, Schoeppenthau M, Kaelberer B, Schlierf G, Kübler W, Schuler G. Am J Cardiol 1994;74:651–656.

Intensive multiple-risk-factor reduction to modify coronary atherosclerosis in men and women with coronary artery disease

William L. Haskell[1,2], Edwin L. Alderman[1], Joan M. Fair[1,2], and the SCRIP Investigators

[1]Division of Cardiovascular Medicine and [2]Center for Research in Disease Prevention, School of Medicine, Stanford University, California, USA

Abstract. To determine if comprehensive multifactor risk reduction favorably alters progression of coronary atherosclerosis, 300 men and women were randomized to usual care or risk reduction, with quantitative arteriograms performed at baseline and 4 years. The rate of narrowing of diseased artery segments was 47% less in the risk-reduction than the usual-care group (change in minimum diameter of –0.024 ± 0.066 vs. –0.045 ± 0.073 mm/year: $p < 0.02$). Disease regression was twice as frequent in the risk-reduction group (20.2 vs. 10.3%, $p = 0.07$) and the number of new lesions per patient tended to be less in the risk-reduction group (0.30 vs. 0.47; $p = 0.06$).

The Stanford Coronary Risk Intervention Project (SCRIP) tested the hypothesis that intensive multifactor risk reduction, including changes in lifestyle and lipid-lowering medications over 4 years, would significantly reduce the rate of narrowing of the minimal diameter of coronary artery segments by angiographically visible atherosclerotic lesions compared with changes in similar segments in subjects receiving usual care from their own physician. Secondary questions included the comparison of changes in the mean diameter and percent stenosis of visibly diseased segments, the minimal and mean diameters of visibly normal segments, the proportion of patients showing disease progression or regression, and the development of new lesions.

Methods

Study design

This study was a randomized trial of 300 men and women with coronary artery disease. Consecutive potentially eligible subjects received arteriography, and, if still eligible, signed an informed consent and completed a comprehensive baseline medical and risk factor evaluation. Subjects were then randomized to the usual care (UC) of their own physician or to an individualized, multifactor, risk reduction (RR) program. All subjects were scheduled for four annual medical/risk factor evaluations and follow-up coronary arteriography at the 4th year.

Subjects

Men and women less than 75 years of age who lived within a 5-h driving distance of Stanford University were eligible if free of severe congestive heart failure, pulmonary disease, intermittent claudication, or noncardiac life-threatening illness and were considered capable of following the study protocol. Subjects were eligible if at least one

Address for correspondence: William L. Haskell PhD, Stanford University School of Medicine, 730 Welch Road, Suite B, Palo Alto, CA 94304-1583, USA. Tel.: +1-415-725-5012. Fax: +1-415-723-7018.

major coronary artery had a segment with lumen narrowing between 5 and 69% that was unaffected by revascularization procedures.

Clinical measurements

At baseline and annual evaluation, measurements included height, weight, skinfold thickness, blood pressure, smoking status by expired CO and plasma thiocyanate, resting ECG, and symptom-limited treadmill exercise test. Physical activity, diet, medication and psychological questionnaire were administered. Fasting lipids and lipoproteins were measured at duplicate visits and included total cholesterol, LDL-C, HDL-C, triglycerides, lipoprotein subfractions, Lp(a) and apolipoprotein B (apoB).

Angiographic measurements

All patients had baseline coronary arteriograms performed in a uniform manner with sublingual nitroglycerin administered 3–5 min prior to angiography. Coronary catheters with tantalum metallic cylindrical markers near their distal end provided a sharp calibration edge for quantitation, which reduces measurement variation when using computer-assisted measurement techniques [1]. Angiographers were blinded to group assignment of subjects. SCRIP required that neither the qualifying segment nor any vessel proximal to it contain a lesion ≥70% in diameter reduction and that no portion of the vessel had been grafted or instrumented by a prior revascularization procedure. Visually normal segments were quantitated, but only those with visible coronary disease on the baseline angiogram were used for testing the primary hypothesis. A secondary analysis was performed on segments that were free of angiographically-determined disease at baseline to assess the influence of the risk-reduction program on new lesion formation.

A computer-assisted quantitation system was designed at Stanford to measure coronary vessels on 35 mm cineangiograms. The system's design, accuracy, precision, and intra- and interobserver variability have been reported [2]. To assess new lesion formation, two experienced angiographic observers (blinded to patient randomization assignment) visually assessed each segment that had an interval reduction in minimum diameter exceeding 0.2 mm within a segment previously considered normal. Using simultaneous side-by-side comparison, the baseline and follow-up angiograms were compared visually. Results of the visual assessment were recorded as three possible outcomes: no apparent change, definite new lesion, or prior disease present with progression.

Risk reduction program

Immediately after randomization, each RR subject met with a SCRIP nurse to design an individualized risk-reduction program based on the subject's risk profile, his/her motivation, and resources for making specific changes. All RR subjects were instructed by a dietitian in a low-fat, low-cholesterol and high-carbohydrate diet with a goal of <20% of energy intake from fat, <6% from saturated fat, and <75 mg of cholesterol per day. A physical activity program was recommended consisting of an increase in daily activities and household chores and a specific endurance exercise training program. Current or recent ex-smokers were provided an individualized stop-smoking or relapse-prevention program by a staff psychologist. A major goal was to decrease LDL-C to <2.84 mmol/l, to decrease Tg below 1.13 mmol/l, and increase HDL-C above 1.42 mmol/l. If the SCRIP staff concluded that it was unlikely that an RR subject would meet the LDL-C goal within the 1st year without drug therapy, a cholesterol-lowering drug regimen was added, starting with a bile-acid-binding resin (colestipol) and, depending on subject response, adding or substituting other drugs including niacin, gemfibrozil, lovastatin and probucol.

The RR subjects were provided verbal and written goals and instructions for their individualized RR plan. To track their progress, contact was maintained with the SCRIP staff using telephone and mail. RR subjects returned every 2 or 3 months to the clinic to evaluate progress and provide additional assistance. During these visits lipids, body weight, and blood pressure were measured; diet, exercise, and smoking program assistance was provided; and hypolipidemic drugs were evaluated and revised as needed.

Statistical analysis

The effect of the RR program on selected risk factors was evaluated by calculating on-study risk factor values for each subject. This on-study value was the average of the values obtained for subjects from the annual evaluations performed between baseline and their follow-up arteriogram, usually 4 years. The primary angiographic endpoint was the change in the minimum artery diameter for coronary artery segments that exhibited visible atherosclerosis (diseased segments) at baseline. The minimum diameter for each diseased segment was measured on the baseline and follow-up arteriogram and the baseline value was subtracted from the value for the follow-up arteriogram to obtain the change in minimum diameter. For analysis by *patient*, the average rate of change for each patient was computed from all eligible diseased segments. The within-group change in the minimum diameter of diseased segments was evaluated by a one-sample paired t-test and between group differences by a two-sample t-test. For analysis by *segment*, analysis of variance was used with segments nested within subjects and subjects nested within groups. We evaluated progression and regression using the threshold of 0.2 mm. The threshold of 0.2 mm was based on a 3-fold multiple of our within-procedure measurement variability (standard deviation = 0.033 mm) (35) and further multiplying by a factor of two to account for between-procedure variation [2]. The relationships between the change in segment diameter of disease segments or the formation of new lesions and selected patient characteristics at baseline, on-study and the change from baseline to on-study were determined using univariate and multivariate regression analysis. Level of significance was set at $p < 0.05$, two-tailed.

Results

Baseline characteristics and dropouts

Of the 300 subjects randomized, 274 (91.3%) had follow-up arteriograms performed and were available for analyses. Of the 274 arteriograms, 28 could not be analyzed for various technical reasons [3]. Thus, most analyses of disease progression or regression include 127 (82%) of the 155 UC subjects and 119 (82%) of the 145 RR subjects randomized. At baseline, significant differences between the usual-care and RR groups include body weight and HDL-C, both due to the usual-care group being comprised of 7.9% women vs. 16.8% women in the RR group (p = 0.03), and the usual-care group having a higher dietary intake of cholesterol and a lower polyunsaturated to saturated fat (P/S) ratio.

Risk-factor reduction

The RR subjects averaged 23.1 ± 7.9 clinic visits during the 4 years. Substantial favorable changes in risk-factor status occurred for patients in the RR group from baseline to on-study compared to the UC group. Significant differences were achieved in body composition, blood pressure, exercise test performance, plasma lipoprotein concentrations, glucose and insulin, and a composite risk score. For example, on-study LDL-C and apoB were reduced by 22%, Tg reduced by 20%, HDL-C increased by 12% and the Framingham risk score decreased by 22%. Mean Lp(a) values (and log Lp(a)) did not change significantly from baseline to year 4 in either group. Among smokers, the reported number of cigarettes smoked per day by smokers decreased by 12.1 per day in RR subjects, not significantly different from UC subjects. Risk-factor changes in the UC group were small, with several showing significant improvement while others became significantly worse. At baseline, 6.3% of the UC and 12.6% of the RR subjects were taking lipid medications. At 1 year, 11.0% of the UC subjects were prescribed lipid medications by their personal physician; in contrast, 70.6% of the RR subjects were placed on lipid medications by SCRIP staff. At the 4-year follow-up, these percentages rose to 22.6% of UC subjects vs. 89.9% for the RR subjects. Antianginal, antiplatelet, and antihypertensive drugs were used equally in both groups at baseline and on-study, with similar reductions in the use of β-blockers and calcium antagonists on-study in both groups.

Angiographic changes

Disease progression

Baseline and follow-up arteriography with good-quality visualization of diseased segments were available for 127 UC and 119 RR subjects, with an average follow-up interval of 3.96 ± 0.43 years for UC and 4.03 ± 0.27 years for RR subjects. Both groups demonstrated net progression of disease defined by the change in minimum diameter of visibly diseased segments. The rate of change in minimum diameter per patient in the RR group was 47% less than for the UC group (p = 0.02). Differences in rates of change in minimum diameter between the UC and RR groups were somewhat greater for women than men (Table 1). There was no association between age and the reduced rate of progression observed in the RR group.

Table 1. Changes in angiographic status over 4 years in the Stanford Coronary Risk Intervention Project (SCRIP)

	Baseline	UC change	RR change	p for Δ UC vs. RR
Minimum diameter, diseased segments (all values in mm)				
By patient (all)	2.35	−0.18	−0.096	0.02
Men (n = 117;99)	2.37	−0.18	−0.104	0.05
Women (n = 10;20)	2.32	−0.184	−0.064	0.27
By segment (all)	2.28	−0.212	−0.084	0.0001
Men (n = 364;316)	2.30	−0.204	−0.092	0.0006
Women (n = 27;63)	2.26	−0.21	−0.044	0.008
Percent of patients with net regression (%)		10.3	20.2	0.02
New lesion formation				
Patients (%)		31.3	23.0	0.16
Segments (%)		7.6	4.7	0.02
Number of new lesions per patient (#)		0.47	0.30	0.06

Disease regression

The distribution of patients between the UC and RR groups into mutually exclusive categories based on segment change exceeding thresholds of 0.2 mm were significant at p = 0.07. There were 10.3% of UC vs. 20.2% of RR patients in the regression category and nearly equal numbers of patients in both groups in the progression category (UC = 49.6%; RR = 50.4%). The patients with no change represented 19.7% of the UC group and 17.6% of the RR group. The mixed-change patients represented 20.5% of the UC and 11.8% of the RR patients.

New lesion formation

For evaluation of new lesion formation, 257 subjects had 1,605 coronary artery segments identified as visually normal (<5% stenosis) at baseline [4]. Among these visually normal segments, 99 new lesions were identified. The percent of all subjects (n = 257; usual care, n = 131, RR, n = 126) with at least one new lesion was lower for the RR group. However, this difference was not statistically significant (UC, n = 41, 31.3% and RR: n = 29, 23.0%, p = 0.16). The average number of new lesions per patient was 0.47 for UC and 0.30 for RR subjects (p = 0.06). Using a per-segment analysis adjusting for within-subject correlation of new lesion formation, the percent of all normal segments with new lesion formation was significantly lower for RR subjects than segments of patients assigned to UC (UC n = 61, 7.6%; RR n = 38, 4.7%; p = 0.02). When the within-patient correlation for new lesion formation is taken into account using a β-binomial model, the level of significance increases to 0.05.

Multivariate analyses

Disease progression

Univariate and multivariate regression analyses were performed to determine if specific patient characteristics were predictive of the rate of change in the minimal diameter of diseased segments. For all subjects (n = 228), the best two-variable model was change in treadmill exercise test performance (max METS) and change in Framingham risk score (consisting of changes in SBP, total cholesterol to HDL-C ratio and cigarette smoking status), with an increase in treadmill exercise performance and a decrease in risk score related to a reduced rate of progression (p = 0.002, R^2 = 0.05). The best three-variable model included change in max METS, change in Framingham risk score and percent of energy from fat at baseline (p = 0.002, R^2 = 0.07), with a higher percentage of fat associated with a greater rate of progression.

New lesions

First, the usual-care and risk-reduction groups were combined and analyzed for clinical correlates (on a per patient basis) for the formation of at least one new lesion vs. no new lesions. Analysis of on-study clinical variables revealed significantly lower values in the no-new-lesion category for percent dietary fat, saturated fat, monounsaturated fat, polyunsaturated fat, and dietary cholesterol. Reductions from baseline to on-study in plasma, total cholesterol, LDL-C, TC:HDL ratio, fasting glucose and the Framingham risk score were also associated with an absence of new lesion development. A logistic regression analysis indicated that patients obtaining 40% of their calories from fat had a 39% chance of developing at least one new lesion, whereas patients who obtained 20% of their calories from fat had a 19% chance of a new lesion developing.

Discussion

SCRIP contributes substantial new information on the success of intensive multifactor risk reduction in decreasing the rate of coronary atherosclerosis progression and clinical cardiac events in men and women with CAD, but not necessarily with elevated blood lipids. Angiographic benefits occurred even in subjects with a relatively low risk profile. For example, the mean LDL-C for RR subjects at baseline at 4.09 mmol/l was generally lower than that in previously reported angiographic trials. Also, the results of the univariate and multivariate regression analyses indicate that the angiographic changes were associated more with the changes in various risk factors than their baseline values.

SCRIP results support the hypothesis that patients with coronary artery disease who sustain substantial improvement in risk factors decrease the rate of progression of their coronary atherosclerosis. The success of SCRIP in managing risk factors over 4 years indicates that greater consideration should be given to including intensive multiple-risk-factor modification in the treatment of patients with coronary artery disease. SCRIP used a "physician supervised, nurse case-manager" model with consultation from other health professionals that could be implemented in a variety of health-care settings.

Acknowledgements

Supported by a research grant from the National Heart, Lung, and Blood Institute (HL-28292) and a gift from the Claude R. Lambe Charitable Foundation.

References

1. Leung WH, Demopulos PA, Alderman EL, Saunders W, Stadius ML. Cathet Cardiovasc Diag 1990;21:148–153.
2. Leung WH, Sanders W, Alderman EL. Cathet Cardiovasc Diag 1991;24:121–134.
3. Haskell WL, Alderman EL, Fair JM, Maron DJ, Mackey SF, Superko HR, Williams PT, Johnstone IM, Champagne MA, Krauss RM, Farquhar JW. Circulation 1994;89:975–990.
4. Quinn TG, Alderman EA, McMillan A, Haskell WL, SCRIP Investigators. J Am Coll Cardiol 1994 (in press).

The monocyte-macrophage in atherosclerosis: historical background and overview

Colin J. Schwartz and Anthony J. Valente

Department of Pathology, Graduate School of Biomedical Sciences, University of Texas Health Sciences Center, San Antonio, Texas, USA

Abstract. Scientific progress in part reflects cyclical episodes of rediscovery. Atherosclerosis is no exception. In 1862 the celebrated Rudolf Virchow noted that atheromatous lesions exhibit morpho-logical evidence of inflammation, coining the term *endarteritis chronica sive nodosa*. The frequent granulomatous foci and the prominent adventitial lymphocytic infiltration of advanced lesions amply validate his early conclusions. Landmark observations reinforcing the inflammatory concept of atherogenesis and implicating the monocyte-macrophage in pathogenesis were those of Duff et al. (1957), and Poole and Florey (1958). With the role of the macrophage as a major progenitor of plaque foam cells no longer in dispute, largely as a result of the recognition of the scavenger-receptor pathway for modified lipoproteins, research interest has shifted substantially, with a current focus on inflammatory cytokines/chemokines and adhesion molecules in intimal monocyte recruit-ment, intimal oxidant stress, the multivalent roles of the macrophage in atherogenesis, and their contribution to plaque rupture and occlusive thrombosis. Salient features of the sequential evolution of atherosclerosis as an inflammatory disorder, and the participation of the monocyte-derived macrophage in pathogenesis are highlighted, together with a review of some unresolved problems.

Contemporary criteria define inflammation as a process characterized by the localized tissue accumulation of blood constituents including plasma and plasma proteins (e.g., lipoproteins, fibrinogen, immune complexes), together with the interstitial or extravascular accumulation of the formed elements of blood (e.g., monocytes, lymphocytes, platelets). Both the early and later stages of atherosclerosis clearly meet many of these criteria. In this necessarily brief review, we present selected facets of the inflammatory nature of atherosclerosis from a historical perspective. Our emphasis is directed specifically to the participation of lymphocytes and peripheral blood monocytes in plaque pathogenesis, and the role of the latter in lesion foam-cell formation. Mechanisms involved in intimal monocyte-macrophage recruitment are examined, together with an assessment of the pathways through which the monocyte-derived macrophage might impact the atherogenic cascades. Finally, we have attempted to identify at least some of the unresolved problems which might provide a basis for future research in this field.

Human and experimental lesions: morphologic evidence of inflammation

Inflammation as a component of human atherosclerosis was clearly recognized by Rudolf Virchow in 1862 [1]. Much later, in 1913, Anitschkow, an early pioneer of experimental atherosclerosis, illustrated macrophage-derived foam cells in the aortas of cholesterol-fed rabbits [2]. Notwithstanding intermittent descriptions implicating macrophages in the pathogenesis of atherosclerosis, it was not until the landmark observations of Duff,

---

Address for correspondence: Department of Pathology, Graduate School of Biomedical Sciences, University of Texas Health Sciences Center, 7703 Floyd Curl Drive, San Antonio, TX 78284-7750, USA.

McMillan & Ritchie in 1957 [3] and Poole and Florey from the Dunn School in Oxford in 1958 [4] that the association between the monocyte-macrophage on the one hand and the development of arterial lesions in the cholesterol-fed rabbit on the other was articulated explicitly. But the significance of these studies eluded the main stream of science, partly because of the emerging dominance of interest in intimal smooth muscle cells (SMC) as the principal progenitor of plaque foam cells. Lipid-containing SMC have a distinct morphology, generally with a bipolar distribution of lipid droplets and fewer lipid inclusions, and usually exhibit the residual markers of their lineage, namely a basement membrane and peripheral dense bodies. While it is not argued that intimal SMC may accumulate lipid, the majority of plaque foam cells are clearly of monocyte-macrophage lineage.

Interest in the monocyte-macrophage-derived foam cell was rekindled some years later when Gerrity et al. in 1979 [5] noted an augmented focal monocyte-macrophage recruitment to the aortic intima of lesion-prone areas in cholesterol–fat-fed pigs. These observations have been subsequently confirmed in a number of species including pigeon [6], rat [7] and nonhuman primates [8]. The detailed studies of Stary in 1987 [9] have clearly established a similar phenomenon in human coronary arteries. In spite of the decisive demonstration of the macrophage scavenger-receptor pathway for modified low-density lipoproteins as a mechanism leading to foam-cell formation (Goldstein et al., 1979) [10], there still remained a need to establish that monocyte-macrophages could become foam cells in vivo. To this end we developed the carrageenan granuloma model in the cholesterol–fat-fed rabbit, which established beyond any doubt a complete sequence of transitions from the monocyte, through the macrophage, to the fully-developed foam cell [11,12]. These developments implicating inflammation, and in particular the monocyte-macrophage, in atherogenesis are selectively summarized in Table 1.

Another aspect of the inflammatory nature of the atherosclerotic process is the presence of aggregates of inflammatory cells, predominantly lymphocytes, in the tunica adventitia of diseased arteries. These have been the subject of a number of reports, some of which were but a passing mention, as summarized in Table 2. The relationship of the degree of lymphocytic adventitial infiltration to atheromatous plaque severity in multiple arterial beds was determined by Schwartz and Mitchell in 1962 [13]. It was concluded that some 80% of arterial sites associated with an advanced stage of atherosclerosis exhibit an adventitial lymphocytosis. The authors suggested that these lymphocytic aggregates probably represent an autoimmune component in the later stages of plaque pathogenesis, as recently reviewed [14]. That a lymphocytic infiltration of the adventitia is relatively inconspicuous in most experimental models of atherosclerosis is intriguing. Further,

Table 1. Inflammation and atherogenesis: a brief selected historical perspective

Year	Author	Topic	Reference
1862	Virchow	Morphologic evidence of inflammation	[1]
1913	Anitschkow	Macrophage-foam cells in rabbit lesions	[2]
1957	Duff, McMillan & Ritchie	Monocyte-macrophages in rabbit lesions	[3]
1958	Poole & Florey	Monocyte-macrophage foam cells in rabbit lesions	[4]
1979	Gerrity et al.	Monocyte-macrophage foam cells in pig lesions	[5]
1982	Lewis et al.	Monocyte-macrophages in pigeon lesions	[6]
1983	Joris et al.	Monocyte-macrophages in hypercholesterolemic rats	[7]
1985	Schwartz et al.	Monocyte-macrophages in nonhuman primates	[8]
1987	Stary	Macrophage-foam cells in human coronary artery lesions	[9]

Table 2. Lymphocytic cells in the tunica adventitia of atheromatous human arteries: an historical overview

Year	Author(s)	Reference
1915	Allbutt	[16]
1933	Ophuls	[17]
1940	Horn & Finkelstein	[18]
1941	Nelson	[19]
1949	von Hausammann	[20]
1956	Gerlis	[21]
1956	Morgan	[22]
1962	Schwartz & Mitchell	[13]
1988	Emeson & Robertson	[15]
1989	Schwartz et al.	[14]

whether certain epitopes of modified lipoproteins might function as neoantigens is a possibility that merits exploration. While lymphocytes are also inconspicuous within most "early" lesions, including the so-called fatty streaks, T-lymphocytes have been observed in the intima of aortic and coronary lesions of young adults using specific markers for their identification [15].

One other inflammatory feature of advanced atherosclerotic lesions is the frequent presence of pleiomorphic granulomatous foci, usually in juxtaposition to the extracellular necrotic plaque lipid, often with polykarions, and sometimes apparently eroding into the subjacent media. Such areas are likely to be foreign body granulomata, developing as a chronic inflammatory response to components of the extracellular necrotic lipid core and cellular debris.

Intimal monocyte-macrophage recruitment in atherogenesis

The mechanisms responsible for both the attachment to and subsequent directed migration through the arterial endothelium to the subendothelium are complex. Any detailed analysis is beyond the scope of this brief overview, but important aspects are presented separately here (pp. 586–592). In Table 3 we summarize some of the key components of this important process. Because of the predictably focal nature of both human and experimental atherosclerotic lesions, there is now a consensus that lesions develop preferentially at sites of low hemodynamic shear stress, otherwise known as lesion-prone areas [23,24]. At such sites blood-monocyte recruitment to the intima is markedly augmented by even short periods of hypercholesterolemia. Further, it is likely that at such low-shear sites, there exist microdomains of reversing blood flow where the residence time of cells such as blood monocytes is prolonged. Additional recent evidence indicates a focal enhancement of the gene expression of both the chemoattractant chemokine MCP-1 and the adhesion molecule VCAM-1 by low relative to high shear-stress levels [23]. Endothelial activation probably also contributes to the recruitment process, and may result from the action of a variety of agents including the cytokines, tumor necrosis factor alpha (TNF-α), interleukin-1ß (IL-1ß), together with thrombin, and oxidatively modified low density lipoproteins (Ox-LDL), as indicated in Table 3. There is clearly a functional interdependence among a number of soluble cytokines on the one hand, and the membrane- or surface-associated adhesion molecules and their ligands on the other, which probably accounts for the mechanisms through which endothelial activation influences leukocyte recruitment. The cytokine families of particular interest in this regard include

Table 3. Blood-monocyte recruitment to the arterial intima

Favorable focal hemodynamic environment: low shear stress, reversing flow

Endothelial activation: TNF-α, IL-1ß, thrombin, Ox-LDL, LPS

Monocyte rolling, arrest, attachment and directed migration:
  (a) Cytokines
      (i)   Interleukins: e.g., IL-1ß
      (ii) Chemokines: e.g., MCP-1, Rantes
      (iii) Interferons: e.g., IFN-γ
      (iv) Colony-stimulating factors: e.g., M-CSF

  (b) Adhesion molecules
      (i)   Selectins: e.g., E-selectin, P-selectin
      (ii) Integrins: e.g., VLA-4
      (iii) Ig superfamily: e.g., ICAM-1, VCAM-1

Activation–differentiation

Migration inhibition: e.g., Ox-LDL

the interleukins, the interferons, chemokines, and colony-stimulating factors, while the three families of adhesion molecules include the selectins, members of the immuno-globulin superfamily, and the integrins, together with their respective ligands. Collectively they modulate the processes of monocyte rolling, arrest, attachment, and directed migration (Table 3). It should be added that C5a, Ox-LDL, and both collagen and elastin peptides may also participate as chemoattractants in the directed migration of monocytes to the subendothelium (Table 3). Other facets of monocyte recruitment include the phenomena of migration inhibition, and so-called activation differentiation.

Mechanisms through which the macrophage may impact the atherosclerotic process

In Table 4 we have listed the protean functions of the monocyte-derived macrophage which might influence either the process of atherogenesis or the development of occlusive complications. Under certain circumstances one could argue that the macrophage has a protective or beneficial role, contributing for example to physiological intimal debride-ment, and protecting the vessel wall from toxic anionic macromolecules. On the other hand the generation of free radicals, and the secretion of metalloproteases which could influence plaque collagen and thus plaque integrity, could be deleterious. As one reviews Table 4, it is obvious that the macrophage may influence vascular immune function, plaque connective tissues, hemostatic mechanisms and possibly thrombolysis, inflammatory mechanisms, and even vasoreactivity. The ultimate biologic significance of each of these potential roles needs explicit clarification.

Some unresolved problems

It is always a useful exercise to attempt to identify questions that remain to be answered. In spite of the explosive growth of information in this field much work has yet to be undertaken. A few of such areas are listed in Table 5, and each has important implications for the development of innovative therapeutic interventions. In concluding, however, we

Table 4. Some putative roles of the monocyte-macrophage in atherosclerosis

Uptake of modified lipoproteins (Ox-LDL, Glyc-LDL)
Foam-cell formation
Phagocytosis: intimal debridement
Free radical generation
Synthesis of complement components
Secretion of connective tissue hydrolases:
  collagenase types I, IV; cathepsin elastase; heparan sulfate endoglycosidase
Secretion of components of hemostasis/coagulation:
  factors II, VII, IX, X, XIII; thromboplastin; prothrombinase; t-PA; u-PA
Secretion of cytokines, chemokines and growth factors:
  colony-stimulating factors G-, M-, GM-CSF
  interleukin-1, interleukin-6
  tumor necrosis factor, TNF- α,
  platelet-derived growth factors, PDGF
  transforming growth factor ß, TGF-ß
  fibroblast growth factors, FGF
  monocyte chemotactic protein-1, MCP-1
Secretion of bioactive lipids:
  platelet activating factors, PAF
  thromboxane B_2
  prostaglandin E_2
  leukotriene B4, C4
Other secretory products:
  nitric oxide, EDRF
  apolipoprotein E
  lipoprotein lipase, LPL
  α_2-macroglobulin

Adapted from Valente and Schwartz [25].

should remember the great contributions of Elie Metchnikoff (1893), the father of the macrophage [26], and Cohnheim (1882) who contributed so greatly to the early studies of inflammation [27].

Acknowledgements

We are grateful to Ms Anna Juiel for help in preparing this manuscript. Some of the work presented was supported by NHLBI grants HL-26890, HL-07446, and HL-41175.

Table 5. Unresolved problems and possible avenues for future research

— Are there subpopulations of monocytes specifically involved?
— Which mechanisms are dominant in monocyte–endothelium attachment and directed migration to the SES?
— Are intimal macrophages a major source of reactive oxygen species?
— How great is the contribution of lipoprotein phagocytosis to foam-cell formation?
— Is foam-cell death necrotic or programmed, i.e., apoptotic?
— What are the pathobiological implications of monocyte-macrophage activation/differentiation?
— What are the biologic implications of retarding intimal monocyte-macrophage recruitment?
— Do macrophages participate in plaque regression?
— Do intimal/adventitial lymphocytes modulate the role of macrophages in atherogenesis?

References

1. Virchow R. In: Phlogose und Thrombose in Gefässsystem. Berlin: Max Hirsch, 1862.
2. Anitschkow N. Beitr Path Anat Allgem Pathol 1913;56:379—404.
3. Duff GL, McMillan GC, Ritchie AC. Am J Pathol 1957;33:845—873.
4. Poole JCF, Florey HW. J Path Bact 1958;75:245—251.
5. Gerrity RG, Naito HK, Richardson M, Schwartz CJ. Am J Pathol 1979;95:775—792.
6. Lewis JC, Taylor RG, Jones ND, St. Clair RW, Cornhill JF. Lab Invest 1982;46:123—138.
7. Joris I, Zand T, Nunnari JJ, Krolikowski FJ, Majno G. Am J Pathol 1983;113:341—358.
8. Schwartz CJ, Sprague EA, Kelley JL, Valente AJ, Suenram CA. Virchows Archiv A 1985;405:175—191.
9. Stary HC. Atherosclerosis 1987;64:91—108.
10. Goldstein JL, Ho YK, Basu SK, Brown MS. Proc Natl Acad Sci USA 1979;76:333—337.
11. Schwartz CJ, Ghidoni JJ, Kelley JL, Sprague EA, Valente AJ, Suenram CA. Am J Pathol 1985;118:134—150.
12. Kelley JL, Suenram CA, Valente AJ, Sprague EA, Rozek MM, Schwartz CJ. Am J Pathol 1985;120:391—401.
13. Schwartz CJ, Mitchell JRA. Circulation 1962;26:73—78.
14. Schwartz CJ, Sprague EA, Valente AJ, Kelley JL, Edwards EH, Suenram CA. In: Glagov S, Newman WP, Schaffer SA (eds) Pathobiology of the Human Atherosclerotic Plaque. New York: Springer-Verlag, 1989;107—119.
15. Emeson EE, Robertson AL. Am J Pathol 1988;130:359—369.
16. Albutt C. Diseases of the Arteries Including Angina Pectoris, vol 1. London: McMillan Co, 1915.
17. Ophuls W. In: Cowdrey EV (ed) Arteriosclerosis: A Survey of the Problem. New York: Macmillan Co., 1933.
18. Horn H, Finkelstein LE. Am Heart J 1940;19:655—682.
19. Nelson MG. J Path Bact 1941;53:105—116.
20. von Hausammann E. Cardiologia 1949;14:225—242.
21. Gerlis LM. Br Heart J 1956;18:166—172.
22. Morgan AD. The Pathogenesis of Coronary Occlusion. Oxford: Blackwell Scientific Publications, 1956.
23. Schwartz CJ, Sprague EA. Nutr Metab Cardiovasc Dis 1992;2:99—100.
24. Schwartz CJ, Valente AJ, Hildebrandt EF. In: Born GVR, Schwartz CJ (eds) New Horizons in Coronary Heart Disease. London: Current Science, 1993;1.1—1.10.
25. Valente AJ, Schwartz CJ. In: Born GVR, Schwartz CJ (eds) New Horizons in Coronary Heart Disease. London: Current Science, 1993;14.1—14.11.
26. Metchnikoff E. Lectures on the Comparative Pathology of Inflammation. London: Kegan Paul, Trench, Trübner and Co., 1893.
27. Cohnheim J. Lectures on General Pathology. London: The New Sydenham Society, 1882, translated 1889.

The macrophage in human and experimental atherosclerosis

Ross G. Gerrity[1], Alexander S. Antonov[1], David H. Munn[1], Frank P. Bell[2], Renu Virmani[3] and Frank Kolodgie[3]
[1]*Medical College of Georgia, Augusta, Georgia;* [2]*The Upjohn Company, Kalamazoo, Michigan; and* [3]*Armed Forces Institute of Pathology, Washington, DC, USA*

Abstract. There is now a large body of evidence showing that specific mechanisms enhancing monocyte recruitment into the arterial intima are activated in atherogenic conditions. These include expression of adhesion molecules, production of monocyte chemotactic and proliferation factors, and preferential production of monocytes by bone marrow. The study described demonstrates that monocyte proliferation is stimulated by adhesion to the endothelium via an endothelial-cell-specific, contact-dependent mechanism, and that intimal macrophages have 4-fold greater proliferative capacity than blood monocytes. These data suggest that the pool of intimal monocytes may be greatly increased by endothelium-induced stimulation of proliferation as monocytes enter the vessel wall.

There is today a consensus that the fatty streak lesion is the precursor of most clinically significant atherosclerotic plaques. Although the foam cell has been considered a hallmark of fatty streaks and atheromatous plaques for over a century, only in the last decade has it been recognized that most of the macrophage foam cells in fatty lesions are derived from circulating blood monocytes, and that recruitment of monocytes is one of the earliest cellular responses in atherogenesis. Once in the intima, macrophage foam cells sequester lipid by activation of scavenger receptors that allow the unregulated uptake of atherogenic lipoproteins, mainly derived from modification of LDL molecules, and by upregulation of lipid metabolic capabilities [1]. In particular, recent interest has focused on the oxidative modification of LDL and its enhanced uptake by macrophages, as well as the role the macrophage itself plays in LDL oxidation through release of active oxygen species. It has been postulated that monocyte-macrophages contribute to plaque development not only by sequestering intracellular lipid, but also by producing oxidized LDL, which has been shown to be cytotoxic to other arterial wall cells in culture. As a result of studies in this area, there is now a growing argument that intervention strategies should be targeted at preventing lipoprotein oxidation, reducing receptor-mediated uptake of modified lipoproteins by macrophages, or preventing recruitment of monocytes into the arterial wall. This reasoning has gained credence by studies showing reduction of atherosclerosis in animal models treated with antioxidants.

If we accept this reasoning, we are faced with a dichotomy and a real and very pressing dilemma. That is, the body appears to activate several defensive mechanisms, all of which promote monocyte recruitment into the arterial wall under atherogenic conditions, and early lesions are capable of regression dependent on this monocyte involvement. Yet current dogma suggests that therapeutic intervention should be aimed

---

Address for correspondence: Ross G. Gerrity, Department of Pathology, BF 223, Medical College of Georgia, Augusta, GA 30912, USA.

at suppressing monocyte involvement and monocyte function. If one accepts the consensus that fatty streaks are the precursors of clinically significant atherosclerotic plaques, and that monocyte-derived macrophages are responsible for lipid removal and regression of lesions, perhaps an alternative strategy should be to *promote* physiological monocyte recruitment mechanisms, particularly in the young. To this end, this article will briefly review mechanisms known to enhance recruitment of monocytes into the arterial wall in atherogenesis and present new evidence indicating that the arterial endothelium stimulates proliferation of blood monocytes as they traverse the endothelium to enter the intima, thus increasing the pool of intimal macrophages.

Monocyte involvement in early atherogenesis

Recruitment of monocytes in early atherogenesis has been extensively documented in the swine, rat, pigeon and monkey (See Gerrity [2], for review). Moreover, recruitment is not random, but occurs preferentially at sites susceptible (S) to atherosclerosis, at stages concurrent with deposition of LDL in these S-regions [2]. Similar S-regions have been demonstrated in humans [3]. There is also evidence from animal models that lipid-laden foam cells leave fatty lesions in large numbers, thus clearing lipid [2]. Monocytes and lymphocytes have been shown to be present in human lesions [4], and recent data from the multicenter PDAY study indicate that, in humans age 15–34, there is preferential recruitment of leukocytes in S-regions of thoracic aorta which may not progress [5]. Some 60–80% of these cells are monocytes, the remainder being T- and B-lymphocytes in relatively equal numbers (Gerrity, unpublished data). Thus there is good correlation between human and animal model data regarding the preferential occurrence of monocytes in S-regions, which suggests that recruitment mechanisms shown to be present in animal models as well as in tissue culture may also be present in human atherogenesis.

Mechanisms promoting monocyte recruitment into arteries

It is now known that adhesion of leukocytes to the endothelial surface is mediated by activation of endothelial-surface adhesion molecules, the expression of which is regulated by cytokines [6]. Furthermore, a monocyte-specific adhesion molecule (Athero-ELAM) has been identified on the endothelium overlying atherosclerotic plaques [7]. A chemotactic factor specific for monocytes from hyperlipemic swine has been shown to be present in S-regions in hyperlipemic swine aorta [8]. This factor appears identical to monocyte chemotactic protein-1 (MCP-1), which is produced by aortic endothelial and smooth muscle cells in culture in response to minimally oxidized LDL [9]. Additionally, PDGF, M-CSF and oxidized LDL have been shown not only to be produced by arterial wall cells but also to be chemotactic for monocytes. There is evidence in the rabbit [10] and swine [11] that preferential monocyte production by bone-marrow progenitor cells is stimulated in hyperlipemic conditions, resulting in a marked leuko- or monocytosis [10,11], thus providing more monocytes available for recruitment. In swine, hyperlipemic serum has been shown to stimulate preferential production of monocytes by cultured bone-marrow progenitor cells [11]. It is evident from these and other studies that the body responds to atherogenic stimuli by expressing monocyte-specific adhesion molecules and chemotactic factors, and by increasing the number of circulating monocytes. All of these mechanisms promote recruitment of monocytes into the arterial wall, particularly at sites known to be susceptible to atherosclerosis.

579

Endothelial-cell-induced monocyte proliferation

It is also feasible that the intimal monocyte pool may be augmented by proliferation of monocytes that have already entered the arterial intima. There has been much speculation, but few data, in the literature regarding proliferation of intimal monocytes. We hypothesized that, since our data in swine show enhanced monocyte proliferation by bone marrow during atherogenesis, recruited monocytes may also continue to proliferate in the intima. The known production of monocyte colony-stimulating factor (M-CSF) by endothelial cells supports this possibility. We therefore examined proliferation of human peripheral blood monocytes cultured on the surface of confluent layers of human aortic endothelial cells and compared it with that of monocytes cultured alone on plastic. In all experiments, M-CSF was present in the medium at concentrations (200 U/ml) shown to stimulate maximal monocyte proliferation. The results demonstrate that peripheral blood monocytes cultured on endothelial cells are induced into sustained proliferative responses with thymidine indexes of 20–60%, i.e., 40- to 100-fold higher than those seen in monocytes cultured alone (Fig. 1). This endothelial cell-mediated stimulation of proliferation results in a 1,000% increase in total monocyte number within 7–8 days of culture compared to a 10% increase in monocytes cultured alone.

Moreover, this proliferation is contact-dependent, since it cannot be reproduced in three-dimensional chambers in which endothelial cell monolayers are grown on coverslips in the same well as monocytes, but physically separated from the monocytes (Table 1). Additionally, conditioned media from either endothelial cell cultures (EC-CM) or endothelial cell cultures with adherent monocytes in coculture (CC-CM) do not elicit monocyte proliferation greater than that seen by monocytes cultured alone in growth medium (GM) containing M-CSF (Table 1). One must conclude from these data that the

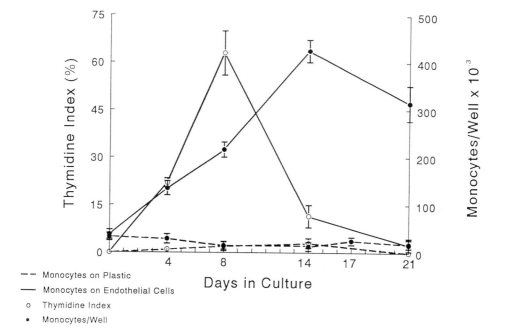

-- Monocytes on Plastic
— Monocytes on Endothelial Cells
o Thymidine Index
• Monocytes/Well

Fig. 1. Endothelial-cell-mediated proliferation of monocytes (μ ± SD).

580

Table 1. Monocyte proliferation is endothelial-cell contact-dependent

Culture condition	Thymidine index[a]
Monocytes/endothelium in contact	35.0 ± 1.8^{b}
Monocytes/endothelium separated	2.0 ± 1.0
Monocytes + EC-CM	3.7 ± 3.1
Monocytes + CC-CM	0.8 ± 0.6
Monocytes + GM	3.0 ± 0.5

[a]Maximal thymidine index between 0–14 days in culture ($\mu \pm$ SD); [b]significantly different ($p < 0.001$) from other conditions.

proliferation is not due to the production of any soluble mediator, including M-CSF.

In other experiments, the proliferation of blood monocytes cultured on endothelial cells was compared to that of monocytes cultured on human aortic intimal cells obtained by enzyme digestion. Intimal cell cultures were shown to consist of approximately 90% smooth muscle cells (SMC) and 10% macrophages by immunohistochemical staining. Additionally, the thymidine index of HAM 56-positive resident intimal macrophages in these intimal cell cultures in the absence of added monocytes was measured. The results (Fig. 2) show that intimal cells do not stimulate monocyte proliferation above that seen in monocytes cultured alone in plastic wells, whereas monocytes cultured on endothelial monolayers showed some 50-fold greater proliferation. Moreover, resident intimal macrophages grown in intimal cell cultures showed a 2–4 times larger thymidine index than blood monocytes grown alone or on identical intimal cell cultures (Fig. 2).

Summary

These results demonstrate that adherence to endothelial cell monolayers stimulates a

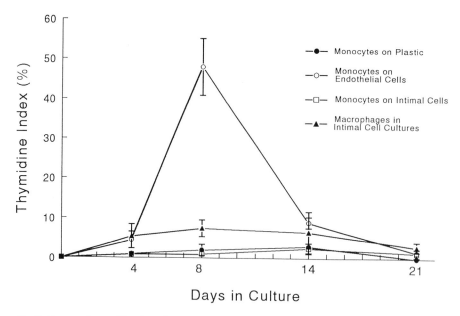

Fig. 2. Comparative proliferation of monocytes and resident intimal macrophages ($\mu \pm$ SD).

sustainable proliferative response in monocytes of a magnitude unobtainable by monocytes alone even under maximal stimulation by M-CSF. This response is endothelial-cell-specific and dependent on endothelial-cell contact. Moreover, the fact that resident intimal macrophages in mixed intimal cell cultures proliferate, but blood monocytes added to intimal cell cultures do not, suggests that the intimal macrophages have been stimulated to proliferate during their adherence to and passage through the endothelium in vivo. If such is the case, not only does the body respond to atherogenic stimuli by production of monocyte chemotactic and growth factors, upregulation of specific adhesion molecules, and stimulation of monocyte production by bone marrow, but also can activate mechanisms inducing proliferation of monocytes as they leave the circulation in the course of becoming intimal macrophages. Although the sustained proliferation in culture induced by continued endothelial-cell contact may not occur in vivo, even a 2- to 4-fold increase in proliferation (Fig. 2) would result in a huge increase in the number of intimal macrophages. Such a response may also explain the presence of clusters of monocytes below the endothelium previously described by ourselves and others in animal models and in humans. Finally, such a proliferative mechanism may also play a role in inflammatory and immune responses.

Acknowledgements

Supported by NIH grant No. HL46312 and Grant-in-Aid No. 193134 from the Juvenile Diabetes Foundation.

References

1. Bell FP, Gerrity RG. Arterioscler Thromb 1992;12:155—162.
2. Gerrity RG. In: Gotto AM Jr (ed) Cellular and Molecular Biology of Atherosclerosis. London: Springer-Verlag, 1992;61—69.
3. Cornhill JF, Herderick EE, Stary HC. Monogr Atheroscler 1990;15:13—19.
4. Gown AM, Tsukada T, Ross R. Am J Pathol 1986;125:191—207.
5. Wissler RW, PDAY Collaborating Investigators. New insights into the pathogenesis of atherosclerosis as revealed by PDAY. Atherosclerosis (in press).
6. Pober JS, Cotran RS. Physiol Rev 1990;70:427—451.
7. Cybulsky MI, Gimbrone MS Jr. Science 1991;251:788—791.
8. Gerrity RG, Goss JA, Soby L. Arteriosclerosis 1985;5:55—66.
9. Cushing SD, Berliner JA, Valente AJ, Territo MC, Navab M, Parhami F, Gerrity R, Schwartz CJ, Fogelman AM. Proc Natl Acad Sci USA 1990;87:5134—5138.
10. Feldman DL, Mogelesky TC, Liptak BF, Gerrity RG. Arterioscler Thromb 1991;11:985—994.
11. Averill LE, Meagher RC, Gerrity RG. Am J Pathol 1989;135:369—377.

582

Adhesion molecules in recruitment of mononuclear cells to the arterial intima

Peter Libby[1], Hongmei Li[1] and Myron I. Cybulsky[2]

[1]*Vascular Medicine and Atherosclerosis Unit, Cardiovascular Division, Department of Medicine and the Vascular Research Division, Department of Pathology, Brigham and Women's Hospital; and* [2]*Harvard Medical School, Boston, Massachusetts, USA*

The adhesion of mononuclear phagocytes to the intact endothelium characterizes the early phase of the arterial response to an atherogenic diet. First recognized by Poole and Florey in rabbit experiments [1], the interaction of monocytes with the endothelium occurs consistently in response to atherogenic diets in other species studied including swine, rats, and nonhuman primates [2–4]. Intimal accumulations of mononuclear phagocytes which transform into lipid-laden foam cells comprise the fatty streak, often a precursor to established atherosclerotic lesions. The process of intimal monocyte recruitment probably occurs in steps. Initially, monocytes must adhere to the endothelium. Until recently, the mechanisms that underlie the process remained elusive. However, recently advances in endothelial biology have suggested plausible explanations for this important initial phase in generation of the atherosclerotic plaque.

The interactions between leukocytes of various classes and the endothelium involve families of selective adhesion molecules expressed on the endothelial surface that recognize cognate ligands on leukocytes of different lineages. The last decade has witnessed the molecular characterization of numerous endothelial-leukocyte adhesion molecules that fall into two broad structural families. One family consists of the selectins, prototypically E-selectin, also known as ELAM-1 (endothelial leukocyte adhesion molecule-1) [5,6]. The other major category of endothelial-leukocyte adhesion molecules includes members of the immunoglobulin superfamily, prototypically ICAM-1 (intercellular adhesion molecule-1) [7].

In the context of monocyte recruitment during atherogenesis, another member of the immunoglobulin superfamily holds particular interest. Vascular cell adhesion molecule-1 (VCAM-1) interacts with very late antigen-4 (VLA-4), an $\alpha_4\beta_1$ integrin expressed on the surface of the very types of leukocytes that accumulate in atheroma, notably monocytes and their derivatives and T-lymphocytes [8,9]. Furthermore, the quest for an atherosclerosis-associated leukocyte adhesion molecule using a monoclonal antibody strategy in rabbits identified VCAM-1 as a structure expressed by endothelial cells overlying established atherosclerotic lesions induced in rabbits by diet or by mutations in the receptor for low density lipoprotein [10]. These various findings suggested VCAM-1 as a likely candidate for an adhesion molecule involved in monocyte recruitment during fatty streak formation.

To determine the potential role of VCAM-1 in this process we studied the early kinetics of VCAM expression after initiation of an atherogenic diet. The endothelial lining of the normal rabbit aorta displays little or no VCAM-1. However, as early as 7 days after

---

Address for correspondence: Peter Libby MD, Brigham & Women's Hospital, 221 Longwood Avenue, Boston, MA 02115, USA. Tel.: +1-617-732-6628. Fax: +1-617-732-6961.

initiation of an atherogenic diet, foci of cells in lesion-prone areas do begin to express VCAM-1 [11]. At this time, the level of hypercholesterolemia is on the order of 300 mg/dl, a level that might be encountered clinically in patients with dyslipidemia. At the next time-point studied, 3 weeks after the atherogenic diet, many macrophages adhered to VCAM-1-bearing aortic endothelial cells. Similar findings regarding VCAM-1 expression have emerged from studies of rabbits with experimentally induced diabetes mellitus with or without concomitant hypercholesterolemia [12]. They support a role for VCAM-1 in leukocyte recruitment, as the expression of VCAM-1 by the endothelium appears to precede substantial macrophage accumulation within the arterial wall.

Almost certainly, molecules other than VCAM-1 must contribute to this process. For example, ICAM-1, although it is more promiscuous in the range of leukocytes with which it interacts, may also participate in monocyte recruitment. Other candidate molecules that may participate in early monocyte–endothelium interactions during fatty streak formation may exist. For example, work from the laboratories of Berman [13], Butcher (McEvoy, unpublished observations), and Berliner [14–16] suggest the existence of such molecules, which remain incompletely characterized at present.

Various types of evidence establish the expression of VCAM-1 by endothelial cells during experimental atherogenesis. However, the signals that elicit this VCAM expression remain unknown. Many cytokines can induce VCAM-1 expression. Notably, interleukin-1 (IL-1) interleukin-4 (IL-4) and tumor necrosis factor-alpha (TNF-α) can all stimulate transcription of VCAM-1 by endothelial cells [17,18]. These mediators also increase expression of VCAM-1 protein by endothelial cells in organoid cultures which maintain endothelial cells in their physiological relationship with matrix and subjacent smooth muscle cells [11]. Cytokines may thus constitute one type of signal that can elicit VCAM-1 expression during atherogenesis in vivo. Other potential triggers for increasing local cytokine expression include oxidatively modified or nonenzymatically glycated lipoproteins. Indeed, components of modified lipoproteins may directly induce VCAM expression. Kume and associates have shown that lysophosphatidyl-choline can induce transcription and translation of VCAM-1 by human endothelial cells in vitro [19,20].

Once monocytes have adhered to the endothelial surface by interaction with VCAM or other adhesion molecules, directed migration must ensue for these cells to accumulate within lesions [21]. Candidate chemotactic molecules in this context include macrophage chemotactic protein-1 (MCP-1), also known as macrophage-activating chemotactic factor-1 or simply as JE (the mouse homolog of MCP-1) [22,23]. Endothelial cells, smooth muscle cells, and macrophages can all express MCP-1 [24–27]. Nelkin and colleagues have documented the presence of MCP-1 transcripts and protein in complicated human atherosclerotic lesions [28]. All these data suggest a role for MCP-1 during atherogenesis.

Once resident within the intima, monocytes differentiate into macrophages and take up lipid, presumably by scavenger receptor-mediated uptake of modified lipoprotein particles. Pathological evidence suggests that human fatty streaks can regress. Therefore, macrophages may leave as well as enter fatty streaks [4,29]. Alternatively, macrophages may undergo necrosis or apoptosis in fatty streaks during their regression [30]. Little is known of the kinetics of leukocyte trafficking during atherogenesis. Various lines of evidence suggest the possibility of bidirectional movement of leukocytes during atherogenesis. However, this remains an area in need of further experimental investigation.

Although many agree that VCAM-1 expression by lesional endothelial cells characterizes early atherogenesis in experimental animals, the analogous role of this molecule in human atherogenesis remains uncertain. Absence of VCAM-1 expression by endothelial cells overlying advanced human lesions does not imply that VCAM-1 did not

584

participate in initial monocyte recruitment earlier in the history of that lesion. During complication of the atherosclerotic plaque numerous microvessels form within the expanding intima [31]. In advanced human lesions such microvessels do express˙VCAM-1 [32]. These plexi of newly formed vessels present a large surface area for leukocyte trafficking compared with the macrovascular luminal endothelium [32,33]. Thus, during the later history of human atheroma, leukocytes may enter or leave the lesions via these plaque microvessels lined with VCAM-1-bearing endothelium.

VCAM-1 induction may actually prove important in vascular diseases other than atherogenesis. For example, after arterial balloon injury, the regenerating vascular endothelial cells express this adhesion molecule [34]. Also, vessels in transplanted organs display augmented VCAM-1 on microvascular endothelial cells during acute rejection, providing a potential portal for leukocyte recruitment during this particular type of immune-mediated inflammatory response [35]. The arteries of transplanted organs commonly develop an accelerated form of arteriosclerosis. The endothelium of affected vessels may also display elevated levels of VCAM-1, in addition to other markers of inflammation or activation [36,37].

Finally, we should note that vascular cells other than endothelium can express VCAM. For example, during the evolution of experimental atheroma in rabbits, we have found [38] a subpopulation of smooth muscle cells that bear VCAM-1. This observation led us to study the regulation of VCAM-gene expression in cultured vascular smooth muscle cells. These experiments formally documented [38] the ability of this cell type to transcribe and translate the VCAM-1 gene. Interestingly, cytokines such as IL-4 and γ-interferon stimulated VCAM expression by both rabbit and human vascular smooth muscle cells. O'Brien and colleagues showed that smooth muscle cells within advanced human atherosclerotic plaques can bear VCAM-1, lending relevance of our experimental observations to human atherogenesis [32].

The functions of VCAM-1 expression by endothelium in acute and chronic vascular response to transplantation, or by smooth muscle cells during atherosclerosis, remain uncertain. In addition to viewing VCAM-1 as an adhesion molecule for leukocytes, we might conceive of a broader role for this molecule [39]. For example, it could participate in nonleukocytic adhesion during development or disease. VCAM-1 might also function as an accessory molecule during antigen presentation in the context of the local vascular immune response. Even in the absence of a defined function, VCAM-1 expression serves as an activation marker indicating the action of inducing stimuli such as cytokines.

Over the last decade many experiments such as those described above have suggested plausible molecular mechanisms for macrophage recruitment. Yet the precise role of individual molecules in vivo remains unproven. Molecular genetic approaches will almost certainly help to answer many of the outstanding questions. For example, study of the kinetics of leukocyte recruitment in mice that bear compound mutations which confer susceptibility to atherogenic diets and interfere with various cytokines will help to define the signals that stimulate expression of adhesion molecules during experimental formation of atherosclerotic lesions. Such experiments though attractive in principle, may prove difficult because of practical considerations that render them harder to perform or interpret than is evident at first glance. For example, animals unable to express certain adhesion molecules may fail to develop. Furthermore, cytokine networks may be so redundant that interruption of any one limb of such a signaling pathway may not produce dramatic effects. Nonetheless, work over the last decade has identified molecular candidates for mediating several of the key initial events in atheroma formation. The advent of modern molecular genetics should permit the testing of many of these mechanisms in critical fashion in the coming years.

Acknowledgements

We thank our colleagues Hiroyuki Tanaka, Michael A. Gimbrone Jr and Michael P. Bevlacqua for their contributions to our work. Experiments described here were supported in part by grants from the National Heart, Lung and Blood Institute of the USA including PO-1 HL-48743 (subsuming RO-1-HL-47840 to P.L. and M.I.C, NIH National Research Service Award F32-HLO9113 to H.L., and HL 45563 to M.I.C.

References

1. Poole JCF, Florey HW. J Pathol Bacteriol 1958;75:245−253.
2. Gerrity RG, Naito HK, Richardson M, Schwartz CJ. Am J Pathol 1979;95:775−786.
3. Joris T, Nunnari JJ, Krolikowski FJ, Majno G. Am J Pathol 1983;113:341−358.
4. Faggiotto A, Ross R, Harker L. Arteriosclerosis 1984;4:323−340.
5. Bevilacqua MP, Nelson RM. J Clin Invest 1983;91:379−387.
6. Bevilacqua MP. Ann Rev Immunol 1993;11:767−804.
7. Springer TA. Nature 1990;346:425−434.
8. Osborn L, Hession C, Tizard R, Vassallo C, Luhowskyj S, Chi-Rosso G, Lobb R. Cell 1989;59:1203−1211.
9. Elices MJ, Osborn L, Takada Y, Crouse C, Luhowskyj S, Hemler ME, Lobb RR. Cell 1990;60:577−584.
10. Cybulsky MI, Gimbrone MA Jr. Science 1991;251:788−791.
11. Li H, Cybulsky MI, Gimbrone MA Jr, Libby P. Arterioscler Thromb 1993;13:197−204.
12. Richardson M, Hadcock SJ, DeReske M, Cybulsky MI. Arterioscler Thromb 1994;14:760−769.
13. Calderon TM, Factor SM, Hatcher VB, Berliner JA, Berman JW. Lab Invest 1994;70:836−849.
14. Territo MC, Berliner JA, Almada L, Ramirez R, Fogelman AM. Arteriosclerosis 1989;9:824−828.
15. Berliner JA, Territo MC, Sevanian A, Ramin S, Kim JA, Bamshad B, Esterson M, Fogelman AM. J Clin Invest 1990;85:1260−1266.
16. Kim JA, Territo MC, Wayner E, Carlos TM, Parhami F, Smith CW, Haberland ME, Fogelman AM, Berliner JA. Arterioscler Thromb 1994;14:427−433.
17. Neish AS, Williams AJ, Palmer HJ, Whitley MZ, Collins T. J Exp Med 1992;176:1583−1593.
18. Collins T. J Vasc Surg 1992;15:923−924.
19. Kume N, Cybulsky MI, Gimbrone MA Jr. J Clin Invest 1992;90:1138−1144.
20. Kume N, Gimbrone M Jr. J Clin Invest 1994;93:907−911.
21. Gerrity RG, Goss JA, Soby L. Arteriosclerosis 1985;5:55−66.
22. Valente AJ, Fowler SR, Sprague EA, Kelley JL, Suenram CA, Schwartz CJ. Am J Pathol 1984;117: 409−417.
23. Navab M, Imes SS, Hama SY, Hough GP, Ross LA, Bork RW, Valente AJ, Berliner JA, Drinkwater DC, Laks H, Fogelman AM. J Clin Invest 1991;88:2039−2046.
24. Rollins BJ, Stier P, Ernst T, Wong GG. Mol Cell Biol 1989;9:4687−4695.
25. Rollins BJ, Yoshimura T, Leonard EJ, Pober JS. Am J Pathol 1990;136:1229−1233.
26. Taubman MB, Rollins BJ, Nadal-Ginard B. Circulation 1989;80(4):II−451.
27. Wang J, Sica A, Peri G, Walter S, Martin-Padura I, Libby P, Ceska M, Lindley I, Colotta F, Mantovani A. Arteriosclerosis 1991;11:1166−1174.
28. Nelken N, Coughlin S, Gordon D, Wilcox J. J Clin Invest 1991;88:1121−1127.
29. Faggiotto A, Ross R. Arteriosclerosis 1984;4:341−356.
30. Libby JP, Clinton SK. Nouv Rev Fr Hématol 1992;34:S47−S53.
31. Barger A, Beeuwkes IR, Lainey L, Silverman K. N Engl J Med 1984;310:175−177.
32. O'Brien K, Allen M, McDonald T, Chait A, Harlan J, Fishbein D, McCarty J, Ferguson M, Hudkins K, Benjamin C, Lobb R, Alpers C. J Clin Invest 1993;92:945−951.
33. Brogi E, Winkles J, Underwood R, Clinton S, Alberts G, Libby P. J Clin Invest 1993;92:2408−2418.
34. Tanaka H, Sukhova GK, Swanson SJ, Clinton SK, Ganz P, Cybulsky MI, Libby P.Circulation 1993;88: 1788−1803.
35. Tanaka H, Sukhova G, Swanson S, Cybulsky M, Schoen F, Libby P. Am J Pathol 1994;144:938−951.
36. Briscoe DM, Schoen FJ, Rice GE, Bevilacqua MP, Ganz P, Pober JS. Transplantation 1991;51:537−539.
37. Tanaka H, Sukhova G, Libby P. Arterioscler Thromb 1994;14:734−745.
38. Li H, Cybulsky MI, Gimbrone MA Jr, Libby P. Am J Pathol 1993;143:1551−1559.
39. Libby P, Li H. J Clin Invest 1993;92:538−539.

Monocyte-macrophage recruitment to the arterial intima: a role for MCP-1 and its receptor

Anthony J. Valente[1], M. Marius Rozek[2], Margaret Abramova[1] and Colin J. Schwartz[1]

[1]The Department of Pathology and the [2]Department of Medicine, University of Texas Health Sciences Center, San Antonio, Texas, USA

Abstract. Monocyte recruitment to the intima is a process which probably occurs throughout all stages of plaque pathogenesis. One mechanism involved in leukocyte accumulation in the tissue is the generation of specific chemoattractants and mediators of leukocyte activation at the site of inflammation. In recent years numerous monocyte chemoattractants of potential importance in the pathogenesis of atherosclerosis have been described, including thrombin, degradation products of matrix proteins, Ox-LDL and members of the C-C subclass of chemokines (e.g., MCP-1, RANTES, MIP-1α and β). MCP-1 is the product of an early response gene and is expressed in a wide variety of tissues. It is induced by cytokines, lipopolysaccharides, modified LDL and thrombin. In human and experimental atherosclerotic lesions, MCP-1 has been identified in smooth muscle cells and in monocyte-macrophages and foam cells. MCP-1 appears to mediate monocyte migration through endothelial cells in vitro and increases the adherence of monocytes to endothelium. Thus MCP-1 may be an important factor in monocyte recruitment in atherogenesis. MCP-1 mediates its effect on monocytes through high-affinity cell-surface receptors. High-affinity binding sites have not been identified on either lymphocytes or polymorphonuclear leukocytes. Recent studies indicate that the chemokine receptors belong to the 7-transmembrane-domain receptor family with G-protein binding activity. Soon after isolation, monocytes lose both chemotactic responsiveness to MCP-1 and MCP-1 binding activity. During this same period, MCP-1 is synthesized and secreted by the cells. Thus as the process of activation-differentiation is initiated, monocytes convert from an MCP-1-responsive to an unresponsive state. This is not inconsistent with the view that a major function of MCP-1 and its receptor is monocyte recruitment from the circulation to the tissue. The spontaneous and prolonged expression of MCP-1 by monocyte-macrophages suggests the presence of specific gene-regulation pathways in these cells. Cloning and sequencing of 1,874 bases of the 5′ flanking region of the human MCP-1 gene has resulted in the identification of cis-acting elements which bind nuclear factors restricted to macrophages and B-cells. Preliminary studies indicate that nuclear proteins from monocytoid cells bind some of these sites specifically.

The migration of leukocytes from the circulation to the tissue involves a complex series of interactions between leukocytes, vascular endothelium and inducible mediators elucidated by both cell types in response to inflammatory stimuli. This complex process has become more clearly defined over the recent years and a consensus view of its underlying mechanisms has evolved [1]. The leukocyte-recruitment process must include contact of the circulating cell with the endothelium, adhesion, induction of locomotion, and migration into the subendothelial space (diapedesis). Leukocyte contact with endothelium is probably influenced by the blood-flow field and in large vessels probably occurs in areas of reversing flow and low fluid mechanical shear, such as occur at bifurcations of major vessels. Leukocyte adhesion to endothelium is perceived as a multistep process involving rolling of the leukocyte along the endothelium, then firm adhesion to

---

Address for correspondence: Anthony J. Valente, 7703 Floyd Curl Drive, San Antonio, TX 78284-7750, USA.

activated endothelium, followed by locomotion and directed migration of the cell into the tissue [1].

It is thought that members of the selectin family of adhesion molecules and selectin/carbohydrate interaction are important in the rolling phenomenon, whereas activation of the endothelium and the expression of ICAM and VCAM molecules and interaction with leukocyte integrins mediate firm adhesion and subsequent migration. Directed migration of the leukocyte through the endothelium is modulated by chemotactic factors elaborated by the tissue. Differential expression by endothelium of specific adhesion molecules and production of specific leukocyte chemoattractants by the inflamed tissue probably account for the type of leukocyte recruited to the site of inflammation. Specific chemoattractants that could potentially stimulate monocyte accumulation in atherogenesis include thrombin, proteolytic fragments of collagen, elastin and fibronectin, oxidatively modified LDL (Ox-LDL) and members of the β (C-C) subfamily of chemokines which includes MCP-1 (Table 1). Although attention will be focused on the role of the chemokine MCP-1 in monocyte migration and recruitment, the importance of the plasma and connective tissue-derived chemoattractants cannot be underestimated, particularly during the later stages of the disease where considerable connective-tissue production and necrosis is present. Some plasma-derived proteins, such as thrombin and oxidatively modified LDL, may also function indirectly by stimulating the synthesis of MCP-1 and other cytokines by vascular cells.

Monocyte chemotactic protein-1 (MCP-1)

MCP-1 is a member of a superfamily of genes called chemokines that act as chemoattractants and modulators of leukocyte function [2]. This large family of small molecular weight proteins (6–12 kDa) is characterized by a similarly spaced motif of 4 cysteine residues and is subdivided structurally into two main groups, the α or C-X-C group and the β or C-C group, dependent on whether a single amino acid intervenes between the adjacent first two cysteine residues. Generally, members of the C-X-C family are chemotactic for and activate granulocytes, whereas the C-C family members act predominantly on monocytes. MCP-1 is currently the most extensively characterized member of the C-C subfamily and its potential role in monocyte recruitment to the tissues will be discussed here. It is becoming evident, however, that within each subgroup there is a degree of overlapping function or redundancy. Therefore in vivo, chemokines of the

Table 1. Potential monocyte chemoattractants mediating intimal monocyte recruitment in atherogenesis

Plasma-derived
    Ox-LDL
    Thrombin
    C5a
Matrix-derived
    Fibronectin peptides
    Collagen peptides
    Elastin peptides
Cell-derived
    MCP-1
    MCP-2
    MCP-3
    RANTES
    MIP-1α and β

same subgroup may act in concert rather than singly.

MCP-1 is expressed by a broad variety of cultured cells, including vascular endo-thelium, smooth muscle cells and monocyte-macrophages. It is rapidly induced by a variety of stimuli including inflammatory cytokines such as 1L-1β, TNF-α and IFN-γ and plasma-derived proteins such as minimally modified LDL and thrombin. Antibody neutralization studies indicate that MCP-1 accounts for most of the monocyte chemotactic activity secreted constitutively by some cells, which suggests that this chemokine is one of the more important mediators of monocyte chemotaxis in tissue injury and inflam-mation. Nevertheless, in some animal models of chronic inflammation, the infusion of neutralizing antibodies to MCP-1 has been shown to inhibit monocyte migration into a site of tissue injury only partially. Thus not unexpectedly, more than one monocyte chemoattractant protein modulates monocyte recruitment in inflammation.

There is indirect evidence that MCP-1 mediates intimal monocyte recruitment in atherogenesis. Firstly, MCP-1 can be identified in human and experimental atherosclerotic lesions (in particular in intimal and medial smooth muscle cells and intimal monocyte-macrophage) but not in normal vascular tissue [3–5]. Secondly, the work of Fogelman and his colleagues has shown that plasma LDL that has undergone a minimal form of oxidative modification (MM-LDL) can be a potent inducer of cytokines and chemokines in vascular endothelial cells [6,7]. Therefore LDL oxidation, believed to be an important mechanism in atherogenesis, may also provide the stimulus for MCP-1 production. Thirdly, Navab and his colleagues have shown that isolated peripheral blood monocytes added to cocultures of smooth muscle cells overlayered with confluent endothelial cells migrated through the endothelial layer to the space below [8]. This migration was augmented by the addition of LDL and inhibited by the antibodies to MCP-1. The fact that monocytes migrated through the endothelial layers at all suggests this process to be an inherent property of both cell types that is initiated possibly by their contact and interaction. Inhibition of migration with antibodies to MCP-1 also suggests that MCP-1 is an important component of this mechanism of migration. These observations together point to a role for MCP-1 in intimal monocyte recruitment in atherogenesis. More direct evidence will require experiments in vivo in which the effect of neutralization of MCP-1 on monocyte accumulation in the intima may be determined.

MCP-1 receptor expression on monocytes

MCP-1 mediates its effect on peripheral blood monocytes through high-affinity cell-surface receptors [9,10]. Equilibrium binding studies have identified the high-affinity sites on monocytes but not on lymphocytes or polymorphonuclear leukocytes, which corresponds to the observed cell specificity of MCP-1 as chemoattractant. MCP-1 also stimulates the release of histamine from basophils. Whether this is mediated by the same receptor protein remains to be determined. To date, cross-competition binding studies have identified three functionally distinct monocyte receptor specificities for the C-C chemokines [11]. One is specific for MCP-1, one appears to be a shared receptor for MIP-1α and MIP-1β, and one a shared receptor for MIP-1α/RANTES/MCP-1. The full physio-logic significance for the shared specificity or promiscuity of the chemokine receptors is not fully understood but in addition to providing the structural basis for functional redundancy between the C-C chemokines, it may also, in combination with differential expression of C-C chemokine genes, provide a more precise modulation of leukocyte function at sites of tissue injury. The genes for two C-C receptor proteins have recently been described [12,13]. The first encodes a protein which binds MIP-1β and RANTES with high affinity and MIP-1α and MCP-1 with low affinity. A second gene, described by Charo and colleagues, selectively binds MCP-1 with high affinity and is expressed in monocytes and monocytic cell lines such as THP-1 and MonoMac 6, but not in polymorphonuclear leukocytes or lymphocytes. Thus at least one C-C receptor protein specific for MCP-1 has been identified. Like all other leukocyte chemoattractant receptor genes, the C-C chemokine receptor genes encode membranous proteins containing seven transmembrane α-helical segments, an extracellular N-terminal domain and an intracellular C-terminal domain. Chemoattractant receptors are coupled to G-proteins which constitute a pertussis toxin-sensitive stimulus-response pathway mediating the biologic response of the leukocytes to the chemotactic ligands [11]. Interaction of the specific receptors with the chemokine ligands leads to chemotaxis as a major biologic response.

In addition, chemokines have also been shown to elicit other biologic activities including increased leukocyte adhesion to endothelium, the stimulation of superoxide anion production and cytokine release, and induction of a pyrogenic response. It is unknown at present whether a single receptor protein is responsible for all these activities or whether they are mediated through separate receptors. This is of potential interest since monocyte responsiveness to MCP-1 is labile and appears to be reduced or absent in cells that have undergone maturation–differentiation into macrophages (e.g., resident peritoneal macrophages). Freshly isolated monocytes show a time-dependent and specific loss of chemotactic reactivity to MCP-1. After 4 h of culture in suspension, chemotactic responsiveness to MCP-1 is significantly reduced, whereas responsiveness to an unrelated chemotactic activity, zymosan-activated serum, remains essentially unchanged (Fig. 1). During this same period we have also observed a reduction in monocyte high-affinity binding activity for MCP-1 (Fig. 2). Incubation of monocytes for 4 h resulted in a 30–70% reduction in specific MCP-1 binding (mean = 49% ± 7.8 SEM, n = 5). This reduction was augmented by treatment of the cells with IFN-γ and lipopolysaccharide

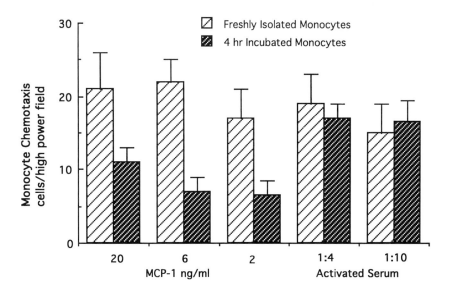

Fig. 1. Effect of culture on monocyte chemotaxis. Freshly isolated monocytes were incubated in teflon vials for 4 h at 5–10 × 10⁵ cells/ml in medium containing 0.5% human serum albumin. The cells were then collected and assayed for chemotactic response to purified human MCP-1 and zymosan-activated serum.

590

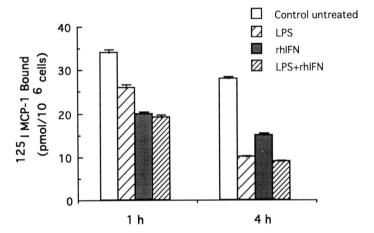

Fig. 2. Influence of culture and activation on monocyte MCP-1-binding sites. Freshly isolated monocytes were incubated in Teflon vials for the indicated times in medium containing 0.5% human serum albumin and 10 ng/ml lipopolysaccharide and/or 250 units/ml recombinant human interferon-γ.

(Fig. 2). This loss of chemotactic responsiveness and receptor-binding activity may be the result of desensitization by monocyte-derived MCP-1. When first isolated, monocytes display very low or undetectable levels of MCP-1 mRNA. After 4-h incubation in suspension, the MCP-1 message is increased and MCP-1 protein is synthesized and secreted. Thus autologous downregulation of the receptors may be taking place. However, an alternative explanation, that MCP-1 receptors are downregulated via an activation pathway independent of MCP-1 production, cannot be ruled out. Whichever mechanism is ultimately determined to be responsible, the loss of MCP-1 responsiveness to MCP-1 and the concomitant upregulation of the MCP-1 gene expression in mononcytes is not inconsistent with the view that the primary function of MCP-1 and its receptor is as mediator of monocyte recruitment from the circulation to the tissue.

MCP-1 expression by monocyte-macrophages

The observation that isolated monocytes rapidly express MCP-1 after isolation and maintain expression for several days even without stimulation [14] suggests a primary role for monocyte-macrophages in the recruitment of further monocytes from the circulation. Studies on human, primate and rabbit atherosclerotic lesions indicate that intimal monocyte-macrophages may be a major source of MCP-1 in the lesion [3–5]. In addition, in some models of chronic inflammatory disease, recently recruited monocyte-macrophages appear to be the dominant source of MCP-1 in the inflamed tissue [15]. Monocytes when isolated from the blood and cultured in the presence of serum adhere to the substrate and undergo morphologic and functional differentiation into mature macrophages. Functional changes include upregulation of cell-surface receptors (e.g., scavenger and C3b receptors) and increased cytokine release. In addition, as outlined above, cultured human monocytes show increased expression of MCP-1 mRNA within 4 h of culture, reach maximal levels of expression by 21 h and continue expression for a number of days. These changes most likely reflect maturation-associated events that take place in vivo. Among the genes that are selectively induced very early after adherence of the cells to a substrate are the proinflammatory cytokines IL-1β and TNF-α, the proto-oncogene c-*fos*, the maturation factor CSF-1, the enzyme superoxide dismutase and members of the C-X-C subfamily of chemokines, IL-8 and GRO [16]. Of particular interest is the parallel induction of a gene termed MAD3 that encodes a protein with the structural and physical properties of IkB, the cytoplasmic inhibitor of the transcription factor NFkB [17]. MAD3 inhibits the DNA binding of the p50/p65 NFkB complex but not of p50/p50 KBF1 or other DNA-binding proteins. It has been suggested that the rapid induction of MAD3/IkB stimulated by adherence provides a potential homeostatic pathway that limits the induction of genes through the cytokine-stimulated NFkB pathway. Thus over-stimulation of the monocyte-macrophage by autologously produced IL-1β and TNF-α may be controlled.

The rapid induction and prolonged expression of the MCP-1 gene in monocyte-macrophages, both in vivo and in vitro, suggest that the transcriptional control of the gene may be modulated by tissue-specific factors. To identify some of the factors regulating transcription of MCP-1 we have cloned and sequenced the 5′-flanking region of the human MCP-1 gene to 1,874 bases from the translational start site, thus extending the previously described sequence [18] by approximately 1,300 bases. Several potential regulatory elements have been identified in this region, but of particular interest is the identification of four copies of the sequence GAGGAA which is recognized by the monocyte/B-cell specific DNA-binding factors PU.1 and Spi-B [19,20]. These factors belong to the ets family of oncogenes which are restricted to hemopoietic tissue. GAGGAA sequences bound by PU.1 have been identified in the promoter regions of the genes for CSF-1 receptor, Ig kappa chain and urokinase plasminogen activator [21—23]. Our preliminary studies using DNAse 1 footprinting and gel-mobility shift assays indicate that at least one of the PU.1 sites in the MCP-1 promoter region binds nuclear proteins isolated from the monocytic cell line THP-1, but not proteins from nonmonocytic HeLa cells. Studies are currently in progress to define the role of these tissue-restricted factors on the transcriptional regulation of the MCP-1 gene in monocytic cells. Identification of such tissue-specific pathways regulating MCP-1 gene expression in monocyte-macrophages will provide insight into one of the basic mechanisms regulating chronic inflammation and the inflammatory component of atherosclerosis.

Acknowledgements

We are grateful to Ms Anna Juiel for help in preparing this manuscript. Some of the work presented was supported by NHLBI grants HL-26890, HL-07446, and HL-41175.

References

1. Lasky LA. Science 1992;258:964—969.
2. Schall TJ. "The Chemokines" In: Thomson A (ed) The Cytokine Handbook. New York: Academic Press, 1994.
3. Yla-Herttuala S, Lipton BA, Rosenfeld ME, Sarkioja T, Yoshimura T, Leonard EJ, Witztum JL, Steinberg D. Proc Natl Acad Sci USA 1991;88:5252—5256.
4. Nelken NA, Coughlin SR, Gordon D, Wilcox JN. J Clin Invest 1991;88:1121—1127.
5. Yu X, Dluz S, Graves DT, Zhang L, Antoniades HN, Hollander W, Prusty S, Valente AJ, Schwartz CJ, Sonenshein GE. Proc Natl Acad Sci USA 1992;89:6953—6957.
6. Cushing SD, Berliner JA, Valente AJ, Territo MC, Navab M, Parhami F, Gerrity R, Schwartz CJ, Fogelman AM. Proc Natl Acad Sci USA 1990;87:5134—5138.
7. Rajavashisth TB, Andalibi A, Territo MC, Berliner JA, Navab M, Fogelman AM, Lusis AJ. Nature 1990; 344:254—257.
8. Navab M, Imes S, Hough GP, Ross LA, Bork R, Valente AJ, Berliner JA, Drinkwater DC, Laks H, Fogelman AM. J Clin Invest 1991;88:2039—2046.
9. Yoshimura T, Leonard EJ. J Immunol 1990;145:292—297.

10. Valente AJ, Rozek MM, Schwartz CJ, Graves DT. Biochem Biophys Res Commun 1991;176:309–314.
11. Murphy PM. Ann Rev Immunol 1994;12:593–633.
12. Neote K, DiGregorio D, Mak JY, Horuk R, Schall TJ. Cell 1993;72:415–425.
13. Charo IF, Myers SJ, Herman A, Franci C, Connolly AJ, Coughlin SR. Proc Natl Acad Sci USA 1994;91: 2752–2756.
14. Cushing SD, Fogelman AM. Arterioscler Thromb 1992;12:78–82.
15. Flory CM, Jones ML, Warren JS. Lab Invest 1993;69:396–404.
16. Sporn SA, Eierman DF, Johnson CE, Morris J, Martin G, Ladner M, Haskill S. J Immunol 1990;144:4434–4441.
17. Haskill S, Beg AA, Tompkins SM, Morris JS, Yurochko AD, Sampson-Johannes A, Mondal K, Ralph P, Baldwin AS. Cell 1991;65:1281–1289.
18. Rollins BJ, Stier P, Ernst T, Wong GG. Mol Cell Biol 1989;9:4687–4695.
19. Klemsz MJ, McKercher SR, Celada A, Van Beveren C, Maki RA. Cell 1990;61:113–124.
20. Ray D, Bosselut R, Ghysdael J, Mattei MG, Tavitian A, Moreau-Gachelin F. Mol Cell Biol 1992;12:4297–4304.
21. Zhang DE, Hetherington CJ, Chen HM, Tenen DG. Mol Cell Biol 1994;14:373–381.
22. Ross IL, Dunn TL, Yue S, Roy S, Barnett CJK, Hume DA. Oncogene 1994;9:121–132.
23. Pongubala JMR, Van Beveren C, Nagulapalli S, Klemsz MJ, McKercher SR, Maki RA, Atchison ML. Mol Cell Biol 1994;12:368–378.

Atherosclerosis X.
F.P. Woodford, J. Davignon and A. Sniderman, editors.

Macrophage adhesion in atherosclerosis: a role for the scavenger receptor?

Willem J.S. de Villiers, Iain P. Fraser, Derralynn A. Hughes and Siamon Gordon
Sir William Dunn School of Pathology, University of Oxford, Oxford, UK

Abstract. We have isolated a rat mAb, 2F8, that inhibits the unique EDTA-resistant ability of macrophages (Mφ) to adhere to tissue-culture plastic (TCP) in the presence of serum [1]. The antibody recognizes both forms of the murine macrophage scavenger receptor (MSR). This receptor, implicated in foam-cell formation in atherogenesis, has previously only been shown to mediate endocytosis. Macrophage-colony stimulating factor (M-CSF) potently upregulates MSR expression and function, including adhesion, in a selective fashion [2]. Vascular endothelial cells and smooth muscle cells produce M-CSF in response to modified lipoproteins, and increased MSR expression and function may be an important mechanism for Mφ recruitment and/or retention in atherosclerotic lesions.

One of the earliest cellular events in atherogenesis is the adherence of monocytes to the endothelium. The macrophage has moved center-stage in our understanding of naturally occurring and experimental atherosclerosis [3,4]. Lipid-laden foam cells interact with other cellular and extracellular constituents of arteries through a variety of receptor and secretory-product mechanisms, establishing a chronic host response to injury. The potential pathways of monocyte recruitment to altered endothelium, migration and retention within lesions, oxidative modification and endocytosis of lipoproteins, stimulation of smooth muscle cell proliferation, as well as the role of the macrophage in inducing coagulation and fibrinolysis, can now be studied in the human and in primate and murine disease models.

The demonstration that acetylated, but not native, LDL could produce foam-cell formation in vitro led to the characterization of the macrophage scavenger receptor (MSR) [5] and its subsequent cloning [6]. Although there is increasing evidence for the importance of the MSR in host defense [7] and adhesion [1,8], its role in atherogenesis remains its best-characterized in vivo function. Oxidation of LDL, and its interaction with endothelial cells (EC), smooth muscle cells (SMC) and monocytes/Mφ, is thought to be a central feature in atherogenesis, and Mφ themselves are capable of oxidizing LDL to form species that are recognized by the MSR. The concept of minimally modified LDL (MM-LDL) has been used to describe LDL that has been mildly oxidized, but insufficiently so for recognition by the MSR. Uptake of MM-LDL by the native LDL receptors on EC has been shown to stimulate monocyte–endothelium interactions as a result of enhanced secretion of monocyte chemotactic factors and increased expression of endothelial adhesion receptors. This effect was specific for monocytes; interactions between neutrophils and endothelium were unaffected by MM-LDL.

This cell specificity was explained, at least in part, by the demonstration that MM-LDL induced secretion by endothelial cells of monocyte chemoattractant protein-1 (MCP-1),

---

Address for correspondence: Dr Willem J.S. de Villiers, Sir William Dunn School of Pathology, University of Oxford, South Parks Road, Oxford, OX2 6UD, UK.

594

as well as secretion of G-, GM-, and macrophage-colony stimulating factor (M-CSF) [9]. The finding that OxLDL inhibited the motility of resident peritoneal Mφ (but not monocytes) in vitro suggested that this may be an important mechanism for Mφ retention in atherosclerotic lesions. Recent work showing that the antioxidant probucol prevented the accumulation of Mφ at atherosclerotic sites in the rabbit provides evidence that this may be an important mechanism in vivo. Our data provide a possible mechanism by which Mφ may use the MSR as an adhesion receptor for their retention within these lipoprotein-rich atherosclerotic plaques.

The regulation of MSR expression and activity may represent an important determinant of the extent of atherogenesis. The interpretation of studies describing regulation of MSR expression and activity has been complicated by: i) the nature of the assays (functional uptake vs. mRNA expression vs. protein expression), ii) the types of cell used (monocytes vs. different Mφ populations), iii) differences in sources and purities of cytokines used to treat cells, and iv) differences between species (murine vs. human vs. bovine). A summary of the major studies published to date are included in Table 1.

It should be noted that dexamethasone has been described as both up- and downregulating MSR activity, an example of the difficulties alluded to above. The inhibitory effect of bacterial LPS on MSR function appears to be mediated via autocrine TNF-α produced by the Mφ. Most of the studies have concentrated on cytokines and regulatory molecules produced by the cells located within the vascular wall and/or in atherosclerotic lesions. Few if any have considered the regulation of MSR in vivo at its many, and apparently highly regulated, nonatherosclerotic locations.

Characterization of MSR regulation and expression has also been hampered by the lack of specific reagents. A novel function for the MSR as an adhesion receptor was recently

Table 1. Factors regulating MSR activity/expression

Upregulation		Downregulation	
Monocyte maturation (phorbol ester, adherence)	Fogelman (1981)	Lymphocyte-conditioned medium	Fogelman (1982)
		LPS/endotoxin	van Lenten (1985)
Serum component(s)	Fogelman (1981)	"Platelet-derived products" (serotonin, ADP, fibrinogen, fibronectin, PDGF)	Aviram (1989)
Dexamethasone	Hirsch (1986)	TGF β₁	Bottalico (1991)
Monocyte-conditioned medium	Aviram (1989)	Protein kinase C inhibitors	Akeson (1991)
Arterial smooth muscle cell-conditioned medium	Aviram (1989)	Poly (I:C)	de Whalley (1991)
		Interferon γ	Fong (1990); Geng (1992)
Fibroplast-conditioned medium	Aviram (1989)	Dexamethasone	Moulton (1992)
1,25-dihydroxyvitamin D3	Jouni (1991)	TNF-α	van Lenten (1992)
M-CSF	Ishibashi (1990); de Villiers (1994)	Prostacyclin agonists	Kowada (1993)

described; this stemmed from the observation that a monoclonal antibody (mAb), 2F8, to the murine MSR inhibited serum-dependent divalent cation-independent Mφ adhesion in vitro. Use of this MSR-specific reagent will greatly facilitate reliable regulatory studies of MSR expression at the protein level.

M-CSF treatment in patients with hematological disease coincides with significant reductions in serum cholesterol levels. As M-CSF enhances acetylated low-density lipoprotein (AcLDL) uptake and degradation in human monocyte-derived Mφ, the MSR pathway has been nonspecifically implicated in this observed reduction. Scavenger receptor activity is, however, also expressed by endothelial, Kupffer and liver parenchymal cells as well as by phorbol ester-induced fibroblasts and smooth muscle cells; molecules other than the macrophage-specific MSR may mediate these properties. Furthermore, other Mφ receptors such as the thrombospondin receptor (CD36) and the IgG Fc receptor (FcγRII-B2; CD32) are capable of mediating uptake of oxidized lipoprotein.

Both human and rabbit atherosclerotic lesions contain M-CSF mRNA and immunoreactive M-CSF. Vascular endothelial cells and smooth muscle cells produce M-CSF in response to a range of stimuli, including modified low-density lipoproteins. By using mAb 2F8 to the murine MSR we showed unequivocally that M-CSF markedly and selectively enhances MSR expression and function in murine peritoneal Mφ [2].

Primary murine Mφ (Biogel-elicited peritoneal macrophages (BgPMφ)) were treated with recombinant human M-CSF, which is known to act on murine cells. Peritoneal Mφ elicited by this means (i.e., Biogel acrylamide beads) are known to be less activated and more responsive to cytokines than those elicited by thioglycollate broth. M-CSF treatment for 48 h markedly upregulated the expression of MSR protein on immunoblot analysis. Recombinant murine GM-CSF, which decreases serum cholesterol to a lesser extent when infused as an adjunct to chemotherapy, caused a noticeable but less marked MSR increase. To exclude effects due to growth factor-induced proliferation, loading of lysates per well was corrected for total cellular protein concentration. Conditioned media from mouse L cells (a rich source of murine M-CSF) or insect cells transfected with murine M-CSF cDNA similarly increased MSR expression and this effect was abrogated by the addition of species-specific antibodies to M-CSF. The increase in MSR expression was dose-dependent and plateaued at concentrations of 500 to 1,000 U/ml M-CSF.

Immunoprecipitation of MSR from metabolically labeled cells confirmed the upregulation by M-CSF. After 48 h of M-CSF treatment MSR protein synthesis increased 2.3-fold (PhosphorImager quantification) at the 0-h chase point; more impressively, 4.5-fold and 6-fold increases in synthesis were seen at 12 and 36 h respectively. This signifies that, in addition to increasing MSR synthesis, M-CSF also markedly prolongs the half-life of synthesized receptor.

Expression of MSR at single-cell level as determined by flow cytometry confirmed that M-CSF upregulated Mφ cell-surface expression of the receptor. However, only a modest increase was seen when intracellular (internal) levels of antigen were assessed by saponin permeabilization. M-CSF may therefore also redistribute the substantial intracellular pool of MSR to the cell surface. This was investigated by biochemically quantifying the fraction of total MSR on the cell surface at steady state. Cells were metabolically labeled to equilibrium followed by surface biotinylation, on ice, by the membrane-impermeant probe sulfo-NHS-SS-biotin. In these experiments M-CSF increased surface MSR expression 13-fold and total MSR protein synthesis nearly 5-fold relative to untreated controls. In addition, M-CSF treatment was associated with a shift of the cellular pool of MSR from a mainly intracellular location (69% of total) to a predominantly surface distribution (82% of total).

596

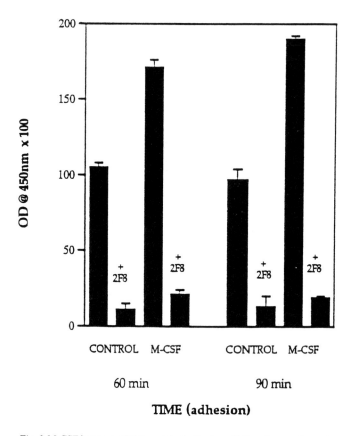

Fig. 1. M-CSF increases EDTA-resistant adhesion of Mϕ to tissue-culture plastic. BgPMϕ were cultured in RPMI plus 10% FCS on tissue-culture plastic (TCP) surfaces in the presence or absence of M-CSF for 48 h. Cell-adhesion assay was performed as described [1]. 2F8 monoclonal Ab was added at a final concentration of 2 μg/ml.

The action of M-CSF on several other Mϕ integral membrane proteins was analyzed. The expression of surface and internal pools of F4/80 (a Mϕ-specific differentiation antigen), type 3 complement receptor, MHC class II antigen and macrosialin (a Mϕ-specific late endosomal membrane molecule) were largely unchanged. Immunoblots of M-CSF-treated BgPMϕ also showed no alteration in expression of macrophage mannose receptor (MMR) or class II MHC. This points to a selective effect of M-CSF on MSR expression in an elicited primary Mϕ population.

The point at which M-CSF mediates its upregulatory effect was investigated by semi-quantitative RT-PCR to detect MSR mRNA changes in response to M-CSF. There was a substantial increase in MSR mRNA and, in addition, levels of mRNA specific for both type I and II MSR mRNA were increased, excluding a type-selective effect for M-CSF. Similar results were obtained after 24 h of M-CSF incubation. M-CSF thus also upregulates MSR expression at mRNA level; whether this is due to transcriptional upregulation or posttranscriptional stabilization was not addressed.

M-CSF therefore increases MSR expression at several different levels: message, protein synthesis, protein stability and shift of mature protein to the cell surface. The significance of these observed differences was tested by relating them to functional MSR studies and, in the first instance, the ability of treated BgPMφ to endocytose and accumulate fluorescent AcLDL (DiI-AcLDL) was assessed. M-CSF-mediated upregulation of murine MSR was associated with an enhanced capacity (1.7–3-fold) of treated Mφ to endocytose AcLDL. A recently described novel function for the MSR is divalent cation-independent adhesion. Human monocytes and macrophages were also shown to adhere to glucose-modified basement membrane collagen IV via their scavenger receptors. This would suggest a new role for the MSR in the accelerated development of diabetic vascular lesions. The ability of M-CSF-treated BgPMφ to adhere to serum-treated tissue culture plastic in an EDTA-independent manner was investigated. M-CSF increased adhesion at 60 min by 63% and at 90 min by 96%; this effect was completely abolished in the presence of mAb 2F8 (Fig. 1). The adherence of M-CSF-treated MØ in vitro was therefore markedly increased in a MSR-dependent (divalent cation-independent, 2F8-inhibitable) fashion.

The LDL receptor is primarily responsible for regulating plasma LDL homeostasis and LDL-cholesterol delivery to tissue and cells by clearing plasma-derived LDL-cholesterol. Hepatic LDL-receptor function, as assayed by LDL binding, is, however, not markedly affected by M-CSF treatment [10]. In contrast, our evidence shows that M-CSF significantly enhances MSR expression and function in vitro. This provides a mechanism whereby production of M-CSF in the atheromatous plaque microenvironment could enhance the recruitment and retention of mononuclear phagocytes and subsequent accumulation of cholesteryl esters and foam-cell formation.

Acknowledgements

We thank R. da Silva for advice and discussion; Cetus Corporation, California for recombinant human M-CSF and E.R. Stanley for antimurine M-CSF polyclonal antibodies. W.J.S. de Villiers is a Nuffield Dominion Medical Fellow. This work was supported by the UK Medical Research Council and Arthritis and Rheumatism Council.

References

1. Fraser I, Hughes D, Gordon S. Nature 1993;364:343–346.
2. de Villiers WJS, Fraser IP, Hughes DA, Doyle AG, Gordon S. J Exp Med 1994;180:705–710.
3. Goldstein JL, Ho YK, Basu SK, Brown MS. Proc Natl Acad Sci USA 1979;76:333–337.
4. Ross R. Nature 1993;362:801–809.
5. Poole JCF, Florey, HW. J Pathol Bacteriol 1958;LXXV:245.
6. Kodama T, Freeman M, Rohrer L, Zabrecky J, Matsudaira P, Krieger M. Nature 1990;343:531–535.
7. Krieger M, Herz J. Ann Rev Biochem 1994;63:611–637.
8. El Khoury J, Thomas CA, Loike JD, Hickman SE, Cao L, Silverstein SC. J Biol Chem 1994;269: 10197–10200.
9. Cushing SD, Berliner JA, Valente AJ, et al. Proc Natl Acad Sci USA 1990;87:5134–5138.
10. Stopeck AT, Nicholson AC, Mancini FP, Hajjar DP. J Biol Chem 1993;268:17489–17494.

Role of recombinant human macrophage colony-stimulating factor (rhM-CSF) in cholesterol metabolism and atherosclerosis

Matthew L. Sherman[1], Evan A. Stein[2], Jonathan Isaacsohn[2], Robert S. Lees[3] and Marc B. Garnick

[1]Genetics Institute, Cambridge, MA 02140; [2]Cardiovascular Research Center, Cincinnati, OH 45219; and [3]Boston Heart Foundation, Cambridge, MA 02141, USA

Abstract. Macrophage colony-stimulating factor (M-CSF) is necessary for the survival, proliferation, differentiation, and activation of cells of the monocyte/macrophage lineage. The gene for this protein has been cloned and expressed. Several studies have demonstrated that rhM-CSF induces significant decreases in plasma cholesterol in normal rabbits, Watanabe heritable hyperlipidemic rabbits (WHHL), and nonhuman primates. Recent studies have also provided insight into the role of rhM-CSF in the modulation of atherosclerosis. rhM-CSF treatment in WHHL rabbits reduced both the aortic cholesterol content and the surface area of aortic lesions as well as carrageenan granuloma foam cell formation. Preliminary studies have demonstrated that rhM-CSF lowers cholesterol in both normocholesterolemic and hypercholesterolemic humans. In phase 1/2 clinical studies, decreases in total cholesterol and LDL-cholesterol were observed in cancer patients. Furthermore, healthy male volunteers receiving rhM-CSF for 7 days by a continuous intravenous infusion or subcutaneous injection showed a maximum decrease from baseline in total cholesterol of 38 and 26%, respectively. To date, seven patients with homozygous familial hypercholesterolemia (FH) have received a total of nine treatment cycles of continuous intravenous infusions of rhM-CSF for 14 days at doses of 10, 20, 40, or 60 μg/kg/day. Dose-dependent decreases in both total cholesterol and LDL-cholesterol were observed. Patients treated at 20 μg/kg/day had a 16 and 18% mean decrease in total cholesterol and LDL-cholesterol, respectively. At the dose level of 40 μg/kg/day, mean decreases of 22 and 24% in total cholesterol and LDL-cholesterol, respectively, were seen. At a dose level of 60 μg/kg/day, mean decreases of 29 and 33% in total cholesterol and LDL-cholesterol, respectively, were seen; one FH patient treated at 60 μg/kg/day had a maximum decrease in LDL-cholesterol of 48%. Taken together, these data suggest that rhM-CSF decreases plasma cholesterol, specifically LDL, concentrations in healthy volunteers and cancer patients, as well as in patients with homozygous FH, and that rhM-CSF may provide a novel approach for the treatment of hypercholesterolemia and atherosclerosis.

Cells of the monocyte/macrophage lineage play an important role in cholesterol homeostasis. Previous studies have demonstrated that macrophage uptake of cholesterol is associated with upregulation of the scavenger receptor and receptor-mediated uptake of modified LDL as well as nonreceptor-mediated mechanisms of LDL removal including pinocytosis and phagocytosis [1—5]. Furthermore, activated macrophages is associated with synthesis of apolipoprotein E (ApoE) [6,7]. ApoE is a major protein component of high density lipoprotein particles and is associated with "reverse cholesterol transport" [8]. Taken together, these data suggest that macrophage activation may lead to a decrease in plasma cholesterol.

rhM-CSF is necessary for the survival, proliferation, differentiation, and activation of cells of the monocyte-macrophage lineage [9,10]. Several studies have demonstrated that rhM-CSF induces significant decreases in plasma cholesterol in normal rabbits, Watanabe heritable hyperlipidemic rabbits (WHHL), and nonhuman primates [11,12]. M-CSF treatment of rabbits is associated with enhanced clearance of lipoproteins by both LDL-receptor-dependent and LDL-receptor-independent mechanisms [13,14]. Furthermore, treatment of WHHL rabbits with rhM-CSF is associated with increases in HDL-cholesterol particle size as well as increases in biliary excretion of cholic acids which suggests that rhM-CSF may stimulate reverse cholesterol transport [12]. The finding that rhM-CSF induces increases in apolipoprotein E gene expression suggests an increase in reverse cholesterol transport [15]. Recent studies have also provided insight into the role of rhM-CSF in the modulation of atherosclerosis. rhM-CSF treatment in WHHL rabbits reduced both the aortic cholesterol content and the surface area of aortic lesions as well as carrageenan granuloma foam-cell formation [16,17]. Preliminary studies have demonstrated that rhM-CSF lowers cholesterol in both normocholesterolemic and hypercholesterolemic humans [18,19]. In phase 1/2 clinical studies in patients with cancer, decreases in total cholesterol and LDL-cholesterol were first observed. Subsequent studies in healthy male volunteers receiving rhM-CSF for 7 days by a continuous intravenous infusion or subcutaneous injection showed a maximum decrease from baseline in total cholesterol of 38 or 26%, respectively [19]. In the present study, we have investigated the effects of rhM-CSF administered by continuous intravenous infusions in patients with homozygous familial hypercholesterolemia.

Materials and Methods

Patients

Seven patients with homozygous familial hypercholesterolemia were entered into this Phase 1/2 dose-ranging study of rhM-CSF. Patients older than 12 and with a calculated plasma LDL-cholesterol >400 mg/dl (on at least one occasion within 8 weeks prior to the initiation of rhM-CSF therapy) and documentation of diagnostic LDL-receptor phenotyping or genotyping were eligible. Patients were excluded from the study if any of the following circumstances were present: (1) unacceptable hematologic function (WBC <4000/µl, hemoglobin <11 g/dl, platelet <150,000/µl), renal function (creatinine >2 mg/dl), or hepatic function (SGOT/SGPT >2.5 upper limits of normal and bilirubin >2 mg/dl); (2) abnormal TSH; (3) triglyceride level >300 mg/dl; (4) congestive heart failure requiring medical intervention, or unstable angina, myocardial infarction or other acute cardiac event within 6 months prior to entry; (5) concomitant lipid-lowering treatment such as LDL apheresis or lipid-lowering agents within 4 weeks of rhM-CSF therapy; and (6) unable to give voluntary, signed informed consent.

Design

The study was an open-label, nonrandomized dose-escalating multicenter study. Patients were instructed to follow a National Cholesterol Education Program (NCEP) Step 2 diet for the duration of the study. Patients discontinued all lipid-lowering therapy at least 4 weeks prior to the initiation of rhM-CSF therapy. Eligibility for entry was determined during this pretreatment stabilization period. During a 4-day run-in period at the end of the stabilization period, a continuous intravenous infusion of 0.9% sodium chloride was administered. At the end of the run-in period, patients were hospitalized for the first 24 h of rhM-CSF administration. rhM-CSF was administered by continuous intravenous infusion for 14 consecutive days, followed by a rest period of 1 week. rhM-CSF was supplied by Genetics Institute, Inc. as a lyophilized product in 4-mg vials [20].

Efficacy and safety measurements

Serum was obtained at the indicated times for determination of total, LDL-, HDL-, and VLDL-cholesterol, and triglycerides. Lipid analyses for cholesterol, HDL and triglycerides were performed at Medical Research Laboratories, Cincinnati, OH, which maintains NHLBI-CDC Part III standardization [21]. HDL-cholesterol was measured after precipitation of apolipoprotein B-containing lipoproteins using heparin–manganese chloride (2 M $MnCl_2$) [22]. LDL-cholesterol was calculated by using the Friedewald equation [23]: LDL = Total – HDL – TG/5.

Blood was also obtained for routine hematology and chemistry laboratory measurements. Subjects were examined clinically daily and any new or continuing adverse experiences were recorded.

Results

Patient characteristics

As shown in Table 1, seven patients were entered onto this study. Two patients were treated at two different dose levels of rhM-CSF; a total of nine treatment cycles were administered. The mean age at the time of treatment was 28 years (range 15–37).

Effect on lipids and lipoproteins

To date, seven patients with homozygous familial hypercholesterolemia have received continuous intravenous infusions of rhM-CSF for 14 days at doses of 10, 20, 40, or 60 µg/kg/day (Table 2). Dose-dependent decreases in both total cholesterol and LDL-cholesterol were observed (Table 3). Patients treated at 20 µg/kg/day had a 16 and 18% decrease in total cholesterol and LDL-cholesterol, respectively. At the dose level of 40 µg/kg/day, decreases of 22 and 24% in total cholesterol and LDL-cholesterol, respectively, were seen; one patient treated at 40 µg/kg/day had a maximum decrease in LDL-cholesterol of 29%. At the dose level of 60 µg/kg/day decreases of 29 and 33% in total cholesterol and LDL-cholesterol, respectively, were seen. One FH patient treated at this dose level had a 48% decrease in LDL-cholesterol after rhM-CSF treatment.

Hematologic effects

Increases in circulating peripheral blood monocytes were noted in homozygous FH

Table 1.

Patient no./initials	Patient age	Gender	Baseline LDL-cholesterol (mg/dl)	Dose (µg/kg/day)
002/BLS	19	M	492	10
003/TEF	15	F	478	10
004/WLF	27	M	594	20
005/RLK	27	M	578	20
006/OCC	37	F	505	40
007/VM	33	F	619	40
008/WLF[a]	28	M	636	60
009/RLK[b]	28	M	648	60
001/RKN	36	M	419	60

[a]Patient 008/WLF is the same individual as 004/WLF; [b]Patient 009/RLK is the same individual as 005/RLK.

Table 2. Summary of fasting lipid profiles

Dose group (µg/kg/day)	Patient no./ Initials	Percent change day 1 vs. day 15			
		Total cholesterol	LDL-C	HDL-C	Triglycerides
10	002/BLS	−2	−2	−19	+12
	003/TEF	−2	−3	−10	+33
20	004/WLF	−24	−28	−20	+30
	005/RLK	−8	−7	−9	−30
40	006/OCC	−16	−19	+6	+39
	007/VM	−27	−29	−17	−4
60	008/WLF	−24	−26	−7	+26
	009/RLK	−23	−25	−12	+42
	001/RKN	−40	−48	−28	+49

patients treated with rhM-CSF. Transient increases of monocytes up to 42% of the WBC differential were observed. In addition, dose-dependent decreases in platelet counts were also noted. Patient 006/OCC treated with 40 µg/kg/day rhM-CSF developed Grade 1 thrombocytopenia with a platelet count of 75,000/µl. Patient 001/RKN treated with 60 µg/kg/day rhM-CSF developed grade 2 thrombocytopenia with a platelet count of 61,000/µl after 12 days of rhM-CSF treatment. These effects were rapidly reversible after rhM-CSF treatment was discontinued.

Toxicity

There were no serious adverse reactions among the seven patients during the nine treatment cycles of rhM-CSF administered. Systemic side effects of rhM-CSF were not observed.

Discussion

The results from this study demonstrated that rhM-CSF treatment of patients with homozygous familial hypercholesterolemia is associated with a dose-dependent decrease in total cholesterol. This decrease was attributable almost entirely to decreases in LDL-cholesterol. The decreases observed were maximal during the 14 days of continuous intravenous infusion and returned to baseline during the 1-week follow-up period. Transient increases in monocyte counts and decreases in platelet counts were noted during rhM-CSF administration; these effects were rapidly reversible after therapy was stopped. No clinical toxicity was observed during this study.

Although the mechanism associated with the cholesterol-lowering effects of rhM-CSF is unknown, certain insights are available. Homozygous FH patients lack functional native

Table 3. Effects of rhM-CSF on cholesterol

Dose group (µg/kg/day)	Mean percent change day 1 vs. day 15	
	Total cholesterol	LDL-cholesterol
10	−2	−3
20	−16	−18
40	−22	−24
60	−29	−33

602

LDL receptors, suggesting alternative mechanisms for cholesterol metabolism. Previous studies have identified macrophage Class A scavenger receptors which bind both acetylated and oxidized LDL [24,25]. Recently, Class B scavenger receptors have been cloned [26]. These scavenger receptors are expressed on adipose tissue and bind both native and modified LDL. Although the effects of rhM-CSF on Class B receptors are unknown, rhM-CSF upregulated expression of the Class A scavenger receptor in human monocytes [15]. Furthermore, LDL-receptor-related protein (LRP) expression is increased by rhM-CSF [27]. Taken together, these studies suggest that alternative receptors are involved in cholesterol homeostasis and that rhM-CSF may play an important role in the metabolism and regulation of lipids. The current human data suggest that rhM-CSF decreases plasma cholesterol, specifically LDL-cholesterol, concentrations in healthy volunteers and cancer patients, as well as in patients with homozygous familial hypercholesterolemia, and that rhM-CSF may provide a novel approach for the pharmacologic treatment of hypercholesterolemia and atherosclerosis.

References

1. Goldstein JL, Ho YK, Basu SK, Brown MS. Proc Natl Acad Sci USA 1979;76:333–337.
2. Traber MG, Kayden HJ. Proc Natl Acad Sci USA 1980;77:5466–5470.
3. Schechter I, Fogelman AM, Haberland ME et al. J Lipid Res 1981;22:63–71.
4. Slater HR, Packard CJ, Shepard J. J Biol Chem 1982;257:307–310.
5. Tabas I, Weiland DA, Tall AR. Proc Natl Acad Sci USA 1985;82:416–420.
6. Basu SK, Brown MS, Ho YK, Havel RJ, Goldstein JL. Proc Natl Acad Sci USA 1981;78:7545–7549.
7. Basu SK, Ho YK, Brown MS et al. J Biol Chem 1982;257:9788–9795.
8. Mahley RW. Science 1988;240:622–630.
9. Tushinski RJ, Oliver IT, Guilbert LJ et al. Cell 1982;28:71–81.
10. Clark SC, Kamen R. Science 1987;236:1229–1237.
11. Stoudemire JB, Garnick MB. Blood 1991;77:750–755.
12. Parker TS, Levine DM, Donnelly TM et al. Circulation 1990;82(suppl III):III–233 (abstract).
13. Shimano H, Yamada N, Ishibashi S et al. J Biol Chem 1990; 265:12869–12875.
14. Yamada N, Ishibashi S, Shimano H et al. Proc Soc Exp Biol Med 1992;200:240–244.
15. Clinton SK, Underwood R, Hayes L et al. Am J Pathol 1992;140:301–316.
16. Inoue I, Inabe T, Motoyoshi K et al. Atherosclerosis 1992;93:245–254.
17. Schaub RG, Bree MP, Hayes LL et al. Arterioscler Thromb 1994;14:70–76.
18. Motoyoshi E, Takaku F. Lancet 1989;735:326–327.
19. Sherman ML, Kaye JA, Schindler J et al. Blood 1993;82(suppl):235a (abstract).
20. Wong GG, Temple PA, Leary AC et al. Science 1987;235:1504–1508.
21. Myers GL, Cooper GR, Winn CL, Smith SJ. Clin Lab Med 1989;9:105–135.
22. Warnick GR, Albers JJ. J Lipid Res 1978;19:65–76.
23. Friedwald WT, Levy RI, Frederickson DS. Clin Chem 1972;18:499–502.
24. Kodama T, Freeman M, Rohrer L et al. Nature 1990;343:531–535.
25. Rohrer L, Freeman M, Kodama T et al. Nature 1990;343:570–572.
26. Acton SL, Scherer PE, Lodish HF, Krieger M. J Biol Chem 1994;269:21003–21009.
27. Hussaini IM, Srikumar K, Quesenberry PJ, Gonias SL. J Biol Chem 1990;265:19441–19446.

Atherosclerosis X.
F.P. Woodford, J. Davignon and A. Sniderman, editors.

603

LDL-induced macrophage toxicity

M.J. Mitchinson, V.C. Reid, S.J. Hardwick, K. Clare, K.L.H. Carpenter and C.E. Marchant

Division of Cellular Pathology, University of Cambridge, Department of Pathology, Tennis Court Road, Cambridge CB2 1QP, UK

Abstract. There is good evidence that the death of macrophage foam cells is an important source of the characteristic acellular lipid core of advanced atherosclerotic lesions. The possibility that foam-cell death might be due to the oxidation of low density lipoprotein (LDL) has therefore been investigated in vitro. Oxidized LDL is toxic to mouse peritoneal macrophages by a mechanism which involves apoptosis. Exposure of human monocyte-macrophages to oxidized LDL and to oxidizable lipid components of LDL also leads to toxicity which is inhibited by antioxidants. The possible contributions to toxicity of different LDL components are discussed.

A striking characteristic of the advanced atherosclerotic plaque is the lipid core. This is an acellular collection of lipid-rich debris containing cholesterol monohydrate crystals, found in the deeper part of the plaque. It is covered by a dense fibrous cap and surrounded by tissue containing variable proportions of fibers and cells, especially smooth muscle cells and macrophage foam cells.

How this core develops is an unanswered question, and an important one, because it is only advanced lesions with a lipid core that give rise to the clinical complications of stenosis and thrombosis. One school of thought is that the lipid deposition is primarily extracellular [1]; although some extracellular lipid deposition is probably occurring, we believe the main source of the lipid core is the death of macrophage foam cells. A recent study here has indeed shown that the lipid core usually originates in the deepest part of the collection of macrophage foam cells in a fatty streak, apparently due to the disintegration of some of these cells. The lipid core also contains two components that, in earlier lesions, are found only in macrophages, namely macrophage antigens, and the lipid pigment, ceroid [2]. Ceroid is produced by the oxidation of lipid–protein mixtures by macrophages, and there is serological evidence that it is largely composed of oxidized LDL [3]. There is little or no evidence of smooth muscle cell death at the edges of the lipid core. We conclude that the lipid core is mainly the result of death of macrophages.

The cause of the death of the macrophage foam cells is unknown. However, in view of the mounting evidence that LDL oxidation occurs in human lesions, and the evidence that oxidation of LDL by macrophages renders it toxic to endothelial and smooth muscle cells in culture [4], we have begun to study the effects of LDL and its oxidizable components upon macrophage integrity.

Materials and Methods

The cells studied have been mouse resident peritoneal macrophages [5], the mouse macrophage-like cell line P388D$_1$ [6] and human monocyte-derived macrophages, using methods previously reported. LDL isolation and artificial oxidation using CuSO$_4$ have also been described previously [5]. Individual lipids were introduced into the cultures as coacervates with bovine serum albumin (BSA), which were readily taken up by the cells [7].

604

Toxicity has been measured by several methods, including trypan blue uptake, leakage of lactate dehydrogenase and release of radioactivity from cells preloaded with tritiated adenine [5,7]. The morphology of the cells has been examined by light and electron microscopy [8].

Results and Discussion

Mouse peritoneal macrophages (MPM) were rapidly damaged by oxidized LDL, but native LDL was toxic only after a time-lag of about 20 h [5]. The MPM exposed to oxidized LDL showed ultrastructural changes of apoptosis at 24 h [8]. Evidence for oxidized LDL-mediated apoptosis was also provided by the P388D$_1$ cell line. In these cells DNA fragmentation was measured using established techniques and internucleosomal chromatin cleavage ('laddering', a biochemical hallmark of apoptosis) was found after exposure to oxidized LDL. These changes occurred prior to enhanced membrane permeability [6].

If oxidation of LDL leads to toxicity for macrophages, it is obviously important to try to assess which of its constituents are responsible. Cholesteryl linoleate (18:2) and arachidonate (20:4), but not oleate (18:1), were first shown to be toxic to MPM, and the toxicity was inhibited by α-tocopherol [7].

The studies have now been extended to human monocyte-macrophages (HMM), but not yet published. It was found that, although oxidized LDL was rapidly toxic, native LDL was not, at any rate during 72 h of culture. HMM maintained in the presence of various artificial lipoproteins containing BSA and individual lipids (cholesteryl esters and triglycerides) showed that the toxicity of the lipids varied. The concentration in the medium was equivalent for each of the lipids, being 900 μM for the cholesteryl esters and 300 μM for triglycerides, because triglycerides possess three fatty acid chains per molecule, whereas cholesterol esters have only one per molecule. Toxicity was assessed as release of radioactivity from HMM preloaded with tritiated adenine. In brief, cholesteryl oleate (18:1) was not toxic, cholesteryl linoleate (18:2) was only slightly toxic, but cholesteryl arachidonate (20:4) led to 30% more leakage of radioactivity than the control at 24 h. Among the triglycerides, triolein (18:1) and trilinolein (18:2) were not toxic, but triarachidonin (20:4), trieicosapentaenoin (20:5) and tridocosahexaenoin (22:6) all led to approximately 75% leakage above that in the no-additions control, at 24 h.

There are a number of reports in the literature of toxicity caused by various oxidized derivatives of cholesterol, mainly for endothelial cells and smooth muscle cells. We have shown previously that cholesterol is oxidized by macrophages in culture if it is esterified to a fatty acid with at least two double bonds; cholesterol itself and cholesteryl oleate do not lead to hydroxycholesterol production [9]. Since this is consistent with the toxicity of these cholesteryl esters for both MPM and HMM, oxysterols are obvious candidates for toxic components of oxidized LDL. Toxicity of certain oxidized derivatives of cholesterol for HMM was therefore tested. Using the same toxicity assay as for the cholesteryl esters and triglycerides, but with a final concentration of 25 μg/ml (62 μM) in the medium, we found all the oxysterols tested toxic, giving at least 33% leakage above that of the control at 24 h. The oxysterols tested were 26-hydroxycholesterol, 25-hydroxycholesterol, 7α-hydroxycholesterol, 7-oxo-cholesterol and 7β-hydroxycholesterol.

We have recently shown that 7β-hydroxycholesterol (cholest-5-en-3β,7β-diol) and 26-hydroxycholesterol (cholest-5-en-3β,26-diol) are relatively abundant in the lipid core of human advanced atherosclerotic lesions but not present in significant amounts in normal artery [10]. Both these oxysterols have also been found in a so far unpublished study of earlier lesions, and are more abundant in lesions rich in macrophages. 7β-Hydroxycholesterol is produced during copper-mediated oxidation and MPM-mediated modification of LDL [11] and of cholesteryl linoleate and arachidonate [9], but 26-hydroxycholesterol, which is an enzymatic product of the cytochrome P-450 sterol 26-hydroxylase, is not [11]. A possible explanation might be that this enzyme is expressed in cells in the lesions but not in macrophages in culture [10,11].

However, because some triglycerides are also toxic when incubated with HMM, cholesterol oxidation products cannot be the whole story. Certain aldehydes, including malondialdehyde and 4-hydroxynonenal, have been reported to be toxic to other cell types [12]; since they are known to be produced during LDL oxidation [12], they may also contribute to the toxicity of these triglycerides, and therefore of LDL, to macrophages, but have not yet been tested in our model.

The different constituents of LDL and oxidized LDL that have been tested are present in LDL in widely different proportions, the exact percentages depending partly upon the diet. Clearly a proper evaluation of their likely differential contribution to the toxicity of oxidized LDL must take into account their relative proportions within the LDL particle. The most toxic lipids, in this model, are relatively minor constituents of LDL. Therefore the (less toxic) cholesteryl linoleate might be most important in vivo because of its much higher concentration in LDL.

Among the limited observations to be made at this stage is that, at least, the findings support the common view that diets containing oleate may be protective. The long-chain polyunsaturated fatty acids (20:5 and 22:6) found in fish oils appear from our results to be potentially quite toxic. Fish oils are, however, reportedly protective against the complications of atherosclerosis. If so, it is perhaps due to their toxicity being outweighed by other properties they possess in vivo, such as inhibition of thrombosis.

The ultrastructural changes found in HMM exposed to oxidized LDL are, as in MPM, characteristic of apoptosis, but definite evidence of the occurrence of apoptosis in human lesions has not yet been reported. The possibility that apoptosis of macrophages is occurring during the development of the lipid core does, however, raise an interesting possibility. There are reports of evidence of DNA synthesis in a minority of foam cells, which has understandably been taken to mean that foam cells undergo mitosis in the lesion [13]. However, cells undergoing apoptosis often enter into an abortive cell cycle and, in these circumstances, DNA synthesis presages cell death. Therefore the foam cells showing evidence of DNA synthesis in the lesions might be about to die rather than to divide. This is, of course, entirely speculative at present, but requires consideration.

In summary, several constituents of LDL, including some whose oxidation products are known to be present in human lesions, are toxic for human monocyte-macrophages in culture. This could theoretically explain the onset and enlargement of the lipid core of the advanced human atherosclerotic lesion.

The fact that the lipid core of both intermediate and advanced lesions has disintegrating macrophages at its edge, and macrophage contents within it, suggests that the mechanism of this macrophage death is important. This is particularly because the presence of the lipid core is associated with the morbidity and mortality of atherosclerosis. Fatty streaks are found in all populations, but the advanced lesions with lipid cores, associated with clinical complications, are found mainly in industrialised societies. It is therefore conceivable that inhibition of macrophage death would hinder this important stage in progression.

606

Acknowledgements

This work has been supported by the U.K. Ministry of Agriculture, Fisheries and Food and by the British Heart Foundation. We are grateful for the collaboration of Dr J.N. Skepper and of N. Law and N. Weeratunge, and the secretarial help of V. Mullins.

References

1. Guyton, JR, Klemp KF. Arterioscler Thromb 1994;14:1305–1314.
2. Aqel NM, Ball RY, Waldmann H, Mitchinson MJ. J Path 1985;146:197–204.
3. Parums DV, Brown DL, Mitchinson MJ. Arch Path 1990;114:383–387.
4. Cathcart MK, Morel DW, Chisolm GM. J Leuk Biol 1985;38:341–350.
5. Reid VC, Mitchinson MJ. Atherosclerosis 1993;98:17–24.
6. Reid VC, Hardwick SJ, Mitchinson MJ. FEBS Letts 1993;332:218–220.
7. Reid VC, Brabbs CE, Mitchinson MJ. Atherosclerosis 1992;92:251–260.
8. Reid VC, Mitchinson MJ, Skepper JN. J Path 1993;171:321–328.
9. Carpenter KLH, Brabbs CE, Mitchinson MJ. Klin Wochenschr 1991;69:1039–1045.
10. Carpenter KLH, Taylor SE, Ballantine JA, Fussell B, Halliwell B, Mitchinson MJ. Biochim Biophys Acta 1993;1167:121–130.
11. Carpenter KLH, Wilkins GM, Fussell B, Ballantine JA, Taylor SE, Mitchinson MJ, Leake DS. Production of oxidised lipids during modification of low-density lipoprotein by macrophages or copper. Biochem J (in press).
12. Esterbauer H, Schaur RJ, Zollner H. Free Rad Biol Med 1991;11:81–128.
13. Ross R. Am J Path 1993;143:987–1002.

©1995 Elsevier Science B.V. All rights reserved.
Atherosclerosis X.
F.P. Woodford, J. Davignon and A. Sniderman, editors.

Secretory group-II phospholipase A2 — a new inducer of foam-cell formation in human atherosclerotic lesions?

Mario Menschikowski[1], Werner Jaross[1], Michael Kasper[2], Peter Lattke[1] and Andrea Schiering[1]

[1]Institute of Clinical Chemistry and Laboratory Medicine; and [2]Institute of Pathology, Faculty of Medicine "Carl Gustav Carus", Technical University of Dresden, Fetscherstraße 74, D-01 307 Dresden, Germany

The processes of atherogenesis and inflammation show a series of similar features that are characterized by leukocytic infiltration, mesenchymal cell proliferation and fibrosis [1,2]. Furthermore, in both cases a large number of proinflammatory mediators are released into the extracellular space, including different growth factors and cytokines such as IL-1 and TNF-α [3]. Besides these agents, a high level of group-II phospholipase A2 (PLA2) was detected in inflammatory fluids, exudates or serum of patients with inflammatory diseases [4,5]. In view of the similarities mentioned and the results of in vitro studies described below, the question arises whether a secretory group-II PLA2 enzyme is also present in human atherosclerotic lesions.

Biological behavior of PLA2-modified lipoproteins

Previously, we found that a modification of the HDL- or LDL-phospholipids by treatment with a porcine pancreatic PLA2 led to an increased level of free and esterified cholesterol in mouse peritoneal macrophages [6]. These data were confirmed indirectly by a simultaneously elevated activity of the cytosolic acylcoenzyme-A:cholesterol acyltransferase (ACAT) after the exposure of cells to PLA2-modified lipoproteins (Fig. 1). The lipid depositions observed in vitro were associated with the formation of numerous intracellular lipid droplets after a 48-h incubation, which indicates a transformation of macrophages into foam-like cells. Similar results were described by Aviram and Maor on the murine macrophage-like cell line J-774 A.1 using a bee venom PLA2 to modify LDL [7].

Modification of lipoproteins by group-II PLA2

To address the question whether a human PLA2 is able to modify lipoproteins in the way mentioned above, we isolated a phospholipase A2 that is synthesized and secreted by human HepG2 hepatoma cells under inflammatory conditions such as after incubation in medium containing the cytokines IL-I, IL-6 and TNF-α [8]. This enzyme is defined as a group-II PLA2 and seems to be identical to the enzymes found in platelets, placenta and rheumatoid synovial fluids [8]. Using a two-step procedure consisting of acidic extraction and ion-exchange chromatography on CM-cellulose, we purified the enzyme 1000-fold. Complete inhibition of the enzyme activity by 1-h incubation at 57°C showed that the entire activity can be related to the group-II PLA2: group-I PLA2 activity was shown to be thermoresistant under the same conditions. The isolated enzyme displayed a molecular weight of 19 kDa in the SDS-gel electrophoresis under nonreducing conditions. The enzyme activity was Ca^{++}-dependent and a pH-optimum was detected at 8.0 [9]. Incubation of HDL and LDL with the purified enzyme resulted in an increased electrophoretic mobility of the lipoproteins and an elevated level of free fatty acids (Table 1). These data

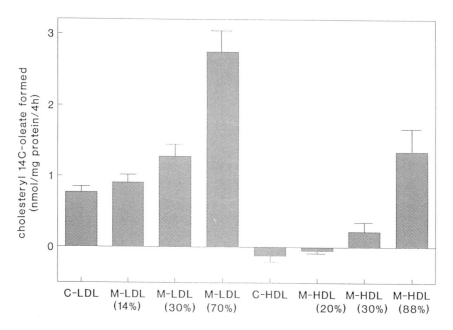

Fig. 1. Determination of ACAT activity in peritoneal macrophages previously incubated in medium containing 200 μg/ml of native (C) or PLA2-modified lipoproteins (M) of which the phospholipids were hydrolyzed to different degrees as indicated. The cholesteryl-ester synthesis rate by cells incubated in medium without additions averaged 0.265 ± 0.016 nmol/mg protein/4 h. Each bar represents the mean ± SE of three different incubations which were run in triplicate.

Table 1. Determination (n = 6) of free fatty acids in HDL and LDL before and after incubation for 12 h with group-II PLA2 (6 U/ml)

Lipoproteins	Free fatty acids (mmol/l)
Control HDL	0.162 ± 0.021
PLA2-modified HDL	0.396 ± 0.046
Control LDL	0.110 ± 0.012
PLA2-modified LDL	0.173 ± 0.010

suggest that human group-II PLA2 leads to the same modification of lipoproteins as was observed with pancreatic or venom PLA2.

Identification of group-II PLA2 in human atherosclerotic plaques

If phospholipase A2 occurs in human atherosclerotic lesions, it could suggest a new mechanism of foam-cell formation in vivo. We therefore analyzed atherosclerotic lesions obtained from 13 patients who had undergone reconstructive procedures. The segments were removed from carotic (n = 6) and femoral (n = 5) arteries, and abdominal aortic aneurysm or stenosis (n = 2). Arteries of patients without atherosclerotic diseases obtained at autopsy served as controls. After fixation and embedding in paraffin, the arterial specimens were analyzed using four monoclonal antibodies recognizing group-II PLA2 of different origin (placenta, sperm, and rheumatoid synovial fluid) and the Vectastain ABC kit. The study demonstrated that in all areas with atherosclerotic lesions a positive immunostaining occurred. In arteries without thickened intima this staining failed completely. By using specific antibodies against macrophages and smooth muscle cells, we identified most PLA2-positive cells as macrophage-derived foam cells. In addition to these cells, extracellular matrix components gave a partially positive reaction with anti-PLA2 antibodies.

Summary and Conclusions

The study has shown for the first time that a group-II PLA2 is present in human athero-sclerotic plaques. Coupled with the biological behavior of PLA2-treated lipoproteins and the in vitro modification of lipoproteins by PLA2 secreted by HepG2 cells, the data suggest that the secretory group-II PLA2 could be involved in atherogenesis. However, whether a causal relation exists in vivo between the expression of group-II PLA2 and foam-cell formation in plaques must be the object of further studies.

Acknowledgements

The authors wish to thank Mrs K. Tzschoppe and Mrs I. Peterson for excellent technical assistance. The work was supported by a grant (Ja 565/2-1) from the Deutsche Forschungsgemeinschaft.

References

1. Joris I, Zand T, Nunnari JJ, Krolikowski FJ, Majno G. Am J Pathol 1983;113:341–358.
2. Ross R. N Engl J Med 1986;314:488–500.
3. Tipping PG, Hancock WW. Am J Pathol 1993;142:1721.
4. Vadas P, Stefanski E, Pruzanski W. Life Sci 1985;36:579–587.
5. Seilhamer JJ, Pruzanski W, Vadas P, Plant S, Miller JA, Kloss J, Johnson LK. J Biol Chem 1989;264: 5335–5338.
6. Jaross W, Menschikowski M, Gorshkova I, Lattke P. Atherosclerosis 1994;109:39 (abstract).
7. Aviram M, Maor I. Biochim Biophys Acta 1992;185:465–472.
8. Crowl RM, Stoller TJ, Conroy RR, Stoner CR. J Biol Chem 1991;266:2647–2651.
9. Menschikowski M, Lattke P, Jaross W. Atherosclerosis 1994;109:48 (abstract).

610

Recent advances in the genetics of atherosclerosis

Kåre Berg

Institute of Medical Genetics, University of Oslo; and Department of Medical Genetics, Ullevål University Hospital, Oslo, Norway

Abstract. The functional candidate gene approach is the method of choice in attempts to identify genes contributing to atherosclerosis risk and led to the detection of lipoprotein(a) as a major genetic risk factor many years ago. Different alleles at the LPA locus may contribute to atherogenesis, placental ischemia or longevity. Lp(a), the LPA gene, disease associations of polymorphisms at candidate loci that are not mediated through levels of traditional risk factors, and the variability-gene concept are major challenges to students of the genetics of atherosclerosis.

Genetic as well as environmental factors contribute to the etiology of coronary heart disease (CHD) and other atherosclerotic or thrombotic diseases and it seems clear that lifestyle, dietary and other environmental factors preferentially cause disease in those with a genetic predisposition. Many risk factors or protective factors with respect to CHD typically exhibit heritability from 0.50 and upwards, and the heritability of Lp(a) concentration is very close to unity. The knowledge that genes contribute to the susceptible state with respect to CHD makes it important to identify genes of major significance so that people at particularly high CHD risk may avail themselves of any known preventive measure from early in adult life.

The functional candidate gene approach

Present attempts to identify genes of importance for CHD or its risk factors most often employ the *functional candidate gene* approach. With respect to CHD, a functional candidate gene is any gene whose protein product is involved in lipoprotein structure, lipoprotein metabolism or lipid metabolism; in thrombogenesis, thrombolysis or fibrinolysis; in regulation of blood flow in coronary arteries; in regulation of blood pressure; in reverse cholesterol transport; in the regulation of growth of atherosclerotic lesions or in the early development of coronary arteries; or is present in atherosclerotic lesions.

The term "candidate gene" is also used for genes which are in an area of the genome where a given gene (for example causing an inherited disorder) must be located. Genes that are candidate genes because of their position in the genome may be referred to as *positional candidate genes* to distinguish them from *functional candidate genes*.

The term "candidate gene" was coined after DNA analyses had become research tools in human and medical genetics. However, the functional candidate gene approach had in fact been successfully applied before variation in DNA could be directly examined. The discovery that a genetically determined high level of Lp(a) [1] is a risk factor for CHD [2] and the demonstration of definite effects on lipid levels of the Ag allotypic

Address for correspondence: Prof Kåre Berg, Institute of Medical Genetics, University of Oslo, P.O. Box 1036, Blindern, N-0315 Oslo, Norway.

polymorphism of low density lipoprotein (LDL) [3] appear to be the first examples of successful uses of the functional candidate gene approach.

Lp(a)

Lp(a) [1] was detected by the use of animal immune sera produced and absorbed according to a strategy aimed at uncovering lipoprotein differences between individuals. It was found even in the earliest studies that Lp(a) is a distinct serum lipoprotein particle, having unique antigenic structures as well as antigens shared with LDL. The long Lp(a) polypeptide chain, apo(a), is attached to apolipoprotein B (apoB) in an LDL-like particle. The successful cloning [4] of cDNA representing the gene for apo(a) (the LPA gene) revealed striking homology to plasminogen, a much smaller protein important in fibrinolytic/thrombolytic processes. Extreme variability in Lp(a) concentration between individuals and very strict genetic control within the individual are striking characteristics of Lp(a). Single-gene control of serum Lp(a) level was postulated when its detection was first reported and has since been confirmed in several studies (for review, see [5]).

The detection by Berg et al. [2] of association between Lp(a) and CHD has been confirmed in numerous studies, including an extensive study of patients and controls where two of the most experienced laboratories examined blindly samples from all participants, as well as repeated split samples, with excellent agreement between split samples and laboratories [6]. On the basis of this study, a population attributable risk of 28% for myocardial infarction before age 60 was calculated for men having an Lp(a) concentration in the top quartile of the population distribution. Correlation analyses have shown that the level of Lp(a) is essentially independent of other known risk factors or protective factors, and the importance of a high serum Lp(a) as a CHD risk factor has recently been confirmed in prospective studies [7] [for review, see 8]. Occasional studies failing to detect the connection between Lp(a) and CHD may have been based on inadequate techniques or reagents (commercial test kits) [9].

Lp(a) is present in atherosclerotic lesions, and some in vitro studies indicate that Lp(a) interferes with thrombolytic/fibrinolytic processes. The discovery [10] that Lp(a) stimulates growth of vascular smooth muscle cells in culture may point to yet another mechanism that could (partly) explain the association between a high serum Lp(a) level and CHD.

The question of the physiological role of Lp(a) is unresolved. In a study of elderly persons we found a much lower proportion of people with very high Lp(a) levels than in the general population. The corresponding excess of people was, however, not found in the lowest quartile of Lp(a) concentrations but in the second to lowest quartile, perhaps indicating that there is some advantage to having a moderate, as opposed to very low, level of Lp(a). This may suggest that genes determining a moderate level of Lp(a) are "longevity genes".

We have recently studied [11] a woman with severe thrombotic disease at age 43 who had given birth to three children with very low birth weights. The placentas had been small and ischemic. Her Lp(a) was above the 99th centile in the general population. This observation could suggest that an exceptionally high Lp(a) may interfere with placental circulation, leading to poor placental development and function.

A recent report [12] of a relationship between endothelial dysfunction and a high Lp(a) level suggests new avenues to explore, as does the suggestion that Lp(a) may be important for repair of vessel damage or wound healing [13] as well as the finding that Lp(a) has vessel-wall affinity in transgenic animals [14] and the detection of a macrophage receptor for apo(a) [15].

Apolipoprotein B polymorphism and CHD

A recent case-control study [16] revealed an association between premature myocardial infarction (MI) and homozygous absence of the restriction site in an XbaI polymorphism at the apoB locus which involves the third base of threonine codon 2488. The association (p = 0.007), which could be detected only through multivariate logistic regression analysis was not mediated via lipid levels. One may speculate that a structural change in apoB might make it more likely to become trapped in arterial walls or assume increased atherogenicity for other reasons.

Effect of normal genes at the ACE locus on CHD risk

The reported association [17] between an insertion/deletion (I/D) polymorphism at the locus for angiotensinogen I converting enzyme (ACE) and MI was not detected in a Norwegian series of patients and controls [18]. However, parental MI was more frequent in homozygotes and heterozygotes for the D-allele than in homozygotes for the I-allele. This confirmation [18] of reports by French workers supports the view that ACE polymorphisms could be important markers of MI risk.

The variability gene concept

We have suggested (for review see [19]) that lipid *variability* may by itself be of clinical importance. It has been known for a great many years that there are important strain differences in the response to dietary lipid intake in several animal species, differences that are almost certainly of a genetic nature. There is now evidence of significant differences between people with respect to response to changes in lipid intake suggesting that "high responders" and "low responders" may exist in man also.

The notion that lipid *variability*, in addition to absolute lipid levels, may contribute to CHD risk was the background for our effort to detect genes that affect lipid variability. The method we have developed to this end utilizes the genetic identity of monozygotic twins. It appears to be a valid instrument to study gene–environment interactions and to detect "variability genes". In addition to our own evidence [19] that variability genes exist at the apoB locus with respect to apoB and at the apoA-I locus with respect to cholesterol, papers from other laboratories confirming the existence of variability genes have started to appear. The variability gene concept could be important for the understanding of genetic predisposition to atherosclerosis since an individual's total genetic risk of CHD may depend on his or her *combination* of *level genes* and *variability genes* (for review see [19]).

Concluding remarks

There is emerging evidence that normal polymorphisms at several *functional candidate loci* are associated with CHD risk or CHD risk-factor level or variability. There is also evidence of gene–gene interactions and of disease associations that may be obliterated by environmental or lifestyle factors such as smoking. Thus, future research must focus not only on level genes and the variability gene concept; on rare genes with large effects and common genes with small effects; but also on a complex tapestry of interactions, including gene–gene interaction, gene–environment interaction, and environmentally caused obliteration of true genetic interrelationships.

Acknowledgements

Work in the author's laboratory is supported by Anders Jahres Foundation for the Promotion of Science, The Norwegian Council on Cardiovascular Diseases, and The Research Council of Norway.

References

1. Berg K. Acta Pathol Microbiol Immunol Scand 1963;59:369−382.
2. Berg K, Dahlén G, Frick MN. Clin Genet 1974;6:230−235.
3. Berg K, Names C, Dahlén G, Frick MN, Krishan I. Proc Natl Acad Sci USA 1976;73:937−940.
4. McLean JW, Tomlinson JE, Kuang W-J, Eaton DL, Chen EY, Fless GM, Scanu AM, Lawn RM. Nature 1987;330,132−137.
5. Berg K. Chem Phys Lipids 1994;67/68:9−16.
6. Rhoads GG, Dahlén G, Berg K, Morton NE, Dannenberg AL. J Am Med Assoc 1986;256:2540−2544.
7. Schaefer EJ, Lamon-Fava S, Jenner JL, McNamara JR, Ordovas JM, Davis CE, Abolafia JM, Lipoel K, Levy RI. J Am Med Assoc 1994;271:999−1003.
8. Berg K. In: Lusis AJ, Rotter JI, Sparkes RS (eds) Molecular Genetics and Coronary Artery Disease. Candidate Genes and Processes in Atherosclerosis. Monogr Hum Genet. Basel: Karger, 1992;189−207.
9. Berg K. Clin Genet 1994;46:57−62.
10. Grainger DJ, Kirschenlohr HL, Metcalfe JC, Weissberg PL, Wade DP, Lawn PM. Science 1993;260:1655−1658.
11. Berg K, Roald B, Sande H. Clin Genet 1994;46:52−56.
12. Sorensen KE, Celermajer DS, Georgakopoulos D, Hatcher G, Betteridge DJ, Deanfield JE. J Clin Invest 1994;93:50−55.
13. Lawn PM. Sci Am 1992;266:26−32.
14. Byrne CD, Lawn PM. Clin Genet 1994;46:34−41.
15. Keesler GA, Li Y, Skiba PJ, Fless GM, Tabas I. Arterioscler Thromb 1994;4:1337−1345.
16. Bøhn M, Berg K. Clin Genet 1994;46:77−79.
17. Cambien F, Poirier O, Lecerf L, Evans A, Cambou J-P, Arveiler D, Luc G, Bard J-M, Bara L, Ricard S, Tiret L, Amouyel P, Alhenc-Gelas F, Soubrier F. Nature 1992; 359;641−644.
18. Berge KE, Bøhn M, Berg K. Clin Genet 1994;46:102−104.
19. Berg K. In: Goldbourt U, de Faire U, Berg H (eds) Genetic Factors in Coronary Heart Disease. Dordrecht/Boston/London, Kluwer Academic Publishers, 1994;373−383.

614

Atherosclerosis X.
F.P. Woodford, J. Davignon and A. Sniderman, editors.

Interpopulation differentiation of the impact of polymorphic susceptibility genes

L.U. Gerdes

Department of Medicine and Cardiology, Aarhus Amtssygehus University Hospital, DK-8000 Aarhus, Denmark

Abstract. If allelic variation at a locus influences the liability to develop ischemic heart disease in synergy with effects of environmental factors or other polymorphic genes, then it cannot have an universally invariant effect at the interindividual level, e.g., in terms of genotype- or allele-specific relative risks. This is illustrated using a relatively simple simulation model, in which the genotype at a locus modifies the effect of "an enviromental factor" on "a biological trait" which in turn influences "risk". Relative risk estimates vary not only because of differential distributions across populations of the environmental factor, but also because of entirely unrelated factors that may cause the incidence of IHD in populations to differ.

Advances in molecular methodology have made it practicable to type individuals at many candidate genes (or marker loci) for ischemic heart disease (IHD) on a mass scale, and thus to map biological meaningful heterogeneities across ethnic groups showing differences in IHD incidence rates that may not appear satisfactorily explained by qualitatively or quantitatively different loads of known environmental risk factors. The aims of such endeavors could be to estimate the relative contributions of specific genetic diversities to interpopulation variation in the burden of IHD, using estimated effects of allelic variation at a candidate gene (or marker locus) at the interindividual level, e.g., in terms of the relative risks associated with different genotypes as determined in follow-up or case-control studies [1].

But does it really make sense to consider the impact of an IHD susceptibility gene at the interpopulation level to be a measurable function of some universally invariant effect at the interindividual level? Is it correspondingly unproblematic for instance to copy genotype-specific relative risk estimates from genetic epidemiologic studies in one ecological setting to evaluate the impact of a gene in another setting?

The answer depends, obviously, on *how* allelic variations at the relevant loci associate with interindividual variability in liability to develop IHD, and the purpose of the present study is to show why *No!* is likely to be the correct answer to the questions above, when we are dealing with the kind of IHD susceptibility genes that presumably play by far the major role in determining interindividual variability in risk [2–4].

Methods

The study is based on examining simulated scenarios of the distribution of incident IHD cases during some observation period of fixed length, in populations of 2,000 healthy individuals of the same age.

The structure of the model used is shown in Fig. 1. Cases were generated in the right side of positively skew distributions of a variable Y, representing a quantitative dynamic-phenotypic characteristic of an underlying pathogenic process, e.g., "lifetime average rate of progression of atherosclerosis" (it can be argued that Y is a biologically meaningful

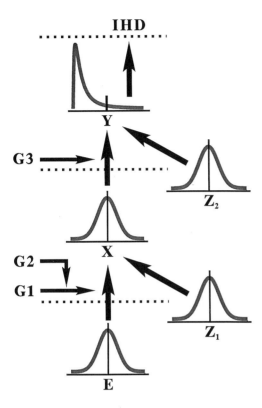

Fig. 1. The structure of the model used for simulations.

physical correlate of the abstraction "individual risk"). The distributions of Y were modeled as:

$$Y = e^a/(1+e^a), \text{ where } a = \alpha_0 + \alpha_1 X^2 + \alpha_2 Z_2,$$

and where X represents a quantitative biological trait external to the pathogenic process per se with a deterministic effect on the process (i.e., an intermediate biological trait [1,2,5]), α_0 and α_2 determine the average and the variance of Y in the population, respectively, due to biological traits (of all kinds) not related to X. Z_2 is randomly sampled from a standardized normal distribution. The distributions of X were generated from:

$$X = \beta_0 + \beta_1 E + \beta_2 Z_1, \text{ with } \beta_1 = 0 \text{ for } E < \delta,$$

where E is a quantitative variable, randomly sampled from a normal distribution to represent an environmental force, and δ is a lower threshold value. β_0 and β_2 determine the average and variance of X in the population, respectively, due to biological traits or environmental forces not related to E. Z_1 was randomly sampled from a standardized normal distribution.

The effects of common allelic variation at three unlinked loci, G1, G2 and G3, were

616

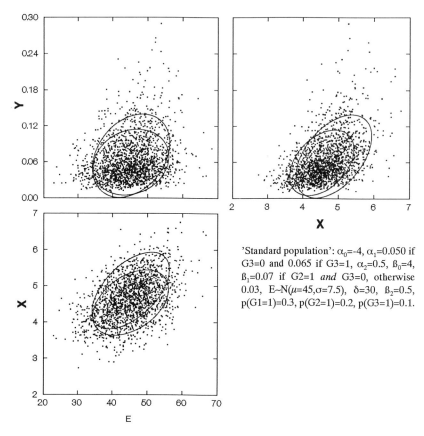

'Standard population': $\alpha_0=-4$, $\alpha_1=0.050$ if G3=0 and 0.065 if G3=1, $\alpha_2=0.5$, $\beta_0=4$, $\beta_1=0.07$ if G2=1 *and* G3=0, otherwise 0.03, E~N($\mu=45,\sigma=7.5$), $\delta=30$, $\beta_2=0.5$, p(G1=1)=0.3, p(G2=1)=0.2, p(G3=1)=0.1.

Fig. 2. An example of simulated distributions of an "environmental factor" (E), the dependent "biological trait" (X) and the resulting "pathogenic process rate" or risk (Y), in individuals with genotype G1 = 0 and in individuals with genotype G1 = 1 (the lower versus the higher 75-percentile ellipses in all panels).

simulated. For simplicity, the effects were assumed to depend only on the presence or absence of a particular allele, Gx = 1 or Gx = 0, i.e., no allele-dose effects etc. were considered. The genotypes could be randomly assigned in varying proportions, p(Gx = 1). The genotype at G1 is the only "measured genotype" and has an effect on the parameter β_1 — its value is higher in individuals with G1 = 1 than in individuals with G1 = 0, i.e., G1 modifies the effect of E on X. The "relative risk" (RR) in G1 = 1 individuals compared to G1 = 0 individuals was estimated from the ratio of the corresponding IHD incidence densities (calculated considering variable losses of observational person-time due to IHD and a 10% loss due to other causes). The effect of G2 = 1 was simulated to eliminate the effect of G1 on β_1, and the effect of the polymorphism at G3 was to modify the effect of X on Y: α_1 is higher in individuals with G3 = 1 than in individuals with G3 = 0.

Simulations were performed using Systat version 5.0 (Systat Inc., Evanston, USA) and Lotus Symphony version 3.0 (Lotus Development Corporation, Cambridge, USA), on an IBM PS/2 model 70 386 equipped with a math coprocessor. All scenarios were simulated in triplicates.

Results and Discussion

Figure 2 shows an example of simulated data pertaining to the "G1 + E → X → Y causal pathway" of the model. The two ellipses are the 75-percentile boundaries of the distributions in individuals with G1 = 0 and G1 = 1, respectively. The "noise" in the data is likely to be realistic, since we are supposed to be looking at versions of high-dimensional influential hyperspaces [5] that are collapsed across levels of only a few measured variables. Also, the evident overlapping of the G1-type-specific distributions of X and Y and the different variances (i.e., $\sigma^2(G1 = 1) > \sigma^2(G1 = 0)$) are realistic findings if G1 is a gene of the kind probably dominating the genetic architecture of IHD, i.e., genes exhibiting common allelic polymorphisms with relatively weak effects on quantitative biological traits [2,3,6]. For instance, the simulated data resemble (and this is not a coincidence) what could have been observed with X = plasma low density lipoprotein

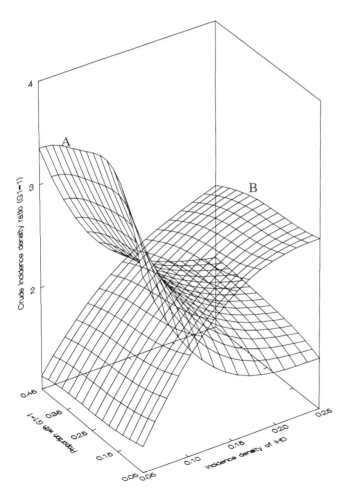

Fig. 3. Associations between p(G1 = 1) and the (total) incidence density of IHD in a population on one hand, and the estimated crude IDR on the other, when the variation in incidence of IHD across populations is made due to differences in either α_0 (profile A), or E (profile B).

(LDL)-cholesterol, E = dietary intake of saturated fatty acids etc., and G1 = the apolipoprotein E (apoE) gene; with G1 = 1 and G1 = 0 corresponding to having or not having an ε4-allele, respectively [7,8].

Figure 3 shows the associations between p(G1 = 1) and the (total) incidence density of IHD in a population on one hand, and the estimated crude IDR on the other (i.e., the RR that would be estimated in a genetic epidemiologic study in the particular population), when the variation in incidence of IHD across populations is due to differences in either α_0 (profile A), or E (profile B). There is a relatively modest influence of p(G1 = 1) on IDR, but marked and evidently very different influences of α_0 and E. Varying p(G2 = 1) or p(G3 = 1) causes additional distortions of the profiles (not shown).

Obviously, when one examines this simple model, it does not make much sense to think of a universally invariant effect of G1 at the interindividual level, and thus try to estimate the contribution of the G1 polymorphism to interpopulation variation in IHD rates, or to use a RR estimate determined in one ecological setting to estimate an impact in another and possibly different setting. This is perhaps not very surprising [9]. However, Fig. 3 may also relate to problems in populations defined in calendar time. If the incidence of IHD is changing in a population, the impact of a gene may increase or decrease, depending on the reasons why the incidence is changing. It may also relate to subpopulations defined by, e.g., age or gender. For instance, since the "unspecific IHD risk" probably tends to increase with age, any specific RR estimate will tend to be lower in studies of older than in studies of younger subpopulations. This seems to be the case in studies of apoE polymorphism and IHD, for instance, and may be one of several reasons why apoE allele-specific RR estimates differ quite substantially among studies [10].

References

1. Sing CF, Moll PP. Int J Epidemiol 1989;18:S183—S195.
2. Sing CF, Haviland MB, Templeton AR, Zerba KE, Reilly SL. Ann Med 1992;24:539—547.
3. Weiss KM. Genetic Variation and Human Disease. Principles and Evolutionary Approaches. Cambridge: Cambridge University Press, 1993.
4. Boerwinkle E, Hallman DM. In: Sing CF, Hanis CL (eds) Genetics of Cellular, Individual, Family, and Population Variability. New York, Oxford: Oxford University Press, 1993;93—105.
5. Sing CF, Reilly SL. In: Sing CF, Hanis CL (eds) Genetics of Cellular, Individual, Family, and Population Variability. New York, Oxford: Oxford University Press, 1993;140—161.
6. Reilly SL, Ferrell RE, Kottke BA, Kamboh MI, Sing CF. Am J Hum Genet 1991;49:1155—1166
7. Davignon J, Gregg RE, Sing CF. Arteriosclerosis 1988;8:1—21.
8. Miettinen TA. Ann Med 1991;23:181—186.
9. Greenland S, Morgenstern H. Int J Epidemiol 1989;18:269—274.
10. Gerdes LU. 3rd Annual Meeting of the International Genetic Epidemiology Society, Paris, 1994 (abstract).

Utility of gene information for predicting atherosclerosis

Eric Boerwinkle

Human Genetics Center, Houston, Texas, USA

Abstract. We have tested the ability of the apolipoprotein E polymorphism to predict the occurrence of carotid artery atherosclerosis in subjects taking part in the Atherosclerosis Risk in Communities Study after considering the contribution of established risk-factor variables. After selecting the set of demographic, anthropometric, and plasma lipid variables, we asked whether any of the apoE genotypes provided additional information for predicting carotid artery atherosclerotic disease status. The ε2/3 genotype provided additional information for predicting carotid-artery atherosclerotic disease (p = 0.078). The odds of being a carotid-artery atherosclerotic disease case for ε2/3 individuals is 2.2 times as high as the odds for ε3/3 individuals, after the effects of the other predictor variables have been accounted for. One possible mechanism of the observed association between the ε2 allele and atherosclerosis is the effect of this allele on postprandial lipemia and the subsequent atherogenic potential of delayed postprandial clearance. The utility of genetic information to predict disease beyond that afforded by traditional risk factors is likely to be greatest when the pathway between a gene and disease is *not* simply reflected in measures of the usual risk-factor variables.

Genes and prediction

The use of genetic information in predicting susceptibility to the common chronic diseases presents several unique problems and opportunities. Mankind is witnessing spectacular advances in the prevention and understanding of several single-gene disorders such as cystic fibrosis. These advances have revolutionized the detection and treatment of many of the rare inborn errors of metabolism. It is the great promise of molecular genetics and the human genome initiative that these advances will also impact on the common chronic diseases. However, once a genetic etiology has been assigned to a disease there is a tendency to oversimplify the relationship between genotype and endpoint when statements are made about risk or treatment. The inevitable interactions between genotypes and environments will confound prediction and treatment of the common chronic diseases. Genetic defects may predispose a patient to coronary heart disease, but the effects of such gene mutations are subject to modification and amelioration by other genetic or environmental factors.

There are many reasons why measures of DNA variation may improve the ability to predict interindividual differences in disease beyond that provided by established risk factors: 1) an individual's genotype does not change throughout life (barring somatic mutation); 2) the genotype is not influenced or changed by the disease process; 3) DNA variation can be measured more accurately than most intermediate predictor traits; 4) measurement of DNA variation is potentially less expensive; 5) measurement of DNA variation is required for assessing genotype-specific responses to environmental challenge (e.g., drug or dietary therapy); 6) the intermediate physiologic traits underlying disease

Address for correspondence: Eric Boerwinkle, Human Genetics Center, P.O. Box 20334, Houston, TX 77225, USA. Tel. +1-713-792-4680.

may be unknown or inaccessible to measurement; and 7) the ability of other traits (e.g., weight) to predict disease may be genotype-dependent.

In this paper, I discuss the utility of gene information to predict atherosclerosis using the common apolipoprotein (apo) E polymorphism as a paradigm.

ApoE

The gene whose effects on normal lipid variation are best understood is apolipoprotein E. ApoE is a structural component of chylomicrons, VLDL lipoproteins and a subset of HDL lipoproteins. ApoE plays a major role in lipid metabolism through cellular uptake of lipoprotein particles by apoE-specific and apoB/E receptors on the liver and other tissues [1]. Human apoE is polymorphic, with three alleles, ε2, ε3, and ε4 coding for three isoforms E2, E3, and E4, respectively. Numerous reports have indicated that the apoE polymorphism influences plasma lipid levels. Hallman et al. [2] have studied the frequency and effects of the apoE polymorphisms among nine ethnically and geographically diverse populations. They concluded that although the frequencies of the apoE alleles are heterogeneous among populations, the effects of this gene are relatively consistent: the average effect of the ε2 allele is to lower plasma cholesterol levels, of the ε4 allele to raise them. Using family data, Boerwinkle and Sing [3] estimated that the apoE polymorphism accounts for 12.5% of the overall polygenetic variance of total serum cholesterol levels.

Even though several reports have described an association between the apoE polymorphism and clinically recognized CHD [4–6], only one previous study [7] has examined the contribution of this gene directly to atherosclerosis and simultaneously considered the effects of more established risk factors. We have tested the ability of the apoE polymorphism to predict the occurrence of carotid-artery atherosclerosis in subjects taking part in the Atherosclerosis Risk in Communities (ARIC) Study [8] after considering the contribution of established risk factor variables [9]. Carotid-artery wall thickness was measured by B-mode ultrasonography. Subjects were designated 'cases' if the maximum carotid arterial intima-media far-wall thickness was greater than 2.5 mm at any site or there was bilateral thickening exceeding 1.7 mm at the internal carotid, 1.8 mm at the bifurcation, or 1.6 mm at the common carotid arteries. Exclusion criteria for case/control selection included: evidence of symptomatic cardiovascular or cerebrovascular disease defined by a history of angina on effort, physician-diagnosed heart attack, transient ischemic attack or stroke, or intermittent claudication.

We selected by stepwise logistic regression the lifestyle variables which were significant predictors of the probability of having carotid-artery atherosclerotic disease (Table 1A). Age, body mass index (BMI), cigarette smoking (CigYears) and hypertension status were the significant risk factors identified by this analysis. Likewise, only those plasma lipid variables which significantly predicted carotid-artery atherosclerotic disease status were included in the prediction equation. These were total cholesterol, Lp[a], and HDL-cholesterol. After selecting this set of demographic, anthropometric, and plasma lipid variables, we asked whether any of the apoE genotypes provided additional information for predicting carotid-artery atherosclerotic disease status. Only the ε2/3 genotype (p = 0.079) provided additional information in predicting carotid-artery atherosclerotic disease at the 0.10 level of significance (Table 1B). According to this analysis, the odds of being a carotid-artery atherosclerotic disease case for ε2/3 individuals is 2.2 times as high as the odds for ε3/3 individuals, after considering the effects of the other predictor variables.

Even though some previous studies in survivors of a myocardial infarction have

Table 1. Prediction of cartoid artery atherosclerotic disease status using a stepwise selection procedure and apoE genotypes

A: Significant lifestyle and plasma lipid variables

Variables	Coefficient	S.E.	p-value	Odds ratio
Age (years)	0.153	0.051	0.003	1.17
BMI (kg/m²)	0.0778	0.0358	0.0297	1.081
CigYears[a]	0.0016	0.0003	0.0001	1.002
Hypertension	0.892	0.407	0.0284	2.440
Cholesterol (mg/dl)	0.0079	0.0037	0.0292	1.008
Lp(a) (µg/ml)	0.0039	0.0017	0.0242	1.004
HDL-cholesterol (mg/dl)	−0.0331	0.0109	0.0025	0.967

B: Significant lifestyle and plasma lipid variables and apoE genotypes

Variables	Coefficient	S.E.	p-value	Odds ratio
Age (years)	0.149	0.0511	0.0036	1.161
BMI (kg/m²)	0.0836	0.0366	0.0224	1.087
CigYears[a]	0.0017	0.0003	0.0001	1.002
Hypertension	0.985	0.406	0.0155	2.68
Cholesterol (mg/dl)	0.0090	0.0037	0.0159	1.009
Lp(a) (µg/ml)	0.0039	0.0018	0.0248	1.004
HDL-cholesterol (mg/dl)	−0.0335	0.0112	0.0026	0.967
ε2/2	2.2	2.56	0.391	9.0
ε2/3	0.8	0.455	0.079	2.23
ε2/4	0.289	1.06	0.785	1.34
ε3/4	−0.0083	0.381	0.983	0.992
ε4/4	0.646	0.790	0.414	1.91

[a]CigYears expressed as number of cigarettes per day × number of smoking years.

suggested an association of the ε2 allele with atherosclerotic disease [10–12], the majority of epidemiologic studies favor an association of the ε4 allele with the occurrence of myocardial infarction or angiographically documented CHD [4–6]. The observed association of the ε2 allele with carotid-artery atherosclerotic disease may, therefore, appear unexpected. However, our study design excluded subjects with known coronary heart disease. Because of an association of carotid intima-media thickness with coronary heart disease, our selection procedure eliminated 3 times as many potential carotid-artery atherosclerotic disease cases as controls from this study. Hence, individuals with more advanced stenotic or occlusive atherosclerotic disease have been excluded, and the associations of the apoE polymorphism with carotid-artery atherosclerotic disease status may have been modified.

What is the possibile mechanism responsible for the observed association between the ε2 allele and atherosclerosis? Because of its recognized importance in remnant clearance, the apolipoprotein [apo] E gene has been targeted for studying postprandial lipid response. It has been argued that prolonged postprandial lipemia promotes the development of atherosclerosis [13,14]. To estimate the contribution of the apoE polymorphism to distinct metabolic aspects of postprandial lipoprotein metabolism, Boerwinkle et al. [15] measured several parameters of postprandial response in a biracial sample of 474 individuals taking part in the Atherosclerosis Risk in Communities (ARIC) Study [8].

The estimated frequencies of the ε2, ε3 and ε4 alleles in the sample of 397 Caucasian subjects were 0.073, 0.802 and 0.125, respectively. Because the inference based on rare

622

classes is limited, the analyses of the effect of the apoE polymorphism on postprandial response are shown only for the three common genotypes — ε2/3s, ε3/3s and ε3/4s. The profile of postprandial triglyceride and retinyl palmitate response for each of the common apoE genotypes is shown in Figs. 1A and B, respectively. The profile of postprandial triglyceride levels was not different among the common apoE genotypes. Postprandial triglyceride concentrations increased from 128.6 (± 75.2) mg/dl at fasting to 270.8 (± 130.5) mg/dl at 3.5 h followed by a decrease to 193.7 (± 137.1) mg/dl at 8 h. The profile

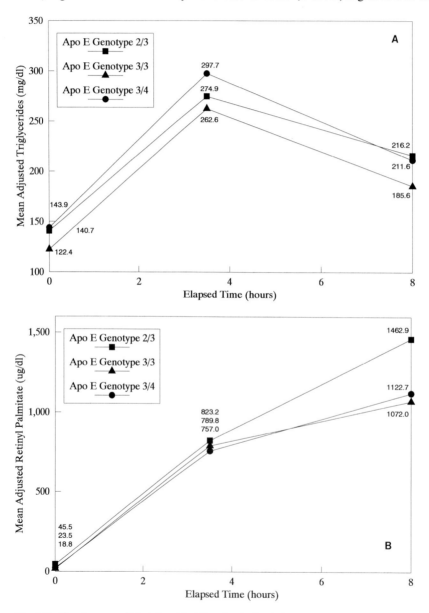

Fig. 1. Profile of postprandial triglyceride (A) and retinyl palmitate (B) levels for each of the common apoE genotypes in 397 Caucasian subjects from the ARIC study.

of postprandial retinyl palmitate, however, was significantly different among apoE genotypes between 3.5 and 8 h after the test meal. Late postprandial retinyl palmitate levels were significantly higher in individuals with the ε2/3 genotype than in the other apoE genotypes. Average late postprandial retinyl palmitate levels were 1,463 (± 737) μg/dl in ε2/3 individuals compared to 1,072 (± 604) μg/dl in the ε3/3s. Reduced binding affinity of the E2 isoform for hepatic lipoprotein receptors [1] and subsequent upregulation of LDL-receptor density have been proposed as the most likely mechanism for the effect of this gene on plasma LDL- and total-cholesterol concentrations. It is also the likely mechanism for the increased late postprandial retinyl palmitate concentrations in ε2/3 subjects observed in the above study. Therefore, one possible mechanism of the observed association between the ε2 allele and atherosclerosis is the effect of this allele on postprandial lipemia and the subsequent atherogenic potential of delayed postprandial clearance.

Summary

The association between the ε2 allele and atheroscleros is not reflected in the effect of this gene on fasting plasma cholesterol: the average effect of the ε2 allele is actually to lower plasma cholesterol levels. The observed association between the ε2 allele and atherosclerosis is probably mediated through the effect of this allele on postprandial lipemia and the impact of postprandial lipid metabolism on HDL-triglyceride [14]. Therefore, the utility of genetic information to predict disease beyond that afforded by traditional risk factors is likely to be greatest when the pathway between a gene and disease is *not* simply reflected in measures of the usual risk-factor variables (e.g., fasting plasma cholesterol).

Acknowledgements

This work was supported by grants HL-40613, and contracts N01-HC55015, N01-HC55016, N01-HC55018, N01-HC55019, N01-HC55020, N01-HC55021, N01-HC55022 with the National Heart, Lung and Blood Institute. Eric Boerwinkle is an Established Investigator of the American Heart Association and the recipient of a Research Career Development Award from the National Institutes of Health (HL-02453).

References

1. Mahley RW, Innerarity TL, Rall Jr SC, Weisgraber KH, Taylor JM. Curr Opin Lipidol 1990;1:87—95.
2. Hallmann DM, Boerwinkle E, Saha N, Sandholzer C, Menzel HJ, Czazar A, Utermann G. Am J Hum Genet 1991;49:338—349.
3. Boerwinkle E and Sing CF Ann Hum Genet 1987;51:211—226.
4. Menzel HJ, Kladetzky RG, Assman G. Arteriosclerosis 1983;3:310—315.
5. Lenzen HJ, Assman G, Buchwalsky R, Schulte HS. Clin Chem 1986;32:778—781.
6. Cumming AM, Roberts FW. Clin Genet 1984;25:310—313.
7. Hixson JE and the Pathobiological Determinants of Atherosclerosis in Youth (PDAY) Research Group. Arterioscler Thromb 1991;11:1237—1244.
8. ARIC Investigators. Am J Epidemiol 1989;129:687—702.
9. de Andrade M, Thandi I, Brown S, Gotto A Jr, Patsch W, Boerwinkle E. Apolipoprotein E genetic polymorphism predicts carotid artery atherosclerosis (submitted).
10. Utermann G, Hardewig A, Zimmer F. Hum Genet 1984;65:237—241.
11. Kameda K, Matsuzawa Y, Kubo M et al. Atherosclerosis 1984;51:241—249.
12. Wilson PWF, Larson MG, Ordovas JM, Schaefer EJ. Circulation 1994;(Suppl I):1—810.
13. Zilversmit DB. Circulation 1979;60:473—485.
14. Patsch JR, Miesenbock G, Hopferwieser T, Muhlberger V, Knapp E, Dunn JK, Gotto Am Jr, Patsch W. Arterioscler Thromb 1992;12:1236—1245.
15. Boerwinkle E, Brown S, Sharrett AR, Heiss G, Patsch W. Am J Hum Genet 1994;54:341—360.

624

Familial combined hyperlipidemia and genetic risk for atherosclerosis

John D. Brunzell[1], Melissa A. Austin[1], Samir S. Deeb[1], John E. Hokanson[1], Gail P. Jarvik[1], David N. Nevin[1], Ellen Wijsman[1], Alberto Zambon[2] and Arno G. Motulsky[1]
[1]University of Washington, Seattle, Washington, USA; and [2]University of Padova, Padova, Italy

Familial combined hyperlipidemia (FCH) was first described in the Seattle Myocardial Infarction Study in 1973 [1]. In this study, the families of individuals who had survived for 3 months after a myocardial infarction were investigated for lipid abnormalities. At least 11% of individuals who were MI survivors, under the age of 60 years, had familial combined hyperlipidemia. This disease was characterized by variable lipoprotein phenotype (increased triglyceride or cholesterol) both in the proband and in the relatives, which could also vary within an individual from time to time. Despite this lipid variability, apoB was found to be significantly elevated [2,3]. FCH was also found in the families of individuals with hypertriglyceridemia, but no coronary artery disease, where relatives of probands with FCH had twice the prevalence of myocardial infarction of relatives of individuals with familial hypertriglyceridemia and the spouse controls [4]. The prevalence of FCH was further estimated in males under the age of 60 who had coronary artery disease by angiography where one-third of males had apoB levels above the 95th percentile of a control population. Of those individuals who were selected for the Familial Atherosclerosis Treatment Study (FATS) with an elevated apoB level [5], 60% of them had FCH by analysis of families, whereas only 15% had familial hypercholesterolemia and 24% had elevations in Lp(a) both in the proband and in the families [6]. Thus it would appear that FCH may contribute to at least 20% of coronary artery disease in males under the age of 60 years, and presumably women 10 years older.

The major lipid abnormalities seen in FCH are an increase in triglyceride and/or cholesterol representing an increase in small VLDL, an increase in intermediate density lipoproteins, and an increase in small, dense LDL [7]. Evaluation of hepatic secretion of VLDL apoB has demonstrated that VLDL apoB secretion is increased in FCH in those who are hypertriglyceridemic, while an increase in LDL apoB turnover can be demonstrated in those who are hypercholesterolemic [8–11].

Genetic epidemiology

Pedigree analysis of the FCH families from the Seattle MI survivors study suggested that FCH was an autosomal dominant disorder [1]. A recent complex segregation analysis of both the Seattle and the new English FCH families indicated that triglyceride, though not cholesterol, is controlled by a single major gene [12]. Other investigators also using complex segregation analysis to evaluate the sources of interindividual variability in apoB in samples of adults have demonstrated that 40% or more of the variation in age- and sex-

Address for correspondence: John D. Brunzell MD, Division of Metabolism, Endocrinology and Nutrition RG-26, University of Washington, Seattle, WA 98195, USA.

adjusted apoB levels can be ascribed to an unmapped, codominant Mendelian locus [13,14]. The predicted phenotype at this putative apoB level locus was also associated with variation in low density lipoprotein and triglyceride levels. Studies by Jarvik et al. have found this locus also to be predictive of the increased apoB levels seen in FCH [15].

Low density lipoproteins are comprised of several distinct subspecies based on density [16] and size [17]. Individuals with small, dense LDL have LDL-subclass phenotype B; those with large, buoyant LDL have phenotype A. Complex segregation analysis in healthy families indicates that small dense LDL (LDL-subclass phenotype B) segregates in a manner consistent with a major gene with a dominant mode of inheritance influencing this trait, with a frequency of this proposed allele of 0.25 [18]. Using nonequilibrium density gradient ultracentrifugation, it can also be shown that there is an increase in VLDL, a decrease in HDL and an increase in the density of the major LDL peak in healthy individuals with phenotype B [19]. Complex segregation analysis of 250 individuals in seven large kindreds with FCH also provided evidence for a dominant major gene with allele frequency of 0.32 [20], against a background of multifactorial inheritance. LDL-subclass phenotype A individuals in the FCH families had elevated apoB levels which were further elevated in the LDL pattern B individuals. This increase in LDL apoB in the phenotype A individuals also suggested something in these families raising apoB in addition to the LDL-subclass phenotype B. Using the technique of commingling analysis, it was demonstrated that there was bimodal distribution of apoB amongst the individuals in these families with phenotype B [21]. Thus it was hypothesized that at least two genes were involved in determining plasma apoB levels in FCH: one common gene with a major influence on LDL subclass phenotypes, and a second gene that results in further elevations of apoB levels.

A recent complex segregation analysis in families with FCH suggests a threshold model for FCH which is influenced by an uncommon major gene controlling the level of apoB [14] interacting with a common gene controlling the small, dense LDL-subclass phenotype B [22]. In this model, these two putative genes were shown to be independent. Homozygote individuals for the putative apoB-elevating allele expressed FCH. Among heterozygotes at this locus, the presence of the proposed allele for LDL-subclass phenotype B increases the probability of being affected with FCHL. Consistent with this model is the bimodal distribution of apoB levels among LDL phenotype B subjects in FCH families, as noted above [21]. The similar depletion of cholesteryl ester, free cholesterol, and phospholipid in small, dense LDL seen both in FCH [23] and in normolipidemic individuals with LDL-subclass phenotype B [19] implies a common determinant of small, dense LDL in both FCH and amongst normolipidemic individuals.

It has been suggested that the small dense LDL seen in FCH might simply be a reflection of the increase in triglyceride seen in this disorder, with an exchange in VLDL-triglyceride for LDL-cholesteryl ester. To evaluate this possibility, we treated individuals with FCH who were hypertriglyceridemic and had small, dense LDL with gemfibrozil for 3 months [7]. Gemfibrozil therapy was associated with a decrease in VLDL-cholesterol (and a compensatory increase in buoyant LDL-cholesterol) but the small, dense LDL persisted in spite of the reduction in triglyceride levels. This suggests that the increase in small, dense LDL was independent of factors that raised triglyceride levels.

Thus we have hypothesized that FCH is due to the combination of a common gene variant (frequency 25–30%) associated with small, dense LDL, and an uncommon gene that also raises apoB and triglyceride levels. Using this oligogenic model for FCH, one can then investigate the candidate genes that might account for these defects.

Candidate genes

An obvious gene that might account for the overproduction of apoB in FCH is the very large apoB gene on chromosome 2. Rauh et al. [24] have found evidence against linkage of the apoB gene with the FCH phenotype. Polymorphism in the AI/CIII/AIV locus has been suggested as segregating with hyperlipidemia and FCH [25], although this has not been confirmed [26].

Another candidate gene with a rare mutation that might contribute to FCH is the lipoprotein lipase gene [6]. It has been reported that one-third of individuals with FCH had one-half the levels of lipoprotein lipase activity of age-matched controls and age-matched individuals with coronary artery disease due to familial hypercholesterolemia or elevated lipoprotein(a) levels. When the structural gene for lipoprotein lipase was investigated in 20 such individuals, six polymorphisms were found among the 40 alleles [27]. One of these was a G to A substitution accounting for Asp9-Asn change. When this polymorphism was expressed in vitro, the protein released had normal activity and mass. Thus Asp9-Asn does not seem to cause a functional defect. Two of the 40 alleles were found to have A to G substitution without changing residue-108 valine. Three of the 40 alleles had a premature stop codon at serine 447 at the end of the LPL gene that does not affect function. Thus, no evidence was found for a structural defect in the LPL gene to account for the decrease in LPL activity seen in the subset of individuals with FCH. Other candidate genes might affect lipoprotein lipase activity, such as the apoC-II gene and the apoC-III gene. No structural abnormalities were found in either of these two genes in these 20 individuals. To rule out regulatory defects in these genes related to the 5′ end of the LPL gene or in intronic sequences, further studies need to be carried out.

It has been suggested that the small, dense LDL may be a marker for insulin resistance [28,29]. We also have found, in normal-weight individuals, that the quantity of intra-abdominal fat is correlated with insulin sensitivity [30] as measured by the Bergman Minimal Model [31], and with LDL size and density [30]. It was proposed that the increase in intra-abdominal fat causes insulin resistance and raises free fatty acid levels. The latter leads to increased apoB secretion from the liver, resulting in elevated apoB levels, by directing apoB from intrahepatic degradation towards secretion. A decrease in intrahepatic free cholesterol would result, increasing the message for the LDL receptor with an increase in removal of LDL, and the message for hepatic lipase and hepatic lipase activity [32] with development of small, dense LDL. Data related to insulin resistance in FCH are somewhat limited, although middle-aged individuals with FCH have been shown to be more obese than their normolipidemic family members [33], and apoB levels have been shown to be moderately correlated with insulin levels in FCH [34].

On the basis of these results, our working hypothesis is that several common genes lead to central/visceral obesity with insulin resistance, elevated free fatty acid levels, and mild dyslipidemia. The small, dense LDL (phenotype B) may be a useful marker for this trait in the population. LDL-subclass phenotype B interacts with one of several additional genes, raising apoB levels to cause the oligogenic disorder, familial combined hyperlipidemia. The candidate genes to account for any of these abnormalities have yet to be identified.

Acknowledgements

Supported in part by NIH grants HL30086 and HL49513. Dr Austin was an Established Investigator of the American Heart Association. Dr Jarvik has a Howard Hughes Medical Institute Physician Research Fellowship. A portion of these studies were performed at the University of Washington Medical Center CRC (RR37).

References

1. Goldstein JL, Schrott HG, Hazzard WR, Bierman EL, Motulsky AG. J Clin Invest 1973;52:1544−1568.
2. Brunzell JD, Albers JJ, Chait A, Grundy SM, Groszek E, McDonald GB. J Lipid Res 1983;24:147−155.
3. Sniderman AD, Shapiro S, Marpole D, Skinner B, Teng B, Kwiterovich PO Jr. Proc Natl Acad Sci USA 1980;77:604−608.
4. Brunzell JD, Schrott HG, Motulsky AG, Bierman EL. Metabolism 1976;25:313−320.
5. Brown G, Albers J, Fisher I, Schaefer S, Lan J, Kaplan C, Zhao X, Bisson B, Fitzpatrick V, Dodge H. N Engl J Med 1989;323:1289−1298.
6. Babirak S, Brown BG, Brunzell JD. Aterioscler Thromb 1992;12:1176−1183.
7. Hokanson JE, Austin MA, Zambon A, Brunzell JD. Arterioscler Thromb 1993;13:427−434.
8. Chait A, Albers JJ, Brunzell JD. Eur J Clin Invest 1980;10:17−22.
9. Janus ED, Nicoll AM, Turner PR, Magill P, Lewis B. Eur J Clin Invest 1980;10:161−172.
10. Kissebah AH, Alfarsi S, Evans DJ. Arteriosclerosis 1984;4:614−624.
11. Venkatesan S, Cullen P, Pacy P, Halliday D, Scott J. Arterioscler Thromb 1993;13:1110−1118.
12. Cullen P, Farren B, Scott J, Farrall M. Arterioscler Thromb 1994;14:1233−1249.
13. Hasstedt SJ, Wu L, Williams RR. Genet Epidemiol 1987;4:67−76.
14. Pairitz G, Davignon J, Mailloux H, Sing CF. Am J Hum Genet 1988;43:311−321.
15. Pairitz GP, Beaty TH, Gallagher PR, Coates PM, Cortner JA. Genet Epidemiol 1993;10:257−270.
16. Fisher WR. Metabolism 1983;32(3):283−291.
17. Krauss RM, Burke DJ. J Lipid Res 1982;23:97−104.
18. Austin MA, King M-C, Vranizan KM, Newman B, Krauss RM. Am J Hum Genet 1988;43:838−846.
19. Capell W, Hokanson JE, Zambon A, Austin MA, Brunzell JD. J Lipid Res 1994 (submitted).
20. Austin MA, Brunzell JD, Fitch WL, Krauss RM. Arteriosclerosis 1990;10:520−530.
21. Austin MA, Horowitz H, Wijsman E, Krauss R, Brunzell JD. Atherosclerosis 1992;92:67−77.
22. Jarvik GP, Brunzell JD, Austin MA, Krauss RM, Motulsky AG, Wijsman E. Arterioscler Thromb (in press).
23. Hokanson JE, Krauss RM, Albers JJ, Austin MA, Brunzell JD. Arterioscler Thromb (submitted).
24. Rauh G, Schuster H, Mueller B, Schewe S, Keller C, Wolfram G, Zoellner N. Atherosclerosis 1990;83: 81−87.
25. Wojciechowski A, Farrall M, Cullen P, Wilson T, Bayliss D, Farren B, Griffin B, Caslake M, Packard C, Shepherd J, Thakker R, Scott J. Nature 1991;349:161−164.
26. Wijsman E, Motulsky AG, Guo S, Yang M, Austin MA, Brunzell JD, Deeb S. Circulation (suppl I) 1992; 86(4):1420.
27. Nevin DN, Brunzell JD, Deeb S. Arterioscler Thromb 1994;14:869−874.
28. Reaven GM, Chen YD, Jeppesen J, Maheux P, Krauss RM. J Clin Invest 1993;92:141−146.
29. Selby JV, Austin MA, Newman B, Zhang D, Quesenberry CP, Mayer EJ, Krauss RM. Circulation 1993; 88:381−387.
30. Fujimoto WY, Abbate SL, Kahn SE, Hokanson JE, Brunzell JD. Obesity Res 1994;2:364−371.
31. Bergman RN, Ider YZ, Bodden CR, Cobelli C. Am J Physiol 1979;236:E667−677.
32. Zambon A, Austin MA, Brown BG, Hokanson JE, Brunzell JD. Arterioscler Thromb 1993;13:147−153.
33. Brunzell JD. Arteriosclerosis 1984;4:180−182.
34. Cabezas MC, de Bruin TWA, de Valk HW, Shoulders CC, Jansen H, Erkelens DW. J Clin Invest 1993; 92:160−168.

628

Interaction between genotype and environmental factors in the development of atherosclerotic-thrombotic disease: the effect of smoking on plasma levels of fibrinogen

S.E. Humphries[1], A. Thomas[1], G. Miller[2], A. Hamsten[3] and F. Green[1]

[1]Cardiovascular Genetics, Department of Medicine, University College London Medical School, London WC1E 6JJ; [2]Wolfson Institute, St Bartholomews, London, UK; and [2]Karolinska Institute, Stockholm, Sweden

Abstract. We have detected several common sequence changes in the promoter region of the β-fibrinogen gene, and healthy nonsmoking men who are carriers (roughly 35% of the population) have slightly higher plasma fibrinogen levels (+5%) than noncarriers, but with much larger genotype-associated effects in smokers (+14%). These sequence changes may affect the affinity of DNA-binding proteins that control the rate of transcription of the gene and hence the amount of mRNA and protein made in and secreted from the liver. One sequence change may affect the binding of a nuclear factor responsive to IL-6, one of the cytokines responsible for the acute phase response, and thus may provide a molecular explanation for the effects on fibrinogen level of genotype–smoking interaction.

The critical role of genes is in coding for structural proteins and enzymes which enable the cell, organ or organism to maintain homeostasis in the face of the environmental challenges experienced. Within a population, genetic variation will mean that individuals will have different abilities to maintain homeostasis when faced with a specific environmental challenge. The clinical features of any disorder with a late age of onset can therefore be thought of as being caused to some extent by the failure of the individual to maintain homeostasis, and this is particularly true for the disorder of coronary artery disease (CAD). Epidemiological studies have identified a number of factors that are associated with increased risk of CAD, including high blood pressure, smoking, high dietary fat intake, and obesity; and a number of plasma risk factors have been identified such as elevated levels of cholesterol carried in low density lipoprotein (LDL) particles, low levels of high density lipoprotein (HDL) particles and high levels of the clotting factor fibrinogen. It is well established that genetic variation determines in part the levels of such lipids and proteins in the blood. Some of the genes involved have been well studied and mutations in these genes have been identified (e.g., the LDL-receptor gene in patients with familial hypercholesterolemia, and the sequence changes that create the common apolipoprotein E isoforms). However, for any selected individual, the level of such risk factors in the blood is also due to an individual's genetically-determined ability to maintain homeostasis in response to environmental factors. Thus the current epidemic of CAD being seen in Western societies is not due to an increase in the frequency of mutations in important genes, but rather to an inability in some individuals to maintain optimum blood levels of these risk-factor components, in the light of the environment experienced as a result of affluent lifestyle changes, such as changes in dietary fat intake and in the proportion of people smoking cigarettes.

Address for correspondence: Cardiovascular Genetics, Department of Medicine, University College London Medical School, London WC1E 6JJ, UK.

Smoking and coronary artery disease

There are many possible mechanisms whereby smoking may lead to CAD [1]. Smoking is chronically associated with a number of potentially atherogenic changes in plasma lipid levels, particularly with lower levels of the protective HDL particles. Smoking increases platelet aggregation, white blood cell count and hematocrit and most markedly fibrinogen levels, and thus results in a significant increase in blood viscosity [2]. Many of the pathophysiological changes seen in response to smoking appear to mimic, albeit at low level, those seen in the acute-phase (AP) response that accompanies severe inflammation. Monocytes play a central role in the AP, and they migrate to sites of tissue damage and respond to various external stimuli by secreting a number of cytokines and growth factors, the most important of which appear to be interleukin-1 (IL-1), IL-6 tumor necrosis factor (TNF) and transforming growth factor-β (TGF-β). For smoking, it is thus believed that damage to the lung tissues results in the recruitment of large numbers of macrophages, and these respond by secreting IL-6, TGF-β etc into the blood, which stimulate the liver to make a low-grade AP response. Hepatocytes have a specific IL-6 receptor on their surface which comprises two proteins, one of which binds IL-6 and through interaction with the second, a transmembrane tyrosine kinase [3], stimulates the phosphorylation of specific cytoplasmic proteins. This initiates a cellular cascade of events which results among other things in the rapid modification of a nuclear transcription factor NF-IL6, which significantly enhances the DNA-binding ability of the protein. NF-IL6 is a leucine-zipper-containing protein which has homology to the transcription factor C/EBP. The transcription of a number of liver-specific genes is controlled by C/EBP binding, due to the presence of a sequence element in the promoter region of both positive and negative AP genes; such an element is found in both the albumin and apoAI promoter. It appears that NF-IL6 competes for C/EBP binding in these genes and this has the effect of suppressing the transcription of negative AP proteins. By contrast, positive AP proteins have related sequence elements which are recognized only by NF-IL6 and binding results in strong transcription; such elements have been identified in the fibrinogen gene promoter, amongst others.

Variability at the fibrinogen locus and plasma fibrinogen levels

Several prospective studies have shown a direct association between plasma fibrinogen concentration and the subsequent incidence of CAD [4,5]. In men in the Northwick Park Heart Study (NPHS), an elevation of one standard deviation in fibrinogen (about 0.6 g/l) was associated with an 84% increase in the risk of CAD within the next 5 years. This association is probably mediated through a number of different pathophysiological processes, including the fact that individuals with elevated fibrinogen levels have an increased propensity for coagulation, and formation of a thrombus in an artery that is already narrowed by atherosclerosis is a frequent cause of myocardial infarction. Fibrinogen is an acute-phase protein, and its plasma level is raised following infection or injury. Because of its sensitivity to environmental factors, the within-individual variation of fibrinogen levels is high, accounting for up to 26% of the sample variance in standardized assays [6]. The extent to which genetic factors may determine the plasma fibrinogen level is unclear, though path analysis has suggested an estimate for heritability of fibrinogen levels of 0.5 [7], while twin studies give a lower estimate of 0.3 [8,9]. To date, there have been no reports of biometrical analysis to investigate the possibility that a major gene determines fibrinogen levels.

Each plasma fibrinogen molecule is composed of two each of the Aα-, Bβ- and γ-

630

fibrinogen polypeptide chains, and the complex is held together by a number of inter- and intra-chain disulfide links. The three fibrinogen genes are in a cluster of less than 50 kb on the long arm of chromosome 4, and each chain is synthesized as a separate mRNA, with the levels of all three mRNAs being co-ordinately controlled. The rate-limiting step in the production of the mature fibrinogen molecule in the human hepatoma cell line HepG2 is the synthesis of the Bβ-polypeptide chain [10], which in turn is influenced by the amount of its mRNA available. It is therefore likely that an alteration in the level of synthesis of the Bβ-chain may have an effect on the amount of fibrinogen secreted by the liver. A cartoon of the β-gene promoter is shown in Fig. 1, and the region from β-150 base pairs to the start of transcription has homology with other AP genes such as α-1-antitrypsin. This region has been reported to contain all the information required to act as a promoter in HepG2 cells and has been shown to bind proteins from a HepG2 cell nuclear extract. The sequence from −89 to −76 contains a conserved liver-specific transcription element which binds hepatic nuclear factor 1 (HNF1), and deletion mapping shows that just upstream lies an IL-6-responsive element, which has been identified in other genes as the motif CTGGGA [11]. It is therefore possible that sequence changes in this region of the gene may have a direct effect on the rate of transcription and thus on plasma fibrinogen levels.

In studies of the β-fibrinogen promoter, a common G/A sequence variation was detected at position −455, the A being present in roughly 20% of alleles examined [12]. In samples of healthy individuals the A-455 allele has been consistently associated with higher fibrinogen levels (Table 1), those with one or more copies of the A-455 allele having for example 0.28 g/l higher fibrinogen levels than those with the genotype G/G in healthy men in the UK [12]. The magnitude of this genotype effect indicates that it is likely to be of biological significance in causing an elevated risk of thrombosis, and by extrapolation from the NPHS data of the relationship between fibrinogen and CAD risk (0.6 g/l associated with 84% greater risk), men with the A allele would be at 40% higher risk of a thrombotic event; this estimate is based on healthy middle-aged men from north London, and may not be the same in other groups. However, in support of the relationship between fibrinogen genotype and risk of disease, polymorphisms at the fibrinogen locus have been reported to be associated with risk of peripheral arterial disease [17], though not with risk of MI in a case-control study [16].

Although the A-455 sequence is outside the region of the reported promoter sequence,

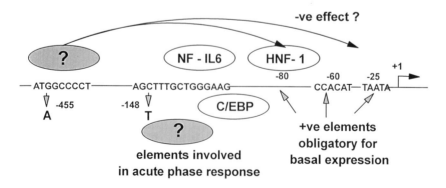

Fig. 1. The promoter region of the β-fibrinogen gene showing the location of the G_{455}-A substitution and C_{-148}-T relative to the transcription initiation site and the IL-6 element and CAAT and TATA boxes (from [11]).

Table 1. Mean of fibrinogen levels in men with different G/A genotypes

Sample (ref)	Genotype	No.	Fibrinogen (g/l)
Healthy men, UK (12)	GG	188	2.71
	GA + AA	101	2.99[a]
PVD + healthy, UK (13)[b]	GG	165	2.92
	GA + AA	82	2.96
MI + healthy, Sweden (14)	GG	44	2.90
	GG + AA	32	3.30[a]
Young males (EARS) (15)	GG	326	2.24
	GG + AA	188	2.34[a]
ECTIM, control group (16)	GG	410	2.97
	GA + AA	238	3.06[a]
ECTIM, MI group (16)	GG	352	3.38
	GA + AA	181	3.54[a]

[a] $p < 0.025$; [b] data not adjusted for the effect of age/smoking etc.

it is possible that it has a direct effect on transcription. Preliminary studies have demonstrated binding of a hepatic nuclear protein to the G but not the A sequence (Green et al., unpublished). However, recently it has been found that in all Caucasian populations studied to date the A-455 sequence change is in complete allelic association with a C-148-T change located close to the consensus sequence of the IL6 element (Fig. 1). This raises the possibility that the G-455-A change is acting as a neutral marker for the C-T change, which is the functional change working through effects on transcription of the β-fibrinogen gene that are mediated by IL6. One possibility is that variation in the IL6-responsive element in the β-promoter may increase the affinity of NF-IL6, leading to enhanced transcription. This hypothesis is supported by recent data from our laboratory [18] using band-shift assays that the T-148 sequence binds a nuclear protein which the C-148 sequence does not. In order to test this hypothesis, experiments are in progress to insert this fragment of the gene into the appropriate vector to test promoter strength.

Interaction between smoking and genotype to determine plasma fibrinogen levels

Individuals who smoke have elevated levels of plasma fibrinogen and have a higher risk of both CHD and stroke, and it is likely that a substantial proportion of the association between smoking and CAD is mediated through the plasma fibrinogen concentration [19]. It is likely that the elevation in fibrinogen experienced in response to a certain degree of smoking will vary between different individuals, and data from two studies are summarized in Fig. 2. Fibrinogen levels were, as expected, higher in the smokers (13% in the Swedish [14] and 9% in the ECTIM study [16]), and in both studies in the nonsmokers, men with one or more A-455 allele had higher levels of fibrinogen than those with only the G-455 allele, although the raising effect associated with the A allele was small (5.2%). In those with only the G-455 allele, the smokers show a smaller than average elevation of fibrinogen levels (9.4 and 6.5%, respectively) while those with one or more A-455 allele show a roughly 2-fold greater effect (elevation of 18.6% and 12.0% respectively). Since these data are cross-sectional they must be interpreted with caution, but they suggest that individuals with the A-455 allele who smoke will experience a greater rise in fibrinogen-associated CAD risk than those lacking this allele. It also predicts that the A-455 individuals will experience a greater than average reduction in fibrinogen levels upon stopping smoking, and this prediction is testable in intervention

632

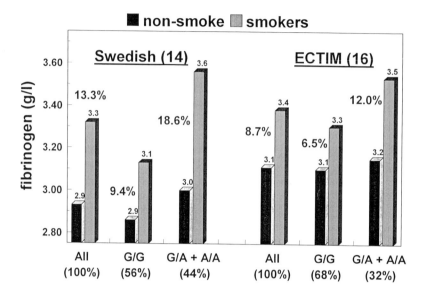

Fig. 2. Bar graph showing mean levels of fibrinogen in men with respect to different genotypes and smoking habits. Data from [14], combining young MI patients and matched controls from Stockholm, Sweden and data from the ECTIM case-control study [16] combining MI cases and controls. Data from cases and controls combined by calculation of the genotype-associated deviation from the sample mean for each group separately and pooling the estimate.

studies. The mechanism of this genotype effect is likely to be mediated through changes in transcription of the β-fibrinogen gene. The IL6-mediated effects on transcription of the gene act through binding of specific nuclear factors to DNA elements, and it may be that these mechanisms or interactions with adjacent elements and/or nuclear factors are disrupted by the sequence changes. If this is the case the precise molecular effects of these polymorphisms will be amenable to study in transfection experiments or in transgenic animal model systems. Once the mechanisms controlling changes in plasma risk factors in response to personal environmental changes are better understood, it may also be possible to develop directed therapeutic strategies that will reduce risk in a genotype-specific manner, an approach which is not possible at present.

Acknowledgements

This work was supported by grants from the British Heart Foundation (RG16 and 86–77).

References

1. Oliver MF. Lancet 1989;i:1241–1243.
2. Lowe GDO. Curr Opin Lipidol 1993;4:283–287.
3. Kishimoto T, Hibi M, Murakami M, Narazaki M, Saito M, Taga T. In: Bock GR, March J, Widdows K (eds) Polyfunctional Cytokines: IL6 and LIF. Chichester: John-Wiley & Sons 1992;5–23.
4. Meade TW, Mellows S, Brozovic M, Miller GJ, Chakrabarti RR, North WRS, Haines AP, Stirling Y, Imeson JD, Thompsom SG. Lancet 1986;ii:533–537.
5. Cook NS, Ubben D. TiPs 1990;11:444–451.
6. Thompson SG, Martin JC, Meade TW. Thromb Haemost 1987;58:1073–1077.
7. Hamsten A, Iselius L, de Faire U, Blomback M. Lancet 1987;ii:998–990.
8. Berg K, Kierulf P. Clin Genet 1989;36:229–235.

9. Reed T, Tracey RP, Fabsitz RR. Clin Genet 1994; (in press).
10. Roy SN, Mukhopadhyay G, Redman CM. J Biol Chem 1990;265:6389−6393.
11. Dalmon J, Laurent M, Courtios G. Mol Cell Biol 1993;13:1183−1193.
12. Thomas A, Kelleher C, Green F, Meade TW, Humphries SE. Thromb Haemost 1991;65:487−490.
13. Conner JM, Fowkes FGR, Wood J, Smith FB, Donnon PT, Lowe GDO. J Med Genet 1992;29:480−482.
14. Green F, Hamsten A, Blomback M, Humphries S. Thromb Haemost 1993;70:915−920.
15. Humphries S, Ye S, Talmud P. Arterioscler Thromb (in press).
16. Scarabin P-Y, Bara L, Ricard S, Poirer O, Cambou JP, Arveiler D, Luc G, Evans AE, Samama MM, Cambien F. Arterioscler Thromb 1993;13:886−891.
17. Fowkes FGR, Conner JM, Smith FB, Wood J, Donnan PT, Lowe GDO. Lancet 1992;339:693−696.
18. Lane A, Humphries SE, Green FR. Thromb Haemost 1993;69:962.
19. Meade TW, Imeson J, Stirling Y. Lancet 1987;ii:986−988.

634

Genetic variation in behavioral risk factors for atherosclerosis: twin-family study of smoking and cynical hostility

J. Kaprio, D.I. Boomsma[2], K. Heikkilä, M. Koskenvuo[3], K. Romanov, R.J. Rose[4], R.J. Viken[4] and T. Winter

[1]*Department of Public Health, P.O. Box 52, FIN-00014 University of Helsinki, Finland;* [2]*Free University, Amsterdam, The Netherlands;* [3]*University of Turku, Turku, Finland; and* [4]*Indiana University, Bloomington, Indiana, USA*

Abstract. Genetic and environmental components of two behavioral risk factors for atherosclerosis, smoking and cynical hostility, were assessed in a twin-family population from Finland. Questionnaire assessment of smoking and MMPI Cook-Medley cynical hostility were obtained from twins aged 16 and their parents, with data on all four family members in 1,228 families. Decomposition of the phenotypic correlation between smoking and hostility, by bivariate twin analysis, found effects of idiosyncratic and common environments in both adolescent sisters and brothers, with additive genetic effects differing across gender. Twin-family analyses indicated a major role of common environmental factors shared by offspring for both variables, but little role for cultural transmission.

Etiological factors for atherosclerosis operate at many different levels such as genetic factors, cellular, organ-specific or societal. At the personal level, behavioral risk factors such as smoking and hostility have been associated with the risk for atherosclerosis and its clinical manifestations. Smokers are more prone to atherosclerosis than nonsmokers and also have an increased risk of CAD, but the mechanisms by which components of cigarette smoke increase the risk of atherosclerosis and CAD are not fully understood [1]. Risk of carotid atherosclerosis in monozygotic twins who smoke is greater than in their nonsmoking cotwins [2]. Data on families and twins show that various aspects of smoking behavior aggregate in families [3] and may have a genetic component.

Epidemiological studies during the last 20 years suggest that individual differences in personality characteristics reflecting various aspects of coronary-prone behavior are related to future risk of cardiovascular illness. This Type A coronary-prone behavior pattern (TABP) was defined by Rosenman and Friedman in 1974. However, subsequent studies support the hypothesis that the hostility/cynicism dimension is the major component of TABP. The Minnesota Multiphasic Personality Inventory (MMPI) Cook-Medley Hostility (Ho) scale is a useful questionnaire-based instrument to measure hostility/anger and shows a stronger effect in relation to coronary atherosclerosis assessed by arteriography than TABP categorization. These findings have been strengthened by results from several prospective studies (see the review by Dembroski and Williams [4]). Although not all prospective studies have found this association, these negative findings may be due to methodological limitations, such as the invalidity of hostility scores resulting from subject selection procedures and the instability of such scores in younger populations. The mechanisms which could explain the deleterious effect of hostility are not clear. It has been suggested that hostile persons respond to some events with more pronounced increases in blood pressure and neuroendocrine levels than do nonhostile persons. Repeated frequently, this phenomenon may have a role in the development and expression on cardiovascular disease. Stronger pathophysiological responses among hostile individuals than in less hostile persons may arise in response to interpersonal challenge or conflict. When assessing various mechanisms for the association of hostility and coronary heart disease, behavioral aspects should be considered. Recently, it has been reported that hostility may contribute to health problems through its influence on other coronary risk factors [5,6].

Genetic determinants of hostility have been analyzed in several studies of twins, and most of them reported that individual differences in Cook-Medley Ho scores have a heritable component [7–9]. Different results may be due to small and selected samples of twins and also due to different measures of hostility. We assessed genetic and environmental components of smoking and cynical hostility in twin-families in Finland.

Materials and Methods

Twin pairs born between 1958 and 1986 have been identified from the Central Population Register of Finland [10]. For twins born in 1974 or after, the number of twins identified from the CPR is practically identical to the number of twins born annually according to birth statistics compiled by the Central Statistical Office of Finland. In February 1991, a health and lifestyle survey of 16-year-old twins was initiated after a pilot study had been carried out to test the questionnaire and mailing procedures. Questionnaires were mailed to twins born in 1975, 1976 and 1977 within 2 months of their 16th birthday. The data reported in these analyses is thus based on 3 years of responses. During this period, 1858 families of twins were contacted. In 1684 families at least one family member replied (91%), while the response rate among individuals was 85% for all boys and 91% for all girls. The parents were also asked to reply separately to a questionnaire on their own health and lifestyle; the response rates for mothers was 85% and 79% for fathers. Among the 1661 families with both twins and both parents alive and with a valid address, all family members replied in 1228 families (74%).

Twin zygosity was determined by the validated questionnaire method, which uses a set of decision rules supplemented by discriminant analysis, to classify the twin pairs as monozygotic (MZ), dizygotic (DZ) or undetermined zygosity [11]. Additional information on zygosity was derived from the family questionnaire filled out by the parents. Uncertainty about zygosity after these procedures remained for 3% of pairs, and these pairs were excluded from these analyses. Sample size in analyses varies, depending on which family members have been included and on the presence of missing data for the dependent variables.

Measures

Three questions were used to assess cigarette smoking status among the adolescents, while adult cigarette smoking was probed using six questions. Because the adolescents' smoking habits are still in their formative stages, the current analyses are based on a dichotomous trait for the presence or absence of some smoking exposure. We defined smokers as those adolescents who had smoked a total of more than 50 cigarettes, whether or not they currently smoked; 32% of sons and 29% of daughters were classified as smokers. For adults (mother and fathers), we applied a similar measure: smokers were defined as those who had smoked more than 100–200 cigarettes – nearly all had been or were regular, daily smokers as adults. Of fathers 71% fulfilled this criterion compared to 46% of mothers, which proportions reflect historical trends in smoking among men and women in Finland. Hostility was assessed using a 17-item cynical hostility subscale of the Cook-Medley Ho scale [9]. The mean score was 10.69 (SD 4.52) for fathers, 10.13 (4.48) for mothers, 11.65 (4.23) for sons and 11.51 (3.98) for daughters.

Statistical methods

To estimate genetic and environmental components of variance, a structural equations model [12] approach using the LISREL [13] program was used. The analysis of twin data alone permits the estimation of three parameters: an additive genetic (a) component, unique environmental (e) components and either effects due to dominance (d) or common (c) environmental components [12]. Familial similarity was estimated by computing polychoric correlations, while parameter estimation was done by using the weighted least squares approach.

A bivariate twin analysis was performed to examine whether the genetic and environmental effects on smoking are correlated with the genetic and environmental effects on hostility. The analysis explores to what extent the observed covariance between smoking and hostility can be accounted for by a correlation between additive genetic effects (r_a), a correlation between common environmental effects (r_c), and a correlation between the unique environmental effects on smoking and hostility (r_e) (p. 269 [12]). Models were fitted separately for male and female twins; opposite-sex twins were excluded from these analyses.

With the inclusion of parental data, other parameters can be estimated from twin-family data. We used a model of phenotypic assortment (p. 334 [12]) to estimate, in addition to a, c and e, the correlation between parental phenotypes (μ), cultural transmission (z), and the correlation (s) between additive genetic and shared environmental effects induced by parental transmission of both genetic and environmental factors to their offspring. The expected correlations under the full phenotypic assortment model are for MZ twins: a^2+c^2+2asc, for DZ twins: $\frac{1}{2}a^2[1 + (a + sc)^2\mu] + c^2 + 2asc$, for spouses ($\mu$), and finally, for mother–offspring and father–offspring: $[\frac{1}{2}a(a + sc) + cz](1 + \mu)$. Chi-square ($\chi^2$) goodness-of-fit statistics were used to assess how well each model fit the data [12].

Results and Discussion

Parent–offspring and spousal correlations for hostility and smoking ranged from 0.11 to 0.42 (Table 1), with the parent–offspring correlations lower than spousal or twin correlations (Table 2). The correlation in the offspring between hostility and smoking was 0.25 with no sex difference. The twin correlations for hostility showed a different pattern from the correlations for smoking in both girls and boys.

The bivariate twin analysis model fitted well in boys ($\chi^2 = 0.87$, df = 4, p = 0.93), yielding estimates that 49% of phenotypic variance in hostility was due to additive genetic effects, 5% to shared environmental effects, and 46% to unique environmental effects.

Table 1. Familial correlations [and standard errors] for hostility (above diagonal) and smoking (below diagonal). Numbers in curved parentheses indicate the number of parent–offspring and spouse pairs

Correlation	Father	Mother	Sons	Daughters
Father	–	0.28 [0.029] (1226)	0.11 [0.047] (1209)	0.12 [0.047] (1314)
Mother	0.42 [0.018] (1317)	–	0.17 [0.043] (1319)	0.16 [0.040] (1473)
Sons	0.22 [0.029] (1290)	0.10 [0.27] (1410)	–	–
Daughters	0.24 [0.28] (1391)	0.30 [0.026] (1537)	–	–

Table 2. Pairwise polychoric correlations (and standard errors) for hostility and smoking among 16-year-old twin pairs

Zygosity and sex	Hostility	Smoking	Pairs
Male MZ	0.54 (0.050)	0.93 (0.032)	176
Male DZ	0.27 (0.058)	0.84 (0.046)	224
Female MZ	0.51 (0.036)	0.93 (0.025)	281
Female DZ	0.40 (0.044)	0.78 (0.056)	225
Opposite-sex	0.26 (0.042)	0.46 (0.063)	513

Corresponding effects for smoking were 17% (additive genes), 75% (shared environment) and 8% (unique environment) respectively. There was no correlation between genetic effects, while the correlation between shared environmental effects was 1.0 (at boundary) and 0.25 for unique environmental effects. The corresponding bivariate twin analysis model for girls also fitted well ($\chi^2 = 2.29$, df = 4, p = 0.68), yielding estimates that 25% of phenotypic variance in hostility was due to additive genetic effects, 26% to shared environmental effects, and 49% to unique environmental effects. Corresponding effects for smoking were 30% (additive genes), 63% (shared environment) and 7% (unique environment) respectively. The correlation between genetic effects was 0.37, between shared environmental effects 0.40, and 0.04 for unique environmental effects.

For each trait, the twin-family data were fitted to the full phenotypic assortment model. In none of the models was the cultural transmission parameter significantly different from zero, and reduced models with this parameter fixed at zero fitted the data well. A similar result was found in analyses of smoking initiation in Dutch twin-families [13]. Compared to the bivariate twin analysis, the family models yielded smaller estimates of additive genetic effects and higher estimates of common environment for hostility, while for smoking the two analyses yielded quite similar results. Spousal correlations were higher for smoking than for hostility. Our results confirm that individual differences in hostility have a heritable basis, while the genetic component in smoking initiation appears to be of lesser importance than common environmental effects shared by children in a family.

Acknowledgements

Support by N.I.H. grant No. AA-08315, Academy of Finland.

References

1. Diana JN. Adv Med Exp Biol 1990;273:1–7.
2. Haapanen A, Koskenvuo M, Kaprio J, Kesaniemi YA, Heikkilä K. Circulation 1989; 80: 10–16.
3. Heath AC, Madden PAF. In: Turner JR, Cardon LR, Hewitt JK (eds) Behavior Genetic Applications in Behavioral Medicine Research, New York: Plenum Publ Corp, 1994 (in press).
4. Dembroski TM, Williams RB. In: Scheiderman N, Weiss SM, Kaufman PG (eds) Handbook of Research Methods in Cardiovascular Behavioral Medicine, New York: Plenum Press, 1989:553–569.
5. Scherwitz LW, Perkins LL, Chesney MA et al. Am J Epidemiol 1992; 136:136–145.
6. Siegler IC, Peterson BL, Barefoot JC, Williams RB. Am J Epidemiol 1992;136:146–154.
7. Rose RJ. J Pers Soc Psychol 1988;55:302–311.
8. Smith TW, McGonigle M, Turner CW, Ford MH, Slattery ML. Psychosom Med 1991;53:684–692.
9. Carmelli D, Swan GE, Rosenman RH. J Soc Behav Pers 1990;5:107–116.
10. Kaprio J, Koskenvuo M, Rose RJ. Acta Genet Med Gemellol (Roma) 1990;39:427–439.
11. Sarna S, Kaprio J, Sistonen P, Koskenvuo M. Hum Hered 1978;28:241–254.
12. Neale MC, Cardon LR. Methodology for Genetic Studies of Twins and Families. Dordrecht: Kluwer Academic Publishers, 1992.
13. Boomsma DI, Koopmans JR, Vandoornen LJP, Orlebeke JF. Addiction 1994;89:219–226.

Alternative genetic strategies for predicting risk of atherosclerosis

Charles F. Sing[1], Martha B. Haviland[1], Alan R. Templeton[2] and Sharon L. Reilly[1]

[1]Department of Human Genetics, University of Michigan Medical School, Ann Arbor, MI 48109-0618; and
[2]Department of Biology, Washington University, St. Louis, MO 63130, USA

Abstract. Twenty years of genetic studies have identified a huge number of genes involved in determining susceptibility to CAD. Establishing which DNA sequences in these genes are responsible for functional effects is proving to be a very difficult task. We propose an iterative cladistic strategy for increasing (or decreasing) the probability that a particular DNA sequence variation has a functional effect. We also propose a non-parametric strategy for modeling the statistical relationships between genome type variation, variation in the agents that are involved in the etiology of disease, and disease phenotypes. This strategy recognizes that there are many biological models that are responsible for the prevalent cases of disease.

The medical problem

Atherosclerosis is a common disease. In the United States nearly 600,000 died from atherosclerosis of the major coronaries of the heart in 1990 [1]. There are more than 6 million alive today in the USA with symptoms of coronary artery disease (CAD) and 1,500,000 are expected to have a myocardial infarct in 1994 [1]. In particular populations, as many as 50% of nuclear families have one or both parents with clinically defined CAD.

CAD is a complex multifactorial disease. None of the signs or symptoms segregate in families as a Mendelian trait. Neither genes nor environments cause disease, i.e., a study of a particular genetic (or environmental) agent cannot hope to reveal the cause of the prevalent cases of disease. Also, full knowledge about an individual's genetic make-up (i.e., genome type) will not be adequate to explain the onset, progression, or severity of disease. Each case is the consequence of interactions between a particular combination of genetic and environmental agents, and interindividual variation in risk of disease is a consequence of interactions between many genome types and many environmental experiences [2].

Most genetic studies have not taken into account the biological complexity of the etiology of CAD. Applications of single-locus Mendelian models ignore the role of interactions with other genes and environments, and do not take into account the fact that interaction effects are translated through quantitative variation of intermediate biological and physiological agents that link discrete genome-type variations and variation in risk of disease. Very few genetic and environmental agents will have independent effects on the determination of susceptibility to disease. The dependency of the effects of a gene on the associated genetic and environmental contexts results in a particular allelic variation being associated with many intermediate phenotypic values and a particular intermediate phenotypic value being associated with variations in many genetic loci. This paper is meant to present a more realistic biological model for CAD, enumerate the genetic strategies that are being used to study the genetic causes of CAD, and suggest alternative research strategies that recognize inherent etiological complexities.

Address for correspondence: Dr Charles F. Sing, Department of Human Genetics, The University of Michigan Medical School, Medical Science II M4708, Ann Arbor, MI 48109-0618, USA.

Modeling coronary artery disease

Figure 1 gives a model, which follows from the results of clinical, epidemiological, and genetic studies, for the relationship between the initial genomic information present at birth and the development of CAD. The biology of coronary-artery health shares properties expected of a complex adaptive system [3].

First, many agents are involved. Second, agents are organized into a hierarchy; the genome in the basement and clinical endpoints at the top floors are connected by intermediate agents involved in the biochemistry and physiology of the whole organism. Third, agents act in a coherent fashion within and between levels of the hierarchy. There are strong forces acting between agents of the same subsystem, e.g., lipid metabolism, and weak forces acting between agents in different subsystems, e.g., lipid metabolism and blood-pressure regulation. Partial decomposability of the etiology of CAD makes possible the distribution of research projects to separate laboratories that specialize in particular subsystems. Fourth, clinical phenotypes are emergent properties of the complex adaptive response of the molecular, biochemical, and physiological hierarchy to environmental inputs indexed by age and ecological position. For example, age of onset of disease is an emergent property not predicted with certainty from knowledge about an individual's genome type. Fifth, the relationship between the initial genetic conditions coded in the genome type and environmental factors is dynamic in time and space. The levels of an individual's intermediate agents and the coherency between them are altered epigenetically by changing influences of genetic and environmental agents throughout the life cycle. Variation in risk of disease is explained in part by interindividual variation in epigenetic patterns [4]. Because not all agents, nor all possible relationships between a particular subset of genetic and environmental agents, can come into play in each individual we expect that different biological explanations (models) will be needed to explain CAD in different individuals.

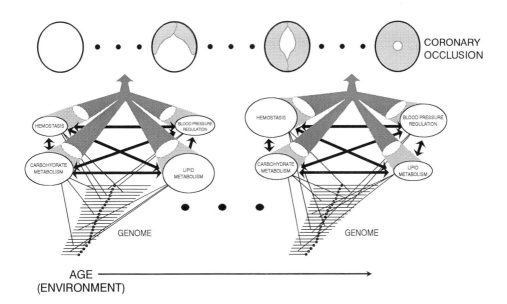

Fig. 1. Modeling coronary artery disease.

Cardinal genetic questions

There are three fundamental questions being asked by geneticists about the genetic architecture of CAD.
(1) How many CAD susceptibility genes are there, and where are they located?
(2) What are the DNA-sequence variations in each susceptibility gene that are responsible for functional effects?
(3) What are the mathematical and biophysical relationships between genome variation, variation in intermediate biochemical and physiological agents, and variation in risk of disease?

With regard to question 1, as many as 200 genes are candidates. The locations of most are known. With regard to question 2, little is known about functional DNA changes in genes which have been implicated in CAD susceptibility. Question 3 involves identifying which subset of genotypes and environments interact to determine disease in which subgroup of patients. The object is to estimate how many biological models, rather than which biological model, are responsible for the prevalent cases of CAD. We address questions 2 and 3 below.

Traditional strategies for addressing genetic questions

Question 2: We previously reviewed the top-down and bottom-up strategies for studying CAD [5–7]. The biometrical top-down approach estimates the genetic component of trait variation but cannot be used to address questions about location of functional DNA sequence variations [8]. The molecular top-down approach involves selecting individuals at the tails of the trait distribution with the ultimate aim of comparing their DNA sequences to determine sequence differences that may be responsible for the extreme phenotypes. This strategy has been used to identify rare mutations with large effects, e.g., Goldstein and Brown [9], but has contributed little to our understanding of the genetic architecture of CAD in the population at large. This strategy gives no information about the penetrance function associated with a particular genome type because the biological complexity of CAD dictates that the probability that a particular genome type will occur in those with a particular phenotype is not equal to the probability that the same phenotype will occur in everyone with that genome type, i.e., $Pr(G|P) \neq Pr(P|G)$.

The bottom-up molecular strategy involves measuring genetic variation and studying its association with phenotypic variation in samples representative of the population at large. Results from single-locus genotype–phenotype studies have been largely inconclusive. Inconsistent findings may be a consequence of unrepresentative sampling, small sample sizes or different coherency, i.e., linkage disequilibria, relationships between marker loci and functional DNA sequence variations in different populations. Although single-locus association studies have confirmed the role of particular candidate genes as being involved in determining susceptibility to CAD, inferences about which DNA sequence variations in these genes are responsible for functional effects are limited [10].

Question 3: Linear regression and linear logistic regression statistical methods have been used to study the biological relationships between variation in risk of disease, variation in risk factor traits, and genotype variation. Although much progress has been made in identifying those intermediate biochemical and physiological agents that are associated with variation in risk of disease, few studies have incorporated genetic predictors. Parametric, linear, statistical methods can give only limited insight into the kind of relationships (many agents organized into a coherent hierarchy, dynamic in time and space) implied by the biological model given in Fig. 1. Furthermore, such an approach is appropriate for asking, which biological model? not the more relevant question, how many biological models are responsible for variation in risk of CAD?

Alternative genetic strategies

Question 2: One of the greatest challenges facing geneticists is to identify the functional DNA-sequence variations that contribute to variation in intermediate risk-factor traits and risk of CAD. Two steps are involved. The first step is to identify DNA-sequence variations in the gene of interest. The second step is to estimate the probability that each particular sequence variation, or combination of sequence variations, is functional. Single-site genotype–phenotype association studies cannot sort out which sites are functional because the variations detected are not independent, they will be in linkage disequilibrium (coherency at the genome level). Thus any statistically significant association may be due to other DNA-sequence variations in linkage disequilibrium with the one under study.

We have proposed an iterative extension (Haviland et al., in preparation) of the cladistic analysis [11–14] to increase or decrease the a priori subjective probability [15] that a particular DNA-sequence variation is functional. This strategy is designed to estimate small marginal effects of DNA-sequence variations. It is illustrated in Fig. 2. In the first iteration the single site difference, A<->a, is associated with a significant phenotypic difference. The second iteration increases the probability that A<->a is the functional change as the F<->f and G<->g changes are not associated with phenotypic differences.

FIRST ITERATION

- Identify DNA sequence variations (A/a, B/b, C/c, D/d, E/e)
- Determine haplotypes
- Estimate cladogram
- Carry out nested phenotype analysis

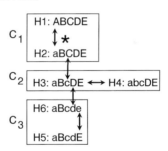

SECOND ITERATION

- Identify *further* DNA sequence variations (F/f, G/g)
- Determine haplotypes
- Estimate *higher resolution* cladogram
- Carry out *higher resolution* nested phenotype analysis

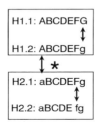

NEXT ITERATIONS

Fig. 2. Iterative cladistic approach.

Results from the application of this strategy can never lead to a probability of one (a particular sequence variation is definitely functional) or a probability of zero (it is definitely not functional). There will always remain the possibility that the genotype–phenotype association is due to an unmeasured functional sequence in disequilibrium with the DNA sequence under study. Also, there will always be the possibility that the size of the effect of the DNA sequence of interest is smaller than can be detected using the available sample size. The goal of the iterative cladistic strategy is to bring the subjective probability of functionality of a particular DNA sequence closer and closer to one, or zero, with each iteration.

Question 3: We have proposed a nonparametric statistical strategy for selecting combinations of genotypes, intermediate risk-factor traits, and environmental agents that are associated with particular subsets of individuals with a disease phenotype [16]. The goal is to estimate how many statistical models are necessary to predict the prevalent cases. We assume that each statistical model reflects a different biological model for CAD. Figure 3 presents an application of this strategy to predicting CAD in fathers using three agents — total cholesterol tertiles, body mass index (BMI) tertiles, and apolipoprotein apoE genotypes — measured on their asymptomatic adult children (Reilly et al., in preparation).

When these agents are considered separately (first three connecting lines, Fig. 3), the odds of having a father with CAD is double for those in the upper tertile of the cholesterol distribution or the BMI distribution, or for those with the ε_{43} genotype. Of the nine statistical models represented by combinations of cholesterol and BMI (4th connecting line, Fig. 3), only the high-cholesterol plus high-BMI model exceeds the odds ratio of 2. When the three common apo genotypes are considered with cholesterol tertiles

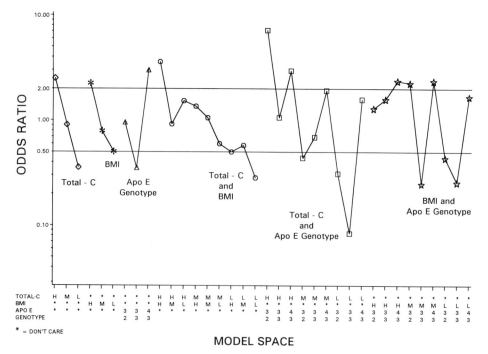

Fig. 3. An illustration of the relationship between different combinations of intermediate risk-factor traits and genotypes and father's history of CAD.

(fifth connecting line), two of the possible nine models gave an increased odds ratio: high cholesterol with either the ε_{32} or the ε_{43} genotypes. Three models with odds ratios greater than 2 were identified when the common apoE genotypes were considered with BMI tertiles. In every case involving the combination of two agents, information about risk is not just the summation of information from each agent considered separately. Extension of this strategy to higher dimensions is straightforward, with the obvious potential for revealing the role of genome-type variation in nonlinear relationships in the hierarchy of many agents involved in CAD (Fig. 1).

Summary

We advocate a model for CAD that considers the development of disease phenotypes as a consequence of the cumulative perturbations of a complex adaptive system. In Kellert's words, when speaking about complexity of causation in meteorology [17], "It is likely that the slight breeze created by a butterfly or the heat of a candle (a polygene effect) will be diluted among the myriad others that affect the environment (development of the organism or control of homeostasis) at every instant". Even if we are in possession of information about the laws of genetics, the initial conditions set forth in each individual's genome type, the particles and constants of biochemistry and physiology, and the exposures to all external environments, we still will not understand the way in which symmetries of these processes have been disguised by the hierarchy of random symmetry breaking (movement of chromosomes at meiosis and mitosis, developmental epigenetic decisions etc.) that occurs during the history of the individual (or the pedigree or the population). Our understanding of etiology will remain seriously incomplete because chance (ignorance?) enters as a powerful force in predicting outcomes. Age of onset, rate of progression and degree of severity of CAD can be defined only as a probability function of the levels and relationships between all agents in the pathways of causation connecting genome type with outcome. These probability statements for the individual must be based on large samples of observations and hence cannot be more than an approximate representation for any particular individual. Until we understand the nature of the universe, complete certainty about etiology and about future CAD events will be beyond our reach [18]. In the meantime, our research goal must be to determine which combinations of genetic and environmental agents can be used to reduce uncertainty about when, and in whom, CAD will emerge.

References

1. American Heart Association. 1994 Heart and Stroke Facts Statistics. Dallas, Texas, 1993.
2. Zerba KE, Sing CF. Curr Opin Lipidol 1993;4:152–162.
3. Waldrop MM. Complexity: the Emerging Science at the Edge of Order and Chaos. New York: Simon & Schuster, 1992.
4. Strohman R. Biotechnology 1994;12:111–164.
5. Sing CF, Boerwinkle E, Moll PP. In: Chakraborty R, Szathmary JE (eds) Diseases of Complex Etiology in Small Populations: Ethnic Differences and Research Approaches. New York: Alan R. Liss, 1985;39–66.
6. Sing CF, Boerwinkle E, Moll PP, Templeton AR. In: Weir B, Eisen EJ, Goodman MM, Namkoong G (eds) Proceedings of the 2nd International Conference on Quantitative Genetics. Sunderland, MA: Sinauer, 1988;250–269.
7. Sing CF, Moll PP. Annu Rev Genet 1990;24:171–187.
8. Moll PP. Curr Opin Lipidol 1993;4:144–151.
9. Goldstein JL, Brown MS. In: Scriver CR, Beaudet AL, Sly WS, Valle D (eds) The Metabolic Basis of Inherited Diseases, 6th ed. New York: McGraw Hill, 1989.

644

10. Kessling AK, Ouellette S, Bouffard O, Chamberland A, Bétard C, Selinger E, Xhignesse M, Lussier-Cacan S, Davignon D. Am J Hum Genet 1992;50:92–106.
11. Templeton AR, Boerwinkle E, Sing CF. Genetics 1987;117:343–351.
12. Templeton AR, Sing CF, Kessling A, Humphries S. Genetics 1988;120:1145–1154.
13. Templeton AR, Crandall KA, Sing CF. Genetics 1992;132:619–633.
14. Templeton AR, Sing CF. Genetics 1993;134:659–669.
15. Murphy EA. A Companion to Medical Statistics. Baltimore: The Johns Hopkins University Press, 1985.
16. Congdon CB, Sing CF, Reilly SL. 13th International Joint Conference on Artificial Intelligence: AI and the Genome Workshop, 1993;107–117.
17. Kellert SH. In the Wake of Chaos: Unpredictable Order in Dynamical Systems. Chicago: University of Chicago Press, 1993.
18. Barrow JD. Theories of Everything: The Quest for Ultimate Explanation. New York: Oxford University Press, 1991.

Apolipoprotein E in remnant lipoprotein metabolism: role of cell-surface heparan sulfate proteoglycans in enhanced hepatic binding and uptake

Robert W. Mahley[1] and Zhong-Sheng Ji[2]

Gladstone Institute of Cardiovascular Disease, Cardiovascular Research Institute, Departments of [1]Pathology and [2]Medicine, University of California, San Francisco, CA 94141-9100, USA

Abstract. Apolipoprotein E (apoE) is a key ligand responsible for the clearance of chylomicron remnants from the plasma by the liver. The initial rapid clearance of remnant lipoproteins from the plasma by the liver may involve sequestration within the space of Disse, where apoE secreted by the hepatocytes may accumulate and interact with the remnants, enhancing their binding and uptake. The enhanced binding of the apoE-enriched remnants appears to be mediated by heparan sulfate proteoglycans (HSPG), which are abundant in the space of Disse. Uptake by hepatocytes may be mediated, at least in part, by the low density lipoprotein (LDL) receptor and by the LDL receptor-related protein (LRP). The HSPG appear to initiate remnant binding and facilitate remnant interaction with the LRP. Subsequently, the LRP may mediate internalization. It remains to be determined whether the remnants are transferred to the LRP from the HSPG or whether the HSPG and LRP form a complex which is internalized.

Several steps may be involved in the uptake and degradation of remnant lipoproteins by the liver [1,2]. The first step appears to be *sequestration* of the remnants within the space of Disse, where apolipoprotein E (apoE) secreted by hepatocytes accumulates and is available to interact with the remnants (Fig. 1). The apoE-enriched remnants appear to bind to heparan sulfate proteoglycans (HSPG), which are abundant in the space of Disse. A second step may involve further *processing* of these lipoproteins by lipases in the space of Disse. Hepatic lipase [3—5] and lipoprotein lipase [6,7] have been implicated in remnant metabolism. Finally, the low density lipoprotein (LDL) receptor [8] and the LDL receptor-related protein (LRP) [9—13] appear to mediate the *uptake* of remnants by hepatocytes. Our recent studies suggest that HSPG may form a complex with the LRP and that this complex may play an important role in the internalization of the remnants [14—17].

Secretion–capture role for apoE in remnant metabolism involves cell-surface HSPG

Previous studies established that apoE-enriched remnant lipoproteins display enhanced binding to and uptake by a variety of cells [18,19]. In these studies, exogenous apoE was added to the remnants (β-VLDL) from cholesterol-fed rabbits.

Our most recent studies showed that apoE secreted locally from the rat hepatoma cell line McA-RH7777 enhanced the binding and uptake of β-VLDL. McA-RH7777 cells were stably transfected with normal human apoE3 or receptor-binding-defective apoE-Leiden [15]. The amount of human apoE secreted from the transfected hepatocytes after a 2-h incubation was 10 times greater than that of the endogenous rat apoE. Rabbit β-VLDL

Address for correspondence: Robert W. Mahley, MD, PhD, Gladstone Institute of Cardiovascular Disease, P.O. Box 419100, San Francisco, CA 94141-9100, USA. Tel.: +1-415-826-7500. Fax: +1-415-285-5632.

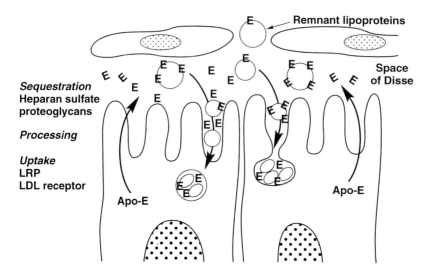

Fig. 1. Hepatocyte secretion of apoE into the space of Disse results in the formation of apoE-enriched remnants which are targeted for uptake.

added to the apoE3-transfected cells displayed enhanced binding and uptake, while much less uptake occurred in the apoE-Leiden-transfected and nontransfected cells. Compared with the apoE-Leiden-transfected and nontransfected cells, the apoE3-secreting cells had a 2- to 3.5-fold enhancement of cell-associated β-VLDL. Furthermore, electron microscopy revealed an abundance of β-VLDL and chylomicron remnants on the cell surfaces and microvilli of apoE3-secreting cells, but not on those of nontransfected or apoE-Leiden-secreting cells. Additionally, chylomicron remnants were observed in abundance within intracellular vesicles and multivesicular bodies of the apoE3-transfected cells.

Heparinase treatment of the cells (3 units/ml) completely abolished the increased association of β-VLDL to apoE3-transfected cells but did not affect the limited association of β-VLDL with apoE-Leiden-transfected and nontransfected cells. These results suggest a secretion–capture role for apoE and indicate an important role for HSPG in remnant lipoprotein metabolism [15].

Role of HSPG in the binding and uptake of apoE-enriched remnant lipoproteins in cultured cells

Detailed studies explored the involvement of HSPG in remnant binding and internalization [14]. Heparinase treatment of LDL receptor-negative familial hypercholesterolemic fibroblasts and human hepatoma cells (HepG2) released 30—40% of newly synthesized cell-surface ^{35}S-labeled proteoglycans. Further, heparinase treatment caused a more than 80% decrease in the binding of β-VLDL + apoE to familial hypercholesterolemic and normal fibroblasts and HepG2 cells. In addition, heparinase caused a significant decrease in the uptake of fluorescently labeled β-VLDL + apoE by HepG2 cells and a 75% decrease in cholesteryl ester synthesis in familial hypercholesterolemic fibroblasts. Heparinase did not affect the binding of β-VLDL (without added apoE) or LDL to these cells or the binding of β-VLDL + apoE to the LRP or to the LDL receptor on ligand blots.

Chinese hamster ovary mutant cells lacking the ability to synthesize either heparan

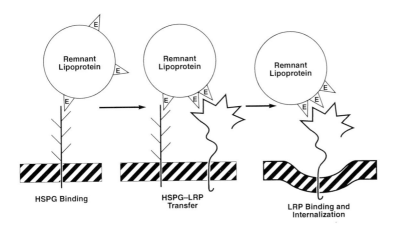

Fig. 2. A theoretical model suggesting how binding by the HSPG and internalization by the LRP may be coupled. The mechanism whereby remnants interact with HSPG and the LRP and are taken up by cells may involve transfer of the remnant to the LRP or inclusion of the HSPG and the LRP in a complex that is internalized with the remnant. Modified from [15] with permission.

sulfate (*pgs*D-677) or all proteoglycans (*pgs*A-745) did not display enhanced binding of β-VLDL + apoE [14]. These findings support a role for cell-surface HSPG in the initial rapid hepatic clearance of remnants from the plasma. The abundance of both HSPG [20] and apoE [21] in the space of Disse may provide the environment necessary for remnant sequestration.

A theoretical model (Fig. 2) depicts the initial binding of apoE-enriched remnant lipoproteins to HSPG, and the subsequent formation of an HSPG–LRP complex [14,15]. The remnants may then be transferred to the LRP for internalization. Alternatively, the HSPG–LRP complex itself may function in the internalization of these lipoproteins. Studies are in progress to distinguish between these possibilities and to extend the observations in vivo.

Variable HSPG binding of apoE variants modulates the expression of type III hyperlipoproteinemia

Studies were undertaken to determine whether variable interactions of mutant forms of apoE with HSPG might account wholly or in part for recessive versus dominant type III hyperlipoproteinemia and whether these interactions might contribute to the impaired uptake of the remnant lipoproteins [16]. The β-VLDL + apoE2 [apoE(Arg$_{158}$→Cys), which is associated with recessive type III hyperlipoproteinemia] bound less avidly than β-VLDL + apoE3 but still displayed significantly enhanced binding (~2- to 2.5-fold compared to β-VLDL without added apoE) to HepG2 and McA-RH7777 cells. In comparison, β-VLDL + apoE(Arg$_{142}$→Cys), β-VLDL + apoE(Arg$_{145}$→Cys), and β-VLDL + apoE-Leiden, all of which are associated with dominant type III hyperlipoproteinemia, bound even less avidly. This hierarchy was confirmed for both binding and uptake by [^{14}C]oleate incorporation into cholesteryl esters in LDL receptor-negative cells (Fig. 3) and by binding of ^{125}I-β-VLDL + apoE3 or + variant apoE forms secreted from McA-RH7777 cells (Fig. 4). Furthermore, enhanced binding of apoE-enriched β-VLDL was almost totally inhibited by heparinase treatment of the cells, and basal binding that remained after heparinase

648

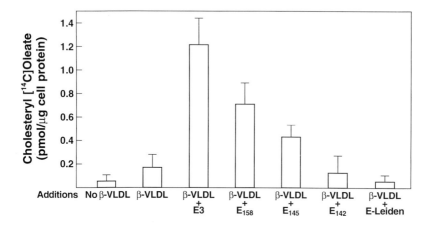

Fig. 3. Cholesteryl ester synthesis stimulated by β-VLDL and various forms of apoE in LDL receptor-negative fibroblasts. The cells were incubated for 3 h at 37°C with β-VLDL (10 mg of protein/ml) or β-VLDL plus various forms of apoE (10 mg of protein/ml + 15 mg of apoE/ml). Then a [^{14}C]oleate–BSA complex was added to the culture medium and the incubation was continued for an additional 2 h. After incubation the cells were washed on ice, the lipids were extracted, and the [^{14}C]cholesteryl oleate was quantitated. Mean ± S.D. was obtained from four separate experiments. Reproduced with permission from [16].

treatment (10–20% of the total binding) was inhibited after addition of an LDL-receptor antibody (Fig. 4). The β-VLDL enriched in the various forms of apoE or apoE/dimyristoylphosphatidylcholine complexes bound to HSPG isolated from McA-RH7777 cells or to the rat liver HSPG on dot blots and to the LRP on ligand blots with a very similar hierarchy, as displayed by the cellular binding and uptake.

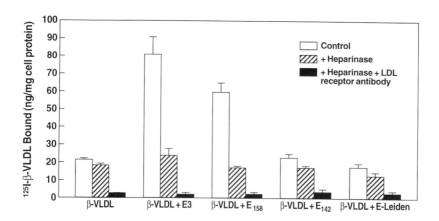

Fig. 4. Effect of heparinase treatment and anti-LDL receptor antibody on binding of [^{125}I]-β-VLDL and [^{125}I]-β-VLDL plus various forms of apoE to nontransfected McA-RH7777 cells. The nontransfected McA-RH7777 cells were treated with 5 units/ml of heparinase at 37°C for 2 h, placed on ice, and washed 3 times with cold Dulbecco's modified Eagle's medium-HEPES. The cells were then incubated with 50 mg/ml of rabbit anti-LDL receptor IgG at 4°C for 1 h. The [^{125}I]-β-VLDL (2 mg of protein/ml) and [^{125}I]-β-VLDL plus various forms of apoE (2 mg of protein/ml + 3 mg of apoE/ml) were added to the incubation medium and the cells were incubated for an additional 1.5 h. Mean ± S.D. is reported from a single experiment repeated in triplicate. Reproduced with permission from [16].

Thus, all of the type III hyperlipoproteinemic apoE variants display defects in enhanced binding to HSPG and in cellular uptake initiated by HSPG. However, the apoE2 variant associated with the recessive form of the disease (apoE(Arg$_{158}$→Cys)) displayed more binding and uptake than variants associated with the dominant form of the disease. The hierarchy of binding and uptake was as follows: apoE3 > apoE2 (apoE(Arg$_{158}$→Cys)) > apoE(Arg$_{145}$→Cys) > apoE(Arg$_{142}$→Cys) ≈ apoE-Leiden (the latter two usually displaying very little, if any, enhanced binding and uptake) [16].

Hepatic lipase-enhanced binding and uptake of remnant lipoproteins

Rat hepatoma cells (McA-RH7777) transfected with a human hepatic lipase (HL) cDNA synthesized and secreted 50–80 ng of human HL/mg of cell protein in 4 h, ~50% of which was bound to cell-surface HSPG [3]. When rabbit β-VLDL and canine chylomicrons or chylomicron remnants were incubated with these HL-secreting cells, remnant binding and uptake were enhanced 3-fold compared to nontransfected cells. Our studies showed that this HL-enhanced binding was mediated by cell-surface HSPG. Heparinase treatment to remove cell-surface HSPG or chlorate treatment to prevent HSPG sulfation of the HL-secreting cells abolished all of the HL-mediated enhanced binding and uptake. Thus, enhanced binding of remnant lipoproteins can be mediated by HL through its interaction with cell-surface HSPG [3]. As binding was not enhanced in the absence of HSPG, an initial HL–HSPG interaction appears essential.

Intravenous heparinase inhibits lipoprotein remnant clearance from the plasma and uptake by the liver in mice

Heparinase (30 units) was infused intravenously into mice to hydrolyze the liver HSPG and to determine the effect of HSPG hydrolysis on remnant clearance by the liver [22]. Intravenous heparinase decreased the amount of ^{35}S-labeled liver HSPG by ~20–40% within 10–15 min. Furthermore, heparinase infusion significantly inhibited the clearance of chylomicrons, chylomicron remnants, chylomicron remnants + apoE, rabbit β-VLDL, and β-VLDL + apoE 1.5- to 2-fold and decreased liver uptake 1.3- to 1.6-fold. Confocal fluorescence microscopy of liver from mice injected with fluorescently labeled β-VLDL + apoE revealed markedly less intense fluorescence from hepatocytes in heparinase-treated animals than from those in saline-treated control animals. Heparinase infusion did not inhibit the clearance of mouse LDL, a ligand for the LDL receptor, and did not affect the clearance of α$_2$-macroglobulin, a ligand for the LRP. These results extend in vitro studies and suggest an important role of the liver HSPG in remnant clearance in vivo [22].

Acknowledgements

This work was supported by National Institutes of Health Program Project Grant HL41633.

References

1. Mahley RW. Science 1988;240:622–630.
2. Mahley RW, Hussain MM. Curr Opin Lipidol 1991;2:170–176.
3. Ji Z-S, Lauer SJ, Fazio S, Bensadoun A, Taylor JM, Mahley RW. J Biol Chem 1994;269:13429–13436.
4. Shafi S, Brady SE, Bensadoun A, Havel RJ. J Lipid Res 1994;35:709–720.
5. Diard P, Malewiak M-I, Lagrange D, Griglio S. Biochem J 1994;299:889–894.
6. Beisiegel U, Weber W, Bengtsson-Olivecrona G. Proc Natl Acad Sci USA 1991;88:8342–8346.

650

7. Chappell DA, Fry GL, Waknitz MA, Muhonen LE, Pladet MW, Iverius P-H, Strickland DK. J Biol Chem 1993;268:14168—14175.
8. Choi SY, Fong LG, Kirven MJ, Cooper AD. J Clin Invest 1991;88:1173—1181.
9. Herz J, Kowal RC, Ho YK, Brown MS, Goldstein JL. J Biol Chem 1990;265:21355—21362.
10. Beisiegel U, Weber W, Ihrke G, Herz J, Stanley KK. Nature 1989;341:162—164.
11. Hussain MM, Maxfield FR, Más-Oliva J, Tabas I, Ji Z-S, Innerarity TL, Mahley RW. J Biol Chem 1991;266:13936—13940.
12. Willnow TE, Sheng Z, Ishibashi S, Herz J. Science 1994;264:1471—1474.
13. Herz J. Curr Opin Lipidol 1993;4:107—113.
14. Ji Z-S, Brecht WJ, Miranda RD, Hussain MM, Innerarity TL, Mahley RW. J Biol Chem 1993;268:10160—10167.
15. Ji Z-S, Fazio S, Lee Y-L, Mahley RW. J Biol Chem 1994;269:2764—2772.
16. Ji Z-S, Fazio S, Mahley RW. J Biol Chem 1994;269:13421—13428.
17. Mahley RW, Ji Z-S, Brecht WJ, Miranda RD, He D. Ann NY Acad Sci 1994;737:39—52.
18. Kowal RC, Herz J, Goldstein JL, Esser V, Brown MS. Proc Natl Acad Sci USA 1989;86:5810—5814.
19. Kowal RC, Herz J, Weisgraber KH, Mahley RW, Brown MS, Goldstein JL. J Biol Chem 1990;265:10771—10779.
20. Stow JL, Kjéllen L, Unger E, Höök M, Farquhar MG. J Cell Biol 1985;100:975—980.
21. Hamilton RL, Wong JS, Guo LSS, Krisans S, Havel RJ. J Lipid Res 1990;31:1589—1603.
22. Ji Z-S, Brecht WJ, Miranda RD, He D, Mahley RW. Circulation 1994;(in press) (abstract).

Atherosclerosis X.
F.P. Woodford, J. Davignon and A. Sniderman, editors.

651

Identification and computer modeling of the functional domains of human apolipoprotein E3

Maryvonne Rosseneu[1], Martine De Pauw[1], Berlinda Vanloo[1], Alexander Dergunov[2], Karl Weisgraber[3] and Robert Brasseur[4]

[1]Department of Clinical Chemistry, A.Z. St-Jan, B-8000 Brugge, Belgium; [2]Institute Preventive Medicine, Moscow, Russia; [3]Gladstone Institute of Cardiovascular Disease, UCSF, San Francisco, CA 94140, USA; and [4]Université Libre Bruxelles, Bruxelles, Belgium

Abstract. Functional domains of apolipoprotein E (apoE) were identified by comparing the properties of two thrombolytic fragments (residues 1−191 and 216−299). Maximal lipid binding and activation of lecithin:cholesterol acyl transferase (LCAT) were observed for the C-terminal fragment of apoE. A new theoretical approach for the calculation of protein folding was applied to the prediction of the structure of the receptor-binding domain of apoE and of the complementary ligand-binding domain of the apoB/E receptor. Ionic interactions can take place between negatively charged residues of the apoB/E receptor repeats and positively charged residues of the apoE142−159 segment. Optimal interactions are predicted to involve GLU-X-SER-ASP-GLU residues, the LDL receptor C-terminal repeats 4 and 5, and residues ARG142 and LYS146 of apoE. Naturally occurring mutations of the receptor and ligand confirm the involvement of these residues.

Apolipoprotein E (apoE) plays an important role in cholesterol metabolism, as a high-affinity ligand for the cellular apoB/E receptor [1]. Like apoA-I and apoA-IV, apoE is able to activate the enzyme lecithin:cholesterol acyl transferase (LCAT).

In order to define the location of the lipid-binding and LCAT-activating domains in apoE3, we compared the behavior of its two major thrombolytic fragments: a 22-kDa (residues 1−191) and a 10-kDa fragment (residues 216−299) [2]. The X-ray crystallographic structure of the 22-kDa fragment shows that it consists of a bundle of four antiparallel helices [3], while three 22-residue helical repeats were predicted to occur in the C-terminal fragment [4].

Naturally occurring mutations of apoE, especially ARG145-CYS, ARG158-CYS and LYS146-GLU, LYS146-GLN substitutions, strongly impair the interaction of apoE with the cellular apoB/E receptor, thus leading to type III dyslipoproteinemia [5]. These observations were confirmed by site-directed mutagenesis of apoE, demonstrating the involvement of apoE residues 140−160 in ligand–receptor interaction.

We carried out a theoretical analysis of the mode of interaction of the repeats of the ligand-binding domain of the LDL receptor [6,7] with the receptor-binding domain of apoE by computer modeling. We could predict the mode of folding of the ligand-binding domain of the apoB/E receptor, its optimal interaction with apoE and the involvement of specific apoE residues. The results are in agreement with naturally occurring mutations in both receptor and ligand.

Experimental procedures

The composition, physicochemical properties and LCAT activation of the complexes prepared with human apoE3, its thrombolytic fragments [2,3] and dipalmitoylphosphatidyl-choline (DPPC) were investigated as described previously [8].

Computational methodology

In the new computational approach applied here, the total energy of the system is considered as the sum of the torsional energies along all axes of the system, plus the van der Waals energy, electrostatic energy and the solvation energy. The classical hydrophobic energy is replaced by the solvation energy between protein atoms and between these atoms and the solvent, which is calculated according to a new semi-empirical equation [9].

The initial secondary structure of the protein, used for the angular molecular dynamics step, is built from the local energy minima calculated for each amino acid during the transition from an ideal α-helix to a β-sheet. The native-like protein structure is finally selected as the structure with the minimal total energy obtained through an angular molecular dynamics process. In this process the length of the atomic bonds and the value of the atomic angles are kept constant [9].

Results

Lipid-binding and LCAT-activating domains of apoE

The composition and size of the complexes generated between apoE, its fragments and DPPC are summarized in Table 1, together with the secondary structure and Trp fluorescence emission of the free and lipid-associated proteins. Electron micrographs demonstrate the discoidal shape of the complexes, and ATR infrared measurements with polarized light indicate that the phospholipid hydrocarbon chains of the complexes are oriented parallel to the apolipoprotein helices surrounding the edge of the discoidal complexes.

The kinetics of the LCAT reaction show the highest percentages of esterification for the PLPC/cholesterol/10-kDa fragment complexes. A reciprocal plot of the initial maximal velocity as a function of the inverse of the cholesterol concentration (Fig. 1) shows that V_{max} (4.9 nmol cholesteryl esters/h) and K_m (3.3 μM) are higher for the complexes generated with the 10-kDa fragment than for those with apoE3 (1.2 nmol/h and 2.6 μM). The substrate efficiency, expressed as V_{max}/K_m, is consequently highest for this fragment. For the 22-kDa fragment, the reaction rate was too low for an accurate determination of the kinetic parameters.

Computer modeling and mode of interaction of apoE with the apoB/E receptor

The N-terminal ligand-binding domain of the apoB/E receptor consists of eight 26-residue homologous repeats between residues 13 and 343 [6,7]. Both a theoretical analysis of the repeat sequences [6] and site-directed mutagenesis experiments [7] suggest that in each repeat, the cluster of C-terminal residues GLU-X-SER-ASP-GLU is involved in ionic

Table 1. Composition and physicochemical properties of the complexes generated between apoE, its fragments and DPPC

Complex	Isolated complex phospholipid/protein (molar ratio)	Diameter GGE/EM (Å)	% helix[a] native protein/complex	λ Trp fluorescence native protein/complex (nm)
DPPC/apoE3	152:1	116/138	46/59	343/337
DPPC/22-kDa	61:1	119/143	56/48	342/341
DPPC/10-kDA	36:1	110–116/167	51/54	341/333

GGE = gradient gel electrophoresis; EM = electron microscopy; [a]determined by circular dichroism.

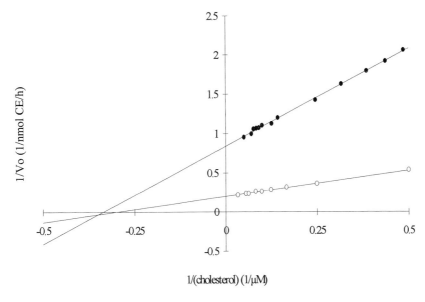

Fig. 1. Lineweaver-Burk plots for the LCAT reaction with PLPC/cholesterol/apolipoprotein complexes: (–●–), PLPC/cholesterol/apoE3; (–O–), PLPC/cholesterol/10-kDa fragment.

interactions. This is further confirmed by the receptor defects observed in patients with familial hypercholesterolemia due to substitutions at these residues [10].

We therefore calculated the mode of folding and the most stable structure for pairs of repeats of the apoB/E receptor. Figure 2 shows an example of the lowest energy structure calculated for repeats 4 (residues 134—159) and 5 (residues 183—208), as these seem most crucial for the interaction with apoB and E [10]. According to the results of the protein folding, each of these repeats consists of two loops, as the proline residues 141 and 150 in repeat 4 and Pro199 in repeat 5 induce β-turns. The clusters of negatively charged

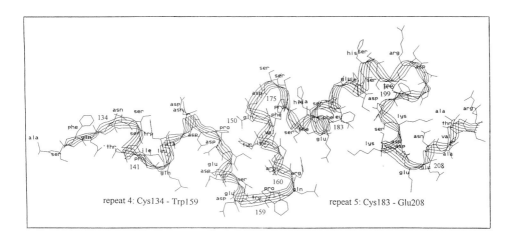

Fig. 2. Skeleton and ribbon representation of the folding of the 130—216 domain of the apoB/E receptor, consisting of repeat 4:C134—W159 and repeat 5:C183—E208 separated by 25 residues.

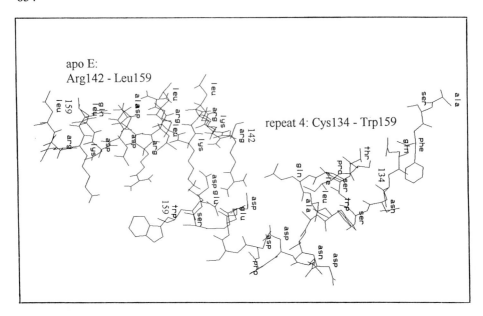

Fig. 3. Skeleton representation of the assembly of apoE142–159 segment with repeat 4 (A130–W159) of the apoB/E receptor.

residues described above are oriented towards the outer face of each repeat and are therefore easily accessible for interactions with the apoE or apoB ligands.

The apoE segment 142–159 was subsequently assembled with the modeled domains of the apoB/E receptor. The predicted conformation of this apoE segment is helical, as confirmed by X-ray crystallography [3]. The minimal energy structure for the receptor–ligand complex between the apoE segment and repeat 4 involves interactions between positively charged R142 and K146 residues of apoE with negatively charged D149, D151, E153, D154, D157, and E158 of the apoB/E receptor (Fig. 3). The distances between positively and negatively charged residues are within 8 Å.

When these calculations are repeated with the naturally occurring mutants of apoE, LYS146-GLU or LYS146-GLN, no stable interactions were observed between receptor and ligand, in agreement with the decreased receptor-binding affinity observed in vivo [5].

Conclusion

Major functional domains of apoE include the lipid-binding and LCAT-activating domains which are located within the 80 C-terminal residues of apoE3, while the receptor-binding domain lies in the N-terminal domain, at residues 142–160. Computer modeling and assembly of the ligand-binding repeats of the apoB/E receptor and of the apoE ligand suggest that ARG142 and LYS146 are critical for an optimal association between apoE and the receptor. This can account for the effect of naturally occurring mutations of apoE leading to dominant type III dyslipoproteinemia.

References

1. Mahley RW, Innerarity TL. Biochim Biophys Acta 1983;737:197–222.
2. Innerarity TL, Friedlander EJ, Rall SC Jr, Weisgraber KH, Mahley RW. J Biol Chem 1983;258:12341–12347.

3. Wilson C, Wardell MR, Weisgraber KH, Mahley RW, Agard DA. Science 1991;252:1817–1822.
4. Brasseur R, Lins L, Vanloo B, Ruysschaert JM, Rosseneu M. Proteins: Structure, Function and Genetics 1992;13:246–257.
5. Talmud P. In: Rosseneu M (ed) Structure and Function of Apolipoproteins. Boca Raton: CRC Press, 1992;123–158.
6. De Loof H, Rosseneu M, Brasseur R, Ruysschaert JM. Proc Natl Acad Sci USA 1986;83:2295–2299.
7. Esser V, Limbird LE, Brown MS, Goldstein JL, Russell DW. J Biol Chem 1988;263:13282–13290.
8. De Pauw M, Vanloo B, Weisgraber K, Rosseneu M. Biochemistry (in press).
9. Brasseur R. In: Cahiers IMABIO 8. Paris: CNRS, 1994;73–76.
10. Hobbs HH, Brown MS, Goldstein JL. Human Mutation 1992;1:445–466.

Effect of expression of apoE mutants in transgenic mice

Louis M. Havekes[1], Bart J.M. van Vlijmen[1], Janine H. van Ree[1], Rune R. Frants[2] and Marten H. Hofker[2]

[1]TNO-PG, Gaubius Laboratory, P.O. Box 430, 2300 AK Leiden; and [2]Department of Human Genetics, Leiden University, P.O. Box 9503, 2300 RA Leiden, The Netherlands

Chylomicron- and VLDL-remnants are atherogenic, nutrition-related lipoproteins. In many different animals and in humans the level of these lipoproteins in the plasma is elevated after excessive calorie and saturated fat intake. It is commonly assumed that in Western societies the high risk of atherosclerosis is mainly due to the presence in plasma of these atherogenic lipoproteins, as in these populations most of the people are in a postprandial state during most of their life span.

Under normal conditions these remnant lipoproteins are cleared from the plasma very efficiently by means of lipoprotein receptors, mainly in the liver. For recognition of these remnants by the receptor, their major protein constituent apolipoprotein E (apoE) plays an important role as ligand. Hence, a defect in apoE as ligand will result in an impaired remnant clearance and, consequently, in an elevated risk for atherosclerosis.

ApoE is a genetically determined polymorphic protein with three commonly occurring isoforms, E2, E3 and E4. E3 and E4 are normally active as ligand for binding to the receptor, whereas E2 is defective in this respect. Patients with familial dysbeta-lipoproteinemia (FD) display strongly elevated plasma levels of chylomicron- and VLDL-remnants concomitantly with strongly increased risk for coronary and peripheral athero-sclerosis. For most FD patients the underlying metabolic defect is a disturbed clearance of the remnant lipoproteins because of E2E2 homozygosity. However, we also found FD patients with heterozygosity for rare apoE variants, like E2(lys146→gln) and apoE3-Leiden. Both for E2E2 homozygous and for heterozygous E3-Leiden FD patients the clinical expression of the disease is highly influenced by age, nutrition and hormonal status (sex and thyroid hormones, insulin).

To understand the factors that influence the metabolism of remnant lipoproteins better, we decided to study the remnant metabolism in transgenic mice carrying the human APOE*3-Leiden gene that codes for a binding-defective apoE and in mutated mice in which the endogenous *Apoe* gene has been disrupted. The use of these mice strains allows us to study the remnant metabolism under highly standardized conditions against a homogeneous genetic and environmental background.

Human APOE*3-Leiden transgenic mice

Because the apoE3-Leiden protein behaves like a dominant trait in the expression of FD in humans, we introduced this dominant APOE*3-Leiden allele in mice by conventional transgenesis, expecting that the presence of endogenous mouse apoE would be overruled by the apoE3-Leiden protein. We generated APOE*3-Leiden transgenic mice by injecting in oocytes a 27-kb DNA construct encompassing both the APOE and the APOC1 gene. Three lines of transgenic mice have been established, #195, #2 and #181. By using Northern blot analyses, we found that these lines exhibited different levels of expression of the transgene, #195 being the lowest and #181 the highest expressor.

All three lines were fed a standard mouse diet (chow), or semisynthetic diets containing sucrose as described by Paigen et al. [1]. Three different types of semisynthetic diets were used: a basic low fat/cholesterol diet (LFC) and a high fat/cholesterol diet (HFC) consisting of the basic diet supplemented with 15% of fat and 1% of cholesterol with either low (0.1%) or high (0.5%) amounts of cholate. The results presented in Table 1 show that all three transgenic mouse lines (#195, #2 and #181) display elevated plasma cholesterol levels, as compared to controls. This increase is positively correlated with the basal plasma level of human apoE3-Leiden (195 << 2 < 181; see Table 1). In addition, plasma cholesterol levels increased with increasing levels of cholate added to the diet (HFC 0.5% > HFC 0.1% > LFC).

In lines #2 and #181 the plasma level of triglyceride was elevated after feeding diet LFC (carbohydrate induction), but this increase was limited upon cholesterol feeding. In control mice and in line #195 the triglyceride levels were lower than values obtained after chow diet, especially at higher amounts of added cholesterol and cholate.

The increase in plasma cholesterol upon cholesterol feeding occurred mainly in the VLDL/LDL-sized fraction both for the control mice and the transgenic lines (not shown). The VLDL/LDL-sized fractions after cholesterol feeding represent cholesterol-rich/triglyceride-poor lipoproteins that resemble the highly atherogenic remnant lipoproteins normally found in patients with severe FD. These observations made us wonder whether these transgenic mice develop atherosclerosis, either without or with cholesterol feeding.

Atherosclerosis in transgenic human APOE*3-Leiden mice

All three transgenic lines and control mice were investigated for atherosclerotic lesions after receiving control diet (chow) or one of the different diets described above (Table 2).

After ingesting a cholesterol-rich diet for 14 weeks, the high expressors (#2 and #181) had developed atherosclerotic lesions. On the contrary, in control mice and in the low expressor (#195) mice atherosclerotic lesions could not be found after cholesterol feeding. The development of atherosclerosis was surprisingly reproducible per diet and per transgenic line (#2 or #181). Semiquantitative evaluation of the atherosclerotic lesions in the aortic arch revealed that the atherogenesis is positively correlated with the amount of cholesterol and cholate in the diet. In addition, line #181 (the highest apoE3-Leiden expressor) appeared to be more sensitive to atherosclerosis than line #2.

The atherosclerotic lesions varied from fatty streaks to atherosclerotic plaques and were localized in the aortic arch, the carotid and myocardial arteries. The fatty streaks were characterized by deposition of foam cells in the intima. The atherosclerotic plaques consisted of foam cells, mononuclear leukocytes and connective tissue in the intima. More severe plaques contained cholesterol crystals and sometimes showed a necrotic calcified center. The latter lesions often extended into the media.

The effect of age and gender on plasma lipid levels in APOE*3-Leiden transgenic mice

At young ages, transgenic mice APOE*3-Leiden #2 display an age-dependent hyperlipidemia, the male mice more pronounced than the females. At a later age (after about 50 days) the plasma lipid levels start to decline to levels slightly higher than in control mice. When fed a high fat/cholesterol diet containing 15% of fat and 0.25% of cholesterol (HFC) the plasma lipid levels increase strongly immediately after weaning, leveling off at about 40 days of age. Thereafter, the cholesterol and triglyceride levels start to

Table 1. Serum lipid and lipoprotein concentrations after 6 weeks of dietary treatment

Mouse line	Chow [TC] mmol/l	Chow [TG] mmol/l	Chow [apoE] mg/dl	LFC [TC] mmol/l	LFC [TG] mmol/l	LFC [apoE] mg/dl	HFC 0.1 % [TC] mmol/l	HFC 0.1 % [TG] mmol/l	HFC 0.1 % [apoE] mg/dl	HFC 0.5 % [TC] mmol/l	HFC 0.5 % [TG] mmol/l	HFC 0.5 % [apoE] mg/dl
#2	3.2 ± 0.7[a]	2.7 ± 0.7[a]	36 ± 18	6.4 ± 0.4[a,b]	5.4 ± 1.1[a,b]	54 ± 13	26.2 ± 1.5[a,b]	3.3 ± 0.4[a]	107 ± 42[b]	39.9 ± 9.0[a,b]	1.6 ± 0.1[a]	68 ± 14[b]
#181	4.8 ± 1.3[a]	2.7 ± 1.0[a]	91 ± 28	13.3 ± 1.9[a,b]	29.4 ± 9.4[a,b]	147 ± 9[b]	43.7 ± 13.2[a,b]	10.5 ± 3.7[a,b]	300 ± 78[b]	59.1 ± 9.8[a,b]	4.5 ± 2.3[a,b]	189 ± 71[b]
#195	2.5 ± 0.4	0.7 ± 0.2	3 ± 1	3.1 ± 1.0	0.5 ± 0.3	4 ± 1[b]	4.1 ± 0.7[a,b]	0.3 ± 0.2	2 ± 1	8.1 ± 1.7[a,b]	0.3 ± 0.4[a,b]	2 ± 1
Control	2.1 ± 0.3	0.5 ± 0.3	–	2.9 ± 0.2[b]	0.6 ± 0.2	–	2.8 ± 0.5[b]	0.1 ± 0.1[b]	-	5.7 ± 1.6[b]	0.1 ± 0.1[b]	–

LFC, low fat/cholesterol diet; HFC, high fat/cholesterol diet 0.1% or 0.5% cholate. TC = total cholesterol (free + esterified); TG = triglyceride; apoE = ApoE3-Leiden. Total cholesterol, triglyceride and ApoE3-Leiden values are the mean serum levels ± SD of five mice per group. [a] $p < 0.05$, indicating the difference between transgenic and nontransgenic groups of mice on the same diet, using nonparametric Mann-Whitney tests; [b] $p < 0.05$, indicating the difference between semisynthetic diet and regular chow within each line, using non-parametric Mann-Whitney.

Table 2. Atherosclerotic lesions in ApoE*3-Leiden transgenic mice on different diets

Mouse line	Chow	LFC	HFC 0.1%	HFC 0.5%
Control	−	−	−	−
#195	−	−	−	−
#2	−	±	+	++
#181	−	−	++	+++

Semiquantitative analysis of atherosclerosis in groups of transgenic and nontransgenic mice was performed after 14 weeks of diet feeding. Each group contained at least three mice. − and + means absence and presence of atherosclerotic lesions.

decrease, in male transgenics more rapidly than in females. The plasma level of apoE3-Leiden protein parallels the cholesterol levels.

We found that the hepatic level of APOE*3-Leiden mRNA was not influenced by gender nor by feeding HFC diet, which implies that the observed age- and gender-related changes in lipid levels are not due to variation in the expression of the transgene. The production of VLDL was determined by measuring triglyceride levels at certain time intervals after Triton WR1339 injection. No differences were found between transgenics and nontransgenics in VLDL production when matched for age. However, young mice displayed a 1.5-fold higher rate of VLDL production than older mice. This strongly suggests that in APOE*3-Leiden transgenic mice a higher VLDL production leads to higher plasma lipid levels, because of a defect in the apoE-mediated plasma clearance of remnants (bottleneck).

Chylomicron-remnant removal was measured by the vitamin A/fat loading test (area under the curve). For both transgenic and control mice, young mice showed a 5-fold lower removal capacity of chylomicron remnants than older mice. In addition, the presence of the APOE*3-Leiden transgene resulted in halving remnant removal as compared to control mice, both at young and older age. Thus, the greater hyperlipidemia in young than in older APOE*3-Leiden mice is due to a combination of increased VLDL production and a more severely impaired plasma clearance of remnants.

The difference between males and females was further investigated by injecting these animals with either estrogen or testosterone. As shown in Fig. 1, injecting male transgenic mice with estrogen leads to a significant increase in plasma triglyceride, while injecting with testosterone leads to a significant decrease in cholesterol. In females the plasma cholesterol and triglyceride increase slightly upon injection of estrogen. Administration of testosterone to females leads to a clearly significant lowering of both plasma lipids. These results sustain the hypothesis that the higher plasma lipid levels in females than in males are due to a different balance between sex hormones. Analyses of the lipoprotein profiles of these animals treated with sex hormones showed that estrogen increases cholesterol and triglyceride levels in the VLDL/LDL-sized lipoprotein fraction, partly because of a shift of these lipids from the HDL to the VLDL/LDL-sized fraction.

Apoe knock-out mice

As Table 3 shows, homozygous *Apoe* knock-out mice are clearly hypercholesterolemic on regular mouse chow, whereas heterozygous *Apoe* knock-out mice do not show higher plasma cholesterol levels than control mice. On the severe atherogenic diet HFC 0.5%, the homozygous mutant mice develop an extreme hypercholesterolemia of about 100

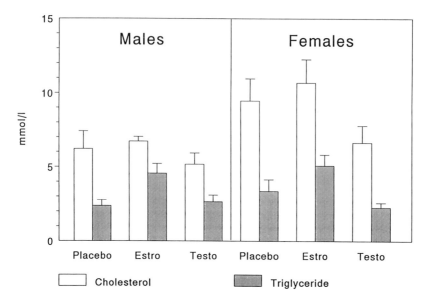

Fig. 1. Mice were injected subcutaneously with estrogen or testosterone twice, with a 2-week interval. After 4 weeks plasma samples were taken and analyzed for lipid levels. Each group of mice consists of 10 mice. Bars represent means ± SD.

mmol/l. Remarkably, heterozygotes also become hypercholesterolemic when compared to controls. This means that one functional *Apoe* allele is not enough to protect against diet-induced hypercholesterolemia. Another striking feature is that female heterozygous apoE-deficient mice are more sensitive to this atherogenic diet than male heterozygotes (Table 3).

As determined by FPLC-superose gel permeation chromatography, all elevations of plasma cholesterol in controls, heterozygous and homozygous *Apoe* knock-out mice upon cholesterol feeding were confined to the VLDL/LDL-sized fractions. The cholesterol-

Table 3. Serum cholesterol levels in apoE-deficient mice after 6 weeks of dietary treatment

Mouse	N		Diet	Serum cholesterol (mmol/l)		
	♂	♀		♂+♀	♂	♀
+/+	26	21	chow	3.1 ± 0.6	3.2 ± 0.5	2.9 ± 0.2
+/−	31	22	chow	2.7 ± 0.7^a	2.9 ± 0.7^c	2.5 ± 0.5^a
−/−	28	19	chow	$19.3 \pm 5.5^{a,b}$	$21.5 \pm 5.0^{a,b,c}$	$16.1 \pm 4.3^{a,b}$
+/+	6	3	HFC 0.5%	4.7 ± 0.8	4.9 ± 0.5	4.4 ± 1.2
+/−	21	11	HFC 0.5%	10.1 ± 4.5^a	$7.4 \pm 1.7^{a,c}$	15.0 ± 3.9^a
−/−	5	2	HFC 0.5%	$102.4 \pm 26.3^{a,b}$	$117.3 \pm 13.9^{a,b}$	65.3 ± 1.4^b

Serum cholesterol levels are given as mean ± SD. N = number of animals analyzed; +/+ = control mice; +/− = heterozygous apoE-deficient mice; −/− = homozygous apoE-deficient mice. [a]Significant difference (p < 0.05) compared with +/+ mice on the same diet using nonparametric Mann-Whitney test; [b]significant difference (p < 0.05) as compared with +/− mice on the same diet using nonparametric Mann-Whitney test; [c]significant difference (p < 0.05) between males and females on the same diet using nonparametric Mann-Whitney test.

rich/triglyceride-poor lipoproteins that accumulate resemble highly atherogenic remnants, as also found in APOE*3-Leiden transgenic mice. Therefore, we again studied whether these mice could develop atherosclerosis.

Homozygous apoE-deficient mice develop massive atherosclerosis, even on a chow diet. However, when heterozygous *Apoe* knock-out mice are fed the HFC 0.5% diet, they also develop atherosclerosis, while control mice do so to a much lesser extent. In addition, female heterozygous apoE-deficient mice are more severely affected than male heterozygotes, reflecting the serum cholesterol levels. Thus, not only does reduced expression of the *Apoe* gene lead to hypercholesterolemia, it also increases the risk of developing atherosclerosis.

Conclusions

Introduction of the APOE*3-Leiden gene into mice results in hyperlipidemia that is positively correlated to the level of expression of the transgene and with diet, age and gender. The elevated plasma lipid levels are mainly confined to the VLDL/LDL-sized lipoprotein fractions. These fractions resemble chylomicron- and VLDL-remnants because of the high cholesterol:triglyceride ratio. The APOE*3-Leiden transgenic mice are susceptible to the development of atherosclerotic lesions, depending on the level of the VLDL/LDL-sized lipoprotein fraction. With this APOE*3-Leiden animal model we are able to modulate the plasma cholesterol and atherosclerotic process in a standardized way. This allows us now to study the effect of subtle (dietary) components on both plasma cholesterol and atherogenesis.

As compared to the APOE*3-Leiden transgenic mice, the *Apoe* knock-out mice are much more severe in their phenotype. They respond extremely to atherogenic diets and develop severe atherosclerosis and atypical deposits of cholesterol in all kinds of tissues. Thus, for studying the effect of environmental factors on plasma cholesterol level and atherogenesis, *Apoe* knock-out mice are less suitable than APOE*3-Leiden mice.

Reference

1. Nishina PM, Verstuyft J, Paigen B. J Lipid Res 1990;31:859–869.

A lipoprotein containing only apoE is present in normal and HDL-deficient plasmas and releases cholesterol from cells

Gerd Assmann[1,2], Arnold von Eckardstein[1], Yadong Huang[2] and Shili Wu[2]

[1]*Institut für Klinische Chemie und Laboratoriumsmedizin, Zentrallaboratorium, Westfälische Wilhelms-Universität Münster, Albert-Schweitzer-Strasse 33, D-48149 Münster; and* [2]*Institut für Arterioskleroseforschung an der Universität Münster, Domagkstrasse 3, D-48149 Münster, Germany*

Abstract. Previous studies have identified a subclass of HDL containing only apolipoprotein A-I (apoA-I) and showing pre-β mobility upon electrophoresis, i.e., preβ_1-lipoprotein A-I (LpA-I), as being the initial acceptor of cell-derived cholesterol in human plasma. The absence of atherosclerosis in some patients with apoA-I deficiency stimulated the search for apoA-I-free Lps which are able to take up cellular cholesterol. Incubation of human plasma with ^{3}H-cholesterol-laden fibroblasts resulted in the identification of just such a lipoprotein. This particle contains apoE as its only apolipoprotein and exhibits γ mobility on electrophoresis. We have therefore called it γ-LpE. It is present in the plasma of normoalphalipoproteinemic subjects and in that of patients with apoA-I deficiency. It acts as the initial acceptor of cell-derived cholesterol which it then transfers to other lipoproteins. In addition, cell culture media from human hepatoma cells and human monocyte-derived macrophages, all of which produce apoE, released ^{3}H-cholesterol from fibroblasts into a γ-migrating lipoprotein. This was not observed for cell culture media of fibroblasts, which do not secrete apoE. In conclusion, our results strongly indicate the presence in normal and HDL-deficient human plasma of a lipoprotein containing only apoE which is a potent acceptor of cell-derived cholesterol. This may indicate a mechanism by which apoE-producing cells from the atherosclerotic plaque, i.e., macrophages, may deplete themselves of cholesterol. Moreover, since apoE2 and apoE4 do not form γ-LpE, the apoE polymorphism may affect the uptake of cell-derived cholesterol into plasma.

Background

Many epidemiological studies have demonstrated the inverse correlation between the concentration of HDL-cholesterol and the risk of myocardial infarction (reviewed in [1]). The antiatherogenicity of HDL is usually explained by its ability to remove excess cholesterol from nonhepatic cells and to transfer this cholesterol to the liver [2]. HDL, however, is heterogeneous and its various subfractions play different roles in reverse cholesterol transport. For example, two-dimensional electrophoresis by means of agarose gel electrophoresis followed by nondenaturing polyacrylamide gradient gel electrophoresis differentiates HDL subfractions by charge and size. After Western blotting of the separate proteins onto immobilizing membranes, HDL are immunodetected using anti-apoA-I antisera. In normal plasma this method discriminates three HDL-subclasses with pre-β mobility, preβ_1-LpA-I, preβ_2-LpA-I, and preβ_3-LpA-I, from the bulk of HDL with α-mobility, which itself can be differentiated into α-LpA-I$_3$ (Stokes diameter 7.2–8.8 nm) and α-LpA-I$_2$ (Stokes diameter 8.8–12 nm) on the basis of size [3,4].

Uptake and transfer of cell-derived cholesterol by apoA-I-containing HDL subfractions

Preβ_1-LpA-I account for less than 5% of HDL in normal plasma, are rich in phospholipids, contain only apoA-I and exhibit pre-β mobility upon agarose gel electrophoresis [5,6].

Using very short pulse-chase incubations of plasma with H-cholesterol-labeled fibroblasts, Castro and Fielding previously identified $preβ_1$-LpA-I as initial acceptors of cell-derived cholesterol into plasma [3]. From these particles, cell-derived cholesterol is transferred to low density lipoprotein (LDL) in the sequence $preβ_2$-LpA-I→$preβ_3$-LpA-I→$α$-LpA-I [7]. A minor portion of cholesterol is esterified in $preβ_3$-LpA-I which contains cholesterol ester transfer protein (CETP), lecithin:cholesterol acyltransferase (LCAT) and apoD [7,8]. The bulk of cholesterol is esterifed in $α$-LpA-I after re-transfer from LDL [7]. Cholesteryl esters are ultimately delivered to the liver, predominantly after transfer to LDL by CETP [2]. In this scheme, apoA-I is the central protein involved in the removal of cholesterol from nonhepatic cells. Deficiency or severe reduction of apoA-I ought therefore to result in HDL deficiency and increased coronary risk. Surprisingly, many of these patients were observed to be free from coronary heart disease at the age of 50 years [9]. Moreover, the family histories of these patients do not indicate an increased frequency of myocardial infarction. This paradox raises the question as to whether proteins other than apoA-I may also be important in the removal of cellular cholesterol. In fact, we have recently identified just such a protein [10].

Demonstration of $γ$-LpE

Skin fibroblasts were loaded with radiolabeled cholesterol and subsequently incubated with plasma. After 1 min of incubation plasma was removed and separated by agarose gel electrophoresis. A proportion of the radiolabel occurred as expected in association with preβ-HDL. An equal amount, however, was associated with proteins with $γ$ mobility. During chase incubation with unlabeled cells the radiolabel was transferred to $α$-HDL, as was the case with preβ-HDL-associated cholesterol. This lipoprotein was anti-apoE-immunoreactive. It was also detectable in plasmas of apoA-I- and LCAT-deficient patients as well as in normal and apoA-I-deficient mice [10,11]. It was absent, however, from the plasma of apoE-deficient mice [10]. On SDS gel electrophoresis, the isolated protein exhibited an apparent molecular weight of 68 or 34 kDa, depending on whether nonreducing or reducing conditions were used [10]. Thus, this lipoprotein appeared to contain apoE as its only lipoprotein. For this reason and because of its electrophoretic mobility, we termed it $γ$-LpE. It is rich in sphingomyelin, contains phosphatidylcholine and is poor in cholesterol. On electron microscopy $γ$-LpE is a homogeneous lipoprotein with a diameter of 12–15 nm. We also identified $γ$-LpE in cell culture media of hepatocytes. Furthermore, in contrast to $preβ_1$-LpA-I, $γ$-LpE is synthesized by macrophages [10]. Since these cells play a major role in atherosclerosis by storing cholesterol and being transformed into foam cells, $γ$-LpE may be very important in protecting against atherosclerosis. $γ$-LpE is not detectable in fibroblast-conditioned cell culture medium. Incubation of lipid-free apoE with fibroblasts, however, helps to generate a particle which has electrophoretic $γ$ mobility and which takes up cell-derived cholesterol. This suggests that lipid-free apoE associates with phospholipids of cell membranes to give rise to $γ$-LPE.

Relative roles of $γ$-LpE and $preβ_1$-LpA-I for the uptake of cellular cholesterol into plasma

After a 1-min incubation of radiolabeled fibroblasts with normal plasma, the amount of ^{3}H-cholesterol accumulating in $γ$-LpE equals that present in $preβ_1$-LpA-I. Incubation of fibroblasts with plasma from an apoA-I-deficient patient led to accumulation of ^{3}H-cholesterol in $γ$-LpE only. This was accompanied by a 55% decrease in the uptake of cellular unesterified ^{3}H-cholesterol after 1-min pulse incubation (submitted for publication). The same reduction in efflux of cellular cholesterol was observed in normal plasmas which had been depleted of apoA- by anti-apoA-I immunoaffinity chromatography [11]. This suggests that apoA-I-free lipoproteins, especially γ-LpE, make a considerable contribution to the uptake of cellular cholesterol into plasma. The importance of γ-LpE for the uptake of cell-derived cholesterol into plasma is also highlighted by the effects of apoE polymorphism on both the formation of γ-LpE and cholesterol efflux. We have found that γ-LpE is present only in plasmas of individuals who carry at least one apoE3 allele (submitted for publication). Plasmas containing apoE3 released ^{3}H-cholesterol from fibroblasts into both γ-LpE and preβ$_1$-LpA-I. Plasmas from homozygotes for apoE2 or apoE4 took up cell-derived ^{3}H-cholesterol into preβ$_1$-LpA-I only. Compared to apoE3-containing plasmas, the ability of samples from individuals homozygous for apoE2 or apoE4 to release cholesterol from cells was 35–40% lower. This shows that γ-LpE is responsible for most of the residual ability of apoA-I-deficient plasma to release cholesterol from cells. Moreover, these data suggest that genetic variation in apoE affects cholesterol efflux from cells.

Possible implications for atherosclerosis

Several studies have shown that apoE4 is associated with increased risk of myocardial infarction [12,13]. Our studies raise the question of whether this increase in risk might be causally linked to the failure of apoE4 to form γ-LpE and the impairment of cholesterol efflux in apoE4 homozygotes. At first sight, the observation that γ-LpE is also lacking in apoE2/2 individuals appears to rule out such a relationship. However, apoE2 binds poorly to apoE and apoB,E receptors. Therefore, macrophages in the arterial wall in apoE2/2 individuals take up less cholesterol via very low density lipoprotein (VLDL) and VLDL-remnants [14]. Consequently, despite impaired efflux of cellular cholesterol due to γ-LpE deficiency, cholesterol homeostasis may be balanced in cells of apoE2-homozygotes, as is the case in apoE3 homozygotes. By contrast, apoE4 does not interfere with cholesterol influx. Hence, decreased efflux of cholesterol may cause intracellular accumulation of cholesterol and increase atherosclerotic risk in apoE4 subjects.

Conclusion

Our findings indicate that the bulk of HDL is not required for effective release of cellular cholesterol into plasma. Rather, minor HDL subfractions such as preβ$_1$-LpA-I and γ-LpE which are present even in HDL-deficient plasmas are functionally important. Moreover, the failure of apoE4 to form γ-LpE may be pathogenically involved in the increased cardiovascular risk of individuals with apoE4.

Acknowledgements

This work is supported by grants to Dr Arnold von Eckardstein from Wissenschafts-minsterium Nordrhein-Westfalen (Bennigsen-Foerder-Preis) and Deutsche Forschungs-gemeinschaft (Ec116,3-1). We are grateful to Dr Paul Cullen for helpful discussion of the manuscript.

References

1. Gordon D, Rifkind BM. N Engl J Med 1989;321:1311–1315.
2. Barter P. Curr Opin Lipidol 1993;4:210–217.
3. Castro GR, Fielding CJ. Biochemistry 1988;27:25–29.

4. Asztalos BF, Sloop CH, Wong L, Roheim PS. Biochim Biophys Acta 1993;1169:291–300.
5. Fielding CJ, Fielding PE. Proc Natl Acad Sci USA 1980;77:3327–3331.
6. Kunitake ST, La Sala KI, Kane JP. J Lipid Res 1985;26:549–555.
7. Huang Y, von Eckardstein A, Assmann G. Arterioscler Thromb 1993;13:445–458.
8. Francone OL, Gurakar A, Fielding CJ. J Biol Chem 1989;264:7066–7072.
9. Assmann G, von Eckardstein A, Funke H. Circulation 1993;87(suppl III):28–34.
10. Huang Y, von Eckardstein A, Wu S, Maeda N, Assmann G. Proc Natl Acad Sci USA 1994;91:1834–1838.
11. Kawano M, Miida T, Fielding CJ, Fielding PE. Biochemistry 1993;32:5025–5028.
12. Davignon J, Gregg RE, Sing CF. Arteriosclerosis 1988;8:1–21.
13. Ordovas JM, Schaefer EJ. Cardiovasc Risk Factors 1994;4:103–107.
14. Mahley RW. Science 1988;240:622–630.

666

Transgenic rabbits that overexpress hepatic lipase have a marked reduction of plasma high density lipoproteins and intermediate density lipoproteins

Jianglin Fan[1], Robert W. Mahley[1,3] and John M. Taylor[1,2]
[1]Gladstone Institute of Cardiovascular Disease, Cardiovascular Research Institute, San Francisco; Departments of [2]Physiology, [3]Medicine and [3]Pathology, University of California, San Francisco, CA 94141, USA

Abstract. A human hepatic lipase (HL) cDNA in a liver-specific expression vector was used to generate transgenic rabbits, an animal that normally has low HL levels. Hepatic lipase activity in plasma was detected only upon administration of heparin, and it was measured at levels up to 80 times greater in transgenic rabbits than in nontransgenic littermates. Transgenic rabbits had 2- to 5-fold lower total plasma cholesterol levels, with substantially lower levels of high density lipoproteins (HDL) and intermediate density lipoproteins (IDL). These results demonstrate the importance of HL in the metabolism of lipoproteins and in plasma cholesterol homeostasis.

Hepatic lipase (HL) functions in the metabolism of chylomicrons, intermediate density lipoproteins (IDL), and high density lipoproteins (HDL) [1,2]. It is produced by hepatocytes and it binds primarily to hepatic cell-surface proteoglycans, exerting a hydrolytic effect upon triglyceride-rich lipoproteins [3]. Hepatic lipase has both triglyceride hydrolase and phospholipase activities, with a high affinity for HDL [1]. Administration of specific antibodies against HL in mammals indicated that it functions in the conversion of VLDL remnants (IDL) to LDL [4,5], in the metabolism of apolipoprotein (apo)B48-containing remnant lipoproteins [6], and in the conversion of the larger triglyceride-rich HDL_2 to the smaller, dense HDL_3 [7,8]. These findings are consistent with the phenotype of HL deficiency in human subjects, a disorder characterized by elevated total plasma triglycerides and cholesterol, an increase in the levels of triglyceride-rich LDL and large HDL [9], and premature atherosclerosis.

To define the precise physiological roles of HL, we expressed the human enzyme in the liver of the rabbit, an animal that normally has only about one-tenth as much HL activity as other mammals [10]. Our results demonstrate that HL is rate-limiting in both IDL and HDL metabolism, affecting the distribution and composition of these particles in plasma, with concomitant effects on plasma cholesterol levels. This is the first study of transgenic rabbits overexpressing an enzyme involved in lipid metabolism.

Constructs designed to express transgenes in only the liver were generated from sequences associated with the human apoE gene: 3 or 5 kb of 5'-flanking sequence, the first exon, the first intron, the first six nontranslated nucleotides of the second exon, a synthetic polylinker for cDNA insertion, the distal 92 noncoding nucleotides of the fourth exon, the proximal 114 nucleotides of 3'-flanking sequence, and the far downstream hepatic control region [11] of the apoE/C-I gene locus. A full-length human HL cDNA was kindly provided by Dr Hans Will (Universität Hamburg, Hamburg, Germany), and the translated portion was inserted into the polylinker.

Address for correspondence: John M. Taylor PhD, Gladstone Institute of Cardiovascular Disease, P.O. Box 419100, San Francisco, CA 94141-9100, USA. Tel.: +1-415-826-7500. Fax: +1-415-285-5632.

For the generation of transgenic rabbits, New Zealand White rabbits were super-ovulated by hormone administration, zygotes were collected from oviducts, and DNA was microinjected essentially as described [11]. Injected zygotes were implanted through the fimbrial end of the oviducts of a pseudopregnant foster mother. Founder (F0) pups were identified by screening genomic DNA, and transgenic founders were mated subsequently with nontransgenic rabbits to produce transgenic F1 progeny. Rabbits were maintained on a high-fiber rabbit chow that contained approximately 1.5% fat, 14% protein, and 25% crude fiber. The effects of transgene expression were similar in male and female rabbits, and the results from females are given here.

Results and Discussion

Six founder rabbits were generated that showed expression of human HL in postheparin plasma. Neither human HL nor rabbit HL was detectable in the preheparin plasma of transgenic rabbits, and rabbit HL was not detectable in nontransgenic rabbit plasma. These findings suggested that the human enzyme in transgenic rabbits is anchored normally to heparan sulfate proteoglycans [1]. Postheparin HL enzymatic activity was 7- to 81-fold higher in transgenic plasma than in control plasma, and partially purified HL from transgenic rabbit plasma had a mean specific activity of $23,000 \pm 8,000$ μeq fatty acids/mg protein/h (mean $\pm$ SD). The transgenic enzyme was similar in amount and specific activity to that in normal human postheparin plasma [12]. Western blot analysis showed that human HL produced by transgenic rabbits was the same size ($\sim$66 kDa) as found in human postheparin plasma. Analysis of total RNA from several different tissues of transgenic F1 progeny by an RNase protection assay showed that transgene expression was found only in the liver. Together, these results demonstrated that transgenic HL of normal specific activity was produced by the appropriate tissue site in the rabbit, a species that is normally deficient in this enzyme.

All transgenic rabbits had decreased levels of total plasma triglyceride and cholesterol, and one of the founder lines (rabbit line 5001) was selected for further study. Analysis of the progeny from this transgenic line (Fig. 1) showed triglycerides 44% lower and cholesterol 58% lower than nontransgenic littermates (Fig. 1). The reduced total cholesterol content of transgenic rabbit plasma was associated with about 5-fold lower HDL-cholesterol in the transgenic animals.

The distribution of transgenic rabbit lipoproteins was compared to that of nontransgenic littermates. Plasma lipoproteins were prepared by density gradient fractionation, resolved further by 1% agarose gel electrophoresis, then detected by staining for neutral lipids with Fat Red 7B (Fig. 2). The most dramatic result of HL overexpression in the transgenic rabbit was the overall reduction in HDL levels. Large HDL particles, including both HDL_2 ($d = 1.06-1.10$ g/ml) and HDL_1 (α-migrating, apoE-containing lipoproteins in the $d = 1.04-1.06$ g/ml fraction) were nearly absent from transgenic rabbit plasma. This reduction in HDL was reflected most notably by a corresponding decrease in antibody-detectable apoE and apoA-I levels in the α-migrating lipoproteins on the agarose gels (Fig. 2). These findings are consistent with the postulated role of HL in the metabolism of triglyceride-rich HDL_2. For example, a role for HL in HDL_2 metabolism is supported by the observation that HL-deficient humans accumulate large, triglyceride-rich HDL [13]. The lack of HL in these individuals appears to prevent the catabolic conversion of HDL_2 to HDL_3.

In the transgenic rabbit, overexpression of HL also resulted in a decrease in HDL_3 ($d = 1.10-1.21$ g/ml). The reduction in apoA-I levels and the lack of immunodetectable apoE in this fraction from transgenic animals relative to controls (Fig. 2) was consistent with

668

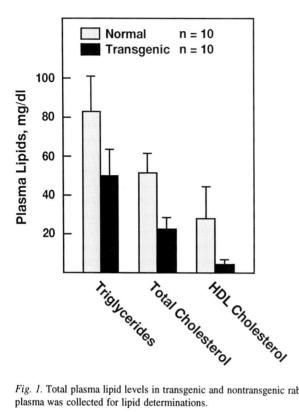

Fig. 1. Total plasma lipid levels in transgenic and nontransgenic rabbits. Rabbits were fasted overnight before plasma was collected for lipid determinations.

this finding. This reduction may be the result of the phospholipase activity of HL on the surface of cholesterol-rich HDL [14], leading to a decrease in the phospholipid content of the lipoprotein surface, thereby facilitating cholesterol efflux from HDL into liver cell

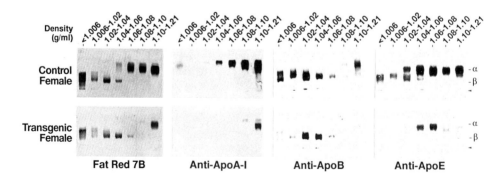

Fig. 2. Effect of human hepatic lipase expression on rabbit lipoproteins. Plasma lipoproteins from fasting nontransgenic (upper panels) and transgenic (lower panels) female rabbits were separated by sequential density ultracentrifugation using the density ranges shown above. An equal volume of each fraction was resolved by electrophoresis in a 1% agarose gel. Then lipoproteins were visualized using Fat Red 7B staining, and apolipoproteins were identified by immunoblotting with specific antibodies to rabbit proteins as described. The arrow denotes the origin; α and β indicate electrophoretic mobility.

membranes. Consistent with this possibility is the finding that humans with increased HL activity have an abnormally low HDL-cholesterol content [13]. This mechanism is supported further by studies of cultured hepatoma cells that were incubated with HL-treated HDL, which resulted in an enhanced uptake of free cholesterol from lipoproteins into the cells [14].

Our data suggest that a reduction in the content of typical IDL has occurred in the transgenic rabbit. For example, the amount of lipoprotein found in the $d = 1.006-1.02$ g/ml fraction is reduced, with most of the apoB-containing lipoproteins found in the $d = 1.02-1.06$ g/ml fractions (Fig. 2) — apoB100 was the only apolipoprotein detected in these fractions (data not shown). The apoB-containing lipoproteins in the $d = 1.02-1.06$ g/ml fractions do not contain significant amounts of apoE, which suggests that the particles are more like LDL than IDL. A modest increase in the quantity of apoB-containing particles was found in the $d = 1.04-1.06$ g/ml fraction, a density characteristic of LDL, and their size and composition was consistent with their identity as LDL (data not shown). These results are consistent with the finding that endogenous HL activity in humans is correlated inversely with LDL size and buoyancy, which is a reflection of IDL catabolism [15]. Thus, our results support a role for HL in the catabolism of IDL, but future studies will be required to determine if the mechanism involves a conversion to LDL or an enhanced clearance of IDL from plasma.

Our results provide the first description of a transgenic rabbit overexpressing an enzyme that regulates lipid metabolism. The analysis provides a consistent picture that implicates HL in the metabolism of HDL and IDL, with concomitant effects on plasma cholesterol and triglyceride levels. These data show that HL plays an important role in HDL and IDL metabolism, thereby mediating plasma cholesterol homeostasis.

Acknowledgements

We thank Jiajin Wang, Dale Newland, and Drs Andre Bensadoun, Stephen J. Lauer, Qi Dang, and David Sanan for their valuable contributions to this project. This research was supported in part by National Institutes of Health Grant HL51588.

References

1. Jansen H, Hülsmann WC. Biochem Soc Trans 1985;13:24–26.
2. Tikkanen MJ, Nikkilä EA. Am Heart J 1987;113:562–573.
3. Doolittle MH, Wong H, Davis RC, Schotz MC. J Lipid Res 1987;28:1326–1334.
4. Grosser J, Schrecker O, Greten H. J Lipid Res 1981;22:437–442.
5. Goldberg IJ, Le N-A, Paterniti JR Jr, Ginsberg HN, Lindgren FT, Brown WV. J Clin Invest 1982;70: 1184–1192.
6. Daggy BP, Bensadoun A. Biochim Biophys Acta 1986;877:252–261.
7. Kuusi T, Kinnunen PKJ, Nikkilä EA. FEBS Lett 1979;104:384–388.
8. Jansen H, van Tol A, Hülsmann WC. Biochem Biophys Res Commun 1980;92:53–59.
9. Hegele RA, Little JA, Vezina C, Maguire GF, Tu L, Wolever TS, Jenkins DJA, Connelly PW. Arterioscler Thromb 1993;13:720–728.
10. Warren RJ, Ebert DL, Mitchell A, Barter PJ. J Lipid Res 1991;32:1333–1339.
11. Simonet WS, Bucay N, Lauer SJ, Taylor JM. J Biol Chem 1993;268:8221–8229.
12. Cheng C-F, Bensadoun A, Bersot T, Hsu JST, Melford KH. J Biol Chem 1985;260:10720–10727.
13. Blades B, Vega GL, Grundy SM. Arterioscler Thromb 1993;13:1227–1235.
14. Bamberger M, Glick JM, Rothblat GH. J Lipid Res 1983;24:869–876.
15. Zambon A, Austin MA, Brown BG, Hokanson JE, Brunzell JD. Arterioscler Thromb 1993;13:147–153.

670

Atherosclerosis X.
F.P. Woodford, J. Davignon and A. Sniderman, editors.

Role of apolipoprotein E in Alzheimer's disease

Karl H. Weisgraber[1,2], Robert E. Pitas[1,2] and Robert W. Mahley[1,2,3]
[1]Gladstone Institute of Cardiovascular Disease, Cardiovascular Research Institute, Departments of [2]Pathology and [3]Medicine, University of California, San Francisco, California, USA

Abstract. Human apolipoprotein E (apoE), a key component in plasma lipoprotein metabolism, was recently linked to Alzheimer's disease (AD). Of the three common apoE alleles (apoE2, apoE3, apoE4), the apoE4 allele was demonstrated to be a major risk factor for AD. This review summarizes the genetic data leading to this conclusion and discusses potential roles for apoE in the pathogenesis of AD based on recent biochemical studies.

Alzheimer's disease (AD) is an irreversible neurodegenerative disorder that results in a progressive dementia characterized by the complete loss of personality. AD is the fourth leading cause of death in developed countries. There are three classifications of the disease: early-onset familial, which occurs before age 60 and is linked to specific mutations or chromosomal loci; late-onset familial, which occurs after age 60; and late-onset sporadic, which occurs after age 60 with no apparent familial association.

Definite diagnosis requires specific neuropathology in the brain, determined at autopsy. This neuropathology includes the presence of both neuritic plaques and neurofibrillary tangles (Fig. 1) [1]. The presence of the plaques and tangles is associated with a profound loss of neurons in the hippocampus and neocortex — up to one-third of these neurons can be lost by the time of death. Neuritic plaques are primarily, if not exclusively, extracellular and comprise classical amyloid deposits [2]. The major component of the plaque is the β-amyloid peptide (Aβ peptide). This peptide arises by cleavage from the amyloid precursor protein (APP). Apolipoprotein E (apoE) has been colocalized with the Aβ peptide in neuritic plaques [3–5].

Neurofibrillary tangles are intracellular and contain structures referred to as paired helical filaments [6]. These filaments are composed of phosphorylated tau, a member of the microtubule-associated protein family that is involved in microtubule assembly and stabilization of the cytoskeleton. ApoE has also been colocalized in these structures [3].

Genetic evidence linking apoE to AD

Considerable effort has gone into identifying genes and genetic markers for AD (for review see [7]). As discussed below, both late-onset familial and sporadic disease is linked to chromosome 19 and the apoE4 allele in a dose-dependent manner. There are also cases of late-onset disease where the apoE gene locus has been excluded, but the relevant chromosome is unknown. Early-onset familial disease has been localized to an unknown gene on chromosome 14, to chromosome 21 in association with APP mutations, and to an unknown gene locus associated with a population of Volga-Germans. AD is thus genetically heterogeneous: several genes can contribute to a common phenotype.

The seminal observation that sparked the explosive interest in apoE and AD was

Address for correspondence: Karl H. Weisgraber PhD, Gladstone Institute of Cardiovascular Disease, P.O. Box 419100, San Francisco, CA 94141-9100, USA.

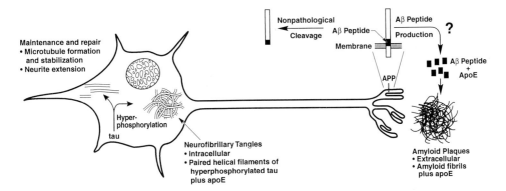

Fig. 1. Model of a nerve cell, highlighting three areas in which apoE might influence the pathogenesis of AD. Indicated are the extracellular amyloid plaques, composed of the Aβ peptide and apoE, and the intracellular neurofibrillary tangles, composed of paired helical filaments (hyperphosphorylated tau) and apoE.

reported by Warren Strittmatter and Alan Roses and their associates [5]. They observed that the apoE4 allele frequency in 83 subjects with late-onset familial disease was greatly overrepresented, compared with age- and sex-matched controls (0.51 vs. 0.15). This observation was extended to late-onset sporadic disease as well [8].

The risk of AD in these late-onset families is affected by the apoE4 allele in a dose-dependent manner, the age of onset of the disease decreasing with an increasing number of apoE4 alleles [9]. A more recent analysis of this population suggests that the apoE2 allele may be protective [10]. The association of the apoE4 allele with AD has been confirmed by several laboratories worldwide and is now universally accepted.

Role of apoE in AD

The role of apoE in lipoprotein metabolism is well established and much is known regarding the structural and functional relationships with respect to lipid metabolism (for reviews see [11] and [12]). With the genetic evidence establishing the apoE4 allele as a major risk factor for AD, the key question has become: how does apoE contribute to the pathogenesis of this disease? Several studies were initiated to answer this question. Three areas where apoE potentially could be involved are introduced in Fig. 1.

Interaction of apoE and the Aβ peptide of amyloid plaques

The Aβ peptide is derived from the APP, which is expressed on the surfaces of a variety of cells as an integral membrane protein with an unknown function. On the cell surface APP undergoes nonpathological cleavage to release a soluble fragment. The Aβ peptide, represented by the shaded area (Fig. 1), varies from 40 to 43 residues, and approximately one-third is contained in the membrane-spanning region of APP. It is not clear how the Aβ peptide is produced or what regulates its production. Normal cleavage destroys the amyloid-forming potential of the Aβ peptide.

When apoE3 or apoE4 were incubated with the Aβ peptide, an SDS-stable complex formed in an isoform-specific manner [13]. Moreover, apoE4 was more effective in complex formation than apoE3. The apoE isoform-specific interaction with the Aβ peptide represented the first potential functional correlation with the genetic evidence. Residues

244–272 in the carboxyl-terminal domain of apoE were demonstrated to be required for peptide binding [13].

In long-term incubations both the apoE3 and apoE4 SDS-stable complexes formed very high molecular weight insoluble fibrils [14]. These complexes were examined by negative-staining electron microscopy. When incubated alone, the Aβ peptide formed twisted ribbons containing two or more strands. Coincubations of apoE and the Aβ peptide led to the formation of monofibrils in an isoform-specific manner. The apoE4 coincubates formed a more dense, more extensive matrix of monofibrils than did the apoE3 co-incubates. In addition, the monofilaments appeared earlier with apoE4 than with apoE3. With both isoforms, immunogold labeling demonstrated that apoE was distributed along the entire length of the monofilaments [14].

Fibrils in amyloid plaques have similar dimensions to monofilaments formed in the apoE and Aβ coincubations. It is reasonable to speculate that in the presence of apoE4, the Aβ peptide produced by neurons or other cells may form monofibrils readily, with the potential to react in a pathological manner. It is known that apoE is abundant in the brain, where it is synthesized and secreted by astrocytes and some microglia [15,16].

Interaction of apoE and tau

The tau protein consists of several isoforms that arise by differential splicing. Depending on the isoform, tau contains three or four imperfect repeats that represent the microtubule-binding region. These repeats are homologous to other microtubule-binding proteins. Tau assists in tubulin polymerization, and it binds to and stabilizes microtubules. The protein contains a number of phosphorylation sites, which when phosphorylated reduce the affinity of tau for microtubules. However, hyperphosphorylation of tau leads to the formation of paired helical filaments in the cytoplasm of neurons.

The interaction of apoE and tau also resulted in the formation of an SDS-stable complex in model studies [17]. However, tau and apoE3 formed a stable complex, but little if any complex was formed with apoE4. After phosphorylation of tau, apoE3 was no longer able to form a stable complex. In binding studies with apoE fragments, the N-terminal domain of apoE3 (residues 1–191) binds to tau. This is in contrast to the interaction with the Aβ peptide where the C-terminal domain of apoE interacts.

These results raise the question of the potential significance of apoE3 binding to tau and the impact of this interaction on AD. It has been speculated that apoE3 binding to tau stabilizes microtubules and the cytoskeleton, and perhaps as a result helps to maintain the structure and function of neurons. Furthermore, it is possible that the interaction of apoE3 with tau might inhibit tau phosphorylation and thus retard the formation of paired helical filaments and the development of neurofibrillary tangles. Consideration of these possibilities led to the hypothesis that apoE4 is associated with AD because it does not have the protective features of apoE3 [17].

Since tau is an intracellular protein, apoE3 too must exist within the cell to modulate tau metabolism. Evidehce that apoE is present in the cytoplasm is emerging. Immunochemical studies suggest that apoE is present in the cytoplasm of hepatocytes [18], in neurons [19], and in the cytoplasm of muscle cells associated with inclusion-body myositis [20]. Interestingly, inclusion-body myositis, a neuromuscular disorder, possesses several features in common with AD, including the presence of amyloid deposits, paired helical filaments, and apoE. If the presence of cytoplasmic apoE in neurons can be firmly established, its origin is unclear. If apoE is internalized via the low density lipoprotein (LDL) receptor or LDL receptor–related protein (LRP), it would have to escape degradation in the endosomal pathway to interact intracellularly with cytoskeletal elements. Alternatively, a fraction of apoE may be bypassing the normal secretory pathway and be shunted into the cytoplasm.

Role of apoE in maintenance and repair of nerves

A significant body of evidence supports a role for apoE in the normal functioning of nerves. In a number of species, brain tissue is second only to the liver in apoE mRNA levels [21]. Astrocytes are the major apoE-producing cells in the brain [15,16]. In cerebrospinal fluid, apoE-containing lipoproteins are present in the high density lipoprotein (HDL) fraction along with apoA-I, which suggests that apoE plays a major role in cholesterol homeostasis in the brain [22]. Unlike the plasma compartment, where apoB-containing lipoproteins (very low density lipoproteins (VLDL) and LDL) are also involved in transport of cholesterol, in cerebrospinal fluid only the apoE-containing HDL possess the ability to bind LDL receptors and to participate in receptor-mediated lipid transport.

The importance of apoE in nerve maintenance was suggested from a peripheral nerve injury model in which it was demonstrated that apoE synthesis was induced 250- to 350-fold by injury [23–26]. Induction of apoE synthesis was also observed in the central nervous system with optic nerve and spinal cord injury [27]. On the basis of these studies a model was developed of peripheral nerve regeneration involving apoE-containing lipoproteins and LDL receptors, in which lipids from degenerating nerves were captured, stored locally, and reused in the process of axon regeneration and remyelinization [27].

This model of nerve regeneration suggested that apoE or apoE-containing lipoproteins might influence neuron growth patterns in cell culture systems. This hypothesis was tested by examining the effects of apoE and lipoproteins on neurite outgrowth from fetal rabbit dorsal root ganglia [28]. Incubation with β-migrating VLDL (β-VLDL), which contain both cholesterol and apoE, increased both neurite extension and branching. Neurite branching was reduced by the addition of purified rabbit apoE together with the β-VLDL, whereas neurite extension was enhanced. This modified growth pattern would be desirable in target-directed axon regeneration.

Recently, an isoform-specific effect of apoE was demonstrated in the dorsal root ganglion cell model system [29]. Compared with cells incubated in medium alone, addition of β-VLDL resulted in more neurite branching, as previously observed [28]. Addition of human apoE3 with the β-VLDL resulted in an increase in neurite extension and a reduction in branching, similar to the effects with rabbit apoE [28]. However, when human apoE4 was added both branching and extension were dramatically reduced, which suggests that apoE3 may promote neuronal growth, whereas apoE4 may inhibit it. Blocking the receptor interaction of apoE with a monoclonal antibody or by chemical modification eliminated the isoform-specific effects [29]. These results suggest that the isoform-specific effects involve binding and/or internalization of the apoE-enriched β-VLDL by lipoprotein receptors and that apoE may interact in an isoform-specific manner with one or more cellular proteins, i.e., cytoskeletal proteins involved in neurite structure and function. These results have clear implications for maintaining and reestablishing synaptic connections, particularly in the sixth and seventh decades of life.

In conclusion, with the establishment of the apoE4 allele as a major risk factor for AD, it is clear that apoE plays a potentially important role in the physiology of the nervous system beyond its known function in lipid metabolism. This suggestion of a dual role for apoE has provided new avenues of research on AD. The link of apoE to AD is obviously of potential clinical significance, particularly with regard to new therapeutic strategies for

674

both treatment and prevention of AD. The challenge for the future is to determine how apoE affects the pathogenesis of AD in an isoform-specific manner.

Acknowledgements

This work is supported in part by the National Heart, Lung, and Blood Institute Program Project Grant HL 41633 and by the L.K. Whittier Foundation. The authors thank Kerry Humphrey for manuscript preparation, Amy Corder and Liliana Jach for graphics, and Lewis DeSimone and Dawn Levy for editorial assistance.

References

1. McKhann G, Drachman D, Folstein M, Katzman R, Price D, Stadlan EM. Neurology 1984;34:939–944.
2. Selkoe DJ. Neuron 1991;6:487–498.
3. Namba Y, Tomonaga M, Kawasaki H, Otomo E, Ikeda K. Brain Res 1991;541:163–166.
4. Wisniewski T, Frangione B. Neurosci Lett 1992;135:235–238.
5. Strittmatter WJ, Saunders AM, Schmechel D, Pericak-Vance M, Enghild J, Salvesen GS, Roses AD. Proc Natl Acad Sci USA 1993;90:1977–1981.
6. Crowther RA. Curr Opin Struct Biol 1993;3:202–206.
7. Roses AD. Curr Neurol 1994;14:111–141.
8. Saunders AM, Strittmatter WJ, Schmechel D, St. George-Hyslop PH, Pericak-Vance MA, Joo SH, Rosi BL, Gusella JF, Crapper-MacLachlan DR, Alberts MJ, Hulette C, Crain B, Goldgaber D, Roses AD. Neurology 1993;43:1467–1472.
9. Corder EH, Saunders AM, Strittmatter WJ, Schmechel DE, Gaskell PC, Small GW, Roses AD, Haines JL, Pericak-Vance MA. Science 1993;261:921–923.
10. Corder EH, Saunders AM, Risch NJ, Strittmatter WJ, Schmechel DE, Gaskell PC Jr, Rimmler JB, Locke PA, Conneally PM, Schmader KE, Small GW, Roses AD, Haines JL, Pericak-Vance MA. Nature Genet 1994;7:180–184.
11. Mahley RW. Science 1988;240:622–630.
12. Weisgraber KH. Adv Protein Chem 1994;45:249–302.
13. Strittmatter WJ, Weisgraber KH, Huang DY, Dong L-M, Salvesen GS, Pericak-Vance M, Schmechel D, Saunders AM, Goldgaber D, Roses AD. Proc Natl Acad Sci USA 1993;90:8098–8102.
14. Sanan DA, Weisgraber KH, Russell SJ, Mahley RW, Huang D, Saunders A, Schmechel D, Wisniewski T, Frangione B, Roses AD, Strittmatter WJ. J Clin Invest 1994;94:860–869.
15. Boyles JK, Pitas RE, Wilson E, Mahley RW, Taylor JM. J Clin Invest 1985;76:1501–1513.
16. Pitas RE, Boyles JK, Lee SH, Foss D, Mahley RW. Biochim Biophys Acta 1987;917:148–161.
17. Strittmatter WJ, Weisgraber KH, Goedert M, Saunders AM, Huang D, Corder EH, Dong L-M, Jakes R, Alberts MJ, Gilbert JR, Han S-H, Hulette C, Einstein G, Schmechel DE, Pericak-Vance MA, Roses AD. Exp Neurol 1994;125:163–171.
18. Hamilton RL, Wong JS, Guo LSS, Krisans S, Havel RJ. J Lipid Res 1990;31:1589–1603.
19. Han S-H, Einstein G, Weisgraber KH, Strittmatter WJ, Saunders AM, Pericak-Vance M, Roses AD, Schmechel DE. J Neuropathol Exp Neurol 1994;53:535–544.
20. Askanas V, Mirabella M, Engel WK, Alvarez RB, Weisgraber KH. Lancet 1994;343:364–365.
21. Elshourbagy NA, Liao WS, Mahley RW, Taylor JM. Proc Natl Acad Sci USA 1985;82:203–207.
22. Pitas RE, Boyles JK, Lee SH, Hui DY, Weisgraber KH. J Biol Chem 1987;262:14352–14360.
23. Skene JHP, Shooter EM. Proc Natl Acad Sci USA 1983;80:4169–4173.
24. Müller HW, Ignatius MJ, Hangen DH, Shooter EM. J Cell Biol 1986;102:393–402.
25. Müller HW, Gebicke-Härter PJ, Hangen DH, Shooter EM. Science 1985;228:499–501.
26. Ignatius MJ, Gebicke-Härter PJ, Skene JHP, Schilling JW, Weisgraber KH, Mahley RW, Shooter EM. Proc Natl Acad Sci USA 1986;83:1125–1129.
27. Boyles JK, Zoellner CD, Anderson LJ, Kosik LM, Pitas RE, Weisgraber KH, Hui DY, Mahley RW, Gebicke-Haerter PJ, Ignatius MJ, Shooter EM. J Clin Invest 1989;83:1015–1031.
28. Handelmann GE, Boyles JK, Weisgraber KH, Mahley RW, Pitas RE. J Lipid Res 1992;33:1677–1688.
29. Nathan BP, Bellosta S, Sanan DA, Weisgraber KH, Mahley RW, Pitas RE. Science 1994;264:850–852.

Atherosclerosis X.
F.P. Woodford, J. Davignon and A. Sniderman, editors.

Regulation of the cellular immune response by apolipoprotein E: mechanism and implications

Judith A.K. Harmony[1], Michael E. Kelly[1], Moira A. Clay[2] and Meenakshi J. Mistry[2]

[1]*Developmental Biology Program and* [2]*Department of Pharmacology and Cell Biophysics, College of Medicine, University of Cincinnati, Cincinnati, Ohio, USA*

Abstract. Apolipoprotein E (apoE) can regulate the proliferation of mitogen/antigen-activated T lymphocytes at two stages in the pathway of clonal or polyclonal T-cell population expansion. Activated lymphocytes incubated with apoE produce interleukin 2 (IL2) with reduced biological activity. As a consequence, activated cells fail to become competent to respond to IL2 in order to proliferate. In addition, apoE blocks IL2-dependent proliferation of fully competent cells; inhibited cells arrest in the G1 phase of the cell cycle. The domain of apoE which is responsible for reduced IL2 bioactivity is localized to the thrombin-derived carboxy-terminal 10-kDa fragment of apoE. That responsible for cell-cycle arrest is localized to the amino-terminal 22-kDa fragment, specifically to residues 141–149.

It is rare for a single protein to be implicated in several diseases. Apolipoprotein E (apoE) is one such protein [1]. ApoE is a 299-amino-acid protein present primarily in plasma, where it is associated with very low density (VLDL) and high density (HDL) lipoproteins. ApoE occurs in humans in three common isoforms: apoE2, -E3 and -E4, which differ by single amino acid substitutions at two loci. The predominant isoform apoE3 has cysteine at position 112 and arginine at position 158. ApoE2 has cysteine at both positions; apoE4, arginine at both positions. The frequency of the apoE alleles varies among different ethnic groups. Individuals homozygous for the apoE2 allele develop hypercholesterolemia and hypertriglyceridemia caused by the accumulation of chylomicron remnants due to inefficient remnant clearance by hepatic chylomicron-remnant receptors. This disorder, type III hyperlipidemia, is correlated with markedly increased risk of atherosclerosis and coronary heart disease. Thus, apoE functions in lipid homeostasis, where it is a structural component of lipoprotein particles and a recognition determinant for lipoprotein receptors.

ApoE is also believed to function in the nervous system. ApoE accumulates extracellularly as well as intracellularly at sites of neurodegeneration [2]. Individuals homozygous for the apoE4 allele are 8 times more likely to develop late-onset familial Alzheimer's disease (AD) than those who lack the apoE4 allele. Moreover, sporadic AD is also associated with apoE4, with onset at a younger age and with increased rate of progression with increased apoE4 allele dosage. In contrast, the apoE2 isoform is associated with decreased risk of AD. This implied role of apoE in neuropathology was suggested by the dramatic induction and secretion of apoE in the central and peripheral nervous systems following nerve injury [1]. Molecular explanations of the role of apoE in neuropathology have yet to be established.

This remarkable protein potentially has a third function: regulation of the immune system [3], particularly of T-lymphocyte proliferative responses to mitogen/antigen. The

Address for correspondence: Prof Judith A.K. Harmony, Department of Pharmacology and Cell Biophysics, University of Cincinnati, College of Medicine, 231 Bethesda Avenue, Cincinnati, OH 45267-0575, USA. Tel.: +1-513-558-2379. Fax: +1-513-558-1169.

production of apoE by macrophages, accessory cells important in the activation of T lymphocytes by antigen, supports the physiological significance of immunoregulation by apoE. The molecular basis by which apoE restricts proliferation of T lymphocytes has been investigated in vitro, using two systems [4,5]: 1) native (Go) T cells activated by polyclonal mitogens, such as plant lectins (phytohemagglutinin, PHA), alone or in combination with tumor promoters (phorbol myristate acetate, PMA) or monoclonal antibodies (mAb) directed against a component (CD3) of the T cell receptor for antigen (TCR); and 2) interleukin 2 (IL2)-dependent T cells arrested in G1 by IL2 deprivation and restimulated with IL2. These systems are related, representing the two sequential stages of clonal or polyclonal expansion of functional T cells. In stage I, TCR activation of naive cells renders them competent to proliferate by inducing IL2 production and expression of IL2 receptors. IL2 receptor-positive competent cells proliferate in stage II consequent on IL2–IL2 receptor engagement. Naive T cells must complete both stages; IL2-dependent cells, only stage II. The mechanism of apoE suppression in the two systems may be the same or different. To address this uncertainty, we compared the effect of apoE on activated naive T cells vs. IL2-dependent T cells and identified structural features of apoE important in regulating proliferation.

Materials and Methods

ApoE was purified from plasma obtained from patients with hyperlipidemia [4]. Some preparations of apoE4 and apoE2 were obtained from Stanley Rall (San Francisco, California). Thrombin-generated apoE 22- and 10-kDa domains were generously provided by Dr Karl Weisgraber (San Francisco, California). ApoE peptides were synthesized and purified as previously described [6]. Cyclosporin A (CsA) was obtained from Roy First (Cincinnati, Ohio). Methyl-[^{3}H]-thymidine (TdR, 6.7 Ci/mmol) was purchased from ICN Biomedicals Inc. AntiCD3 and antiCD25 were purchased from Ortho Diagnostics. TU27, a monoclonal antibody (Mab) specific for the p75 subunit of the human IL2R, was provided by Kuzuo Sugamura, Sendai, Japan. Anti-IL2R β-subunit (p75) Mab was purchased from Endogen, Inc. Collaborative Biomedical Products was the source of human recombinant IL2 (rIL2). FITC-conjugated goat antimouse F(ab)$_2$ and purified goat antimouse Fc-specific antibodies were purchased from Cappel Labs.

Cells were maintained at 37°C in a humidified 5% CO_2 incubator. Cell viability was assessed by trypan blue exclusion or by ^{45}Cr release [6]. Naive human T cells (>90% CD3-positive) were obtained from peripheral blood mononuclear cells (PBM) [4]. T cells (1 × 10^5/0.24 ml) were stimulated for 72 h with 1.0 μg/ml of PHA alone, 0.5 ng/ml of PMA + 50 ng/ml of PHA, or 0.5 ng/ml of PMA + 0.5 ng/ml of OKT3. Cells were pulsed with 1 μCi/well of TdR 8 h prior to harvest. Primary IL2-dependent human T cells (98—99% CD3-positive) were isolated from PBM and incubated (2.5 × 10^6 cells/ml) without IL2 for 24 h prior to addition of rIL2 [5,6]. Cells (1 × 10^5/0.24 ml) were cultured with 4 U/ml of IL2 for 24—72 h and pulsed with 1 μCi of TdR per well 7—8 h prior to harvest. Mouse IL2-dependent CTLL-15G T cells, obtained from Kendall Smith (Hanover, New Hampshire), were maintained in DMEM-SFM plus 5% rat spleen factor [5]. CTLL-15G cells (4 × 10^3) were cultured in 0.24 ml of SFM with growth factor and harvested after 26 h; 1 μCi of TdR was added to each well at least 4 h prior to harvest.

Expression of cell-surface proteins was analyzed by the indirect immunofluorescence procedure of Cantrell and Smith [7], 10,000 cells per sample being analyzed.

Incorporation of TdR into DNA was determined by liquid scintillation counting of triplicate cultures maintained in SFM in flat-bottomed microtiter plates. DNA synthesis data are represented as the mean and standard deviation of the mean. The effect of apoE, as a percentage of control value, was calculated: {[cpm(-apoE)-cpm(+apoE)] ÷ (cpm(-apoE)} ×100 = % change.

IL2 bioactivity was quantitated by measuring the proliferation of mouse IL2-dependent CTLL-2 cells [4]. Binding of radiolabeled IL2 was determined by the procedure of Robb et al. [8]. T lymphocytes (3×10^6/ml) in SFM were activated for 72 h in the absence or presence of 2.8 µM apoE, washed 2 times with SFM, followed by incubation (1×10^6/ml) at 37°C in IL2-free SFM for two 1-h intervals to promote dissociation of endogenous IL2. ^{125}I-IL2 (sp. act. 1×10^6 cpm/pmol) was added to $1-2 \times 10^6$ cells/0.2 ml SFM. Nonspecific binding was determined in the presence of a 150-fold molar excess of unlabeled IL2. Scatchard [9] analysis of equilibrium binding data was used to calculate the number and the affinity of IL2 receptors expressed by activated T cells. The lower limit of detection was 50 sites/cell.

Results

Naive T cells and IL2-dependent T cells differ in sensitivity to apoE. To ascertain whether naive TCR-activated T cells and primary IL2-dependent T cells are equally sensitive to apoE suppression, we established cultures of each from PBM obtained from five different donors. ApoE suppressed the proliferation of mitogen-activated naive T cells to a significantly greater extent (~2.3 times) than that of the IL2-dependent cells (Fig. 1).

Suppression of T-cell proliferation by apoE isoforms. To compare the suppressive potency of apoE isoforms, naive T cells were activated with PHA in the absence or presence of

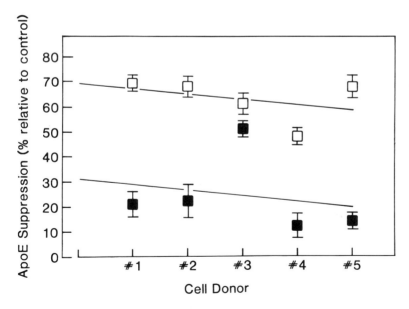

Fig. 1. Naive, activated T cells are more sensitive to apoE suppression than IL2-dependent T cells. Purified T cells and IL2-dependent T cells, generated from PBM obtained from the same individual, were activated with PHA+PMA, and cultured for 72 h in the absence or presence of apoE (100 µg/ml). IL2-dependent T cells were cultured with rIL2 for 24 h. The DNA replication data represent the mean ± SD of five experiments, each using cells isolated from a different individual.

Table 1. ApoE isoforms differentially suppress IL2-dependent cell proliferation but not proliferation subsequent to mitogen activation

System	ApoE (μM)	ApoE isoform		
		E2	E3	E4
			% suppression	
PHA-activated T cells[a]	0.7	38 ± 9	20 ± 3	17 ± 8
	1.4	66 ± 11	43 ± 6	56 ± 11
	2.8	86 ± 21	71 ± 10	88 ± 16
CTLL-15G cells[b]	2.2	8 ± 2	71 ± 1	79 ± 1
IL2-dependent human T cells[c]	2.8	26 ± 3	61 ± 3	ND
	5.6	48 ± 4	79 ± 1	ND

[a]Peripheral blood T lymphocytes (1×10^5/well) were cultured with 1 μg/ml of PHA. TdR incorporation, measured at 72 h in three experiments with each performed in triplicate, was $12,100 \pm 675$ cpm; [b]CTLL-15G cells (4×10^3/well) were washed and cultured in SFM with 4 U/ml of IL2, pulsed with TdR then harvested at 26 h. TdR incorporated in the absence of apoE was $18,340 \pm 970$; [c]primary human T cells (1×10^5/well), incubated without IL2 for 48 h, were cultured in SFM with 4 U/ml of IL2. Cells were pulsed with TdR then harvested at 72 h. TdR incorporated in the absence of apoE was $10,620 \pm 835$ cpm. ND = not determined.

the three apoE isoforms (Table 1). ApoE2, -E3, and -E4 equally suppressed cell-cycle progression. In contrast, suppression of IL2-dependent CTLL-15G cell proliferation was isoform-specific. ApoE4 was slightly more suppressive than apoE3, and both were significantly more suppressive than apoE2. ApoE suppression of human primary IL2-dependent T cells demonstrated similar isoform selectivity to the CTLL-15G cells. These results were confirmed by using each isoform of apoE purified from at least two different donors.

ApoE suppression of activated naive T cells is associated with reduced IL2 activity. Differential sensitivity of naive and IL2 receptor-positive T cells to apoE concentration and isoform suggests that apoE has independent effects on the induction of competent T cells (stage I) and the progression of these cells through the cell cycle (stage II). Since competent cells produce and secrete IL2, apoE's effect on IL2 activity was established. To obtain measurable IL2 in PHA-stimulated cultures, cells were cultured at high density (3×10^6 cells/ml) and IL2 utilization was blocked with antiCD25. Under these conditions 1.4 and 2.8 μM apoE decreased IL2 activity by 40 and 65%, respectively; 0.7 μM apoE had only a minor effect (Table 2). In contrast, we [4] previously demonstrated that apoE did not reduce IL2 mRNA or alter IL2 size and isoelectric point. ApoE therefore did not antagonize signals required for IL2 gene activation, but appeared to interfere with event(s) required for full expression of IL2 biological activity. Lower IL2 activity was also not due

Table 2. ApoE inhibits the production of active IL2

PHA + antiCD25	Bioactive IL2, pM
no apoE	13.1 ± 0.9
+0.7 μM apoE	11.7 ± 0.9
+1.4 μM apoE	7.6 ± 0.8 (p = 0.01)
+2.8 μM apoE	4.5 ± 0.6 (p = 0.002)

IL2 activity in medium conditioned by T cells (3×10^6/ml) was determined by using IL2-dependent mouse CTLL-2 cells [4].

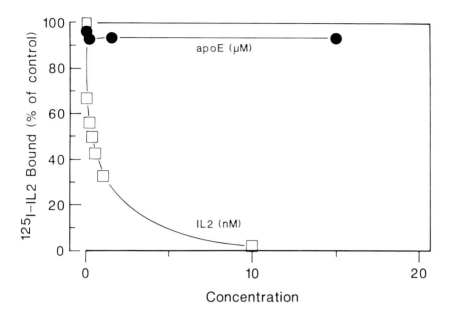

Fig. 2. ApoE does not compete with IL2 for binding to IL2. T lymphocytes were stimulated with immobilized OKT3 in SFM containing 10% FBS. Activated T cells (2 × 10⁶) were incubated with 100 pmol of ¹²⁵I-IL2 in the absence or presence of apoE (●) or IL2 (□). IL2 binding is expressed as a percentage of ¹²⁵I-IL2 bound after subtraction of nonspecific binding.

to direct inactivation of IL2 by apoE or to an effect of apoE on IL2 binding to high-affinity IL2 receptors (Fig. 2). Unlabeled rIL2 competed with ¹²⁵I-IL2 for binding to high-affinity receptors, whereas apoE had no effect.

Suppressive activity is located in the carboxy terminus of apoE. Cleavage of apoE by thrombin results in two major fragments, corresponding to the independently folded 22-kDa amino terminus of residues 1–199 and 10-kDa carboxy terminus of residues 216–299 [10]. Both fragments can inhibit mitogen-induced T cell proliferation [21]. We compared the ability of these fragments to reduce IL2 activity in order to localize the bioactive apoE domain responsible (Table 3). The 22-kDa fragment had little effect on IL2 activity; in contrast, the 10-kDa fragment was potently suppressive. The localization of IL2-suppressive activity to the carboxy terminus is consistent with the lack of apoE isoform specificity in inhibiting mitogen induction of competent T cells (Table 1).

Table 3. Localization of apoE's IL2 inhibitory activity

ApoE fragment	Concentration (µM)	IL2 activity (pM)	Inhibition (%)
None	–	92	–
22-kDa	2.8	80	13
	5.6	76	17
10-kDa	2.8	52	43
	5.6	30	67

Table 4. ApoE causes similar suppression of IL2 binding and proliferation

Experiment	^{125}I-IL2 bound (pmol/10^6 cells)	DNA synthesis cpm of TdR
PHA	3.75 ± 0.35	25885 ± 2235
PHA + 1.4 μM E	2.45 ± 0.55 (35%)	9285 ± 2370 (64%)
PHA + 2.8 μM E	1.90 ± 0.35 (50%)	6235 ± 1820 (76%)

T lymphocytes (1 × 10^6/ml SFM) were activated with PHA ± apoE for 72 h. The results depict mean pmol of IL2 bound (100 pmol ^{125}I-IL2 added) or cpm of TdR incorporated ± SEM for three experiments performed in triplicate. Percentage suppression is indicated in parentheses.

ApoE causes suppression of IL2 receptors. To determine the effects of apoE on high-affinity IL2 receptor induction, we activated T cells for 72 h with PHA in the absence or presence of apoE, and quantitated DNA replication and IL2 binding (Table 4). ApoE suppressed IL2 binding and DNA replication to similar extents. Since the lower IL2 binding may be due to decreased number and/or affinity of the IL2 receptors, ^{125}I-IL2 binding was analyzed in further detail. Unstimulated T cells did not bind measurable IL2, in contrast to activated T cells. Results from five different experiments with mitogen-stimulated T cells (Table 5) indicated that apoE reduced the number but not the affinity of high-affinity IL2 receptors. The number and affinity of high-affinity IL2 receptors on activated T cells were within the reported range [11,12]. On the basis of flow cytofluorimetric analysis, apoE had no effect on the number of p55- and p75-positive cells or on the density of these IL2 receptor subunits per cell (not shown).

ApoE can enhance the potency of immunosuppressive drugs. The data suggest that apoE suppresses proliferation of mitogen-activated T cell proliferation by interfering with the production of fully active IL2 and with the assembly of high-affinity IL2 receptors. That is, apoE inhibits the production of competent, IL2-responsive T cells. Since the activity but not the presence of the growth factor and its receptor are both affected, the mechanism of apoE suppression most probably involves an alteration in post-translational modification of both nascent and/or trafficking IL2 and its receptor subunits.

The immunosuppressive drug cyclosporin A (CsA) is noted for its ability to inhibit IL2 gene transcription [13]. Since apoE and CsA apparently inhibit IL2 production at distinct

Table 5. ApoE affects IL2-receptor expression

Experiment	High-affinity IL2 receptors (sites/cell)			
	PHA	PHA + E	PMA + PHA	PMA + PHA + E
1	560	420	235	150
2	365	220	150	55
3	640	290	190	110
4	360	245	350	245
5	250	160	190	140
Mean ± SEM	435 ± 72	267 ± 43[a]	223 ± 34	140 ± 31[b]

T lymphocytes (3 × 10^6/ml SFM) were activated with or without 2.8 μM apoE with PHA or PMA + PHA for 72 h. ApoE suppressed proliferation by an average of 65% in the five experiments. The p values were determined by ANOVA analysis. Dissociation constants (Kd, mean pM ± SEM; n = 5) were as follows: PHA, 5.0 ± 2.6; PHA + apoE, 4.0 ± 3; PMA + PHA, 2.0 ± 0.6; PMA + PHA + apoE, 2.0 ± 0.5. [a]p = 0.02; [b]p = 0.001.

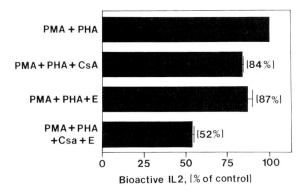

Fig. 3. ApoE and cyclosporin A act cooperatively to inhibit IL2 induction. T cells were activated with PMA + PHA for 24 h in the absence or presence of CsA (0.5 ng/ml) or apoE (0.7 μM), alone or in combination. IL2 activity was determined in cell-conditioned media. The mean values of IL2 activity in PMA + PHA culture supernatants for three experiments were 111, 125 and 240 pmol.

points, namely at the post-translational level vs. the transcriptional level, respectively, we predicted that they would additively reduce the level of IL2 produced by mitogen-activated T cells. T cells were stimulated with PMA + PHA in the presence of apoE (0.7 μM) or CsA (1 ng/ml), either alone or in combination, and IL2 in cell-conditioned medium was quantitated by bioassay (Fig. 3). These concentrations of apoE or CsA alone had minimal effects on IL2. When combined, however, apoE and CsA reduced IL2 activity by 50%; this compared to a calculated value of 27% suppression of IL2 if the effects of these agents were strictly additive. Thus apoE and CsA can act cooperatively to inhibit IL2 produced by activated T cells.

ApoE inhibits IL2-induced proliferation. In spite of the apparent association between apoE-suppressed DNA replication and apoE-reduced IL2 activity and high-affinity IL2 receptor number, apoE suppression of proliferation was independent of its effect on IL2 receptors. Fully active rIL2 restored high-affinity IL2 receptor expression but did not alleviate suppression of DNA replication (Table 6), indicating a separate effect of apoE on IL2-induced proliferation. This conclusion is supported by the fact that apoE inhibited proliferation of primary (Fig. 1) as well as long-term [5] lines of IL2-dependent T lymphocytes. The apoE concentration which inhibited IL2-induced proliferation by 50% is 2.3–2.8 μM, compared to the approximately 1 μM apoE required for 50% suppression of naive T cell activation [4,5]. IL2-dependent cells incubated with apoE are arrested in early G1, at or before the $G1_A/G1_B$ transition [5]. Since apoE does not interfere with

Table 6. IL2 restores high-affinity IL2 receptor expression but not proliferation

Experiment	High-affinity IL2 receptors		DNA synthesis
	sites/cell	Kd, pM	cpm of TdR
PHA + PMA	1063	2.7	17716 ± 612
PHA + PMA + ApoE	688 (35%)	2.3	9414 ± 456 (47%)
PHA + PMA +IL2	975	2.5	18890 ± 799
PHA + PMA + ApoE + IL2	875 (10%)	2.3	8860 ± 646 (53%)

Percentage suppression is indicated in parenthesis.

IL2–IL2 receptor interaction (Fig. 2), it may block IL2 signalling or a subsequent process essential for G1 progression. The fact that IL2-dependent T cell-mediated lysis of target cells is insensitive to apoE [5] argues that the site of its action is subsequent to IL2 signal transduction.

Identification of a suppressive apoE domain. Cummulative data suggested that independent domains of apoE suppress induction of T cell competence and IL2-dependent proliferation. Since the 22-kDa apoE fragment inhibited IL2-dependent cell proliferation (not shown), peptides corresponding to residues within the apoE sequence 130–169, encompassing both the low density lipoprotein (LDL)-receptor and heparin-binding sites [1], were synthesized and tested for their ability to suppress DNA replication (Table 7). Peptides representing sequences in the 10-kDa apoE fragment served as controls. Activity was localized to the region encompassed by residues 130–169. In contrast, peptides representing the carboxy-terminal 10-kDa apoE fragment were devoid of suppressive activity.

Remarkably, the IC_{50} of peptide 130–169 was only about twice that of native apoE. A comparison of the IC_{50}'s of the active peptides identified indicates that suppressive potency was confined to residues 141–149. However, the potency of this sequence was influenced by the context in which it exists. For example, in peptide 130–169 the substitution of Cys for Arg at position corresponding to residue 158 of intact apoE significantly increased the IC_{50}, consistent with the relative potencies of the native apoE isoforms (Table 1). Moreover, the density of positive charge at the amino terminus of 141–149 markedly increased bioactivity. This is evident from comparison of activities of peptides which start at residue 130 and those which start at 141. Moreover, potency is greatly increased when peptides contain two copies of the 141–149 region, possibly due

Table 7. Suppression by apoE peptides

Peptide	IC_{50} (μM)	Amino acid sequence
$E_{130\text{-}169}$	5.8 ± 0.6	`   +  +    +  ++ +++   +       ++        +` `TEELRVRLASHLRKLRKRLLRDADDLQKRLAVYQAGAREG`
$E_{130\text{-}169}$	26.6	`   +  +    +  ++ +++   +       +         +` `TEELRVRLASHLRKLRKRLLRDADDLQKCLAVYQAGAREG`
$E_{130\text{-}149}$	15.1 ± 1.9	`   +  +    +  ++ +++   +` `TEELRVRLASHLRKLRKRLLR`
$E_{130\text{-}155}$	22.0	`   +  +    +  ++ +++   +` `TEELRVRLASHLRKLRKRLLRDADDL`
$E_{141\text{-}169}$	>30	`++ +++   +          ++        +` `LRKLRKRLLRDADDLQKRLAVYQAREG`
$E_{150\text{-}169}$	NS	`+          ++          +` `RDADDLQKRLAVYQAGAREG`
$E_{141\text{-}155}$	NS	`++ +++   +` `LRKLRKRLLRDADDL`
Tandem $E_{(141\text{-}155)2}$	1.9 ± 0.2	`++ +++   +          ++ +++   +` `LRKLRKRLLRDADDL-LRKLRKRLLRDADDL`
$E_{211\text{-}243}$	NS	` +  +  +       +  +       +       +  +` `GERLRARMEEMGSRTRDRKDEVKEQVAEVRAKL`
$E_{263\text{-}286}$	NS	`               +        +` `SWFEPLVEDMQRQWAGLVEKVQAA`

IC_{50} = concentration required to inhibit DNA replication by 50%; NS = not suppressive at concentrations up to 40 μM.

to the contribution of positive charge density provided by one unit at the amino terminus of the other unit in the tandem repeat.

Discussion

ApoE has fascinating, multifunctional regulatory activity toward mitogen-activated and lymphokine-induced T lymphocytes. ApoE can block proliferation of activated naive T cells, in part, by causing production of less active IL2, but can also restrict IL2-initiated proliferation of IL2-receptor-positive T cells in G1. It remains to be determined whether apoE's effects are limited to cells of the immune system, such as the T lymphocytes featured here. However, absence of growth factor specificity [5] suggests that, at least in suppressing cell-cycle progression, other cell types will be susceptible to the inhibitory potency of apoE. Vogel et al. [14] recently reported the apoE inhibition of endothelial and breast carcinoma cell proliferation, supporting a broad cellular target range for apoE.

Against T lymphocytes, apoE uses the full extent of its structural capacity. The two independently folded domains of apoE, identified by solution and crystallographic studies, can be separated by thrombin into the 22- and 10-kDa amino and carboxy terminii, respectively. The 10-kDa fragment contains the apoE motif which suppresses competence induction; the 22-kDa fragment, the motif which restricts cell-cycle progression in G1. These dual suppressive mechanisms make apoE unique among known regulators of T lymphocyte clonal expansion. It is interesting to reflect on the known biochemical properties of these two apoE domains. The region of apoE which is associated with production of defective IL2 also contains the site of interaction with the amyloid β protein [15], potentially explaining the accumulation of apoE in AD plaques. In addition, the major lipid-binding region of apoE, responsible for determining the lipoprotein distribution of apoE [16], is within this domain. The apoE motif responsible for cell-cycle inhibition is also important in apoE binding to members of the LDL-receptor gene family and to glycosaminoglycans [1]. In addition, this motif may be responsible for apoE's interaction with tau (KH Weisgraber, personal communication), a microtubule-associated protein abundant in intracellular neurofibrillary tangles in brains of AD patients.

The chemical details which account for both suppressive mechanisms are unknown, as are the interactions between apoE and lymphocytes responsible. The absence of isoform specificity in apoE suppression of activated naive T cells, combined with the unexpected and dramatic differences between apoE isoform potencies in suppressing T-cell responses to the autocrine hormone IL2, complicates the "immunoregulatory receptor" issue, implying that the apoE immunoregulatory receptors on fully activated, IL2-responsive and activated naive T cells are distinct. The differential sensitivity of the two populations of T cells to apoE suppression supports this conclusion. Our work implicates a heparin-like glycosaminoglycan, or a receptor comprised of a similar distribution of negative charge, such as the LDL receptor or the LDL receptor-related protein, in mediating apoE's suppressive action on IL2-dependent T cells. This hypothesis is based on the fact that the sequence 141–149 is critical in the suppressive mechanism. No specific sequence in the 10-kDa fragment has yet been identified which alters IL2 bioactivity. The apoE–lymphocyte interaction responsible for the fact that newly activated naive T cells fail to become fully competent to proliferate is even less well defined at this time.

From a cell biology perspective, apoE offers a unique opportunity to define biochemical pathways and activator proteins that participate in the retrieval of nonproliferating Go cells into the cell cycle and the events distal to growth-factor signalling required for the $G1_A$ transition. From a physiological perspective, apoE is likely to be an important

684

natural modulator of cell proliferation, particularly in the immune system. Not only is apoE expressed in diverse tissues in the body, it is a product of an important accessory cell, the monocyte/macrophage, necessary to initiate and sustain T lymphocytes in the activated state. ApoE accumulates in atherosclerotic plaque [17,18]. Activated T lymphocytes are present in both human plaque and in experimentally induced lesions [19], and immune mechanisms play an important role in atherosclerosis and myocardial injury in ischemia. ApoE, by effectively suppressing both stages of induction required for clonal expansion of activated lymphocytes, may limit the rate of lesion progression. Notably, mice in which the apoE gene has been ablated spontaneously develop arterial lesions which progress from fatty streaks to advanced fibrous cap lesions [20].

Acknowledgements

This project was supported by NIH grant HL27333 (MERIT Award to JAKH). Moira Clay received support from the NIH Program of Excellence HL41496, and Michael Kelly was sponsored by NIH Training Grant HL07527.

References

1. Mahley RW. Science 1988;240:622–630.
2. Roses AD. J Neuropathol Exp Neurol 1994;53:429–437.
3. Harmony JAK, Akeson AL, McCarthy BM, Morris RE, Scupham DW, Grupp SA. Biochemistry and Biology of Plasma Lipoproteins. New York: Marcel Dekker Inc., 1986;403–452.
4. Kelly ME, Clay MA, Mistry MJ, Hsieh-Li H-M, Harmony JAK. Cell Immunol 1994 (in press).
5. Mistry MJ, Clay MA, Kelly ME, Steiner MA, Harmony JAK. Cell Immunol 1994 (in press).
6. Clay MA, Anantharamaiah GM, Mistry MJ, Balasubramaniam A, Harmony JAK. J Biol Chem 1995 (in press).
7. Cantrell DA, Smith KA. J Exp Med 1983;158:1895–1911.
8. Robb RJ, Munck A, Smith KA. J Exp Med 1981;154:1455–1474.
9. Scatchard G. Ann NY Acad Sci 1949;51:660–662.
10. Wilson C, Wardell MR, Weisgraber KH, Mahley RW, Agard DA. Science 1991;252:1817–1822.
11. Herzberg VL, Smith KA. J Immunol 1987;139:998–1004.
12. Krause DS, Deutsch C. J Immunol 1991;146:2285–2294.
13. Kronke M, Leonard WJ, Depper SK, Arya F, Wang-Stahl F, Gallo RC, Waldman TA, Greene WC. Proc Natl Acad Sci USA 1984;81:5214–5218.
14. Vogel T, Guo N, Guy R, Drezlich N, Krutzsch NC, Blake DA, Panet A, Roberts DO. J Cell Bochem 1994;54:299–308.
15. Strittmatter WJ, Weisgraber KH, Huang D, Dong L-M, Salvesen GS, Pericak-Vance M, Schmechel D, Saunders AM, Goldgaber DM, Roses AD. Proc Natl Acad Sci USA 1993;90:8098–8102.
16. Westerlund JA, Weisgraber KH. J Biol Chem 1993;268:15745–15750.
17. Badimon JJ, Kottke BA, Chen TC, Chan L, Mao SJT. Atherosclerosis 1986;61:57–66.
18. Rosenfeld ME, Butler S, Ord VA, Lipton BA, Dyer CA, Curtiss LK, Palinski W, Witztum JL. Arterioscler Thromb 1993;13:1382–1389.
19. Hansson GK, Johasson L, Seifert PS, Stemmer S. Arteriosclerosis 1989;9:567–578.
20. Reddick RL, Zhang SH, Maeda N. Arterioscler Thromb 1994;14:141–147.
21. Kelly MA. PhD Thesis, University of Cincinnati 1991.

Remodeling after angioplasty: a new target for prevention

David P. Faxon and Jesse W. Currier
University of Southern California School of Medicine, Division of Cardiology, 1355 San Pablo Street, Suite 117, Los Angeles, CA 90033, USA

Abstract. Restenosis continues to be the major limitation of angioplasty. The commonly accepted paradigm of the pathophysiology of restenosis is a process of neointimal hyperplasia in response to balloon injury. Despite more than 50 randomized trials, no pharmacological agent has been clearly shown to be effective. Arterial remodeling is well described in de novo atherosclerosis. We hypothesized that remodeling, not intimal hyperplasia, was responsible for restenosis. In an established atherosclerotic rabbit model of restenosis, we have demonstrated that the area circumscribed by the internal elastic lamina (IEL) increased by 20% from acute to 4-week follow-up after angioplasty, and this compensation was able to accommodate nearly 60% of the neointimal formation. When the chronic group was divided into restenotic and nonrestenotic subgroups, the intimal areas in the two subgroups were virtually identical. The difference in the lumen area between restenotic and nonrestenotic vessels was due to the significantly greater IEL area in the nonrestenotic subgroup. In the restenotic arteries, the slope of the correlation between IEL and intimal area was less than 1, while on the nonrestenotic vessels, the slope was greater than 1, such that a given increase in intimal area was associated with preservation of the lumen area. These data and other studies suggest that vascular remodeling is more important than intimal formation in determining chronic lumen diameter. Preliminary clinical studies confirm these findings. These studies suggest that vascular remodeling and extensive intimal formation are responsible for restenosis and may in part account for the paucity of success in clinical trials to date.

Angioplasty remains the most frequently preformed revascularization procedure in the United States. Despite its enormous acceptance as an effective therapy, it continues to be complicated by restenosis in 30–40% of patients, necessitating a repeat procedure in 20% [1]. Despite remarkable advances in technology with a high acute success and low mortality, the incidence of restenosis has changed little since the introduction of the procedure nearly 18 years ago by Dr Andreas Gruentzig. Part of the reason for the lack of success in the past has been the limited understanding of the pathophysiology of restenosis. Extensive experimental studies have extended our knowledge of the process considerably.

Balloon angioplasty, as well as other interventional devices, causes severe vascular damage to the blood vessel wall in the process of enlarging the vessel lumen. Balloon angioplasty enlarges the vessel by stretching the wall and in the process, tears the inner layers of the vessel wall, creating localized dissections. The process that follows this injury and results in restenosis is analogous to generalized wound healing and occurs in nearly all patients [2].

Pathophysiology

Angioplasty results in immediate removal of the endothelial lining with exposure of the subendothelium to circulating blood elements. Experimental studies indicate that platelets immediately adhere and aggregate, with the greatest propensity for thrombus formation at the site of the neointimal tears [2,3]. While thrombosis is not a prominent feature of the acute injury, in the presence of a severe dissection it can lead to abrupt closure and may contribute to restenosis. The stretch injury, as well as the thrombotic and inflammatory response to injury, results in release of growth factors and mitogens, such as platelet-derived growth factor, fibroblast growth factor, and transforming growth factor beta (TGF-β). These powerful mitogenic stimuli activate quiescent smooth muscle cells to change from a contractile phenotype to a secretory phenotype, capable of migrating into the damaged neointima in a manner similar to the migration of fibroblasts into a wound. Proliferation of the smooth muscle cell occurs with secretion of a large amount of extracellular matrix proteins including fibronectin, vitronectin, glycosaminoglycans, collagen and elastin. This granulation phase is then followed by re-endothelialization, return of the smooth muscle cell to a quiescent state, and further organization of the extracellular matrix. This wound-healing process probably occurs in nearly all patients and is a desired outcome, as long as it does not result in significant renarrowing of the lumen. Most pharmacological trials have been based upon the paradigm that restenosis is mainly due to excessive intimal hyperplasia.

Pharmacological trials

Pharmacological efforts to reduce restenosis by inhibition of platelet deposition, thrombosis, and smooth muscle cell proliferation have been remarkably unrewarding in clinical trials, despite considerable experimental data to support the pathophysiological role of these processes in restenosis [4]. Antiplatelet agents have been the most studied to date, with 15 clinical trials reported. Aspirin, both in high and low dose and in combination with dipyridamole, the prostacyclin analogue ciprostene, the serotonin antagonist ketanserin, and thromboxane A2 antagonists have all been tried unsuccessfully. Recently, the EPIC trial using the glycoprotein-receptor antibody GP IIb/IIIa reported a 30% reduction in a composite clinical endpoint and was the first antiplatelet drug to show benefit. Previous studies of coumarin and fish oils have also been unrewarding. Likewise, a number of calcium antagonists have been studied with negative results. The greatest promise had been for antiproliferative agents, but clinical trials of ACE inhibitors, lovastatin, steroids, and angiopeptin (a growth hormone analogue) have also been unsuccessful. Finally, a recent study reported the results of a nitric oxide donor drug, melsidomine, which showed significant clinical and angiographic benefit and suggested a new approach to therapy. Overall, however, the results of these 45 clinical trials studying over 1,200 patients have been remarkably disappointing.

Importance of intimal hyperplasia

There are numerous explanations for the lack of success in the prevention of restenosis pharmacologically. One potential explanation is that intimal hyperplasia is not the principal process responsible for restenosis. Pathological studies have shown that intimal hyperplasia is not a uniform finding in patients at autopsy [5]. Intimal hyperplasia occurred in only 60% of 32 cases in a series by Waller et al., while other studies have shown the incidence to range from 40 to 80% [5]. Pathological analysis of atherectomy specimens also have shown complex atheroma and have not uniformly demonstrated intimal hyperplasia (IH). Garrett et al. reported that IH was evident in 40% of specimens from restenotic native arteries and 60% from restenotic saphenous vein grafts [6]. They also found a significant incidence of IH in de novo lesions of both native and saphenous vein grafts. IH may be a process that occurs spontaneously in atherosclerosis and is not a specific marker of restenosis. Further evidence that IH is not prominent in restenosis comes from the report of O'Brien et al., who reported a low proliferative rate, as determined by anticyclin antibody staining, in over 60 atherectomy specimens [7]. Regardless of when the specimen was obtained (2—24 weeks), the proliferation index was less than 5%, with many samples showing no proliferation and only a few showing proliferation of more than 30%. Not all studies agree with these findings, and higher degrees of proliferation have been reported. Nevertheless, taken together, these findings raise the possibility that mechanisms other than thrombosis and intimal hyperplasia are primarily responsible for restenosis.

Compensatory enlargement

Enlargement of coronary and peripheral vessels during the development of atherosclerosis was first described in primate studies. The enlargement was capable of maintaining lumen patency during the development of atherosclerosis [8]. In 1987, Glagov et al. described compensatory enlargement in man. These investigators demonstrated that in 136 hearts obtained at autopsy the left main coronary artery enlarged during the development of atherosclerosis [9]. They showed that the area circumscribed by the internal elastic lamina enlarged in proportion to the increase in plaque area until the stenosis reached 40%. Plaque area was most important, but other factors including age and heart weight also had an influence. Subsequent pathological and intravascular ultrasound studies have also shown that compensatory enlargement occurs in all the coronary vessels, as well as peripheral vessels [10]. In 44 consecutive patients, Hermiller showed that compensatory enlargement occurred in all three coronaries, with a close relationship between internal elastic lamina area and plaque area [11]. As had been shown by Glagov, when the area stenosis exceeded 30%, lumen patency was not preserved and instead narrowed in response to increases in plaque volume. The ubiquitous nature of this finding is shown by similar observations in peripheral vessels [12].

Remodeling after angioplasty

Recently, experimental data from our laboratory and others have also confirmed that compensatory changes in vessel size occurs in restenosis [13—15]. Utilizing an atherosclerotic New Zealand white rabbit model, we demonstrated that arteries compensatively dilate following angioplasty [13]. Morphometric analysis of histological cross-sectional areas of vessels from animals killed 4 weeks after angioplasty (n = 37) had a significantly greater vessel circumference and more plaque than those examined immediately after angioplasty (n = 11). Because of a 20% increase in vessel size, lumen area diminished only moderately (48%). The impact of this compensation is illustrated in Fig. 1, where the effect of lesser degrees of compensation is shown. If no compensation had occurred, the lumen would have been totally occluded. When the arteries from the chronic group were analyzed separately, a range of stenosis was seen. The groups with restenotic arteries and nonrestenotic arteries had identical plaque area. The nonrestenotic vessels, however, had a larger vessel circumference than the stenotic vessels. Surprisingly, the minimal lumen diameter did not correlate with the plaque area, but did so strongly with the internal elastic laminal area. The slope of the correlation for the restenotic group was less than 1, while it was greater than 1 for the nonrestenotic group, indicating that for any degree of intimal hyperplasia the artery enlarged to a lesser degree. In addition, those arteries that developed minimal intimal hyperplasia after angioplasty developed constriction of the artery rather than dilation. Thus, these studies in the atherosclerotic rabbit indicate that restenosis is more related to the degree of compensation than to the degree of intimal

688

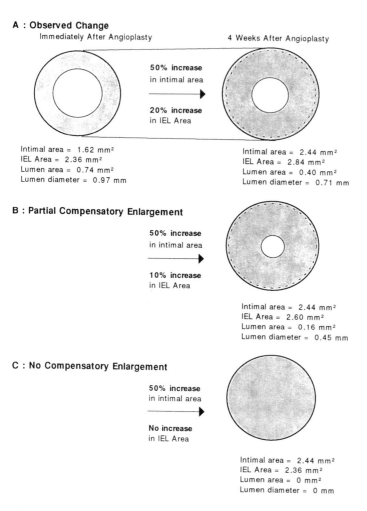

A : Observed Change

Immediately After Angioplasty   4 Weeks After Angioplasty

50% increase
in intimal area

20% increase
in IEL Area

Intimal area = 1.62 mm²
IEL Area = 2.36 mm²
Lumen area = 0.74 mm²
Lumen diameter = 0.97 mm

Intimal area = 2.44 mm²
IEL Area = 2.84 mm²
Lumen area = 0.40 mm²
Lumen diameter = 0.71 mm

B : Partial Compensatory Enlargement

50% increase
in intimal area

10% increase
in IEL Area

Intimal area = 2.44 mm²
IEL Area = 2.60 mm²
Lumen area = 0.16 mm²
Lumen diameter = 0.45 mm

C : No Compensatory Enlargement

50% increase
in intimal area

No increase
in IEL Area

Intimal area = 2.44 mm²
IEL Area = 2.36 mm²
Lumen area = 0 mm²
Lumen diameter = 0 mm

Fig. 1. Restenosis in a rabbit model resulted in a 50% increase in intimal area. However, the 20% increase in internal elastic lamina (IEL) prevented the lumen from narrowing beyond 48% (A). If no compensatory dilation had occurred with an equal degree of internal growth, the lumen would have been totally occluded (C). Reproduced from [13] with permission.

hyperplasia [13]. In a similar experimental study in rabbits and swine, Post showed that following balloon or laser injury, constriction of the dilated vessel segment occurred that was more responsible for the final lumen diameter than intimal hyperplasia [14]. A similar observation has been reported by Lafont et al. in an atherosclerotic rabbit model [15]. All of these experimental studies support the concept that restenosis is not primarily the result of intimal hyperplasia with lumen encroachment from an expanding plaque, but the result of either lack of compensatory enlargement or inappropriate constriction of the artery.

Changes in vessel size after angioplasty also occur in man. Intravascular ultrasound studies in the coronary arteries confirm similar changes. Mintz et al. showed that the change in external elastic laminal area was more responsible for lumen narrowing than plaque area, when ultrasound images from before, immediately after, and after 6 months or at restenosis were compared [16]. In this study, vessel constriction occurred more often than vessel enlargement. A preliminary study from our laboratory by Beer et al. has shown that restenotic lesions are less dilated than de novo lesions in vessels of similar size with an equal degree of stenosis [17].

The mechanism of remodeling remains poorly defined. In a series of studies, Glagov et al. were able to demonstrate that compensatory enlargement was greater when blood flow and wall shear were high [10]. Conversely, when flow was diminished constriction occurred that was partially regulated by endothelial mechanisms. Regression studies in primates resulted in greater degrees of vessel dilation, often exceeding the degree of plaque growth and resulting in overcompensation.

Changes in deposition and organization of the extracellular matrix (ECM) may also play an important role. Collagen is the major structural protein in the ECM and is in part regulated by the growth factor TGF-β [18]. Degradation of ECM is controlled by a family of melanoproteinases which in turn are regulated by inhibitors (TIMPS) [19]. TGF-β is also important in regulating this tightly controlled proteinase system.

While the mechanisms responsible for the compensatory enlargement remain to be elucidated, these studies suggest an important new direction for intervention that may lead to a reduction in this major clinical problem.

References

1. Nobuyoshi M et al. J Am Coll Cardiol 1991;17:433−439.
2. Forrester JS et al. J Am Coll Cardiol 1991;17:758−769.
3. Ip JH et al. J Am Coll Cardiol 1991;17:77B−88B.
4. Franklin SM, Faxon DP. Cor Artery Dis 1993;4:232−242.
5. Waller BF et al. J Am Coll Cardiol 1991;17:58B−70B.
6. Garratt KN et al. J Am Coll Cardiol 1991;17:442−448.
7. O'Brien et al. Circ Res 1993;73:223−231.
8. Kaplan JR et al. Arterioscler Thromb 1993;13:254−262.
9. Glagov S et al. N Engl J Med 1987;316:1371−1375.
10. Glagov S. Circulation 1994;89:2888−2891.
11. Hermiller JB et al. Am J Cardiol 1993;71:665−668.
12. Losorda DW et al. Circulation 1994;89:2570−2577.
13. Kakuta T et al. Circulation 1994;89:2809−2815.
14. Post MJ et al. Circulation 1994;89:2816−2821.
15. Lafont AM et al. J Am Coll Cardiol 1994;23:137A (abstract).
16. Mintz GS et al. J Am Coll Cardiol 1994;23:138A (abstract).
17. Bier JD et al. J Am Coll Cardiol 1994;23:139A (abstract).
18. Amemto EP et al. Arterioscler Thromb 1991;11:1223−1230.
19. Woessner JF. FASEB J 1991;5:2145−2154.

Cellular activation in restenosis following angioplasty

Peter Libby[1], Galina Sukhova[1], Roger Kranzhöfer[1] and Hiroyuki Tanaka[1,2]

[1]Vascular Medicine and Atherosclerosis Unit, Cardiovascular Division, Department of Medicine, Brigham and Women's Hospital, and Harvard Medical School, Boston, Massachusetts, USA; and [2]Department of Cardiothoracic Surgery, Tokyo Medical and Dental University, Tokyo, Japan

Each new advance with respect to the technique of angioplasty, from simple balloons to laser-assisted angioplasty and atherectomy by various devices, has raised hopes that the new technique would obviate restenosis. With more judicious assessment, each such innovation in turn has yielded rates of restenosis at least equal to those after simple balloon techniques. Recently, the possibility that intravascular stents might avoid restenosis has received much attention. Indeed, because a greater luminal diameter is achieved immediately after the procedure, patients receiving coronary artery stents usually have a greater luminal diameter at follow-up than patients treated with balloon angioplasty alone [1,2]. However, the percentage decline of the minimum luminal diameter (determined by quantitative coronary angiography) in the stent-treated patient is even greater than that in the patients receiving simple balloon angioplasty (Table 1). A similar situation may pertain to aggressive atherectomy. These two technical modifications illustrate the principle that "bigger is better", but do not show that these interventions actually reduce the biological process that underlies restenosis.

Indeed, the problem of hyperplastic responses to vascular interventions extends well beyond angioplasty. Failure of vein grafts and of small-caliber arterial prosthetic grafts commonly results from formation of a hyperplastic lesion, often at the distal anastomosis site. These anastomotic lesions share many characteristics of restenotic vessels. The long-term solution to avoiding these complications of interventional and operative therapies for occlusive vascular disease will evidently require mastery over the biology of the arterial wall rather than increasing our armamentarium of interventional devices.

The restenosis problem has proven quite intractable to "shotgun" therapy with various pharmacologic regimens based on supposed, but unproven, biological mechanisms. For example, in the early days of coronary angioplasty, thrombosis and its sequelae were

Table 1. Late loss of acute gain in two clinical trials comparing balloon angioplasty with stent placement

	Minimum luminal diameter (mm)		
	Immediately after	Δ 6 months later	% loss
"BENESTENT" [1]			
Balloon	0.97 ± 0.39	0.32 ± 0.47	33
Stent	1.40 ± 0.44	0.65 ± 0.57	46
"STRESS" [2]			
Balloon	1.23 ± 0.48	0.38 ± 0.66	31
Stent	1.72 ± 0.46	0.74 ± 0.58	43

Address for correspondence: Peter Libby MD, Brigham and Women's Hospital, 221 Longwood Avenue, Boston, MA 02115, USA. Tel.: +1-617-732-6628. Fax: +1-617-732-6961.

considered the most likely instigators of restenosis. This conjecture led to several trials with various anticoagulant and antithrombotic regimens, none of which yielded worthwhile advances against restenosis. Most recently, interest has centered on encouraging initial results with administration of antibodies directed against platelet glycoprotein IIb/IIIa [3]. This therapy does decrease acute thrombotic events following angioplasty, and had some longer-term clinical success [3,4]. However, to date, there is no evidence that any antiplatelet or anticoagulant regimen actually retards restenosis measured by accepted quantitative angiographic parameters. Thus, our best attempts at interfering with thrombosis and coagulation have met with frustration.

Another difficulty with inculpating thrombosis as the sole pathogenic process in restenosis rests on the disparity between the time course of restenosis (which peaks somewhere after 3 months in humans after coronary angioplasty) and platelet deposition (which subsides within days after the acute intervention). Faced with these facts and in the spirit of enhancing our knowledge of the biology of the events that ensue after arterial injury, we embarked some years ago on studies aimed at evaluating the more chronic aspects of cellular activation following restenosis. We reasoned that by examining the longer time course and characteristics of the cellular response to injury we might gain insight into types of signals leading to the delayed cellular responses in restenosis.

For this purpose we selected the rabbit as an experimental animal. The characterization of certain convenient markers and the ability eventually to study injury to atherosclerotic vessels led to this choice. We produced a balloon injury to the infrarenal abdominal aorta using standard techniques, and monitored indices of cellular activation over 1 month following injury. The markers we used (Table 2) were chosen not so much because of the interesting functions of the molecules scrutinized but because of their well-defined structure and regulation and ready availability of reagents for their detection in rabbits.

Within the first few days after balloon-withdrawal injury, endothelial regeneration began at the border zone of the injured area with the uninjured proximal aorta. The regenerating endothelial cells, rigorously identified by cell-typing reagents and by incorporation of proliferation marker (BrdU), bore all three markers of activation studied [5]. By 10 days after injury, endothelial healing had progressed. Endothelial expression of the activation markers began to subside in the more distantly healed regions near the border zone while the leading edge of endothelial regrowth contained cells bearing these activation markers. More strikingly, the neointimal smooth muscle cells exhibited floridly expressed intercellular adhesion molecule 1 (ICAM-1), a molecule expressed normally at almost undetectable levels on vascular smooth muscle cells by the techniques employed.

Most noteworthy and interesting to us were the results obtained 1 month after balloon injury. Although detectable local platelet deposition and acute thrombosis ceased nearly 4 weeks before this time, we found that endothelial cells at the leading edge of regrowth still expressed activation markers and residual augmented ICAM-1 expression in neointimal smooth muscle cells (although to a lesser extent than at 10 days after injury). Astonishingly, we saw many cells bearing Class II histocompatibility antigens at this late time-point. This observation has interesting implications as the only signal we know that

Table 2. Activation markers studied in rabbit aorta after balloon injury

Vascular cell adhesion molecule-1 (VCAM-1)
Intercellular adhesion molecule-1 (ICAM-1)
Class II major histocompatibility antigen (MHC II)
Tumor necrosis factor alpha (TNF-α)

elevates Class II histocompatibility molecule expression by vascular smooth muscle cells is immune interferon (interferon γ), a product of activated immunocytes such as T lymphocytes, a cell type present even in this previously normal vessel after injury [6]. Thus, we found unexpected and surprising evidence for immune activation long after balloon injury in this experimental preparation.

The ultimate message to us from these studies was that vascular cells display signs of activation even a month after acute balloon injury. Since cytokines regulate each of the markers that we studied, we inferred the possibility that prolonged cytokine signaling may contribute to the ongoing activation of cells in the injured artery long after the injury.

Other studies focused on the expression of one particular cytokine, tumor necrosis factor-α (TNF-α), because it can induce expression of two of the markers studied: ICAM-1 and vascular cell adhesion molecule-1 (VCAM-1). TNF can also simulate smooth-muscle proliferation, a process thought by some to contribute to restenosis [7,8]. We found substantial evidence for TNF expression at least 10 days after injury. Extracts of injured portions of aorta at this time contained higher levels of messenger RNA encoding TNF-α than did control uninjured portions of the aorta, as determined by reverse transcriptase, polymerase chain reaction technology. Moreover, immunodetectable TNF-α localized to smooth muscle cells in the injured, but not uninjured zones. Previous studies from our laboratory had established that smooth muscle cells can express the TNF-α gene [9]. Interestingly, double immunohistochemical labeling studies indicated colocalization of markers of proliferation and TNF-α expression. We concluded that TNF-α expression provides yet another marker of continuing vascular activation after balloon injury. Our observations also raised the intriguing possibility that TNF-α may participate as a mitogenic signal or inducer of mitogens in smooth muscle cells of injured arteries.

These studies indicated that smooth muscle cells themselves may be a source of an autocrine regulator, TNF-α. However, in terms of cytokine production, intrinsic vascular wall cells are generally considered much less abundant sources of cytokines than "professional" phagocytic cells such as macrophages. Atherosclerotic lesions contain abundant macrophages, a feature not replicated in usual animal models for restenosis after injury, including those experiments just described. Therefore, we postulated some years ago that macrophages may furnish an amplification loop for maintaining and propagating cytokine signals after injury to atherosclerotic vessels [10].

We have also been intrigued by the possibility that thrombin, a stimulus clearly activated in the acute phases of arterial injury, might elicit subsequent signals from macrophages and play a principal role as initiator of a cytokine cascade following vascular injury. Although thrombin has been known for decades to activate proliferation of smooth muscle cells, scant data in the literature substantiate its effect as a macrophage activator. Accordingly, we undertook a more detailed study of the effect of thrombin on macrophage functions. Having hypothesized an important role for macrophages in amplifying thrombin signals, we were disappointed to find that it took extraordinarily high concentrations of thrombin to elicit very weak signs of activation from macrophages. For example, we found that it took micromolar concentrations of thrombin to induce macrophages to produce amounts of the cytokines IL6 and TNF-α several orders of magnitude below those readily achievable by endotoxin stimulation. We also found that human blood monocytes did not develop calcium transients following thrombin stimulation whereas they readily reacted to formyl-Met-Leu-Phe. Moreover, we could not document by fluorescent activated cell sorting or by Northern blotting the expression by human monocytes of the protein or mRNA for the cloned thrombin receptor (reagents generously supplied by Dr Shaun Coughlin) [11].

As a control for these studies of the effect of thrombin on activation of mononuclear phagocytes, we studied human vascular smooth muscle cells, and found that human smooth muscle cells readily responded to nanomolar concentrations of thrombin to release IL6. Our laboratory had previously noted the ability of vascular smooth muscle cells to express the IL6 gene inducibly [12,13]. Such low concentrations of thrombin also elicited calcium transients from smooth muscle cells, which did bear the thrombin receptor determined as described above.

Thus, although we had initially hypothesized that macrophages within lesions played an important role as an amplifier of thrombin signals, our data indicate that smooth muscle cells themselves respond directly to thrombin by producing cytokines, and may act as important transducers of thrombin's effects as initiator of vascular injury.

These studies have convinced us that chronic activation of vascular cells, particularly smooth muscle cells, persists long after injury. We have yet to work out the molecular stimuli that maintain this prolonged activation. However, cytokines, including those produced by smooth muscle cells, remain intriguing candidates. Recent data indicate that the previous focus on cell proliferation as a major mechanism for production of the restenotic lesion may not pertain to human coronary arteries after angioplasty [14]. Furthermore, extracellular matrix rather than cells comprises much of the volume of restenotic lesions. Thus, future research into the cell biology of restenosis must focus on the signals for matrix accumulation, much as past research has considered proliferation.

Acknowledgements

This work was supported by a grant to Peter Libby, MD, from the National Heart, Lung and Blood Institute of the USA, PO-1 HL-48743 subsuming RO-1-HL-47840. Roger Kranzhöfer is a fellow of the Deutsche Forschungsgemeinschaft.

References

1. Serruys PW, de Jaegere JP, Kiemeneij F, Macaya C, Rutsch W, Heyndrickx G, Emanuelsson H, Marco J, Legrand V, Materne P et al. N Engl J Med 1994;331:489−495.
2. Fischman DL, Leon MB, Baim DS et al. N Engl J Med 1994;331:496−501.
3. The EPIC Investigation. N Engl J Med 1994;330:956−961.
4. Topol EJ, Califf RM, Weisman HF, Ellis SG et al. Lancet 1994;343:881−886.
5. Tanaka H, Sukhova GK, Swanson SJ et al. Circulation 1993;88:1788−1803.
6. Warner SJC, Friedman GB, Libby P. Arteriosclerosis 1989;9:279−288.
7. Sawada H, Kan M, McKeehan WL. Cell Dev Biol 1990;26:213−216.
8. Palmer H, Libby P. Lab Invest 1992;66:715−721.
9. Warner SJC, Libby P. J Immunol 1989;142:100−109.
10. Libby P, Schwartz D, Brogi E, Tanaka H, Clinton SK. Circulation 1992;86(III):47−52.
11. Vu TK, Hung DT, Wheaton VI, Coughlin SR. Cell 1991;64:1057−1068.
12. Loppnow H, Libby P. Lymphokine Res 1989;8:293−299.
13. Loppnow H, Libby P. J Clin Invest 1990;85:731−738.
14. O'Brien ER, Alpers CE, Stewart DK et al. Circ Res 1993;73:223−231.

©1995 Elsevier Science B.V. All rights reserved.
Atherosclerosis X.
F.P. Woodford, J. Davignon and A. Sniderman, editors.

Role of plasminogen activators and their inhibitor PAI-1 in pericellular proteolysis of smooth muscle cells and endothelial cells

Victor W.M. van Hinsbergh, Paul H.A. Quax, Pieter Koolwijk and Jan H. Verheijen

Gaubius Laboratory TNO-PG, P.O. Box 430, 2300 AK Leiden, The Netherlands

Abstract. Cell accumulation in the thickened intima largely depends on migration of blood monocytes and medial smooth muscle cells into the intima, a process that is accompanied by considerable changes in the composition of the extracellular matrix. Plasminogen activators, plasmin and matrix-degrading metalloproteinases play a role in matrix remodeling. Plasminogen activators are both involved in fibrinolysis and pericellular proteolysis. While fibrinolysis within the vessel lumen is regulated by tissue-type plasminogen activator secreted by endothelial cells, receptor-bound urokinase-type plasminogen is involved in the migration of smooth muscle cells, monocytes and endothelial cells and in angiogenesis.

Alterations in the arterial intima depend largely on lipid deposition and migration of cells from the blood (monocytes) and from the arterial media (smooth muscle cells) into the intima. Both the formation of an arteriosclerotic intima and the rapid intimal hyperplasia causing restenosis are accompanied by considerable changes in cell and matrix composition of the intima. It is generally believed that proteases are involved in cell migration and in matrix remodeling. A number of proteases including plasmin, plasminogen activators (PAs), stromelysin, collagenase and gelatinases are involved in matrix remodeling. Stromelysin-1 has also been demonstrated in the human arteriosclerotic vessel wall [1]. In addition, most of the components of the fibrinolytic system, i.e., PAs, their inhibitor PAI-1, and a receptor for urokinase-type PA (uPAR) have been encountered in specimens of human arteriosclerotic tissue and in experimental animals during intimal proliferation induced by balloon injury. The fibrinolytic system or components thereof is not only involved in lysis of fibrin and in recanalization of mural thrombi, but also in the migration of monocyte-derived macrophages, smooth muscle cells and endothelial cells. It probably participates in the activation of stromelysin and other matrix-degrading metalloproteinases.

Role of endothelial PAs in fibrinolysis and pericellular proteolysis

PAs produced by endothelial cells are involved both in the regulation of fibrinolysis and in pericellular proteolysis (Fig. 1). t-PA released from endothelial cells plays a key role in the dissolution of fibrin within the vessel lumen. Both the t-PA synthesis rate and the acute release of t-PA from a cellular storage pool after stimulation of the endothelial cells by vasoactive substances or thrombin are important in the regulation of intravascular fibrinolysis [2]. Fibrinolytic activity is modulated by PAI-1, a specific inhibitor of both PAs. PAI-1 synthesis is absent or very low in normal endothelial cells, but its synthesis is markedly induced after exposure of the endothelium to the inflammatory mediators endotoxin, tumor necrosis factor-α (TNFα) or interleukin-1 (IL-1).

At the albuminal side of the endothelial cell PAs, in particular urokinase-type PA (u-PA), are involved in pericellular proteolysis accompanying cell migration and angiogenesis. u-PA, which is induced in human endothelial cells by endotoxin and the cytokines TNFα and IL-1 [3], binds immediately after secretion to a specific cellular receptor (uPAR) and is converted from its inactive single-chain form into its active two-chain

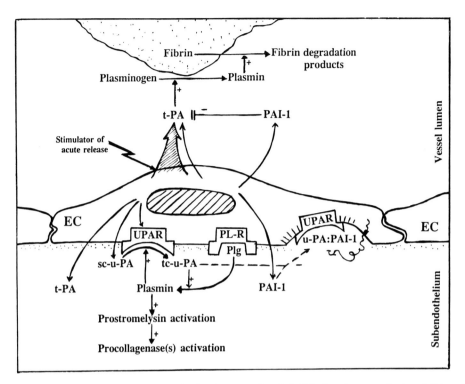

Fig. 1. Schematic representation of the involvement of endothelial plasminogen activators (t-PA, u-PA), plasminogen activator inhibitor (PAI-1) and receptors (uPAR, PL-R) in fibrinolysis and pericellular proteolysis accompanying cell migration. Abbreviations: PA, plasminogen activator; t-PA, tissue-type PA; u-PA, urokinase-type PA; sc-u-PA, single chain u-PA; tc-u-PA, two-chain u-PA; Plg, plasminogen; UPAR, u-PA receptor; PL-R, plasmin(ogen) receptor; PAI-1, PA inhibitor-1; EC, endothelial cell. +, stimulation –, inhibition. (From [7], with permission.)

form. The u-PA:uPAR complex has been localized at focal attachment sites and in areas of cell–cell contacts [4]. It is believed that active receptor-bound u-PA can convert cell-bound plasminogen into plasmin and causes proteolysis of matrix proteins [5,6], by which cell-matrix contacts are disrupted, a process required for cell movement. Active u-PA is rapidly inhibited by PAI-1. The receptor-bound u-PA:PAI-1 complex is subsequently internalized, after which the u-PA:PAI-1 complex detaches from the uPAR and is degraded, while the empty uPAR returns to the plasma membrane. It is likely that the primary function of the induction of PAI-1 by TNFα and IL-1 is to protect the cell environment against uncontrolled u-PA activity.

The expression of uPAR in endothelial cells in vitro is enhanced by basic fibroblast growth factor (bFGF), vascular endothelial cell growth factor (VEGF) or activation of protein kinase C. When a confluent monolayer of human microvascular endothelial cells on a fibrin gel is incubated with bFGF, VEGF and TNFα simultaneously, its cells grow in capillary-like tubular structures into the fibrin gel. This process is inhibited by simultaneous addition of soluble uPAR, anti-u-PA antibodies or trasylol. This suggests that the proteolytic activity of u-PA bound to uPAR plays an essential role in capillary outgrowth into a pure fibrin gel. Whether the u-PA–uPAR interaction additionally transduces signals into the endothelial cell, as for other cell types [8], is not known.

696

Role of u-PA and uPAR in smooth muscle cell and monocyte migration

A role of u-PA and uPAR in the migration of monocytes and smooth muscle cells has also been demonstrated. Estreicher et al. [9] reported the presence of receptor-bound u-PA activity on the invading pseudopodia of monocytes. u-PA and uPAR have been demonstrated immunohistochemically associated with monocyte-derived macrophages in human atherosclerotic plaque. When a culture of smooth muscle cells derived from arterial intima was wounded by removal of a strip of smooth muscle cells, the cells adjacent to the wound migrated into the gap. This was accompanied by an increase in u-PA activity on the cells. The migration was inhibited by the addition of anti-u-PA antibodies, which blocked the enzymatic activity of u-PA, by trasylol, which inhibits plasmin generation, and by soluble uPAR. Whether t-PA can perform a similar role is not yet certain. Clowes et al. [10,11] reported that t-PA expression in the injured vessel wall is associated with smooth muscle migration in the rat carotid artery. On the other hand, it has recently been reported that t-PA can stimulate the proliferation of human smooth muscle cells in vitro [12]. Important questions to be answered are: (a) is this effect direct or the consequence of the liberation of growth factors from the cellular matrix [13]; (b) what makes smooth muscle cells respond to t-PA?

PAs and PAI-1 in arteriosclerosis and restenosis

An enhanced expression of PAs and PAI-1 has been found in specimens of human arteriosclerotic blood vessels and during smooth muscle migration and proliferation in injured animal blood vessels [14,15]. Strong support for a contributing role of the fibrinolytic system in intimal thickening was recently reported by Carmeliet and Collen [16], who showed that intimal thickening after vascular injury was impaired in u-PA-deficient mice and exacerbated in PAI-1-deficient mice. These observations further strengthen the suggestion that the increased expression of PAI-1 in arteriosclerotic blood vessels is also a response to protect the blood vessel against uncontrolled PA activity. Other proteases, such as stromelysin and occasionally gelatinase B, are also expressed in human arteriosclerotic plaque [1]. Because PA/plasmin is able to activate stromelysin and subsequently other matrix-degrading metalloproteinases, it is possible that PA activity may also contribute to remodeling of the collagenous matrix of the vessel wall. Such remodeling may make certain areas of the arteriosclerotic plaque more prone to rupture.

References

1. Henney AM, Wakeley PR, Davies MJ et al. Proc Natl Acad Sci USA 1991;88:8154–8158.
2. Emeis JJ. Ann NY Acad Sci 1992;667:249–258.
3. van Hinsbergh VWM, van den Berg EA, Fiers W, Dooijewaard G. Blood 1990;75:1991–1998.
4. Conforti G, Dominguez-Jimenez C, Rønne E, Høyer-Hansen G, Dejana E. Blood 1994;83:994–1005.
5. Niedbala MJ, Stein Picarella M. Blood 1992;79:678–687.
6. Sperti G, van Leeuwen RTJ, Quax PHA, Maseri A, Kluft C. Circ Res 1992;71:385–392.
7. van Hinsbergh VWM, Hanemaaijer R, Koolwijk P. In: Maragoudakis ME, Gullino P, Lelkes P (eds) Angiogenesis: Molecular Biology, Clinical Aspects. London: Plenum Publishing Company Ltd, 1994;171–182.
8. Dumler I, Petri T, Schleuning W-D. FEBS Lett 1994;343:103–106.
9. Estreicher A, Mühlhauser J, Carpentier J-L, Orci L, Vassalli J-D. J Cell Biol 1990;111:783–792.
10. Clowes AW, Clowes MM, Au T, Reidy MA, Belin D. Circ Res 1990;67:61–67.
11. Clowes AW, Clowes MM, Kirkman TR, Jackson CL, Au YPT, Kenagy R. Circ Res 1992;70:1128–1136.
12. Herbert JM, Lamarche I, Prabonnaud V, Dol F, Gauthier T. J Biol Chem 1994;269:3076–3080.
13. Falcone DJ, McCaffrey TA, Haimovitz-Friedman A et al. J Biol Chem 1993;268:11951–11958.
14. Schneiderman J, Swadey MS, Keeton MK et al. Proc Natl Acad Sci USA 1992;89:6998–7002.
15. Lupu F, Bergonzelli GE, Heim DA et al. Arterioscl Thromb 1993;13:1090–1100.
16. Carmeliet P, Collen D. VIIIth Int Symp Biology of the Vascular Cell, Heidelberg, Sept 1994.

Analysis of recombinant gene expression and function in arteries following direct gene transfer

Elizabeth G. Nabel

University of Michigan, Medical Center, Ann Arbor, MI 48109-0644, USA

Direct gene transfer is the introduction of recombinant genes into host cells and represents a new approach to the investigation of gene expression and function. Our laboratory has been interested in examining the function of growth-factor genes during the development of vascular lesions in vivo using direct gene transfer.

Gene expression and function

We have investigated the mechanisms of cellular proliferation following the expression of three growth-factor genes in porcine arteries in vivo. These recombinant growth-factor genes include platelet-derived growth factor B (PDGF B), a secreted form of fibroblast growth factor-1 (FGF-1), and a secreted form of active transforming growth factor-β (TGF-β1). Data from human atherosclerosis specimens and gene-targeting studies suggest a role for these growth factors in the pathogenesis of vascular lesions, but their direct effects in vivo have been difficult to analyze. Gene transfer permits the analysis of gene expression and function within target tissues. Therefore, to explore the function of these growth factors in situ, we constructed plasmid expression vectors and tested them in vitro in porcine endothelial and smooth muscle cells (SMC). Gene-transfer experiments were then performed in vivo by transfection of the plasmid expression vector into focal segments of porcine peripheral arteries using cationic liposomes. Control experiments were performed by transfection of a reporter gene into porcine arteries. Gene expression and biological function were analyzed 21 days later. Arteries transfected with a PDGF B gene showed intimal thickening, characterized by increased smooth muscle cell proliferation during the first 14 days after gene transfer [1]. Continued expansion of the intima after 14 days was observed, and resulted from increased procollagen synthesis. Intimal lesions were stable from 21 to 60 days following transfer of the PDGF B gene.

Intimal thickening was also present in arteries transfected with a FGF-1 gene; however, in contrast to PDGF B gene-transfected arteries, intimal angiogenesis was observed [2]. This formation of capillaries in the intima was most prominent in vessels with advanced intimal lesions. Immunohistochemical studies suggested that capillary endothelial cells are derived from luminal endothelium. Current studies are investigating whether other cofactors, such as VEGF and FGF-2, may contribute to the intimal angiogenesis in addition to FGF-1. Porcine arteries transduced with a TGF-β1 gene showed intimal thickening characterized by increased procollagen synthesis [3]. This increase in extracellular matrix was apparent within the first 4 days after gene transfer.

These studies suggested that expression of PDGF B, FGF-1 and TGF-β1 genes have distinct effects on arterial morphology, including different effects on the proliferation of SMCs, angiogenesis, and extracellular matrix synthesis. Intimal thickening after vascular injury is a complex process, resulting from the expression of several growth-factor and cytokine genes.

Modification of cell proliferation

Several strategies might be employed to inhibit these consequences of vascular injury. Targeting of single growth factors could be performed, although our earlier studies suggested that inhibition of a single growth factor may be insufficient to limit intimal thickening. Another approach is to target nuclear cell-cycle regulatory pathways in SMC. Some of these factors might include cell-cycle genes, such as cdc and cdc kinases [4,5]; proto-oncogenes c-myb and c-myc [6,7]; proliferating cell nuclear antigen [4,8]; or suppressor genes, such as p53 and p21 [9,10]. A third approach is the selective elimination of dividing cells using cytotoxic agents.

We [11] and others [12] have taken the latter approach in order to examine the role of a herpes-virus thymidine-kinase (HSV-tk) gene and ganciclovir treatment in limiting the cell proliferation that follows vascular injury. Since the accumulation of vascular SMCs constitutes a major feature of vascular proliferative disorders, we hypothesized that transfection of an antiproliferative gene into an injured arterial segment during the peak of SMC division might limit intimal hyperplasia. One common approach to the selective elimination of dividing cells is to express a HSV-tk gene in SMCs. HSV-tk converts the nucleoside analog ganciclovir into a phosphorylated form in transduced cells, and the subsequent incorporation of phosphorylated ganciclovir into cellular DNA induces cell death [13]. Thymidine-kinase gene expression and ganciclovir treatment have been explored in several tumor models where HSV-tk gene expression renders cells susceptible to ganciclovir, resulting in the elimination of dividing tumor cells [14,15].

We initiated experiments to examine the feasibility of using a HSV-tk gene and ganciclovir approach to limit smooth muscle cell proliferation in porcine arteries following balloon injury [11]. We first conducted experiments in vitro in porcine SMCs and endothelial cells which demonstrated the presence of a bystander effect in these vascular cells. Subsequent experiments in porcine arteries established that after balloon injury, SMC proliferation increased rapidly during the first week and declined by the end of 2 weeks. In addition, infection of injured porcine arteries with an adenoviral vector encoding an alkaline-phosphatase reporter gene resulted in gene expression in SMCs in the intima and luminal region of the media, exactly the pool of SMCs which proliferate and produce intimal lesions. We introduced adenoviral vectors encoding HSV-tk (ADV-tk) or a control vector (ADV-ΔE1) into balloon-injured porcine arteries, and treated the animals with ganciclovir (+GC) or saline (–GC). Introduction of the tk gene into intimal and medial SMCs in vivo rendered them sensitive to treatment with ganciclovir. A 40% reduction in cell proliferation, measured by BrdC labeling, was detected 7 days after gene transfer in ADV-tk/+GC vs. ADV-tk/-GC arteries. Lower intima:medial (I/M) area ratios were observed in ADV-tk/+GC arteries than in ADV-tk/-GC arteries at 3 weeks (59%) and 6 weeks (48%) after gene transfer or in arteries infected with a control vector treated with ganciclovir (ADV-ΔE1/+GC) (54%) or saline (ADV-ΔE1/–GC) (57%). These studies suggest that direct gene transfer of a HSV-tk gene in injured arteries allows sufficient conversion of ganciclovir at the site of pathology to limit cellular proliferation in vivo. Gene transfer of an antiproliferative gene into arteries after balloon injury may provide insight into the pathogenesis and treatment of vascular diseases.

References

1. Nabel EG, Yang Z, Liptay S, San H, Gordon D, Haudenschild CC, Nabel GJ. J Clin Invest 1993;91:1822–1829.

2. Nabel EG, Yang Z, Plautz G, Forough R, Zhan X, Haudenschild CC, Maciag T, Nabel GJ. Nature 1993;362:844–846.
3. Nabel EG, Shum L, Pompili VJ, Yang ZY, San H, Shu HB, Liptay S, Gordon D, Derynck R, Nabel GJ. Proc Natl Acad Sci USA 1993;90:10759–10763.
4. Morishita R, Gibbons GH, Ellison KE, Nakajima M, Zhang L, Kaneda Y, Ogihara T, Dzau VJ. Proc Natl Acad Sci USA 1993;90:8474–8478.
5. Morishita R, Gibbons GJ, Ellison KE, Nakajima M, von der Leyen H, Zhang L, Kaneda Y, Ogihara T, Dzau VJ. J Clin Invest 1994;93:1458–1464.
6. Simons M, Edelman ER, DeKeyser JL, Langer R, Rosenberg RD. Nature 1992;359:67–70.
7. Shi Y, Fard A, Galeo A, Hutchinson HG, Vermani P, Dodge GR, Hall DJ, Shaheen F, Zalewski A. Circulation 1994;90:944–951.
8. Simons M, Edelman ER, Rosenberg RD. J Clin Invest 1994;93:2351–2356.
9. Yonish-Rouach E, Resnitzky D, Lotem J, Sachs L, Kimchi A, Oren M. Nature 1991;352:345–347.
10. Waga S, Hannon GJ, Beach D, Stillman B. Nature 1994;369:574–578.
11. Ohno T, Gordon D, San H, Pompili VJ, Imperiale MJ, Nabel GJ, Nabel EG. Science 1994;265:781–784.
12. Guzman RJ, Hirschowitz EA, Brody SL, Crystal RG, Epstein SE, Finkel T. Proc Natl Acad Sci USA 1994; (in press).
13. Smith KO, Galloway KS, Kennell WL, Ogilvie KK, Radatus BK. Antimicrob Agents Chemother 1982;22:55–61.
14. Culver KW, Ram Z, Wallbridge S, Ishii H, Oldfield EH, Blaese RM. Science 1992;256:1550–1552.
15. Chen S-H, Shine HD, Goodman JC, Grossman RG, Woo SLC. Proc Natl Acad Sci USA 1994;91:3054–3057.

Vascular smooth muscle cell proliferation: basic investigations and new therapeutic approaches

Robert D. Rosenberg

Beth Israel Hospital and Harvard Medical School, Boston, Massachusetts; and Massachusetts Institute of Technology, Cambridge, Massachusetts, USA

The smooth muscle cells (SMC) of the blood vessel wall are normally present in a relatively quiescent state. However, arterial injury or vascular disease induces a proliferative response. The mitogens involved in inducing SMC growth include PDGF, IGF-1, bFGF, EGF and IL-1 [1]. The interactions of these growth factors with their specific SMC receptors induce a complex series of biochemical reactions involving protein kinase C, receptor-linked tyrosine phosphorylation, and cAMP-dependent kinases which culminate in the activation of DNA-binding proteins and the initiation of DNA replication as well as cell division. The signal-transduction pathway which links receptor activation with SMC proliferation includes induction of c-myc and c-fos mRNA at 30 min to 2 h with a decline to normal by 12 h; expression of c-myb at 8–12 h with a decline to normal by 16 h; transcription of histone H3 message at 16–20 h with a decline to normal by 24 h; and the appearance of nonmuscle myosin message relatively late in the cell cycle. However, it is unclear whether any of the above intracellular events are critical for SMC proliferation.

The oncogene c-myb is a DNA-binding protein which may play an important role in SMC growth. The oncogene is homologous to the transforming gene of the avian myeloblastosis virus and was originally thought to be present only in hematopoietic cells. However, c-myb is synthesized by chick embryo fibroblasts as well as proliferating SMC and may also be produced by other cell types. The expression of the proto-oncogene is growth-dependent; it occurs at low levels in quiescent cells, increases rapidly as cells begin to proliferate and peaks in the late G_1 phase of the cell cycle. The oncogene appears to regulate cellular growth. Thus, expression of the oncogene in fibroblasts directly or indirectly induces the appearance of DNA polymerase alpha, histone H3, as well as PCNA mRNAs by a posttranscriptional mechanism and permits the cells to enter the S phase. Heparin, as well as the closely related heparan sulfate proteoglycans, suppress SMC proliferation in vivo as well as in vitro [2]. The block occurs in the late G_1 phase of the cell cycle and is associated with a decrease in c-myb levels [2] as well as a partial return of expression of SMC-specific contractile proteins. The observation that heparin's suppression of SMC growth is associated with a decrease in c-myb message level and the known effects of the proto-oncogene suggest an important role for c-myb in SMC proliferation. We confirmed the above hypothesis by adding c-myb antisense oligonucleotides to SMC under in vitro conditions and observing decreased levels of c-myb mRNA and protein as well as suppression in growth [3]. In the section below, we summarize recent data from our laboratory which outline the mechanism of action of the proto-oncogene as a regulator of calcium influx at the G_1/S interface of the cell cycle.

Address for correspondence: Department of Biology, Massachusetts Institute of Technology, 68-480, 77 Massachusetts Avenue, Cambridge, MA 02139, USA.

The intracellular levels of calcium are involved in controlling cell-cycle progression and cell growth. It is widely appreciated that transient increases of intracellular calcium occur early in mitosis and during anaphase [4]. These elevations appear to be required for disappearance of the nuclear envelope, condensation of chromosomes, breakdown of mitotic spindles and activation of the contractile ring [5,6]. The regulation by intracellular calcium concentrations of the G_1 to S-transition is less thoroughly documented. For the above reasons, we measured the intracellular ionized-calcium concentrations of SMC early in the cell cycle and then ascertained whether c-myb which is differentially expressed at this time might be responsible for the observed variations [7].

We employed SV40LT-SMC (a large T-transformed smooth muscle cell line) to investigate changes in intracellular calcium levels during cell cycle progression. To this end, SMC were growth-arrested and then stimulated by addition of media containing growth factor. The concentrations of intracellular ionized calcium were determined at 8-h intervals. The data obtained by full-field image analysis of representative cells using Fura-2 demonstrate that intracellular calcium levels are unchanged for the first 8 h, decline at 16 h, rise to the initial levels at 24 h, and drop back again at 32 h. Flow cytometric analysis of cellular DNA shows partial cell-cycle synchronization and reveals that increased intracellular calcium levels occur at 24 h as the cell population enters S phase. Identical experiments have been carried out with primary rat aortic SMC, isolated as previously described, with similar changes in intracellular levels of ionized calcium [7].

The concentrations of c-myb mRNA in SV40LT-SMC were then determined by dot-blot analysis with normalization to GAPDH mRNA which demonstrate that message levels are low in growth-arrested cells (0 h), increase significantly at 16 h (late G_1), and reach a maximum at 24 h (G_1/S interface). Thus, the increased concentrations of proto-oncogene mRNA precede the elevation in intracellular calcium levels. The measurements of intracellular calcium in SV40LT-SMC were repeated after addition of antisense or missense c-myb oligonucleotides prior to serum stimulation. The concentrations of antisense oligonucleotide selected had previously been shown to inhibit proto-oncogene expression and block S-phase progression in this cell-culture system [3]. These experiments show that addition of antisense c-myb oligonucleotide, as compared to missense c-myb oligonucleotide, almost completely suppresses elevated $[Ca^{2+}]_i$ levels seen at 24 h, but not at 0 h [7]. Therefore, the increased concentrations of intracellular calcium at the G_1/S interface appear to be under the control of c-myb, whereas the molecular events responsible for increased concentrations of intracellular calcium at G_0 and decreased intracellular calcium levels at G_1 are unknown. However, c-myb might function in a very indirect manner to raise intracellular calcium levels by allowing cells to progress to a point in the cell cycle which is associated with elevations of divalent cation.

To exclude this possibility, we determined whether expression of c-myb could directly elevate intracellular calcium concentrations independent of growth state. We accomplished this by stably transfecting SV40LT-SMC with the proto-oncogene, demonstrating that the levels of c-myb mRNA as well as the oncoprotein were elevated 2- to 4-fold and then measuring the concentrations of intracellular calcium [7]. Full-field imaging with Fura-2 shows that growth-arrested transfected cells, as compared to growth-arrested untransfected cells, exhibit an elevated but relatively homogeneous distribution of calcium concentrations. The measurements reveal a substantial increase in Fura-2 ratios which correspond to an average 1.8-fold increase in the levels of intracellular calcium (158 ± 15.6 nM vs. 92 ± 9.6 nM, p < 0.05) [7].

We also exposed the growth-arrested transfected and untransfected cells to antisense c-myb oligonucleotide or antisense two-base-pair mismatch c-myb oligonucleotide. The treatment of growth-arrested transfected cells with antisense c-myb oligonucleotide, but not two-base-pair mismatch oligonucleotide, completely abolishes elevated concentrations of intracellular calcium while the treatment of similarly designated untransfected control cells with antisense c-myb oligonucleotide had no effect on the levels of intracellular calcium [7]. Northern analysis showed a 2.5-fold reduction in the concentrations of c-myb message in growth-arrested transfected cells after exposure to antisense c-myb oligonucleotide, as well as the lack of effect on proto-oncogene message with antisense two-base-pair mismatch c-myb oligonucleotide.

We then attempted to determine whether elevated concentrations of intracellular calcium induced by c-myb are secondary to altered influx from extracellular sources or altered efflux from intracellular compartments. To resolve this issue, we measured the levels of $[Ca^{2+}]_i$ in growth-arrested transfected and similarly designated untransfected control cells placed for 5 min in 1 mM calcium-containing buffer, calcium-free buffer, and phosphate-buffered saline supplemented with 2 mM EGTA. The growth-arrested transfected and untransfected control cells exhibited a decline in the concentrations of intracellular ionized calcium to the same final levels. Thus the c-myb-dependent elevations of intracellular calcium are likely to be generated by increased influx of the cation from the external environment rather than increased efflux of the cation from an internal compartment. However, the increased entry of calcium does not appear to occur via L-type channels since nifedipine is unable to suppress the observed alterations and is unlikely to take place via T-type channels since these structures are not usually present in vascular SMC.

The augmented calcium influx could be due to a direct effect of c-myb on a novel calcium channel or an unknown calcium transporter. It is also possible that the proto-oncogene could exert an indirect effect on well-characterized calcium exchangers or antiporters. The structure of c-myb is similar to a typical DNA-binding protein with an N-terminal helix–loop–helix domain as well as a C-terminal leucine zipper motif. The proto-oncogene binds to specific DNA sequences and regulates transcription of known genes such as c-myc and mim-1 [8–9]. Therefore, c-myb is likely to increase concentrations of intracellular calcium by a transcriptional mechanism which alters synthesis of a component of a cation-transport system or which changes production of a protein that modifies activity of a cation-transport system.

We believe that elevated concentrations of intracellular calcium at the G_1/S interface produced by increased expression of c-myb may be essential for cell-cycle progression. Prior investigations have demonstrated that calcium deprivation of many eukaryotic cells, including yeast, induces a temporary growth arrest in late G_1 [6,10]. In preliminary experiments, we have reversed the G_1 arrest of SMC induced with antisense c-myb oligonucleotide by adding small amounts of the calcium ionophore, 4-bromo-A23187, 16 h after serum stimulation. Thus, the normal transition of cells from G_1 to S phase appears to be dependent upon threshold levels of intracellular calcium. On the basis of the available evidence, we suggest that the proto-oncogene elevates intracellular calcium concentrations at late G_1 which regulates S-phase progression of SMC as well as other cell types. This novel mechanism would provide a specific growth-regulatory function for c-myb and might also explain the effects of the proto-oncogene on cell differentiation.

References

1. Ross R, Raines EW, Bowen-Pope DF. Cell 1986;46:155–169.
2. Reilly CF, Kindy MS, Brown KE, Rosenberg RD, Sonenshein GE. J Biol Chem 1989;264:6990–6995.
3. Simons M, Rosenberg RD. Circ Res 1992;70:835–843.

4. Poenie M, Alderton J, Steinhardt R, Tsien R. Science 1986;233:886–889.
5. Steinhardt RA, Alderton J. Nature 1988;332:364–366.
6. Pardee AB, Dubrow R, Hamlin JL, Kletzien RF. Ann Rev Biochem 1978;47:715–750.
7. Simons M, Morgan KG, Parker C, Collins E, Rosenberg RD. J Biol Chem 1993;268:627–632.
8. Evans JL, Moore TL, Kuehl WM, Bender T, Ting JP. Mol Cell Biol 1990;10:5747–5752.
9. Dudek H, Tantravahi RV, Rao VN, Reddy ES, Reddy EP. Proc Natl Acad Sci USA 1992;89:1291–1295.
10. Iida H, Sakaguchi S, Yagawa Y, Anraku Y. J Biol Chem 1990;265:21216–21222.

704

Absence of replication of vascular smooth muscle

Stephen M. Schwartz[1] and Edward R.M. O'Brien[2]

[1]*Department of Pathology SJ-60, University of Washington School of Medicine, Seattle, Washington, USA; and*
[2]*Division of Cardiology, University of Ottawa Heart Institute, Ottawa, Ontario, Canada K1Y 4E9*

History

As long ago as the time of Virchow, pathologists equated the cellularity of atherosclerotic plaques with some form of proliferation of vascular smooth muscle. This idea was reinforced when Ross and others first put smooth muscle into culture and found that the cells could be stimulated by factors thought to be present in plaques, i.e., growth factors released by platelets [1]. Our topic is smooth muscle proliferation. We have compiled a long list of growth factors and growth inhibitors for smooth muscle cells [2]. Aside from such traditional polypeptide growth factors as platelet-derived growth factor (PDGF), this list includes proteases, vasoactive amines, and neuropeptides as well as a list of growth inhibitors including heparin and somatostatin. The existence of all these in vitro growth factors, however, does not prove that growth occurs. The questions addressed in the present review include whether smooth replication occurs in vascular lesions and where antiproliferative approaches may have therapeutic value.

For the most part, our interest in smooth muscle proliferation is confined to the intima. French offered a seminal review describing the unique properties of the arterial intima over 20 years ago [3]. His major points, given the technology of the day, were that the smooth muscle cells of the intima had a unique morphology as seen by either light or electron microscopy. Moreover, intimal formation appeared to be the characteristic response of arteries to almost any imaginable injury, as well as occurring during normal development and aging. Finally, French emphasized the importance of the intima as the unique soil for the development of atherosclerosis. As we will review, there have been two different but not mutually exclusive hypotheses about why the intima is such a unique soil. The Campbells and others have published extensively on the loss of differentiation when smooth muscle cells are placed in culture. These authors call the loss of differentiation "modulation" to a "synthetic" phenotype and suggest that similar adaptive changes explain the lack of smooth muscle markers in cells of the normal or atherosclerotic intima [4,5]. In contrast, this laboratory has suggested that intimal cells may belong to a distinct smooth muscle subset characterized by expression of its own unique set of genes. Of course, both ideas may be correct; however, the question of smooth muscle replication may have become especially confused by claims that proliferative smooth muscle cells have a characteristic "smooth muscle phenotype" and that replicating cells are synthetic. It is important to realize that this is not the case. Despite pathologists' use of the term "proliferative" or "hyperplasia" [6], there is no distinctive morphology, other than mitosis itself, that allows one to identify smooth muscle cells as being in the cell cycle. To our knowledge, there are no experimental data showing that smooth muscle cells must dedif-

---

Address for correspondence: Stephen M. Schwartz MD, PhD, Department of Pathology SJ-60, University of Washington School of Medicine, Seattle, WA 98195, USA. Tel.: +1-206-543-0258. Fax: +1-206-685-3662.

ferentiate before replication. In our own work we have seen smooth muscle cells in vivo replicate within 24 h of injury, before any loss of smooth muscle α-actin at an immunocytochemical level. Similarly, newborn smooth muscle cells are actually more stable in their expression of smooth muscle-specific proteins than are typical adult cells [7—9] and, at least for the PDGF isoforms, there is a confusing dissociation between loss of phenotype and ability to stimulate smooth muscle replication. Again, the important point is that loss of phenotype, "modulation", in the terminology used by the Campbells and others, is not necessary for, nor does it imply, cell replication.

Not much is known about the time course of intimal formation. The absence of an intima in some arteries has been essential to studies identifying molecules critical to neointimal formation after injury. In human coronary arteries, the intima grows rapidly after birth until about 6 months of age [10,11]. Unfortunately, replication has never been directly measured in this artery at this early age.

Another site where spontaneous intimal formation has been studied is the ductus arteriosus [12,13]. Contrary to conventional wisdom, the ductus forms an intima spontaneously before birth. This event may be essential for ductus closure rather than a result of injury occurring during closure. Indeed, the characteristic stenosis seen in the ductus suggests that the function or malfunction of the intima could play a key role in control of vascular lumen size — a key issue in atherosclerosis, restenosis and hypertension. Again, we lack direct measures of cell replication at this site.

The only direct evidence for intimal replication was written two decades ago and is based on a very unusual concept. In 1973, Benditt reported that atherosclerotic plaques were monoclonal. He used G6PD (glucose-6-phosphate dehydrogenase) as an allotypic marker in plaques of Black females [14]. The original observation has been reproduced by two other groups [15—17]. Because G6PD isoforms can only be identified in blocks of tissue, the original studies did not provide direct evidence that the cell type being studied was the smooth muscle cell type. The remaining cells in these lesions are lymphocytes, macrophages, and endothelial cells. Hansson later showed that lymphocytes in lesions are polyclonal [18]. While plaque macrophage and endothelial cells do replicate, there are no known examples of these cell types forming monoclonal growths other than in neoplasms [1,19]. Thus, Benditt's observation implies that substantial smooth muscle replication must have occurred at some time during the origin of the lesions. Given the high rate of intimal growth in infants before frank lesion formation, it is tempting to ask whether the bulk of smooth muscle replication in a monoclonal lesion may not have occurred in the first weeks of life, perhaps before the lesion has developed a fatty core [20].

Neointimal formation: a generic response of vessels to injury?

If intima is the natural layer that forms between the endothelium and the internal elastic lamina, a similar structure, the "neointima", is the intima that forms in response to injury. We recognize neointima because many arteries, especially smaller ones, either do not form an intima at all, or do so only slowly as the animal ages [3,21]. Neointimal formation, however, occurs in all arteries as a response to a wide variety of injuries, including irradiation, application of turpentine to the adventitia, wrapping the vessel, and electrical stimulation, as well as mechanical injuries, including placement of a suture, scratching with a probe, or dilatation of the common carotid artery with an embolectomy balloon catheter [3,22—31]. These changes are seen in large arteries, small arteries and even in transplanted veins that undergo arterialization.

The important point is that the vessel wall is a very special tissue. Unlike almost any other tissue, the normal vessel wall is composed almost entirely of smooth muscle cells; thus, the typical response to injury will be somewhat different from the classical response seen in a skin wound. The brain, too, has a unique cellular composition and responds to injury by gliosis. Similarly, we may consider neointimal formation as the peculiar response of vessels to injury. The most obvious questions about this process are:

1. To what extent does the neointima form by migration of cells from the media vs. replication of cells in the intima?
2. Does neointimal formation require medial smooth muscle replication?
3. How does neointimal formation relate to spontaneous development of an intima?
4. Are intimal or neointimal cells, like glia, a distinct cell type?
5. What molecules control neointimal formation?

Pharmacology of neointimal formation

While the last 20 years have seen the identification of a large number of molecules that stimulate smooth muscle replication in vitro [2], the central theme of this article is the relevance of smooth muscle replication to pathology in vivo. We will begin by discussing the best studied model for in vivo replication: neointimal formation in the response of the rat carotid artery to balloon angioplasty [24,27,32]. It is important to realize that this model is much simpler than the same response in larger, more complex human arteries which already are diseased. First, as previously discussed, the rat carotid artery has only rare intimal cells [33]. Even normal arteries in larger animals have a pre-existing intima [34,35]. Second, unlike the response of arteries in larger animals, including rabbits, swine, and nonhuman primates, the response of rat arteries to most injuries involves platelets, but there is no deposition of fibrillar fibrin or adherence of leukocytes [36–45]. The simplicity of the rat model has made it possible to develop methods for detailed kinetic analyses of the processes leading to neointimal formation and to define four waves of response to injury with the molecules responsible for each of these waves [22,46–50].

The balloon injury model begins with complete destruction of the endothelium as well as extensive death of medial smooth muscle cells [32]. The first response to balloon injury, called "first wave", consists of medial smooth muscle cell proliferation and begins about 24 h after the injury. In elegant studies, Reidy et al. have shown that this wave of replication can be completely accounted for by release of basic fibroblast growth factor (bFGF) from dying smooth muscle cells [51,52]. Among other candidate molecules, studies with infused PDGF, as well as studies with anti-PDGF antibodies, have shown that this molecule does not play a significant role as a mitogen [53,54]. In addition, other molecules may be active, as more limited data suggest that α-adrenergic antagonists and angiotensin II (AII) antagonists can block medial replication [55–57].

The migration of smooth muscle cells across the internal elastic lamina to form the intima constitutes the "second wave". Smooth muscle cells are readily observed on the luminal side of the internal elastic lamina 4 days after injury [32]. The duration of the second wave is not known. Several molecules can contribute to smooth muscle migration, including PDGF, transforming growth factor-β (TGF-β), bFGF and AII. The relative contributions of these different molecules are not known, nor do we know whether other molecules are involved [52,57,58]. Interestingly, the effects of angiotensin-converting enzyme (ACE) inhibitors may result from the ability of these drugs to elevate bradykinin levels by preventing its degradation rather than the expected effect of these agents on lowering levels of AII. ACE inhibitors are not specific for the conversion of AI to AII [59–62]. Among other effects, these drugs inhibit degradation of bradykinin, and there is evidence from studies involving bradykinin antagonists that elevation of bradykinin can explain part of the effect of ACE inhibitors on neointimal formation [59] (deBlois and Schwartz, unpublished results). The effect of PDGF is noteworthy, given the emphasis from in vitro studies that this molecule is a mitogen, despite the apparent lack of mitogenicity in vivo [53].

Once smooth muscle cells arrive in the intima, they may replicate for weeks to months [63]. This replication is called the "third wave". As of the time of writing this review, no specific molecular antagonist has been shown to inhibit this replication. Even antibodies to bFGF, which are so effective in inhibiting the first wave, are impotent against third-wave replication [52]. Therefore, although we cannot say that any specific molecule has definitively been identified as a third-wave mitogen, a few potential candidates appear to be present in the intima. For example, PDGF-A chain is overexpressed in the intima, but will not stimulate replication if infused, nor do antibodies to PDGF suppress third-wave replication [53,64,65]. Other growth-control molecules that appear to be overexpressed in the rat neointima include the AII receptor and TGF-β [58,66]. Insulin growth factor-1 (IGF-1) is also overexpressed following injury; however, it is overexpressed in the media [67]. While we cannot identify the critical molecules that sustain elevated replication in the third wave, we do know that the neointima can be stimulated to show a further increase of replication by infusion of other molecules. This increased responsiveness to mitogens can be called a "fourth wave", and involves at least TGF-β, bFGF, or AII as agonists [51,55,58]. Again, PDGF does not appear to be mitogenic [53]. Table 1 summarizes the molecules that control the three waves.

Clinical targets

The rat carotid model has led to a focus on specific molecules as possible mediators of intimal hyperplasia and therefore as clinical targets. The renin–angiotensin system has received a great deal of attention. The principal AII receptor, AT1, is elevated in the neointima, although both AT1 and AT2 receptors are also present in the normal wall [66].

Table 1. Likely mediators of neointimal formation

	Description	Mediators	Inhibition		Stimulation
			Antibody	Antagonist	Agonist
First wave (0-3 d)	Replication of SMC within the media	FGF	+	NA	+
		PDGF	±	NA	–
		TGF-β	NA	ND	±
		AII	ND	+	ND[a]
Second wave (3-14 d)	Migration of SMC from the media into the intima	PDGF	+	NA	+
		AII	ND	+	ND
		FGF	+	NA	+
Third wave (7 d-mo)	Proliferation of SMC within the neointima	FGF	–	NA	±
		PDGF	–	NA	–
		TGF-β	NA	NA	+[b]
		AII	ND	–	+[b]

AII = Angiotensin II; PDGF = platelet-derived growth factor; FGF = basic fibroblast growth factor; TGF-β = transforming growth factor β; ND = not done; NA = not available. + = supporting evidence; – = evidence against hypothesis; ± = weak response. [a]AII does stimulate medial smooth muscle; [b]"Restimulation" experiments [52–55,58,68].

The source of AII in the wall may be local activation. Angiotensinogen is available from the circulation. Kininase II (ACE) has been found in the normal vessel wall, even in the absence of its highest source, the endothelium [69]. Finally, the possibility that the vessel wall contains angiotensinogenases with renin-like activity has been raised [70].

AII is able to stimulate the first wave and it is also able to restimulate replication in the neointima. First-wave replication, migration into the intima, and intimal thickening can be prevented by angiotensin-receptor antagonists as well as converting-enzyme inhibitors [71,72]. Furthermore, the persistence of replication after injury and the elevated replicative response of the neointima to infused angiotensin, compared to uninjured media, could be due to increased intimal expression of angiotensin I receptors [55]. Thus, it is quite reasonable to interpret the effects of ACE inhibitors in blocking neointimal formation as being the result of blocking formation of AII [68]. In summary, there is sufficient evidence for components of the angiotensin system in the injured vessel wall and for this complex system to play a role in intimal hyperplasia. Despite all of these data, why did the clinical studies fail? A full discussion is beyond our purpose here. Suffice it to say that existing studies with ACE inhibitors are inconclusive in part because higher drug doses are needed to achieve significant suppression of intimal thickening (3—30 mg/kg/day) than to obtain a maximal (20%) reduction of blood pressure in the same strain of normotensive rats (3 mg/kg/day) [73]. It is also important to consider the possibility that the endpoint in the animal studies, intimal thickening, is not the critical process in the renarrowing of human vessels, and this will be discussed below.

TGF-β may also play an important role in third- and fourth-wave replication. As already noted, we found that infused TGF-β was a mitogen and there is an accumulation of TGF-β in the neointima [58]. These in vivo data are at odds with studies in vitro in which TGF-β is sometimes seen as a growth stimulant and at other times as an inhibitor. Some of the variability may reflect the strain of smooth muscle cells studied and their state of confluence [74—76]. A particularly intriguing hypothesis for a role for TGF-β as a growth inhibitor comes from a recent report by Grainger et al. These authors propose a link between TGF-β as an endogenous growth inhibitor and elevated atherosclerosis risk due to elevated lipoprotein (a) (Lp(a)) [77]. A recent study suggests that apolipoprotein (a) (apo(a)) levels correlate with increased incidence of restenosis [78,79]. The mechanism of action of apo(a) is believed to be due to its homology with plasminogen and its ability to inhibit the formation of plasmin [80,81]. Atherosclerosis may then depend on inadequate clot lysis [80,81]. Plasmin, in addition to its role in fibrinolysis, is essential to the activation of TGF-β [82]. Grainger et al. found that apo(a) is mitogenic for smooth muscle cells in culture. They were also able to attribute the mitogenic effect to inhibition of an autocrine growth inhibitor, TGF-β. Apo(a), they propose, blocks formation of plasmin and subsequent ability of the cells to activate TGF-β [77,83,84]. In this view, the predominant role of TGF-β would be as an endogenous inhibitor of lesion formation at sites of active coagulation and apo(a) would enhance lesion formation by diminishing the production of activated TGF-β. Perhaps in contradiction to Grainger's hypothesis, a recent study of atherectomy specimens found elevated levels of TGF-β in restenotic lesions [85].

Finally, anticoagulants and antithrombotics may play a major clinical role. Heparin has been widely studied as an inhibitor of intimal formation in animal models [86]. While much attention has been focused on the potential role of heparin on c-myb, this molecule is expressed in late G1 of the cell cycle, and likely represents only one of several defects when growth is inhibited [87]. Equally intriguing is the role of heparin in inhibiting migration and suggestions from Lindner et al. that heparin's major action may be to wash bFGF out of the injured vessel wall after the mitogen is released from dying cells [51].

Unfortunately, clinical trials using heparin to prevent restenosis have been disappointing [88,89]. Ellis et al. administered intravenous heparin to patients over the first 18—24 h after angioplasty and found no difference in the restenosis rates of patients treated with heparin compared to those given a dextrose infusion (41 vs. 37%, respectively, p = NS) [88]. Similarly, a subsequent attempt to limit restenosis with a single daily subcutaneous injection of 10,000 IU of heparin was halted prematurely due to higher rates of restenosis and clinical events in the heparin treatment group than in the usual-care group [89]. This lack of clinical benefit is difficult to explain; however, Edelman and Karnovsky suggest that differences in heparin dose scheduling may be critical [90]. For example, the antiproliferative effect of heparin requires that the drug be administered for at least 4—7 days after injury in the rat carotid balloon injury model [32]. Furthermore, cell proliferation and the intima:media area ratio are made worse when rats are treated with heparin dosages and administration schedules similar to those used clinically [90]. Low-molecular-weight heparins also appear to be ineffective for the prevention of restenosis [91].

Finally, recent attention has been focused on clinical trials using monoclonal antibodies or antagonists to the platelet glycoprotein IIb-IIIa receptor [92—94]. For example, as part of the EPIC study, the chimeric monoclonal antibody Fab fragment, which is directed against the platelet glycoprotein IIb/IIIa receptor, was administered to patients undergoing angioplasty or atherectomy who were at high risk for ischemic complications [94]. This therapy resulted in a reduction in acute ischemic complications (e.g., nonfatal myocardial infarction, emergency revascularization procedures), although at the risk of increased bleeding complications. While it is easy to imagine that these trials are affecting only platelets, these antagonists to Gp IIb-IIIa, a platelet adhesive protein, may also affect a closely related integrin, $\alpha_v\beta_{III}$. Antagonists to $\alpha_v\beta_{III}$ have recently been shown to block smooth muscle migration in vitro and intimal formation in vivo [95]. Moreover, we have found that this same receptor is required for movement of smooth muscle cells in response to osteopontin, an abundant and specific marker of intimal smooth muscle cells (Liaw, Schwartz, and Giachelli, unpublished data). In summary, there is an increasing body of circumstantial data suggesting that the second wave, i.e., migration, is a critical step in neointimal formation and possibly in restenosis.

The role of the intimal replication in the formation of an atherosclerotic lesion

The role of intimal replication in atherosclerosis is confusing. Is intimal thickening a result of atherosclerosis or a cause? Does it precede or follow formation of the atherosclerotic lesion?

Before answering these questions, it is important to point out a major, practical difference between studies of replication in animals, where it is practical to use labeled analogs of thymidine, either BUdR or [^{3}H]TdR, and studies in humans where this is generally not possible in vivo. Figure 1 illustrates the ways replication can be measured in human tissues. [^{3}H]TdR or BUdR can be used in vitro. Spagnoli used this method with plaque specimens and found very low levels of replication, less than 1%. This method has one major source of error: the tissue in vitro is likely to be deteriorating during the incubation and the labeled material may not penetrate to a cell of interest until that cell has died. Thus one might expect in vitro incubation studies to underestimate the levels of replication [96]. The first alternative procedure used in the vessel wall was staining for "proliferating cell nuclear antigen" (PCNA). This is a bit confusing, since PCNA will stain cells that are generally replicating, rather than identifying cells in a specific part of the cell cycle. Thus, PCNA tends to overestimate levels of replication. Nonetheless, studies of plaque show low

710

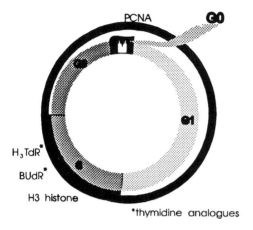

Fig. 1. Cell cycle with labeling by different methods.

levels of PCNA. The one confusing exception is a report [97] of high levels of PCNA in primary lesions sampled by atherectomy. The reasons for these high values is unclear, but the simplest possibility is that PCNA is easily overstained. The best control is a piece of gut or tonsil, since these tissues have been independently studied with labeled analogs and we know what to expect. When this was done, two labs found low levels of replication, under about 1% [19,98]. Finally, a new and appealing cell cycle marker is histone H3. The RNA for this protein is present at extremely high levels during S phase and only during S phase. Thus in situ hybridization for H3 may be a very good substitute for use of labeled analogs in human tissue. We have recently confirmed the PCNA studies of primary atherosclerotic lesions using H3 (Shoval et al., unpublished data).

Of course, one might not expect to see proliferation in advanced lesions. Fatty streaks, however, form at many sites in humans as well as in other fat-fed animals [99–101]. Many investigators regard these as early lesions and one can see higher levels of replication in fat-fed animals [102]. Nonetheless, when PCNA was used to look at human fatty streaks, again the PCNA levels were very low [98].

The absence of evidence for smooth muscle replication needs to be considered in terms of the natural history of the atherosclerotic lesion. We have already noted that the monoclonality of lesions implies that proliferation must occur at some time during lesion development. Perhaps the simplest way to understand the critical issues is to consider some of the terminology used by the World Health Organization. Stary et al. state that intimal thickening is not the early lesion of atherosclerosis because intimal thickening is not lipid-rich and is a normal developmental change at specific vascular sites in our species [101]. These authors do note, however, that lipid accumulation can occur deep in the wall, within the pre-existing intimal mass. This sequence of events, with a localization and initiation of atherosclerosis, is reminiscent of experiments in balloon-injured animals in which lesions develop selectively at sites of previous injury and intimal formation [33]. Thus, the initiation of atherosclerosis, or at least the form of atherosclerosis that leads to classical lesions in humans, may begin in the "soil" of the intima and most of the replication of the plaque may exist in the intima prior to lipid accumulation.

This point of view conflicts with a popularly held hypothesis. However, smooth muscle cell proliferation as a component of the advanced lesion or even the fibrous streak is not supported by cell kinetic studies measuring either the frequency of cells able to incorporate labeled thymidine ex vivo or the number of cells identified as replicative on the basis of staining for a cell cycle-specific marker [19,103]. On the other hand, monoclonality implies that smooth muscle proliferation must occur during the formation of the lesion and that the initial group of cells giving rise to the lesion must be very small. Such an early expansion of intimal smooth muscle mass has been described in the proximal anterior descending coronary artery (LAD), a common site for occlusive coronary artery lesions in adults [10,11]. If the increase in mass described in the newborn LAD is correlated with smooth muscle replication, very few further doublings may be required to account for the mass of smooth muscle seen in an adult lesion. The low replicative rates seen in advanced lesions correlate with studies of cells cultured from lesions. Moss and Benditt were the first to culture these cells [104]. They found that plaque smooth muscle cells have a much shorter life span than normal medial cells. This observation has been reproduced by others [105,106].

Of course, even if monoclonality is an early event, very few doublings would be required to convert the mass of the normal intima into the mass of an occlusive lesion over the several decades before lesions are full-grown. Such doublings might occur at rare intervals, intervals too rare to detect by the random samplings we now have. These doublings might even occur in bursts, consistent with angiographic studies that demonstrate rapid growth, or at least loss of lumen, at sites that are initially relatively normal [107].

Finally, we also need to consider proliferation of cells other than smooth muscle cells. A recent study from this laboratory shows focal levels of endothelial replication as high as 10% [108]. This may be evidence that angiogenesis is a very active and chronic process adding to plaque mass. Finally, while most studies have focused attention on the smooth muscle cell, Gordon et al. found more impressive evidence for macrophage replication than for smooth muscle replication [19].

In summary, the available direct evidence suggests that smooth muscle replication occurs very early in the formation of atherosclerotic lesions [10,11]. It is also likely that monoclonality precedes or occurs early in lesion formation. Unfortunately, testing this hypothesis would require novel methods for serial study of clonality at a histological level in human tissue. We also cannot rule out the possibility that smooth muscle replication occurs at a very low rate over several years or that replication occurs at a high rate in an episodic fashion.

Plaque-specific gene expression by smooth muscle cells

Whether or not plaque smooth muscle cells are rapidly proliferating, it is clear that smooth muscle cells in human plaques overexpress a large number of genes that are generally not seen in the normal wall. Some of these are also associated with replicating smooth muscle or with the "modulation" described by the Campbells.

Among the more interesting genes shown to be overexpressed in plaques are:

Tissue factor

The normal vessel wall contains little or no tissue factor at a level demonstrable by in situ hybridization or immunocytochemistry [109]. High levels of tissue factor seen in plaque may promote coagulation, a factor that is probably important to both plaque progression and the final morbid outcome [109,110]. The time course for the appearance of tissue factor in plaques is not known; however, Davies and others have suggested that thrombosis is a critical event in plaque progression, and it is likely that accumulation of this molecule is critical to the morbidity of lesions [111–113].

Pdgf chains

PDGF-A chain is found in the plaque, and, as already discussed, it is not a potent smooth muscle mitogen in vitro. Nonetheless, antibodies to this mitogen will inhibit replication induced by other molecules, including TGF-β and bFGF [74,75,114,115]. Interestingly, PDGF-A chain synthesis is induced in cultured cells by a number of molecules likely to be present in advanced plaques, including thrombin, angiotensin, and phenylephrine [116–118]. In vivo, PDGF mRNA levels may be lowered by antagonists to thrombin [116] or phenylephrine [64].

PDGF-B chain is also seen in plaque macrophage and endothelial cells, although from in situ hybridization studies the latter cells are probably the major source of synthesis [1,114]. The failure to detect PDGF-B chain in plaque smooth muscle, however, may be misleading. Recent studies of rat neointima show that PDGF-B chain mRNA is confined to about 10% of the most superficial cells in the neointima (Lindner, Giachelli, Reidy and Schwartz, unpublished data). Such a low percentage would be difficult to detect if a similar low frequency were confined to a portion of primary or restenotic human lesions.

MCSF/GMSCF

The presence of these leukocyte growth factors, as well as receptors for leukocyte factors is of special importance because of growing evidence that plaque macrophages, rather than plaque smooth muscle cells, may comprise the only unique proliferative element in the plaque [19,103]. The unique properties of the proliferative plaque macrophage have yet to be explored.

Osteopontin and bone morphogenic protein

Osteopontin and bone morphogenetic protein 2a have both been found in smooth muscle cells of atherosclerotic plaques [119–121]. The presence of these molecules is supportive of the hypothesis that plaques are derived from unique subsets of smooth muscle cells because osteopontin was first found in neointimal cells of the rat pup artery as part of the π phenotype [122]. Bone morphogenetic protein 2a, on the other hand, is also seen in plaques. Intriguingly, cells found to express bone morphogenetic protein 2a also express immunocytochemical markers associated with a special form of smooth muscle cell, the pericytes seen around small vessels, again suggesting a unique lineage for plaque smooth muscle as compared with medial smooth muscle [121]. The association of osteopontin and bone morphogenetic protein 2a with areas of calcification in the plaque also suggests that the mechanisms of bone mineralization may also play a role in vessel wall calcification.

Constitutive nitric oxide (NO) synthase

An excellent example of the difference between a vessel with only a media and one with an atherosclerotic intima is the issue of vascular contractility. Normally the vessel wall exists in a relaxed state because of the endogenous production of NO by endothelium. NO-dependent relaxation, however, is greatly impaired in atherosclerotic vessels [123]. This loss of NO function has been attributed to endothelial injury or to the inactivation of NO by free radicals produced in the plaque [124]. In contrast, Joly et al. described the appearance of the inducible form of NO synthase following balloon injury [125]. Similarly, as described above, the neointima overexpresses angiotensin receptors and the plaque has been shown to overexpress endothelin [126]. While to this point we have not distinguished effects of atherosclerosis from those of the more general appearance of the neointima, our point is simply that we might expect the vasomotor activity of a diseased artery with an intima to be very different from vasomotor regulation in a normal artery. The contribution of this altered pharmacology to the ability of the vessel wall to maintain a normal lumen caliber is largely unexplored.

Mechanism of lumen occlusion in atherosclerosis

Until this point, we have focused on the formation and properties of the arterial intima. We have assumed that increased intimal mass occludes the lumen.

The experimental data supporting the assumption that intimal mass obstructs the lumen of large vessels is unclear. For example, Glagov et al. noted that human vessels can undergo massive accumulations of atherosclerotic mass without lumen narrowing [127]. The vessel wall compensates for the new mass by dilating to permit a normal level of blood flow until an adaptational limit is exceeded. This limit appears to occur when approximately 40% or more of the area bounded by the internal elastic lamina is occupied by intimal mass. The compensatory dilation is a structural change in the vessel wall and is usually called "remodeling." Decreased lumen size probably does not occur until Glagov's limit is exceeded and may depend on pharmacological mechanisms associated with the neointima or the plaque that cause a failure of normal remodeling events.

If the correlation of intimal (or plaque) mass with lumen caliber is not a simple one, how do we account for angiographic changes seen after aggressive lipid-lowering therapy [128–130]? The actual degree of improvement of stenosis diameter in these studies is small (e.g., 0.7–5.3%, or an increase of 0.003 to 0.117 mm in minimum absolute diameter). To put these results in perspective, one should note that 6 months after percutaneous coronary angioplasty, there is an average improvement of 16% diameter stenosis units and a 0.47 mm increase in minimum absolute diameter [131]. It is critical to realize that angiographic studies provide no insight into the mechanisms that may account for loss of lumen caliber. Thus, it is possible that apparent changes in mass reflect changes in adherent thrombotic material or state of vasospasm rather than in the extent of lumen narrowing due to accumulation of lipid and necrotic material in the atherosclerotic intima [132].

These angiographic regression studies showed only a modest change in lumen caliber compared to the beneficial change in clinical events [128,130]. This raises the intriguing possibility that lipid-lowering therapies may improve clinical outcome by stabilizing the lesion rather than by altering the lumen. Davies and others have suggested that the formation of fissures in plaques is the critical step leading to vascular occlusion [111–113]. They propose that fissuring results from a combination of biochemical events that weaken the fibrous cap over lesions and may include the expression of certain proteases [133]. Another group has added to this concept by proposing that accumulation of TNF-α may lead to necrotic changes that result in plaque rupture [134]. While Arbustini et al. were unable to find a clear correlation of fissuring with acute ischemic heart disease, Davies et al. found a high incidence of fissuring in atherosclerotic "control" arteries of patients dying of noncoronary events, hypothesizing that the control patients may have had undetected myocardial infarctions and these fissures may simply represent the sequelae of advanced atherosclerosis [112,134,135]. Davies' hypothesis would imply that we may be able to develop diagnostic tests, based on plaque composition as assessed by magnetic resonance imaging (MRI), intravascular ultrasound (IVUS), or even gene expression patterns in atherectomy specimens, that might indicate lesion prognosis or the effectiveness of drugs targeted at stabilizing the lesion.

It is important to emphasize the potential value of new modalities for imaging human coronary artery lesions (e.g., MRI or IVUS) in testing the impact that plaque fissuring and subsequent thrombosis may have on eventual lumen diameter. Animal models with rare and spontaneous occlusive atherosclerotic arterial diseases, even with fat feeding, are poorly characterized. Human data, as of now, however, are confusing. As just discussed, it is difficult to define a control population if one depends on autopsy material. Serial angiographic studies in humans, moreover, suggest that the majority of myocardial infarctions may occur because of thrombotic occlusion of arteries that previously did not contain significant stenoses (e.g., <50%) [136,137]. However, postmortem studies do not bear this out. For example, Qiao et al. have reported that in both native coronary arteries and saphenous venous bypass grafts, atherosclerotic plaque rupture with thrombosis most commonly occurred at sites with severe narrowing (e.g., >90% area stenosis) [138,139]. Possibly, this is just another example of the inability of angiography to estimate the extent of atherosclerotic disease.

The nature of restenosis following angioplasty

Surprising as the absence of replication in atherosclerosis may be, it is at least equally surprising to look at replication values following angioplasty. As discussed above, we have used immunocytochemical labeling for PCNA to determine the proliferative profile of atherosclerotic lesions and found only very low levels of smooth muscle replication. We have used the same method to study 100 restenotic coronary atherectomy specimens [140]. To our surprise, the vast majority of the restenotic specimens (74%) had no evidence of PCNA labeling. Moreover, in those specimens with proliferation, only a modest number of PCNA-positive cells were present per slide (typically <50 cells per slide). PCNA labeling was detected over a wide time interval after the initial procedure (e.g., 1–390 days), with no obvious proliferative peak. There were no differences in the proliferative profiles of restenotic specimens collected in the first 3 months, 4–6 months, 7–9 months or >9 months after the initial interventional procedure (Spearman rank correlation coefficient = 0.081, p = 0.43). Furthermore, only 12 of 30 specimens obtained within 60 days of the initial coronary interventional procedure had one or more PCNA-positive nucleus per slide (including nine specimens collected within 6 days of the initial procedure, only three of which had immunolabeling of one, seven and 20 cells per slide). In support of these findings, a recent preliminary study using in vitro bromodeoxyuridine labeling also found low levels of proliferation in restenotic atherectomy specimens [141]. Similarly, Strauss et al. found no PCNA-positive cells in atherectomy specimens from seven restenotic stented coronary artery lesions [142].

As already discussed, these results and those of Strauss [142] contrast with a recent report by Pickering et al. [97]. Overall, the labeling indices reported by Pickering et al. seem exceptionally high (e.g., as many as 59% of cells being PCNA-positive), and resemble those of malignant neoplasms [143]. It is important, however, to realize that PCNA is not a direct measure of replication (Fig. 1). Thus, the detection of differences in the frequency of PCNA-positive cells in the Pickering study should raise concerns that differences between primary and restenotic tissue in Pickering's study could reflect changes specific to peripheral arterial lesions, a tissue not included in our study.

These data on replication force us to reconsider the relevance of animal models to the human problem. Almost all animal studies, particularly those performed in the rat, measure a decrease in lumen size from the initially normal situation. This can rightly be called "stenosis". In contrast, the clinical problem is defined by the extent of dilatation that is lost after an atherosclerotic vessel has been dilated to achieve what the interventional cardiologist believes is an optimal diameter. The loss of this optimal diameter, rather than the pre-existing vessel caliber, is rightly called "restenosis" (a popular clinical definition of restenosis is >50% loss of initial luminal diameter gain). By current angiographic criteria, even a return of the human vessel to its predilation diameter would be defined as restenosis, despite no change in intimal mass. Thus, stenosis, as seen in most animal models of arterial injury, is very different from the clinical process called restenosis and may not be useful in predicting the result of restenosis therapies. This statement is especially true of studies that equate intimal hyperplasia with restenosis. The relationship of intimal mass to loss of lumen caliber is unclear even within animal models. For example, luminal narrowing after injury to the rat carotid artery is more pronounced after 2 weeks (75%) than after 12 weeks (35%), implying that early stenosis may be due to smooth muscle contraction of the vessel. Loss of lumen caliber could depend more on the extent of remodeling of the vessel wall to compensate for a change in mass than on the intimal mass itself [127]. Therefore, it may be more appropriate to define "stenosis" as a decrease in lumen size from the caliber existing prior to angioplasty. Unfortunately, such an incremental change in diameter is difficult to measure with existing quantitative angiography.

Using these definitions, we would consider the response of the rat carotid artery as stenosis. To the best of our knowledge, angiographic studies in humans do not show that angioplasty produces stenoses similar to those seen in animal models. This, of course, would be difficult to demonstrate angiographically as the initial lesion usually already has a critical stenosis. Furthermore, animal models, perhaps by design, require that all manipulated arteries show narrowing, i.e., stenosis, as shown in Fig. 2. There is no animal model in which 50% (or any significant percentage) of manipulated arteries remain dilated beyond their initial, unmanipulated caliber; yet this 50% rate (or higher) is the success rate seen when atherosclerotic human arteries are dilated with an angioplasty balloon. Perhaps, with more than 50% of human arteries remaining free of restenosis months after angioplasty, we may want to ask whether we have a sufficient animal model that allows us to explain why angioplasty is ever successful in the first place.

Another way of thinking about this problem is to ask whether restenosis is the result of an increase in wall mass due to intimal hyperplasia, remodeling of the vessel wall to re-establish its preangioplasty caliber, or a combination of these processes. Our ability to evaluate human vessels is changing because of new technologies; in particular, the use of intravascular ultrasound (IVUS) to image the affected wall and atherectomy to biopsy the same tissue. Previous data, based on histologic and imaging studies, suggested that plaque compression, disruption with fracture and dissection of the intima and media, and stretching of the more normal portions of the media, are involved in creating a bigger lumen [144–151]. However, newer concepts are emerging. For example, Losordo et al. used IVUS to study 40 patients immediately before and after iliac artery angioplasty [152]. The areas of the arterial wall, plaque, lumen, and neolumen resulting from the procedure were examined. Over 70% of the increase in luminal area immediately after angioplasty was contained within the plaque fracture (the so-called neolumen). Plaque cross-sectional area decreased by approximately one third, but total artery cross-sectional area increased only minimally (approximately 5%) with the dilatation. Thus, the major effects of angioplasty may be to redistribute the components of the wall. Conversely, loss of lumen, i.e., "restenosis", might be due to healing of the fissure rather than formation of new mass.

The emphasis on neointimal formation as the cause of restenosis is not simply by

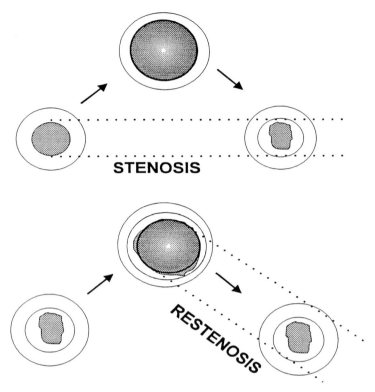

Fig. 2. Comparison of stenosis, i.e., loss of lumen following injury to normal vessel, with restenosis, i.e., loss of gain produced by dilation of a pathologic vessel.

analogy with animal models. The original studies on the pathology of human restenosis emphasized a histologic change called intimal hyperplasia. For example, Nobuyoshi et al. examined 39 dilated lesions from the postmortem coronary arteries of 20 patients who had undergone angioplasty [153]. The extent of "intimal proliferation" was defined by the histologic appearance of stellate, fibroblast-like cells with a myxomatous appearance. It is essential to note that the term "proliferative" as used here is a morphological term, not a measure of replication such as thymidine index or mitotic frequency. Cells having this "proliferative" morphology are not unique to restenosis. Similar cells are commonly seen beneath the endothelium in areas of nonatherosclerotic intimal thickening as well as in primary atherosclerotic coronary artery lesions that have never been exposed to an interventional device [6,154]. While the myxomatous tissue seen in atherosclerotic or restenotic lesions does not appear to be actively proliferative, most observers agree that there is an increase in the amount of this tissue in restenotic vs. primary lesions [6,19,140,154–156].

We do not know whether the increase in amount of "proliferative" tissue represents a redistribution of the components of lesions due to compression by the catheter or some reaction such as formation of extracellular matrix, migration or cell proliferation at a low level not measured by current methods. Postmortem examination of stented coronary arteries supports the idea that this is not simply a redistribution of pre-existing plaque components, yet to date has failed to show evidence of replication [142]. Perhaps the wires push into the wall or wall components migrate around the wires.

Preliminary intracoronary ultrasound studies suggest that increases in plaque area with restenosis following angioplasty are actually small (e.g., 5—7%) [157]. The clinical significance of this small increase in plaque mass in an artery that is already severely diseased is unknown. The authors speculate that intimal hyperplasia may not be a dominant factor in the restenotic lesion, and that instead, "chronic recoil" or remodeling may account for approximately 60% of late lumen loss [158]. This concept of "chronic recoil" is similar to the phenomenon of vascular remodeling or to the wound-healing model discussed above.

In summary, the available data do not demonstrate that cell proliferation is a major component of coronary restenosis. If this is true, antiproliferative approaches to therapy with the elegant use of molecular biology to inhibit growth may be irrelevant [87]. It is intriguing to note that a recent study in the swine-stent model actually showed an increase in restenosis when an injured wall was irradiated to prevent cell proliferation [159]. As ultrasound technology improves, it will be possible to test these hypotheses based on serial measurements of changes in vessel wall mass. The kinetics of those changes may be useful in estimating the expected rate of cell replication in tissues undergoing restenosis.

Summary

Before ending this article, it is important to state clearly that smooth muscle proliferation does occur, although perhaps not as dramatically as had been suggested by data based on studies in vitro. Moreover, while we have concentrated on the proliferation associated with atherosclerosis and restenosis [140], there is much better evidence for proliferation in hypertensive vascular injury [97,98,160—165], transplant atherosclerosis [166], AV shunt grafts [167] and, of course, in animal models of angioplasty [168,169]. Whatever the case for angioplasty and replication, these other forms of smooth muscle replication are important in their own right.

We have also attempted to distinguish between proliferation and phenotypic changes. In atherosclerosis it is the intima that accumulates fat, becomes calcified, expresses tissue factor, and ultimately breaks down, leading to occlusive vascular disease. Restenosis, of course, would not be a problem if we did not need to treat atherosclerosis. Moreover, any mechanism likely to account for restenosis is probably going to depend on new tissue formed after injury. This new tissue is important, and may be the result of replication, migration or extracellular matrix accumulation. Furthermore, this new tissue may contribute to lumen narrowing by occupying space, causing tissue contraction or geometric remodeling of the vessel wall. Thus, whether or not advanced lesions are proliferative, the special and pathologic properties of intimal smooth muscle are central to atherosclerosis. The observation of monoclonality remains unchallenged and, if true, obliges us to explain how the intima is formed.

Finally, theories of both atherosclerosis and restenosis place smooth muscle replication in a central role. These hypotheses simplistically assume that an increase in mass of the intima is the cause of loss of lumen caliber. We know that this is not simply true, but we lack a more comprehensive hypothesis. Terms like "late loss", "chronic recoil", or "remodeling" simply put names on poorly understood processes. Concepts of plaque enlargement by mural thrombosis or breakdown of plaque with critical fissuring offer a tantalizing prospect of molecular targets for therapy that again depend on our knowing why these events occur in the progressing plaque. One can guess where advances are likely to occur. Better, preferably noninvasive, imaging methods are needed to give us

718

more precise definitions of the clinical problems. This, in turn, will hopefully lead to the development of better animal models. In turn, tissue from humans and from better animal models should help us learn how to control expression of the molecules that lead to plaque narrowing and ultimately death.

References

1. Ross R. Nature 1993;362:801–813.
2. Jackson CL, Schwartz SM. Hypertension 1992;20:713–736.
3. French JE. Int Rev Exp Pathol 1966;5:253–354.
4. Chamley-Campbell JH, Campbell GR, Ross R. J Cell Biol 1981;89:379–383.
5. Campbell GR, Campbell JH. Ann NY Acad Sci 1990;598:143–158.
6. Miller MJ, Kuntz RE, Friedrich SP, Leidig GA, Fishman RF, Schnitt SJ, Baim DS, Safian RD. Am J Cardiol 1993;71:652–658.
7. Desmouliere A, Rubbia-Brandt L, Abdiu A, Walz T, Macieira-Coelho A, Gabbiani G. Exp Cell Res 1992;201:64–73.
8. Bochaton-Piallat ML, Gabbiani F, Ropraz P, Gabbiani G. Differentiation 1992;49:175–185.
9. Clowes AW, Clowes MM, Kocher O, Ropraz P, Chaponnier C, Gabbiani G. J Cell Biol 1988;107:1939–1945.
10. Velican D, Velican C. Atherosclerosis 1976;23:345–355.
11. Sims FH, Gavin JB, Vanderwee MA. Am Heart J 1989;118:32–38.
12. Slomp J, Van Munsteren JC, Poelmann RE, DeReeder EG, Bogers AJJC, Gittenberger-de Groot AC. Atherosclerosis 1992;93:25–39.
13. Boudreau N, Turley E, Rabinovitch M. Dev Biol 1991;143:235–247.
14. Benditt EP, Benditt JM. Proc Natl Acad Sci USA 1973;70:1753–1756.
15. Pearson TA, Solez K, Dillman J, Heptinstall R. Lancet 1979;1:7–11.
16. Pearson TA. Science 1979;206:1423–1425.
17. Thomas WA, Reiner JM, Janakidevi K, Florentin RA, Lee KT. Exp Molec Pathol 1979;31:367–386.
18. Hansson GK, Holm J, Holm S, Fotev Z, Hedrich HJ, Fingerle J. Proc Natl Acad Sci USA 1991;88:10530–10534.
19. Gordon D, Reidy MA, Benditt EP, Schwartz SM. Proc Natl Acad Sci USA 1990;87:4600–4604.
20. Stary HC. Atheriosclerosis 1989;9(suppl 1):119–132.
21. Chobanian AV, Prescott MF, Haudenschild CC. Exp Molec Pathol 1984;41:153–169.
22. Friedman RJ, Stemerman MB, Wenz B, Moore S, Gauldie J, Gent M, Tiell ML, Spaet TH. J Clin Invest 1977;60:1191–1201.
23. Bjorkerud S, Bondjers G. Part 5. Atherosclerosis 1973;18:235–255.
24. Schwartz SM, Stemerman MB, Benditt EP. Am J Pathol 1975;81:15–42.
25. Clowes AW, Reidy MA, Clowes MM. Lab Invest 1983;49:208–215.
26. Betz E, Schlote W. Basic Res Cardiol 1979;74:10–20.
27. Baumgartner HR. Z Ges Exp Med 1963;137:227.
28. Stemerman MB, Spaet TH, Pitlick F, Clintron J, Lejneks I, Tiell ML. Am J Pathol 1977;87:125–142.
29. Nomoto A, Hirosumi J, Sekiguchi C, Mutoh S, Yamaguchi I, Aoki H. Atherosclerosis 1987;64:255–261.
30. Haudenschild C, Studer A. Eur J Clin Invest 1971;2:1–7.
31. Baumgartner HR. Haemostasis 1979;8:340–352.
32. Clowes AW, Clowes MM, Reidy MA. Lab Invest 1983;49:327–333.
33. Salisbury BG, Hajjar DP, Minick CR. Exp Molec Pathol 1985;42:306–319.
34. Vesselinovitch D. Arch Pathol Lab Med 1988;112:1011–1017.
35. Anderson PG. Cardiovasc Pathol 1992;1:263–278.
36. Schwartz SM, Haudenschild CC, Eddy EM. Lab Invest 1978;38:568–580.
37. Bjorkerud S. Virchows Arch 1969;347:197–210.
38. Reidy MA, Yoshida K, Harker LA, Schwartz SM. Arteriosclerosis 1986;6:305–311.
39. Richardson M, Hatton MWC, Buchanan MR, Moore S. Am J Pathol 1990;137:1453–1465.
40. Reddick RL, Read MS, Brinkhous KM, Bellinger D, Nichols T, Griggs TR. Arteriosclerosis 1990;10:541–550.
41. Weidinger FF, McLenachan JM, Cybulsky MI, Fallon JT, Hollenberg NK, Cooke JP, Ganz P. Circulation 1991;84:755–767.
42. Scott RF, Imai H, Makita T, Thomas WA, Keiner JM. Exp Molec Pathol 1980;33:185–202.

43. Stadius ML, Rowan R, Fleischhauer JF, Kernoff R, Billingham M, Gown AM. Arterioscler Thromb 1992;12:1267–1273.
44. Groves HM, Kinlough-Rathbone RL, Richardson M. Lab Invest 1979;40:194–206.
45. Nichols TC, Bellinger DA, Reddick RL, Read MS, Koch GG, Brinkhous KM, Griggs TR. Circulation 1991;83(suppl 6):IV56–IV64.
46. Clowes AW, Schwartz SM. Circ Res 1985;56:139–145.
47. Schwartz SM, Reidy MA, Clowes A. Ann NY Acad Sci 1985;454:292–304.
48. Miano JM, Vlasic N, Tota RR, Stemerman MB. Arterioscler Thromb 1993;13:211–219.
49. Majesky MW, Schwartz SM, Clowes MM, Clowes AW. Circ Res 1987;61:296–300.
50. Hanke H, Strohschneider T, Oberhoff M, Betz E, Karsch KR. Circ Res 1990;67:651–659.
51. Lindner V, Reidy MA. Proc Natl Acad Sci USA 1991;88:3739–3743.
52. Olson NE, Chao S, Lindner V, Reidy MA. Am J Pathol 1992;140:1017–1023.
53. Jawien A, Bowen-Pope DF, Lindner V, Schwartz SM, Clowes AW. J Clin Invest 1992;89:507–511.
54. Ferns GAA, Raines EW, Sprugel KH, Motani AS, Reidy MA, Ross R. Science 1991;253:1129–1132.
55. Daemen MJAP, Lombardi DM, Bosman FT, Schwartz SM. Circ Res 1991;68:450–456.
56. Van Kleef EM, Smits JFM, DeMey JGR, Cleutjens JPM, Lombardi DM, Schwartz SM, Daemen MJAP. Circ Res 1992;70:1122–1127.
57. Prescott M, Webb R, Reidy MA. Am J Pathol 1991;139:1291–1302.
58. Majesky MW, Lindner V, Twardzik DR, Schwartz SM, Reidy MA. J Clin Invest 1991;88:904–910.
59. Farhy RD, Carretero OA, Ho K, Scicli AG. Circ Res 1993;72:1202–1210.
60. Kauffman RF, Bean JS, Zimmerman KM, Brown RF, Steinberg MI. Life Sci 1991;49:PL223–PL228.
61. Dzau VJ, Gibbons GH, Pratt RE. Hypertension 1991;18(suppl 4):II100–II105.
62. Bunning P, Holmquist B, Riordan JF. Biochem 1983;22:103–110.
63. Clowes AW, Clowes MM, Reidy MA. Lab Invest 1986;54:295–303.
64. Majesky MW, Reidy MA, Bowen-Pope DF, Wilcox JN, Schwartz SM. J Cell Biol 1990;111:2149–2158.
65. Jackson CL, Raines EW, Ross R, Reidy MA. Arterioscler Thromb 1993;13:1218–1226.
66. Viswanathan M, Stromberg C, Seltzer A, Saavedra JM. J Clin Invest 1992;90:1707–1712.
67. Cercek B, Fishbein MC, Forrester JS, Helfant RH, Fagin JA. Circ Res 1990;66:1755–1760.
68. Powell J, Clozel J, Muller R, Kuhn H, Hefti F, Hosang M, Baumgartner H. Science 1989;245:186–188.
69. Rogerson FM, Chai SY, Schlawe I, Murray WK, Marley PD, Mendelsohn FA. J Hypertension 1992;10:615–620.
70. Rosenthal J, Thurnreiter M, Plaschke M, Geyer M, Reiter W, Dahlheim H. Hypertension 1990;15:848–853.
71. Pan X, Nelken N, Colyvas N, Rapp JH. J Vasc Surg 1992;15:693–698.
72. Laporte S, Escher E. Biochem Biophys Res Commun 1991;187:1510–1516.
73. Powell JS, Muller RKM, Rouge M, Kuhn H, Hefti F, Baumgartner HR. J Cardiovasc Pharmacol 1990;16(suppl 4):S42–S49.
74. Majack RA, Majesky MW, Goodman LV. J Cell Biol 1990;111:239–247.
75. Battegay E, Raines E, Seifert RA, Bowen-Pope DF, Ross R. Ceil 1990;63:515–524.
76. Gibbons G, Pratt R, Dzau V. J Clin Invest 1992;90:456–461.
77. Grainger DJ, Kirschenlohr HL, Metcalfe JC, Weissberg PL. Science 1993;260:1655–1658.
78. Tenda K, Saikawa T, Maeda T, Sato Y, Niwa H, Inoue T, Yonemochi H, Maruyama T, Shimoyama N, Aragaki S. Japan Circ J 1993;57:789–795.
79. Hearn JA, Donohue BC, Ba'albaki H, Douglas JS, King SBI, Lembo NJ, Roubin GS, Sgoutas DS. Am J Cardiol 1992;69:736–739.
80. Ezratty A, Simon DI, Loscalzo J. Biochemistry 1993;32:4628–4633.
81. Etingin OR, Hajjar DP, Hajjar KA, Harpel PC, Nachman RL. J Biol Chem 1991;266:2459–2465.
82. Sporn MB, Roberts AB, Wakefield LM, De Crombrugghe B. J Cell Biol 1987;105:1039–1046.
83. Kirschenlohr HL, Metcalfe JC, Weissberg PL, Grainger DJ. Am J Physiol 1993;265:C571–C576.
84. Grainger DJ, Weissberg PL, Metcalfe JC. Biochem J 1993;294:109–112.
85. Nikol S, Isner JM, Pickering JG, Kearney M, Leclerc G, Weir L. J Clin Invest 1992;90:1582–1592.
86. Au YP, Kenagy RD, Clowes MM, Clowes AW. Haemostasis 1993;23(suppl 1):177–182.
87. Simons M, Edelman ER, DeKeyser J, Langer R, Rosenberg RD. Nature 1992;359:67–70.
88. Ellis SG, Roubin GS, Wilentz J, Douglas JS, King SB. Am Heart J 1989;117:777–782.
89. Lehmann KG, Doria RJ, Feuer JM, Hall PX, Hoang DT. J Am Coll Cardiol 1991;17:181A.
90. Edelman ER, Karnovsky MJ. Circulation 1994;89:770–776.
91. Faxon D, Sprio T, Minor S, Douglas J, Cote G, Dorosti K, Gottlieb R, Califf R, Topol E, Gordon J. J Am Coll Cardiol 1992;19:258A.

92. Tcheng JE, Topol EJ, Kleiman NS, Ellis SG, Navetta FI, Fintel DJ, Weisman HF, Anderson K, Wang AL, Miller JA, Sigmon KN, Califf RM, EPIC Investigators. Circulation 1993;88:I–506 (abstract).
93. Tcheng JE, Ellis S, Kleiman NS, Harrington RA, Mick MJ, Navetta FI, Worley S, Smith JE, Kereiakes DJ, Kitt MM, Miller JA, Sigmon KN, Califf RM, Topol EJ. Circulation 1993;99:I–595.
94. EPIC Investigators. N Engl J Med 1994;330:956–1007.
95. Choi ET, Engel L, Callow AD, Sun S, Trachtenberg J, Santoro S, Ryan US. J Vasc Surg 1994;19:125–134.
96. Villaschi S, Spagnoli LG. Atherosclerosis 1983;48:95–100.
97. Pickering JG, Weir L, Jekanowski J, Kearney MA, Isner JM. J Clin Invest 1993;91:1469–1480.
98. Katsuda S, Coltrera MD, Ross R, Gown AM. Am J Pathol 1993;142:1787–1793.
99. McGill HC. Lab Invest 1968;18:560–564.
100. Moon HD, Rinehart JF. Circulation 1952;6:481–488.
101. Stary HC, Blankenhorn DH, Chandler AB, Glagov S, Insull WJ, Richardson M, Rosenfeld ME, Schaffer SA, Schwartz CJ, Wagner WD. Circulation 1992;85:391–405.
102. Rosenfeld ME, Ross R. Arteriosclerosis 1990;10:680–687.
103. Ross R. Am J Pathol 1993;143:987–1002.
104. Moss NS, Benditt EP. Am J Pathol 1975;78:175–190.
105. Ross R, Wight TN, Strandness E, Thiele B. Am J Pathol 1984;114:79–93.
106. Dartsch PC, Voisard R, Bauriedel G, Hofling B, Betz E. Arteriosclerosis 1990;10:62–75.
107. Waters D, Higginson L, Gladstone P, Kimball B, LeMay M, Boccuzzi SJ, Lesperance J. Circulation 1994;89:959–968.
108. O'Brien ER, Garvin MR, Dev R, Stewart DK, Hinohara T, Simpson JB, Schwartz SM. Angiogenesis in human coronary atherosclerotic plaque. Am J Pathol 1994 (in press).
109. Wilcox JN, Smith KM, Schwartz SM, Gordon D. Proc Natl Acad Sci USA 1989;86:2839–2843.
110. Edgington TS, Mackman N, Brand K, Ruf W. Thromb Haemostas 1991;66:67–79.
111. Constantinides P. J Atheroscler Res 1966;6:1–17.
112. Davies MJ, Thomas AC. Br Heart J 1985;53:363–373.
113. Falk E. Am J Cardiol 1989;63:114E–120E.
114. Wilcox JN, Smith KM, Williams LT, Schwartz SM, Gordon D. J Clin Invest 1988;82:1134–1143.
115. Lindner V, Majack RA, Reidy MA. J Clin Invest 1990;85:2004–2008.
116. Okazaki H, Majesky MW, Harker LA, Schwartz SM. Circ Res 1992;71:1285–1293.
117. Majesky MW, Daemen MJAP, Schwartz SM. J Biol Chem 1990;265:1082–1088.
118. Itoh H, Mukoyama M, Pratt RE, Gibbons GH, Dzau VJ. J Clin Invest 1993;91:2268–2274.
119. Giachelli C, Bae N, Almeida M, Denhardt D, Alpers CE, Schwartz SM. J Clin Invest 1993;92:1686–1696.
120. O'Brien ER, Garvin MR, Stewart DK, Hinohara T, Simpson JB, Schwartz SM, Giachelli CM. Osteopontin is synthesized by macrophage, smooth muscle and endothelial cells in primary and restenotic human coronary atherosclerotic plaques. Arterioscler Thromb 1994 (in press).
121. Bostrom K, Watson KE, Horn S, Wortham C, Herman IM, Demer LL. J Clin Invest 1993;91:1800–1809.
122. Giachelli CM, Bae N, Lombardi DM, Majesky MW, Schwartz SM. Biochem Biophys Res Commun 1991;177:867–873.
123. Ludmer PL, Selwyn AP, Shook TL, Wayne RR, Mudge GL, Alexander RW, Ganz P. N Engl J Med 1986;315:1046–1051.
124. Flavahan NA. Circulation 1992;85:1927–1938.
125. Joly GA, Schini VB, VanHoutte PM. Circ Res 1992;71:331–338.
126. Winkles JA, Alberts GF, Brogi E, Libby P. Biochem Biophys Res Commun 1993;191:1081–1088.
127. Glagov S, Weisenberg E, Zarins CK, Stankunavicius R, Kolettis GJ. N Engl J Med 1987;316:1371–1375.
128. Brown BG, Albers JJ, Fisher LD, Schaefer SM, Lin JT, Kaplan CK, Zhao XQ, Bisson BD, Fitzpatrick VF, Dodge HT. N Engl J Med 1990;323:1289–1298.
129. Blankenhorn DH, Nessim SA, Johnson RL, Sanmarco RE, Azen SP, Cachin-Hamphill L. J Am Med Assoc 1987;257:3233–3240.
130. Watts GF, Lewis B, Brunt JN, Lewis ES, Coltart DJ, Smith LD, Mann JI, Swan AV. Lancet 1992;339:563–569.
131. Gould KL. J Am Coll Cardiol 1992;19:946–947.
132. Kragel AH, Reddy SG, Wittes JT, Roberts WC. Circulation 1989;80:1747–1765.
133. Henney AM, Wakeley PR, Davies MJ, Foster K, Hembry R, Murphy G, Humphries S. Proc Natl Acad Sci USA 1991;88:8154–8158.

134. Arbustini E, Grasso M, Diegoli M, Pucci A, Bramerio M, Ardissino D, Angoli L, de Servi S, Bramucci E, Mussini A. Am J Cardiol 1991;68:36B—50B.
135. Davies MJ. Circulation 1992;85(suppl 1):I19—I24.
136. Little WC, Constantinescu M, Applegate RJ, Kutcher MA, Burrows MT, Kahl FR, Santamore WP. Circulation 1988;78(5 Pt 1):1157—1166.
137. Ambrose JA, Tannenbaum MA, Alexopoulos D, Hjemdahl-Monsen CE, Leavy J, Weiss M, Borrico S, Gorlin R, Fuster V. J Am Coll Cardiol 1988;12:56—62.
138. Qiao JH, Walts AE, Fishbein MC. Am Heart J 1991;122(4 Pt 1):955—958.
139. Qiao JH, Fishbein MC. J Am Coll Cardiol 1991;17:1138—1142.
140. O'Brien ER, Alpers CE, Stewart DK, Ferguson M, Tran N, Gordon D, Benditt EP, Hinohara T, Simpson JB, Schwartz SM. Circ Res 1993;73:223—231.
141. Leclerc G, Kearney M, Schneider D, Rosenfield K, Losordo DW, Isner JM. Clin Res 1993;41:343A (abstract).
142. Strauss BH, Umans VA, VanSuylen RJ, deFeyter PJ, Marco J, Robertson GC, Renkin J, Heyndrickx G, Vuzevski VD, Bosman FT. J Am Coll Cardiol 1992;20:1465—1473.
143. Garcia RL, Coltrera MD, Gown AM. Am J Pathol 1989;134:733—739.
144. Dotter CT, Judkins MP. Circulation 1964;30:654—670.
145. Gruentzig AR, Myler RK, Hanna EH, Turina MI. Circulation 1977;84(suppl II):II-55—II-56.
146. Lee G, Ikeda RM, Joye JA, Bogren HG, Demaria AN, Mason DT. Circulation 1980;61:77—83.
147. Block PC, Myler RK, Stertzer S, Fallon JT. N Engl J Med 1981;305:382—385.
148. Castaneda-Zuniga WR, Formanek A, Tadavarthy M, Vlodaver Z, Edwards JE, Zollikofer C, Amplatz K. Radiology 1980;135:565—571.
149. Baughman KL, Pasternak RC, Fallon JT, Block PC. Am J Cardiol 1981;48:1044—1047.
150. Waller BF. Human Pathol 1987;18:476—484.
151. Mizuno K, Jurita A, Imazeki N. Br Heart J 1984;52:588—590.
152. Losordo DW, Rosenfield K, Pieczek A, Baker K, Harding M, Isner JM. Circulation 1992;86:1845—1858.
153. Nobuyoshi M, Kimura T, Ohishi H, Horiuchi H, Nosaka H, Hamasaki N, Yokoi H, Kim K. J Am Coll Cardiol 1991;17:433—439.
154. Schnitt SJ, Safian RD, Kuntz RE, Schmidt DA, Baim DS. Hum Pathol 1992;23:415—420.
155. Orekhov AN, Ankarpova II, Tertov VV, Rudchenko SA, Addreeva ER, Krushinsky AV, Smirnov RN. Am J Pathol 1984;115:17—24.
156. Andreeva ER, Rekhter MD, Romanov YA, Antonova GM, Antonov AS, Mironov AA, Orekhov AN. Tissue Cell 1992;24:697—704.
157. Mintz GS, Douek PC, Bonner RF, Kent KM, Pichard AD, Satler LF, Leon MB. J Am Coll Cardiol 1993;21:118A (abstract).
158. Mintz GS, Kovach JA, Javier SP, Ditrano CJ, Leon MB. Circulation 1993;88(4 Pt 2):I—654 (abstract).
159. Schwartz RS, Koval TM, Edwards WD, Camrud AR, Bailey KR, Browne K, Vlietstra RE, Holmes DR, Jr. J Am Coll Cardiol 1992;19:1106—1113.
160. Owens GK, Rabinovitch PS, Schwartz SM. Proc Natl Acad Sci USA 1981;78:7759—7763.
161. Owens GK, Schwartz SM. Circ Res 1982;51:280—289.
162. Owens GK, Schwartz SM. Circ Res 1983;53:491—501.
163. Owens GK, Schwartz SM, McCanna M. Hypertension Dallas 1988;11:198—207.
164. Lee RM, Gzik DJ. Basic Res Cardiol 1991;86(suppl 1):55—64.
165. Leitschuh M, Chobanian AV. Hypertension (Dallas) 1987;9(suppl III):III-106—III-109.
166. Masuda J, Ogata J, Yutani C. Stroke 1993;24:1960—1967.
167. Rekhter M, Nicholls S, Ferguson M, Gordon D. Arterioscler Thromb 1993;13:609—617.
168. Isik FF, McDonald TO, Ferguson M, Yamanaka E, Gordon D. Am J Pathol 1992;141:1139—1149.
169. Gordon D. J Heart—Lung Transplant 1992;11:S7.

Drug prevention of restenosis after angioplasty: an update

Guy Leclerc, Pierre Voisine, Martin Bouchard, Angelica Fleser and Rémi Martel

Molecular Cardiology Laboratory, Louis-Charles Simard Research Center, Notre-Dame Hospital, Montreal, Canada

Abstract. New strategies in pharmacological interventions are being developed to prevent the occurrence of postangioplasty restenosis, in terms both of drug design and of drug delivery. As the pathophysiological process underlying restenosis becomes better understood, drugs are tailored to interfere with specific events involved in the complex interaction of platelet aggregation, thrombus formation, cellular proliferation and matrix deposition. Platelet-inhibitor agents and anticoagulants have been used without success to reduce the rate of restenosis after coronary interventions. Newer drugs, such as the thrombin inhibitor hirudin or monoclonal antibodies directed against platelet glycoprotein IIb/IIIa receptor, may help to interfere with restenosis. Other classes of drugs, from antiproliferative agents to lipid regulators, have been tried in the prevention of restenosis, but none has yet demonstrated any clear clinical benefit. Local drug delivery may improve our ability to develop a strategy to interfere with this phenomenon. Several devices have been designed to effect either short-term or long-term delivery at a specific site in the vasculature. With this approach, conventional drugs and even "genetic" drugs such as antisense oligonucleotides could be delivered to the vessel wall to control the healing process that follows angioplasty.

Restenosis is a complex vascular response to balloon catheter-induced injury that occurs mainly in the first 3 months after angioplasty, affecting 35—45% of patients undergoing this type of revascularization procedure. Dissection of the various elements causing this phenomenon has led to the identification of local smooth muscle proliferation, thrombosis, mononuclear cell infiltrates, extracellular matrix deposition, elastic recoil and vascular remodeling as important events leading to restenosis.

Contribution of stents

Whereas pharmacological strategies have for the most part failed to prevent restenosis, recent progress was accomplished in this field by the use of intravascular stent implantation at the site of angioplasty [1,2]. Stents are small stainless steel scaffolds that can be implanted at the time of dilatation. Current recommendations stipulate that they should be placed in arteries having at least 3.0 mm in diameter. In the first study, Benestent, 520 patients were randomized to revascularization by conventional balloon angioplasty with or without stent placement. At follow-up angiography, restenosis was found in 22% of patients with stents and in 32% of patients randomized to conventional angioplasty alone (p = 0.02). In a similar study, Stress, the restenosis rate for patients receiving a stent was 31.6 vs. 42.1% in the conventional group (p = 0.046). Although these results are encouraging, they do not imply any effect on phenomena such as smooth muscle cell proliferation, thrombosis or extracellular matrix deposition. It is proposed that the stent effect resides in its physical ability to obtain an initial greater luminal diameter during the angioplasty procedure. Coupling a stent with drugs having the potential to

Address for correspondence: Guy Leclerc MD, Louis-Charles Simard Research Center, Cardiovascular Research, Notre-Dame Hospital, 1560 Sherbrooke east, Montreal, Quebec, Canada H2L 4M1.

affect biological processes that are not tackled by the prosthesis could eventually yield a stronger approach to this complex problem.

Past clinical trials

Over 30 drugs have been tried in human clinical trials to prevent the occurrence of restenosis. If some of them have yielded encouraging results, none has been shown conclusively to reduce the restenosis rate. Five families of drugs have been explored as potential "magic bullets" to prevent the recurrence of stenosis postangioplasty: antithrombotic, antiproliferative, anti-inflammatory, antivasospastic and hypolipemic drugs. No agent from any of these families has been shown to be successful in reducing restenosis rates. Results of human trials with some of these drugs have been encouraging, but study design or patient population have not permitted strong conclusions. Several new clinical trials are either under way or about to start and should provide better evidence for the role of several candidate molecules in the prevention of restenosis.

Promising candidates

Several new candidates, from DNA to peptides, have recently been proposed to prevent restenosis. From the anticoagulant family of drugs, glycoprotein IIb/IIIa receptor blockers were recently studied in a randomized, multicenter, double-blind trial [3]. The end-point of the study was to determine the efficacy of a monoclonal Fab fragment (c7E3) directed against the platelet glycoprotein IIb/IIIa to reduce the need for repeat angioplasty or surgical coronary revascularization and the occurrence of ischemic events. In this study, patients receiving c7E3 bolus/c7E3 infusion had less need for revascularization (16.5%), either percutaneous or surgical, than patients receiving the placebo drug (22.3%, p = 0.007) at 6-month follow-up. It is important to note that the criteria for need of revascularization were based on clinical symptoms and not on systematic repeat angiography to determine the extent of renarrowing in the treatment groups. Also, an increase in bleeding events and transfusion requirements was noted in the c7E3 bolus/c7E3 infusion group.

Another candidate drug in the anticoagulant category is hirudin. This agent is a 65-amino-acid polypeptide that prevents fibrinogen clotting and activation of factors V, VIII, XIII, protein C and platelets by binding to thrombin at several sites. Although no clinical studies aiming at restenosis prevention have thus far been reported with hirudin, it was recently used successfully to reduce restenosis in a rabbit model by Sarembock et al. [4].

Antiproliferative drugs have received a lot of attention in studies designed to prevent restenosis. Among this family of drugs, the latest to be tried in large human trials are ACE inhibitors, angiopeptin and very recently, NO donors. Although there seems to be no role for ACE inhibition in restenosis prevention, as shown in the MARCATOR trial [5], new classes of drugs such as angiotensin II receptor blockers will soon be tried to inhibit smooth muscle cell proliferation. Angiopeptin, a somatostatin analog, was seen as a promising candidate to prevent restenosis. This agent has been effective in animal studies, including pigs [6], in reducing restenosis rates. However, in a recently completed human trial of angiopeptin [7], the drug showed no effect on angiographic parameters measured 6 months later.

Nitric oxide donors are a novel group of vasodilators that have potent antiproliferative effects in animal models of angioplasty. A recent French trial compared restenosis rates in patients receiving either diltiazem or NO donors (SIN-1 and molsidomine) before and for 6 months after PTCA [8]. Restenosis rates in the NO-donor and diltiazem groups were

724

respectively 38 and 46.5%. The level of significance of this finding was borderline (p = 0.052). Other clinical studies will be needed to confirm these findings.

Another important family of drugs tried in human angioplasty studies is lipid regulators. The efficacy of fish oil in preventing restenosis after PTCA has been the subject of a long debate. Recently, a double-blind, placebo-controlled trial randomized a total of 503 patients to receive either high doses (8 mg/day) of ω-3 fatty acids or corn oil, with pretreatment for a minimum of 12 days prior to PTCA [9]. Restenosis rate, assessed by angiography, was no different between groups (52 vs. 46%) whether analyzed as a discrete or continuous variable. Two trials involving an HMG-CoA reductase inhibitor, lovastatin, have yielded conflicting results on restenosis rates. Another major clinical trial (Fluvastatin Angioplasty Restenosis (FLARE)) is under way to test the ability of fluvastatin to reduce restenosis rates. Basic studies have suggested that fluvastatin may exert a greater direct inhibitory effect on proliferating vascular myocytes than other HMG-CoA reductase inhibitors, independent of any lipid-lowering action.

The concept of gene therapy was put forward in the past few years as a new strategy to prevent restenosis. With the demonstration that direct gene transfer could be performed in normal and atherosclerotic arteries [10,11], different new approaches to prevent restenosis were proposed. Rosenberg et al. [12] initially studied in vitro the effects of antisense oligonucleotides directed against c-myb and nonmuscle myosin mRNA and showed that they inhibited proliferation of smooth muscle cells. They then applied this concept to a rat model of intimal hyperplasia and obtained a significant reduction in luminal narrowing after angioplasty in arteries treated with antisense oligonucleotides delivered by a pluronic gel [13]. Similar experiments were conducted in other laboratories, aiming at other genetic targets implicated in smooth muscle cell proliferation such as c-myc and PCNA mRNA; they obtained in vitro and more recently in vivo an inhibition of smooth muscle cell proliferation. Human trials involving the use of antisense molecules to prevent restenosis will probably be proposed to the FDA in the coming year.

A potential caveat of this gene-transfer strategy resides in the ability to deliver the genetic material to the vessel wall efficiently. Adenoviruses have recently been suggested as an efficient vector and have been used with success by Nabel et al. in a recent publication [14]. Injured porcine arteries were transfected with adenoviral vectors encoding herpesvirus thymidine kinase, which rendered infected cells expressing the tk gene sensitive to the nucleoside analog gancyclovir. Intimal hyperplasia of treated arteries was significantly lower during the gancyclovir treatment.

References

1. Serruys PW et al. N Engl J Med 1994;331:489–495.
2. Fishman DL et al. N Engl J Med 1994;331:496–501.
3. Topol EJ et al. Lancet 1994;343:881–886.
4. Sarembock IJ, Gertz SD, Gimple LW, Owen RM, Powers ER et al. Circulation 1991;84:232–243.
5. Santoian EC, Foegh M, Gravanis MB, Ramwell PW, Kot PA. J Am Coll Cardiol 1992;19:164A.
6. Faxon DP et al. Circulation 1992;86:1–53.
7. Emanuelsson H et al. J Am Coll Cardiol 1994;23:59A.
8. ACCORD Study Investigators. J Am Coll Cardiol 1994;23:59A.
9. Jacobs AK et al. J Am Coll Cardiol 1994;23:59A.
10. Nabel EG, Plautz G, Nabel GJ. Science 1990;249:1285–1288.
11. Leclerc G et al. J Clin Invest 1992;90:937–945.
12. Simons M, Rosenberg RD. Circ Res 1992;70:835–843.
13. Simons M et al. Nature 1992;359:67–70.
14. Ohno T et al. Science 1994;265:781–784.

An overview of reverse cholesterol transport

Alan Tall

Division of Molecular Medicine, Department of Medicine, Columbia University College of Physicians and Surgeons, New York, NY 10032, USA

Abstract. In mammalian species a major portion of cholesterol synthesis occurs in peripheral tissues, which lack enzymes to degrade cholesterol. Thus there is a large daily flux of cholesterol from peripheral tissues back to the liver, a process called reverse cholesterol transport. The reverse transport of cholesterol is mediated by HDL particles which carry cholesterol in free or esterified forms. The transfer of cholesterol from peripheral cells into HDL probably occurs by diffusion or during transient binding to cell membranes. The net movement of cholesterol into HDL is stimulated by cholesterol esterification by LCAT, and both processes may occur preferentially in specific subclasses of HDL. There appear to be several poorly understood processes mediating the uptake of HDL-cholesterol and HDL-cholesteryl ester in the liver. In addition, large, apolipoprotein E (apoE)-enriched HDL particles may be taken up by hepatic LDL receptors. In some species a plasma cholesterol ester transfer protein (CETP) mediates the movement of cholesteryl esters from HDL to VLDL or chylomicrons, which are subsequently removed by the liver as cholesteryl ester-enriched remnant particles. The relationship of reverse cholesterol transport to atherosclerosis is poorly understood. Although changes in HDL levels appear to have direct effects on atherogenesis, genetic deficiency states of LCAT and CETP do not necessarily predispose to premature atherosclerosis. This paper will emphasize the role of CETP in reverse cholesterol transport, with discussion of recently described human genetic deficiency states of CETP, and studies of CETP physiology and gene regulation in transgenic mice.

In mammalian species the major part of cholesterol biosynthesis occurs in the periphery. Since cholesterol synthesized or deposited in the periphery cannot be degraded, it must be transferred from the periphery back to liver for reutilization or excretion. The movement of cholesterol from peripheral tissues back to the liver is termed reverse cholesterol transport.

The initial step of reverse cholesterol transport involves the net transfer of cholesterol from peripheral cell membranes into HDL, in a process most likely involving both aqueous diffusion of cholesterol as well as nonspecific binding of HDL to the plasma membrane. Small phospholipid-rich HDL containing apoA-I (of pre-β mobility by agarose gel electrophoresis) is the preferred initial acceptor of cellular cholesterol. The activity of lecithin:cholesterol acyltransferase (LCAT) within the HDL provides a driving force for the net transfer of cholesterol from peripheral cells into HDL. The cholesteryl ester (CE) formed by LCAT may either be transferred to other lipoproteins by plasma cholesterol ester transfer protein (CETP) or it may remain within the HDL. The continued action of LCAT on HDL results in the formation of larger HDL particles that become enriched in apoE. There are two well-defined pathways for the removal of HDL-CE from plasma: 1) the direct clearance of apoE-enriched, CE-rich large HDL particles by hepatic LDL receptors, and 2) the transfer of HDL-CE to triglyceride-rich lipoproteins, and subsequent removal by the LDL-related receptor protein (LRP), or conversion to smaller particles with eventual removal by hepatic LRP or LDL receptors. Although both the direct and indirect pathways of reverse cholesterol transport result in the return of cholesterol to the liver, the two pathways could have different consequences for atherogenesis, since the

726

pathway involving lipid transfer results in enrichment of remnant lipoproteins with CE.

Studies in our laboratory have focused on the role of CETP in reverse cholesterol transport and atherogenesis. The role of CETP in these processes has been elucidated by the discovery of human genetic deficiency states of CETP, as well as by the development of CETP transgenic mice. There are two well-characterized genetic deficiency states involving the CETP gene, an intron-14 splicing defect, caused by a G:A transition of the first nucleotide of intron 14, and an exon-15 missense mutation, changing amino acid 442 of CETP (476 amino acids) from aspartic acid to glycine. Both mutations cause moderate to marked increases in HDL-CE and apoA-I in the homozygous state, and moderate increases in HDL-CE and apoA-I in the heterozygous state. In addition, there are reciprocal decreases in VLDL- and IDL-CE in both homozygotes and heterozygotes. The intron-14 splicing defect is a null allele with co-dominant expression. The exon-15 missense mutation results in reduced amounts of partially defective CETP, and appears to have dominant expression.

These genetic deficiency states were discovered in the Japanese population. Remarkably, general surveys of subjects of Japanese ancestry reveal that about 6–7% of the Japanese population are heterozygous for genetic CETP deficiency, with the intron-14 splicing defect present in 1–2%, and the exon-15 missense mutation in 4–5% of the general population. Although the first subjects who came to the attention of researchers were those with very high HDL levels and low rates of coronary artery disease, the effects of genetic CETP deficiency on atherosclerosis in the general population have still to be determined.

Another informative approach to the study of CETP has involved the creation of transgenic mice. Mice normally lack CETP activity in plasma. The expression of the CETP transgene results in human-like levels of plasma CETP (2 μg/ml) and modest reductions in HDL-cholesterol levels (about 25%). More dramatic reductions in HDL were achieved by crossing human-CETP transgenic mice with human-apoA-I transgenic mice. Compared to apoA-I transgenic animals, those expressing both transgenes show about 40% lower HDL-cholesterol, as well as more marked decreases in apoA-I and HDL size. These studies indicate that the human-like HDL formed in apoA-I transgenic mice is a better substrate for human CETP in vivo than mouse HDL. By further crossing with apoC-III transgenic mice we examined the interaction of hypertriglyceridemia with CETP. CETP expression in mice containing apoA-I and apoC-III transgenes results in about 70% lower HDL-cholesterol as well as profoundly lower apoA-I levels and HDL size. Even though the mice show markedly lower HDL, preliminary investigation of the development of aortic fatty streak lesions in response to a high-cholesterol atherogenic diet indicates that CETP expression results in fewer lesions than in controls or in mice expressing apoC-III alone. These findings suggest that the dynamics of reverse cholesterol transport may be more important than HDL levels in the development of atherosclerosis.

Atherosclerosis X.
F.P. Woodford, J. Davignon and A. Sniderman, editors.

LCAT activity and the risk of coronary heart disease: relationship to HDL subspecies, sex, hyperlipidemia and coronary artery disease

Jiri Frohlich[1], P. Haydn Pritchard[1] and Milada Dobiasova[2]
[1]*Department of Pathology and Laboratory Medicine, University of British Columbia, Vancouver, British Columbia, Canada; and [2]Institute of Physiology, Czech Academy of Sciences, Prague, Czech Republic*

Abstract. We introduce the notion that the esterification of plasma cholesterol alone may not promote reverse cholesterol transport. We have developed a new assay to measure cholesterol esterification rates in plasma. This estimation, called FER_{HDL}, measures the fractional rate of esterification in plasma from which VLDL and LDL has been removed by precipitation. Our preliminary data suggest that FER_{HDL} is increased in those individuals who are at risk of CAD as a consequence of hyperlipidemia or hypertension. More importantly, FER_{HDL} is markedly higher in patients with angiographically proven CAD than in appropriate controls. Finally, we believe that changes in FER_{HDL} reflect the structural and metabolic heterogeneity within the HDL pool and, as such, may be of use as a prognostic indicator of the risk to CAD.

Is esterification of cholesterol an atherogenic process?

Reverse cholesterol transport (RCT) is a hypothetical pathway by which cholesterol from peripheral tissues may be esterified in plasma and transported to the liver for disposal. Estimates of cholesterol clearance by the liver predict that up to 1 g of cholesterol may be transferred by this process each day and so the biochemistry, pathology, and genetics of each individual step of this theoretical pathway have been studied in great detail (for reviews see [1,2]). Since HDL appears to play a central role in RCT, it has been proposed that this pathway is the mechanism by which high levels of HDL in plasma result in a decreased risk of coronary artery disease (CAD). It is also possible, however, that this pathway may not always be protective. Indeed, the process of cholesterol efflux, esterification and transfer may be atherogenic if the generated esters are not efficiently cleared from the plasma compartment, or if they are not incorporated in the nonatherogenic HDL class of lipoproteins.

In this paper, we outline some of our data on the relationship between cholesterol esterification by lecithin:cholesterol acyl transferase (LCAT) in plasma and the risk of CAD. Specifically, we are testing the hypothesis that increased esterification of cholesterol in plasma by LCAT is potentially atherogenic. The term *potentially* must be used since our studies cannot yet directly relate the atherogenic process to cholesterol esterification in plasma. There are three lines of evidence in support of this hypothesis:
1. Patients with familial LCAT deficiency have only a moderate risk of developing premature CAD, even in the absence of LCAT activity and a lifelong severe deficiency of plasma HDL. Thus, we may conclude that the esterification of cholesterol by LCAT is not *required* for RCT.
2. Cholesterol in different lipoprotein pools is esterified at different rates. The complexity

Address for correspondence: Dr Jiri Frohlich, Atherosclerosis Specialty Laboratory, 950 W 28th Ave, Room 375, Vancouver, BC, Canada V5Z 4H4.

of cholesterol transport in the interstitial space in plasma has been studied extensively by Fielding et al. [3]. They have observed that the rate of esterification of cholesterol in pre-β HDL is distinctly different from that of cholesterol derived from plasma lipoproteins. It appears that the latter occurs independently of the esterification of cholesterol in pre-β HDL which generates the chemical concentration gradient that presumably regulates cholesterol efflux from peripheral tissues. Since esterification of cholesterol in plasma lipoproteins can result in the synthesis of several hundred milligrams of cholesteryl esters per day, we believe that this contribution to the total pool of plasma cholesteryl ester is detrimental.

3. It is also our contention that the transfer of newly synthesized CE to LDL, rather than its retention within the HDL pool, is atherogenic. Evidence for this comes from early studies from our laboratory in which we studied the equilibration of cholesteryl esters in plasma. We showed that the rate of transfer of cholesteryl esters from HDL to the endogenous plasma lipoproteins is variable [4]. In normal individuals approximately half the transferred CE was retained within the HDL pool, whereas in individuals at risk of CAD from dyslipidemia significantly larger amounts were transferred to LDL/VLDL, with significantly less CE retained within the HDL pool, particularly in those individuals with hypo-α-lipoproteinemia.

Is the rate of esterification in plasma higher in those individuals who have CAD or who are at risk of CAD?

To test our hypothesis we have examined the relationship between esterification rate and disease status. Since virtually all cholesteryl ester in plasma is synthesized by the enzyme LCAT, it is important to note some of the salient features of this plasma protein. LCAT is found in association with HDL. The factors that regulate the binding of LCAT to HDL are not well understood although it is generally well established that apolipoprotein A-I (apoA-I) in HDL is required for full LCAT activity in vivo [5].

Various methods have been used to study the regulation of cholesterol esterification by LCAT. For example, an exogenous proteoliposome substrate prepared from human apoA-I:phospholipid and unesterified cholesterol is routinely used to estimate LCAT activity. Incubation of the substrate containing known amounts of unesterified cholesterol with a sample of plasma permits calculation of a molar esterification rate, which is expressed as nmol/h/ml. We feel, however, that this assay reflects the concentration of LCAT protein in plasma rather than the endogenous cholesterol esterification rate since the endogenous lipoproteins do not affect the observed activity of LCAT as they do in vivo.

A new assay to determine the cholesterol esterification rates in plasma: FER$_{HDL}$

Over the last few years, we have utilized measurement of the cholesterol esterification rate to estimate the net synthesis of CE in whole plasma. This assay utilizes both the endogenous LCAT and the endogenous lipoproteins present in an essentially unmodified sample of plasma. Determination of the fractional esterification rate (FER) together with knowledge of the concentration of unesterified cholesterol in the sample enables us to define the net plasma esterification rate.

These two measurements have been particularly useful in defining differences in the phenotypic expression of LCAT deficiency syndromes. However, the differential utilization of cholesterol from VLDL and LDL as compared to cholesterol from HDL means that not all cholesterol in the plasma is equally available for esterification by LCAT.

We have developed a novel assay in which the VLDL and LDL are removed from the patient's plasma by precipitation with phosphotungstic acid prior to determination of the esterification rate [6]. The remaining sample is then incubated at 4°C overnight with a filter disc which has been impregnated with sufficient [^{3}H]cholesterol to label the lipoproteins present to an appropriate specific radioactivity. The filter disc is removed and the sample is incubated for 30 min at 37°C. The synthesis of [^{3}H]cholesteryl esters occurs in a linear manner during this time. After stopping the reaction and extracting the lipids, we used TLC to separate cholesterol from cholesteryl esters and determined the radioactivity in each fraction. This permits an estimation of the fraction (or proportion) of the cholesterol in plasma that was esterified during the incubation.

Using this assay, we have studied the rate of cholesterol esterification in the HDL of several patient groups. Specifically, we looked at a cohort of healthy men and compared their fractional esterification rate in HDL (FER$_{HDL}$) to that a cohort of healthy women and apparently healthy septuagenarian men [6,7]:

- FER$_{HDL}$ was significantly higher in the men than in women of similar age but there were no significant differences between healthy old and young men.
- Men and women with various degrees of hypertension had higher FER$_{HDL}$ than controls.
- Men with proven CAD had significantly higher FER$_{HDL}$ than male controls.
- Women with proven CAD had a FER$_{HDL}$ that was not significantly different from the men with CAD but was 3 times higher than in female controls.

The limitations of this relatively small study must be considered in interpreting these results. Further cross-sectional and longitudinal studies are required before we can use FER$_{HDL}$ as a quantitative prognostic indicator of the risk of CAD. On the whole, however, these data support our contention that high rates of esterification of HDL-cholesterol are associated with increased risk of CAD rather than being protective.

What is the mechanism of differences in FER$_{HDL}$?

We have studied the correlation between FER$_{HDL}$ with several lipid and lipoprotein parameters in 56 normal and hypertensive individuals [6,7]. The age range was 29–79 but age was not correlated with FER$_{HDL}$. Positive correlations with body mass index, total cholesterol, and a negative correlation with HDL-cholesterol were observed. However, the strongest correlation was with triglyceride levels. Since high triglycerides are associated with a decrease in HDL particle size, we studied the correlation between FER$_{HDL}$ and the distribution of HDL subclasses. There was a significant negative correlation between FER$_{HDL}$ and the larger HDL particles (namely HDL2b and HDL3a) and a highly significant positive correlation with small dense HDL3b.

Since the cohort investigated in the correlation study comprised hypertensive and normal individuals, we studied the heterogeneity of the HDL pool by gradient gel electrophoresis. Here we see that increasing severity of hypertension is associated with an increase in the smaller HDL (HDL3b) and a decrease in the larger HDL subclasses.

How does a change in the average size of HDL cause the observed increase in FER$_{HDL}$?

We have shown that the Km of LCAT for HDL substrates is regulated by particle size [8]. The greater the diameter of the reconstituted spherical HDL, the lower the Km of LCAT for unesterified cholesterol in the lipoprotein. How then does this relate to our observations? If we were to measure the fractional rate of esterification in individual subclasses of all lipoproteins, we would observe that the lowest rate of esterification is with the larger particles. This is not unexpected. However, we believe that differences in the overall fractional rate of esterification result from the relative increases in the proportion of small HDL compared to other lipoproteins. This would explain why higher levels of FER_{HDL} are observed when there is a relatively high proportion of the HDL_{3b} subclass in the HDL pool. We are impressed by the strength of the relationship between these two parameters and we have proposed therefore that FER_{HDL} may represent a novel method by which we can estimate the particle size distribution of the HDL pool within a sample of plasma. However, before we can fully elucidate the potential of FER_{HDL} to predict HDL heterogeneity, we must understand all of the factors that regulate this activity.

Particle size is clearly the most important factor in determining the FER_{HDL}. In addition, we can exclude simple explanations such as isotope dilution at the level of unesterified cholesterol in the HDL, since we observed only a weak correlation between FER_{HDL} and unesterified HDL-cholesterol. More convincing is the observation that widely differing FER_{HDL} results are seen in patients who have identical levels of unesterified HDL-cholesterol.

What is the potential for FER_{HDL} as a prognostic tool?

There is now a great deal of research interest in HDL heterogeneity and risk of CAD. However, there is no consensus on the best method to be used to assess this heterogeneity. Historically, differential precipitation or ultracentrifugation have been used to quantitate relative HDL subclasses. These methods are poorly reproducible from lab to lab and consequently are of little value to the routine lipid clinic laboratory. More recently, gradient gel electrophoresis and immunoelectrophoresis have been used to study the size and apoprotein heterogeneity of HDL, respectively. We believe that our assay has the potential to be a single numerical reflection of the overall structural and metabolic heterogeneity of the HDL pool. Specifically, we believe that the biological sensitivity of LCAT to select preferred substrates permits us to define a composite of the biological and structural heterogeneity that may exist within HDL in plasma.

Acknowledgements

This work was supported by grants from the Medical Research Council of Canada and the Heart and Stroke Foundation of BC and Yukon.

References

1. Barter P. Curr Opin Lipidol 1993;4:210—217.
2. Carlson LA. Disorders of HDL. London: Smith Gordon, 1990.
3. Fielding CJ. Curr Opin Lipidol 1991;2:376—378.
4. Sparks DL, Frohlich J, Lacko AG, Pritchard PH. Atherosclerosis 1989;77:183—189.
5. Glomset JA. J Lipid Res 1968;9:155—167.
6. Dobiasova M, Stribrna J, Sparks DL, Pritchard PH, Frohlich JJ. Arterioscler Thromb 1991;11:64—70.
7. Dobiasova M, Stribrna J, Pritchard PH, Frohlich JJ. J Lipid Res 1992;33:1411—1418.
8. Sparks DL, Pritchard PH. Biochem Cell Biol 1989;67:358—364.

Roles of hepatic lipase and cholesterol ester transfer protein in HDL metabolism

P.J. Barter, H.-Q. Liang, M.A. Clay and K.-A. Rye

Department of Medicine, Royal Adelaide Hospital, Adelaide, South Australia, Australia

Abstract. Much of the regulation of HDL is achieved by factors operating within the plasma compartment. Two such factors are hepatic lipase and cholesterol ester transfer protein (CETP). These factors both deplete HDL of core lipids. They also promote a reduction in HDL size and dissociation of apolipoprotein A-I (apoA-I) from HDL. This dissociated apoA-I is free of lipid and has a pre-β electrophoretic mobility. The lipid-free apoA-I may subsequently re-enter the HDL fraction by: (i) associating with phospholipids to form discoidal HDL or (ii) reassociating with existing HDL particles, the size of which is being increased by lecithin:cholesterol acyltransferase. These processes of dissociation and reassociation have obvious implications in terms of the regulation of plasma apoA-I concentration.

The importance of high density lipoproteins (HDL) relates both to their fundamental role in the process of reverse cholesterol transport and to the fact that their concentration in plasma is a powerful inverse predictor of the development of premature coronary heart disease. Like all plasma lipoproteins, HDL consist of a core of hydrophobic lipids (cholesteryl esters and triglyceride) which is enclosed by a surface monolayer of phospholipids, unesterified cholesterol and proteins. The HDL fraction in human plasma includes a number of subpopulations which differ in size, density and both lipid and apolipoprotein composition. Several factors which operate in plasma (lecithin:cholesterol acyltransferase (LCAT), cholesterol ester transfer protein (CETP) and the endothelial lipases, lipoprotein lipase and hepatic lipase) have been shown to influence the size, density and lipid composition of HDL [1]. In this report, we describe how hepatic lipase, CETP and LCAT also play a role in the regulation of the main HDL apolipoprotein, apoA-I.

Role of hepatic lipase in dissociating apoA-I from HDL

The first evidence that hepatic lipase may have a role in modulating the apoA-I content of HDL was provided by studies of the plasma of rabbits [2], a species with a naturally high level of CETP combined with a very low level of activity of hepatic lipase. CETP acts to deplete HDL of cholesteryl esters while enriching them with triglyceride. In human plasma the HDL triglyceride is readily hydrolyzed by hepatic lipase. In rabbit plasma, however, the low activity of hepatic lipase results in an HDL fraction which is triglyceride-rich. When rabbit plasma is incubated in vitro in mixtures containing hepatic lipase, much of the HDL triglyceride is hydrolyzed, leading to a depletion of the core lipid content of HDL. The consequent reduction in HDL particle size is accompanied by the dissociation of a proportion of the apoA-I from the HDL. This dissociation of apoA-I from rabbit HDL has been demonstrated both by ultracentrifugation and by the much

---

Address for correspondence: Prof P.J. Barter, Department of Medicine, Royal Adelaide Hospital, North Terrace, Adelaide, South Australia 5000, Australia.

gentler technique of nondenaturing gradient gel electrophoresis with immunoblotting for apoA-I [2].

Hepatic lipase has also been shown to dissociate apoA-I from human HDL [3]. When the HDL in human plasma are depleted of cholesteryl esters and enriched in triglyceride by the action of CETP in vitro, hydrolysis of the HDL triglyceride by hepatic lipase reduces the HDL size and dissociates a proportion of the apoA-I from the HDL. This effect of hepatic lipase is not mimicked either by phospholipase A_2, which hydrolyzes HDL phospholipids, or by lipoprotein lipase, which generates lipolytic products following its interaction with triglyceride-rich lipoproteins. It is probable that the hepatic lipase-mediated dissociation of apoA-I from HDL is secondary to a reduction in HDL size which in turn is secondary to a reduction in the core lipid content of the HDL.

The time course of the hepatic lipase-mediated dissociation of apoA-I from HDL in incubations of human plasma is complex. When human plasma is supplemented in vitro with additional CETP and additional very low density lipoproteins (VLDL), the triglyceride enrichment of HDL is enhanced. Under these circumstances, activity of hepatic lipase results in an initial dissociation of apoA-I from HDL followed by a subsequent reappearance of the apoA-I in the HDL fraction [4]. During the first 2—3 h of incubation there is a loss of up to 30% of the apoA-I from HDL; this apoA-I is recovered ultracentrifugally in the lipoprotein-free fraction of the plasma. Continuation of the incubation beyond 3 h results in a progressive return of apoA-I to the HDL density range such that by 8 h there is no longer any evidence of dissociation. The return of apoA-I to the HDL fraction is accompanied by the electron-microscopic appearance of discoidal HDL which are subsequently converted to small, spherical particles [4]. These findings have been interpreted in terms of: (i) an initial dissociation of apoA-I from HDL which follows the hydrolysis of HDL-triglyceride by hepatic lipase and the consequent reduction in HDL size; (ii) the formation of discoidal HDL resulting from an interaction of the dissociated apoA-I, with phospholipids being released from triglyceride-rich lipoproteins which are undergoing lipolysis; and (iii) a conversion of the discoidal HDL to spherical particles by the action of LCAT. This complex sequence of events makes it difficult to determine either the form in which the apoA-I initially dissociates from the HDL or the factors which regulate the dissociation. These issues have been addressed in subsequent studies conducted under conditions in which dissociation of apoA-I from HDL is promoted by CETP in the absence of lipase activity [5]. While this CETP-mediated dissociation of apoA-I is much slower than that which occurs in the presence of hepatic lipase, the dissociated apoA-I does not return to the HDL fraction. Rather, it remains in the form in which it initially dissociates and can thus be quantitated and characterized.

Role of CETP in the dissociation of apoA-I from HDL

When HDL and VLDL are incubated with CETP there are net mass transfers of cholesteryl esters from HDL to VLDL and of triglyceride from VLDL to HDL. However, the triglyceride transfer is less than that of cholesteryl esters. As a result, there is a reduction in the core lipid content and particle size of the HDL [5,6]. Similarly, incubation of HDL and LDL in the presence of CETP results in a reduction in HDL core lipids and particle size [5]. Coincident with the reduction in size of HDL, there is a dissociation of apoA-I which is demonstrable by ultracentrifugation, by size exclusion chromatography and by nondenaturing gradient gel electrophoresis with immunoblotting for apoA-I [5]. The extent of the dissociation is quantifiable as the loss of apoA-I from the ultracentrifugal fraction of d < 1.25 g/ml.

When HDL are incubated at 37°C for 24 h in the absence of other additions, there is no dissociation of apoA-I from HDL. Nor does apoA-I dissociate during incubations of HDL either in the presence of CETP in the absence of other lipoprotein fractions, or in the presence of other lipoproteins in the absence of CETP. However, when mixtures of HDL and CETP are incubated for 24 h in the presence of physiological concentrations of either VLDL or LDL, there are time-dependent reductions in HDL core lipids and particle size and a dissociation of up to one-third of the apoA-I from the HDL fraction. This dissociation of apoA-I is linear with time up to 24 h of incubation. The percentage of apoA-I which dissociates from HDL correlates positively with the concentrations of VLDL, LDL and CETP in the incubation mixture and negatively with the concentration of HDL [5].

The dissociated apoA-I has been isolated as the ultracentrifugal fraction of d > 1.25 g/ml and also as the lower molecular weight fractions recovered after size exclusion chromatography [5]. In each case the dissociated apoA-I is essentially free of cholesterol and phospholipids and is not associated with other apolipoproteins. Furthermore, when subjected to agarose-gel electrophoresis, the dissociated apoA-I migrates to a pre-β position which is identical to that of purified, lipid-free apoA-I and is clearly distinct from the α migration of unmodified HDL.

It is not known whether lipid-free apoA-I dissociates from HDL in vivo, although it is well documented that a small proportion of the apoA-I in human plasma exists as a component of small, pre-β migrating particles that are distinct from any of the major lipoprotein fractions [7]. Furthermore, the concentration of this pre-β apoA-I is increased in subjects with hypertriglyceridemia [8]. Although the pre-β apoA-I found in human plasma is associated with a small amount of phospholipid and unesterified cholesterol, it is possible that it originates as lipid-free apoA-I which has dissociated from HDL in a process comparable to that demonstrated in vitro.

If lipid-free apoA-I does dissociate from HDL in vivo, it has several potential fates (Fig. 1). (i) The apoA-I may enter the interstitial space where it has the capacity to function as an acceptor of cellular cholesterol. (ii) It has also been suggested that it may be excreted through the kidney. (iii) It may interact with the phospholipids released from triglyceride-rich lipoproteins undergoing lipolysis to form apoA-I–phospholipid discs within the plasma. (iv) Finally, just as apoA-I dissociates from HDL when they lose core lipids and become smaller, it is possible that apoA-I reincorporates into HDL which are increasing in size as a consequence of acquiring additional cholesteryl esters generated by LCAT. This final possibility has been tested in vitro by measuring the net mass incorporation of purified, lipid-free apoA-I into HDL during the interaction of HDL with LCAT.

Role of LCAT in the incorporation of lipid-free apoA-I into HDL

HDL were first reduced in size during 37°C incubation of the human plasma lipoprotein fraction (d < 1.21 g/ml) with CETP. After 24 h of such incubation, the modified lipoproteins were separated from both the CETP and any dissociated apoA-I by ultracentrifugation at 1.21 g/ml. The modified lipoproteins were then subjected to a further 12 h of incubation at 37°C in either the absence or the presence of LCAT and either the absence or the presence of purified, lipid-free apoA-I. When the modified lipoproteins were kept at 4°C or incubated at 37°C in the absence of LCAT, the addition of purified apoA-I did not increase the apoA-I concentration in the subsequently reisolated HDL. However, when the incubation was conducted at 37°C in the presence of LCAT, the increase in HDL size was accompanied by a substantial incorporation of the added apoA-I

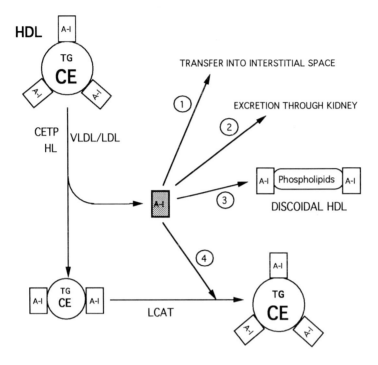

Fig. 1. Potential fates of lipid-free apoA-I following its dissociation from HDL. 1) It may enter the interstitial space and function as an acceptor of cellular cholesterol. 2) It may be excreted through the kidney. 3) It may interact with phospholipids released from triglyceride-rich lipoproteins during lipolysis to form discoidal complexes within the plasma; such complexes are likely to be converted rapidly into spherical HDL by LCAT. 4) It may be reincorporated into pre-existing HDL which are increasing in size as a result of acquiring additional cholesteryl esters generated by LCAT.

into the HDL fraction, such that the concentration of HDL apoA-I increased by more than 30% (Liang and Barter, unpublished observation). This LCAT-mediated appearance of lipid-free apoA-I in the HDL fraction does not occur if HDL are not present in the incubation mixture, indicating that the apoA-I is incorporated into pre-existing HDL rather than being formed into new HDL particles.

Conclusion

The studies outlined above suggest the existence of a cyclic process in which lipid-free apoA-I dissociates from and reassociates with HDL depending on whether the HDL are decreasing or increasing in size. The balance between factors which decrease and those which increase HDL size will therefore influence not only the particle-size distribution of the HDL but also the concentration of HDL apoA-I.

The fact that lipid-free apoA-I has not been identified in human plasma is not surprising since this apolipoprotein has a high affinity for phospholipids and that there is an abundant supply of phospholipids in plasma. For example, any lipid-free apoA-I which dissociates from HDL in vivo is likely to interact rapidly with phospholipids released from VLDL and chylomicrons which are undergoing lipolysis. Such an interaction of dissociated, lipid-free apoA-I with phospholipids may well be the origin of the pre-β migrating, apoA-I–phospholipid complexes which have been implicated as the initial plasma acceptors of cell cholesterol in the first step in the pathway of reverse cholesterol transport [9]. Of potentially greater importance, however, is the possibility that dissociation of apoA-I from HDL is of importance in determining the concentration of apoA-I in plasma.

Such a proposition is supported by the observation that subjects with elevated concentrations of triglyceride-rich lipoproteins have not only decreased concentrations of plasma apoA-I but also increased concentrations of pre-β migrating apoA-I [8]. It has been suggested that the pre-β apoA-I in such subjects has its origin as a dissociation of apoA-I from HDL and that a subsequent rapid clearance of the pre-β apoA-I by the kidney is the reason why the plasma concentration of apoA-I is low in these subjects [10]. Such a suggestion is totally consistent with the in vitro results described above.

References

1. Barter PJ. In: Carlson L (ed) Disorders of HDL. London: Smith-Gordon, 1990;150–156.
2. Clay MA, Rye K-A, Barter PJ. Biochim Biophys Acta 1990;1044:50–56.
3. Clay MA, Newnham HH, Barter PJ. Arterioscler Thromb 1991;11:415–422.
4. Clay MA, Newnham HH, Forte TM, Barter PJ. Biochim Biophys Acta 1992;1124:52–58.
5. Liang H-Q, Rye K-A, Barter PJ. J Lipid Res 1994;35:1187–1199.
6. Barter PJ, Chang LBF, Rajaram OV. Biochim Biophys Acta 1990;1047:294–297.
7. Kunitake ST, LaSala KJ, Kane JP. J Lipid Res 1985;26:549–555.
8. Neary RH, Gowland E. Clin Chem 1987;33:1163–1169.
9. Castro GR, Fielding CJ. Biochemistry 1988;27:25–29.
10. Horowitz, BS, Goldberg IJ, Merab J, Vanni T, Ramakrishnan R, Ginsberg, HN. In: Miller NE, Tall AR (eds) High Density Lipoproteins and Atherosclerosis. Amsterdam, London, New York, Tokyo: Excerpta Medica, 1992;215–222.

Cholesterol ester transfer protein and cardiovascular disease

Yuji Matsuzawa, Shizuya Yamashita, Naohiko Sakai, Ken-ichi Hirano and Masato Ishigami

The Second Department of Internal Medicine, Osaka University Medical School, 2-2 Yamadaoka Suita, Japan

Abstract. The antiatherogenicity of HDL may be attributed to the fact that HDL has a key role in reverse cholesterol transport (RCT), which is assumed to be protective against cholesterol accumulation. RCT may be impaired when there are genetic defects in enzymes, functional proteins or HDL. Deficiency of cholesterol ester transfer protein (CETP) is one such disorder which causes marked elevation of plasma HDL-C. We found patients with two types of deficiency, one a point mutation at the 5' splice donor site of the CETP gene and the other a CETP missense mutation (442D:G). In these patients, cholesteryl ester accumulates in the HDL2 fraction and the HDL particles become very large. In addition, LDL particles were cholesterol-poor and TG-rich and showed marked polydispersity. We discuss the physiological role of CETP and the atherogenicity of CETP deficiency on the basis of data on the interaction between these abnormal lipoproteins and cells such as macrophages and fibroblasts, as well as the results of epidemiological studies in a city in northern Japan where the gene deficiency is extremely prevalent.

Introduction

During the last decade, patients with marked hyper-HDL-cholesterolemia have been reported from several institutes in Japan [1–4]. The molecular mechanism for the increase of HDL-cholesterol in most of these patients has now been clarified as a deficiency of cholesterol ester transfer protein. This genetic defect is important, since the analysis of the patients gives us important information not only about physiological roles of CETP but also about the molecular mechanism of cholesterol transport in man. In this paper, clinical profiles, molecular basis and lipoprotein abnormalities in this disease are reviewed, and atherogenicity is also discussed.

Clinical profile and plasma lipids

About 40 homozygous cases, including 20 cases from our institute, have been found in Japan. At least one case originated in Korea. Most of the cases were found by chance because at a regular health examination they were found to have markedly elevated HDL-cholesterol in plasma. Two cases were associated with corneal opacifications, and coronary artery disease is present in one proband. A relatively high frequency of cerebrovascular disease was observed in two families (Fig. 1). In two homozygous cases, corneal opacities were observed. As shown in Table 1, total cholesterol was moderately elevated, while HDL-cholesterol is markedly high, up to 3–6 times normal levels. Triglyceride levels are widely distributed and the average value is higher than controls. Apolipoprotein A-I (apoA-I) is markedly elevated, apoC-III and E higher than control and apoB slightly lower than average.

Lipoprotein abnormalities

Analytical ultracentrifugation of lipoproteins showed that the increase of HDL-cholesterol is due to the increase of cholesterol in the HDL2 fraction (d = 1.063–1.125); the

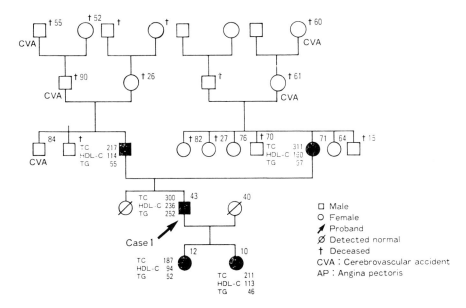

Fig. 1. Family pedigree of case with CETP deficiency.

cholesterol content in HDL3 fraction is not increased. Cholesterol levels are relatively high in the ultracentrifugally separated LDL fraction (d = 1.019–1.063), but this does not mean an increase of cholesterol in ordinary LDL. In this fraction, apoE-rich HDLs which migrate with a slow α-mobility in agarose electrophoresis were detected as well as apoB-containing LDL [5]. HDL particles are richer in cholesteryl ester and poorer in triglyceride than those of control, while the cholesteryl ester content is decreased and triglyceride is increased in VLDL and LDL particles. Bisgaier et al. suggested [6] that the cholesteryl esters of VLDL and its catabolic product LDL may derive predominantly from intracellular acyl-CoA:cholesterol acyltransferase; they deduced this from the class composition of fatty acids in cholesteryl esters. Polyacrylamide gradient gel electrophoresis showed a marked enlargement of HDL2 which is due to their lipid content (Fig. 2). Not only HDL, but also LDL particles in patients show striking abnormalities: marked polydispersity ranging in size from 230 to 290 Å. When the distribution of cholesterol mass and total protein was determined among the density gradient subfractions prepared

Table 1. Serum lipids and apolipoproteins in homozygous CETP deficiency

	(n = 15)	CETP deficiency	Control
TC	(215–358)	285 ± 57	170 ± 17
HDL-C	(119–281)	202 ± 56	52 ± 11
TG	(55–505)	163 ± 142	86 ± 29
ApoA-I	(175–262)	217 ± 33	134 ± 16
ApoA-II	(33–55)	41 ± 8	33 ± 4
ApoB	(50–94)	64 ± 13	83 ± 16
ApoC-II	(4.2–10.6)	7.0 ± 2.4	3.0 ± 1.0
ApoC-III	(12–44)	27 ± 12	6.8 ± 0.9
ApoE	(4.5–21.6)	13 ± 5	3.5 ± 0.9

Note: Values are given as mean ± SD (range), mg/dl.

738

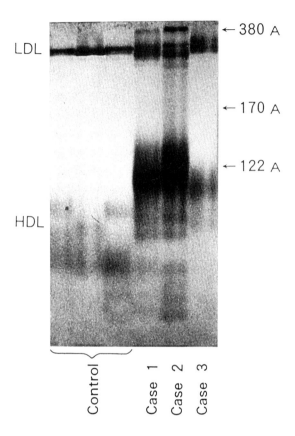

Fig. 2. Polyacrylamide gel electrophoresis (2–16%) of lipoproteins.

by equilibrium density gradient ultracentrifugation, a wide distribution without a prominent peak was observed over subfractions 1–13 (1.023 < d < 1.053 g/ml). In contrast, the control LDL-cholesterol was distributed around a narrow range from 1.030 to 1.046 g/ml, with a single sharp peak. Polyacrylamide gel electrophoresis showed that there are two species of LDL particles with different sizes in each LDL subfraction (Fig. 3). In contrast, each control LDL subfraction contained relatively homogeneous lipoprotein particles, which became progressively smaller with the increase in density. In patients, all the subfractions are rich in triglycerides and poor in cholesteryl ester [7].

From these lipoprotein abnormalities, the following hypothesis concerning the physiological roles of CETP arose. VLDL is secreted by the liver as two species of lipoprotein particles different in size, and each type of VLDL is successively metabolized to LDL through IDL by a separate pathway. Various modulations might be involved in producing cholesterol-rich LDL, which possesses a high affinity for LDL receptors. The hydrolysis of triglycerides by lipoprotein lipase (LPL) and hepatic triglyceride lipase (HTGL) has been known to be important in this process. In addition, an alteration of lipoprotein metabolism in CETP-deficient patients clearly showed that CETP may also play an important part in converting small TG-rich LDL particles to large, CE-rich and homogeneous LDL particles by transferring cholesteryl ester from HDL (Fig. 4).

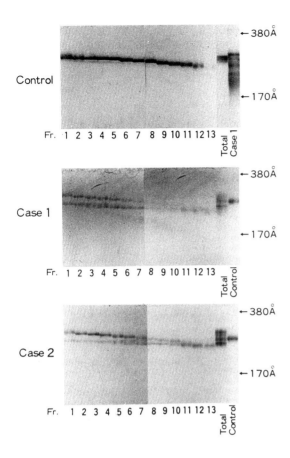

Fig. 3. Polyacrylamide gradient gel electrophoresis (2–16%) of LDL in density gradient subfractions.

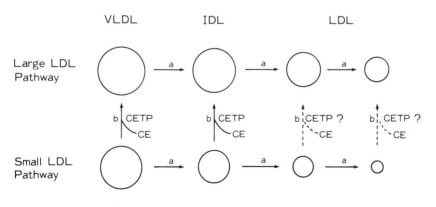

Fig. 4. Two proposed metabolic pathways for LDL formation.

740

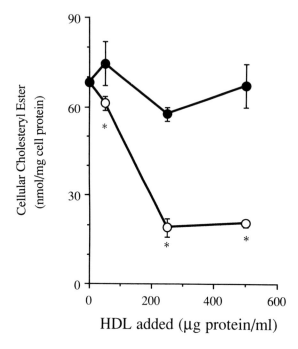

Fig. 5. Effect of HDL2 on intracellular cholesteryl ester content in macrophages incubated with acetylated LDL. (● = HDL2 from a CETP-deficient patient; ○ = HDL2 from normal control.)

Interaction of abnormal lipoproteins with cells

HDL has been shown to prevent or reduce cholesterol accumulation in macrophages incubated with acetylated LDL and to enhance cholesterol efflux from cholesteryl ester-rich large HDL. However, HDL2 particles from CETP-deficient patients are not able to prevent acetylated LDL-induced cholesterol accumulation in macrophages (Fig. 5), although HDL3 particles from the same patients do so [8]. LDL particles from the patients are, like HDL2, functionally abnormal. Unlabeled LDLs from the patients are less effective than normal LDL in competing with normal ^{125}I-LDL for binding, internalization and degradation. These observations suggest that CETP deficiency causes functional abnormalities of both HDL and LDL as well as compositional abnormalities of these lipoproteins [9].

Molecular basis of CETP deficiency and the frequency of gene defects

Alan Tall and his group first described a G-A mutation in the 5′-splice donor site of intron 14 in one Japanese patient with CETP deficiency which may cause impaired splicing of pre-messenger RNA [10]. Subsequent molecular analysis has shown that this mutation is relatively common in Japanese subjects with hyper-HDL-cholesterolemia [11]. Thus, out of 171 patients with marked hyper-HDL-cholesterolemia whose HDL-cholesterol is more than 100 mg/dl, 6 subjects (3.5%) were homozygous and 48 (28.1%) heterozygous for this mutation [12]. Furthermore, in unrelated healthy Japanese subjects, 5 (0.98%) were identified as heterozygous for the G-A mutation. In addition, we reported two cases

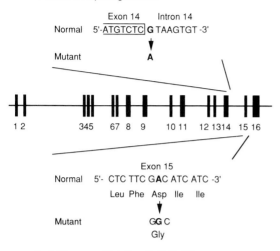

1. Intron 14 Splicing Defect

Exon 14   Intron 14

Normal   5'- ATGTCTC G TAAGTGT -3'

Mutant   A

1 2   345   67 8 9   10 11   12 1314 15 16

Exon 15

Normal   5'- CTC TTC GAC ATC ATC -3'

          Leu Phe Asp Ile   Ile

Mutant   GG C
                      Gly

2. A Missense Mutation (442 D: G)

Fig. 6. Two common gene defects in CETP deficiency.

also heterozygous for this mutation but totally lacking both activity and protein mass of CETP, and with lipoprotein patterns similar to those of homozygotes [11]. Recently, cases with a novel mutation (442 D-G) in exon 15 were found in Japan by a group at Chiba University and by our group independently. Although the subjects are heterozygous for the mutation, they have 3-fold increases in HDL concentration and markedly decreased plasma CETP activity and mass, which suggests that the mutation has a dominant effect on CETP and HDL in vivo [13]. The frequency of this mutation is calculated to be 0.5% in the general population. Both mutations (Fig. 6) have been found only in Japanese and Korean subjects. Recently, we have found an area in northern Japan, Ohmagari City, where the prevalence of a splice defect in intron 14 is enormously high, reaching 27 times that elsewhere in Japan, such as Osaka or Tokyo. The reason for the accumulation of the gene defect in this area remains to be elucidated.

Atherogenicity of CETP deficiency

Since antiatherogenicity of HDL is generally accepted, hyperalphalipoproteinemia has been believed to be an antiatherogenic state. However, there has been no previous study of the atherogenicity of marked hyperalphalipoproteinemia in which HDL-cholesterol levels exceed 100 mg/dl. As we mentioned above, lipoprotein abnormalities in CETP-deficient patients are pronounced in terms of both composition and function. We can say at least that the reverse cholesterol transport system is impaired in CETP-deficient patients. Epidemiological studies in the area where the splice defect accumulates suggest that CETP-deficient subjects are never long-lived, since the prevalence of the splice defect decreases markedly in subjects over 80 years old (paper submitted). More systematic studies in this area on the correlation between prevalence of ischemic heart disease and CETP-gene defects may give an answer to the question whether hyperalphalipoproteinemia is atherogenic or not.

742

References

1. Matsuzawa Y, Yamashita S, Kameda K. Atherosclerosis 1984;53:207—212.
2. Kurasawa T, Yokoyama S, Miyakc Y, Yamaura T, Yamamoto A. J Biochem 1985;98:1499—1508.
3. Koizumi J, Mabudri H, Yoshimura A, Michishita I, Takeda M, Itoh H, Sakai Y. Atherosclerosis 1988;58:175—186.
4. Yamashita S, Matsuzawa Y, Okazaki M, Kato H, Yasugi T, Tarui S. Atherosclerosis 1988;70:7—12.
5. Yamashita S, Sprecher DL, Sakai N, Matsuzawa Y, Tarui S, Hui DY. J Clin Invest 1990;86:688—695.
6. Bisgaier CL, Siebenkas M, Brown ML, Inazu A, Koizumi J, Mabuchi H, Tall AR. J Lipid Res 1991;32:21—32.
7. Sakai N, Matsuzawa Y, Hirano K, Yamashita S, Nozaki S, Ueyama Y, Kubo M, Tarui S. Arterioscler Thromb 1991;11:71—79.
8. Ishigami M, Yamashita S, Sakai N, Arai T, Hirano K, Hiraoka H, Takemura K, Matsuzawa Y. J Biochem 1994;116:257—262.
9. Hirano K, Sakai N, Hiraoka H, Ueyama Y, Funahashi T, Matsuzawa Y. Clin Biochem 1992;25:357—362.
10. Brown ML, Inazu A, Hesler CB, Agelon LB, Mann C, Whitlock MT, Marcel YL, Milne RW, Koizumi J, Mabuchi H, Takeda R, Tall AR. Nature 1989;342:448—451.
11. Yamashita S, Hui DY, Watterau JR, Sprecher DL, Harmony JAK, Matsuzawa Y, Tarui S. Biophys Biochem Res Commun 1990.
12. Hirano K, Sakai N, Yamashita S, Kameda-Takemura K, Matsuzawa Y. Atherosclerosis 1993;100:85—90.
13. Takahashi S, Jiang XC, Sakai N, Yamashita S, Hirano K, Bujo H, Yamazaki H, Kusunoki J, Miura T, Kussie P, Matsuzawa Y, Saito Y, Tall AR. J Clin Invest 1993;2060—2064.

HDL vs. triglycerides: which is important in cardiovascular disease?

Norman E. Miller

Department of Cardiovascular Biochemistry, St Bartholomew's Hospital Medical College, Charterhouse Square, London EC1M 6BQ, UK

Abstract. Plasma triglycerides and HDL-cholesterol are both risk factors for coronary heart disease (CHD), but on multivariate analysis usually only HDL has remained independent. However, in view of the negative correlation between triglycerides and HDL, and the greater intrasubject variance of triglycerides, such statistical analyses may not reflect causality. There is evidence that HDL might inhibit atherogenesis via effects on cholesterol transport, fibrinolysis, platelet aggregation and/or LDL oxidation. The existence of a direct antiatherogenic effect has been supported by effects of drugs, selective breeding, genetic engineering and HDL or apolipoprotein A-I (apoA-I) infusions in animals, by clinical disorders of HDL metabolism, and by clinical trials of LDL-lowering/HDL-raising drugs in hypercholesterolemic men. But not all hypoalphalipoproteinemias in humans or animals, nor all genetically engineered alterations of HDL-cholesterol, have reciprocal effects on atherogenesis. Many humans with low HDL-cholesterol have prolonged postprandial lipemia, probably leading to activation of the blood coagulation system and/or increased uptake of remnant particles by arterial macrophages. On present evidence the high risk of CHD in the hypertriglyceridemia/low-HDL syndrome probably reflects several pathogenic mechanisms involving both lipoprotein classes. Furthermore, delayed lipolysis may itself diminish reverse cholesterol transport.

On univariate analysis HDL-cholesterol concentration is negatively correlated with coronary heart disease (CHD) prevalence, CHD incidence, extent of coronary artery disease (CAD) as quantified by coronary angiography, extent of CAD at autopsy, and rate of progression of CAD on repeated quantitative angiography. The association is present in both sexes, over a wide range and in all industrialized communities, with the possible exception of Russia [1,2]. Recently, incidence of nonhemorrhagic stroke was also found to be negatively correlated with HDL-cholesterol [3]. In most of these studies plasma triglycerides were positively associated with each of these clinical and epidemiological endpoints, though the correlations were usually weaker. Both fasting and nonfasting triglycerides have been found to be predictive [4], and the extent of postprandial lipemia after a standardized oral fat load has shown analogous associations [5].

On multivariate analysis these associations of HDL-cholesterol and triglycerides with disease have generally been found to be independent of other established risk factors, including plasma total or LDL-cholesterol. When both HDL-cholesterol and triglycerides were included in a multivariate analyses, plasma triglycerides usually lost their significant association with disease, while HDL-cholesterol has consistently retained a strong negative association [4].

In cross-sectional epidemiological studies HDL-cholesterol is consistently negatively associated with fasting plasma triglycerides, nonfasting triglycerides and the extent of postprandial lipemia after a standardized oral fat load. Statistically about 40% of the variance of HDL-cholesterol can be explained by variation in plasma triglyceride. Overall, therefore, the accumulated epidemiological evidence suggests that HDL-cholesterol is a major independent predictor of the development of coronary atherosclerosis and its complications in humans, and that plasma triglycerides are associated positively with the disease only by virtue of their negative correlation with HDL-cholesterol.

This epidemiological evidence for the importance of HDL as a risk factor has been strengthened by several other lines of evidence from clinical studies. A number of genetic disorders producing low levels (severe defects of the apoA-I-C-III-A-IV gene cluster) or very high levels (overproduction of apoA-I or CETP deficiency) of HDL-cholesterol are associated with a high or low susceptibility to CHD within affected families [6]. In hypercholesterolemic men, drugs which have several effects on lipoproteins (resins, nicotinic acid, gemfibrozil) have been found, alone or in combination, to reduce CHD incidence or CAD progression to an extent which is correlated not only with the decrease in LDL-cholesterol but also independently with the increment in HDL-cholesterol [7—9]. In contrast, on multivariate analyses clinical outcome appeared to be unrelated to change in triglycerides. There is evidence that oral estrogens in postmenopausal women (which tend to lower LDL-cholesterol while raising both HDL-cholesterol and triglycerides in such subjects) is associated with a reduction of CHD prevalence to an extent which is correlated positively with the increment in HDL-cholesterol [10].

Studies in experimental animals have supported a direct antiatherogenic effect of HDL. Susceptibility to diet-induced atherosclerosis in rabbits has been found to be correlated negatively with the response of HDL-cholesterol to dietary cholesterol [11]. The development of arterial fatty lesions in inbred strains of mice is correlated negatively with HDL-cholesterol but not with triglycerides, and the gene loci have been mapped [12]. And the extent of atherosclerosis in different nonhuman primates has been shown to be related to apoA-I synthesis rate and apoA-I gene expression in liver [13]. Diet-induced athero-sclerosis in rabbits has been reported to be inhibited by infusions of rabbit HDL or apoA-I [14,15]. Two drugs which are powerful HDL-raising drugs (BRL26314, NO-1880) have been shown also to inhibit atherogenesis in rabbits or rats [16,17]. BRL 26314 had little or no effect on other lipoproteins. Although NO-1880 also lowered triglycerides (by increasing lipoprotein lipase (LPL) activity), on multivariate analyses the beneficial effect on atherosclerosis was correlated with the change in HDL, not with that in triglycerides. Support has also been provided by the results of genetic engineering. Human apoA-I gene transfer inhibited the development of diet-induced fatty lesions in cholesterol-fed mice [18], inhibited vascular smooth muscle cell proliferation in rats [19] and inhibited atherogenesis in apoE knock-out mice [20]. Simian CETP gene transfer decreased HDL-cholesterol in mice and increased their susceptibility to arterial fatty lesions [21].

Several plausible mechanisms by which HDL could exert an antiatherogenic effect have been suggested by studies in vitro. It is now well established that the HDLs play a critical role in the reverse transport of cholesterol from peripheral tissues to the liver [22]. In vitro observations have also provided evidence that HDL may inhibit the oxidative modification of LDL [23], may promote fibrinolysis [24], may stimulate prostacyclin synthesis [25], and may inhibit platelet aggregation [26]. Different subclasses of HDL appear to be more effective in some of these processes than in others.

Notwithstanding the consistency of these experimental observations, proof of a direct antiatherogenic effect of HDL in humans awaits the outcome of appropriate clinical trials. In the absence of such trial results, the possibility remains that the epidemiologic and clinical associations of HDL with disease may reflect, at least in part, an atherogenic effect of triglyceride-rich lipoproteins or their remnants. In this context it is noteworthy that in a few studies both HDL-cholesterol and -triglycerides have been found to be independent predictors of CHD risk [27]. Furthermore, interpretation of the outcome of multivariate regression analyses involving HDL and triglycerides in any circumstances is complicated by the fact that plasma triglycerides are much more variable within subjects than is HDL-cholesterol [28]. In consequence, a single measurement of HDL-cholesterol is a better estimate of its mean value in a given subject than is a single measurement of triglycerides. We drew attention to the impact this might have on multivariate analyses of plasma triglycerides and HDL-cholesterol as CHD risk factors [28]. This theme has since been developed and refined by epidemiologists and statisticians. Others have drawn attention to the characteristics of LDL commonly found in subjects with high triglyceride/low HDL-cholesterol, small dense LDL predominating in such subjects, and have suggested that they might be particularly atherogenic [29].

It seems clear from the absence of premature CHD in conditions such as LPL absence, apoC-II absence and familial hypertriglyceridemia that large, newly secreted triglyceride-rich lipoproteins in themselves are not directly atherogenic. However, their cholesterol-rich remnants almost certainly are a source of cholesterol in the lesions. Evidence for the atherogenicity of remnant lipoproteins comes from several sources: in mice and rabbits fed a cholesterol-rich diet chylomicron remnants, not LDL, are the predominant cholesterol-rich lipoproteins; mice in which remnant clearance is defective as a result of genetic engineering of the apoE gene (apoE knock-out mice) develop atherosclerosis [30]; humans with delayed remnant clearance due to certain apoE genotypes or, more rarely, to apoE absence (type III hyperlipoproteinemia) are prone to premature atherosclerosis, though more strikingly in lower limb vessels than in coronary arteries; and remnant lipoproteins are rapidly endocytosed by macrophages, leading to foam-cell formation, in tissue culture. There is increasing evidence that partially lipolyzed triglyceride-rich lipoproteins may also promote thrombosis by activation of Factor VII [31].

In addition to the evidence for a direct atherogenic effect of triglyceride-rich lipoprotein remnants, other observations have questioned a direct causal role of HDL. Though apoA-I absence in humans is associated with premature atherosclerosis [32], no arterial fatty lesions developed in apoA-I gene knock-out mice [33]. Likewise, no atherosclerosis develops in chicks with a naturally occurring mutation that produces very low HDL levels [34]. In clinical studies, not all genetic disorders associated with reduction of HDL levels produce premature CHD [35]. The apoA-I$_{Milano}$ mutation, though associated with a modest reduction of HDL-cholesterol, appears to be characterized by a reduction of CHD [36]. In Tangier disease, in which accelerated apoA-I catabolism appears to underlie the low HDL-cholesterol, CHD incidence, though raised, is not increased to the extent that might be expected [37]. Although this might be explained by the very low LDL levels in Tangier patients, and/or by the fact that the apoA-I-containing particles in Tangier plasma are avid cholesterol acceptors [38,39], it suggests at least that not all HDL subclasses are antiatherogenic. This conclusion accords with the reports that familial apoA-II absence in humans has no effect on HDL-cholesterol or CHD prevalence [40], and that increasing HDL-cholesterol levels by apoA-II gene overexpression in mice increased, rather than decreased, susceptibility to arterial fatty lesions [41].

In international comparisons, attention also been drawn to the fact that non-Western communities consuming very little saturated fat or cholesterol have much lower CHD rates and lower mean HDL-cholesterol levels than Western societies. It has been suggested that the low HDL-cholesterols in such communities are a consequence of their low cholesterol consumption, and that in Western societies CHD risk is greatest in those individuals who develop the smallest increments in HDL in response to a high-cholesterol/high-fat diet [42]. However, this remains an untested hypothesis.

In the light of these apparent inconsistencies in the HDL literature, could the HDL–triglycerides–atherosclerosis triad in humans even be explained entirely by an atherogenic or procoagulant effect of partially lipolyzed triglyceride-rich lipoproteins? This seems unlikely for several reasons. First, the weight of the experimental evidence that HDL is at least potentially antiatherogenic is now considerable. Second, many subjects with low HDL-cholesterol have normal triglycerides, yet are at greatly increased risk of CHD. Third, although such subjects sometimes exhibit prolonged postprandial lipemia, this is not invariably the case [43–47].

While the central role of HDL in reverse cholesterol transport is now well established, the question of whether or not plasma HDL-cholesterol concentration reflects the efficiency of the process in humans has not been answered. The cholesterol in HDL is derived from several sources, only one of which is peripheral tissues, and several processes can affect HDL-cholesterol concentration apart from its rate of uptake of cholesterol: transfer of cholesteryl esters to other lipoproteins; clearance of HDL particles from plasma; and direct removal of cholesteryl esters by the liver. Negative correlations have been reported between body cholesterol pool size and HDL-cholesterol in humans [48] and baboons [49], but not in a larger second study of humans [50]. Though explanations for this apparent discrepancy have been suggested [48], even if these are correct, associations can never establish causality, and even when subjected to multivariate analysis, suffer from the same problems, created by the differing biological variabilities of plasma triglycerides and HDL-cholesterol, as the epidemiological studies already discussed. Schwartz et al. [51] have estimated reverse cholesterol transport in HDL by multicompartmental analysis of cholesterol-specific radioactivity time curves, but have not as yet related their data to plasma HDL-cholesterol concentration in a large number of subjects. Others have presented evidence that the ability of human plasma to promote efflux of cholesterol from cultured cells is a positive function of plasma HDL-cholesterol concentration [52]. We are currently attempting to quantify reverse cholesterol transport in humans by comparing the distribution and cholesterol content of size subclasses of HDL in peripheral lymph and plasma from the same individuals. Comparisons of such lymph–plasma differences in hyper- and hypoalphalipoproteinemic subjects may allow the association of plasma HDL-cholesterol concentration with reverse cholesterol transport to be examined in vivo [53].

More clinical and experimental work will be needed to dissect the relative impacts of triglyceride-rich lipoproteins and HDL on the atherogenic process, and to understand the nature of their effects. Such studies will require inter alia further genetic engineering in mice, and other species, of enzymes and apolipoproteins involved in the metabolism of HDL, triglyceride-rich lipoproteins and remnant particles. Quantification of reverse cholesterol transport in relatively large numbers of subjects is needed, as also are clinical trials with drugs which have clearly defined effects on HDL metabolism or triglyceride transport. Increasingly we need to think in terms not of the effects of drugs on lipoprotein levels, but of effects on different aspects of the metabolism of lipoproteins: a drug which increases apoA-I synthesis, for example, might have a different effect on atherogenesis from one which slows apoA-I clearance. No study has yet examined the association of CHD with the putative primary cholesterol acceptor particles, pre-β lipoprotein A-I (LpA-I) [54].

Clinical trials are in progress to examine the effects of HDL-raising drugs on CHD incidence or angiographic evidence of CAD progression in subjects with normal total cholesterol but low HDL-cholesterol levels. These will answer an important clinical question, and contribute significantly to the future management of this category of patients. However, only if changes in other lipoproteins are small will they provide unequivocal evidence for or against a direct causal association between HDL and human atherosclerosis. Because of the close interrelationships between the metabolism of different classes of lipoproteins, drugs which affect HDL without altering others may be difficult, or indeed impossible, to develop.

Whatever the outcome of further research, on present evidence it seems clear that the high incidence of CHD and the hypertriglyceridemia/low-HDL syndrome, now recognized as at least as important as hypercholesterolemia, probably reflects many pathogenetic mechanisms involving both lipoprotein classes. In the case of triglyceride-rich lipoproteins, it seems clear that it is their lipolysis, not production rate, which matters, producing particles which may be both atherogenic and thrombogenic: the slower the rate of lipolysis the greater the exposure of arterial tissues to these potentially damaging effects. It is also a low lipolytic rate, not a high production rate, of triglyceride-rich lipoproteins, which lowers HDL-cholesterol. Three processes appear to underlie this: the transfer of surface material, including unesterified cholesterol and phospholipids, from partially lipolyzed triglyceride-rich lipoproteins to HDL; the transfer of cholesteryl esters from HDL, where they are produced by the lecithin:cholesterol acyltransferase (LCAT) reaction, to triglyceride-rich lipoproteins; and an as yet unexplained reduction in the fractional catabolic rate (FCR) of apoA-I which accompanies lipolysis [55]. Each of these processes could in different ways influence reverse cholesterol transport, sluggish lipolysis reducing its efficiency. First, a prolonged residence time of partially lipolyzed particles increases the extent of transfer of cholesteryl esters to them from HDL, thereby recycling tissue-derived cholesterol en route to the liver back to the periphery [56]. Second, the increase in apoA-I FCR produced by sluggish lipolysis reduces the pool size of apoA-I, the principal apoprotein of cholesterol acceptor particles. Third, there is evidence that slow lipolysis may reduce cholesterol efflux from tissues by other mechanisms [57–59].

Thus, in many subjects with the hypertriglyceridemia/low HDL-cholesterol syndrome, low LPL activity, by reducing the rate of lipolysis, may increase the delivery of cholesterol to arterial macrophages (in remnant particles), increase blood coagulation tendency, and reduce the efficiency of reverse cholesterol transport — a potent proathero-genic combination, even in the presence of normal LDL concentrations. Many subjects with low HDL-cholesterol levels and normal triglycerides may have a similar lipolytic problem, but one which is concealed by a low triglyceride production rate. Others will have primary disorders of HDL metabolism, unrelated to triglyceride transport. The precise nature of these is probably critical, and not all disorders which lower HDL-cholesterol increase CHD. On current evidence, disorders which reduce the concentration and availability of small apoA-I-containing cholesterol acceptors are probably powerfully atherogenic.

References

1. Miller NE. High Density Lipoproteins and Atherosclerosis II. Amsterdam: Elsevier Science Publishers, 1989.
2. Miller NE, Tall AR. In: Miller NE, Tall AR (eds) High Density Lipoproteins and Atherosclerosis III. Amsterdam: Excerpta Medica, 1992.
3. Lindenstrom E, Boysen G, Nyboe J. Br Med J 1994;309:11.
4. Criqui MH, Heiss G, Cohn R et al. N Engl J Med 1993;328:1220.
5. Miesenböck G, Patsch JR. Cardiovasc Risk Factors 1991;1:293.
6. Breslow JL. Circulation 1993;87(suppl III):III–16.
7. Gordon DJ, Knoke J, Probstfield JL et al. Circulation 1986;74:1217.
8. Manninen V, Elo MO, Frick H et al. J Am Med Assoc 1988;260:641.
9. Brown G, Albers JJ, Fisher LD et al. N Engl J Med 1990;323:1289.
10. Bush TL, Barrett-Connor E, Cowan LD. Circulation 1987;75:1102.
11. Adams CWM, Miller NE, Morgan RS et al. Atherosclerosis 1982;44:1.

12. Nishina PM, Wang J, Toyofuku W et al. Lipids 1993;28:599.
13. Sorci-Thomas M, Prack MM, Dashti N et al. J Biol Chem 1988;263:5183.
14. Badimon JJ, Badimon L, Galvez A et al. Lab Invest 1989;60:455.
15. Beitz J, Beitz A, Antonov IV et al. Prostaglandins Leukotriencs Essen Fatty Acids 1992;47:149.
16. Fears R, Ferres H, Tyrrell AWR. In: Fears R, Levy RI, Shepherd J et al. (eds) Pharmacological Control of Hyperlipidemia. Barcelona: Prous Science Publishers, 1986:353.
17. Tsutsumi K, Inoue Y, Shima A et al. J Clin Invest 1993;92:411.
18. Rubin EM, Kraus RM, Spangler EA et al. Nature 1991;353:265.
19. Swanson ME, Hughes TE, St Denny I et al. Transgenic Res 1992;1:142.
20. Pászty C, Maeda N, Verstuyft J et al. J Clin Invest 1994;94:899.
21. Marotti KR, Castle CK, Boyle TP et al. Nature 1993;364:73.
22. Reichl D, Miller NE. Arteriosclerosis 1989;9:785.
23. Steinberg D, Parthasarathy S, Carew et al. N Engl J Med 1989;320:915.
24. Saku K, Ahmad M, Glas-Greenwalt P et al. Thromb Res 1985;39:1.
25. Fleisher LN, Tall AR, White LD et al. J Biol Chem 1982;257:6653.
26. Higashihara M, Kinoshita M, Teramoto T et al. FEBS Lett 1991;282:82.
27. Bainton D, Miller NE, Bolton CH et al. Br Heart J 1992;68:60.
28. Mjos OD, Rao SN, Bjoru L et al. Atherosclerosis 1979;34:75.
29. Krauss RM, Williams PT, Brensike J et al. Lancet 1987;11(7):62.
30. Qiao J-H, Xie P-Z, Fishbein MC et al. Arterioscler Thromb 1994;14:1480.
31. Mitropoulos KA, Miller GJ, Watts GF et al. Atherosclerosis 1992;95:119.
32. Ng DS, Leiter LA, Vezina C et al. J Clin Invest 1994;93:223.
33. Li H, Reddick RL, Maeda N. Arterioscler Thromb 1993;13:1814.
34. Poernama F, Subramanian R, Cook ME et al. Arterioscler Thromb 1992;12:601.
35. Assmann G, von Eckardstein A, Funke H. Circulation 1993;87(suppl III):III−28.
36. Gualandri V, Franceschini G, Sirtori CR et al. Am J Hum Genet 1985;37:1083.
37. Serfaty-Lacrosniere C, Civeira F, Lanzberg A et al. Atherosclerosis 1994;107:85.
38. Duchatwau P, Rader D, Duverger N et al. Biochim Biophys Acta 1993;1182:30.
39. Cheung MC, Mendez AJ, Wolf AC et al. J Clin Invest 1993;91:522.
40. Deeb SS, Takata K, Peng R et al. Am J Hum Genet 1980;46:822.
41. Warden CH, Hedrick CC, Qiao J-H et al. Science 1993;261:469.
42. Miller GJ, Miller NE. Lancet 1982;4(12):1270.
43. Edelstein C, Fredenrich C, Schuelke JC et al. Metabolism 1993;42:247.
44. Miller M, Kwiterovich Jr PO, Bachorik PS et al. Arterioscler Thromb 1993;13:385.
45. Karpe F, Bard J-M, Steiner G et al. Arterioscler Thromb 1993;13:11.
46. Lamarche B, Després J-P, Pouliot M-C et al. Arterioscler Thromb 1993;13:33.
47. Miesenböck G, Hölzl B, Föger B et al. J Clin Invest 1993;91:448.
48. Miller NE. Atherosclerosis 1987;67:163.
49. Flow BL, Mott GE. J Lipid Res 1984;25:469.
50. Palmer RH, Nichols AV, Dell RB et al. J Lipid Res 1986;27:637.
51. Schwartz CC, Zech LA, VandenBroek JM et al. J Clin Invest 1993;91:923.
52. Llera Moya de la M, Atger V, Paul JL et al. Arterioscler Thromb 1994;14:1056.
53. Miller NE, Nanjee MN, Lucas J et al. In: Witte MH, Witte CL (eds) Lymphology. Tucson: International Society of Lymphology, 1994:44.
54. Kawano M, Miida T, Fielding CJ et al. Biochem 1993;32:5025.
55. Magill P, Rao SN, Miller NE et al. Eur J Clin Invest 1982;12:113.
56. Hayek T, Azrolan N, Verdery RB et al. J Clin Invest 1993;92:1143.
57. Castro GR, Fielding CJ. J Clin Invest 1985;75:874.
58. Miller NE, Nanjee MN. FEBS Lett 1991;285:132.
59. Miller NE. In: Miller NE, Tall AR (eds) High Density Lipoproteins and Atherosclerosis III. Amsterdam: Excerpta Medica, 1992:235.

Diabetes and atherosclerosis: epidemiology and intervention trials

George Steiner
WHO Collaborating Center for the Study of Atherosclerosis in Diabetes, and the Department of Medicine, at the Toronto Hospital (General Division) and the University of Toronto, Toronto, Ontario, Canada

Atherosclerosis in diabetes

Atherosclerosis is the major complication of diabetes [1]. Mortality figures from a number of studies indicate that those with diabetes have 2–4 times the cardiovascular death rate of those without diabetes [2–4]. The relative increase in the risk of peripheral arterial disease, manifesting as intermittent claudication, is even greater [3]. This increase in the relative risk of atherosclerotic cardiovascular disease in diabetes appears to be universal. It is found in countries both with high and with low rates of atherosclerosis [5].

Clinically diabetes has been divided into insulin-dependent (or type I) diabetes and non-insulin-dependent (or type II) diabetes. The relative risk of atherosclerosis is increased in both. However, in insulin-dependent diabetes, it does not generally start to become apparent until after age 30 years [6]. Although myocardial infarction at a young age is a very dramatic and tragic event, the disease burden imposed by atherosclerosis in those with insulin-dependent diabetes is not as great as in those with type II diabetes. The reason for this is that 80% of diabetes is of the non-insulin-dependent type and that the absolute prevalence of coronary artery disease increases with age. In those with insulin-dependent diabetes it appears that there is an association of coronary disease with the duration of diabetes [6]. However, such a relationship could not be clearly established for those with non-insulin-dependent diabetes. In fact, many of them already have coronary disease when their diabetes is first diagnosed. This may reflect the fact that most patients with type II diabetes are older and that the incidence and prevalence of atherosclerosis increase with age. Even more, it probably reflects the difficulty in timing the onset of diabetes. In many, type II diabetes is asymptomatic and is diagnosed only when the patient is found to have hyperglycemia on "routine" blood testing. They may therefore already have had diabetes for some time.

It is well known that there is a great difference in the proportion of diabetes that is insulin-dependent and in the incidence and prevalence of atherosclerosis in various parts of the world, but the higher incidence of atherosclerotic cardiovascular disease in diabetics is observed throughout the world [5].

One other feature that sets diabetes apart with respect to atherosclerosis is the incidence of the disease in women. Prior to menopause, women have a lower incidence of coronary artery disease than men. However, in diabetes this relative "immunity" in women is lost. In fact, because women start from a lower incidence in those without diabetes, the relative increase in risk in those with diabetes is even greater than that in men [7].

Address for correspondence: Dr George Steiner, DAIS Project Office, Room NUW 9-112, The Toronto Hospital (General Division), 200 Elizabeth Street, Toronto, Ontario, Canada M5G 2C4. Tel.: +1-416-340-4538. Fax: +1-416-340-3473.

Atherogenic factors in diabetes

Many factors could account for the increase in atherosclerosis in diabetes. These include abnormalities in blood clotting and clot lysis, hypertension, dyslipoproteinemias, nonenzymatic glycation and advanced glycation endproduct accumulation, and alterations in vessel-wall metabolism and physiology. The pieces of evidence supporting these possibilities come from a variety of approaches ranging from studies conducted in cell cultures to epidemiologic studies. Many of these experiments have been conducted in nondiabetic models and the data extrapolated to diabetics. This may be reasonable where conditions such as hypertension are more prevalent or more severe in individuals with diabetes. However, such extrapolations do not actually prove that a given factor is also atherogenic in diabetes. In addition, some atherogenic factors may be unique to diabetes. An example of both of these situations can be seen in the data from the Multiple Risk Factor Intervention Trial (MRFIT) [2]. That study provided prospective data demonstrating that the incidence of coronary mortality in those with diabetes followed a curvilinear relationship with plasma cholesterol that had a shape similar to that seen in those without diabetes. However, the curve in those with diabetes was set about 4 times higher in those with diabetes. This can be extrapolated to indicate that in diabetes hypercholesterolemia is an atherogenic risk factor, just as it is in the general population. However, the fact that the incidence of coronary mortality at any given cholesterol level in diabetes is 4 times greater than that in the general population suggests that there may be some other factor(s) that are special in those with diabetes.

Hyperglycemia and atherosclerosis

One example of a special factor in diabetes that might be atherogenic is hyperglycemia. On pathophysiologic grounds, support for the potential atherogenicity of hyperglycemia comes from several studies. Hyperglycemia can result in the intracellular accumulation of sorbitol, with consequent changes in cellular sodium and water balance and in cellular metabolism [8]. If this happens in the arterial wall, it has the potential to be atherogenic. Another potential mechanism for atherogenesis is by nonenzymatic glycation of a variety of proteins. High glucose concentrations have been shown to result is glycation of lipoproteins with consequent alterations in their metabolism that could lead to atherosclerosis [9–11]. A number of structural proteins, such as collagen, can also be glycated. If this is sufficient in both extent and duration, cross-linking of the proteins can occur that produces advanced glycation endproducts (AGEs). The accumulation of these in the artery wall could also result in increased susceptibility to atherogenesis [12]. However, against that pathophysiologic background one must recognize that epidemiologic evidence supporting the atherogenicity of hyperglycemia in humans is not clear-cut [13]. The recently completed Diabetes Control and Complications Trial provided data that suggested that improving glycemic control in diabetes might reduce the risk of coronary disease [14]. However, although suggestive, the data were not statistically significant.

Hyperinsulinemia and atherosclerosis

Another special factor that may be atherogenic in diabetes is hyperinsulinemia. There are three prospective studies in general populations that suggest that the incidence of coronary artery disease is positively related to the level of insulin in the fasting or post-glucose-challenge plasma [15–17]. Prevalence data suggest that this is also the case in diabetic populations [18]. Such information has raised questions about the optimum treatment for hyperglycemia in diabetes. Almost 25 years ago it was suggested that diabetic patients taking either of two oral hypoglycemic agents, tolbutamide and phenformin, may be more prone to cardiovascular death than those patients treated with insulin [19]. Two more recent studies have suggested that the prevalence of coronary atherosclerosis is higher in those taking higher doses of insulin [20], and that long-term post-myocardial infarct prognosis in those taking insulin was worse than that in those on oral hypoglycemics or those on diet alone [21]. However, one must beware of a number of problems and limitations in interpreting any of these three studies.

Dyslipoproteinemias and atherosclerosis in diabetes

In the patient with diabetes it is more appropriate to speak of dyslipoproteinemias than of hyperlipoproteinemias. This is because such individuals may have changes not only in the quantity but also in the quality of lipoproteins. The most frequently observed quantitative abnormality is hypertriglyceridemia [22]. The Paris Prospective Study found that hypertriglyceridemia, independently of several other atherogenic factors, is associated with increased coronary mortality in men with impaired glucose tolerance or diabetes [23]. Unfortunately, that study did not assess HDL levels. HDL levels in those with diabetes may be elevated, normal, or reduced [24]. This depends on the presence or absence of other coexisting factors such as obesity, inactivity, etc., and on the patient's treatment regimen. In any event, it may be very difficult to separate the epidemiologic impact on atherosclerosis of hypertriglyceridemia from that of a low HDL and it may be more appropriate to think of the combination of a high triglyceride and a low HDL concentration together.

The cholesterol concentration in a diabetic population is similar to that in the general population. As noted earlier, the relationship between serum cholesterol and coronary mortality has a curvilinear relationship that is similar in diabetics and nondiabetics, but with 4 times greater incidence. This raises the possibility that any given amount of LDL in the diabetic person is more atherogenic than the same amount of LDL normally would be. There are three possible ways in which LDL in diabetes could be more atherogenic. One, already mentioned, is that in the presence of high glucose concentrations LDL can be nonenzymatically glycated. Another is that in diabetes LDL may be more oxidized than normally. The third is that in those with diabetes LDL particles may be smaller and more dense than in those without [25]. The presence of such small dense LDL has been associated with an increased risk of atherosclerosis.

Lipid intervention studies in diabetes

From the above summary one can conclude that a number of lipoprotein abnormalities exist in diabetes and many of them may contribute, at least in part, to the increase in this population's atherosclerosis risk. Despite this, to date, there is no clear demonstration that correcting these abnormalities will reduce the risk of atherosclerosis. The Diabetes Intervention Study has shown that an intensive multifactorial approach can reduce a number of coronary risk factor in diabetes, but it has not produced conclusive information with respect to dyslipoproteinemias [26]. The Helsinki Heart Study did a subgroup analysis of those few diabetic patients who happened to be entered into the study [27]. Although their data suggested that triglyceride reduction might be associated with a reduction in coronary disease, this was a subgroup analysis and it did not reach significance. Against this background, the Diabetes Atherosclerosis Intervention Study (DAIS) has been started. DAIS is a study being conducted in cooperation with the World

752

Health Organization. It is examining whether correcting the dyslipoproteinemias of diabetes with fenofibrate will reduce the risk of coronary disease, as assessed by quantitative coronary angiography, in a population of men and women aged 40–65 with non-insulin-dependent diabetes. DAIS, being conducted at 12 clinical sites in Canada, France, Sweden and Finland, is currently in its recruitment phase and should be completed 3 years after the last entrant is randomized. Until its data are available, the rationale for treating the dyslipoproteinemias of diabetes must be based on extrapolation from studies that have investigated primarily nondiabetic populations.

References

1. Steiner G. In: Vranic M, Hollenberg CH, Steiner G (eds) Comparison of Type I and Type II Diabetes. New York: Plenum Publishing Corp., 1985;277–297.
2. Stamler J, Vaccaro O, Neaton JD, Wentworth D. Diabetes Care 1993;16:434–444.
3. Wilson PF, Kannel WB. In: Ruderman N, Williamson J, Brownlee M (eds) Hyperglycemia, Diabetes and Vascular Disease. Oxford: Oxford University Press, 1992;21–29.
4. Haffner SM, Stern MP, Rewners M. In: Draznin B, Eckel RH (eds) Diabetes and Atherosclerosis. Amsterdam: Elsevier Science Publishers, 1993;229–254.
5. Diabetes Drafting Group. Diabetologia 1985;28:615–640.
6. Krolewski AS, Kosinski EJ, Warram JH et al. Am J Cardiol 1987;59:750–755.
7. Barret-Conner E, Wingard DL. Am J Epidemiol 1983;118:489–496.
8. Greene DA, Lattimer SA, Sima AAF et al. N Engl J Med 1987;316:559–606.
9. Mamo JCL, Szeto L, Steiner G. Diabetologia 1990;33:339–345.
10. Duell PB, Oram JF, Bierman EL. Diabetes 1991;40:377–384.
11. Reaven PD, Picard S, Witztum JL. In: Draznin B, Eckel RH (eds) Diabetes and Atherosclerosis. Amsterdam: Elsevier Science Publishers, 1993;17–38.
12. Brownlee M. Annu Rev Med 1991;42:159–166.
13. Stamler R, Stamler J. J Chronic Dis 1979;32:683–837.
14. The Diabetes Control and Complications Trial Research Group. N Engl J Med 1993;329:977–986.
15. Welborn TA, Wearne K. Diabetes Care 1979;2:154–160.
16. Pyorala K, Savolainen E, Kaukola S et al. Acta Med Scand 1985;70(suppl):38–52.
17. Fontbonne A, Charles MA, Thilbult N et al. Diabetologia 1991;34:356–361.
18. Ronnemaa T, Laakso M, Pyorala K et al. Arterioscler Thromb 1991;11:80–90.
19. Goldner MG, Knatterud GL, Prout TE. J Am Med Assoc 1971;218:1400–1410.
20. Standl E, Janka HU. Horm Metab Res Suppl 1995;15:46–51.
21. Orlander P, Goff D, Ramsey D et al. Diabetes 1994;43(suppl 1):214A.
22. Steiner G. The dyslipoproteinemias of diabetes. Atherosclerosis 1995 (in press).
23. Fontbonne A, Eschwege E, Cambien F et al. Diabetologia 1989;32:300–304.
24. Nikkila EA. Diabetes 1981;30(suppl 2):82–87.
25. Feingold KR, Grunfeld C, Pang M et al. Arterioscler Thromb 1992;12:1496–1502.
26. Hanefeld M, Fischer S, Schmechel H. Diabetes Care 1991;14:308–317.
27. Koskinen P, Manttari M, Huttenen JK et al. Diabetes Care 1992;15:820–825.

Insulin, lipoproteins and hemostatic function

Anders Hamsten, Per Eriksson, Fredrik Karpe and Angela Silveira
Atherosclerosis Research Unit, King Gustaf V Research Institute, Department of Medicine, Karolinska Hospital, Karolinska Institute, Stockholm, Sweden

Abstract. Interest has increased considerably in the past few years in possible interactions between insulin, insulin propeptides and lipoproteins, and several components of the hemostatic system. There is now consistent epidemiological, clinical and experimental evidence that hypertriglyceridemia represents a procoagulant state involving derangements of both blood coagulation and fibrinolysis. Furthermore, elevated plasma plasminogen activator inhibitor-1 (PAI-1) activity should be included as a component of the insulin resistance syndrome along with hyperinsulinemia, hypertriglyceridemia, hypertension and abdominal obesity. Experimental studies are now needed to elucidate the molecular basis for the relationships between apolipoprotein B (apoB)-containing lipoproteins, insulin and insulin resistance on the one hand and plasma PAI-1 activity on the other and between apoB-containing lipoproteins and factor VII activity. Basic research on the link between hemostasis and atherosclerosis should be given high priority, since modulation of hemostatic function is likely to be a potent complementary approach to the prevention of coronary heart disease (CHD).

Many interactions have been described in the past few years between insulin, lipoproteins and components of the hemostatic system that influence clotting activity and fibrinolytic function. These effects are likely to be of clinical importance, since imbalance in the hemostatic system secondary to increased clotting activity, impaired fibrinolytic function, or a combination thereof, could be expected to influence the growth and final size of evolving thrombi and predispose to arterial occlusion. This might be of particular significance in the coronary circulation, where a hypercoagulable state is likely to promote thrombosis at the site of a suddenly ruptured atherosclerotic plaque. Furthermore, the hemostatic system is indicated to play a part in plaque formation and plaque growth. As early as 1852 Carl von Rokitansky suggested that thrombotic processes are involved in atherogenesis [1]. This hypothesis revived again when biochemical analyses of arterial wall specimens indicated that fibrin is deposited in developing atherosclerotic lesions [2,3]. Several potentially important interactions between the hemostatic system, lipoproteins, insulin and insulin propeptides, and cells present in the normal and atherosclerotic arterial wall have subsequently been proposed based on studies using cell and molecular biological techniques.

This brief review will focus on recent advances in our understanding of how insulin resistance, insulin and insulin propeptides, and apolipoprotein B (apoB)-containing lipoproteins participate in the regulation of blood coagulation and fibrinolysis and influence the risk of primary and recurrent manifestations of coronary heart disease (CHD). The emphasis is placed on interactions with fibrinogen, coagulation factor VII (FVII) and plasminogen activator inhibitor-1 (PAI-1), the components of the hemostatic system which have been consistently linked to CHD in epidemiological and clinical studies.

Address for correspondence: Anders Hamsten MD, King Gustaf V Research Institute, Karolinska Hospital, S-171 76, Stockholm, Sweden. Tel.: +46-8-7293201. Fax: +46-8-311298.

Associations with insulin and insulin propeptides in the epidemiological and clinical perspective

Hyperinsulinemia secondary to insulin resistance could explain a major proportion of the plasma PAI-1 activity elevation seen in several clinical conditions such as obesity, non-insulin-dependent diabetes mellitus (NIDDM), hypertriglyceridemia, angina pectoris and myocardial infarction. In fact, plasma insulin has been proposed as a major physiological regulator of PAI-1 levels in plasma and thereby of fibrinolytic activity [4]. In the European Concerted Action on Thrombosis and Disabilities (ECAT) study on 1,484 patients with angina pectoris, a strong relation was, indeed, found between plasma insulin and PAI-1 levels [5]. However, most studies of the link between insulin and fibrinolytic function have used conventional radioimmunoassays for insulin which may overestimate plasma insulin concentrations because of cross-reaction with insulin propeptides. This raises the possibility that proinsulin-like molecules might have confounded the relationships of plasma insulin to PAI-1, other hemostatic proteins and CHD observed in recent studies and that this might be particularly true in patients with NIDDM. It is notable that the one study of patients with NIDDM in which insulin propeptides were determined along with insulin indicated that des31,32 proinsulin, but not insulin, relates to plasma PAI-1 activity [6]. Similarly, insulin treatment of patients with NIDDM has been shown to suppress the plasma concentrations of insulin propeptides and to reduce plasma PAI-1 activity [7].

Studies using conventional radioimmunoassays for plasma insulin have also shown significant positive correlations between fasting or postload insulin levels and plasma fibrinogen concentration [8,9]. Furthermore, plasma fibrinogen has been inversely associated with insulin action as measured by euglycemic hyperinsulinemic clamp experiments [10]. The mechanism underlying the associations between insulin resistance, hyperinsulinemia and raised plasma fibrinogen concentration are largely unknown. Free fatty acids (FFA) might be implicated along with inflammatory reactions accompanying atherosclerosis which induce increased hepatic synthesis of fibrinogen through cytokine effects. In contrast, limited clinical and experimental data are currently available concerning the role of hyperinsulinemia and insulin resistance in contributing to elevated FVII protein and activity levels in plasma.

Insulin and insulin propeptides enhance PAI-1 synthesis and secretion

Strong support for the role of insulin and its precursors as determinants of plasma PAI-1 activity comes from cell biology studies. Both PAI-1 mRNA and secretion of PAI-1 increase in HepG2 cells exposed to insulin [11–13], the mechanism being mRNA stabilization [14]. Proinsulin may also impair endogenous fibrinolysis by stimulating the secretion of PAI-1 from endothelial cells through an insulin- and IGF-1-independent pathway [15]. In contrast to insulin, proinsulin increases PAI-1 mRNA expression and PAI-1 synthesis concordantly in porcine aortic endothelial cells [13]. Time- and concentration-dependent effects of split products of proinsulin (des31,32 proinsulin and des64,65 proinsulin) on PAI-1 synthesis in HepG2 cells have also been documented, stimulation being at least in part transduced by the insulin receptor and mediated at the level of PAI-1 gene expression [16]. Furthermore, Anfosso et al. have demonstrated increased PAI-1 synthesis on insulin stimulation in HepG2 cells after induction of an insulin-resistant state [17]. Metformin inhibited this effect by acting at the cellular level. However, glucose at concentrations encountered in patients with NIDDM also induces PAI-1 secretion from arterial endothelial cells, which means that the increase in plasma

PAI-1 activity seen in patients with NIDDM may be attributable to direct effects of glucose on the endothelium [18,19].

Hypertriglyceridemia and hypercoagulability

A striking feature of PAI-1 is its positive association with the VLDL triglyceride concentration [20]. However, there is heterogeneity in the association between hypertriglyceridemia and plasma PAI-1 elevation. A study of patients with endogenous hypertriglyceridemia has suggested that insulin resistance is the common cause of hypertriglyceridemia and elevated plasma PAI-1 activity in obese subjects, whereas other mechanisms operate in alcohol-related hypertriglyceridemia [21].

Triglyceride-rich lipoproteins have also been implicated in the regulation of FVII activity. Activation of FVII was recently demonstrated during alimentary lipemia [22,23] and shown to relate to lipolysis of triglyceride-rich lipoproteins and generation of FFA from intestinal lipoproteins [23]. Furthermore, long-term increase in FVIIc activity, as in hypertriglyceridemia, appears to be associated with a rise in factor FVII protein concentration [24]. On the basis of in vitro experiments and studies of the hypercholesterolemic rabbit it has been hypothesized that large triglyceride-rich lipoprotein particles, such as chylomicrons, VLDL and their remnants, carrying the appropriate FFA at a sufficient density of negative charge, activate FVII through the intrinsic coagulation pathway and activated FXII (XIIa) [25–27]. The generation and subsequent transfer of FFA from the triglyceride core to the phospholipid surfaces of large triglyceride-rich lipoproteins through the action of lipoprotein lipase plays an important role in this sequence of events [28].

Activation of FVII is generally achieved by tissue factor, with formation of a complex with the activated FVIIa molecule, and initiates blood coagulation by subsequent activation of factors IX and X. Activation of blood coagulation by formation of a FVIIa/tissue factor complex is counteracted by a serine protease inhibitor now named tissue factor pathway inhibitor (TFPI) [29]. TFPI specifically binds to the activated FX and induces feedback inhibition of the tissue factor-induced coagulation pathway by complex formation with the VIIa/tissue factor complex. TFPI is present in vivo in three separate pools, one being blood platelets, one probably of endothelial cell origin, and one associated with plasma lipoproteins. The anticoagulant activity of TFPI in human plasma is preferentially associated with small, dense LDL subspecies, with the densest HDL subclasses and with lipoprotein (a) (Lp(a)) [30]. Plasma TFPI activity is enhanced in hyperlipoproteinemic young postinfarction patients [31] and in subjects with heterozygous familial hypercholesterolemia [32], findings which may reflect a compensatory mechanism to prevent activation of blood coagulation. However, it is currently not known whether lipoprotein-bound and free TFPI have identical capacity for inactivating the VIIa/tissue factor complex. Binding of TFPI to plasma lipoproteins might impair the anticoagulant activity of TFPI in hyperlipidemic subjects by attracting TFPI from the endothelial surface. The role of TFPI in thrombosis and atherosclerosis remains to be established. Whether increase in LDL-associated TFPI may prevent local thrombosis on atheromatous plaques or merely indicates impaired antithrombotic properties of endothelial cells that have been depleted of TFPI is open to speculation.

Effects of VLDL and oxidized LDL on PAI-1 secretion

In vitro, VLDL induces a dose-dependent increase in PAI-1 secretion from endothelial cells [33,34] and liver cells [34]. In addition to VLDL, LDL oxidized by ultraviolet light

756

stimulates the synthesis and secretion of PAI-1 from cultured endothelial cells [35], whereas LDL subjected to more drastic peroxidation does not induce PAI-1 secretion [33]. The molecular mechanisms underlying the effect of mildly oxidized LDL include hydrolysis of membrane phosphatidyl inositol through activation of phospholipase A_2 [36]. However, native and acetylated LDL also induce increased PAI-1 synthesis and secretion by endothelial cells in culture [37]. The effect of normal LDL appears not to be dependent on interactions with the specific LDL receptor, and the PAI-1-releasing capacity of both normal and acetylated LDL is lost after extensive oxidation of the lipoprotein [40]. The mechanism(s) by which VLDL and LDL initiate secretion of PAI-1 from endothelial and liver cells need(s) further clarification. A possible role of the LDL receptor-related protein (LRP) should be considered. In fact, LRP has been proposed to mediate the clearance of plasminogen activator–inhibitor complexes [38–40]. In addition, nonreceptor-mediated mechanisms should be explored.

Conclusions

There is now consistent epidemiological, clinical and experimental evidence that hypertriglyceridemia represents a procoagulant state involving derangements of both blood coagulation and fibrinolysis. Elevated plasma PAI-1 activity should also be included as a component of the insulin-resistance syndrome along with hyperinsulinemia, hypertriglyceridemia, hypertension and abdominal obesity. Experimental studies are now needed to disentangle the molecular mechanisms for these associations. Basic research on the link between hemostasis and atherosclerosis should be given high priority, since modulation of hemostatic function is likely to be a potent complementary approach to the prevention of CHD.

References

1. Von Rokitansky C. A Manual of Pathologic Anatomy. London: The Sydenham Society 1852;265–275.
2. Smith EB, Staples EM, Dietz HS, Smith RH. Lancet 1979;ii:812–816.
3. Bini A, Fenoglio JJ, Mesa-Tejada R, Kudryk B, Kaplan KL. Arteriosclerosis 1989;9:109–121.
4. Juhan-Vague I, Alessi MC, Vague P. Diabetologia 1991;34:457–462.
5. Juhan-Vague I, Thompson SG, Jespersen J, on behalf of the ECAT Angina Pectoris Study Group. Arterioscler Thromb 1993;13:1865–1873.
6. Nagi DK, Hendra TJ, Ryle AJ, Cooper TM, Temple RC, Clark PMS, Schneider AE, Hales CN, Yudkin JS. Diabetologia 1990;33:532–537.
7. Jain SK, Nagi DK, Slavin BM, Lumb PJ, Yudkin JS. Diabet Med 1993;10:27–32.
8. Juhan-Vague I, Alessi MC, Joly P, Thirion X, Vague P, Declerck PJ, Serradimigni A, Collen D. Arteriosclerosis 1989;9:362–367.
9. Landin K, Stigendal L, Eriksson E, Krotkiewski M, Risberg B, Tengborn L, Smith U. Metabolism 1990;39:1044–1048.
10. Landin K, Tengborn L, Smith U. J Intern Med 1990;227:273–278.
11. Alessi MC, Juhan-Vague I, Kooistra T, Declerck PJ, Collen D. Thromb Haemost 1988;60:491–494.
12. Kooistra T, Bosma PJ, Töns HAM, van den Berg AP, Meyer P, Princen HMG. Thromb Haemost 1989;62:723–728.
13. Schneider DJ, Sobel BE. Proc Natl Acad Sci USA 1991;88:9959–9963.
14. Fattal PG, Schneider DJ, Sobel BE, Billadello JJ. J Biol Chem 1992;267:12412–12415.
15. Schneider DJ, Nordt TK, Sobel BE. Diabetes 1992;41:890–895.
16. Nordt TK, Schneider DJ, Sobel BE. Circulation 1994;89:321–330.
17. Anfosso F, Chomiki N, Alessi MC, Vague P, Juhan-Vague I. J Clin Invest 1993;91:2185–2193.
18. Maiello M, Boeri D, Podesta F, Cagliero E, Vichi M, Odetti P, Adezati L, Lorenzi M. Diabetes 1992;41:1009–1015.
19. Nordt TK, Klassen KJ, Schneider DJ, Sobel BE. Arterioscler Thromb 1993;13:1822–1828.
20. Hamsten A, Wiman B, de Faire U, Blombäck M. N Engl J Med 1985;313:1557–1563.

21. Raccah D, Alessi MC, Scelles V, Menard C, Juhan-Vague I, Vague P. Fibrinolysis 1993;7:171–176.
22. Salomaa V, Rasi V, Pekkanen J, Jauhiainen M, Vahtera E, Pietinen P, Korhonen H, Kuulasmaa K, Ehnholm C. Atherosclerosis 1993;103:1–11.
23. Silveira A, Karpe F, Blombäck M, Steiner G, Walldius G, Hamsten A. Arterioscler Thromb 1994;14:60–69.
24. Scarabin PY, Bara L, Samama M, Orssaud G. Br J Haematol 1985;61:186–187.
25. Mitropoulos KA, Esnouf MP, Meade TW. Atherosclerosis 1987;63:43–52.
26. Mitropoulos KA, Esnouf MP. Biochem J 1987;244:263–269.
27. Mitropoulos KA, Martin JC, Reeves BEA, Esnouf MP. Blood 1989;73:1525–1533.
28. Mitropoulos KA, Miller GJ, Watts GF, Durrington PN. Atherosclerosis 1992;95:119–125.
29. Broze Jr GJ. Sem Hematol 1992;29:159–169.
30. Lesnick P, Vonica A, Guérin M, Moreau M, Chapman MJ. Arterioscler Thromb 1993;13:1066–1075.
31. Moor E, Hamsten A, Karpe F, Båvenholm P, Blombäck M, Silveira A. Thromb Haemost 1994;71:707–712.
32. Sandset PM, Lund H, Norseth J, Abildgaard U, Ose L. Arterioscler Thromb 1991;11:138–145.
33. Stiko-Rahm A, Wiman B, Hamsten A, Nilsson J. Arteriosclerosis 1990;10:1067–1073.
34. Mussoni L, Mannucci L, Sirtori M, Camera M, Maderna P, Sironi L, Tremoli E. Arterioscler Thromb 1992; 12:19–25.
35. Latron Y, Chautan M, Anfosso F, Alessi MC, Nalbone G, Lafont H, Juhan-Vague I. Arterioscler Thromb 1991;11:1821–1829.
36. Chautan M, Latron Y, Anfosso F, Alessi M-C, Lafont H, Juhan-Vague I, Nalbone G. J Lipid Res 1993; 34:101–110.
37. Tremoli E, Camera M, Maderna P, Sironi L, Prati L, Colli S, Piovella F, Bernini F, Corsini A, Mussoni L. Arterioscler Thromb 1993;13:338–346.
38. Orth K, Madison EL, Gething M-J, Sambrook JF, Herz J. Proc Natl Acad Sci USA 1992;89:7422–7426.
39. Bu G, Williams S, Strickland DK, Schwartz AL. Proc Natl Acad Sci USA 1992;89:7427–7431.
40. Nykjaer A, Petersen CM, Moller B, Jensen PA, Moestrup SK, Holtet TL, Etzerodt M, Thogersen HC, Munch M, Andreasen PA, Gliemann J. J Biol Chem 1992;267:14543–14546.

Postprandial lipemia and lipoprotein lipase

M.-R. Taskinen, H. Hilden, N. Mero and M. Syvänne

Third and First Departments of Medicine, University of Helsinki, Helsinki, Finland

The concept that atherosclerosis is a postprandial phenomenon was introduced by Zilversmit 15 years ago [1]. The recognition of the fact that man is feasting more of the 24 h than he is fasting has caused an upsurge of interest in the postprandial metabolism of triglyceride-rich particles. Several recent studies have provided consistent evidence that exaggerated postprandial lipemia is a risk factor for cardiovascular diseases [2–4]. Interestingly, the delayed clearance of chylomicron remnants is also a predictor for the angiographically defined progression of coronary atherosclerosis [5]. One major regulator of postprandial lipemia is the fasting concentration of triglycerides [6,7]. Since the constellation of hypertriglyceridemia and low HDL-cholesterol is frequent in NIDDM it would be expected that postprandial lipemia is exaggerated in NIDDM patients.

Metabolism of postprandial triglyceride-rich particles

Chylomicrons are the particles transporting exogenous fat from the intestine to tissues. Following the consumption of a fat-rich meal, absorbed triglycerides and cholesterol are packaged together with apolipoprotein B48 (apoB48), which is synthesized in the intestinal cells, into large triglyceride-rich particles, the chylomicrons. The catabolism of chylomicrons includes two steps. First, the circulating chylomicrons encounter lipoprotein lipase attached to the vascular endothelium. The rapid hydrolysis of chylomicron triglycerides is due to the cooperative action of several LPL molecules on each chylomicron [8]. Recent data suggest that in this process LPL is released from the endothelium and binds to the triglyceride-rich remnants which are generated during the lipolysis. In the next step LPL attached to the remnants acts as a ligand for the binding of remnant particles to LDL receptor-related protein (LRP) which participates in the uptake of remnants by the liver [9]. This function of LPL is not correlated with its activity but is closely dependent on the structure of the enzyme. There is evidence that FFA derived from the hydrolysis of triglycerides in chylomicrons can dissociate LPL from its binding sites. Karpe et al. [10] demonstrated an increase of plasma concentration of LPL activity during an oral fat tolerance test which paralleled that of plasma (free) linoleic acid. There was a positive correlation between AUICs (area under the incremental curve) of LPL activity and plasma free linoleic acid levels. In conclusion, LPL seems to have a dual function in the metabolism of chylomicron particles. First, it is the rate-limiting enzyme in the lipolysis of chylomicrons and second, it acts as the ligand for the removal of remnant particles in the liver.

Postprandial lipemia and lipoprotein lipase

The importance of LPL activity is evidenced by the inverse correlation observed between

Address for correspondence: Prof Marja-Riitta Taskinen, Third Department of Medicine, University of Helsinki, Haartmaninkatu 4, 00290 Helsinki, Finland. Fax: +358-0-471-4012.

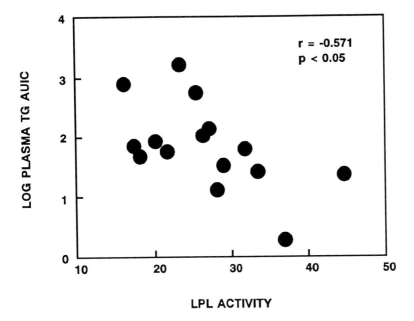

Fig. 1. Relationships between plasma incremental plasma triglyceride responses (AUIC, mmol/l·h⁻¹ log transformed) and postheparin plasma LPL activities (μmol free fatty acids·h⁻¹·ml⁻¹) in normolipidemic, nondiabetic men.

incremental responses (AUIC) of plasma triglycerides and postheparin plasma LPL activity in healthy normolipidemic men (Fig. 1). The relationships between incremental responses of triglycerides in chylomicrons (Sf > 400) and VLDL1 (Sf 60–400) were comparable. Likewise, Weintraub et al. [11] reported that chylomicron levels correlated inversely with lipoprotein lipase activity. The critical role of LPL in the initial lipolytic process is further evidenced by the accumulation of chylomicrons after a fat load in patients with familial type I hyperlipidemia [12]. Chylomicrons were found for prolonged periods in the circulation and the patients still had clearly elevated chylomicron retinyl palmitate levels at 24 h. The baseline level was not returned to until 48 h. In contrast, there was very little accumulation of remnant particles in nonchylomicron fractions. The data suggest that remnants are not formed other than under the action of LPL [12]. Likewise in heterozygotes with lower LPL activity, postprandial lipemia was greater than in control subjects [12]. Recently Miesenböck et al. [13] reported that heterozygous carriers of an LPL mutation in codon 188 have fat intolerance although their baseline values of lipids and lipoproteins were within the normal range. All carriers of this mutation had LPL activity averaging 38% of the normal values. The phenotype of the carriers was characterized by pronounced postprandial lipemia, elevation of IDL, lower HDL2, small dense LDL and compositional changes of both VLDL and HDL fractions. The detection of these abnormalities, however, requires sensitive analysis and they cannot be found if only routine lipid parameters are measured. The lipoprotein phenotype closely resembled the constellation observed in the metabolic syndrome and NIDDM. Consequently, heterozygous LPL deficiency may be more frequent than previously expected among these cohorts.

Postprandial lipemia and lipoprotein lipase in metabolic disorders

As expected, several studies have demonstrated that postprandial lipemia is greater in NIDDM patients than in nondiabetic subjects [14–16]. To define more precisely the metabolism of triglyceride-rich particles in NIDDM subjects we used retinyl palmitate as a marker of intestinally derived particles and followed the responses of triglycerides and RP in different lipoprotein fractions separated by density gradient ultracentrifugation [16]. The exaggerated response of plasma triglyceride was due to increases of triglycerides in chylomicrons as well as in Sf 60–400 particles, which consist of large VLDL particles and remnants. No consistent changes were observed in triglyceride responses in Sf 20–60 and Sf 12–20 between NIDDM patients and controls.

The inverse correlations between the AUIC of triglycerides in plasma, chylomicrons and Sf 60–400 and postheparin plasma LPL activity in nondiabetic men were less strong and not significant in NIDDM patients. Likewise in NIDDM men with angiographically defined CAD we found no correlation between AUIC of triglycerides and LPL activity. The fact that we observed no substantial differences in the LPL activity between NIDDM patients with and without CAD and controls (21 ± 1, 23 ± 2 vs. 27 ± 2 µmol FFA·ml·h, $p < 0.05$ vs. controls) suggests that chylomicrons of NIDDM patients are less good as a substrate for LPL than "normal" chylomicrons.

Accordingly we observed only a weak association between the response of postprandial triglycerides and postheparin plasma LPL activity in nondiabetic men with low HDL, mild hypertriglyceridemia and CAD verified angiographically ($n = 50$, $r = -0.282$, $p < 0.05$). In conclusion, unknown factors disrupt the normal interaction of LPL with chylomicrons in metabolic disorders.

The curves of both triglycerides and retinyl palmitate in plasma, chylomicrons and Sf 60–400 were closely parallel in the two diabetic groups. The fact that the response of retinyl palmitate in the Sf 60–400 fraction was much larger in the two diabetic groups than in control subjects matched for age and BMI suggests that the removal of remnants was also impaired in NIDDM patients, independently of the presence or absence of CAD. Of note is that the magnitude of postprandial lipemia did not distinguish NIDDM patients with CAD in our cohorts. Thus, dual defects in processing of triglyceride-rich particles characterize NIDDM.

Effect of gemfibrozil on postprandial lipid metabolism

Since evidence is increasing that postprandial triglyceride-rich particles and their remnants are potentially atherogenic the clinical problem becomes how to reduce postprandial lipemia. Gemfibrozil is known to lower VLDL-triglyceride levels and to increase HDL-cholesterol effectively. The lowering of VLDL-triglycerides by gemfibrozil is partly explained by the increase of LPL activity. Recently we have studied the postprandial effects of gemfibrozil in subjects with mild hypertriglyceridemia. Twenty NIDDM patients [17] and 20 nondiabetic subjects with fasting triglyceride levels between 1.5 and 4.5 mmol/l were randomly allocated to receive either 600 mg gemfibrozil twice daily or placebo over 12 weeks. The double-blind medication period was preceded by a 6-week run-in period with placebo. The oral fat load consisted of 200 ml of cream (38% fat) with 760 kcal energy and 345,000 IU of vitamin A [17]. At randomization the groups were similar with respect to age and BMI and had similar concentrations of serum triglycerides (Table 1). The two diabetic groups also had similar glycemic control (HbA$_{1C}$ 7.6 ± 0.3 vs. $7.8 \pm 0.2\%$). The responses of both triglycerides and retinyl palmitate in plasma (Fig. 2) as well as in chylomicrons and Sf 40–600 fractions after a fat load were markedly

Table 1. Baseline characteristics of the subjects

	NIDDM+		NIDDM–	
	Gemfibrozil (n = 10)	Placebo (n = 10)	Gemfibrozil (n = 10)	Placebo (n = 10)
Age (yr)	60 ± 2	52 ± 3	52 ± 7	53 ± 7
BMI (kg/m²)	27.1 ± 0.7	27.4 ± 0.7	28.6 ± 1.5	26.4 ± 1.6
HbA$_{1C}$ (%)	7.6 ± 0.3	7.8 ± 0.2	5.4 ± 0.4	5.4 ± 0.4
Triglycerides (mmol/l)	2.99 ± 0.37	3.14 ± 0.40	3.34 ± 1.13	3.08 ± 1.65
HDL-cholesterol (mmol/l)	1.15 ± 0.06	1.24 ± 0.06*	0.99 ± 0.19	1.00 ± 0.17

reduced by gemfibrozil in both diabetic and nondiabetic subjects. The AUICs of triglycerides and retinyl palmitate in Sf 60–400 were reduced on averaged by 40 and 47%, respectively. No major differences were observed in any parameters measured in the two placebo groups. Although gemfibrozil increased postheparin plasma LPL activities the actual changes were trivial, averaging +17 and +18% in the two gemfibrozil-treated

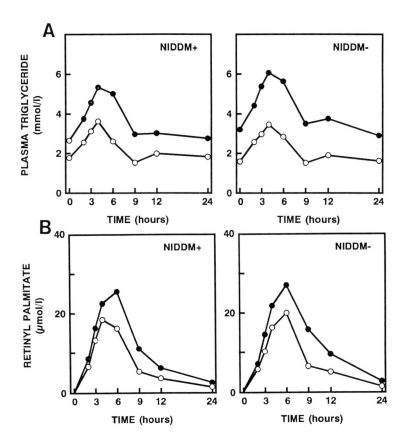

Fig. 2. Responses of triglycerides (A) and retinylpalmitate (B) in plasma to oral fat load at baseline (●) and after 12 weeks' therapy of gemfibrozil (O) in NIDDM and nondiabetic subjects with mild hypertriglyceridemia (with permission, [17]).

groups. The fact that we observed no correlations between the changes of LPL activities and the postprandial triglyceride and retinyl palmitate measures disputes the hypothesis that enhanced lipolysis of triglyceride-rich particles due to an increase of LPL is the major mechanism behind the marked lowering of postprandial lipemia and remnant particles. Our tentative proposal is that the suppression of endogenous VLDL transport by fibrates may leave more catabolic sites available for catabolism of triglyceride-rich particles and their remnants. This concept is supported by recent observations that VLDL particles contribute significantly to postprandial hyperlipidemia [18,19].

Summary

Lipoprotein lipase plays a dual role in the metabolism of postprandial triglyceride-rich particles and their remnants. LPL is the key enzyme in the lipolysis of chylomicrons. The role of LPL is evidenced by fat intolerance in heterozygotes with LPL deficiency. The inverse relation between postprandial lipemia and LPL is disrupted in metabolic disorders like NIDDM and low HDL/mild hypertriglyceridemia. Substantial evidence indicates that LPL bound to circulating lipoproteins also acts as a ligand for their removal by liver. However, our understanding of the regulation of these two processes is incomplete.

References

1. Zilversmit DB. Circulation 1979;50:473–485.
2. Simons J et al. Atherosclerosis 1987;65:181–189.
3. Groot PHE, Stiphout WAHJ, Krauss XH et al. Arterioscler Thromb 1991;11:653–662.
4. Patsch JR, Miesenböck J, Hoplerwieser T et al. Arterioscler Thromb 1992;12:1336–1345.
5. Karpe F, Steiner G, Uffelman K, Olivecrona T, Carlson LA, Hamsten A. Atherosclerosis 1994;106:83–97.
6. Cohn JS, McNamara JR, Cohn SD, Ordovas JM, Schaefer EJ. J Lipid Res 1988;29:925–936.
7. O'Meara NM, Lewis GF, Cabana VG, Iverius PH, Getz GS, Polonsky KS. J Clin Endocrinol Metab 1992;75:465–471.
8. Olivecrona T, Bengtsson-Olivecrona G. Curr Opin Lipidol 1993;4:187–196.
9. Beisiegel U, Weber W, Bengtsson-Olivecrona G. Proc Natl Acad Sci USA 1991;88:8342–8346.
10. Karpe F, Olivecrona T, Walldius G, Hamsten A. J Lipid Res 1992;33:975–984.
11. Weintraub MS, Eisenberg S, Breslow JL. J Clin Invest 1987;79:1110–1119.
12. Sprecher DL, Knauer SL, Black DM, Kaplan LA, Akeson AA, Dusing M, Lattier D, Stein EA, Rymaszewski M, Wiginton DA. J Clin Invest 1991;88:985–994.
13. Miesenböck G, Hölzl B, Föger B, Brandstätter E, Paulweber B, Sandhofer F, Patsch JR. J Clin Invest 1993;91:448–455.
14. Lewis GF, O'Meara NM, Soltys PA. J Clin Endocrinol Metab 1991;72:934–944.
15. Ida Chen Y-D, Swami S, Skowronski R, Coulston A, Reaven GM. J Clin Endocrinol Metab 1993;76:172–177.
16. Syvänne M, Hilden H, Taskinen M-R. J Lipid Res 1994;36:15–26.
17. Syvänne M, Vuorinen-Markkola H, Hilden H, Taskinen M-R. Arterioscler Thromb 1993;13:286–295.
18. Schneeman BO, Kotite L, Todd KM, Havel RJ. Proc Natl Acad Sci USA 1993;90:2069–2073.
19. Cohn JS. Curr Opin Lipidol 1994;5:185–190.

Cholesteryl ester transfer in diabetes mellitus

John D. Bagdade and Mary C. Ritter

Department of Medicine, Rush Medical College, Chicago, Illinois, USA

Cholesteryl ester transfer (CET) is an integral step in reverse cholesterol transport that is facilitated by a specific cholesteryl ester transfer protein (CETP) [1]. In mediating the transfer of CE from HDL to apolipoprotein B (apoB)-containing lipoproteins, CETP not only is one of the major determinants of plasma HDL-cholesterol levels, but it is also a modulator of the core lipid composition of the plasma lipoproteins. The fact that both the activity and mass of CETP appear to be directly related to atherosclerosis susceptibility in humans [2] and experimental animals [3] has led to the current belief that the actions of CETP enhance the atherogenicity of the apoB-containing lipoproteins. The accelerated atherogenesis in diabetes mellitus is clearly multifactorial [4]. We provide evidence here (some of which has been accumulated in my laboratory) indicating that CET is abnormally increased in both IDDM and NIDDM and this abnormality can be added to the list of new, recently recognized cardiovascular risk factors in diabetes.

Castro and Fielding first showed that CET is normally stimulated in humans during the postprandial state [5]. Subsequent work by others has revealed that maximal CET activity in plasma is normally synchronous with physiologic increases in other postprandial enzyme activities (lipoprotein and hepatic lipases and lecithin:cholesterol acyl transferase (LCAT)) [6]. This temporal association between CET, the putative atherogenesis-enhancing actions of the CETP on the apoB-containing lipoproteins, and the perception that the postprandial state is inherently atherogenic, are highly relevant to understanding the pathophysiology of lipoprotein transport in diabetes because insulin levels and these activities are normally maximal and synchronous postprandially. Tall et al. were the first to show that exposure of TG-rich lipoproteins to lipoprotein lipase (LpL) enhanced their interaction with CETP and stimulated CET [7].

CET in IDDM

Since insulin is a key hormonal regulator of LpL, which in turn appears to be an important modulator of CET in vivo, we hypothesized that the unphysiologic sustained hyperinsulinemia that is present in conventionally treated insulin-requiring diabetic patients may simulate the postprandial state. As a result, we queried whether this iatrogenic form of hyperinsulinemia might stimulate both LpL and CET in the fasting state and thereby promote the production of CE-enriched postprandial-like apoB-containing lipoproteins. To assess this possibility, we studied CET in plasma obtained after an overnight fast from a group of otherwise healthy normolipidemic IDDM subjects. Consistent with our prediction, we found that CET measured by both mass and isotopic transfer assays was abnormally increased [8]. This enhanced CET activity of plasma was found in recombination experiments with isolated lipoprotein fractions from IDDM and control subjects to

Address for correspondence: John D. Bagdade MD, Rush-Presbyterian St. Luke's Medical Center, Section of Endocrinology and Metabolism, 1653 West Congress Parkway, Chicago, IL 60612, USA. Tel.: +1-312-942-7459.

be due to dysfunction of the VLDL subfraction even though the mass of CETP present in a small subset of the IDDM group was somewhat higher than in controls (IDDM 2.19 ± 1.08 vs. controls 1.46 ± 0.42 mg/ml; p < 0.1) (measurements generously performed by Dr Ruth McPherson's laboratory). In more recent studies we have found [9] that the extent of the abnormality in CET in whole plasma correlated directly with glycemic control. However, even in very well-controlled IDDM subjects, CET was still pathologically increased.

If iatrogenic hyperinsulinemia resulting from subcutaneous insulin injection plays a pathogenic role in the activation of CET by stimulating LpL, one would predict that lowering systemic insulin levels in IDDM patients by administering insulin into the portal circulation from an implanted pump with an intraperitoneal catheter would reduce LpL and secondarily lower CET. This hypothesis was tested in a series of collaborative experiments performed with Dr Frederick Dunn at Duke University Medical Center, where the feasibility of intraperitoneal insulin delivery (IP) was being conducted in a small group of IDDM patients. Consistent with the earlier observation of Nikkila et al. [10] in postheparin plasma, we found that basal LpL activity was also increased in conventionally treated IDDM patients. When systemic insulin levels measured over 24 h were lowered by IP treatment, LpL and CET both declined to normal [11]. These observations indicated that the pathologic increase in systemic insulin levels in IDDM did in fact simulate the postprandial state by stimulating both LpL and CET.

CET after pancreas transplantation

If systemic hyperinsulinemia triggers CET through its stimulatory effects on LpL, CET should be: 1) increased in IDDM patients who have undergone successful pancreas transplantation and have persisting hyperinsulinemia because their allografts have been placed in the pelvis and drain systemically [12]; and 2) normal in recipients in whom the grafted pancreas is anastomosed to the portal vein which allows the normal hepatic extraction of insulin to take place. Indeed, consistent with the hypothesis assigning a central role to systemic hyperinsulinemia in the pathogenesis of accelerated CET in IDDM, we found in collaboration with workers at the University of Chicago and the University of Tennessee that CET was increased in IDDM transplant recipients with pelvic grafts and normal in those with portal vein anastomoses [13]. All subjects were euglycemic and received no insulin treatment. Combined with the data in the IP-treated patients, these findings indicated that accelerated CET in IDDM patients was attributable to iatrogenic systemic hyperinsulinemia in both conventionally treated and successfully transplanted IDDM patients. This disturbance in CET in the transplant population could be a factor that contributes to their accelerated atherogenesis and premature cardiovascular morbidity and mortality [14].

CET in IDDM

One obvious related question is whether the degree of endogenous hyperinsulinemia present in NIDDM patients is sufficient to stimulate LpL and CET. We have found that CET is also increased in non-insulin-treated normolipidemic NIDDM patients, and as in IDDM this abnormality also appears to relate to dysfunction of VLDL [15]. In contrast to the IDDM subjects in whom CETP mass was measured and found to be somewhat higher than in nondiabetic controls, no difference was found between NIDDM and control CETP concentration in plasma (NIDDM 1.63 ± 0.36 vs. control 1.33 ± 0.36 mg/ml). The situation in NIDDM appears to be more complex than in IDDM, however, since LpL and hepatic lipase in NIDDM do not show the same profile of changes observed in IDDM. However, preliminary studies in insulin-requiring NIDDM subjects [16] performed as part of a Veterans Administration Collaborative study indicate that IP insulin delivery has the same beneficial effect on CET that we observed in IDDM subjects. As predicted by the correlation described earlier between CET and glycemic control in IDDM patients, we found that intensive conventional subcutaneous treatment did improve CET commensurate with the degree of reduction of glycated hemoglobin attained. Thus, accelerated CET appears to be present in both IDDM and NIDDM.

Pharmacologic modification of CET

If accelerated CET is an unavoidable proatherogenic consequence of conventional subcutaneous insulin treatment that persists in the face of excellent glycemic control, what can be done to correct this abnormality? While IP insulin delivery appears to reverse this disturbance in both IDDM and insulin-requiring NIDDM subjects, this form of pump treatment in the United States at least is not yet an approved therapy for diabetes. The therapeutic approach we have taken to reduce CET without altering systemic insulin levels takes advantage of the fact that the affinity of lipoproteins for CETP appears to be influenced by their composition [1]. Enhanced affinity for CETP is perhaps demonstrated best by the behavior of chylomicrons and VLDL following exposure to LpL. We sought a therapy that would instead *reduce* the interaction of lipoproteins with CETP. Our findings earlier that altering the composition of lipoproteins in nondiabetic hypercholes-terolemic patients with marine lipids [17] and that the antioxidant probucol [18] normalized their accelerated CET suggested that a similar effect on CET might be achieved in IDDM patients. Preliminary studies show that administration of n-3 fatty acids (6 g/day) containing 3.6 g eicosapentaenoic and 2.4 g docosahexaenoic acid together with probucol (1 g twice daily) to eight normolipidemic IDDM subjects normalized both the net mass and isotopic CE transfer in all subjects, with no deterioration in glycemic control.

The precise changes in the apoB-containing lipoproteins induced by CETP that render them more atherogenic are not yet clear, though Chait et al. found that LDL exposed to CETP was avidly internalized by cultured human arterial smooth muscle cells [19]. Nevertheless, there is sufficient evidence in humans showing that cardiovascular risk increases when CET is elevated to warrant pharmacologic interventions such as marine lipids and probucol. There is no evidence that the increase in LDL-C that results from n-3 fatty acid treatment [20] increases risk. In fact, studies in primates fed marine lipids show that the resulting changes in LDL composition and physical properties may in fact reduce their potential atherogenicity [21]. The additional salutary effects of n-3 fatty acids on blood pressure, plasma triglycerides, and hemostasis make them an especially appealing therapeutic option in NIDDM. With its potent antioxidant properties, probucol on the other hand may be a rational choice in IDDM subjects in whom there is evidence of increased biological oxidation [22].

Acknowledgement

This work was supported by a grant from the National Institutes of Health (NHLBI RO1 DK 43227).

References

1. Tall AR. J Lipid Res 1993;34:1255–1274.
2. Inazu A, Brown ML, Hesler CB, Agellon LB, Koizumi J, Takata K, Maruhama Y, Mabuchi H, Tall AR.

N Engl J Med 1990;323:1234—1238.

3. Quinet E, Tall A, Ramikrishnan R, Rudel L. J Clin Invest 1991;87:1559—1566.
4. Bierman EL. Arterioscler Thromb 1992;12:647—656.
5. Castro GR, Fielding CJ. J Clin Invest 1985;75:874—882.
6. Marcel YI, McPherson R, Hogue M, Czarnecka H, Zawadzki Z, Weech PK, Whitlock ME, Tall AR, Milne RW. J Clin Invest 1990;85:10—17.
7. Tall AR, Sammett D, Vita GM, Deckelbaum R, Olivercrona T. J Biol Chem 1984;9587—9594.
8. Bagdade JD, Subbaiah PV, Ritter MC. Eur J Clin Invest 1991;21:161—167.
9. Ritter MR, Bagdade JD. Influence of acceptor lipoproteins, cholesteryl ester transfer protein, and glycemic control on cholesteryl ester transfer in IDDM. Eur J Clin Invest 1994 (in press).
10. Nikkila EA, Huttunen JK, Enholm C. Diabetes 1977;26:11—21.
11. Bagdade JD, Dunn FL, Eckel RH, Ritter MC. Intraperitoneal insulin therapy corrects abnormalities in cholesteryl ester transfer and lipoprotein lipase activities in insulin-dependent diabetes mellitus. Arterioscler Thromb 1994 (in press).
12. Diem P, Abid M, Redmon JB, Sutherland DER, Robertson RP. Diabetes 1990;39:534—540.
13. Bagdade J, Ritter M, Eckel R, Thistlewaite R, Fellner S. Accelerated cholesteryl ester transfer (CET) in pancreas allograft recipients. 643a (211) Program and Abstracts Endocrine Society 75th Annual Meeting, Las Vegas, Nevada, 1993.
14. Lemmers MJ, Barry JM. Diabetes Care 1991;14:295—301.
15. Bagdade JD, Lane JT, Subbaiah PV, Otto ME, Ritter MC. Atherosclerosis 1993;104:69—77.
16. Bagdade JD, Kelly DE, Henry RR, Ritter MC. Intraperitoneal insulin improves cholesteryl ester transfer (CET) in insulin-requiring patients with NIDDM. 776c (394) Program and Abstracts Endocrine Society 76th Annual Meeting, Anaheim, CA, 1994.
17. Bagdade JD, Ritter MC, Davidson M, Subbaiah PV. Arterioscler Thromb 1992;12:1146—1152.
18. Bagdade JD. Unpublished observations.
19. Chait AS, Eisenberg S, Steinmetz A, Albers JJ, Bierman EL. Biochim Biophys Acta 1984;795:314—325.
20. Connor WE, DeFrancesco CA, Connor SL. Ann NY Acad Sci 1993;683:16—34.
21. Parks JS. In: Yasugi T, Nakamura H, Soma M (eds) Advances in Polyunsaturated Fatty Acid Research. Amsterdam: Elsevier Science Publishers, 1993.

Atherosclerosis X.
F.P. Woodford, J. Davignon and A. Sniderman, editors.

767

Lipoprotein abnormalities in diabetes

Richard W. James and Daniel Pometta

Division of Diabetology, Department of Medicine, University Hospital, Geneva, Switzerland

Cardiovascular disease is one of the principal complications of diabetes mellitus. This has focused particular attention on blood lipids and lipoproteins for several reasons. Firstly, they constitute one of the major risk factors for vascular disease in the nondiabetic population. Secondly, conditions associated with diabetes (hyperglycemia, raised free fatty acids, insulin resistance) can influence blood lipids. Thirdly, insulin interacts with the lipoprotein metabolic system at many points, influencing plasma concentrations of the major endogenous subclasses (VLDL, LDL, HDL) as well as chylomicrons. Finally, dyslipidemias are common in poorly controlled diabetic patients [1].

In recent years greater attention has been paid to what have been described as qualitative modifications to the blood lipid and lipoprotein profile [2]. These include compositional changes that may compromise the role of lipoproteins in blood lipid transport and modifications to the lipoprotein distribution profile which influence relative, but not necessarily absolute, lipoprotein concentrations. A corollary of the latter point is the growing awareness that the major lipoprotein subclasses are themselves heterogeneous not only with respect to composition and metabolism but probably as regards their role in the atherogenic process. These qualitative modifications can therefore give rise to a more atherogenic lipid profile which may not be reflected by routine blood lipid measurements.

Hypertriglyceridemia would appear to be one of the principal sources of both compositional and distributional anomalies of the blood lipid profile [3]. It is also the most frequently encountered lipid disorder in poorly controlled diabetic subjects. This brief overview examines some aspects of the association between triglycerides and the lipoprotein profile in patients with non-insulin-dependent diabetes (NIDDM) and underlines potential differences between male and female subjects.

VLDL in NIDDM

The hypertriglyceridemia prevalent in poorly controlled diabetic patients leads to alterations to the lipoprotein pattern within VLDL. This is illustrated in Fig. 1 which shows VLDL subfraction concentrations in hypertriglyceridemic diabetic men and women as well as normotriglyceridemic, nondiabetic controls. It demonstrates that in both diabetic groups, the hypertriglyceridemia is due to overproduction of triglyceride-enriched large VLDL particles (1 and 2) relative to the small VLDL particles (VLDL-3) which predominate in the control subjects. This has important metabolic implications, as there is clear evidence of divergent metabolism between large and small VLDL [4]. The clinical implications are less well defined. The patients comprising the diabetic groups were carefully matched for plasma triglyceride and cholesterol levels (men: triglycerides 2.93 ± 1.15, cholesterol 5.89 ± 1.20 mmol/l; women: triglycerides 2.85 ± 1.25, cholesterol 6.01 ± 1.12 mmol/l). Nevertheless there was a tendency for men to have higher plasma concentrations of larger VLDL-1 and 2 but lower concentrations of denser VLDL-3 than in women. This is illustrated by the ratios of the plasma concentrations of large to small

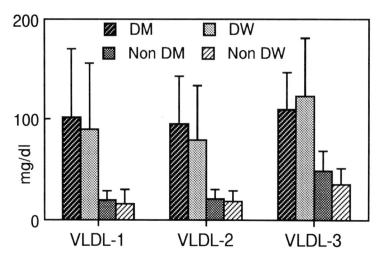

Fig. 1. Plasma concentrations (shown in mg/dl) of VLDL subfractions from NIDDM men (DM, n = 14, plasma triglycerides, 2.93 ± 1.15 mmol/l) and women (DW, n = 14, plasma triglycerides, 2.85 ± 1.25 mmol/l) and normolipemic control men (non-DM, n = 23; plasma triglycerides, 1.00 ± 0.28 mmol/l) and women (non-DW, n = 20, plasma triglycerides, 0.94 ± 0.30 mmol/l).

VLDL (diabetic men 1.72 ± 1.00, diabetic women 1.22 ± 1.49; p < 0.05). This tendency to higher concentrations of small VLDL particles in women reflects underlying differences in the association between triglycerides and VLDL subfractions. Table 1 gives the correlation coefficients for the combined diabetic population and male and female patients separately. In all cases, there was a highly significant positive correlation between triglycerides and the three VLDL subfractions, underlining their roles as triglyceride transport vehicles. The strong correlations with large VLDL-1 and 2 are maintained for VLDL-3 in women, but the coefficient is weaker in men (p < 0.05 comparing men and women for VLDL-3). Improved glycemic control with concomitant normalization of plasma triglyceride levels also largely corrects the VLDL distribution profile. Figure 2 gives the subfraction concentrations in male and female NIDDM patients before and after short-term treatment. The groups had similar plasma triglyceride levels (men 3.09 ± 0.87; women 3.01 ± 1.40 mmol/l) at entry and underwent similar decreases in these con-

Table 1. Correlations between fasting triglycerides and lipoprotein subfraction concentrations in male (n = 14) and female (n = 14) NIDDM patients

Subfraction	Correlation		
	Combined	Male	Female
VLDL-1	0.88[a]	0.88[a]	0.86[a]
VLDL-2	0.90[a]	0.90[a]	0.97[a]
VLDL-3	0.71[a]	0.56[b]	0.85[a]
LDL-1	0.45[b]	0.36	0.59[b]
LDL-2	−0.41[b]	−0.37	−0.62[b]
LDL-3	0.50[a]	0.64[b]	0.36
LDL-2/LDL-3	−0.73[a]	−0.70[a]	−0.71[a]

[a]p < 0.0001; [b]p < 0.005.

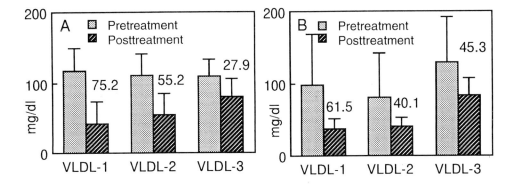

Fig. 2. Plasma concentrations of VLDL subfractions in NIDDM diabetic men (A) and women (B) before and after short-term therapy to improve glycemic control. The values above the post-treatment bars indicate the mean decreases (mg/dl) in plasma concentrations.

centrations (men 1.69 ± 0.50; women 1.83 ± 0.35 mmol/l: NS). Significant reductions of all three VLDL subfractions were noted but these were more marked for the larger subfractions in men and the smaller VLDL-3 in women. The mean decrease in each subfraction is indicated (in mg/dl) above the post-treatment bar on the graphs.

Thus, male and female NIDDM patients show qualitatively similar modifications to the VLDL profile with the onset of hypertriglyceridemia, the increases in larger triglyceride-rich particles being notable. In female patients, raised triglyceride levels also correlate strongly with increased levels of the most dense VLDL subfraction. Improved glycemic control and subsequent correction of hypertriglyceridemia are associated with a more marked reduction of VLDL-1 and 2 in men, and of VLDL-3 in women.

LDL in NIDDM

As VLDL are precursors of low density lipoproteins, any modification to VLDL metabolism will have repercussions on LDL. This is clearly portrayed by the correlation coefficients given in Table 1 which illustrate the association between fasting triglycerides and subfractions covering the LDL density range. Correlations do not prove direct interactions, but there is abundant metabolic and clinical evidence of the links between VLDL and LDL. Triglycerides are negatively correlated with LDL-2, which is the predominant subfraction in control subjects, and positively correlated with small dense LDL-3. Again, male and female patients show qualitatively similar associations between triglycerides and the individual subfractions, but there are quantitative differences. Women showed highly significant correlations with LDL-1 and 2, but the association did not reach significance (p = 0.065) for LDL-3. Conversely, men showed highly significant, positive correlations between triglycerides and LDL-3 whereas the correlations failed to attain significance (at p ≤ 0.05) for the larger LDL subfractions. Thus, the highly significant, negative association between triglycerides and the LDL2/LDL3 mass ratio exhibited by both groups of patients (Table 1) seems to arise from somewhat different associations of triglycerides with the subfractions.

The LDL2/LDL3 mass ratio is an indication of the tendency to produce smaller, denser LDL particles. As Table 1 shows, this is greatly influenced by plasma triglyceride levels.

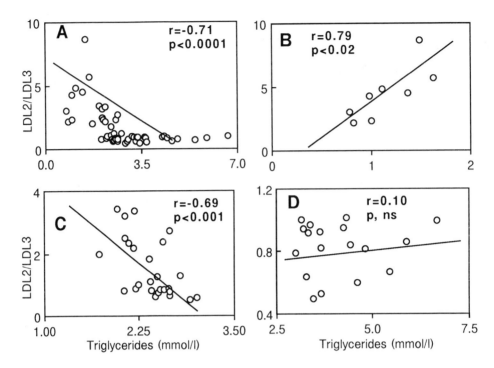

Fig. 3. Correlations between fasting triglycerides and the LDL2/LDL3 mass ratio in male and female NIDDM patients. A: total population (triglycerides 0.7–6.6); B: triglycerides up to 1.7; C: triglycerides between 1.7 and 3.0; and D: triglycerides > 3.0.

This relationship is shown graphically in Fig. 3 for male and female patients with a range of fasting triglyceride levels. It is quite clearly a complex relationship, as shown for the whole population in Fig. 3A. Indeed, the association can be broken down into three subgroups where the apparent impact of triglycerides on the LDL2/LDL3 ratio is strikingly different, as illustrated in Fig. 3B–D. For patients with fasting plasma triglyceride concentrations up to 1.6 mmol/l, the association is positive and highly significant. Under these conditions, the VLDL–LDL metabolic cascade favors production of larger, LDL-2 particles. Between 1.6 and 3.0 mmol/l this trend is reversed; production of smaller, denser LDL particles now predominates (Fig. 3C) giving rise to a highly significant, negative correlation between triglycerides and the LDL2/LDL3 ratio. Beyond 3.0 mmol/l there is no longer a significant association between the two parameters (Fig. 3D). These results indicate that the impact of triglycerides on the LDL profile is apparent at values considerably lower than currently proposed "normal" levels of 2.0–2.3 mmol/l. Similar conclusions have been reached by other groups studying essentially nondiabetic populations [5,6].

Conclusions

Modifications to plasma triglyceride levels have clear implications for the lipoprotein profile and, as a consequence, blood cholesterol transport. Accumulating data suggest that overproduction of triglycerides occasions a more atherogenic lipoprotein profile, thus providing one avenue by which they could pathologically influence the atherogenic process [5,7]. The impact of triglycerides on the LDL profile is already apparent at concentrations below those currently considered to be clinically important. This implies that strict control of triglyceride levels should be a consideration in diabetic patients who are particularly prone to hypertriglyceridemia. Finally, potential gender differences in the association between triglycerides and lipoprotein subfractions may help to explain the greater relative increase in the incidence of vascular disease in diabetic women.

Acknowledgements

Supported by grants from the Swiss National Research Foundation (Nos. 32-9484.88 and 32-30782.91) and from the Foundation Suisse de Diabète.

References

1. Taskinen M-R. Clin Endocrinol Metab 1990;4:743—775.
2. Taskinen M-R. Diabetes 1992;41(suppl 2):12—17.
3. Deckelbaum RJ, Granot E, Oschry Y, Rose L, Eisenberg S. Arteriosclerosis 1984;4:225—231.
4. Packard CJ, Munro A, Lorimer AR, Gotto AM Jr, Shepherd J. J Clin Invest 1984;74:2178—2192.
5. Richards EG, Grundy SM, Cooper K. Am J Cardiol 1989;63:1214—1220.
6. Griffin BA, Freeman DJ, Tait GW, Thomson J, Caslake MJ, Packard CJ, Shepherd J. Atherosclerosis 1994; 106:241—253.
7. Austin MA, Breslow JL, Hennekens CH, Buring JE, Willett WC, Krauss RM. J Am Med Assoc 1988;260: 1917—1922.

Insulin and hypertension

Steven M. Haffner

Department of Medicine, University of Texas Health Science, Center of San Antonio, San Antonio, Texas, USA

Michaela Modan initially suggested that insulin concentrations were associated with hypertension independently of glucose tolerance or obesity [1]. This concept was furthered by Ferrannini et al. [2] who showed a decrease in insulin sensitivity in normoglycemic subjects with hypertension relative to normotensive controls [2]. Several mechanisms have been suggested to explain the association of insulin resistance and blood pressure including increased sympathetic nervous system activity, proliferation of vascular smooth muscle cells, altered cation transplant, and increased sodium reabsorption [3]. Insulin resistance and hyperinsulinemia has also been linked to dyslipidemia (especially low HDL cholesterol and elevated triglyceride concentrations) and impaired glucose tolerance in syndrome X [4].

The relationship between insulin resistance and hypertension remains the most controversial part of syndrome X [5]. Cross-sectional studies have supported an association between insulin concentrations and hypertension [1,6–8] although other epidemiological studies have not found such a relationship [9–11]. Relatively few studies have examined the association between insulin resistance and hypertension [2,12–16]. These studies have been limited by selection by level of obesity [2,13], diabetic status [12] and race [15,16].

Unfortunately only in a few studies has the association between insulin concentrations and the incidence of hypertension been examined prospectively. Only in these studies can the temporal relationship between insulin and hypertension be elucidated. This is an important issue since Julius et al. have suggested a hemodynamic basis for insulin resistance in hypertension [17]. In three prospective studies insulin concentrations predicted the incidence of hypertension [18–20] while in the fourth study, insulin predicted the incidence of hypertension in lean subjects but not in obese subjects [21].

In this brief review we will examine some of the issues that may obscure the relationship of insulin and hypertension such as antihypertensive therapy, obesity, racial differences, acute vasodilatory effects of insulin and the issue of proinsulin.

Pharmacological therapy of hypertension

Pharmacological therapy may affect insulin sensitivity. Beta blockers and thiazides may worsen insulin resistance, and angiotension converting enzyme inhibitors may decrease insulin resistance [22]. For example, if an investigator included hypertensive subjects on thiazides, they might observe a spurious association between insulin and hypertension. However, this problem is now widely recognized. Clinically, the effect of pharmacologic agents on insulin resistance may have important implications since insulin resistance and

Address for correspondence: Steven M. Haffner MD, Department of Medicine, University of Texas Health Science, Center of San Antonio, 7703 Floyd Curl Drive, San Antonio, TX 78284-7873, USA. Tel.: +1-210-567-4737. Fax: +1-210-567-6955.

hyperinsulinemia are strong predictors of non-insulin-dependent diabetes mellitus (NIDDM) [23], and hypertensive subjects have an increased risk of developing NIDDM [24,25]. Indeed, antihypertensive therapy with β blockers and thiazides has been associated with an increased risk of NIDDM in some studies [24] but not in others [25].

Obesity

It is not surprising that obesity may be an important confounder since obesity both strongly predicts the development of hypertension [21,26] and is associated with hyperinsulinemia [1] and insulin resistance [27]. Several studies have found associations between insulin levels and blood pressure which disappeared after adjustment for obesity [9,11]. More interesting is the possibility that the effect of insulin and blood pressure may differ according to the level of obesity. Laakso et al. [12] have suggested that lean subjects with NIDDM and hypertension were more insulin-resistant than lean normotensive subjects, but obese hypertensive and nonhypertensive NIDDM subjects were equally insulin-resistant. In another study [21] in lean subjects, the incidence of hypertension for those in the highest tertile of insulin concentrations compared with those in the other two was 10.0 vs. 4.5% (relative risk (RR) = 2.24; p = 0.0321); in subjects with BMI between 25 and 30 kg/m^2 the incidence of hypertension was 15.0 vs. 11.5% (RR = 1.32; p = NS); and in obese subjects the incidence of hypertension in corresponding categories was 12.1 vs. 17.3% (RR = 0.70; p = NS). Consistent with this outlook is a strong relationship between insulin resistance and hypertension in lean subjects [2] but not in obese subjects [13]. However, in one report, a strong relationship between insulin resistance and hypertension was found in both lean and obese subjects [14].

Ethnic differences

Saad et al. [15] have reported an association between insulin resistance and blood pressure in Caucasians but not in Blacks or Pima Indians. In contrast, Falkner et al. [16] have reported that young hypertensive Black males are more insulin-resistant than lean normotensive Black males. The discrepancy might be explained by the greater obesity of Blacks in the Saad et al. study (BMI = 31 vs. 24 kg/m^2, respectively). In a prospective study [23], the relationship of fasting insulin to the incidence of hypertension was equally strong in Mexican Americans and non-Hispanic whites.

Vasodilatory effects of insulin

Rowe et al. have reported that insulin infusion increases catecholamine levels and blood pressure [28]. In a more recent study, acute hyperinsulinemia was associated with an increase in norepinephrine levels but also with vasodilation and a fall in blood pressure [29]. In normotensive subjects, whole body glucose disposal and the ability of insulin to increase blood flow was inversely related to basal blood pressure [30]. Thus, the decreased insulin sensitivity in normotensive subjects with higher blood pressure was related to a decrease in insulin-induced vasodilation. Recently Baron et al. [31] have suggested that the impaired insulin-induced vasodilation associated with insulin resistance may act as a predisposing factor for the development of hypertension.

Proinsulin

Most of the studies describing the association of hyperinsulinemia to hypertension have been limited by the fact that insulin was measured with an assay that cross-reacts with

774

proinsulin. Temple et al. [32] have suggested that proinsulin and split 32–33 proinsulin may comprise the majority of circulating immunoreactive insulin in subjects with NIDDM. Other studies have also suggested disproportionate increases in proinsulin in subjects in NIDDM [33–35] and perhaps impaired glucose tolerance as well [35,36]. Proinsulin was more strongly associated with blood pressure than was insulin in diabetic subjects [37] and in nondiabetic subjects [38]. In a recent report, fasting insulin (measured by a radio-immunoassy that does not recognize proinsulin), fasting proinsulin and the fasting proinsulin/insulin were all associated with hypertension in nondiabetic subjects [39]. The latter study suggests that hypertension may be associated not only with insulin resistance but with a degree of β-cell dysfunction as well.

Conclusion

The area of insulin resistance and hypertension remains very controversial. I believe that the major confounding variable is the presence of obesity. If there is a strong relationship between insulin and blood pressure, it is most likely to be found in lean subjects. It is not known whether the relationship between insulin and blood pressure varies in different ethnic groups.

References

1. Modan M, Halkin H, Almog S, Lusky A, Eshkol A, Shefi A, Shitrit A, Fuchs Z. J Clin Invest 1987;75: 809–817.
2. Ferrannini E, Buzzigoli G, Bonadonna R, Giorico MA, Oleggini M, Graziadei L, Pedrinielli R, Brandi L, Bevilacqua S. N Engl J Med 1987;317:350–357.
3. DeFranzo RA, Ferrannini E. Diabetes Care 1991;14:173–194.
4. Reaven GM. Diabetes 1988;37:1595–1607.
5. Haffner SM. J Clin Endocrinol Metab 1993;76:541–543.
6. Ferrannini E, Haffner SM, Stern MP, Mitchell BD, Natali A, Hazuda HP, Patterson JK. Eur J Clin Invest 1991;21:280–287.
7. Wing RR, Bunker CK, Kuller LK, Mathews RW. Arteriosclerosis 1989;9:473–484.
8. Every NR, Marshall JA, Boyko FJ, Rewers M, Keane EM, Hamman RF. Diabetes Care 1993;16:1543–1550.
9. Cambien F, Warnet J, Eschwege E, Jacqueson A, Richard JL, Rosselin G. Arteriosclerosis 1987;7:197–202.
10. Dowse CK, Collins VR, Alberti KGMM, Zimmet PZ, Tuomilehto J, Chitsan P, Gareebo H. J Hypertension 1993;11:297–307.
11. Miller DC, Elahi D, Pratley RE, Tobin JD, Andres R. J Clin Endocrinol Metab 1993;76:544–548.
12. Laakso M, Sarlund K, Mykkänen L. J Clin Invest 1989;19:518–526.
13. Bonora F, Moghetti P, Zenere M, Tusi F, Travi D, Muggeo M. Intl J Obesity 1990;14:735–742.
14. Pollare T, Lithell H, Berne C. Metabolism 1990;39:167–174.
15. Saad MF, Lillioja S, Nyomba BL, Castillo C, Ferraro R, De Gregorio M, Ravussin E, Knowler WC, Bennett PH, Howard BV, Bogardus C. N Engl J Med 1991;324:733–739.
16. Falkner B, Hulman D, Tannenbaum J, Kushner K. Hypertension 1990;16:706–711.
17. Julius S, Gudbrandssan T, Jamerson K, Shahab ST, Andersson O. J Hypertension 1991;9:983–986.
18. Niskanen LK, Usitupa MI, Pyörälä K. J Hum Hypertension 1991;5:155–159.
19. Skarfors ET, Lithell KO, Selenius I. J Hypertension 1991;9:217–223.
20. Lissner L, Bengtsson C, Lapidus L. Kristjansson K, Wedel H. Hypertension 1992;20:707–801.
21. Haffner SM, Ferrannini E, Hazuda HP, Stern MP. Hypertension 1992;20:38–45.
22. Lithell HO. Diabetes Care 1991;14:203–209.
23. Haffner SM, Valdez RA, Hazuda HP, Mitchell BD, Morales PA, Stern MP. Diabetes 1992;41:715–722,
24. Skafors ET, Lithell KO, Selinus I, Aberg H. Br Med J 1989;289:1495–1497.
25. Morales PA, Mitchell BD, Valdez RA, Hazuda HP, Stern MP, Haffner SM. Diabetes 1993;42:154–161.
26. Dyer AR, Stamler J, Shekelle RB, Schonberger JR, Stamler R, Shekelle S, Berkson DM, Paul O, Lepper MK, Lindberg HA. J Chronic Dis 1982;35:897–908.
27. Olefsky JM, Kolterman OG, Scarlett JA. Ann J Med 1982;243:E15–E30.

28. Rowe JW, Young JB, Minaker KL, Stevens AL, Pallotta J, Landsberg L. Diabetes 1981;30:219—225.
29. Anderson GA, Hoffman RP, Balon TW, Sinkey CA, Mark AL. J Clin Invest 1991;87:2246—2252.
30. Baron AD, Brechtel G. Am J Physiol 1993;265:E61—E67.
31. Baron AD, Brechtel-Hock G, Johnson A, Hardin D. Hypertension 1993;21:129—135.
32. Temple RC, Carrington CA, Luzio SD, Owens DR, Schneider AE, Sobey WJ, Hales CN. Lancet 1989;1: 293—295.
33. Ward WK, La Cava FE, Paquette TL, Beard JC, Wallum BJ, Porte D. Diabetologia 1987;30:698—702.
34. Saad MF, Rahm SE, Nelson RG, Pettitt DJ, Knowler WC, Schwartz MW, Kowalyk J, Bennett PH, Porte D. J Clin Endocrinol Metab 1990;20:1247—1253.
35. Haffner SM, Bowsher RR, Mykkänen L, Hazuda HP, Mitchell BD, Valdez RA, Gingerich R, Monterossa A, Stern MP. Proinsulin and specific insulin concentrations in high and low risk populations from non-insulin dependent diabetes mellitus. Diabetes (in press).
36. Davies M, Rayman G, Gray IP, Day GL, Hales CN. Diabetes Med 1993;10:313—320.
37. Nagi DK, Hendra TJ, Ryle HJ, Cooper TM, Temple RC, Clark PMS, Schneider AE, Hales CN, Yudkin JS. Diabetologia 1990;33:532—537.
38. Haffner SM, Mykkänen L, Stern MP, Valdez RA, Heisserman JA, Bowsher RR. Diabetes 1993;92:1297—1302.
39. Haffner SM, Mykkänen L, Valdez RA, Stern MP, Holloway DL, Monterrosa A, Bowsher RR. Disproportionately increased proinsulin levels are associated with the insulin resistance syndrome. J Clin Endocrinol Metab (in press).

Treatment of hyperlipidemia in diabetes

Rafael Carmena

Department of Medicine, Endocrine Division, Hospital Clinico Universitario, 17 Blasco Ibanez, 46010-Valencia, Spain

Abstract. Dietary therapy, proper weight maintenance, exercise programs, and good glycemic control should be used before considering lipid-lowering drugs in the treatment of diabetic dyslipidemias. Fibrates are a first-choice therapeutic option, since they may correct hypertriglyceridemia and low HDL-C. The HMG-CoA reductase inhibitors are indicated in diabetic patients with elevated LDL-C. Indications to use resins are restricted by their triglyceride-raising effects and frequent gastrointestinal side effects, aggravated if diabetic autonomic neuropathy is present.

Abnormalities of plasma lipids and lipoproteins are frequent in both insulin-dependent (IDDM) and non-insulin-dependent diabetes mellitus (NIDDM) and may contribute to the increased risk of coronary heart disease (CHD) observed in these patients [1]. No prospective intervention studies are yet available in diabetic patients to prove that treatment of dyslipidemias reduces the risk of CHD, and current policy and practice are based on studies conducted in nondiabetic populations.

The high cardiovascular risk of diabetic patients has been addressed in recent guidelines in Europe and the USA [2,3], emphasizing that such patients may be candidates for aggressive intervention. The American Diabetes Association (ADA) recently convened a Consensus Development Conference on the Detection and Management of Lipid Disorders in Diabetes [1] including recommendations for the management of dyslipidemia in this population. All three panels noted that the most common lipid abnormalities in diabetes, particularly NIDDM, are increased plasma triglyceride and decreased high density lipoprotein cholesterol (HDL-C); elevated low density lipoprotein cholesterol (LDL-C) may also be present. Patients with diabetes tend to have small, dense LDL, which may be associated with insulin resistance and show higher susceptibility to oxidation [1,4]. Diabetic nephropathy aggravates the lipoprotein disturbances and is associated with rising Lp(a) levels [5].

Lipid metabolism in diabetes is modulated by factors such as type and treatment of diabetes, degree of glycemic control, degree of insulin resistance, and presence of nephropathy. The independent coexistence of diabetes and genetic hyperlipidemias, a not uncommon occurrence, should also be considered.

Action limits for treatment of dyslipidemia in diabetes vary according to whether macrovascular disease is present or not (Table 1).

Hygienic treatment and glycemic control

Reduction of overweight, a low-fat diet, physical activity, control of other CHD risk factors, and glycemic control are fundamental to lipid management in the diabetic population. The ADA consensus panel called for an aggressive approach to weight control, individualized increases in physical activity, and referral to a dietitian for customized diet planning and appropriate nutrition education. In addition, control of hyperglycemia may greatly improve abnormal lipid values, particularly in IDDM [6,7].

Dietary recommendations [1] regarding total fat, saturated fat, cholesterol and carbo-

Table 1. Treatment of dyslipidemia in adults with diabetes mellitus (ADA Consensus Development Conference [1])

No macrovascular disease present	Macrovascular disease present	Treatment
If LDL-C >130 or TG >200 or HDL-C <35	If LDL-C >100 or TG >150 or HDL-C <35	Treat vigorously by: Glucose control Diet Exercise program
If after 6 months of hygienic therapy: LDL >160 or LDL-C >130 + >1 other major RF[a] or TG >400 or TG >200 + >1 other major RF[a]	If after adequate trial of above measures: LDL-C >100 or TG >150	Consider use of lipid-lowering drugs
Treatment goals: LDL <130 TG <200	LDL <100 TG <150	

[a]Other major CHD risk factors: HDL <35, smoking, hypertension, family history of premature CHD. All lipid values in mg/dl.

hydrate intake for lipid lowering are those set forth in the NCEP Step I and Step II Diets. They advise intakes of carbohydrates up to 55–60% of total energy and restriction of total fat to <30% of total energy, limiting saturated fatty acids to <10% of total energy and cholesterol to <300 mg/day; the use of fiber-rich carbohydrates is encouraged. For diabetic patients with hyperlipidemia, the ADA recommends further restriction of dietary fats to 20% of total energy intake and cholesterol to 100–150 mg/day. The wisdom of recommending high-carbohydrate diets to all diabetics has been questioned because of their potentially harmful effects on lipoprotein levels [8]. An alternative diet, with partial replacement of carbohydrates with monounsaturated fatty acids, has been shown to be beneficial for NIDDM patients with hypertriglyceridemia and low HDL-C [8].

Ingestion of soluble fiber may have additional beneficial effects on total and LDL-C levels as well as the glycemic index. Restriction of alcohol use and, if hypertension is present, limitation of sodium intake, are also advised. Recommendations for increased physical activity should take into account that many diabetic patients have a low level of fitness. In addition, smoking cessation is imperative.

Achieving and maintaining glycemic control is the first step in the treatment of diabetic dyslipidemia. In most IDDM patients, intensive insulin therapy corrects both hyperglycemia and dyslipidemia, although the composition of some lipoproteins may remain abnormal [7]. In NIDDM, dietary therapy with emphasis on weight reduction if necessary should be continued for 3–6 months. In our experience [9], a mean weight loss of 9.2 kg during a 5-month period with a hypocaloric diet significantly improved glycemic control, insulin resistance and lipid disturbances in obese NIDDM patients. If optimal glycemic control is not achieved, treatment with oral sulfonylureas and/or biguanides is necessary. Metformin has been shown to improve insulin sensitivity and favorably influence the dyslipidemic profile in obese NIDDM patients [10]. In many NIDDM patients, institution of insulin therapy is required to improve glycemic control and has been shown to have multiple beneficial effects on lipid metabolism in these patients [6]. In practice, however, there are many patients in whom good glycemic control is not achieved and lipid levels remain abnormal. In these cases, therapy with lipid-lowering drugs becomes necessary.

Treatment of diabetic dyslipidemia with lipid-lowering drugs

When an adequate trial of diet, exercise, and improved glucose control fails to produce an acceptable lipid response, lipid-lowering agents are the next therapeutic step. As in the treatment of any dyslipidemic patient, lipid-lowering pharmacotherapy supplements rather than replaces nonpharmacological measures.

No firm recommendations exist regarding the use of antioxidants (probucol, vitamins E and C, β-carotenes) in the diabetic patient. On the other hand, postmenopausal diabetic women can be considered candidates for estrogen replacement therapy. In markedly hypertriglyceridemic patients, however, estrogen should be used in minimal doses and with careful follow-up evaluation. Alternatively, in such patients the percutaneous estrogen patch can be used.

Fibric acid derivatives

They include bezafibrate, ciprofibrate, clofibrate, etofibrate, fenofibrate and gemfibrozil. Fibrates lower triglyceride and increase HDL-C levels, the characteristic dyslipidemia in NIDDM. The effect on LDL-C is variable but generally small, although the prevalence of slowly metabolized, dense LDL particles may be reduced [11,12].

The effect of a fibrate on carbohydrate metabolism seems to depend on the degree of glycemic control prior to its administration. In hypertriglyceridemic NIDDM patients with fasting blood sugar (FBS) >160 mg/dl, fibrates have been shown to improve glucose tolerance and insulin sensitivity [13]. In patients with FBS <160 mg/dl, the effects of fibrates on glucose tolerance are more variable. In NIDDM hypertriglyceridemic patients with FBS and 2 h postprandial BS <200 mg/dl, ciprofibrate corrected the lipid disorders and lowered serum fibrinogen without adversely influencing glucose tolerance and insulin sensitivity (unpublished observation). Fibrates may increase the risk of cholelithiasis. They are excreted by the kidney and should not be used in patients with diabetic nephropathy or chronic renal insufficiency because of increased risk of myopathy.

HMG-CoA reductase inhibitors

Reductase inhibitors (fluvastatin, lovastatin, pravastatin and simvastatin) effect substantial reduction in LDL-C levels. They also have beneficial effects on triglyceride and HDL-C, but the effects may be marginal when both values are abnormal. They are well tolerated and have been used successfully to treat elevated LDL-C in both IDDM and NIDDM patients [6,8,14]. Combination with a fibrate increases the risk of myopathy but, in selected cases, it may control severe dyslipidemia in NIDDM [14]. Glycemic control is not affected by these drugs. The liver is their primary route of excretion and they can be used to treat dyslipidemia in the presence of diabetic nephropathy, including the nephrotic syndrome [15,16].

Bile-acid sequestrants (resins)

Bile-acid sequestrants (cholestyramine and colestipol) cause a significant fall in plasma LDL-C, but stimulate liver VLDL production. They can increase VLDL triglyceride levels and have little effect on HDL-C. Small doses may be used in combination with a fibrate in patients with elevated LDL-C and VLDL triglyceride [8]. Resins commonly produce indigestion and constipation; they must be used with great care if at all in the diabetic patient with gastrointestinal autonomic neuropathy. They have no adverse effects on glucose control and, not being absorbed systemically, they are the safest lipid-lowering agents for patients with diabetic nephropathy and elevated LDL-C levels, provided triglyceride levels are monitored. For hypercholesterolemic children and adolescents with IDDM resins are the drugs of choice [7].

Nicotinic acid

Although it substantially lowers total and LDL-C and triglyceride and raises HDL-C, treatment with nicotinic acid is not usually recommended in diabetes because it increases insulin resistance and fasting and postprandial hyperglycemia and hyperinsulinemia.

References

1. American Diabetes Association. Diabetes Care 1993;16(suppl 2):106–112.
2. Recommendations of the European Atherosclerosis Society and the International Task Force for Prevention of Coronary Heart Disease. Nutr Metab Cardiovasc Dis 1992;2:113–156.
3. Expert Panel on Detection, Evaluation, and Treatment of High Blood Cholesterol in Adults (ATP II). J Am Med Assoc 1993;269:3015–3023.
4. Stewart MW, Laker MF, Dyer RG, Game F, Mitcheson J, Winocour PH, Alberti KG. Arterioscler Thromb 1993;13:1046–1052.
5. Jenkins AJ, Steele JS, Janus ED, Best JD. Diabetes 1991;40:787–790.
6. Taskinen MR. Nutr Metab Cardiovasc Dis 1991;1:201–206.
7. Garg A. Diabetes Care 1994:17:224–234.
8. Garg A, Grundy SM. Diabetes Care 1990;13:153–169.
9. Carmena R. In: Stein O, Eisenberg S, Stein Y (eds) Atherosclerosis IX. Tel Aviv: R & L Creative Comm, 1992;485–488.
10. Wu M–S, Johnston P, Sheu WH-H, Hollenbeck CB, Jeng C-Y, Goldfine ID, Chen Y-DI, Reaven GM. Diabetes Care 1990;13:1–8.
11. Lahdenpera S, Tilly-Kiesi M, Vuorinen-Markkola H, Kuusi T, Taskinen MR. Diabetes Care 1993;16:584–592.
12. Caslake MJ, Packard CJ, Gaw A, Murray E, Griffin BA, Vallance BD, Shepherd J. Arterioscler Thromb 1993;13:702–711.
13. Shen DR, Fuf MMT, Shieh S-M, Chen Y-I, Reaven GM. J Clin Endocrinol Metab 1991;73:503–510.
14. Garg A, Grundy SM. Diabetes 1989;38:364–372.
15. Hommel E, Andersen P, Gall M-A, Nielsen F, Jensen B, Rossing P, Dyerberg J, Parving HH. Diabetologia 1992;35:447–451.
16. Nielsen S, Schmitz O, Moller N, Porksen N, Klausen IC, Alberti KG, Mogensen CE. Diabetologia 1993;36:1079–1086.

Blood coagulation: linkage between thrombosis and atherosclerosis, an overview

Kenneth G. Mann

Department of Biochemistry, University of Vermont, College of Medicine, Room C401 Given Building, Burlington, VT 05405, USA

Abstract. The response to vascular damage results in the focal generation of α-thrombin, which produces a fibrin/platelet clot at the site of vascular injury. The regulated coagulation response derives from the assembly and activity of enzyme complexes which are localized to surfaces presented by the vascular damage. The product of each enzymatic complex provides the serine protease component required for the assembly and activity of each successive enzyme complex, ultimately leading to the formation of thrombin. When one limits attention to those complexes clearly associated with hemostatic or thrombotic risk, the significance of the vitamin K-dependent enzyme complexes becomes apparent. Each of these complexes involves a serine protease and a cofactor protein which assemble on a membrane surface in the presence of Ca^{++}. The expression of an active complex involves, besides activation of zymogen to an enzyme, the presentation or activation of a cofactor protein and the provision of the appropriate membrane to support the reaction. Since the membrane plays an essential part in the formation and expression of vitamin K-dependent complexes, its regulation is vital in the expression of procoagulant activity.

The blood coagulation response is a complex array of processes which collectively respond to vascular injury. If the vascular injury is of a perforating nature we term the process "hemostasis" and the resulting blockage of blood flow represents a desirable endpoint for the host. The generation of the equivalent blood clotting response in an intact but partially occluded blood vessel in response to an interluminal vascular injury may have catastrophic consequences which can be collectively termed "thrombosis". Stedman's medical dictionary [1] differentiates between the processes of thrombosis and hemostasis in the context of desirable and undesirable events. In part, this is a reflection of the historical development of the clinical and basic science interests in the field of hemostasis and thrombosis. Unfortunately, these two events are often separated in the clinical training arena. It is probably time to merge the intellectual property of thrombosis and hemostasis on the cell biological, biochemical, and clinical levels.

The interluminal vascular injury presented by a disease like atherosclerosis is intimately related to thrombosis on both a mechanistic and the pathologic basis. The combination of these two processes is, by far, the major cause of death in the human population. The pathologic representation of the combination of atherosclerosis and thrombosis is primarily achieved when the resulting vascular occlusion significantly influences the function of a major organ. It is likely that throughout life, the processes of luminal vascular damage associated with atherosclerosis are followed by hemostatic responses relevant to the extent of these injuries. The resulting cycle of vascular injury/thrombosis may be clinically silent until a vascular occlusion occurs on a scale that produces significant end-organ pathology.

It is logically desirable to represent the hemostatic response to vascular injury in the form of a cycle in which a chronologically distinct series of events associated with vascular damage, platelet adherence, coagulation, fibrinolysis and wound healing can be considered (Fig. 1) [2]. This sort of paradigm, while intellectually satisfying, is very

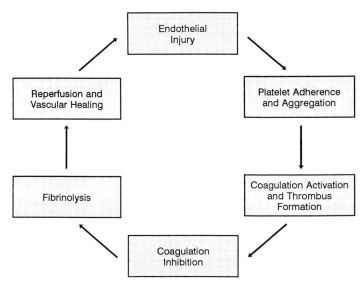

Fig. 1. Endothelial injury cycle.

misleading. All of the processes represented in the "cycle" of Fig. 1 are extraordinarily interconnected. If, for example, we take the process of platelet aggregation, feedback-feedforward events occur with respect to every other event in the repair "cycle" (Fig. 2). Similarly the endothelial injury process itself is directly connected to every other event in the "cycle" represented in Fig. 1 (Fig. 3). The diagram resulting for the major known interactions among the various "cycle" compartments represents a highly interactive network (Fig. 4) rather than a cyclic process. At present we really have no idea of the extent which this injury/repair process is continuously occurring in the human vascular

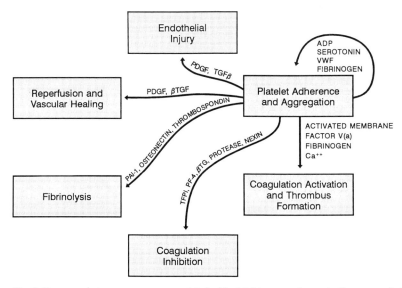

Fig. 2. Crossover between processes associated with platelet aggregation and adherence and other compartments of the injury cycle.

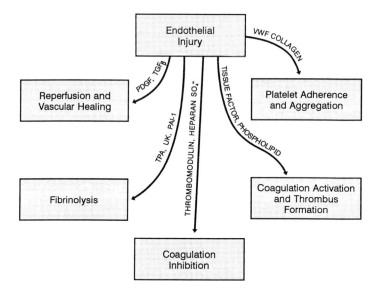

Fig. 3. Crossover between direct consequences of endothelial injury and other compartments of the endothelial injury cycle.

system, although data from several laboratories suggest that a process is always ongoing to some extent.

The principal focus of research in my laboratory has been to understand the relationship between the plasma coagulation system and the activated cell membranes and/or membrane particles that participate in the activation of the coagulation cascade and the formation of the fibrin–platelet thrombus. Our studies and those of many other laboratories

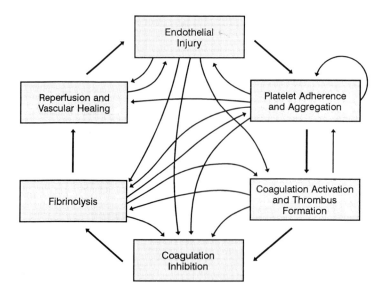

Fig. 4. The endothelial injury network.

have led to the elucidation of the multiprotein complex enzymes of the vitamin K-dependent proteolytic cascade [3,4]. The common feature of each of these complex enzymes is the association of a membrane-binding, vitamin K-dependent, serine protease (factor VIIa, factor IXa, factor Xa, factor IIa) with a companion membrane-bound cofactor (factor Va, factor VIIIa, tissue factor thrombomodulin) on an activated membrane surface. These protein membrane complexes in turn convert membrane-bound protein substrates (factor X, factor IX, factor II, protein C) to their final products (Fig. 5).

The primary events associated with complex catalyst formation include: 1) the activation of a vitamin K-dependent zymogen to its respective enzyme by proteolytic cleavage; 2) the activation of a soluble procofactor protein (factor V, factor VIII) or the presentation of membrane-bound cofactor (tissue factor, thrombomodulin); and 3) the generation of the appropriate activated membrane. The membrane provides for catalyst localization, which is vital to a regional injury response, and the membrane ultimately regulates the extent of the coagulation response which can occur. Numerous feedback and crossover reactions occur in the coagulation process and the sort of network described in the vascular injury cycle of Fig. 1 is also appropriate for the network of highly interactive reactions associated with α-thrombin formation. The α-thrombin formation process is not unidirectional, and enormous enhancement of the various reactions occurs because of feedback of product enzymes which contribute to their own formation. The inhibition processes involving activated protein C thrombomodulin are also proteolytically regulated.

Most investigators today believe that the initiating point of a coagulation reaction, whether resulting in hemostasis or thrombosis, is associated with the presentation of tissue factor either from the perivascular tissue or from the surface of a cytokine-activated endothelial cell or derived from an activated blood monocyte. A primary contribution of the vascular injury of Fig. 1 toward development of a thrombus is the presentation of

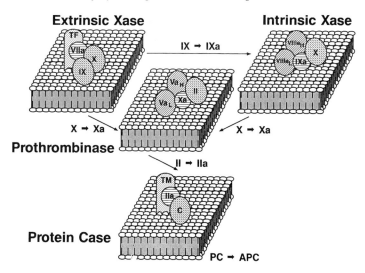

Fig. 5. A schematic representation of the vitamin K-dependent blood coagulation enzyme complexes. Each complex is represented assembled on a phospholipid surface. The cofactors, tissue factor (TF), thrombomodulin (TM) factor VIIIa, and factor Va are represented associated with their respective complementary serine proteases, factor VIIa, factor Xa, factor IXa, and thrombin (IIa). The substrates of the complexes, factor IX, factor X, prothrombin (II), and protein C (C), are also represented; APC corresponds to the activated form of protein C. The reactants and products associated with each reaction complex are also represented. From [4], reprinted by permission (Academic Press, Inc.).

tissue factor and the presentation of the appropriate activated membrane surface to flowing blood. Recent studies in our laboratory have attempted to recapitulate all the known actions of the plasma coagulation system initiated by the tissue-factor pathway [5]. These studies have made use of synthetic mixtures of the known coagulation factors at plasma concentrations. These studies reveal that in the absence of inhibitors, the maximal expression of procoagulant activity in the form of α-thrombin is achieved with only trivial activation of the other vitamin K-dependent zymogens, factor IX and factor X but with massive activation of the procofactors factor V and VIII to their respective active forms. Work in progress also includes the inhibitors antithrombin III, tissue-factor-pathway inhibitor, and the protein C/thrombomodulin system. In general, the reaction profile associated with the tissue-factor-dependent generation of α-thrombin is categorized by a lag phase in which small amounts of factor X and factor IX (<1%) are activated and nearly quantitative conversion of the procofactors factor V and factor VIII takes place. During the lag or "initiation" phase very little thrombin is produced. This phase is followed by a "propagation" phase in which large amounts of α-thrombin are produced. The duration of the initiation phase is largely a function of the extent of membrane expressed and tissue factor presented while the rate of the expression of α-thrombin activity during the propagation phase is almost a constant, dependent only upon the concentrations of active membrane and the plasma blood clotting factors. In many respects, the blood clotting reaction can be seen as a threshold-limited reaction, in which, once certain levels of intermediate activities have been accumulated, the reaction proceeds independently of the initiator concentration. In this regard, the response of the coagulation system is decidedly nonlinear and reminiscent of an explosion. In this analogy, the concentration of the factor VIIa–tissue factor complex corresponds to the fuse, which describes the duration of the initiation phase, while the propagation phase corresponds to an explosion whose dimensions are determined by the plasma concentrations of the coagulation factors.

The complexity of the biological coagulation system makes empirical modeling of the system both technically arduous and expensive. We have attempted to develop computer models of the clotting system which can act as surrogates to aid us in the design of hypotheses regarding how the coagulation system might respond to a given insult. Kinetic modeling of the blood clotting system also permits valuable insights into how one might intervene to alter a coagulation response [6]. On the basis of the preliminary results already obtained it is likely that the most effective interventions occur during the early phases of the generation of the blood clotting response and the application of the feedback reactions which amplify thrombin generation.

Acknowledgements

The research in this laboratory has been supported by grant awards HL34575 and HL 46703 of the National Institute of Health.

References

1. Stedman T. Stedman's Medical Dictionary. Baltimore/London, Williams & Wilkins, 1982;638,1449.
2. Mann KG. In: Kelley W. Textbook of Internal Medicine, 2nd edn. New York: J.B. Lippincott Co., 1992; 1240−1245.
3. Mann KG, Nesheim ME, Church WR, Haley P, Krishnaswamy S. Blood 1990;76:1.
4. Mann KG and Lorand L. Methods in Enzymology. San Diego, CA:Academic Press, 1993;1−10.
5. Lawson JH, Kalafatis M, Stram S and Mann KG. J Biol Chem 1994;269:23357−23366.
6. Jones KC and Mann KG. J Biol Chem 1994;269:23367−23373.

The 'fibrinogen hypothesis': is elevated plasma fibrinogen a major cardiovascular risk factor?

E. Ernst and K.L. Resch

University of Exeter Postgraduate Medical School, Barrack Road, Exeter EX2 5DW, UK

Abstract. Epidemiological studies have produced a sizable body of prospective data identifying elevated fibrinogen as a major, independent cardiovascular risk factor. Cross-sectional results show strong associations between fibrinogen and conventional cardiovascular risk factors and clinical endpoints. Clinical cohort studies demonstrate that increased fibrinogen might also be a risk factor for the sequelae of cardiovascular disease. At present, knowledge about the determinants of the (highly variable) plasma level of fibrinogen in health and disease is incomplete. Understanding of the mechanisms that might be involved in the atherogenic action of fibrinogen is also fragmentary. Fibrinogen strongly affects blood coagulation, blood rheology and platelet aggregation, it has direct effects on the vascular wall and is a prominent acute phase reactant. All these phenomena might provide some insight into the pathophysiological mechanisms involved in the association between fibrinogen and cardiovascular events. Even though many crucial questions await conclusive answers, the published evidence leaves little doubt that fibrinogen represents a major, independent risk factor.

Our knowledge of "accepted" risk factors has become widespread and its application to clinical practice may have promoted a considerable reduction of cardiovascular mortality and morbidity, particularly in the USA. It is tempting, therefore, to forget that our understanding is still highly incomplete. Only about 30% of all cardiovascular events can be extrapolated on the basis of "accepted" risk factors [1]. Additional determinants may therefore exist; more and more evidence suggests that fibrinogen is a potential candidate [2].

Human fibrinogen is a long protein of a molecular mass of 340,000 daltons predominantly synthesized in the liver. It consists of three different polypeptide chains. 80—90% of the body's fibrinogen is found in the blood plasma. "Normal" plasma levels range from 2 to 4.5 g/l; the molecule's half-life is 3—6 days. Its synthesis is believed to be under the feedback control of its plasma degradation products, and of cytokines produced by activated macrophages.

Fibrinogen is well known as an acute-phase protein and a clotting factor but it has numerous other functions [3]. It is an essential cofactor for platelet aggregation, a determinant of the rheological behavior of blood, and a stimulant of smooth muscle cell migration and proliferation. These and other circumstances may be involved in its ability to act as a cardiovascular risk factor.

Epidemiological evidence

Prospective analyses

In the Northwick Park Heart Study, 1510 white men aged 40—64 years were randomly recruited and tested for a range of clotting factors, including fibrinogen. At 4-year follow-up, 49 individuals had died, 27 from cardiovascular diseases [4]. There was a significant association between cardiovascular deaths and fibrinogen which was independent of other risk factors and stronger than the corresponding association for total cholesterol. Other causes of death were *not* related to fibrinogen levels. 15 of the 25 patients who died of ischemic heart disease were in the highest tertile of fibrinogen (<3.2 g/l). At 10-year follow-up [5], 109 men had suffered a first coronary event. Multiple regression analyses showed an association between fibrinogen and ischemic heart disease, which was again independent of conventional risk factors. Approximately half of all the incident coronary events occurred in the upper tertile of fibrinogen.

About 2,000 men aged 45—64 years were recruited for the Speedwell Study [6]. Baseline fibrinogen was positively associated with prevalent ischemic heart disease. When the study was expanded into the Caerphilly/Speedwell Study it involved more than 4,700 men [7]. Its baseline data revealed a significant association of smoking with fibrinogen. The prospective evaluation of the Speedwell and Caerphilly/Speedwell Studies, with an average follow-up of 5.1 and 3.2 years respectively, included a total of 251 major coronary events [8]. A multivariate analysis demonstrated that fibrinogen was an independent risk factor for ischemic heart disease. Its predictive power was stronger than that of accepted coronary risk factors like total cholesterol, blood pressure or body mass index.

In the Gothenborg Study, fibrinogen, blood pressure, total cholesterol and smoking habits were recorded for a random sample of 792 men, all of them born in 1913 [9]. After a mean follow-up period of 13.5 years, there were 92 cases of myocardial infarction, 37 strokes, and 60 deaths of noncardiovascular causes. Univariate analyses identified smoking, cholesterol and fibrinogen as risk factors for myocardial infarction, while blood pressure and fibrinogen were risk factors for stroke. In a multivariate analysis the association between fibrinogen and cardiovascular events weakened, but was still statistically significant for stroke. When the study was extended to 21 years, 119 myocardial infarctions, 81 strokes and 333 deaths from other causes had occurred [10]. In the multivariate evaluation, stroke and total mortality were significantly associated with fibrinogen.

In a relatively small prospective study 297 men aged 40—69 years, initially free of coronary heart disease, were recruited from one general practice in the UK [11]. After a mean follow-up period of 7.3 years, 40 cases of heart infarction had occurred, and fibrinogen was positively correlated with its incidence. In hypertensive patients the incidence was 6 times higher when fibrinogen levels exceeded 3.5 g/l than in the subpopulation with values below this threshold. Multivariate analyses showed that the predictive power of all variables, in descending order were: fibrinogen, age, systolic blood pressure, total cholesterol, obesity, number of cigarettes smoked per day, VLDL.

The tenth biannual examination of the Framingham Study analyzed the interrelation of fibrinogen with smoking [12]. During a 14-year follow-up period, the risk of cardiovascular disease in men and women increased as a function of initial fibrinogen levels. The age-adjusted incidence in male smokers with high fibrinogen levels was twice that of a low-fibrinogen subgroup. As in the Northwick Park Heart Study [4,5], the effect was more pronounced in younger males. Fibrinogen was demonstrated to be a risk factor for coronary heart disease, independent of smoking or other accepted risk factors [13]. In women, the magnitude of the fibrinogen-mediated risk declined with age. Fibrinogen was also a risk factor for stroke in men, but not in women. The relative impact of fibrinogen was similar to those of blood pressure, obesity, smoking and diabetes. A more recent analysis of the Framingham material [14] revealed that in men the fibrinogen risk ratio was greatest for stroke and smallest for peripheral vascular disease. For women the risk ratio was greatest for coronary heart disease.

The PROCAM study [15] examined 1,674 men aged 40—65 years without a history of myocardial infarction or stroke. 15 cardiovascular events were observed during 2 years of follow-up 10 of which fell into the high fibrinogen tertile. When this trial was extended to 2,116 men, followed for 6 years, 82 coronary events had occurred. The incidence of coronary events in the upper tertile of fibrinogen was 2.4 times higher than in the lower tertile [16]. The combination of high fibrinogen and elevated LDL levels led to an increase of coronary risk by a factor of 6.1.

This cumulative evidence is highly suggestive, yet it also shows weaknesses. For instance, the above studies either do not consider LDL-cholesterol in their multivariate models or quantify this variable by inadequate methods. As LDL-cholesterol is one of the strongest predictors of coronary heart disease known to date, previous results might have overestimated the predictive power of fibrinogen. The GRIPS Study [17], a prospective cohort study of 5,239 men aged 40–60 initially free of cardiovascular disease, attempted to overcome this drawback. 107 myocardial infarctions had occurred after 5 years of follow-up. Fibrinogen was a strong predictor in an univariate model. Its average level (± SD) was 3.6 ± 0.8 g/l in the nonevent and 4.2 ± 1.0 g/l in the event group. Using a multivariate regression model, which accounted for LDL-cholesterol, the relationship weakened, yet remained statistically significant. In the final model the rank order of predictors was as follows: LDL-cholesterol, familial predisposition, Lp(a), HDL-cholesterol, fibrinogen, age, smoking, glucose, blood pressure.

Cross-sectional analyses

According to one MONICA study center [18], fibrinogen was raised in male and female smokers. In another center [19] plasma viscosity (strongly influenced by fibrinogen) was raised in males with hypercholesterolemia, untreated hypertension or in smokers, as well as in females with hypercholesterolemia or obesity. In the Scottish Heart Health Study 8,824 men and women were examined. Women had higher fibrinogen levels than men [20]. Fibrinogen was positively associated with age, smoking, cholesterol and body mass index and negatively linked to alcohol consumption. Female menopause also coincided with higher fibrinogen levels. A Danish study [21] of 439 men aged 51 showed positive associations of fibrinogen with low social class, psychological variables, smoking, physical inactivity, low HDL-cholesterol, low physical fitness and high LDL-cholesterol.

The largest (n = 15,803) epidemiological study to include fibrinogen so far is the ARIC study [22]. Its baseline data showed fibrinogen to be 22 mg/dl higher in blacks than in whites. It also confirmed higher values in women than in men. Fibrinogen furthermore increased with age, smoking, body size, diabetes, fasting serum insulin, LDL, Lp(a), leukocyte count and menopause. It was lower with ethanol intake, exercise, HDL and post menopausal female hormone use.

These epidemiological studies are of adequate sample size (several thousand participants and several hundred with major cardiovascular events) and sample composition (several random samples of the population with different genetic, occupational, social and geographical backgrounds). They leave little doubt as to a strong link between fibrinogen and atherothrombotic diseases and demonstrate that fibrinogen is an important, *independent* risk factor. Its relative impact is roughly as strong as that of total cholesterol or other "accepted" risk factors. Fibrinogen is also related to most other risk factors. Theoretically this could suggest that its relationship to cardiovascular endpoints is indirect, and confounded merely by associations with true risk factors. However, most of the above studies did consider these "confounders" and fibrinogen remained of significant predictive value. Therefore the cumulative data suggest that fibrinogen represents one mechanism by which various other risk factors lead to atherothrombotic events.

Clinical evidence

Coronary heart disease

It has long been appreciated that an acute myocardial infarction leads to transient hyperfibrinogenemia (review [23]). Fibrinogen increases progressively with the severity of coronary atherosclerosis [24–26]. This can be interpreted in terms of an acute phase response, yet fibrinogen (or plasma viscosity) remains elevated for years after an infarction [27]. Recent evidence links this fact to chronic *Helicobacter pylori* infections which affect about half the adult population and seem to predispose to coronary heart disease and simultaneously elevate fibrinogen levels [28]. A prospective study investigated fibrinogen levels in 120 survivors of a myocardial infarction [29]. Reinfarction occurred only in cases where the initial fibrinogen level exceeded 750 mg/dl during the acute phase of the disease. A prospective study followed 1,716 men for 2 years who, 6 months before, had suffered a myocardial infarction [30]. During this period 126 had suffered a second ischemic event. Fibrinogen was significantly elevated in this subgroup. Statistically significant differences in fibrinogen also existed between patients who survived and those who died. The relative odds for death showed an approximately linear relationship to fibrinogen levels.

Stroke

Similarly, fibrinogen levels increase after an acute stroke [31]. This has also been attributed to an acute-phase reaction subsequent to brain-tissue necrosis. However, plasma viscosity is significantly increased in TIA patients, suggesting that fibrinogen levels are elevated *before* the stroke [32,33]. In a prospective study of stroke survivors, fibrinogen was significantly higher in patients who suffered a second cardiovascular event during the 2 years after the initial stroke. The effect was independent of concomitant risk factors [34]. These results are in accordance with data showing that patients with a progression of carotid artery lesions had significantly higher fibrinogen levels than those with nonprogressing lesions in the angiogram [35].

Peripheral arterial disease

In peripheral arterial occlusive disease (PAOD) fibrinogen is significantly increased [36,37]. A large-scale study [38] demonstrated that fibrinogen is independently associated with peripheral arterial narrowing. In claudicants it is often highly abnormal in the absence of gross angiographic narrowing of the arteries, a finding that led to the concept of "rheologic claudication" [37]. Longitudinal data of PAOD patients showed that high fibrinogen was a predictor for reocclusion of femoro-popliteal vein grafts [39]. Recently it was demonstrated that PAOD patients have a high incidence of variation of the β-fibrinogen locus leading to elevated plasma levels [40].

   These clinical findings suggest that fibrinogen is elevated in overt atherosclerotic disease, which might be interpreted in terms of a hematological stress syndrome [36]. Longitudinal data identify fibrinogen as a valuable prognostic indicator in several clinical situations, suggesting that it also represents a risk factor for the sequelae of cardiovascular disease.

Determinants of the fibrinogen level

Associations with other risk factors

A *genetic* determination of fibrinogen levels undoubtedly exists [41,42]. However, it does not fully account for its wide physiologic variability. Some reports have shown that fibrinogen levels increase with *age* [43–45]. Others have suggested that fibrinogen (or plasma viscosity) is not age-dependent [46]. The apparent contradiction may be due to confounding by disease status: in elderly subjects there is a higher prevalence of unrecognized diseases associated with elevated fibrinogen, causing spuriously high mean values. If strict criteria for health are applied, individuals with hidden diseases are excluded and the age dependence disappears [46].

Fibrinogen levels are elevated in patients with type II *hyperlipoproteinemia* [47], familial hypercholesterolemia [48] and hypertriglyceridemia [49]. In a large population sample, plasma viscosity correlated positively with total cholesterol and apoprotein B [50]. The baseline data from the GRIPS Study [17] show that fibrinogen levels are associated positively with total cholesterol, triglycerides, LDL-cholesterol and HDL-cholesterol, but not with Lp(a).

Smoking is known to increase fibrinogen levels in healthy individuals (see above). The effect is dose-related [51] and reversible upon cessation of smoking [52]. There is a significant correlation between fibrinogen and carboxyl hemoglobin levels [53]. Plasma viscosity was found to be raised in male but not in female smokers [54]. The most detailed analysis of the interrelationship of fibrinogen with smoking and CVD is probably the one from Framingham [12–14]. Its authors estimated that 50% of the cardiovascular harm done by chronic smoking is mediated through its effect on fibrinogen.

In patients with essential *hypertension*, fibrinogen levels are higher than in normotensive controls [55]. Similarly, plasma viscosity is elevated in hypertensive subjects, and blood-pressure readings are positively correlated with plasma viscosity [56]. Even when hypertension is only mild, patients have higher fibrinogen levels than normotensive controls [57].

Fibrinogen is raised in *diabetics* [58]. Patients with microvascular involvement have higher fibrinogen levels than diabetics free from such complications. The Framingham data revealed a correlation between blood-sugar levels and fibrinogen [59]. Fasting glucose correlates with fibrinogen even in normal individuals [19]. In diabetics with albuminuria fibrinogen is higher than in diabetics without this complication [60], and fibrinogen has been shown to be an independent predictor of vascular complications in type II diabetes [61]. Fibrinogen is also raised in obese individuals and increases with *skinfold thickness* [62].

Dietary influences

Diets low in fat and rich in carbohydrates lower fibrinogen slightly [63]. Diets containing large amounts of n-3 and n-6 polyunsaturated fatty acids may reduce fibrinogen [64,65], and apparently so does moderate alcohol intake [16].

Other influences

Fibrinogen is related to social class [66], which has in part been attributed to different levels of emotional stress [67,68]. Controlled trials have shown that fibrinogen levels increase in women taking oral contraceptives [69]. Recently it has been demonstrated that fibrinogen is lower in adults who had low infant weight [70]. It has also been shown to be higher in individuals with poor dental health [71].

This list of determinants partly confirms the above epidemiological results. The pathophysiological mechanisms behind these associations need to be evaluated in much more detail.

Pathophysiological mechanisms

The mechanisms by which fibrinogen may promote atherothrombosis are still uncertain. Fibrinogen strongly affects coagulation, blood flow, platelet aggregation and endothelial function. A hypercoagulable state would seem to favor the thrombotic aspects of atherothrombosis. Fibrinogen is a major determinant of plasma viscosity and induces reversible red cell aggregation. Both phenomena limit the blood's fluidity. Blood rheology might act at various levels, by reducing flow, by predisposing to thrombosis, or by enhancing atherogenesis [2,68].

Platelet hyperaggregation plays an accepted role in the genesis of an atherosclerotic lesion. Fibrinogen binds to receptors on the platelet membrane, a phenomenon which in turn is a precondition for aggregation in flow [72]. Furthermore, fibrinogen is also integrated directly into arteriosclerotic vascular lesions, where it is converted to fibrin and fibrinogen degradation products; it binds low density lipoproteins and sequesters more fibrinogen. Both fibrinogen and fibrinogen degradation products have been shown to stimulate smooth-muscle proliferation and migration [73,74]. By these effects it seems to be involved in the earliest stages of plaque formation.

The fact that fibrinogen is an acute-phase reactant also deserves consideration [75]. Atherosclerosis bears similarities to an inflammatory process [76]. For instance, white cell counts are significantly elevated in the presence of active atherosclerosis [77]. Thus it is theoretically possible that early atherosclerosis itself leads to a mild inflammatory response which slightly elevates acute-phase proteins [37] and other variables of the acute-phase response [78].

It is likely that the above clinical and epidemiological findings are the result of complex interactions between these and possibly other phenomena, which we still need to understand more completely. The intense research activities in respect to the pathophysiological mechanisms involved are discussed in more detail elsewhere [72,73].

Therapeutic implications

The final test for the hypothesis that fibrinogen is a causal cardiovascular risk factor would be a randomized trial to lower it therapeutically in patients and determine the subsequent cardiovascular outcome. An essential precondition for doing so would be the availability of a drug which reduces fibrinogen levels safely and selectively. Unfortunately no such a substance is yet known [79]. Several medications have been shown to decrease fibrinogen in various clinical settings [80]. All of these are known primarily for other pharmacological actions on the cardiovascular system. Fibrates, for example, have been reported to induce relatively large fibrinogen reductions [81]. Yet they primarily reduce blood lipids, which makes them unsuitable for a trial of the independent fibrinogen effect. Monoclonal antibodies against platelet glycoprotein IIb/IIIa receptor may be a decisive step forward in clinical terms [82], yet it does not solve the above problem. Thus the value of reducing fibrinogen in an attempt to reduce the cardiovascular risk is unknown, and the ultimate test for the validity of the 'fibrinogen hypothesis' is not readily available.

Conclusions

A link between fibrinogen and athero-thrombogenesis is likely and plausible. A meta-analysis [83] of prospective data indicates that a plasma fibrinogen level above 3.5 g/l is a powerful, independent risk factor for brain and/or heart infarction. Clinical findings suggest that increased fibrinogen may also be a risk factor for the sequelae of CVD. Time would seem right to test the 'fibrinogen hypothesis' by controlled intervention trials. Yet the ideal drug to lower fibrinogen exclusively has not (yet?) been found. Future research on arteriothrombotic diseases should attempt to solve the many questions which remain to be answered.

References

1. Heller RF, Chinn S, Tunstall-Pedoe HD, Rose G. Br Med J 1984;288:1409−1411.
2. Ernst E. J Int Med 1990;227:365−372.
3. Dang CV, Bell WR. Am J Med 1989;87:567−576.
4. Meade TW, Chakrabarti R, Haines AP, North WRS, Stirling Y, Thompson SG. Lancet 1980;1:1050−1053.
5. Meade TW, Mellows W, Brozovic M, Miller GJ, Chakrabarti R, North WR, et al. Lancet 1986;2:533−537.
6. Baker LA, Eastham R, Elwood PC, Etherington M, O'Brian JR, Sweetham PM. Br Heart J 1982;47:490−494.
7. Yarnell JWG, Sweetnam PM, Rogers S, Elwood PC, Bainton D, Baker IA, et al. J Clin Pathol 1987;40:909−913.
8. Yarnell JWG, Baker JA, Sweetnam PM, Bainton D, O'Brian JR, Whitehead PJ, Elwood PC. Circulation 1991;83:836−844.
9. Wilhelmsen L, Svärdsudd K, Korsan-Bengtsen K, Larsson B, Welin L, Tibblin G. N Engl J Med 1984;311:501−505.
10. Eriksson H, Korsan-Bengtsen E, Welin L, Svärdsudd K, Larsson B, Tibblin G, Wilhelmsen L. In: Ernst E, Keonig W, Lowe GDO, Meade TW (eds) Fibrinogen, a "New" Cardiovascular Risk Factor. Oxford: Blackwell, 1992;115−119.
11. Stone MC, Thorp JM. J Roy Coll Gen Prac 1985;35:565−569.
12. Kannel WB, D'Agnostino RB, Belanger AJ. Am Heart J 1987;113:1006−1010.
13. Kannel WB, Wolf PA, Castelli WP, D'Agostino RB. J Am Med Assoc 1987;258:1183−1186.
14. Kannel WB. In: Ernst E, Koenig W, Lowe GDO, Meade TW (eds) Fibrinogen, a "New" Cardiovascular Risk Factor. Oxford: Blackwell, 1992;101−109.
15. Balleisen L, Schulte H, Balleisen L, Assmann G, Van De Loo J. Lancet 1987;1:461.
16. Heinrich J, Balleisen L, Schulte H, Assmann G, Van De Loo J. Arterioscler Thromb 1995;14 (in press).
17. Cremer P, Nagel D, Labrot B, Mann H, Muche E, Elster H, Seidel D. Eur J Clin Invest 1994;24 (in press).
18. Lowe GDO, Smith WCS, Tunstall-Pedoe HD, Crombie IK, Lennie SE, Anderson J, Barbenel JC. Clin Hemorheol 1988;8:517−524.
19. Ernst E, Koenig W, Matrai A, Keil U. Clin Hemorheol 1988;8:507−515.
20. Lee AJ, Smith WCS, Lowe GDO, Turnstall-Pedow H. J Clin Epidem 1990;43:913−919.
21. Möller L, Kristensen TS. Arterioscler Thromb 1991;11:344−350.
22. Folsom A. In: Ernst E, Koenig W, Lowe GDO, Meade TW (eds) Fibrinogen, a "New" Cardiovascular Risk Factor. Oxford: Blackwell, 1992;124−129.
23. Dormandy J, Ernst E, Matrai A, Flute P. Am Heart J 1982;104:1364−1367.
24. Lowe GDO, Drummond MM, Lorimer AR, Hutton I, Forbes CD, Prentice CRM, Barbenel JC. Br Med J 1980;1:673−674.
25. Handa K, Kiono S, Saku K. Atherosclerosis 1989;77:209−213.
26. Broadhurst P, Kelleher C, Hughes L, Imeson JD, Raftery EB. Atherosclerosis 1990;85:169−173.
27. Ernst E, Resch KL, Krauth U, Paulsen HF. Br Heart J 1990;64:248−250.
28. Patel P, Carrington D, Strachan DP, Leatham E, Goggin P, Northfield TC, Mendall MA. Lancet 1994;343.
29. Fulton RM, Duckett K. Lancet 1976;2:1161−1164.
30. Martin JF, Bath PMW, Burr ML. Lancet 1992;338:1409−1411.
31. Eisenbert S. Circulation 1966;33/34(suppl 2):10−14.
32. Ernst E, Matrai A, Marshall M. Stroke 1988;19:634−636.
33. Coull BM, Beamer N, de Garmo P, Sexton G, North F, Knox R, Seaman GVF. Stroke 1991;22:162−168.
34. Resch KL, Ernst E, Matrai A, Paulsen HF. Ann Int Med 1992;177:371−375.

35. Grotta JC. Neurology 1989;39:1325—1331.
36. Stuart J, George AJ, Davies AJ, Aukland A, Hurlow RA. J Clin Pathol 1981;34:464—467.
37. Dormandy JA, Hoare E, Colley J, Arrowsmith DE, Dormandy TL. Br Med J 1973;4:576—581.
38. Lowe GDO, Fowkes FGR, Dawes J, Donnan PT, Lennie SE, Housley E. Circulation 1993;87:1915—1920.
39. Wiseman S, Kenehington G, Dain R. Br Med J 1989;299:643—646.
40. Fowkes FGR, Connar JM, Smith FB, Wood J, Donnan PT, Lowe GDO. Lancet 1992;339:693—696.
41. Hamsten A, Iseluis L, de Faire U, Blomback M. Lancet 1987;2:988—990.
42. Humphries SE, Cook M, Dubowitz M, Stirling Y, Meade TW. Lancet 1987;1:1452—1455.
43. Hamilton PJ, Dawson AA, Ogston D, Douglas AS. J Clin Pathol 1974;27:326—329.
44. Meade TW, Chakrabarti R, Haines AP, North WRS, Stirling Y. Br Med J 1979;1:153—156.
45. Bongrand P, Barolin R, Bouvenot G, Arnaud C, et al. J Clin Lab Immunol 1984;15:45—50.
46. Ernst E, Koenig W, Matrai A, Keil U. VASA 1986;15:365—372.
47. Lowe GDO, Drummond MN, Third JLH, Bremer WF et al. Thromb Haemost 1979;42:1503—1507.
48. Di Minno G, Silver MJ, Cerbone AM, Rainone A, Postliglione A, Mancini M. Arteriosclerosis 1986;6:203—211.
49. Eikeles RS, Chakrabarti R, Vickers M, Stirling Y, Meade TW. Br Med J 1980;281:973—974.
50. Koenig W, Sund M, Ernst E, Mraz W, Doring A, Keil U, Hombach V. Biorheology 1989;26:601.
51. Ernst E, Matrai A, Schölzl C, Magyarosy I. Br J Haematol 1987;65:485—487.
52. Ernst E, Matrai A. Atherosclerosis 1987;64:75—77.
53. Powell JT, Sian M, Wiseman S, Grennhalgh RM. Lancet 1988;1:121.
54. Ernst E, Koenig W, Matrai A, Filipiak B, Stieber J. Arteriosclerosis 1988;8:385—388.
55. Letcher RL, Chien S, Pickering TG, Sealey JE, Laragh JH. Am J Med 1981;70:1195—1202.
56. Koenig W, Sund M, Ernst E, Matrai A, Keil U, Rosenthal J. Angiology 1989;40:153—163.
57. Landin K, Tengborn L, Smith U. J Int Med 1990;227:273—278.
58. Barnes A, Willars E. In: Chien S, Dormandy J, Ernst E, Matrai A, (eds) Clinical Hemorheology. Dordrecht: M. Nijhoff, 1987;275—309.
59. Kannel WB, D'Agostino RB, Wilson PW, Belanger AJ, Gagnon DR. Am Heart J 1990;120:672—676.
60. Schmitz A, Ingerslev J. Diabetic Med 1990;7:521—525.
61. Ganda, Arkin F. In: Ernst E, Koenig W, Lowe GDO, Meade TW (eds) Fibrinogen, a "New" Cardiovascular Risk Factor. Oxford: Blackwell, 1992;254—258.
62. Meade TW. In: Bloom AL, Thomas DP (eds) Haemostasis and Thrombosis. Edinburgh: Churchill Livingstone, 1987;575—592.
63. Mehrabian M, Peter JB, Barnard RJ, Lusis A. Atherosclerosis 1990;84:25—32.
64. Wojenski CM, Silver MJ, Walker J. Biochim Biophys Acta 1991;1081:33—38.
65. Racack K, Deck C, Huster G. J Am Coll Nutr 1990;9:352—357.
66. Markowe HLJ, Marmot MG, Shipley MJ, Bulpitt CJ et al. Br Med J 1985;291:1312—1314.
67. Ernst E, Weihmayr T, Schmid M, Baumann M, Matrai A. Atherosclerosis 1986;59:263—269.
68. Rosengren A, Wilhelmsen L, Welin L, Tsipogianni A, Teger—Nilsson AC, Wedel H. Br Med J 1990;300:634—638.
69. Ernst E. Atherosclerosis 1992;93:1—5.
70. Fall CHD, Barker DJP, Meade TW. In: Ernst E, Koenig W, Lowe GDO, Meade TW (eds) Fibrinogen a "New" Cardiovascular Risk Factor. Oxford: Blackwell, 1992;330—335.
71. Lowe GDO, Kweider M, Murray GD, Kinane D, McGowan DA. In: Ernst E, Koenig W, Lowe GDO, Meade TW (eds) Fibrinogen a "New" Cardiovascular Risk Factor. Oxford: Blackwell, 1992;336—337.
72. Cook NS, Ubben D. TIPS 1990;11:444—451.
73. Thompson WD, Smith EB. J Pathol 1989;159:97—106.
74. Smith EB, Keen GA, Grant A, Stirk CH. Arteriosclerosis 1990;10:263—275.
75. Ernst E. Eur Heart J 1993;14(suppl):K82—K87.
76. Spodick DH. Ann Int Med 1985;102:699—702.
77. Ernst E, Hammerschmidt DE, Bagge U, Matrai A, Dormandy J. J Am Med Assoc 1987;257:2318—2324.
78. Kannel WB, Anderson K, Wilson PWF. J Am Med Assoc 1992;267:1253—1256.
79. Machin SJ, Mackie IJ. Br Med J 1993;307:882—883.
80. Ernst E. Clinical Pharmacy 1992;11:986—971.
81. Farnier M, Bonnefous F, Debbas N, Irvine A. Arch Int Med 1994;154:441—449.
82. The EPIC Investigators. N Engl J Med 1994;330:956—961.
83. Ernst E, Resch KL. Ann Int Med 1993;118:956—963.

Detection of a prethrombotic state

Kenneth A. Bauer

Beth Israel Hospital and Brockton-West Roxbury Department of Veterans Affairs Medical Center, Harvard Medical School, Boston, Massachusetts, USA

Abstract. Advances in our understanding of the blood coagulation mechanism have permitted the development of immunoassays for activation peptides that monitor the biochemically defined pathways of enzyme generation. Studies employing these markers indicate that a biochemical imbalance between procoagulant and anticoagulant mechanisms can be detected in the blood of humans prior to the appearance of thrombotic phenomena. Properly designed prospective studies will be required to determine whether these assay techniques will enable us to identify individuals who are entering a clinically relevant hypercoagulable state, and intervene with appropriate therapy prior to the onset of overt thrombotic disease.

For years, clinicians have sought to employ blood tests to predict thrombotic events in high-risk patients. Advances in our knowledge of the biochemistry of coagulation have facilitated the development of sensitive and specific assays that detect the generation of coagulation enzymes, and products of intravascular fibrin formation. As it is not possible to measure most hemostatic enzymes in vivo directly, immunochemical assays have been developed for activation peptides that are liberated with the activation of zymogens (factor IX, factor X, prothrombin, and protein C) or with substrate consumption (fibrinopeptide A). Most of these assays were initially developed in research laboratories, but some are now available commercially.

Establishing a relationship between measurements of activation peptides in blood and thromboembolic disease requires studies that are carefully designed and executed. First, assays must be properly standardized to perform in a reproducible manner. Second, preanalytic variables such as the quality of the venipuncture procedure and the choice of anticoagulant for blood samples should be carefully controlled to minimize the occurrence of artifactual elevations in marker levels [1,2]. Third, objective endpoints must be used to establish thrombotic endpoints. Fourth, appropriate control groups are required and studies should have sufficient power to detect significant differences between thrombosis cases and controls.

Assays for activation peptides

The activation of factor IX can be monitored by measuring the levels of the factor IX activation peptide [3]. This assay reflects the action of factor XIa or the factor VII–tissue factor complex upon factor IX. Factor X activation mediated by the extrinsic or intrinsic pathways can be monitored by measuring the factor X activation peptide [4]. Under physiologic conditions, thrombin generation takes place at an appreciable rate in the presence of factor Xa, factor Va, calcium ions, and activated platelets. This results in cleavage of the amino terminus of the prothrombin molecule and liberation of the F_{1+2}

Address for correspondence: Kenneth A. Bauer MD, Beth Israel Hospital, 330 Brookline Avenue, Boston, MA 02215, USA.

fragment. A second bond scission generates thrombin, which converts fibrinogen into fibrin and releases fibrinopeptide A. Immunoassays have been developed for the F_{1+2} fragment [5–8] and fibrinopeptide A [9] that can be used as markers of prothrombin activation and thrombin generation in vivo, respectively.

Thrombin can also rapidly activate protein C by binding to thrombomodulin on vascular endothelial cells and an activation peptide assay has been developed to monitor this transformation [10].

Coagulation factor deficiencies

The investigation of patients with hereditary coagulation factor deficiencies has generated information regarding the pathways responsible for coagulation activation in vivo under basal conditions (i.e., the absence of thrombosis or provocative stimuli). Patients with factor VII deficiency but not factor XI deficiency have lower levels of factor IX activation [3], whereas patients with deficiencies of factor VIII or factor IX have normal levels of factor X and prothrombin activation [4]. The infusion of relatively small doses of recombinant factor VIIa (10–20 μg/kg of body weight) in factor VII-deficient patients results in substantial elevations in the plasma concentrations of the factor IX activation peptide, factor X activation peptide, and prothrombin fragment F_{1+2} [11]. Thus these data demonstrate that the factor VII–tissue factor pathway is largely responsible for the activation of factor IX as well as factor X in the basal state [3,4,11].

Administration of highly purified factor IX concentrates to hemophilia B patients increases their plasma factor IX activation peptide levels that are initially greatly decreased, but does not change factor X activation peptide or F_{1+2} measurements [11]. The infusion of highly purified factor VIII concentrates into hemophilia A patients does not change the plasma concentrations of factor X activation peptide and F_{1+2} [11]. These observations indicate that the factor IXa–factor VIIIa–cell surface complex is unable to activate factor X under basal conditions. In response to vascular injury or thrombotic stimuli, it is surmised that increased formation of free thrombin or factor Xa via the action of the factor VII–tissue factor pathway generates factor VIIIa or a natural surface (e.g., activated platelets) on which assembly of the factor IXa–factor VIIIa complex takes place. This hypothesis is consistent with the severe bleeding tendency of most patients with factor VIII or factor IX deficiency, and the insensitivity of the factor X activation peptide and F_{1+2} assays to deficiencies of these two proteins.

The above mechanistic findings derived from studies of patients with coagulation factor deficiencies have significant potential implications with regard to the utility of basal coagulation system markers in diagnosing prethrombotic patients. It follows that the conversion of a prethrombotic state to a thrombotic event occurs due to small increases in the generation rates of hemostatic enzymes that exceed the inhibitory threshold of an individual's endogenous anticoagulant mechanisms as well as the sequestration of these proteases on specialized cell surfaces. It remains to be determined whether persons with elevated basal levels of coagulation system markers are more likely to respond in a hypersensitive fashion to environmental stimuli. Because the activity of the blood coagulation mechanism in such individuals is closer to the threshold of normal inhibitory processes, such individuals may generate slightly more thrombin via the factor VII–tissue factor mechanism via the extrinsic pathway. This thrombin could then be used to ignite the dormant intrinsic cascade, which could ultimately result in the generation of large amounts of free thrombin and the development of arterial or venous thrombosis.

Hereditary prethrombotic disorders

Hereditary deficiencies of protein C, protein S, antithrombin III, and resistance to activated protein C have all been associated with hypercoagulable states. In asymptomatic people with heterozygous deficiencies of protein C, protein S, and resistance to activated protein C, the mean F_{1+2} concentration is significantly higher than age-matched controls [12–14]. Approximately one-third of patients have levels greater than the upper normal limit of normal controls (defined as the mean + 2 standard deviations) [12,13]. Fibrinopeptide A levels are elevated in approximately 20% of subjects [12,13]. Protein C activation as measured by the protein C activation peptide assay is reduced to about 50% of normal in patients with heterozygous protein C deficiency [12].

Asymptomatic patients with hereditary antithrombin III deficiency have levels of F_{1+2} and fibrinopeptide that are not significantly different from age-matched controls [2,13].

Coronary artery disease

Elevated levels of fibrinopeptide A are present soon after the onset of acute transmural myocardial infarction and then decrease over the next 24 h [15–17]. Using assays for F_{1+2} as well as fibrinopeptide A, coagulation activation has been measured in patients presenting with unstable angina or acute myocardial infarction and compared to those in control patients with stable angina or normal individuals matched for age and sex [18]. At the onset of acute coronary syndromes, patients with unstable angina or acute myocardial infarction have significantly elevated concentrations of both markers. At 6 months, patients who did not experience additional cardiac events including silent ischemia were reinvestigated and found to manifest increased concentrations of F_{1+2} with virtually normal plasma levels of fibrinopeptide A.

The initial elevations in patients presenting with unstable angina or myocardial infarction reflect the presence of ongoing intracoronary thrombosis. The normalization of fibrinopeptide values in most patients has been interpreted as showing that coagulation-system hyperactivity is restricted to the period during which the coronary thrombus is generated. However, the persistent elevations in F_{1+2} several months after the assay at acute presentation support the view that abnormalities of the hemostatic mechanism frequently occur in patients with acute coronary syndromes long after clinical stabilization [18]. The occurrence of a persistent hypercoagulable state in patients with unstable angina or myocardial infarction as well as stable angina is independent of the severity of coronary artery atherosclerosis. These findings raise the interesting possibility that increased activity of the hemostatic mechanism may predate the onset of acute coronary syndromes, and this hypothesis is currently under examination in a large prospective trial (Northwick Park Heart Study II).

Anticoagulants

In most patients with venous thromboembolism, treatment with adequate doses of heparin rapidly inhibits thrombin action upon fibrinogen and lowers elevated fibrinopeptide A levels into the normal range [9]. Prothrombin activation as measured by the F_{1+2} assay declines gradually over the first several days of heparin treatment, but can often remain higher than in healthy controls after even a week of treatment [19]. This may reflect the fact that factor Xa in the prothrombinase complex is relatively protected from inhibition by heparin bound to plasma antithrombin III [20].

Therapy with oral anticoagulants such as warfarin suppresses prothrombin activation

796

in vivo as measured by the F_{1+2} assay [21–23]. In patients with prior thrombotic histories and high F_{1+2} levels, stable anticoagulation at moderate intensity as reflected by International Normalized Ratios (INRs) of 2.5–3.5 produces 5- to 10-fold reductions in the extent of prothrombin activation [21]. It has also been shown that F_{1+2} values decrease in parallel with the intensity of warfarin therapy and INRs as low as 1.3–1.6 result on average in a 50% reduction in prothrombin activation from baseline levels [24]. It is important to note that these findings cannot currently be translated into clinical practice as the F_{1+2} level that confers antithrombotic protection has yet to be determined.

While F_{1+2} levels are often suppressed below normal in stably anticoagulated patients on oral agents, this has not been found for fibrinopeptide A. Plasma fibrinopeptide A concentrations increase above the normal range in patients with a prior history of myocardial infarction several weeks after the cessation of the drug [25].

Acknowledgements

Supported in part by National Institutes of Health Grant No. HL 33014.

References

1. Miller GJ, Bauer KA, Barzegar S et al. The effects of quality and timing of venipuncture on markers of blood coagulation in healthy middle-aged men. Thromb Haemost (in press).
2. Bauer KA, Barzegar S, Rosenberg RD. Thromb Res 1991;63:617–628.
3. Bauer KA, Kass BL, ten Cate H, Hawiger JJ, Rosenberg RD. Blood 1990;76:731–736.
4. Bauer KA, Kass BL, ten Cate H, Bednarek MA, Hawiger JJ, Rosenberg RD. Blood 1989;74:2007–2015.
5. Lau HK, Rosenberg JS, Beeler DL, Rosenberg RD. J Biol Chem 1979;254:8751–8761.
6. Teitel JM, Bauer KA, Lau HK, Rosenberg RD. Blood 1982;59:1086–1097.
7. Pelzer H, Schwart A, Stuber W. Thromb Haemost 1991;65:153–159.
8. Hursting MJ, Butman BT, Steiner JP et al. Clin Chem 1993;39:583–591.
9. Nossel HL, Yudelman I, Canfield RE et al. J Clin Invest 1974;54:43–53.
10. Bauer KA, Kass BL, Beeler DL, Rosenberg RD. J Clin Invest 1984;74:2033–2041.
11. Bauer KA, Mannucci PM, Gringeri A et al. Blood 1992;79:2039–2047.
12. Bauer KA, Broekmans AW, Bertina RM et al. Blood 1988;71:1418–1426.
13. Mannucci PM, Tripodi A, Bottasso B et al. Thromb Haemost 1992;67:200–202.
14. Martinelli I, Faioni EM, Monzani ML, Mannucci PM. Ann Int Med (in press).
15. van Hulsteijn H, Kolff J, Briet E, van der Laarse A, Bertina R. Am Heart J 1984;107:39–45.
16. Eisenberg P, Sherman LA, Schechtman K, Perez J, Sobel BE, Jaffee AS. Circulation 1985;71:912–918.
17. Mombelli G, Im Hof V, Haeberli A, Straub PW. Circulation 1984;69:684–689.
18. Merlini PA, Bauer KA, Oltrona L et al. Circulation 1994;90:61–68.
19. Estivals M, Pelzer H, Sie P, Pichon J, Boccalon H, Boneu B. Br J Haematol 1991;78:421–424.
20. Teitel JM, Rosenberg RD. J Clin Invest 1983;71:1383–1391.
21. Conway EM, Bauer KA, Barzegar S, Rosenberg RD. J Clin Invest 1987;80:1535–1544.
22. Mannucci PM, Bottasso B, Tripodi A. Thromb Haemost 1991;66:741.
23. Elias A, Bonfils S, Daoud-Elias M et al. Thromb Haemost 1993;69:302–305.
24. Millenson MM, Bauer KA, Kistler JP, Barzegar S, Tulin L, Rosenberg RD. Blood 1992;79:2034–2038.
25. Harenberg J, Haas R, Zimmermann R. Thromb Res 1983;29:627–633.

Triglycerides and the fibrinolytic system: in vitro regulation of the synthesis of plasminogen activator type 1 by triglyceride-rich lipoproteins in HepG2 cells

Elena Tremoli, Luigi Sironi, Marina Camera, Livia Prati, Cristina Banfi, Damiano Baldassarre and Luciana Mussoni

Enrica Grossi Paoletti Center, Institute of Pharmacological Sciences, University of Milan, Via Balzaretti 9, 20133 Milan, Italy

Abstract. Clinical studies have demonstrated an association between elevated triglyceride levels and reduced fibrinolytic activity. Moreover, the levels of tissue plasminogen activator inhibitor type 1 (PAI-1) have been reported to correlate directly with plasma triglycerides. We have investigated the in vitro effects of very low density lipoproteins (VLDL) on PAI-1 biosynthesis in human umbilical vein endothelial cells and in HepG2 cells. The results indicate that VLDL (10–100 µg protein/ml) incubated for 14–16 h with either endothelial or HepG2 cells are able to double the level of PAI-1 in conditioned medium of cells. In addition, studies in HepG2 cells indicate that the increase in PAI-1 biosynthesis induced by VLDL is consequent on an enhancement in the accumulation of mRNA for PAI-1. Specifically, VLDL increase the accumulation of the 2.2-kb PAI-1 mRNA, with only minor effects on the 3.2-kb PAI-1 mRNA transcript.

The fibrinolytic system is devoted to the removal of fibrin clots and it constitutes a physiological mechanism against the deposition of thrombi within the vascular tree [1]. Plasmin, the central enzyme of the fibrinolytic system, is generated from its precursor plasminogen through the action of tissue-type (t-PA) and urinary-type (U-PA) plasminogen activators [1]. The activity of plasminogen activators is regulated by several inhibitors, e.g., α-2-antiplasmin and plasminogen activator inhibitor type 1 (PAI-1) [2].

PAI-1 is a single-chain glycoprotein and a member of the serin protease inhibitor (SERPIN) family [2]. PAI-1 is synthesized by several cell types, e.g., endothelial and smooth muscle cells and liver cells [3], and its levels increase in response to acute-phase stimuli, which suggests that the liver is the major source of PAI-1.

Elevated levels of PAI-1 in blood have been reported in patients with venous thrombosis, and plasma PAI-1 levels have been proposed as having pathogenetic importance in arterial thrombosis [4]. Indeed, the elevated levels of PAI-1 reported in young patients who survive myocardial infarction have been shown to be an independent risk of recurrent infarction in the same individuals [5]. Moreover, PAI-1 levels are associated with the major features of Syndrome "X" and with hyperinsulinemia, the biological marker of insulin resistance, thus providing a plausible mechanism for the atherothrombotic occlusions associated with the syndrome [6].

An association between elevated triglyceride levels and alterations of the fibrinolytic system has been previously reported [7,8]. Specifically, it has been demonstrated that PAI-1 levels are elevated in plasma of hypertriglyceridemic patients, and a direct correlation between plasma triglycerides and PAI-1 has been documented in the general population [9,10].

To explore the link between plasma triglycerides and PAI-1 biosynthesis by competent cells, we have performed in vitro studies on endothelial cells and HepG2 cells.

Effect of very low density lipoproteins on PAI-1 biosynthesis by endothelial cells and HepG2 cells

To assess whether triglyceride-rich lipoproteins influenced PAI-1 biosynthesis by competent cells, we conducted studies in human umbilical vein endothelial cells. To this end, cells between the second and the fourth passages were incubated for 14–16 h in vitro with medium containing increasing concentrations (10–100 µg protein/ml) of very low density lipoproteins (VLDL) isolated from plasma of normolipidemic subjects and of patients with diagnosis of hypertriglyceridemia. At the end of the incubation, the supernatants were removed and the levels of PAI-1 were determined using a commercially available ELISA kit (F1-5 Monozyme, Copenhagen, Denmark). Levels of PAI-1 were significantly greater in conditioned medium of VLDL-treated cells than in cells incubated with medium alone (Table 1). The effect of VLDL on PAI-1 release was shown to be concentration-dependent and specific for this protein, because levels of tissue plasminogen activator determined in the same samples were not affected by VLDL treatment [9]. These data agree with those reported by Stiko Rahm et al. [11], who showed that VLDL increase PAI-1 antigen synthesis in endothelial cells because of binding of the lipoprotein to the apolipoprotein B/E (ApoB/E) receptor present on the cell surface [11].

In similar experiments, VLDL were incubated with HepG2 cells, a human hepatoma cell line that possesses most of the characteristics of human hepatocytes. The results indicate that VLDL also increase the release of PAI-1 by HepG2 cells. Specifically, at 100 µg protein/ml concentration VLDL doubled PAI-1 antigen levels in conditioned medium of HepG2 cells (Table 1). In parallel, VLDL increased PAI-1 activity in the conditioned medium of treated cells from 5.9 ± 1.0 to 10.8 ± 2.3 IU (n = 5). Interestingly, in HepG2 cells the enhancement of PAI-1 antigen release exerted by VLDL isolated from hypertriglyceridemic patients was more pronounced than that of VLDL isolated from normolipidemic donors [9].

Thus, VLDL are able to induce PAI-1 release by competent cells, possibly directly influencing synthesis of this inhibitor of the fibrinolytic system. In an attempt to elucidate the mechanisms by which VLDL influence the synthesis of PAI-1, further studies were performed in HepG2 cells.

Effect of VLDL on PAI-1 mRNA expression in HepG2 cells

The human PAI-1 gene encodes for two distinct mRNA species, one of 3.2 kb and one of 2.2 kb [12,13]. The two PAI-1 mRNAs have an identical coding region, but they differ

Table 1. Effect of VLDL (100 µg protein/ml) isolated from normolipidemic donors on PAI-1 release by human endothelial and HepG2 cells

	PAI-1 antigen (ng/ml)	Statistical significance
Endothelial cells		
Control cells (n = 7)	11.8 ± 1.6	
VLDL-treated cells (n = 7)	18.0 ± 1.6	$p < 0.01$
HepG2 cells		
Control cells (n = 7)	15.2 ± 1.6	
VLDL-treated cells (n = 7)	33.4 ± 4.6	$p < 0.01$

Cells were incubated with medium alone or with medium containing the lipoprotein fraction for 16 h. At the end of the incubation supernatants were removed and processed for PAI-1 determination. Values are the means ± SEM. Number of experiments in parentheses.

in the length of the 3' untranslated region that results from alternative polyadenylation [14]. The 3' end of the larger transcript contains an AU-rich sequence homologous to sequences implicated in mRNA stability; absence of this sequence in the small transcript suggests that the two mRNAs are specifically regulated by different agents [15].

In vitro studies have shown that PAI-1 synthesis is regulated by a variety of agents including glucocorticoids, cytokines, bacterial lipopolysaccharide and insulin. We have investigated the mechanism responsible for the increase in PAI-1 release induced by VLDL in HepG2 cells. In particular, we have evaluated whether the increase in PAI-1 release induced by VLDL in HepG2 cells was accompanied by concomitant accumulation of PAI-1 mRNA. Northern analysis showed that VLDL incubated for 16 h with HepG2 cells at the 100 µg protein/ml concentration doubled the accumulation of total PAI-1 mRNA (Fig. 1). Interestingly, VLDL increased specifically the accumulation of the shorter PAI-1 mRNA transcript (2.2 kb), with only minor effects on the 3.2-kb transcript (Fig. 1). The effect of VLDL on PAI-1 mRNA was shown to be specific for this lipoprotein subfraction, since neither high density nor low density lipoproteins (100 µg protein/ml) influenced PAI-1 mRNA accumulation.

So far, agents that induce PAI-1 mRNA accumulation have been shown to act at transcriptional (phorbol esters) and post-transcriptional (insulin) levels [15]. To assess whether VLDL influenced PAI-1 gene transcription, nuclear run-on experiments were performed. To this end, HepG2 cells were incubated for various times with 100 µg protein/ml VLDL isolated from normal donors. Isolation of nuclei, transcription run-on and isolation of nascent transcripts were performed according to Greenberg and Ziff with minor modification [16]. VLDL did not increase the transcription rate of the PAI-1 gene (data not shown), nor did it affect transcription of GAPDH gene, and no detectable signal

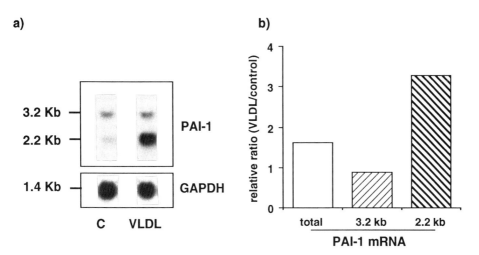

Fig. 1. Effect of VLDL on PAI-1 mRNA expression in HepG2 cells. Confluent HepG2 cells (3–4 × 10⁶ cells) were incubated for 16 h with serum-free medium in the absence or presence of VLDL. Total RNA was extracted and analyzed by Northern blotting (10 µg of RNA/lane) and hybridized with PAI-1 and GADPH probes. Relative amounts of PAI-1 mRNA were normalized against the corresponding glyceraldehyde-3-phosphate dehydrogenase (GAPDH) mRNA. Bands were quantitated by densitometric scanning. Panel a: Representative Northern blot of untreated (C) and HepG2 cells treated (VLDL) with 100 µg protein/ml of VLDL isolated from a normolipidemic donor. The top two bands are 3.2 and 2.2-kb PAI-1 mRNA and the bottom band is 1.4-kb GAPDH mRNA. Panel b: ratio between relative amounts of PAI-1 mRNA of VLDL-treated cells and control cells.

800

was given by the pBR322 used as negative control. These data tend to exclude the possibility that VLDL act at gene level and suggest that, possibly, these lipoproteins influence PAI-1 mRNA turnover, inducing PAI-1 mRNA stabilization. Stabilization of PAI-1 mRNA has been previously described for insulin, a known inducer of PAI-1 biosynthesis [17]. The effect of VLDL on PAI-1 mRNA accumulation, however, differs from that of insulin. Indeed, VLDL induce specific accumulation of the 2.2-kb PAI-1 mRNA transcript, whereas insulin has been shown to induce stabilization of the 3.2-kb PAI-1 mRNA transcript. Further studies will define the molecular mechanisms responsible for the described effect of VLDL on PAI-1 mRNA.

Conclusions

VLDL induce PAI-1 biosynthesis not only in endothelial cells but also in HepG2 cells. These data strongly support a role for this lipoprotein fraction in modulating PAI-1 antigen levels in in vivo conditions in which plasma triglycerides are elevated. Studies on the mechanisms by which VLDL exert such an effect indicate that this lipoprotein subfraction influences PAI-1 mRNA accumulation, with complex mechanism(s) involving the specific accumulation of the shorter PAI-1 mRNA transcript. Interestingly, the half-lives of the two PAI-1 mRNA transcripts are largely different, the longer transcript being more unstable with a half life of ~60 min. Thus, the specific effect of VLDL on the accumulation of the shorter PAI-1 mRNA transcript may have functional significance. Indeed, the accumulation of the 2.2-kb PAI-1 mRNA transcript induced by VLDL (half-life ~180 min) may result in more prolonged PAI-1 biosynthesis.

In conclusion, the data discussed above reveal that triglyceride-rich lipoproteins at concentrations that occur in plasma of normolipidemic subjects regulate PAI-1 biosynthesis. Further studies will define the molecular mechanism(s) responsible.

Acknowledgements

This work was supported by National Research Council targeted project "Prevention and Control of Disease Factors" (No 91.00257.PF41).

References

1. Bachman F. In: Colman RW, Hirsh J, Marder VJ, Salzman EW (eds) Haemostasis and Thrombosis: Basic Principles and Clinical Practice. Philadelphia: J.B. Lippincott Co., 1994;1592–1622.
2. Sprengers ED, Kluft C. Blood 1987;69:381–387.
3. Emeis JJ, Kooistra T. J Exp Med 1986;163:1260–1264.
4. Dawson S, Henney A. Atherosclerosis 1992;95:105–117.
5. Hamsten A, Walldius G, Szamosi A et al. Lancet 1987;2:3–9.
6. Juhan-Vague I, Alessi MC, Vague P. Diabetologia 1991;34:457–462.
7. Mehta J, Mehta P, Lawson D, Saldeen T. J Am Coll Cardiol 1987;9:263–268.
8. Aznar J, Estelles A, Tormo G, Sapena P, Tormo V, Blanch S, Espana S. Br Heart J 1988;59:535–541.
9. Mussoni L, Mannucci L, Sirtori M et al. Arterioscler Thromb 1991; 12:19–27.
10. Tremoli E, Mannucci L, Sironi L et al. In: Crepaldi G, Tiengo A, Manzato E (eds) Diabetes, Obesity and Hyperlipidemia: V. The Plurimetabolic Syndrome. Amsterdam: Excerpta Medica, 1993;291–298.
11. Stiko Rahm AB, Wiman A, Hamsten A, Nilsson J. Arteriosclerosis 1990;10:1067–1073.
12. Ginsburg DR, Zeheb AY, Rafferty UM et al. J Clin Invest 1986;78:1673–1680.
13. Ny T, Sawdey M, Lawrence D, Millan JM, Loskutoff DJ. Proc Natl Acad Sci USA 1986;83:6776–6780.
14. Loskutoff DJ, Linders M, Keijer J et al. Biochemistry 1987; 26:3763–3768.
15. Loskutoff DJ. Fibrinolysis 1991;5:197–206.
16. Greenberg M, Ziff B. Nature 1984;311:433–438.
17. Fattal PG, Schneider DJ, Sobel DJ, Billadello JJ. J Biol Chem 1992;267:12412–12415.

Risk of thrombosis and the prethrombotic state

G.J. Miller

MRC Epidemiology and Medical Care Unit, Medical College of St. Bartholomew's Hospital, Charterhouse Square, London EC1M 6BQ, UK

Abstract. The Northwick Park Heart Study (NPHS) revealed an increased risk of fatal coronary heart disease (CHD) in men with a high factor VII activity (VII$_c$), possibly indicative of a prethrombotic state. This suggestion is supported by preliminary analysis of data for subgroups of men entering a second prospective cardiovascular survey (NPHS-II), which has provided evidence for increased basal activity throughout the coagulation pathway when VII$_c$ is raised and in men at high risk of CHD according to conventional risk-factor status. A state characterized by increased subclinical thrombin generation and activity has also been revealed.

The first prospective cardiovascular survey designed to identify a prethrombotic state related to risk of CHD commenced in the late 1960s in Göteborg, Sweden [1]. This was soon followed by the Northwick Park Heart Study (NPHS) of hemostatic factors and CHD [2]. Extended follow-up to 16 years in NPHS has shown that a high fibrinogen concentration is predictive of both nonfatal and fatal forms of the disease [3], and that a high factor-VII coagulant activity (VII$_c$) is predictive of fatal CHD [4].

The Second Northwick Park Heart Study (NPHS II)

The main purpose of NPHS II is to provide a more detailed profile of the hemostatic system in men at high risk of CHD. Subsidiary aims are to describe the relations between markers of hemostatic activity at several steps in the coagulation pathway in healthy middle-aged men, the extent to which this activity varies with conventional risk-factor status, and the influence of genotype on hemostatic risk of CHD. Just under 3,000 men aged 50–61 years registered with nine participating medical practices and free of clinical CHD are eligible for recruitment. So far, about 9,500 person-years of follow-up have accrued. As the study progresses several substudies are being performed, two of which are reported here.

Markers of basal coagulant activity and risk factors for CHD

A first attempt to determine the interrelations between markers of basal coagulant activity was made in a sample of 263 men. Measurements were made of activated factor VII (VIIa) as described by Morrissey et al. [5], factor IX activation peptide [6] and factor X activation peptide [7] as markers of factor IXa and factor Xa generation, respectively, VIIc, factor VII antigen (VIIag), prothrombin fragment 1+2 (F_{1+2}) [8], fibrinopeptide A and fibrinogen concentration. Table 1 presents the mean values ± SD.

Table 2 is a correlation matrix of these hemostatic variables plus serum cholesterol, nonfasting triglyceride, and body mass index (weight/height^2). There is a cluster of statistically significant positive associations between the markers of basal coagulant activity to the upper left of the matrix; in particular, F_{1+2} is correlated with all other markers, including VII$_c$. A second cluster of significant positive associations exists between the established risk factors plasma fibrinogen, triglyceride, cholesterol and body

Table 1. Mean (SD) values of hemostatic characteristics relevant for cardiovascular disease in a subsample (n = 263) of the study population

Prothrombin fragment 1+2 (nM)	0.67 (0.29)
Fibrinopeptide A (nM)	1.35 (0.74)
Factor X activation peptide (pM)	121 (30)
Factor IX activation peptide (pM)	205 (59)
Activated factor VII (ng/ml)	2.62 (1.56)
Factor VII activity (% standard)	111 (26)
Factor VII antigen (% standard)	131 (38)
Fibrinogen (mg/dl)	258 (49)

mass index (BMI). Apart from a weak positive association between factor IX activation peptide and triglyceride concentrations, the main links between the indices of hemostatic activity and the established risk factors are VIIa, VII_c and VIIag. The absence of associations of VII_c (and VIIa) with factor IX activation peptide and factor X activation peptide concentrations, and the negative associations of VIIag with both of these peptides, were unexpected. However, a very recent and internally consistent analysis of data for 621 men in two participating practices on samples taken at baseline and after 1 year of follow-up has revealed highly significant positive correlations for both VII_c and VIIag with factor X activation peptide, and a positive association between VII_c and factor IX activation peptide (VIIa results are not yet available). Thus these preliminary findings confirm the increases of all measures of factor VII in the hyperlipidemic states, and are suggestive of increased basal activity throughout the coagulation pathway in the presence of elevated levels of VII_c and VIIa. Final conclusions must, however, await formal analysis of the complete data set.

The 263 men were given a risk score for CHD based upon their smoking status

Table 2. Correlation matrix of hemostatic variables, plasma lipids and body mass index in 263 middle-aged men

	F_{1+2}	FPA	Xp	IXp	VIIa	VII_c	VIIag	FIB	TRIG	CHOL	BMI
F_{1+2}		0.23	0.40	0.32	0.24	0.17					
FPA			0.15			0.15					
Xp				0.55			−0.20	−0.17			
IXp							−0.12		0.13		
VIIa						0.67	0.39			0.13	0.13
VII_c							0.50		0.22	0.32	0.18
VIIag								0.18	0.25	0.22	
FIB									0.16		0.16
TRIG										0.35	0.30
CHOL											

VII_c = factor VII coagulant activity; VIIa = activated factor VII; VIIag = factor VII antigen; IXp = factor IX activation peptide; Xp = factor X activation peptide; F_{1+2} = prothrombin fragment 1+2; FPA = fibrinopeptide A; FIB = fibrinogen; CHOL = serum cholesterol; TRIG = serum triglyceride; BMI = body mass index. Statistical significance of correlation coefficients: 0.12, p = 0.05; 0.16, p = 0.01; 0.21, p = 0.001.

Table 3. Classification of 1,732 men according to quintiles of the distribution of prothrombin fragment 1+2 (F_{1+2}) and fibrinopeptide A (FPA) at baseline and at 1 year

	Baseline		
	Lowest fifth of FPA Lowest fifth of F_{1+2}	Middle fifth of FPA Middle fifth of F_{1+2}	Highest fifth of FPA Highest fifth of F_{1+2}
1 Year			
Lowest fifth of FPA Lowest fifth of F_{1+2}	20 (3)[a]	50 (65)	1 (3)
Middle fifths of FPA Middle fifths of F_{1+2}	56 (69)	1456 (1429)	58 (72)
Highest fifth of FPA Highest fifth of F_{1+2}	0 (3)	71 (83)	20 (4)[a]

Note: The analysis is confined to men with satisfactory venepunctures on both occasions. Numbers expected by chance alone are given in parentheses. [a]$p < 0.0001$.

(current smoker or otherwise), a family history of CHD, BMI, serum cholesterol concentration, fibrinogen concentration and systolic blood pressure at baseline. The score was given by an equation derived from NPHS, where risk referred to fatal CHD. A significant trend was found to increasing levels of VII_c ($p = 0.0004$), VIIag ($p = 0.0001$) and F_{1+2} (borderline significance; $p = 0.06$) across the quintiles of the distribution of this risk score, together with a statistically nonsignificant trend to increasing levels of VIIa ($p = 0.09$). Factor IX and factor X activation peptide levels were unrelated to the risk score. These findings are preliminary evidence for increased hemostatic activity at the levels of factor VII and prothrombin in men at high risk of CHD.

Plasma F_{1+2} and FPA as markers of a hypercoagulable state

To search for evidence of a state in which thrombin generation and its activity were persistently or recurrently raised, we classified all men in NPHS-II according to their F_{1+2} and FPA concentrations both at baseline and at 1 year. Table 3 shows that so far, of 1,732 men with satisfactory venepunctures on both occasions, 20 had F_{1+2} and FPA concentrations consistently within the highest quintiles of the distributions, as compared with 4 expected by chance alone ($p < 0.0001$). Similarly, 20 had both concentrations consistently in the lowest quintiles of the distributions, as compared with 3 expected ($p < 0.0001$). This was good evidence for the existence of two states, one with persistent or recurrent increases in basal hemostatic activity and the other with persistent or recurrent decreases in activity. The true period prevalences of these conditions are likely to be considerably higher than 20/1732 (1.2%), and improved estimates will be obtained when the number of days of measurements is increased. For this reason, F_{1+2} and FPA are being measured in NPHS-II annually for 5 years.

Acknowledgements

The collaboration of Prof R.D. Rosenberg, Dr K.A. Bauer, Mr S. Barzegar, Dr J.H. Morrissey, Mrs Y. Stirling, Mr D. Howarth, Miss J.P. Mitchell, Miss A. Foley and Miss J.A. Cooper is gratefully acknowledged.

804

References

1. Wilhelmsen L, Svärdsudd K, Korsen-Bengtsen K, Larsson B, Welin L, Tibbin G. N Engl J Med 1984;311: 501–505.
2. Meade TW, North WRS, Chakrabarti R, Stirling Y, Haines AP, Thompson SG, Brozovic M. Lancet 1980;1: 1050–1054.
3. Meade TW, Ruddock V, Stirling Y, Chakrabarti R, Miller GJ. Lancet 1993;342:1076–1079.
4. Ruddock V, Meade TW. Quart J Med 1994;87:403–406.
5. Morrissey JH, Macik BG, Neuenschwander PF, Comp PC. Blood 1993;81:734–744.
6. Bauer KA, Kass BL, ten Cate H, Hawiger JJ, Rosenberg RD. Blood 1990;76:731–736.
7. Bauer KA, Kass BL, ten Cate H, Bednarek MA, Hawiger JJ, Rosenberg RD. Blood 1989;74:2007–2015.
8. Teitel JM, Bauer KA, Lau HK, Rosenberg RD. Blood 1982;59:1086–1097.

Gene–environment interactions and the risk of thrombosis

F.R. Green[1], A. Lane[1], A.E. Thomas[1], S. Dawson[1], G. Miller[2], A. Hamsten[3] and S.E. Humphries[1]

[1]Cardiovascular Genetics, Department of Medicine, University College London Medical School, Rayne Institute, London; [2]Epidemiology & Medical Care Unit, Medical College of St Bartholomew's Hospital, London, UK; and [3]King Gustaf V Research Institute, Karolinska Hospital, Stockholm, Sweden

Abstract. This paper describes an example of gene–environment interaction as an indicator of thrombosis risk. Common genetic variation in the factor VII (fVII) gene determines not only the plasma level of factor VII coagulant activity (fVIIc), but also the relationship of fVIIc with plasma triglyceride level in the population. This provides a possible explanation for the differential response of different individuals to their environment and may be of potential prognostic and/or therapeutic value.

It is becoming increasingly clear that genetic factors play a role in thrombotic disease, but it is equally clear that such factors cannot act in isolation from their environment. It is therefore the interaction of genetic and environmental factors that will determine an individual's risk of thrombosis. This paper describes one such gene–environment interaction: the interaction of plasma triglyceride level, a somewhat controversial risk factor for atherosclerotic disease, with the factor VII aminoacid-353 arginine/glutamine polymorphism (fVII Arg/Gln$_{353}$) [1–3] in determining plasma factor VII coagulant activity (fVIIc). Elevated fVIIc has recently been shown to be a strong predictor of fatal ischemic heart disease events presumably precipitated by thrombosis [4,5]. In the 16-year follow-up of the Northwick Park Heart Study (NPHS), the increase in risk associated with a fVIIc level one standard deviation above the mean was associated with a 45% increase in risk of fatal ischemic heart disease events overall and a 54% increase among men aged 55–64 years [4]. Epidemiological studies have also shown a positive correlation between plasma levels of fVIIc and of lipids, particularly very low density lipoproteins (VLDL) and chylomicrons and their triglyceride constituents (for example see [6,7]). It is now believed that it is the lipolysis of VLDL particles and chylomicrons by lipoprotein lipase (LPL) that generates a negatively charged lipid surface that promotes activation of fVII, with factor XII implicated as a possible intermediary [8]. The sustained fVII activation that accompanies chronic hypertriglyceridemia is thought to increase prothrombin $F_{1.2}$ generation which, in turn, causes increased fVII production from the liver [9]. Thus plasma triglyceride and fVII levels are intimately linked and may provide at least part of the explanation for the association between hypertriglyceridemia and ischemic heart disease.

The fVII Arg/Gln$_{353}$ polymorphism has been shown to be consistently associated with highly statistically significant differences in plasma fVIIc and fVII antigen (fVIIag) level in various population samples including both men and women, healthy individuals and myocardial infarction patients and different ethnic groups [1–3,10], around 20% of the population being heterozygous for this polymorphism [1]. Carriers of the Gln$_{353}$ allele have fVIIc and fVIIag levels consistently 20–25% below those of the majority who possess

---

Address for correspondence: F.R. Green, Cardiovascular Genetics, Department of Medicine, University College London Medical School, Rayne Institute, 5 University Street, London WC1E 6JJ, UK.

only the Arg_{353} allele. For example, in one recent study of healthy middle-aged men the 301 men homozygous for the Arg_{353} allele had a mean fVIIc 99% of standard (95% confidence interval 95–100%), whilst the 63 carriers of the Gln_{353} allele (57 heterozygotes and six Gln_{353} homozygotes) had a mean fVIIc of 78% (74–83%), $p < 0.01$ for the difference [3].

Computer modeling of the three-dimensional structure of fVII suggests that amino acid 353 is on the opposite side of the molecule to the active site (EGD Tuddenham, personal communication). The peripheral location of amino acid 353 suggests that the Arg-Gln_{353} substitution probably does not affect enzyme activity directly, although the active-site serine at position 344 is close in terms of the primary sequence. However, in view of the charge change ensuing from the substitution of the positively charged arginine by a neutral glutamine, it may influence interactions of fVII with lipid surfaces or cofactors, thereby affecting factor VII activation or activity indirectly. Since the Gln_{353} allele is associated with lower levels of both fVIIc and fVIIag, it seems likely that the amino acid substitution may also affect secretion or catabolism of the fVII molecule [2,3].

In addition to this strong and consistent association of fVII genotype with fVIIc and fVIIag levels, it became apparent that there was a difference in the relationship between fVIIc and triglyceride level according to Arg/Gln_{353} genotype. In one small study, the 25 Arg_{353} homozygotes showed the positive correlation as expected, $r = 0.23$, while the 24 Gln_{353} carriers showed no correlation, although the differences were not statistically significant [2]. This has since been confirmed in a larger study of healthy middle-aged men, with the 301 Arg_{353} homozygotes showing a positive correlation, $r = 0.14$ ($p < 0.0001$), whilst there was no correlation in the 63 Gln_{353} carriers $r = -0.15$ ($p = 0.8$) [3]. A similar trend was also observed, although less pronounced, for the relationship between plasma triglyceride and fVIIag levels. In this study, the difference in mean fVIIc and fVIIag level between men homozygous for the Arg_{353} allele and carriers for the Gln_{353} allele was much greater in the group whose triglyceride levels were in the highest tertile [3]. This interaction between fVII Arg/Gln_{353} genotype and plasma triglyceride level in determining fVIIc level was highly statistically significant ($p = 0.007$) [3] and suggests that at least some of the effect of genotype on fVIIc levels may be mediated through differential, allele-specific effects of plasma lipids on fVII activation and/or production. Although all of this is strong evidence for the polymorphism being functional, we are currently testing this assumption by expression of the two allelic fVII molecules in vitro followed by a comparison of their biosynthetic and kinetic properties, together with biochemical analysis of possible interactions with plasma lipoproteins.

The 20–25% reduction in fVIIc associated with heterozygosity for the Arg/Gln_{353} polymorphism is comparable with the one standard deviation (25% of standard in NPHS as a whole) increase in fVIIc associated with a 45% increase in risk of fatal ischemic heart disease found in NPHS [4]. This suggests that carriers of the Gln_{353} allele may be protected, to some extent, from arterial thrombotic disease. Conversely, those individuals who are both homozygous for the Arg_{353} allele and who have elevated plasma triglyceride levels may be at increased risk of disease: in the study of Humphries et al. [3], those particular individuals had fVIIc levels from 13 to 32% higher than the others, suggesting a 25–50% associated increase in risk of fatal thrombotic events.

The predictive value and clinical relevance of gene–environment interactions is only just beginning to be appreciated. Knowledge of an individual's genotype may be more predictive of an individual's future risk of arterial thrombosis than a single measurement of a plasma protein level, either because of intrinsic variability in the protein level that is controlled genetically or because of a genetically determined differential response to environmental factors. The polymorphism described above provides an example where individuals identified by simple genetic tests could be targeted for more frequent monitoring and given appropriate advice on lifestyle changes, such as adoption of a low-fat diet, which would reduce the possibility of their entering into a high-risk group. It also opens up the possibility of identifying individuals who would most benefit from drug therapy. Once the precise molecular mechanisms of the genetically determined variability and differential response to environment have been determined, simple tests can be developed that will have a considerable degree of accuracy and diagnostic potential.

Acknowledgements

The financial support of the British Heart Foundation is gratefully acknowledged.

References

1. Green F, Kelleher C, Wilkes H, Temple A, Meade T, Humphries SE. Arterioscler Thromb 1991;11:540–546.
2. Lane A, Cruickshank JK, Stewart J, Henderson A, Humphries S, Green F. Atherosclerosis 1992;94:43–50.
3. Humphries SE, Lane A, Green FR, Cooper J, Miller GJ. Atherosclerosis 1994;14:193–198.
4. Meade TW, Ruddock V, Stirling Y, Chakrabarti R, Miller GJ. Lancet 1993;342:1076–1079.
5. Heinrich J, Balleisen L, Schulte H, Assmann G, van de Loo J. Arterioscler Thromb 1994;14:54–59.
6. Miller GJ, Cruickshank JK, Ellis LJ, Thompson RL, Wilkes HC, Stirling Y, Mitropoulos KA, Allison JV, Fox TE, Walker AO. Atherosclerosis 1989;78:19–24.
7. Mitropoulos KA, Miller GJ, Reeves BEA, Wilkes HC, Cruickshank JK. Atherosclerosis 1989;76:203–208.
8. Mitropoulos KA, Miller GJ, Watts GF, Durrington PN. Atherosclerosis 1992;95:119–125.
9. Mitropoulos KA, Esnouf MP. Thromb Res 1990;57:541–545.
10. Green FR, Humphries SE. Bailliere's Clin Haematol 1994;7(3):675–692.

Antithrombotic agents in coronary artery disease

S. Janssens[1], F. Van de Werf[1], P. Zoldhelyi[1] and M. Verstraete[2]
[1]Cardiac Unit and [2]Center for Molecular and Vascular Biology, University Hospital Gasthuisberg, University of Leuven, 49 Herestraat, B-3000 Leuven, Belgium

Abstract. Acute ischemic coronary syndromes are caused by ruptured atherosclerotic plaques with partial or occlusive coronary artery thrombosis. Antithrombotic aspirin therapy reduces mortality in unstable angina and in myocardial infarction as adjunctive therapy during thrombolysis. Recently developed platelet glycoprotein IIb/IIIa receptor blockade improves infarct vessel patency and significantly reduces clinical restenosis following angioplasty. In contrast, extended heparin use after thrombolysis is no more effective than adequate antiplatelet therapy in maintaining vessel patency and in reducing residual thrombus, but hirudin, a direct antithrombin, may be advantageous. Finally, the role of prolonged oral anticoagulation in unstable angina and in secondary prevention after infarction needs further study.

The basic process of atherosclerosis and thrombosis in coronary artery disease

During the last decade new insights in the pathogenesis of coronary artery disease have led to changing concepts in the treatment of patients with acute and stable coronary syndromes. The understanding of the pathophysiology of coronary atherosclerosis, and the role of thrombosis in its acute complications, have spurred numerous clinical trials focusing on antiplatelet, anticoagulant, and thrombolytic drugs for this condition.

There is now ample evidence both in experimental animals and in patients that coronary artery disease involves a close relationship between atherosclerosis and thrombosis. Fatty streaks or focal collections of lipid-filled foam cells represent the first macroscopically recognizable atherosclerotic lesions and may develop into raised fibrous plaques, the archetypal atherosclerotic lesions that may ultimately lead to clinical coronary syndromes. Depending on size, cellular content, and local rheological conditions, these plaques may exhibit intramural hemorrhage and mural platelet aggregation as in unstable angina or may rupture with subsequent occlusive thrombosis as in myocardial infarction. We will briefly review here the role and potential benefits of antiplatelet agents and anticoagulants in both conditions.

Platelet inhibitors in coronary artery disease: aspirin

The major antithrombotic effect of aspirin is due to its irreversible inhibition of the platelet cyclo-oxygenase pathway which prevents formation of proaggregatory and vasoconstrictive thromboxane A2. A number of large clinical trials has unequivocally confirmed the beneficial effects of aspirin in patients with both unstable angina [1] and myocardial infarction. In the landmark ISIS-2 trial [2] on 17,187 patients with suspected myocardial infarction, aspirin conferred an impressive 21% mortality reduction at 5 weeks' follow-up. This was most probably related to a reduction of the early platelet-mediated reocclusion following endogenous or pharmacologic thrombolysis, as the drug also significantly reduced nonfatal reinfarction and stroke rates with no significant difference in major bleeding from placebo. The impressive early mortality benefit achieved with aspirin in patients with acute coronary syndromes persists for at least 4 years. Moreover, in fully anticoagulated patients undergoing percutaneous transluminal coronary angioplasty (PTCA) aspirin significantly reduced the incidence of acute thrombotic reocclusion and periprocedural infarction.

Aspirin has therefore become standard adjunctive therapy in acute myocardial infarction, and any new justifiable adjunctive agent tested after the results of ISIS-2 must improve on the efficacy of full-dose aspirin combined with thrombolysis. In addition, in stable coronary syndromes aspirin also has a favorable effect with regard to the secondary prevention of myocardial infarction and protection against cardiac mortality.

Thrombin inhibitors in coronary artery disease

Antithrombin III-dependent thrombin inhibitors: heparin

Because aspirin only interferes with the thromboxane A2-dependent pathway of platelet activation and not with platelet adhesion to exposed subendothelial structures or platelet aggregation induced by collagen or thrombin, it is not surprising that it cannot completely prevent platelet-mediated thrombosis in acute coronary syndromes. Indeed, thrombin-mediated thrombus formation is of primordial importance in the development of partial or complete coronary occlusion and justifies more aggressive antithrombotic therapy combining antiplatelets and thrombin inhibitors. Theoretically, this combination may offer better results in these conditions than either agent alone. In contrast to antiplatelets, antithrombin therapy by heparin as sole adjunctive treatment to thrombolysis in myocardial infarction has not been assessed in large, randomized clinical mortality trials. Only in a subgroup of approximately 400 patients in the SCATI trial [3] the effect of subcutaneous heparin after thrombolysis was studied in the absence of aspirin, and was associated with a gain in short-term survival.

The recent GUSTO trial provided important information on the risks and benefits of combined administration of heparin, aspirin, and thrombolytics in myocardial infarction patients [4]. Overall, no net clinical additional benefit was observed when heparin was added to streptokinase plus aspirin. In contrast, when added to accelerated-dose t-PA a significant reduction in combined death and nonfatal stroke rate was observed which was related to the more rapid and complete restoration of coronary flow through the infarct-related artery. The concept that earlier reperfusion leads to better survival is now generally accepted, as the reduction in early mortality in patients treated with t-PA plus heparin also accounted for more than 50% of the absolute reduction in overall mortality. Antithrombotics, therefore, should be given simultaneously or at least very early after thrombolysis, when thrombin burden is very high and patients are at risk of reocclusion. Extending the use of heparin in this setting more than 24 h after thrombolytic therapy was no more effective than adequate antiplatelet therapy alone in maintaining coronary artery patency and reducing the presence of residual thrombus [5]. Taken together, these findings suggest that the use of heparin to improve further the effect of full-dose aspirin plus thrombolysis seems limited to shorter-acting and more fibrin-specific agents like t-PA.

In unstable angina, treatment is ultimately directed towards keeping the coronary arteries open to prevent recurrence of ischemic episodes. This is most effectively achieved by combined antithrombotic therapy with aspirin and heparin [6], although the precise role of heparin in this setting is still debated, especially since withdrawal of the compound was shown to induce rebound thrombin generation. In any case, the combined treatment regimen of aspirin and heparin necessitates careful attention to the partial thromboplastin time as it probably increases the risk of bleeding.

Antithrombin III-independent thrombin inhibitors: hirudin

Antithrombotic treatment with heparin, however, suffers from several considerable drawbacks: it requires antithrombin III as a cofactor and the heparin–antithrombin III complex is unable to inactivate clot-bound and subendothelial matrix-bound thrombin. Moreover, heparin is inactivated by a variety of serum proteins and by platelet factor IV. These important deficiencies have spurred great interest for novel antithrombin III-independent treatment strategies. Hirudin, a potent and specific thrombin inhibitor, is the prototype of this class of inhibitors. It inhibits both clot-bound and matrix-bound thrombin, is well tolerated in humans, nonimmunogenic, and resistant to agents that degrade heparin. It has recently been studied in several pilot studies as adjunctive antithrombotic therapy in acute coronary syndromes with encouraging results.

The TIMI-5 trial [7] on 246 patients with myocardial infarction receiving t-PA plus aspirin, plus either heparin or hirudin at one of four ascending doses for 5 days, showed a significant angiographic benefit of hirudin compared with heparin at 18–36 h and a significant reduction in hospital death and reocclusion. No significant bleeding complications were reported. Similarly, in unstable angina patients hirudin treatment was associated with better angiographic improvement than with heparin [8]. Given the relatively small number of patients in both studies, GUSTO II was designed as a large, randomized, double-blind, multinational trial comparing heparin with a fixed dose of recombinant hirudin (0.6 mg/kg bolus followed by a 0.2 mg/kg/h infusion for 3–5 days) to test the hypothesis that direct antithrombin therapy is superior to heparin in both unstable angina and acute myocardial infarction. The trial was stopped prematurely after 2,564 patients were enrolled because of excess intracerebral bleeding in the hirudin group, which was significant in patients receiving thrombolytic therapy [9]. We have conducted a European GUSTO-2A Hemostasis substudy on these acute trial patients and found significantly higher aPTT 24-h-to-baseline ratios during hirudin infusion in patients receiving thrombolysis compared to nonlysis, unstable angina patients. After the bolus-induced early overshoot in plasma hirudin levels, no significant differences were observed from predicted pharmacokinetics in volunteers with stable coronary artery disease (P. Zoldhelyi, S. Janssens et al., unpublished observations). Excess bleeding may therefore have been related to the combined effects of thrombolysis, antiplatelet treatment, and hirudin concentrations previously found safe in pilot studies. Indeed, excessive prolongation of the activated thromboplastin time was predictive of hemorrhagic stroke in GUSTO IIa (C. Granger et al., unpublished observations). These findings once again underscore the compelling need for scrupulous monitoring of the activated thromboplastin time, especially in myocardial infarction patients receiving thrombolysis, and favor subsequent downward adjustment of the hirudin dose to avoid serious bleeding complications.

Monoclonal antibodies against platelet glycoprotein IIb/IIIa receptor

As aspirin is not able to block all the different pathways of platelet activation, several other platelet inhibitors have been characterized and studied in experimental models. Most interesting among these are antagonists to the receptor in the platelet membrane that binds fibrinogen and von Willebrand factor, the glycoprotein IIb/IIIa receptor. This integrin plays a pivotal role in the final common pathway of platelet aggregation and specific antibodies can thus theoretically produce substantial prolongation of the bleeding time. Pilot studies, however, have confirmed safety and efficacy of a chimeric monoclonal antibody (c7E3) and initial results so far in two large multicenter trials in refractory

811

unstable angina patients [10] and in high-risk angioplasty patients [11] are promising, although bleeding complications still remain a concern. The results indicate that effective glycoprotein IIb/IIIa blockade decreases major adverse effects in unstable angina, including myocardial infarction and need for urgent interventions, and that it has favorable long-term effects on clinical restenosis following PTCA, as indicated by the smaller number of major ischemic events and the reduced need for target vessel revascularization at 6-month follow-up.

Oral anticoagulants in coronary artery disease: warfarin

While the net benefit of antiplatelet therapy in acute coronary syndromes is clearly documented and has led to profound changes in patient management, that of anticoagulant therapy is less clear, partly because of the higher risk of bleeding. It has been suggested that unstable patients need prompt and aggressive antithrombotic therapy with platelet inhibition plus anticoagulation, which may offer more benefit than either agent alone. A recently conducted open-label, randomized multicenter trial on combination antithrombotic therapy in unstable rest angina and non-Q-wave infarction in nonprior aspirin users conveyed a significant clinical benefit over combination therapy with aspirin and oral warfarin (international normalized ratio 2−3), while bleeding complications were slightly more common [12]. Whether this aggressive medical treatment regimen also improves long-term survival compared with urgent revascularization deserves further study in prospective trials. So far the only indication of a long-term beneficial effect from oral anticoagulant therapy is the substantial risk reduction of cerebrovascular events and recurrent myocardial infarction in low-risk patients after myocardial infarction [13].

References

1. Lewis HD, Davis JW, Archibald DG, Steinke WE, Smitherman TC, Doherty JE, Schnaper HW, Le Winter MM, Linares E, Pouget JM, Sabharwal SC, Chesler E, DeMots H. N Engl J Med 1983;309:396−403.
2. ISIS-2 (Second International Study of Infarct Survival) Collaborative Group. Lancet 1988;2:349−360.
3. The SCATI Group. Lancet 1989;334:182−186.
4. The GUSTO (Global Utilization of Streptokinase in Occluded arteries) angiographic investigators. N Engl J Med 1993;329:1615−1622.
5. Thompson PL et al. for the Australian National Heart Foundation trial. Circulation 1991;83:1534−1542.
6. Theroux P, Ouimet H, McCans J, Latour J, Joly P, Levy G, Pelletier E, Juneau M, Stasisk J, Deguise P, Pelletier G, Rinzler D, Waters D. N Engl J Med 1988;319:1105−1111.
7. Canon CP et al. for the TIMI 5 investigators. J Am Coll Cardiol 1994;23:993−1003.
8. Topol E, Fuster V, Harrington RA, Califf RM, Kleiman NS, Kereiakes DJ, Cohen M, Chapekis A, Gold HK, Tannenbaum MA, Rao AK, Debowey D, Schwartz D, Henis M, Chesebro J. Circulation 1994;89:1557−1566.
9. The GUSTO IIa Investigators. A randomized trial of intravenous heparin versus recombinant hirudin for acute coronary syndromes. Circulation 1994 (in press).
10. Simoons ML, de Boer MJ, van den Brand M, van Miltenburg A, Hoorntje J, Heybndrickx G, van der Wieken R, De Bono D, Rutsch W, Schaibe T, Weisman H, Klootwijk P, Nijssen K, Stibbe J, de Feyter P for the European Cooperative Study Group. Circulation 1994;89:596−603.
11. Topol EJ, Califf RM, Weisman HF, Ellis SE, Tcheng JE, Worley S, Ivanhoe R, George BS, Fintel D, Weston M, Sigmon K, Anderson KM, Lee KL, Willerson JT on behalf of the EPIC investigators. Lancet 1994;343:881−886.
12. Cohen M et al. for the Antithrombotic Therapy in Acute Coronary Syndromes Research Group. Circulation 1994;89:81−88.
13. ASPECT (Anticoagulants in the Secondary Prevention of Events in Coronary Thrombosis) Research Group. Lancet 1994;343:499−503.

Hemodynamics, the endothelium and atherosclerosis

Robert M. Nerem

Bioengineering Center, Georgia Institute of Technology, Atlanta, GA 30332-0405, USA

Abstract. The hemodynamic environment within a blood vessel plays an important role in the regulation of the pathobiologic processes leading to atherosclerosis and the cellular participants in these events. The vascular endothelium, as the interface between flowing blood and the underlying vessel wall, is influenced directly by the local hemodynamics, with much of the evidence for this coming from cell-culture studies. However, the vascular smooth muscle cell and the monocyte-macrophage also reside in an environment influenced by the hemodynamics of the vascular system, and available information on this suggest a potentially important role of hemodynamics in the regulation of the biology of each of these cellular participants. The behavior of both the vascular smooth muscle cell and the monocyte-macrophage, in addition to direct mechanical effects, may be modulated by hemodynamic influences on vascular endothelium. Thus, the endothelial cell may be involved in the hemodynamic regulation of other cellular participants in atherogenesis.

Atherosclerosis is a disease resulting from a complex cascade of events involving the endogenous cells of the arterial wall, connective tissue elements, the formed elements of blood, and plasma proteins. The disease is one which is focal in nature, in particular in its early stages, and the interaction among the above-noted participants is modulated by the local environment.

An important ingredient locally is the mechanical environment in which the cellular participants reside. This environment is imposed by the hemodynamics of the vascular system, and although hemodynamics may not be directly causative of atherosclerosis, there is general acceptance that hemodynamics contributes to the local environment and as such can enhance the predilection for disease in localized regions (for a review see [1,2]). Some insight into how this takes place may be gained by recognizing the influence of hemodynamics on the mechanical environment in which some of the major cellular participants reside.

The vascular endothelium

The endothelial cell, once thought to be a passive, nonthrombogenic barrier, is actually a dynamic participant in vascular biology and pathobiology, capable of being activated and of synthesizing a variety of biologically active molecules. The endothelium is the interface between the flowing blood and the underlying vessel wall components, and thus it is strategically located to play a critical role in the genesis of atherosclerosis.

The vascular endothelium is acted on directly by the hemodynamic stress imposed by flowing blood. This stress has two components, one acting normal to the vessel surface, i.e., pressure, and the other acting tangentially to the surface, a frictional force per unit area, i.e., wall shear stress. The pressure is pulsatile, and the endothelium is both acted on directly by pressure and "rides" on a basement membrane being cyclically stretched. The endothelium is also acted on directly by the time-varying wall shear stress associated with the pulsatile flow. The result is that an endothelial cell resides in a very complicated mechanical environment.

The shear stress is orders of magnitude smaller than that due to pressure; however, research over the past decade has demonstrated the important influence of shear stress on vascular endothelial biology. Although there is some confirmation of this from in vivo animal studies [1], our knowledge of shear-stress effects on endothelial cells has largely been obtained through in vitro cell-culture studies [2]. These studies have indicated that shear stress alters cell morphology, cytoskeletal localization and cell mechanical properties, cell proliferation, and the synthesis and secretion of biologically active molecules [3]. Such studies have recently been extended to include the regulation by flow the expression of cell-adhesion molecules [4]. Cyclic stretch studies of cultured endothelial cells have also been conducted, and here again there is a wide range of effects. It thus is clear that the biology of the vascular endothelial cell is altered by the mechanical environment in which it resides. What is unclear are the signaling mechanisms involved in the recognition and transduction of a mechanical stimulus. A variety of studies are in progress, with a number of laboratories, including our own, focusing on intracellular calcium as a second messenger [5].

The vascular smooth muscle cell

The vascular smooth muscle cell (SMC) resides within the vessel wall, normally within the media, but invades the intima as part of the intimal thickening process. Though linked with atherosclerosis, this process may be viewed as an adaptation of the vessel wall to its hemodynamic environment. The role of the SMC in this involves intimal migration and proliferation, and associated with this may be a phenotypic change. SMCs also synthesize extracellular matrix components and other molecules, e.g., the monocyte-specific chemoattractant MCP-1. In the early stages of disease, the endothelium is intact; thus the hemodynamically imposed mechanical environment of the smooth muscle cell is one where it does not see flow directly, but experiences the cyclic stretching of the arterial wall as the pressure pulses. Cell-culture studies provide supporting evidence for a cyclic stretch effect on smooth-muscle-cell function [2,6]. There also is a school of thought which correlates the focal nature of the disease with enhanced internal wall stresses [7].

In addition, there is the possibility of an indirect hemodynamic effect. This is one where hemodynamic alterations in endothelial biology might be communicated to the underlying vessel wall through interactions between endothelial and smooth muscle cells. An example of this is NO, i.e., endothelial-derived relaxing factor, which is known to be regulated by shear stress [8,9]. In addition to its role as a vasodilator, NO has a number of other properties, including that of being an inhibitor of smooth muscle cell proliferation. It may act in some way as an antiatherogenic molecule [10], perhaps as an antioxidant.

The monocyte-macrophage

The monocyte-macrophage is a major participant in the disease process, a cell which experiences an interesting series of hemodynamic environments. The word "series" is used because in going from a monocyte being carried by flowing blood to a lipid-laden foam cell within the vessel wall, it experiences fundamentally different hemodynamically imposed environments. The first of these is the environment experienced as a blood cell circulating through the vascular system. Here it sees the same type of hemodynamic, mechanical environment as any other blood cell, e.g., the erythrocyte or the platelet. Once adherent to the endothelium, the monocyte resides in another type of hemodynamic environment, one like that of the endothelial cell. A third type of environment occurs

814

when the monocyte invades the intima and becomes a macrophage, residing now within the vessel wall and experiencing an environment similar to that of the smooth muscle cell, i.e., a cyclic stretch environment.

In an initial study, Matsumoto et al. [11] have demonstrated an influence of cyclic stretch on the morphology of both rat peritoneal macrophages and the monocyte-like cell line, the U937. Since the effects of a cell's mechanical environment seem to be wide-ranging, it is not surprising that there would be cyclic stretch effects on the monocyte-macrophage; however, here there is still much more to be learned.

The endothelium here also may play an important role, influencing the involvement of the monocyte-macrophage in the disease process. This is particularly true of the recruitment process, and there are in vivo observations of enhanced adherence of monocytes in Evans-blue-stained, lesion-prone regions of the pig aorta which are believed to represent low-shear regions. In cell-culture studies there is evidence of reduced adherence under conditions of high-shear flow as opposed to those corresponding to low shear [12]. Cell-culture studies also provide evidence of a differential regulation of adhesion-molecule mRNA expression by shear stress. In our own research, confluent human umbilical vein endothelial monolayers, preconditioned for 24 h with a shear stress of 5 dynes/cm^2 and then incubated with the cytokine IL-1β, have been shown to exhibit an inhibition of VCAM-1 expression as compared to nonpreconditioned, statically cultured EC [13]. Flow cytometry verified that this decrease in IL-1β-induced VCAM-1 message is coupled with a reduction in cell-surface expression [14]. Furthermore, these effects of shear stress are strikingly similar to those of the thiol antioxidant pyrrolidine dithiocarbamate.

Hemodynamics and lesion initiation

The genesis of atherosclerosis is believed, at least by many, to start with the focal infiltration of LDL into the vessel wall, where it becomes trapped in the extracellular matrix of the subendothelial space [1]. In general, these focal regions exhibit a thickened intima, one which may not be due to the atherogenic process itself but rather the result of an earlier adaptation to the local hemodynamic environment, thus predisposing that region to the genesis of the disease. Also, this infiltration could be modulated by the hemodynamic environment through its influence on endothelial permeability.

Important to this initial phase is the modification of LDL, e.g., its oxidation. As noted previously, there is an important influence of hemodynamics on endothelial biology, and it seems reasonable to believe that, as part of this, the oxidative environment of the endothelial cell and related processes might be modulated by the local hemodynamic events. An aspect of this discussed previously could be the role of hemodynamic shear stress in regulating the secretion of nitric oxide, there being an inhibition of NO secretion in low-shear regions.

Whatever the mechanism, the result is the enhanced recruitment of blood monocytes in these regions. Whether this is due to an effect of the oxidatively modified LDL on the endothelium or is associated with a direct influence of hemodynamics on monocyte recruitment and adherence is not known. As already noted, however, cell-culture studies have demonstrated greater adherence of monocytes in low-shear regions than high-shear regions and the differential regulation of cell-adhesion molecules. Once adherent, monocytes migrate to within the vessel wall and differentiate into monocyte-macrophages. There are various cytokines which could play an important role in such processes, and these in turn could be modulated by hemodynamic events. Furthermore, macrophage products can additionally modify LDL into a highly oxidized form, which is then recognized by the macrophage scavenger receptor, resulting in foam-cell formation. Ultimately, the foam cells become overwhelmed by the lipid, which itself is cytotoxic, and there then results a significant amount of extracellular lipid. In this series of events it is not unreasonable to believe that there might be additional hemodynamic influences.

In the recruitment into the intima of monocytes, chemoattractants are believed to play an important role. One of these chemoattractants is the monocyte chemotactic protein MCP-1, which is synthesized and secreted by both smooth muscle and endothelial cells. The generation of MCP-1 by endothelial cells has been demonstrated in cell-culture studies to be hemodynamically regulated [15].

An important feature of atherosclerosis is the frequent co-localization of lesion development and regions of adaptive intimal thickening. However, advanced lesions are not confined to regions of adaptive intimal thickness, and in the absence of any such adaptation, intimal SMCs may still be present, having migrated from the media, through the internal elastic lamina, and into the intima. The hemodynamic regulation of smooth muscle cell synthesis of extracellular matrix proteins may be important, and the modification of smooth muscle cell connective tissue protein synthesis due to cyclic stretch has been demonstrated in cell-culture experiments as discussed earlier.

Although the endothelium is intact through these early events, as the disease progresses it will be disrupted, at which time platelet adherence occurs. Through these events, as well as others, the fatty streak begins its progression into a more advanced lesion. In all of this there are undoubtedly various hemodynamic influences, where the effects of hemodynamics may be very different in the later disease stages from those associated with the initiation of the disease.

Discussion

Finally, there are two points to be emphasized. First is the fact that there is little information on how the hemodynamic environment regulates the specific events involved in the atherogenic process. Without an understanding of the role of the hemodynamic environment, there cannot be a total understanding of the disease process.

Secondly, there has been considerable focus on the role of wall shear stress in atherosclerosis. As already noted, cell-culture studies have clearly demonstrated shear-stress effects on endothelial monolayers. There also is in vivo evidence of the importance of wall shear stress in atherosclerosis. However, data from the latter represent largely "guilt by association", and thus whether it is truly low shear which causes an enhanced predilection for disease occurrence, or some other feature of these low-shear regions, e.g., oscillatory shear or a prolonged residence time, is not known.

Even so, much progress has been made in understanding the role of hemodynamics, not only in vascular biology, but also in atherosclerosis. As a result, there is little doubt about the importance of hemodynamics as an influence on pathobiologic processes. However, it must be emphasized that it is not just wall shear stress which is important; it is the influence of the total mechanical environment, one imposed by the hemodynamics of the vascular system, on the structure and function (or dysfunction) of the various participating cells which must be understood as part of any further advancement in our knowledge of atherosclerosis.

Acknowledgements

This work was supported by National Institutes of Health Grants PO1 HL-48667 and NSF Grant BCS-9111761 and BES-9412010. The author thanks R.W. Alexander, D. Harrison,

D.N. Ku, T. Matsumoto, R. Medford, C.J. Schwartz, E.A. Sprague, W.R. Taylor, and T.M. Wick for the many discussions which have led to the ideas reflected in this paper and for their participation as collaborators in the study of this subject.

References

1. Schwartz CJ, Valente AJ, Sprague EA, Kelley JL, Nerem RM. Clin Cardiol 1991;14:I-1—16.
2. Nerem RM. ASME J Biomech Eng 1992;114:274—282.
3. Nerem RM. ASME J Biomech Eng 1993;11:510—514.
4. Nagel T, Resnick N, Atkinson WJ, Dewey CF Jr, Gimbrone MA Jr. J Clin Invest 1994;94:885—891.
5. Helmlinger G, Berk BC, Nerem RM. In: Liepsch D (ed) Biofluid Mechanics, Proceedings of 3rd International Symposium. Düsseldorf: VDI-Verlag GmbH 1994;509—521.
6. Grande JP, Glagov S, Bates SR, Horwitz AL, Mathews MB. Arteriosclerosis 1989;9:446—452.
7. Thubrikar MJ, Baker JW, Stanton PN. Arteriosclerosis 1988;8:410—420.
8. Taylor WR, Harrison DG, Nerem RM, Peterson TE, Alexander RW. FASEB J 1991;56(6):A1727 (abstract).
9. Nishida K, Harrison DG, Navas JP, Fisher AA, Dockery SP, Uematsu M, Nerem RM, Alexander RW, Murphy TJ. J Clin Invest 1992;90:2092—2099.
10. Cooke JP. Arterioscler Thromb 1994;14:653—654.
11. Matsumoto T, Delafontaine P, Schnetzer KJ, Tong BC, Nerem RM. In: Langrana NA, Friedman MH, Grood ES (eds) Bioengineering Conference. New York: ASME 1993;24:123—126.
12. Sprague EA, Levesque MJ, Rozek MM, Schwartz CJ, Nerem RM. In: Goldstein SA (ed) Advances in Bioengineering. New York: ASME 1990;17:357—360.
13. Varner SE, Chappell D, Offerman MK, Nerem RM, Alexander RW, Medford RM. Laminar shear stress regulates VCAM-1 gene expression and transcription in human vascular endothelial cells. Ann Biomed Eng (Abstract) (in press).
14. Chappell DC, Nerem RM, Alexander RW. Adhesion molecule expression on vascular endothelial cells in response to flow. Ann Biomed Eng (Abstract) (in press).
15. Shyy Y-J, Hsieh H-J, Usami S, Chien S. Proc Natl Acad Sci 1994:91:4678—4682.

Hemodynamics, modeling of the artery wall and atherosclerosis

Seymour Glagov[1], Hisham S. Bassiouny[1], Christopher K. Zarins[2] and Don P. Giddens[3]

[1]*Department of Pathology, University of Chicago, Illinois;* [2]*Stanford University, Palo Alto, California; and* [3]*Johns Hopkins University, Baltimore, Maryland, USA*

Abstract. Artery size, structure and composition correspond to imposed levels of wall shear and tensile stress. Adaptive modeling changes continue in the presence of atherogenesis and account for localizing as well as some of the structural compensatory features noted in atherosclerotic plaques. Resistance or susceptibility of lesions to the development of symptomatic disruptions may depend on structural features and strains induced by mechanical stresses as well as upon metabolic determinants of plaque progression. Interventional plaque disruptions also induce proliferative adaptive reactions which may proceed to restenosis if baseline levels of wall stress are not restored.

Modeling of the artery wall in response to tension and flow

Arteries develop, grow and subsequently adapt to changes in flow or wall tension in such a manner as to establish or restore baseline values of tensile stress and wall shear stress. The relevant tissue processes result in modifications of both dimension and composition. Evidence has accrued that hemodynamic and tensile forces are also determinants of atherosclerotic plaque localization, composition and organization and may play a role in lesion complication. In the present communication, we review some of the principal features of these adaptive modeling responses.

Artery wall tension is considered mainly as the reaction to the tangential force acting in the direction of the vessel circumference. It is estimated by applying the law of Laplace and is proportional to the product of distending pressure and radius. Burton, in a review published in 1954 [1], called attention to the relationship between wall thickness and artery radius. Large arteries have relatively thick walls while small arteries have relatively thin walls, although mean pressure may be the same at both levels. He also proposed that the major matrix fibers, i.e., collagen and elastin, differed in relative proportion depending on artery size, thereby determining the particular physical properties of the wall at each level. The component smooth muscle cells were seen as modifiers of the mechanical properties by virtue of their contractile properties. Both the relative proportion of cells to fibers and the likelihood that matrix fiber orientation could be modified by smooth muscle cell contraction were considered to be the major contributing factors.

Roach and Burton [2] treated arteries with collagenase or elastase and subjected them to increasing stress and showed that elastin and collagen contributed contrasting mechanical properties to the artery wall. The combination in the intact artery wall accounted for the shape of the pressure–volume curves. Subsequent morphologic studies of the mammalian aorta [3] confirmed this concept and showed that in the range between nondistention and diastolic distending pressure, as diameter increased markedly and wall thickness diminished, aortic elastic fibers straightened progressively and stretched.

Address for correspondence: Dr S. Glagov MD, Department of Pathology, University of Chicago, 5841 S. Maryland Ave., Chicago, IL 60637, USA.

Collagen fibers were progressively oriented circumferentially and once taut, prevented further diameter increase at pressures beyond systolic levels. Since vessels grow and are maintained under conditions corresponding to the interval between diastolic and systolic pressure, vessel wall organization and component configuration need to be evaluated under these conditions. Studies of suitable preparations of mammalian aortas indicated that the transmural structure consists of uniform layers proportional in number to radius and therefore to circumferential tension [4]. The layers can be further resolved into units comprised of fascicles of similarly oriented smooth muscle cells surrounded by a common basal lamina and fine collagen fibers and by similarly oriented elastic fibers [5]. Intervening collagen fiber bundles tend to be located between adjacent elastic fiber groups. The musculoelastic fascicles are oriented in the presumed direction of tensile stress. These structural features suggest a role for wall tension as inducer and modulator of vessel wall structure and composition. Support for such relationships was forthcoming from experiments relating increasing wall tension during early growth to matrix fiber accumulation [6] and to matrix biosynthesis in response to in vitro cyclic stretching of arterial smooth muscle cells [7].

Wall shear stress is proportional to volume flow and is inversely proportional to the third power of vessel radius. Computations have indicated that the lumen surface of most mammalian arteries is normally subjected to a mean wall shear stress of about 15 dynes/cm^2 [8]. Animal experiments as well as observations of human vessels suggested to earlier investigators such as Rodbard [9] that volume flow was a determinant of vessel diameter. Recent experimental manipulations indicate that decreased wall shear stress result in reduction in diameter [10] while increases in flow results in artery enlargement [8]. These changes stabilize when normal baseline wall shear stress is restored. An increase in radius under these conditions results in an increase in wall tension and in corresponding modifications of artery wall structure and composition. During growth, vessel adaptation to normal or abnormal changes in flow or tension appears to be confined to the media. Later adaptations may include participation of the intima such that intimal thickening may narrow the lumen to increase wall shear stress and/or thicken the wall to decrease mural tensile stress, tending to restore these stresses to baseline values. Thus, the vessel wall may be considered to undergo a self-limiting adaptive-reactive modeling tissue response designed to maintain or establish a stable state with respect to wall shear and tensile stress.

Mechanical determinants of modeling in atherogenesis

Mechanical factors related to shear stress and/or wall tension are also determinants of plaque location, composition, organization and complication during atherogenesis.

Plaque localization. Intimal thickening in human arteries occurs selectively in regions of relatively low wall shear stress and flow separation and where shear stress reverses in direction during the cardiac cycle [11]. Much of the data which relates intimal thickening to low wall shear stress is based on observations of the localization of intimal thickening, both atherosclerotic and nonatherosclerotic, in human arteries and on flow-field studies in corresponding models. The position of the regions at highest risk for intimal thickening is determined mainly by geometric configuration. Thus, intimal reactive effects are observed on the inlet side of aortic branch ostia [12], the dorsal aspect of the aorta or the region opposite the flow divider at the carotid bifurcation [11]. As a result of reduced wall shear and cyclic flow reversal these susceptible regions are subject to delayed clearance of circulating particles, which suggests that these regions are likely to have relatively prolonged exposure to circulating atherogenic agents compared to regions of high, unidirectional flow [13]. Increased particle residence time has indeed been demonstrated in these locations in experimental models. The co-localization of nonatherosclerotic intimal thickening and atherosclerosis suggests that the nonatherosclerotic form, though not necessarily an inevitable or necessary precursor of atherosclerosis, favors plaque deposition possibly by delaying or inhibiting transmural clearance or by direct capture of infiltrating lipids by intimal matrix elements [14].

Plaque modeling during plaque evolution. During early phases of plaque enlargement, plaque components become stratified [15]. The lipid core is segregated to a zone between outer and inner fibrocellular regions. The outer intimal region is often associated with atrophy of the underlying media and outward bulging of the wall. At early stages, lipid core material and foam cells may be associated with erosion of the underlying media. With continued lesion progression, several presumably defensive features become apparent which effectively act to preserve stable and adequate flow. The innermost subendothelial region of fibrocellular tissue differentiates into a layered, more or less well-defined zone or fibrous cap with morphologic features recalling the structure of the media and often of a thickness comparable to the uninvolved opposite media wall. A new internal elastin lamina frequently forms beneath the structurally intact endothelium. Unless there is plaque disruption, ulceration or thrombosis, the lumen remains very nearly circular despite the outward bulging which may render the outer vessel contour oval [16]. These features indicate that the physical forces which determine vessel lumen size and shape and artery wall composition and structure are probably operative during plaque formation. Thus, tissue modeling responses are elicited which tend to preserve a lumen configuration consistent with stable flow and to sequester the lesion away from the lumen. The outward bulging is associated with artery enlargement so that lumen cross-sectional area may remain close to normal even in the presence of relatively large plaques [17]. These modeling and organizing responses therefore have the effect of preserving or approximating normal vessel function in the face of evolving disease.

Plaque disruption of function. Despite these adaptive, defensive modeling reactions, plaques may progress to cause stenosis and obstruction to flow, to modify artery wall structure and artery wall reactivity, and to predispose to plaque disruption. Although large and stenosing plaques tend to be both complex and complicated, recent considerations have placed new emphasis on plaque fragility and have emphasized that plaques not associated with severe degrees of stenosis may nevertheless be prone to disruption, thrombus formation and significant clinical events [18,19]. In these instances, the adaptive modeling processes have presumably been inadequate or blunted. The interaction among plaque composition, mechanical stresses, and the elicited remodeling responses which determine plaque stability or vulnerability to disruption may be related to rapidity of plaque formation, changing prevalence of various clinical risk factors and individual tissue reactivity. Detailed studies of plaque composition and breakdown as well as the distribution of strains corresponding to long-acting forces as well as to sudden changes in shear and/or tensile stresses are indicated. Mechanical properties of plaques of various composition are under investigation in many laboratories.

Intimal hyperplasia and restenosis. Methods for direct interventions on stenosing plaques

820

are now in widespread use. These include angioplasty, atherectomy, application of laser energy, drilling and the deployment of stents. Although reopening of stenoses is often achieved by these maneuvers, reocclusion often occurs after several months, appearing as a characteristic proliferative response termed intimal hyperplasia or neointima formation. A good deal of attention has been focused on inhibiting the proliferative response by the administration of pharmacological agents which have been shown to inhibit the healing proliferative response after experimental balloon injury. None of these strategies as yet has had a significant effect on the incidence of restenosis. The balloon injury denudation model has produced new knowledge concerning mediators of smooth muscle cell migration and proliferation, but it does not reproduce conditions prevailing at angioplasty or atherectomy sites and has not provided information of preventive or therapeutic value. Although direct mechanical interventions elicit a proliferative healing response, these disruptions also result in redistributions of wall shear and tensile stresses and elicit modeling responses in intima, media, and plaque.

It is reasonable to suppose that if local levels of wall shear stress and tensile stress are prevented from reaching or re-establishing normal baseline stress conditions, the intimal proliferative reaction would be expected to continue and result in restenosis [20]. Should normal baseline wall shear stress conditions be restored before the reactive intimal hyperplastic process results in occlusion, the reaction would be expected to stop and stabilize, with maintenance of a patent lumen. The initial predominantly proliferative intimal hyperplasia phase would then differentiate to form a layered intimal fibrocellular hypertrophic response, most probably modulated by local tensile-stress conditions similar to those which previously determined the formation and structure of the fibrous cap. Factors preventing stabilization and persistence of a patent lumen would therefore include the presence or creation of irreducible deformities as well as the persistence of low-flow states due to proximal or distal atherosclerotic stenoses or to reduced cardiac output. Measurements of flow and lesion configuration before and periodically after intervention are likely to provide insights into the critical mechanical determinants of the modeling reactions underlying restenosis or persistence of patency.

Since plaques include several cell types and are living tissues, it should not be surprising that modeling reactions are prominent features of plaque development. Since exposure to mechanical stress underlies artery wall and morphogenesis at all stages one should not be surprised that the modeling reactions of plaques are also closely linked to the mechanical stimuli associated with wall shear and tension. The natural history of atherosclerosis and its complications will not be fully understood until the effects of mechanical forces on artery wall and plaque organization and adaptation are elucidated.

References

1. Burton AC. Physiol Rev 1954;34:619–642.
2. Roach M, Burton AC. Can J Biochem Physiol 1957;35:681–690.
3. Wolinsky H, Glagov S. Circ Res 1964;14:400–413.
4. Wolinsky H, Glagov S. Circ Res 1967;20:99–111.
5. Clark JM, Glagov S. Arteriosclerosis 1985;5:19–34.
6. Leung DYM, Glagov S, Mathews MB. Circ Res 1977;41:316–323.
7. Leung DYM, Glagov S, Mathews MB. Science 1976;191:475–477.
8. Zarins CK, Zatina MA, Giddens DP, Ku DN, Glagov S. J Vasc Surg 1987;5:413–420.
9. Rodbard S. Perspect Biol Med 1970;13:507–527.
10. Langille BL, Bendeck MP, Keeley FW. Am J Physiol 1989;256:H931–H939.
11. Glagov S, Zarins CK, Giddens DP, Ku DN. Arch Path Lab Med 1988;112:1018–1031.
12. Caro CG, Fitzgerald JM, Schroter RC. Proc Roy Soc Lond B 1971;117:109–159.

13. Ku DN, Giddens DP. Arteriosclerosis 1983;3:31—39.
14. Frank JS, Fogelman AM. J Lipid Res 1989;30:967—978.
15. Stary HC, Chandler AB, Glagov S, Guyton JR, Insull W Jr, Rosenfeld ME, Schaffer SA, Schwartz CJ, Wagner WD, Wissler RW. Circulation 1994;89:2462—2478.
16. Glagov S, Zarins CK. In: Bond MG, Insull W, Glagov S, Chandler AB, Cornhill F (eds) Clinical Diagnosis of Atherosclerosis. New York: Springer-Verlag, 1983;11—35.
17. Glagov S, Weisenberg E, Zarins CK, Stankunavicius R, Kolettis G. N Engl J Med 1987;316:1371—1375.
18. Fuster V, Badimon L, Badimon JJ, Chesebro JH. N Engl J Med 1992;326:242—249,310—317.
19. Glagov S, Zarins CK, Giddens DP, Ku DN. In: Yoshida Y, Yamaguchi T, Caro CG, Glagov S, Nerem RM (eds) Role of Blood Flow in Atherogenesis. New York: Springer-Verlag, 1988;3—10.
20. Glagov S. Circulation 1994;89:2888—2891.

822

Mechanical stimulation affects phenotype features of vascular smooth muscle cells

Vladimir P. Shirinsky[1], Konstantin G. Birukov[1], Olga V. Stepanova[1], Vsevolod A. Tkachuk[1], Alfred W.A. Hahn[2] and Terese J. Resink[2]

[1]Laboratory of Molecular Endocrinology, Cardiology Research Center of the Russian Academy of Medical Sciences, Moscow 121552, Russia; and [2]Department of Research, Basel University Hospitals, Basel CH-4031, Switzerland

Abstract. We investigated the effect of mechanical stimulation on proliferation of rabbit aortic smooth muscle cells and expression of contractile phenotype protein markers h-caldesmon, calponin and smooth muscle myosin. Cyclic stretch was applied using a Flexercell Strain unit. Strain potentiated proliferation in serum-activated cells but not in quiescent cultures. It induced a reversible accumulation of h-caldesmon but not of calponin or myosin in the cells, and this effect was inhibited by Gd^{3+}. Stretch-induced h-caldesmon expression was more prominent in cells grown on laminin than on collagen type I and IV. Our findings suggest that cyclic mechanical stimulation contributes to the restoration and maintenance of the features of differentiated vascular smooth muscle cell phenotype.

Periodic mechanical stretching is a naturally occurring stimulus affecting all types of muscles in the organism. Heart and arteries are perhaps the most prominent examples where strain is developed regularly at comparatively high frequencies throughout the lifetime of muscle cells. It might therefore be expected that mechanical stimulation, like humoral and neural influences, is an essential determinant of myocyte biology. Indeed, stretching of cardiomyocytes was shown to induce a hypertrophic response manifested by increased expression of c-fos gene, skeletal alpha-actin and atrial natriuretic factor [1]. However, in contrast to cardiac cells the evidence collected so far with respect to smooth muscle cells (SMC) shows that stretching favors secretion of platelet-derived growth factor (PDGF) [2] and the proliferation [2] and production of extracellular matrix components [3], i.e., it promotes features opposite to differentiated quiescent phenotype which these cells maintain in the vessel wall. Results presented in this study may help to overcome this discrepancy as they show that stretching of profoundly modulated SMC selectively induces accumulation of h-caldesmon, a regulatory protein peculiar to differentiated smooth muscle [4].

Materials and Methods

Enzymes for SMC isolation were purchased from Boehringer Mannheim AG (Switzerland). Tissue culture reagents were obtained from GIBCO (Basel, Switzerland) and tissue culture plasticware was purchased from Costar (Tecnomara AG, Switzerland). Other reagents were of analytical grade. Rabbit polyclonal affinity-purified antibodies against

Address for correspondence: Vladimir P. Shirinsky, Cardiology Research Center, 3rd Cherepkovskaya St. 15A, Moscow 121552, Russia. Tel.: +7-95-414-6713; Fax: +7-95-414-6719; Email: shirinsk@cardio.med.msu.su.

chicken gizzard caldesmon, calponin, and myosin have been characterized previously [5—7].

Sodium dodecyl sulfate polyacrylamide gel electrophoresis (SDS-PAGE), quantitative immunoblotting and SMC isolation from rabbit aorta were accomplished as described in [8]. Cells were cultured in minimal essential medium (MEM) supplemented with 10% fetal calf serum (FCS), 20 mM L-glutamine, 10 mM TES-NaOH/HEPES-NaOH (pH 7.3), 100 U/ml penicillin, 100 µg/ml streptomycin in a humidified atmosphere (37°C; 5% CO_2). Primary SMC and subcultures between passages 2 to 5 were used. Cell counting was accomplished using an electronic counter (Coulter, Instrumenten-Gesellschaft AG, Basel, Switzerland).

SMC were seeded onto Flex culture plates (Flexcell Corp., McKeesport, USA) coated with collagen type I, if not specified otherwise, in MEM supplemented with FCS at an initial density of $2—8 \times 10^4$ cells/cm^2 and subjected to cyclic stretch (30 cycles/min; 15% elongation at the periphery of the culture plate bottom) for up to 8 days using a computerized Flexercell strain unit. At the end of the stretch session SMC were counted and samples for SDS-PAGE and immunoblotting were prepared.

Statistical analysis was carried out by unpaired Student's t test and a value of $p < 0.05$ was considered to be statistically significant. The data points in Figs. 1—4 represent mean ± SD of data obtained in 3—4 separate experiments, in each of which quadruplicate determinations were made.

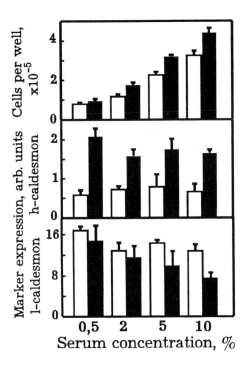

Fig. 1. Effect of CS on SMC proliferation and caldesmon isoform expression at various FCS concentrations. SMCs were cultured for 6 days in the presence of indicated concentrations of FCS without (open bars) or with (solid bars) application of CS.

824

Results and Discussion

Application of CS increases the proliferation rate of SMC grown at different FCS concentrations by about 30% (Fig. 1, top panel). These results agree with the findings of Wilson et al. [2], who demonstrated that stretching stimulates expression and secretion of PDGF by SMC and thus promotes their proliferative activity in the absence of serum. On the other hand, our results indicate that CS potentiates the action of mitogens on SMC since the enhancement of cell proliferation is observed over a broad range of FCS concentrations, including those where stretch-induced secretion of endogenous PDGF should not make a significant contribution (Fig. 1, top panel). We suggest that this potentiating effect of CS is due to its action on cytosolic Ca^{2+} turnover. By imposing regular Ca^{2+} oscillations via stretch-activated Ca^{2+} channels CS favors Ca^{2+}-dependent processes which cells are tuned to execute. Therefore, modulated SMC of synthetic phenotype (used in all stretch experiments reported in the literature) will probably respond to CS by division and secretion of extracellular matrix proteins and growth factors, while differentiated SMC (in mature smooth muscle tissue) will react by contraction [9]. From this point of view CS reveals analogy with Ca^{2+}-mobilizing vasoactive substances such as epinephrine, norepinephrine, endothelin, PDGF. All these agents are capable of inducing contraction of differentiated smooth muscle whereas in noncontractile modulated SMC they cause or potentiate proliferation (for a review see [10]).

Another effect of CS was a 2- to 3-fold increased expression of h-caldesmon, a high molecular weight caldesmon isoform peculiar to SMC of contractile phenotype (Fig. 1,

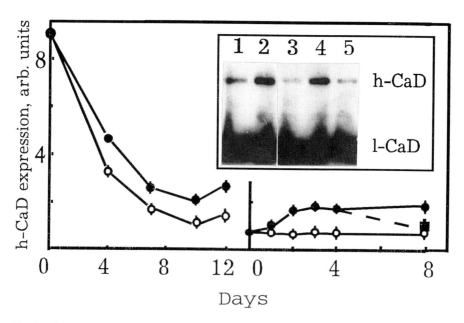

Fig. 2. Effect of CS on h-caldesmon expression in primary and passaged SMC. Cells were cultured in the presence of 0.5% FCS for the indicated periods of time without (open circles) or with (closed circles) application of CS. Left panel, primary SMC culture; right panel, passaged SMC culture. Separate Flex plates stretched for 4 days were then left without agitation for days 5–8 of the experiment (right panel, filled box). Inset represents anticaldesmon immunoblots used to generate data points in right panel. SMC were cultured for 4 days without (lane 1) or with CS (lane 2), for 8 days without (lane 3) or with CS (lane 4), or for 4 days with CS followed by 4 days in stationary conditions (lane 5). h-CaD, h-caldesmon; l-CaD, l-caldesmon.

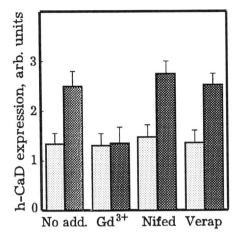

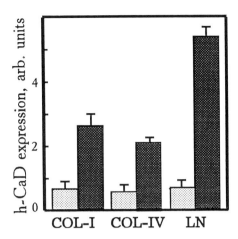

Fig. 3. Effect of Ca²⁺-channel blockers on CS-induced h-caldesmon expression in SMC. Passaged SMC were maintained in 0.5% FCS for 4 days in the presence of stretch-activated Ca²⁺-channel blocker Gd³⁺ (0.8 μM) and voltage-operated Ca²⁺-channel blockers nifedipine (4 μM) and verapamil (4 μM) in stationary (gray bars) and CS (black bars) conditions.

Fig. 4. CS-activated h-caldesmon expression in SMC grown on various extracellular matrices. Cells were seeded on matrix-coated Flex plates and maintained in the presence of 0.5% FCS under stationary (gray bars) or CS (black bars) conditions for 6 days. Col-I and Col-IV, collagen types I and IV, respectively; LN, laminin.

middle panel). This effect was independent of the proliferative status of SMC and the state of their confluency (Fig. 1, top and middle panel). By contrast, the expression of l-caldesmon, a low molecular weight caldesmon isoform which is predominantly expressed in modulated SMC and nonmuscle cells [4], demonstrated no dependence on CS but was rather inhibited in dense cultures (Fig. 1, top and bottom panel). CS partially prevented the loss of h-caldesmon in enzymatically isolated primary SMC and stabilized its content on the higher level throughout the experiment (Fig. 2, left panel). In passaged cells subjected to CS the increase in h-caldesmon expression matched that achieved in primary SMC at basal level and reverted to the control unstretched level when CS was omitted (Fig. 2, right panel and inset). The expression of smooth muscle myosin and calponin was insensitive to mechanical stimulation of SMC (data not shown). The selective accumulation of h-caldesmon in mechanically agitated SMC might be related to a unique role ascribed to this protein in smooth muscle. h-Caldesmon is considered a key Ca²⁺-dependent actomyosin cross-linker and a regulator of smooth-muscle contraction and tone [4]. Stretching of the artery by blood pulsation is a physiological trigger for a contractile response of the vessel wall and this event is mediated by intracellular Ca²⁺ elevation. Perhaps the major "tonic protein" of smooth-muscle h-caldesmon is regulated by the stretch-induced Ca²⁺ rise both functionally and at the level of expression. Indeed, blocking of Ca²⁺ influx via stretch-activated channels with Gd³⁺ prevents stretch-induced increase of h-caldesmon expression in SMC (Fig. 3).

Strain-dependent h-caldesmon expression was reproduced at comparable degree in SMC grown on collagen type I and IV (Fig. 4), gelatin and poly-L-lysine (data not shown). This indicates that the reception of a mechanical signal occurs via several cell–matrix interactions and the underlying substrate merely transduces mechanical strain to the cell body. In the case of laminin, however, the increase in h-caldesmon content was

826

several-fold higher than on other matrices (Fig. 4). These findings correspond well to a prodifferentiating action of laminin reported by others (for a review see [10]). Apparently, activation of laminin receptors enhances CS-induced intracellular signaling via positive cross-talk mechanisms. The biochemical nature of this interference remains to be elucidated.

In brief, repetitive mechanical agitation of vascular SMC results in accumulation of h-caldesmon, a protein marker of a differentiated contractile SMC phenotype. This effect is consistently reproduced even in profoundly modified SMC, indicating that CS may contribute to smooth-muscle differentiation in normal vessel wall as well as in the regions of vessel injury and in development. The enhancement by CS of quite diverse cellular events such as differentiated phenotype marker expression and proliferation, contraction and growth-factor secretion may be related to its ability to synchronize intracellular Ca^{2+} oscillations and thus to support various Ca^{2+}-dependent processes.

Acknowledgements

Financial support from the Russian Fundamental Research Foundation, the International Science Foundation (grant no. M33000), the Swiss National Foundation (grants nos. 31-29275.90 and 32-30315.90), the Swiss Cardiology Foundation and the European Cardiology Society is gratefully acknowledged.

References

1. Sadoshima J, Jahn L, Takahashi T, Kulik T, Izumo S. J Biol Chem 1992;267:10551–10560.
2. Wilson E, Mai Q, Sudhir K, Weiss RH, Ives HE. J Cell Biol 1993;123:741–747.
3. Leung DY, Glagov S, Mathews MB. Science (Wash. DC) 1976;191:475–477.
4. Sobue K, Sellers JR. J Biol Chem 1991;266:12115–12118.
5. Shirinsky VP, Biryukov KG, Vorotnikov AV, Gusev NB. FEBS Lett 1989;251:65–68.
6. Birukov KG, Stepanova OV, Nanaev AK, Shirinsky VP. Cell Tissue Res 1991;266:579–584.
7. Nanaev AK, Shirinsky VP, Birukov KG. Cell Tis Res 1991;266:535–540.
8. Shirinsky VP, Birukov KG, Koteliansky VE, Glukhova MA, Spanidis E, Rogers JD, Campbell JH, Campbell GR. Exp Cell Res 1991;194:186–189.
9. Barany K, Ledvora RF, Mougios V, Barany M. J Biol Chem 1985;260:7126–7130.
10. Thyberg J, Hedin U, Sjolund M, Palmberg L, Bottger BA. Arteriosclerosis 1990;10:966–990.

Influence of flow on the endothelial tight junction and extracellular matrix

Yoji Yoshida, Masako Mitsumata, Su Wang, Tetsu Yamane, Mitsuji Okano, Tomoyuki Arisaka and Masahiko Kawasumi

Department of Pathology, Yamanashi Medical University, Tamaho, Yamanashi 409-38, Japan

Abstract. Laminar unidirectional high shear stress stimulated the synthesis of tight junction (TJ)-related proteins ZO-1 and 7H6 and of glycosaminoglycans by porcine aortic endothelial cells in vitro. These data support in vivo findings of the rabbit aorta that zonular-typed TJ and thick glycocalyx as antiatherosclerotic structures developed better in high-shear regions than in low-shear regions.

Atherosclerosis, both in humans [1,2] and in experimental animals [3], occurs preferentially at low mean shear stress regions and hardly develops at high shear stress regions in the arterial wall. High-stress regions such as the leading edges of flow dividers at branchings of the rabbit aorta show little lipid deposition even if hypercholesterolemia is present, and endothelial cells there develop more zonular tight junctions (TJs) [3] and thicker glycocalyx [4] than low-shear regions.

To obtain direct evidence of the beneficial effects of laminar high shear stress induced by blood flow on the production of TJ and glycocalyx by the endothelial cells, which possibly function as synthesizers of the TJ-related proteins 7H6 [5] and ZO-1 [6], we studied the synthesis of glycosaminoglycans by endothelial cells in vitro.

Materials and Methods

Cell

Confluent porcine aortic endothelial cells (ECs), cultured on polyester sheets in DMEM supplemented with 10% fetal calf serum, were placed at the bottom of rectangular flow chambers to be exposed to a laminar and unidirectional flow of the culture medium at a speed which was controlled by the height of an upper reservoir and a speed regulator. The flow loop, reservoirs and chamber were filled with the medium kept at 36°C and saturated with 5% CO_2 and 95% air. The fluid was recirculated by a roller pump. Arrow-shaped flow chambers (Fig. 1) were used to get both high-speed laminar and stagnation flows. Static control ECs were cultured in the same way as the sheared ECs except for being kept in dishes in an incubator for given experimental periods.

Tight junction

Anti-ZO-1 and -7H6 mABs conjugated with FITC were used for histochemical and flow cytofluorometric analysis. Fine structures of junctional complexes of ECs were investigated by a freeze-fracture and replica method under an electron microscope.

Glycosaminoglycans (GAGs)

GAG biosynthesis by ECs was measured by a modified method of Shimada et al. [7].

828

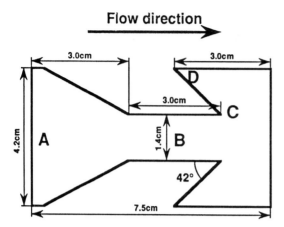

Fig. 1. Arrow-shaped conduit in the flow chamber.

Immediately after exposure to shear stress, ECs were incubated with 30 µCi/ml of [^{35}S]sulfate in the fresh medium for 12 or 24 h for metabolic labeling. Conditioned medium (medium fraction), trypsin-extractable substances of cell layers (trypsinated fraction), and a cell pellet (cell fraction) were obtained to detect [^{35}S]GAGs. After pronase digestion, GAGs were extracted with cetylpyridinium chloride (CPC). Aliquots of pronase digests were treated with chondroitin ABC lyase before CPC precipitation.

[^{3}H] leucine and thymidine uptake on sheared cells were studied in parallel with rates of GAG biosynthesis.

Statistical analysis

Triplicate determinations were averaged for each experiment, expressed as the mean ± SD and analyzed by *t*-test and variance. Statistical significance was assumed as $p < 0.05$.

Results

Tight junction

The anti-ZO-1 and -7H6 fluorescent immunolabeling was hardly visible in the static cells even after culture for 72 h, but a significant increase of fluorescence was recognized at the cell boundaries in the confluent monolayer subjected to 30 dyn/cm^2 for 24 h. The frequency of cells stained with anti-7H6 antibody increased in proportion to the magnitude and duration of shear stress applied. When 30 dyn/cm^2 is applied at the entry of an arrow-shaped conduit, approximately 90 dyn/cm^2 operates on the cells in the narrowest segment (B in Fig. 1), but the shear stress is very low on the cells in the angle (D in Fig. 1) in which the flow stagnates. In this condition, the cells in B showed an elongated form (an average shape index: 0.24) parallel to the flow direction and were stained strongly with 7H6 and ZO-1 antibodies, while those in the angles were polygonal (average shape index: 0.73) and were hardly stained by those antibodies after 72 h of exposure (Fig. 2). Expression of mRNA for ZO-1 synthesis was proven by RT-PCR (using a 522-bp fragment of mouse ZO-1 cDNA) in the cells subjected to 30 dyn/cm^2 after 2 h, but not in the static cells.

In freeze-fractured samples, the static cells in a completely confluent layer had only

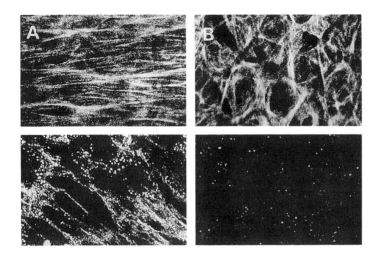

Fig. 2. Shapes (upper) and TJ-related proteins (lower) of endothelial cells in B and D of the conduit (Fig. 1). Actin filaments stained with fluorescent phalloidin run in parallel with boundaries of elongated cells in B(A) whereas cells are polygonal in D(B). More TJ protein stained with 7H6 mAb was observed in B than D.

a few gap junctions, without any ridges of membranous protein particles forming tight junctions. The cells placed under 30 dyn/cm^2 for 24 h developed continuous ridges of protein particles resembling the macular type of TJ. These ridges were short and widely spaced at 24 h of this shear stress. They increased in length and number of strands with an increase in exposure time at the same magnitude of shear stress.

GAGs

In the static culture, the amount of newly synthesized GAGs produced in the trypsinated fractions increased with culture time up to 48 h. This increase was in inverse proportion to the amount of DNA synthesis. On the basis of these findings, the cells were exposed to shear stress for 24 h on day 3 after seeding and to [^{35}S]sulfate on day 4 for 12 h.

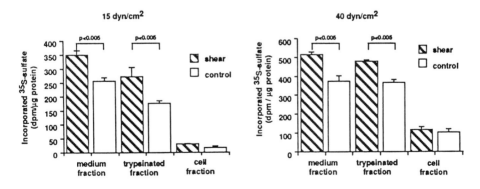

Fig. 3. Incorporation of [^{35}S]sulfate into fractions prepared from the endothelial cells either under sheared or static (control) conditions. Incorporation rates of ^{35}S into both the medium and trypsinated fractions were higher in either shear stress condition than in the static condition.

The amount of [^{35}S]sulfate incorporated was significantly enhanced in the sheared cells. Synthesized GAGs in both medium and trypsinated fractions of the EC were significantly increased by exposure to either 15 or 40 dyn/cm^2 shear stress for 24 h (Fig. 3) or more. GAGs increased in the medium by shear stress were digestible with chondroitin ABC lyase, but those in the trypsinated fractions were not. These results suggest that major portions of sulfated GAGs in the medium and on the surface of ECs consist of chondroitin or dermatan sulfate and heparan sulfate respectively.

To determine the correlations between GAG synthesis, cell growth and protein synthesis, we incubated the cells with [^{3}H] thymidine or [^{3}H] leucine immediately after exposure to 40 dyn/cm^2 shear stress for 24 h. The DNA and protein syntheses of sheared cells were altered to 56 and 150% of control, respectively.

Discussion

In normolipidemic rabbit endothelial cells at laminar high shear stress regions of aortic bifurcations had well-developed zonular-type tight junctions, thicker glycocalyx, fewer vesicles labeled with horseradish peroxidase or ferritin [4], and thicker basement membrane than those in low shear stress regions. These can be expected to reduce the permeability of endothelial cells to macromolecular serum constituents.

To investigate whether laminar high shear stress produces antiatherosclerotic structures on ECs such as TJ and glycocalyx, we subjected ECs in culture to laminar shear stress ranging from 15 to 90 dyn/cm^2 for 2–72 h. These in vitro studies revealed that ECs synthesized TJ-related proteins and structured ridges of proteins, though incompletely. The ECs also synthesize GAGs which were deposited on the cell surfaces and released into the culture medium.

Details of protein synthesis of TJ under laminar shear stress are still obscure. Since elongated endothelial cells with an organized assembly of stress fibers induced by laminar high shear stress had many TJ-related proteins, there would appear to be a strong relationship between stress fibers and TJ.

The RT-PCR method showed expression of ZO-1 mRNA induced in the ECs exposed to shear stress. The higher the magnitude and the longer the duration of shear stress, the longer the ridges of protein particles of interendothelial junctions became.

GAGs synthesized by ECs exposed to laminar and unidirectional shear stress were heparan sulfate and chondroitin/dermatan sulfate. Heparan sulfate was secreted and deposited mainly on the cell surface and/or into the extracellular matrix, and chondroitin/dermatan sulfate was secreted into the medium.

More than 24 h of shear stress is required to stimulate GAG synthesis in EC. GAG synthesis of EC under static conditions also did not appear until 24 h of culture. These results suggest that shear stress does not shorten the period between incorporation of [^{35}S]sulfate into cells and the secretion of synthesized GAGs, but it does increase the amount of GAGs synthesized.

The transmission and transduction mechanisms of mechanical stress in ECs have previously been assumed [8], but the mechanisms for augmenting syntheses of TJ-related proteins and GAGs induced by shear stress have never till now been determined.

The antiatherosclerotic structure of ECs observed in the area exposed to laminar high shear stress such as the tight junction and glycocalyx were constructed progressively in vitro under unidirectional high shear stress. These functional and structural alterations may determine the location of atherosclerosis.

Acknowledgements

We are grateful to Dr Robert M. Nerem for kindly providing an original model of the flow chamber, and to Dr Michio Mori with the 7H6 mAb. This work was supported by research grants from the Ministry of Education, Science and Culture of Japan, and from the Ministry of Health and Welfare of Japan.

Reference

1. Caro CG, Fitz-Gerald JM, Schroter RC. Proc Roy Soc Lond (Biol) 1971;177:109—159.
2. Ku DN, Giddens DP, Zarins CK, Glagov S. Arteriosclerosis 1985;5:293—302.
3. Okano M, Yoshida Y. Frontiers Med Biol Eng 1993;5:95—120.
4. Wang S, Okano M, Yoshida Y. J Jpn Atheroscler Soc 1991;1089—1100.
5. Zhong Y, Saitoh T, Manase T, Sawada N, Enomoto K, Mori M. J Cell Biol 1993;120:477—483.
6. Stevenson BR, Siliciano JD, Mooseker MS, Goodenough DA. J Cell Biol 1986;103:755—766.
7. Shimada K, Ozawa T. J Clin Invest 1985;75:1308—1316.
8. Davies PF, Tripathi SC. Circ Res 1993;72:239—245.

Effects of shear stress on endothelial cells: cell-surface dynamics using atomic force microscopy and tandem scanning confocal microscopy

Peter F. Davies[1], Kenneth A. Barbee[1], Andre Robotewskyj[1] and Melvin L. Griem[2]

Departments of [1]Pathology and [2]Radiation Oncology, Pritzker School of Medicine, The University of Chicago, Department of Pathology MC 6079, 5841 S. Maryland Avenue, Chicago, IL 60637, USA

Abstract. The mechanisms of hemodynamic mechanotransduction are poorly understood. However, the initial interaction is of hemodynamic forces with an intact cell that is already maintained under tension, and the nature of that interaction is closely related to the geometry of the endothelial cell surface. By mechanical and optical imaging methods, we have documented changes in the topography of both the luminal and abluminal endothelial cell surfaces in response to a flow environment that principally embodies forces due to shear stress. We demonstrate altered topography of the endothelial luminal surface as a consequence of exposure to flow, and estimate the surface distribution of shear stress. The abluminal surface topography, particularly at focal attachment sites, is also flow-responsive as imaged in the living cell in real time.

At the interface between flowing blood and the vascular wall, the endothelium responds to hemodynamic forces by a range of electrophysiological, biochemical, cell biological, gene regulatory, and morphological changes [1] that influence not only endothelial cell structure and function but also the biology of the underlying vessel wall. There is convincing evidence that the endothelium in vivo transduces mechanical forces into biochemical pathways that have profound consequences for the regulation of arterial diameter and for the pathological development of cardiovascular diseases [2,3]. When adherent to an extracellular matrix, tension generated by the maintenance of cell shape is distributed throughout the cell via the cytoskeleton. In a confluent endothelial monolayer, the cells are attached to each other at intercellular junctions as well as at focal attachment sites on the abluminal surface. During flow, the internal cellular tension changes to equalize the external force. Onset of flow is accompanied by a series of biological responses in endothelial cells that range from rapid ion fluxes to long-term gene regulatory and morphological changes [1]. The sites of conversion of the physical force to bioresponses are unknown but several candidates include: (a) the luminal cell surface where frictional shear stress may act directly on a "mechanosensor", or (b) elsewhere in the cell, tension being transmitted to a remote mechanosensing system via the cytoskeleton. Two prominent possibilities are the sites of interactions of cytoskeletal components with numerous plasma-membrane proteins at the lateral boundaries of the cell [4], and the focal adhesion sites on the abluminal surface of the cell [5]. Cytoskeletal interactions with nuclear membrane proteins may also transmit forces directly to the nucleus [6]. In addition to direct forces acting to displace cellular components, blood flow also influences the local concentrations of labile agonists at the cell surface by altering the rates of delivery from the bulk fluid and/or the rates of degradation at the cell surface to cause modification of ligand–receptor coupling [7].

Lumenal surface

Cellular geometry, and particularly the luminal surface topography, influences the spatial variations of shear stress during flow. Thus, shear-stress forces may be transmitted either locally to mechanosensors at the luminal surface or across the plasma membrane to other sensing sites throughout the cell. It follows therefore that the geometry of the endothelial cell will be important in determining the subcellular distribution of shear-stress forces acting on the cell surface. In order to model the detailed real-flow behavior very close to the cell surface we obtained images of the geometry of living endothelial cells in tissue culture by the use of atomic force microscopy (AFM) [8]. In AFM, a fine stylus is moved over the surface of the cell in a raster in which the distance between the stylus tip and cell proteins is kept constant by compensating for the varying intermolecular attraction between them. The X, Y, and Z (height) positions are known for all positions on the raster (which encompasses an entire cell or group of cells). Endothelial cells were polygonal in shape in a confluent monolayer that was not exposed to flow. AFM images (Fig. 1) showed undulations from the nuclear bulge to the intercellular junctions of approximately 6 μm. The cell surface was smooth. After exposure to unidirectional shear stress at 12 dynes/cm^2 for 24 h, the cells in the monolayer aligned in the direction of flow (Fig. 2). This was accompanied by a streamlining of the endothelial cell surface such that the incline between the lowest positions (at intercellular junctions) to the top of the nuclear bulge decreased. Elongation of the cell resulted in a more shallow gradient both upstream and downstream from the nuclear bulge than in nonaligned cells. The implications of this altered cell-surface geometry became evident when computational methods were applied to calculate the effects upon flow near the surface.

Using hybrid spectral element analyses, flows were simulated over endothelial surface geometries of living cells that had been defined by AFM [9]. Flow perturbations due to the undulating surface produced cell-scale variations of shear-stress magnitude in the nonaligned, no-flow monolayer that included large shear-stress gradients. When the cell surface was reorganized in response to steady flow, there were significantly lower peak shear stresses and shear stress gradients than in no-flow control cells. Microscopic

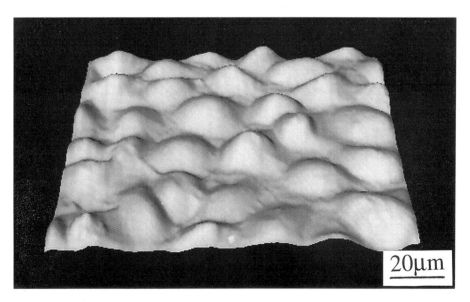

20μm

Fig. 1. Atomic force microscopic (AFM) image of the luminal surface of a living confluent bovine aortic endothelial-cell monolayer. The cells were not exposed to flow.

834

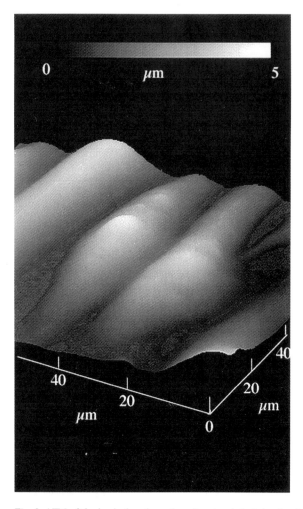

Fig. 2. AFM of the luminal surface of confluent endothelial cells after exposure to flow (laminar shear stress, 12 dynes/cm², 24 h).

departures from a flat boundary due to the presence of the endothelial cells were shown to cause a localized perturbation of the macroscopic flow field. One implication of these studies is that the position of a putative mechanosensor relative to shear stress on the luminal cell surface may be critical in determining its response to the applied force. For example, responses in an aligned cell may occur only at a higher flow rate because the shear-stress magnitude or shear-stress gradient remains below the critical threshold required to trigger a mechanosensor, whereas in a nonaligned cell where the topography is different, higher local shear-stress values that activate mechanosensing systems may render the cells more responsive (Fig. 3). Furthermore, the location of a sensor upstream or downstream or on the steepest part of the cell surface may influence its sensitivity to flow. If a mechanosensor is located other than at the luminal cell surface but is connected to it via the cytoskeleton, bioresponsiveness may be critically influenced by the location(s) of cytoskeleton–cell surface interactions.

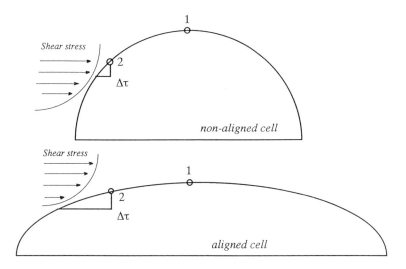

Fig. 3. Hypothetical effect of endothelial-surface topography upon the sensitivity of a putative mechanosensor (O) at the luminal cell surface following cell alignment by shear stress. At position 1, the shear stress will be similar, but at position 2 the shear stress gradient ($\Delta\tau$) will be markedly reduced in the aligned cell. Cell responses may depend both on the distribution of mechanosensors (or surface elements linked to them) and on the altered topography.

Abluminal surface

Adhesion is maintained at the abluminal surface of the cell at sites of focal attachment to the extracellular matrix. Transmembrane integrins adhere to extracellular matrix-adhesion proteins on the exterior of the cell and associate with filamentous actin microfilaments on the inner side of the membrane. However, the cytoskeletal–integrin association is indirect, being mediated by a series of linker proteins that include vinculin, paxillin, α-actinin, tensin, talin, and p125[FAK] (a tyrosine kinase). The sites are also enriched in other kinases (with serine, threonine, and tyrosine substrates) and with proteins containing an src-homology binding region (SH-2 domain). Focal adhesion sites in endothelial cells are dynamic, forming and rearranging over a period of minutes as shown by tandem scanning confocal microscopy imaging (TSCM) [10]. The spatial relationships between the abluminal cell surface and adhesion proteins of the substratum were observed in three dimensions by image reconstruction (Fig. 4). When endothelial cells were exposed to flow (i.e., defined shear stress acting at the luminal surface of the monolayer), the focal adhesion sites underwent complex rearrangements that included remodeling in the direction of flow and the formation of elongated focal adhesion regions that were aligned in the direction of the flow. We concluded from these studies that shear-stress signaling at the luminal surface influenced adhesion-related events at the abluminal membrane, suggesting the participation of focal adhesion sites in shear-stress signaling. One such mechanism is the transmission of stress forces to focal adhesion sites via the cytoskeletal elements, principally filamentous actin. However, it is impossible to rule out adhesion-site rearrangement secondary to a primary biochemical signaling event originating at the luminal surface.

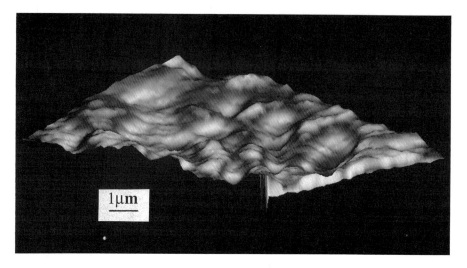

Fig. 4. Reconstructed three-dimensional image of the abluminal surface of a living confluent endothelial cell observed by tandem scanning confocal microscopy. The substratum has been removed from the image to expose the surface topography. Membrane projections represent focal adhesion sites where the cell is attached to the underlying (invisible) extracellular matrix.

Mechanical signaling at focal adhesions?

If focal adhesion sites participate in the early stages of mechanical signaling, one might expect to be able to identify localized biochemical changes at these sites. Preliminary evidence in support of such a mechanism has recently been obtained. Immunoprecipitation of paxillin, a linker protein involved in the structural continuity between the β-subunit of integrins and filamentous actin, revealed increased tyrosine phosphorylation within 20 min of exposure to 10 dynes/cm^2 of shear stress. Paxillin phosphorylation increased 2-fold within 2 h of exposure to unidirectional laminar flow. In contrast, p125^{FAK} phosphorylation, an event which is greatly inhibited when cell adhesion is compromised, was not significantly changed. Both groups of proteins were predominantly phosphorylated (= basal levels) in adherent endothelium in the absence of flow. Recently, tyrosine phosphorylation of both paxillin and p125^{FAK} has been demonstrated to be obligatory for cytoskeleton assembly and fibroblast adhesion to fibronectin-coated surfaces. Adhesion, as defined by an integrated measurement of the area of focal adhesions combined with the separation distances between the membrane and the substrata at focal adhesions [11], remained unchanged during flow-induced directional remodeling of focal attachment sites [10]. This measurement is consistent with an unchanged level of p125^{FAK} phosphorylation, which is known to be adhesion-sensitive.

Other evidence suggests convergence of signaling pathways at the integrin-rich focal adhesion sites. A heterotrimeric G protein γ subunit, γ_5, has been reported to be localized to these sites and to adjacent stress fibers in a variety of cells [12]. The subunit distribution was similar to that of zyxin, a protein that binds α-actinin and is considered to be involved in focal adhesion signal transduction. When G protein-linked receptors for endothelin and bombesin were stimulated by agonist binding, there was immediate phosphorylation of p125^{FAK}, again suggesting localization of these receptors to focal adhesion sites. The co-localization of G protein γ_5 is consistent with convergence of signaling pathways involving two families of transmembrane proteins: G protein-linked receptors of the serpentine superfamily and integrins. Heterotrimeric G proteins may therefore also be involved in integrin-receptor signaling at focal adhesion sites. Pertussis-toxin inhibition of G protein activation interfered with cell adhesion-activated K^+ channels that have been linked to integrin–extracellular matrix binding [13]. Considering the dynamic rearrangement at focal adhesion sites both under flow (directional remodeling) and no-flow (random remodeling) conditions, and the involvement of filamentous actin in mechanical responses of endothelial cells to shear stress, we suggest that both phosphorylation and G protein-linked pathways may be involved in mechanical signaling at focal adhesions, as well as locally at the luminal plasma membrane.

Acknowledgements

Supported by NIH grants HL15062 and American Heart Association Grant-In-Aid 91-15570.

References

1. Davies PF. Flow-mediated endothelial mechanotransduction. Physiol Rev 1994 (in press).
2. Pohl U, Holtz J, Busse R, Bassenge E. Hypertension 1986;8:37—47.
3. Cornhill JF, Roach MR. Atherosclerosis 1976;23:489—499.
4. Takeichi M. Development 1988;102:639—655.
5. Burridge K, Fath K, Kelly T, Nuckolls G, Turner C. Ann Rev Cell Biol 1988;4:487—525.
6. Pienta KJ, Coffey DS. J Cell Biochem 1992;49:357—365.
7. Dull RO, Davies PF. Am J Physiol 1991;261:H149—H156.
8. Barbee KA, Davies PF, Lal R. Circ Res 1994;74:163—171.
9. Barbee KA, Mundel T, Lal R, Davies PF. Subcellular distribution of shear stress at the surface of flow-aligned and nonaligned endothelial monolayers. Am J Physiol 1994 (in press).
10. Davies PF, Robotewskyj A, Griem ML. J Clin Invest 1994;93:2031—2038.
11. Davies PF, Robotewskyj A, Griem ML. J Clin Invest 1993;91:2640—2652.
12. Hansen CA, Schroering AG, Carey DJ, Robishaw JD. J Cell Biol 1994;126:811—829.
13. Arcangeli A, Becchetti A, Mannini A, Mugnani G, Philippi P, Tarone G, Del Bene M, Barletta E, Wanke E, Olivotto M. J Cell Biol 1993;122:1131—1143.

Endothelial gene regulation by biomechanical forces

Nitzan Resnick[1], Sumpio E. Bauer[2], Wei Du[2] and Michael A. Gimbrone Jr.[1]

[1]*Vascular Research Division, Department of Pathology, Brigham and Women's Hospital, Boston, Massachusetts; and* [2]*Department of Vascular Surgery, Yale University, New Haven, Conneticut, USA*

Abstract. Hemodynamic forces generated by the pulsatile flow of blood through the circulatory system have been shown to influence the structure and function of vascular endothelium. Several groups, using in vitro systems, have demonstrated that defined biomechanical forces, including wall shear stress and cyclic strain, can modulate endothelial gene expression. In particular, our group has demonstrated that PDGF B-chain gene transcription is induced by exposure of cultured endothelial cells to a physiologic level of laminar shear stress. We have defined a region within the PDGF B-chain promoter that is responsible for this shear-induced gene expression, and have called this the "Shear Stress Response Element" (SSRE). This promoter element binds nuclear proteins extracted from shear-stressed endothelial cells. A core sequence (GAGACC) within the SSRE is also present in the promoters of several other endothelial genes that are responsive to shear stress. This core sequence was shown by electromobility shift assays to be a nuclear-protein binding site. Moreover, hybrid promoters containing the SSRE sequence (as present in the PDGF B-chain promoter) were inducible by shear stress when transfected into bovine aortic endothelial cells, thus confirming that this element is both necessary and sufficient for gene induction by laminar shear stress. We have recently extended these studies to another physiologically relevant hemodynamic force, cyclic strain, induced by biaxial stretching. Interestingly, the SSRE binds to nuclear proteins extracted from endothelial cells, but not from smooth muscle cells, exposed to the same level of cyclic strain (10% average strain, 60 cycles/min). These results suggest that different biomechanical forces may act on the endothelium through a common, but cell-type-specific, mechanism to activate gene transcription.

Introduction

Vascular endothelial cells in direct contact with flowing blood bear the frictional forces imparted by this fluid, and also transmit wall tension derived from systolic–diastolic pressure changes acting perpendicular to the vessel lining. In vivo, these hemodynamic forces appear to affect endothelial structure and function, and have been implicated in the changes in macromolecular permeability, lipoprotein accumulation and cell damage that are associated with branch points and bifurcations [1—4]. In vitro systems have been developed to study the mechanisms of these physical effects on endothelial cells [5,6], and have confirmed the direct cellular actions of both fluid shear stresses and cyclic strains. More recently, a number of these hemodynamic effects have been shown to involve changes in endothelial gene expression [7,8]. Using a well-characterized fluid mechanical system, the cone and plate apparatus developed in collaboration with Prof. C.F. Dewey (Fluid Mechanics Laboratory, Massachusetts Institute of Technology, Cambridge, MA), we have studied the regulation of several pathophysiologically relevant genes after exposure of cultured endothelial monolayers (bovine, human) to defined fluid shear stresses. Our experimental approach was: (a) to identify candidate genes that are

Address for correspondence: Dr Nitzan Resnick, Vascular Research Division, Department of Pathology, Brigham and Women's Hospital, 221 Longwood Ave. (LMRC-4), Boston, MA 02115-5817, USA.

transcriptionally regulated by laminar shear stress in cultured endothelial cells; (b) to examine the 5′ flanking regions of these genes for "shear-stress response elements"; and (c) to extend these studies to other types of biomechanical forces, e.g., cyclic strain.

Our initial studies have focused on the human PDGF B-chain gene [9]. This gene is transcriptionally upregulated as early as 30 min after the exposure of cultured endothelial cells to a physiological level of laminar shear stress (10 dynes/cm^2). We identified a 50-bp region within the PDGF B-promoter responsible for the inducibility of this gene by shear stress, using deletion constructs of the PDGF B promoter. Using electromobility shift assays (EMSA), a 12-bp shear-stress response element (SSRE) was further defined. This element binds nuclear proteins from endothelial cells exposed to laminar shear stress, but does not encode a consensus binding site for any of the known transcription factors. Database analyses revealed that several promoters of endothelial genes responsive to shear stress contain the same 6-bp core sequence (GAGACC) present in the SSRE in the PDGF B gene. Further studies in our group [10] have demonstrated a selective pattern of induction of endothelial–leukocyte adhesion molecules (ICAM-1, but not VCAM-1 or E-selectin) that is correlated with the presence or absence of this SSRE core sequence in their promoters.

Recently, it has been demonstrated that cyclic strain can also regulate endothelial-cell gene expression in vitro, and that several endothelial genes are responsive to both cyclic strain and shear stress [11]. Here, we will review data demonstrating that: (a) the SSRE core sequence is the binding site for nuclear proteins induced by laminar fluid shear stress; (b) SSRE is both necessary and sufficient for gene induction by shear stress in endothelial cells; and (c) nuclear proteins extracted from endothelial, but not from smooth muscle cells, subjected to cyclic strain bind to the SSRE. These results suggest a cell-type-specific mechanism for endothelial gene induction by various types of hemodynamic forces.

Materials and Methods

Shear stress apparatus

The design of the cone and plate flow apparatus has been described [5]. In all the following experiments endothelial cells (bovine aortic endothelial cells (BAEC) or human umbilical vein endothelial cells (HUVEC)) were grown under standard culture conditions [5,9] on polystyrene tissue-culture coated coverslips, and were exposed to a physiologic level of laminar shear stress (10 dynes/cm^2), or incubated under static (no-flow) conditions.

Cyclic strain

BAEC or HUVEC were exposed to biaxial stretching on a Flexercell system (FLEXER-CELL Inc. Corp., McKeesport PA), as described elsewhere [6]. Both cell types were exposed to the same 10% average strain (60 cycles/min) for various time intervals.

Nuclear extracts and EMSA

Nuclei were extracted from cells exposed to shear stress, cyclic strain, or static (control) conditions, as described previously [9]. Nuclear proteins were incubated with ^{32}P-labeled oligonucleotide probes (30 mer) at room temperature under low-salt conditions [9], and then analyzed on 4% acrylamide gels.

Hybrid promoters

SSRE hybrid promoters were constructed using an enhancerless SV40/CAT vector (Promega, Madison, WI). The various constructs were transfected into BAEC by the modified calcium phosphate method [9]. Transfected cells were either grown under static conditions or exposed to flow, and CAT activity was measured and normalized to transfection efficiency.

Results

SSRE core sequence is a binding site for shear-stress-inducible nuclear proteins in endothelial cells

Nuclei were extracted from BAEC exposed to laminar shear stress (10 dynes/cm^2) or incubated under static conditions for 1 h. Nuclear protein binding was assayed with a set of oligonucleotide probes encoding various permutations of the SSRE. An inducible DNA–protein complex was consistently observed (Fig. 1) with the probe carrying the 3′ part of the SSRE (GAGACC), but not with the 5′ part (CTCTCA) or with a mutated SSRE (CTCTCAGTGTCC). This inducible complex was demonstrable with nuclear extracts from cells exposed to shear for only 15 min, and was still evident after 4 h (data not shown).

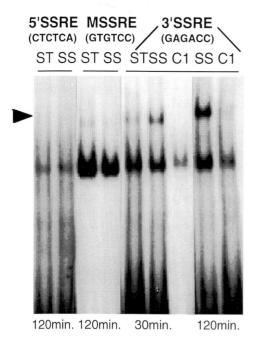

Fig. 1. Characterization of the DNA binding site within the SSRE: Nuclear extracts derived from BAEC incubated under static conditions (ST), or subjected to laminar shear stress (10 dynes/cm^2) (SS) were incubated with three SSRE-derived probes (30 mer each). Binding and EMSA conditions are described elsewhere [9]. The SSRE probes included the 5′SSRE (noncore) (CTCTCA), a mutated SSRE (MSSRE)(CTCTCAGTGTCC) and the SSRE core sequence (3′SSRE)(GAGACC). The latter probe was incubated with nuclei extracted from cells exposed to shear stress for either 30 min (left) or 120 min (right). Specificity of formation of complex (arrow) was tested by the addition of unlabeled identical probe (C1).

SSRE is sufficient for gene induction by laminar shear stress

As revealed by database analyses, several genes responsive to shear stress contained the SSRE core sequence (GAGACC), or its complementary sequence (GGTCTC), in their promoters [9]. To test the role of the SSRE in conferring shear responsiveness directly, we constructed a vector containing a SV40 enhancerless promoter and the CAT reporter gene, which was itself uninducible by shear stress, and then added the SSRE or its complementary sequence. Specifically, the following hybrid reporter gene constructs were made: (a) the SSRE (CTCTCAGAGACC) in the context of flanking sequences from the human PDGF-B promoter (SV-SSRE/CAT); (b) the complementary sequence (alternate strand) of the SSRE (CTCTCAGGTCTC) [SV-(C)SSRE/CAT)]; and (c) the 5′ (nonbinding) part of the SSRE (CTCTCA) [SV-(5′)SSRE/CAT]. Each oligonucleotide was coupled to the SV/CAT construct in the ECO RI-BglII site. BAEC transfected with these constructs were exposed to shear stress for 2 h, or incubated under static conditions. As seen in Table 1, the addition of the SSRE or its complementary sequence, but not the 5′ part of the SSRE, converted the SV/CAT-uninducible backbone vector into a fluid shear-stress-responsive one.

Nuclear proteins from endothelial cells exposed to cyclic strain bind to the SSRE

To test whether similar mechanisms are involved in gene induction by both shear stress and cyclic strain, we exposed BAEC or HUVEC to 10% average biaxial cyclic stretching (60 cycles/min) for various time intervals. Nuclear proteins were then extracted and tested for their ability to bind the SSRE probe. As can be seen in Fig. 2, nuclear proteins from HUVEC (as well as from BAEC, data not shown) formed a specific inducible complex with the SSRE probe, which was strongly evident at 30 min but rapidly declined to below control (unstretched) levels by 2 h. This kinetic profile thus differs from that obtained with nuclei of endothelial cells exposed to fluid shear stress in which a positive gel-shift was still evident at 4 h. Similar nuclear proteins/SSRE complexes did not form in cultured human aortic smooth muscle cells exposed to cyclic strain for various time intervals (data not shown).

Table 1. Hybrid promoters containing the SSRE core sequence (GAGACC) or its complementary sequence (GGTCTC) are shear-stress responsive

Construct	CAT activity		Fold induction
	Static	Shear	
CMV/CAT	275	261	1
SV/CAT	14	14	1
SV-SSRE/CAT	9	34	3.6
SV-(C)SSRE/CAT	11	40	3.8
SV-(5′)SSRE/CAT	12	15	1.3

BAEC were transfected with various reporter genes containing: the cytomegalovirus (CMV) promoter, the SV40 enhancerless promoter, the SV40 promoter coupled to the SSRE taken from the PDGF B promoter (SV-SSRE/CAT), the SV40 promoter coupled to the SSRE complementary sequence (SV-(C)SSRE/CAT), and the SV40 promoter coupled to the 5′ portion (non-core) of the SSRE (SV-(5′)SSRE/CAT). The transfected cultures were either subjected to shear stress (10 dynes/cm^2, 2 h) or incubated under static conditions. CAT activity was normalized to the efficiency of transfection.

842

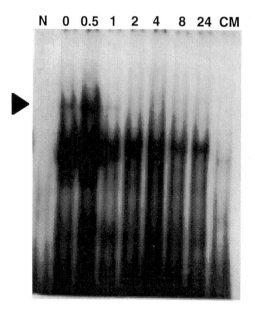

Fig. 2. Endothelial cells exposed to cyclic strain contain nuclear proteins that bind to the SSRE. HUVEC were exposed for various time intervals (0.5–24 h) to cyclic stretching (10% average strain, 60 cycles/min) in a FLEXERCELL system (FLEXERCELL Inc. Corp., McKeesport, PA) and their nuclei were extracted and incubated under conditions previously described [9] with a 30-mer PDGF B SSRE probe (containing the sequence CTCTCAGAGACC). A specific complex (arrow) was strongly induced 30 min after the exposure of the cells to cyclic strain but then declined to below control (unstretched) levels. N = no nuclear proteins, CM = competition with a 50-fold excess of a identical unlabeled probe.

Discussion

Hemodynamic forces acting on the vascular endothelium play an important role in the structural remodeling of the vasculature and in the development of atherosclerotic lesions [1–4,12,13]. Although the effects of these forces on vessel wall components have been studied both in vitro and in vivo, the molecular mechanisms mediating these changes are far from understood. In the studies summarized here, we have focused on the human PDGF B-chain gene, as a model, and have examined the molecular mechanisms regulating its expression at the level of transcription. These studies have led to the identification and characterization of a "shear-stress response element, SSRE", a cis-acting transcriptional regulatory element, which appears to be necessary for induction of this gene by physiological levels of shear stress. The insertion of this element into a minimal promoter construct generates a "hybrid promoter" that is shear-responsive and is sufficient to mediate induction of a reporter gene transfected into cultured endothelial cells. Although this SSRE does not encode a consensus binding site for known transcription factors, it does form specific complexes with nuclear proteins extracted from endothelial cells stimulated by exposure to physiological levels of laminar shear stress. The nature of these putative transcriptional factors that are activated by shear stress and interact with the SSRE in vascular endothelium is the subject of ongoing investigation.

In preliminary studies described here, we have examined the potential role of this molecular system in mediating gene regulation in response to a second type of hemodynamically generated force, cyclic strain. Unlike shear stress, which is a frictional force imparted selectively to the endothelial lining, cyclic strain results from the stretching of the vessel wall induced by arterial pulsatile flow and acts on both endothelium and smooth muscle. Interestingly, cyclic stretching of endothelial cells, but not smooth muscle cells, upregulates SSRE-nuclear protein binding, after only 30 min. These findings suggest that the SSRE may mediate endothelial responses to different types of biomechanical forces, and that this mechanism may be specific to cell type. Further studies are required to elucidate the biomechnical transduction and second-messenger coupling cascades that are activated in endothelial cells by these hemodynamic forces.

In conclusion, the discovery of a "shear stress response element (SSRE)" in the promoter of several endothelial genes provides a potential genetic regulatory mechanism to explain various biomechanically induced changes in endothelial function. Consideration of this mechanism, as well as other effector systems in the vessel wall, leads to a working concept of the endothelial cell as an important transducer and integrator of the local pathophysiologic milieu.

Acknowledgements

The authors thank D. Fenner for assistance in apparatus design and maintenance and Wm. Atkinson for assistance in the flow experiments. This research was supported primarily by grants from the National Institutes of Health (P01-HL36028; R01-HL51150).

References

1. Bell FP, Gallus AS, Schwartz CJ. Exp Mol Pathol 1974;20:281–287.
2. Caplan BA, Schwartz CJ. Atherosclerosis 1973;17:401.
3. Nerem RM, Levesque MJ, Cornhill JF. J Biochem Eng 1981;103:172–178.
4. Zarins CK, Giddens DP, Bharadvaj BK, Sottiurai VS, Mabson RF, Glagov S. Circ Res 1983;53:502–514.
5. Dewey CF, Bussolari SR, Gimbrone MA Jr, Davies PF. J Mechan Eng 1981;103:177–185.
6. Mills I, Cohen RC, Sumpio BE. In: Sumpio BE (ed) Hemodynamic Forces and Vascular Cell Biology. Austin, Texas: R.G. Landes Company, 1993;66–89.
7. Panaro NJ, McIntire LV. In: Sumpio BE (ed) Hemodynamic Forces and Vascular Cell Biology. Austin, Texas: R.G. Landes Company, 1993;47–65.
8. Davies PF, Tripathi SC. Circ Res 1993;72:239–245.
9. Resnick N, Collins T, Atkinson W, Bonthron DT, Dewey CF, Gimbrone MA Jr. Proc Natl Acad Sci 1993;90:4591–4595.
10. Nagel T, Resnick N, Atkinson WJ, Dewey CF, Gimbrone MA Jr. J Clin Invest 1994;94:885–891.
11. Isales C, Rosales O, Sumpio BE. In: Sumpio BE (ed) Hemodynamic Forces and Vascular Cell Biology. Austin Texas, R.G. Landes Company, 1993;90–115.
12. Ross R. Nature 1993;362:801–809.
13. Malek AM, Jackman R, Rosenberg RD, Izumo S. Circ Res 1994;174:852–860.
14. Gibbons GH, Dzau VJ. N Engl J Med 1994;330:1431–1438.

Arterial remodeling in response to altered blood flow

B. Lowell Langille and Avrum I. Gotlieb

Vascular Research Laboratory, Department of Pathology, Banting and Best Diabetes Centre, University of Toronto, The Toronto Hospital, Toronto, Ontario, Canada

Abstract. Vascular structures readily remodel in response to changes in intraluminal blood flows. This remodeling is invoked in the course of many developmental, physiological and pathological phenomena. Current work is providing novel clues concerning flow sensing by endothelial cells, the signal-transduction pathways that translate flow detection into endothelial responses, and some of the signals that are transmitted to the effector cells, namely the vascular smooth muscle cells in the media. Endothelial cells respond by altering their structure, both in terms of gross cell morphology and in terms of ultrastructure, especially the cytoskeleton. They also respond by altering their production of many mediators that affect other endothelial cells, smooth muscle cells and matrix to ultimately remodel the vessel. However, there is very little information on the processes that accomplish "remodeling" beyond evidence that modulation of new tissue synthesis occurs.

Structural remodeling of mature arteries in response to changes in perfusion probably contributes substantially to vessel growth and atrophy in many physiological situations including pregnancy and reproductive cycles, as well as to all vascular pathologies that alter arterial blood flow rates. Remodeling involves an acute vasomotor response followed by medial restructuring that entrenches diameter changes [1]. Both phases of remodeling are endothelium-dependent [2]. Vasodilation with increased flow is due to release of endothelium-derived relaxing factor (EDRF) in large arteries [3]. The extent to which arterial remodeling is secondary to chronic vasomotion versus a direct response to shear stress is unknown.

Endothelial structural responses to altered blood flow (shear stress)

Endothelial cells are directly exposed to the shear stresses produced by flowing blood. To maintain endothelial integrity, the cells must adhere firmly to their substratum and they must form tight junctions with adjacent cells. They must also adapt to changes in shear stress.

The sensitivity of endothelial cells to shear stress is evident from the gross morphology of the cells. Endothelial cells exposed to blood flow are long, thin and oriented in the direction of shear stress [4]. Experimentally induced changes in local flow conditions cause the cells to change shape and to reorient in a manner consistent with the altered flow pattern, or to lose any preferred orientation if flow is eliminated. There is also evidence of major intracellular adaptations of the cell cytoskeleton. For example, endothelial F-actin redistribution varies according to local patterns of shear stress [5]. Although in vivo shear-stress distribution is complex, there is a consensus that zones immediately downstream from branch sites are exposed to high shears. Endothelial cells in these areas do not exhibit the concentration of F-actin at the cell periphery seen at other

Address for correspondence: B. Lowell Langille PhD, The Toronto Hospital Research Institute, 200 Elizabeth Street, Toronto, ON, Canada M5G 2C4.

sites; instead, F-actin is redistributed into very long, thick stress fibers [5]. Other factors at branch sites could influence F-actin distribution; however, manipulations that elevate shear stress far from branch sites in vivo yield F-actin distribution that replicates that seen downstream from branches, and normal patterns are restored if shears are renormalized. Stress fibers are thought to protect the integrity of the endothelial lining when it is exposed to high shear forces.

The influences of shear stresses on the other major component of the cytoskeleton, the microtubules, is less well-defined. The microtubule-organizing centers from which microtubules emanate are predominantly on the heart side of the endothelial cell nucleus, but since this is true in veins (in which the heart is downstream) and arteries (in which the heart is upstream) [6], this interesting phenomenon is probably unrelated to shear stress.

We recently reported that decreased shear stress on endothelium led to monocyte adherence and transmigration across the endothelial monolayer of rabbit carotid arteries in vivo. This finding was intriguing given that low shear and monocyte uptake are both associated with early atherosclerotic lesions. It was possible that low shear favored monocyte uptake simply by reducing forces that would disrupt endothelial–monocyte adhesion. On the other hand, Li et al. [7] recently reported increased expression of vascular cell adhesion molecule type 1 (VCAM-1), a molecule that mediates endothelium–monocyte adhesion, at sites where atherosclerotic lesions form in hypercholesterolemic rabbits. We have shown that the expression of VCAM-1 is enhanced dramatically by reductions in blood flow rates [8], which suggests a possible causal mechanism linking low shear to monocyte uptake. VCAM-1 expression was also increased slightly by doubling of shear, thus a minimum in expression was observed at resting levels of shear stress. The response of VCAM-1 to reduced shear was selective. ICAM-1 expression was downregulated by decreased shear stress and upregulated by increased shear.

Our observations on in vivo expression of endothelial cell adhesion molecules are, in some ways, inconsistent with observations made in vitro. Shear caused no change in VCAM-1 expression in cultured endothelial cells [8]. Possibly this difference is due to secondary effects of arterial remodeling on VCAM-1 in vivo, or it may be due to modulating effects of blood constituents or matrix. ICAM-1 expression by endothelium in vitro was upregulated by shear only at very low shear stresses, below 2.5 dynes/cm^2. The graded responses that we saw over a more physiological shear range in vivo may again be secondary to mechanisms other than direct responses to shear.

The direct sensitivity of ICAM-1 expression only to very low shears has been reported for the PDGF B-chain [9] gene, whose promoter also possesses a shear-stress-responsive element [10]. Possibly other conditions modulate this shear sensitivity to yield a graded response in vivo. Failing this, modulation of expression only at very low shear stresses may be more relevant to conditions that induce stasis than to normal variations in blood flow rates.

Remodeling of the arterial media

Critical questions concerning how arterial remodeling is achieved remain unanswered. How is it possible, for example, for the smooth muscle cells that make all medial tissues to deliver newly synthesized tissue (elastin, matrix constituents, daughter cells) in the radial direction to thicken the wall when pressure rises, but to deliver these tissues in the circumferential direction to increase diameter when flow increases? Is this what happens? How are changes in smooth muscle and endothelial cell populations controlled? What communications between these cells are involved in regulating remodeling? These questions are central to our understanding of normal and abnormal arterial growth. Since cells of the vessel wall synthesize all constituents, local changes in this cell population are critical to all aspects of remodeling.

Remodeling of elastin

Elastin is one of the most important constituents in determining wall mechanical properties and geometry at physiological pressures, because elastin bears much of the total wall tension at physiological pressure. Elastin synthesis may therefore be critical to flow-induced remodeling processes. This has been proven in developing arteries, since both increased and decreased flow rates through carotid arteries of immature rabbits dramatically affect subsequent elastin accumulation in these vessels.

Regulation of elastin synthesis is complex. The elastin gene has been well characterized [11]. It is a single-copy gene of about 45 kb containing 35 (human) exons that are subject to alternative splicing of unknown significance. Transcription yields a 3.5-kb mRNA. The promoter region contains several SP-1- and AP2-binding sites as well as putative elements responsive to glucocorticoid, cAMP, and TPA. Expression is modulated by cortisol [12], insulin-like growth factor-1 (IGF-1) [13] and transforming growth factor type beta (TGF-β) [14]. TGF-β induces transcription of elastin after binding to a responsive element at -138 to -127 in the human gene [15], and it appears to regulate stability of elastin mRNA, at least in fibroblasts [16]. TGF-β is potentially very important because of growing evidence that this factor is critically important in regulating the synthesis of many constituents of the extracellular matrix. Furthermore, the promoter region of the TGF-β gene contains a putative shear-stress-responsive element [17].

Remodeling of elastin involves more than synthesis. Thus, Prosser et al. have shown that a distinct subpopulation of smooth muscle cells expresses elastin in pulmonary arteries of calves during experimental pulmonary hypertension [18] and we have demonstrated a similar subpopulation in normal aorta of lambs (Courtman, Koopmans and Langille, unpublished results). Thus, spatial variations in elastin accumulation can alter ultimate structure. No evidence pertains to the effects of changing blood flow on these subpopulations of smooth muscle.

There are additional mechanisms that restructure elastin in developing arteries. Elastin in large arteries forms concentric lamellae separated by single layers of smooth muscle cells. We have examined lamellar morphology at various ages in the rabbit carotid artery, using laser-scanning confocal microscopy to section optically whole-mount arterial preparations, and found that elliptical fenestrae through lamellae increase in size and number when blood flow rates are increased, at least in developing arteries (unpublished data). Thus enlarging lamellae when arteries increase in size involves, in part, enlarging fenestrae through the lamellae. The contribution of this phenomenon to remodeling of mature arteries is unknown.

Role of cell proliferation and cell death in arterial remodeling

The endothelial cell population of large arteries adjusts to changes in blood flow and subsequent arterial remodeling, so that there is a loss of these cells when blood flow decreases, such that the density of cells on the vessel surface (cells/mm^2) remains at control levels [1]. We did not detect a change in smooth muscle cell number in adult arteries when blood flow was chronically decreased for 1 month, but this may simply reflect the very slow turnover rate for these cells under normal conditions. With slow turnover it may take a very long time for mature vascular populations to be altered.

However, amplified or accelerated responses in immature arteries, in which cell replication rates are high, may provide insights into long-term remodeling. We have shown that smooth muscle cell populations in immature rabbit carotid arteries are sensitive to experimental changes in blood flow rates, especially decreases in flow rates [1]. We initially assumed that cell replication rates were being affected, but other mechanisms may be involved. Thus, we subsequently observed that increases in cell populations in neonatal lamb abdominal aortas were well below those predicted by cell replication rates [19] and we postulated, and now have evidence, that apoptosis (programmed cell death) may contribute to vascular remodeling. Apoptosis is cell suicide that can be induced by both physiological stimuli and toxic or traumatic insults. It differs from necrosis in that cells die singly, and then are phagocytosed by neighboring cells. Apoptosis is important in the embryonic morphogenesis of many tissues, but its role in later development or after maturation is poorly understood for most tissues.

Regulation of remodeling induced by hemodynamics

Both acute and chronic vascular responses to altered blood flow (shear stress) are mediated by endothelial cells. Shear-induced changes in endothelium include cell-shape changes and redistribution of cytoskeleton and organelles, cell proliferation, expression of cell-adhesion molecules, production of matrix constituents such as fibronectin, transport of macromolecules, and release of vasoactive substances, growth factors and modulators of thrombogenicity. The diversity of responses to shear stress may indicate that many signal-transduction pathways are activated. Signal transduction appears to involve G proteins [20] and the inositol pathway [21], and shear stimuli have been associated with opening of K^+ channels [22,23], hyperpolarization of the cell membrane [24,25] and increases in intracellular Ca^{2+} [26]. Shear-induced NO release activates guanylyl cyclase. Resulting cGMP production causes relaxation in smooth muscle and inhibits endothelin production in endothelium [27].

Both vasomotor and remodeling responses to altered shear require signaling between endothelium and medial smooth muscle. Vasoactive agents released by endothelium under shear stress include NO and PGI_2. Evidence concerning release of agents involved in growth and remodeling is limited. Release of both PDGF-B [9] and FGF [28] is shear-sensitive, and Resnick et al. [10] recently demonstrated a shear-sensitive response element in the PDGF-B chain promoter that also is found in other shear-sensitive genes including tissue-type plasminogen activator (tPA), TGF-β-1 and intercellular adhesion molecule type 1 (ICAM-1). These agents may contribute to remodeling both by changing cell proliferation/apoptosis rates and by altering matrix synthesis/degradation.

Acknowledgements

This work was supported in part by grant MI 6485, and MA 10029 from the Medical Research Council of Canada, grant T1259 from the Heart and Stroke Foundation of Ontario. B. Lowell Langille is a Career Investigator of the Heart and Stroke Foundation of Ontario.

References

1. Langille BL, Bendeck MP, Keeley FW. Am J Physiol 1989;256:H931–H939.
2. Langille BL, O'Donnell F. Science 1986;231:405–407.
3. Kaiser L, Hull SS Jr, Sparks HV Jr. Am J Physiol 1986;250:H974–H981.
4. Langille BL, Adamson SL. Circ Res 1981;48:481–488.

848

5. Kim DW, Langille BL, Wong MKK, Gotlieb AI. Circ Res 1989;64:21–31.
6. Rogers KA, Kalnins VI. Lab Invest 1983;49:650–654.
7. Li H, Cybulsky MI, Gimbrone MA Jr, Libby P. Arterioscler Thromb 1993;13:197–204.
8. Walpola PL, Gotlieb AI, Cybulsky MI, Langille BL. Arterioscler Thromb 1994 (in press).
9. Hsieh H-J, Li N-Q, Frangos JA. Am J Physiol 1991;260:H642–H646.
10. Resnick N, Collins T, Atkinson W, Bonthron DT, Dewey CF Jr, Gimbrone MA Jr. Proc Natl Acad Sci USA 1993;90:4591–4595.
11. Bashir MM, Indik Z, Yeh H, Ornstein-Goldstein N, Rosenbloom JC, Abrams W, Fazio M, Uitto J, Rosenbloom J. J Biol Chem 1989;264(15)8887–8891.
12. Keeley FW, Johnson DJ. Connect Tis Res 1987;16:259–268.
13. Rich CB, Ewton DZ, Martin BM, Florini JR, Bashir M, Rosenbloom J, Foster JA. Am J Physiol Lung Cell Mol Physiol 1992;263:L276–L282.
14. Kähäri V-M, Olsen DR, Rhudy RW, Carrillo P, Chen YQ, Uitto J. Lab Invest 1992;66:580–588.
15. Marigo V, Volpin D, Vitale G, Bressan GM. Biochem Biophys Res Commun 1994;199:1049–1056.
16. Kahari V-M, Olsen DR, Rhudy RW, Carillo P, Chen YQ, Uitto J. Lab Invest 1992;66:580–588.
17. Dive C, Gregory CD, Phipps DJ, Evans DL, Milner AE, Wyllie AH. Biochim Biophys Acta Mol Cell Res 1992;1133:275–285.
18. Prosser IW, Stenmark KR, Suthar M, Crouch EC, Mecham RP, Parks WC. Am J Pathol 1989;135:1073–1088.
19. Bendeck MP, Langille BL. Circ Res 1991;69:1165–1169.
20. Berthiaume F, Frangos JA. FEBS Lett 1992;308:277–279.
21. Prasad ARS, Logan SA, Nerem RM, Schwartz CJ, Sprague EA. Circ Res 1993;72:827–836.
22. Olesen SP, Clapham DE, Davies PF. Nature Lond 1988;331:168–170.
23. Cooke JP, Rossitch E Jr, Andon NA, Loscalzo J, Dzau VJ. J Clin Invest 1991;88:1663–1671.
24. Schwarz G, Droogmans G, Nilius B. Pflügers Arch 1992;421:394–396.
25. Berthiaume F, Frangos JA. Biochim Biophys Acta Bio Memb 1994;1191:209–218.
26. Mo M, Eskin SG, Schilling WP. Am J Physiol 1991;260:H1698–H1707.
27. Kuchan MJ, Frangos JA. Am J Physiol Heart Circ Physiol 1993;264:H150–H156.
28. Malek AM, Gibbons GH, Dzau VJ, Izumo S. J Clin Invest 1993;92:2013–2021.

Intermediate phenotypes in early primary hypertension: the Dutch Hypertension and Offspring Study

Diederick E. Grobbee, Ingrid M.S. van Hooft and Albert Hofman

Department Epidemiology and Biostatistics, Erasmus University Medical School, Rotterdam, The Netherlands

Hypertension is a state of chronic elevation of blood pressure (BP) associated with a well-demonstrated elevated risk of cardiovascular disease [1,2]. Many causes of high BP have been determined, yet in the vast majority of hypertensive patients a single etiologic factor cannot be found. Rather, in these cases of so-called 'primary hypertension' complex interactions between constitutional and environmental factors eventually result in sustained blood-pressure elevation. 'The cause' of hypertension, therefore, does not exist and it seems likely that the relative importance of specific factors in the etiology of primary hypertension varies across subgroups of patients. For certain subgroups, distinct genetic abnormalities may set the stage for subsequent deviations in mechanisms that regulate blood pressure. Such deviations may become apparent only under particular environmental conditions such as a high sodium intake. As a consequence of the complex and multi-factorial origin of hypertension, BP distributions in populations tend to be unimodal, with hypertension arbitrarily defined as the upper region [3]. Similarly, the cardiovascular risk related to BP elevation increases continuously and steadily across the range of BP values. Any subdivision of a population in normotensive and hypertensive subjects is thus subjective and based on pragmatic rather than physiologic considerations.

There is persuasive evidence that the roots of primary hypertension are to be found in childhood [4,5]. A gradual departure from the normal BP track during growth and maturation may eventually lead to a position of an individual's BP in the 'hypertensive' part of the distribution. Even small changes in the slope of BP with age, when maintained, may have profound consequences for the eventual adult BP level. In view of this, it is of interest to study hypertension in its early phase, early in life, in order to explore etiologic factors and mechanisms. There is yet another reason why the early phase of primary hypertension is of special interest in research. When hypertension is more marked and has been present for a prolonged period of time, the cardiovascular system will adapt to the chronic elevation of BP and several compensatory mechanisms may be activated. This may obfuscate the view on the underlying causal patterns. Indeed, in adult established hypertensive subjects the characteristics of BP regulation and circulatory adaptation tend to become ever more similar. In the search for the genetic basis of hypertension, the potential number of genes involved is overwhelming. BP level per se, as a phenotype, is inadequate as a means of delineating etiologically comparable subgroups of patients. Rather, mechanistic clusters that may characterize such subgroups need to be defined in order to indicate the underlying genetic abnormalities. In view of the above, these 'intermediate phenotypes' are the focus of research in the Dutch Hypertension and Offspring Study.

Address for correspondence: Prof D.E. Grobbee, Department of Epidemiology and Biostatistics, Erasmus University Medical School, P.O. Box 1738, 3000 DR Rotterdam, The Netherlands.

The Dutch Hypertension and Offspring Study

The Dutch Hypertension and Offspring Study was designed to describe mechanisms of potential etiological importance in primary hypertension [6]. With the support of the Netherlands Heart Foundation a group of Dutch investigators set out to list mechanisms likely to play a part in chronic BP elevation that could be studied in vivo in non-hospitalized subjects. For reasons described above, the population to be studied needed to be as 'prehypertensive' as possible, which implied a study group of relatively young subjects. Yet, given that prehypertensive subjects are normotensive by definition, an alternative means of finding future hypertensive and future normotensive subjects was needed and selection was based on familial risk [7].

There is a substantial body of data demonstrating the familial aggregation of elevated BP. Less certainty, however, exists as to the magnitude of risk of hypertension associated with a parental history of hypertension in a young individual [8]. This uncertainty has several explanations. First, the definition of hypertension is arbitrary and the degree of BP elevation in a parent is likely to be a major determinant of offspring risk. Next, a family history is but a crude indicator of familial risk. It often relies on recall of a diagnosis of hypertension without further specification. Moreover, the presence of one versus two hypertensive parents makes a clear difference. Even more problematic is the use of a history to define a group with normotensive parents. Inadequate recall and nondiagnosed hypertension, also in relation to the age and gender of the parent, may result in substantial misclassifaction. It is highly preferable to rely only on measured parental BP data in the selection of offspring at increased familial risk. Obviously, as in any diagnosis of hypertension, many readings over time are necessary to solidify the estimation of usual parental BP. Improved categorization of subjects with and without familial risk also has a drawback. As the difference in risk increases, so does the difference in BP level among the offspring. Differences in BP between subjects with hypertensive and normotensive parents are already present at birth and gradually become larger. In some studies involving groups with a different parental history of hypertension, the BP difference was considerable whereas in others hardly any dissimilarity in BP was observed. It has been shown that many of the discrepancies between studies of offspring of hypertensive and normotensive parents in group differences in BP may be traced back to differences in quality of parental classification and the resulting contrast in risk [9].

In the Dutch Hypertension and Offspring Study, subjects were selected on the basis of parental BP measured in a large population-based BP survey.

Methods

From 1975 to 1978, all the residents of two districts of the town of Zoetermeer, The Netherlands, were invited for measurement of BP and other cardiovascular risk factors as part of a study on determinants of chronic disabling disease [10]. Blood pressure was measured in 10,532 of the 13,462 eligible residents (78%). This group included 1,642 couples with children. A stringent selection procedure was applied to these couples to select groups whose children would have a maximal contrast in familial predisposition to hypertension. Individual parents with both systolic and diastolic BP in the upper (hypertensive) or lower (normotensive) quartile of the age- and sex-specific BP distribution were selected. Those who were receiving antihypertensive medication were included in the hypertensive group. Three groups of couples with children were invited for repeat measurement of BP for this study after a period of approximately 10 years: couples of which both members were normotensive, those with one normotensive and one hypertensive member, and those of which both members had hypertension. At the time of repeat measurement, the same criteria for hypertension and normotension were applied as at the initial screening. Of 250 couples that were remeasured (80% of those invited), 121 were still in the BP category to which they had originally been assigned: 35 couples of which both members were normotensive, 35 with one normotensive and one hypertensive member, and 51 of which both members were hypertensive. These 121 couples had 291 healthy biological children, all of whom were invited to take part in this study. Of these children, who ranged from 7 to 32 years of age, 154 participated: 41 with two normotensive parents, 52 with one normotensive and one hypertensive parent, and 61 with two hypertensive parents. The BP values and other characteristics of the parents and their children (subjects) at the time of enrolment are shown in Table 1. The study protocol was approved by the ethics committee of the University Hospital Dijkzigt, and informed consent was obtained from the subjects and their parents.

The participants visited the Dutch Hypertension and Offspring Study Research Centre for a series of sessions at which various measurements were performed. These ranged from simple BP measurement and collection of blood and urine samples to ultrasound evaluation of the heart and carotid arteries and electrolyte challenge. Also, 24-h ambulatory BP was recorded and the groups underwent protocols in which they were submitted to physical and psychological stresses. For the purpose of this paper, by way of example, findings on renal hemodynamics are given in some detail [11].

Table 1. Blood pressure and related characteristics of subjects and their parents, according to study group[a]

Characteristic	Two normotensive parents	One normotensive and one hypertensive parents	Two hypertensive parents
Parents			
No. of couples	29	30	38
Age (yr)	46.7 ± 8.8	50.9 ± 8.9	52.1 ± 8.3
Blood pressure (mmHg)			
Systolic	111.3 ± 6.3	133.0 ± 11.4	151.8 ± 14.1
Diastolic	68.5 ± 5.4	80.6 ± 6.9	89.8 ± 6.4
Drug treatment for hypertension (%)	0	23.3	38.2
Subjects			
Sex (M/F)	25/16	27/25	37/24
Age (yr)	21.3 ± 7.0	22.1 ± 6.1	23.4 ± 5.9
Height (cm)	170.0 ± 17.8	172.8 ± 13.3	175.2 ± 11.4
Weight (kg)	62.5 ± 19.2	63.6 ± 13.5	68.2 ± 13.5
Blood pressure (mmHg)			
Systolic	117.7 ± 11.2	124.8 ± 13.1	128.0 ± 10.6
Diastolic	71.1 ± 8.7	75.8 ± 9.7	78.8 ± 7.8
Adjusted blood pressure (mmHg)[b]			
Systolic	119.3 ± 9.3	125.4 ± 9.4	126.5 ± 9.4
Diastolic	71.6 ± 8.6	75.8 ± 8.6	78.4 ± 8.6
Serum sodium (mmol/l)	141 ± 2.0	141 ± 2.3	141 ± 2.3
Urinary sodium (mmol/24 h)	126 ± 51	136 ± 65	135 ± 49
Serum potassium (mmol/l)	4.1 ± 0.3	4.2 ± 0.3	4.2 ± 0.3
Urinary potassium (mmol/24 h)	67.7 ± 27.1	68.3 ± 25.5	63.8 ± 22.3

[a]Values are mean ± SD.
[b]Adjusted for differences among the groups in age, height, weight, and proportion of males.

852

All the subjects collected a 24-h urine sample during the day before their visit to the Research Centre. Their usual diet was not altered, but they were asked to refrain from smoking and from drinking coffee. At the examination centre, BP was measured at the left arm with a random-zero sphygmomanometer. Before the beginning of the renal-function tests, an intravenous cannula was inserted: the subject then remained supine in a quiet room for 30 min, after which fasting venous blood samples were collected for measurement of immunoreactive angiotensin II, plasma renin activity and renin, prorenin, and aldosterone concentrations. For the renal-function tests, a second intravenous cannula was inserted in the opposite arm. The effective renal plasma flow and glomerular filtration rate were calculated on the basis of measurements of the clearance of para-aminohippuric acid and inulin with use of a constant-infusion technique and timed collections of urine. Urine samples were collected by active voiding before and 1.5 and 2.5 h after the beginning of the infusion. Blood samples were collected just after voiding. Clearance rates were calculated from both the rate of intravenous infusion and the rate of urinary excretion for the 1-h period between 1.5 and 2.5 h after the beginning of the infusion.

Results

The findings on renal hemodynamics are given in Table 2. The mean renal blood flow was lower in the subjects with two hypertensive parents than in those with two normotensive parents (mean difference $\pm$SE, 198 $\pm$ 61 ml/min per 1.73 m^2 of body-surface area; p = 0.002). Moreover, both the filtration fraction and renal vascular resistance were higher in the subjects with two hypertensive parents (filtration fraction: mean difference, 3.0 $\pm$ 1.1 percentage points; p = 0.006; renal vascular resistance: mean difference, 2.7 $\pm$ 0.8 mmHg/dl/min per 1.73 m^2; p = 0.006). The subjects with two hypertensive parents had lower plasma concentrations of renin (mean difference, 3.3 $\pm$ 1.6 mU/l; p = 0.03) and aldosterone (mean difference, 111 $\pm$ 36 pmol/l; p = 0.003) than those with two normotensive parents. The values in the subjects with one hypertensive and one normotensive parent fell between those for the other two groups.

Conclusion

The findings on renal hemodynamics in the Dutch Hypertension and Offspring Study suggest renal vasoconstriction in young persons at risk for hypertension. These findings support the hypothesis that alterations in renal hemodynamics occur at an early stage in the development of primary hypertension. Moreover, the hemodynamic alterations are accompanied by reduced renin and aldosterone secretion. Renal vasoconstriction and changes in the renin–angiotensin–aldosterone system may demarcate a subgroup of prehypertensive subjects with a congruous etiologic abnormality, potentially of genetic origin. The importance of the kidney in BP as a long-term regulator of blood volume and BP is well recognized [12]. From elegant kidney transplant experiments in animals and humans it appears that 'hypertension goes with the kidney'. In humans, essential hypertensive patients with nephrosclerosis who received a kidney from a normotensive donor became normotensive [13]. Kidney transplant recipients with a negative family history of hypertension receiving a kidney from a normotensive donor with a positive family history of hypertension needed more antihypertensive treatment after transplantation than did recipients of a kidney from a normotensive donor with a negative family history of hypertension [14]. The renal findings in the Dutch Hypertension and Offspring Study, as intermediate phenotypes of primary hypertension, are compatible with the presence of a genetic abnormality leading to these hemodynamic changes in subgroups of hypertensive patients.

Table 2. Renal hemodynamics in the offspring groups participating in the Dutch Hypertension and Offspring Study

Characteristic	Two normotensive parents	One normotensive and one hypertensive parent	Two hypertensive parents
Urine method			
Effective renal plasma flow (ml/min/1.73 m²)	709 ± 30	584 ± 25[a]	591 ± 21[a]
Renal blood flow (ml/min/1.73 m²)	1132 ± 50	934 ± 41[2]	934 ± 35[a]
Glomerular filtration rate (ml/min/1.73 m²)	147 ± 6	127 ± 5[b]	137 ± 4
Filtration fraction (%)	20.9 ± 0.9	22.0 ± 0.7	23.9 ± 0.6[a]
Renal vascular resistance (mmHg/dl/min/1.73 m²)	7.6 ± 0.6	9.5 ± 0.5[b]	10.3 ± 0.4[a]
Plasma method			
Effective renal plasma flow (ml/min/1.73 m²)	566 ± 18	516 ± 14[b]	531 ± 13
Renal blood flow (ml/min/1.73 m²)	903 ± 29	828 ± 23[b]	847 ± 20
Glomerular filtration rate (ml/min/1.73 m²)	119 ± 3	114 ± 2	121 ± 2
Filtration fraction (%)	21.8 ± 0.7	22.3 ± 0.6	23.1 ± 0.5
Renal vascular resistance (mmHg/dl/min/1.73 m²)	9.1 ± 0.4	10.5 ± 0.3[a]	10.4 ± 0.3[a]

Values are mean ± SE, adjusted for differences in age and sex.
[a] $p < 0.01$ for the comparison with the subjects with two normotensive parents;
[b] $p < 0.05$ for this comparison.

The mechanisms responsible for the decrease in renal blood flow, the increase in renal vascular resistance and the filtration fraction, and the decrease in the plasma renin and aldosterone levels in the early phase of essential hypertension remain to be established. Increased renal vasoconstriction may reduce renal blood flow if the BP and cardiac output remain normal. The combination of reduced renal blood flow with an increased filtration fraction and a reduced plasma renin concentration might point to an increase in resistance in renal efferent arterioles. Dluhy and co-workers proposed the presence of 'non-modulators' in subjects with a family history of hypertension [15], who are characterized by an inability to modulate normally the responsiveness of the renal arteries and adrenal gland to angiotensin II at different levels of sodium intake. Such nonmodulation could reflect increased renal vasoconstriction. In the Dutch Hypertension and Offspring Study several characteristics of the normotensive subjects with hypertensive parents were compatible with nonmodulation. In particular, the reduced renal blood flow in subjects with hypertensive parents resembled the reduced renal blood flow observed in non-modulators with a high salt intake [16,17], and the reduced ratio of plasma aldosterone to plasma angiotensin II is analogous to the diminished responsiveness of aldosterone to infused angiotensin II. However, we found differences between the groups of subjects in our study without the infusion of vasoactive substances, perhaps because of the large contrast in familial predisposition to hypertension among the groups, which resulted from the strict selection criteria.

854

It has been postulated that a primary defect residing in the kidney decreases water and sodium excretion [18]. Many mechanisms in the kidney contribute to its sodium excretion capacity [19], both intrinsic mechanisms such as a redistribution of blood flow between cortical and juxta-medullary nephrons [20], the glomerulo-tubular balance, the tubulo-glomerular feedback, and the renin–angiotensin system may be important. Major extra-renal mechanisms include renal perfusion pressure and flow. A reduced sodium excretory capacity in certain individuals at risk for high BP is likely to express itself in particular under high sodium intake.

Our findings on renal hemodynamics serve to illustrate the potential of the family history approach in research on the etiology of hypertension. The use of BP measurements in parents to select offspring at contrasting risk of high BP provides for the study of intermediate phenotypes at a time when the mechanistic characteristics of the hypertensive circulation have not yet been modified by a prolonged BP elevation. However, even in this approach a predictable consequence of careful selection is the presence of BP differences across the groups of offspring. Paradoxically, the better the selection the larger the difference. Such difference cannot be circumvented, at whatever age the offspring is studied [21]. An artificial way to deal with this problem to some extent is to adjust differences in characteristics for the difference in BP. Our findings on renal hemodynamics were not affected when statistical adjustments were made for the BP's potential confounding effects. A hazard of this procedure is over-adjustment, as those subjects with familial risk who have the highest age-specific BP may be those with the clearest abnormalities. At present no satisfactory solution for this problem is available.

In addition to the kidney, the Dutch Hypertension and Offspring Study has explored central hemodynamics [22,23], the sympathetic nervous system, sodium- and volume-regulating hormones [24,25], calcium homeostasis [26] and various other mechanisms potentially involved in the etiology of primary hypertension. The availability of DNA samples of the participants allows targeted exploration of genetic polymorphisms [27]. Follow-up of the participants in the study as they develop sustained hypertension or remain normotensive with age, will add further to the knowledge to be gained from the data collected in the groups. Finally, the general approach adopted in the study may similarly be used for research on other chronic conditions, such as COPD, that express their morbid consequences in the middle-aged and the elderly but have their roots early in life.

Acknowledgements

Supported by grant No. 35.004 from the Netherlands Heart Foundation.

References

1. MacMahon S, Peto R, Cutler J, Collins R, Sorlie P, Neaton J, Abbott R, Godwin J, Dyer A, Stamler J. Lancet 1990;335:765–774.
2. Bots ML, Grobbee DE, Hofman A. Epidemiologic Rev 1991;13:294–314.
3. Swales JD, ed. Platt versus Pickering: An episode in recent medical history. London: The Keyness Press, 1986.
4. Hofman A, Grobbee DE, Schalekamp MADH, eds. The Early Pathogenesis of Primary Hypertension. Amsterdam: Elsevier, 1987.
5. Launer LJ, Hofman A, Grobbee DE. Br Med J 1993;307:1451–1454.
6. van Hooft IMS, Grobbee DE, Hofman A, Valkenburg HA. Int J Epidemiol 1988;17:228–229.
7. Watt G. J Hypertens 1986;4:1–7.
8. Grobbee DE. J Am Coll Nutr 1992;11:55S–9.

9. De Visser DC, Mulder PGH, van Doornen LJP, Grobbee DE. In: Stress-reactivity in the Dutch Hypertension and Offspring Study: An Epidemiological Approach to the Psychophysiology of Early Hypertension (Dissertation). Rotterdam, The Netherlands: Erasmus University Rotterdam, 1994;17—48.
10. Hoes AW, Grobbee DE, Valkenburg HA, Lubsen J, Hofman A. Eur J Epidemiol 1993;9:285—292.
11. van Hooft IMS, Grobbee DE, Derkx FHM, Leeuw PW de, Schalekamp MADH, Hofman A. N Engl J Med 1991;324:1305—1311.
12. Mizell HL, Montani JP, Hester RL, Didlake RH, Hall JE. Hypertension 1993;22:102—110.
13. Curtis JJ, Luke RG, Dustan HP, Kashgarian M, Whelchel JD, Jones P, Diethelm AG. New Engl J Med 1983;309:1009—1015.
14. Guiddi E, Bianchi G, Rivolta E, Ponticelli C, Quarto di Palo F, Minetti L, Polli E. Nephron 1985;41:14—21.
15. Dluhy RG, Hopkins P, Hollenberg NK, Williams GH, Williams RR. J Cardiovasc Pharmacol 1988;12 (suppl 3): 149—154.
16. Shoback DM, Williams GH, Moore TJ, Dluhy RG, Podolsky S, Hollenberg NK. J Clin Invest 1983;72: 2115—2124.
17. Hollenberg NK, Moore T, Shoback D, Redgrave J, Rabinowe S, Williams GH. Am J Med 1986;81:412—418.
18. De Wardener HE, MacGregor GA. Kidney Int 1980;18:1—9.
19. Bianchi G. In: Zanchetti A, Tarazi RC (eds) Handbook of Hypertension, Vol 8: Pathophysiology of Hypertension — Regulatory Mechanisms. Amsterdam: Elsevier, 1986;278—294.
20. Britton KE. Lancet 1981;ii:900—902.
21. van Hooft IMS, Hofman A, Grobbee DE, Valkenburg HA. J Hypertens 1988;6:S594—S596.
22. van Hooft IMS, Grobbee DE, Waal-Manning HJ, Hofman A. J Hypertens 1989;7(suppl 6):S66—S67.
23. van Hooft IMS, Grobbee DE, Waal-Manning HJ, Hofman A. Circulation 1993;87:1100—1106.
24. van Hooft IMS, Grobbee DE, Hofman A, Schiffers P, de Pont JJHHM. N Engl J Med 1988;320:867—868.
25. van Hooft IMS, Schiffers P, Grobbee DE, Rahn KH, Hofman A. J Hypertens 1989;7(suppl 1):S43—S44.
26. van Hooft IMS, Grobbee DE, Frölich M, Pols HAP, Hofman A. Alterations in calcium metabolism in young people at risk for primary hypertension. Hypertension.
27. Schmidt S, van Hooft IMS, Grobbee DE, Ganten D, Ritz E. J Hypertens 1993;11:345—348.

Finding the genes for human hypertension

Roger R. Williams[1], Steven C. Hunt[1], Paul N. Hopkins[1], Sandra J. Hasstedt[2], Lily L. Wu[1,3] and Jean Marc Lalouel[2,4]

[1]*Department of Internal Medicine, Cardiology Division;* [2] *Department of Human Genetics;* [3]*Department of Pathology; and* [4]*Howard Hughes Medical Institute, University of Utah Medical School, Salt Lake City, UT 84132, USA*

Abstract. This is a brief review of studies suggesting specific genetic traits that may be related to essential hypertension in humans. Pedigree analysis suggests six segregating major gene traits (low urinary kallikrein excretion, high fasting plasma insulin level, high sodium–lithium countertransport, a fat pattern index, dense LDL subfractions, and body mass index). 22 candidate genes localized on 15 different chromosomes are also listed. Two of them (GRA and AGT) are well established. Glucocorticoid-remediable aldosteronism (GRA) is caused by a mutation on chromosome 8q21 that leads to high levels of abnormal adrenal steroid hormones and early stroke deaths from early severe hypertension unresponsive to ordinary medications but very responsive to glucocorticoid hormone treatment. The angiotensinogen (AGT) locus on chromosome 1q42 has been consistently related to hypertension in several sibship linkage studies. In some but not all studies a specific AGT variant was associated with hypertension and with higher angiotensinogen levels. Genes at this locus seem to promote both essential hypertension and pre-eclampsia.

High blood pressure (HBP) has a significant genetic component, but a lack of phenotypic specificity, multifactorial determination and etiological heterogeneity contribute to a confused picture eluding conventional approaches of classical Mendelian genetics. The consensus has emerged, however, that there is a reasonable likelihood that such genetic determinants can be identified by a combination of molecular marker technology and robust, model-independent methods to infer genetic linkage and association.

Different subgroups of hypertension

Because HBP is heterogeneous, the search for genes should begin with the definition of informative subtypes based on clues to pathophysiology. Several subgroups are quite intuitive: severe hypertension, early age at onset, thin versus obese, those with or without strong family history of coronary disease or stroke. Others are more complex and described below.

Dyslipidemia, hyperinsulinemia and hypertension

A clustering of HBP with metabolic factors has been reported using a variety of titles including familial dyslipidemic hypertension (FDH), insulin-resistance syndrome (IRS), plurimetabolic syndrome, and Syndrome X [1]. Dyslipidemic hypertension seems to represent a subset with much stronger coronary risk. In the NHLBI twin study, dyslipidemic hypertensives had a 16-year coronary mortality rate 4 times as great as persons with either dyslipidemia or hypertension alone or with neither factor [2]. In Utah about one-fifth of population-based families with early CHD had FDH [1].

Address for correspondence: Cardiovascular Genetics Research Clinic, 410 Chipeta Way, Room 161, Salt Lake City, UT 84108, USA.

Nonmodulation of the renin–angiotensin system

A blunted response of renal blood flow change and aldosterone secretion after intravenous infusion of angiotensin II aggregates strongly in families and seems to identify a subset of patients with hypertension who respond particularly well to inhibitors of angiotensin converting enzyme (ACE) [3]. It has also been suggested that these 'nonmodulators' have sodium-sensitive hypertension.

Interactions of electrolyte and energy metabolism

Several studies show that fasting insulin predicts 'sodium sensitivity' [4]. Obesity-induced hyperinsulinemia potentiates increase of blood pressure with sodium loading, and weight reduction abolishes both hyperinsulinemia and sodium sensitivity [4].

Hypertension in American Blacks

It has been suggested that 'selective survival' led to the enrichment of genes promoting hypertension among Black Americans [5]. Several characteristics reported to be prominent in this group include increased 'sodium sensitivity', lower urinary kallikrein excretion and plasma renin activity, different means for cation-flux test rates, good response to diuretics but poorer response to ACE inhibitors, higher frequency of AGT variants reported in some studies associated with HBP, stronger familial correlations for urinary aldosterone levels, and association of HBP with MNS blood type and haptoglobin.

Segregating traits and hypertension

Mendelian models (recessive, additive or dominant inheritance) combined with a poly-genic background ('mixed model'), age and environmental factors affecting penetrance have been tested using likelihood analysis [4]. The results for several traits possibly related to hypertension are summarized in Table 1. The predominantly 'recessive' results may reflect the presence of two or more common segregating 'HBP genes' in persons with hypertension (i.e., persons with hypertension being compound heterozygotes rather than true homozygotes).

Low urinary kallikrein excretion

Kallikrein, a vasodilating substance, was excreted in lower amounts in offspring of

Table 1. Candidate traits from segregation analysis

Traits	Mode	Heritability (%)		
		Total	Major gene	Polygenic
1. SLC	Recessive	80	34	46
2. Urinary kallikrein	Additive	78	51	27
3. High fasting insulin	Recessive	44	33	11
4. Fat pattern index	Recessive	52	42	10
5. Dense LDL	Dominant	29	?	?
6. Body Mass Index	Recessive	70	37	33

The total heritability (percent of variance attributable to all genetic factors) has been partitioned into single-gene effects (major gene) and blended multiple-gene effects (polygenic) using maximum likelihood analysis.

hypertensive parents than in offspring of normotensive parents [4]. It has also been found to segregate as a monogenic trait [4] and to show significant interactions with urinary potassium excretion (a good indirect measure of dietary potassium intake). High and low kallikrein homozygotes should respectively have low and high risk of hypertension. Approximately 50% of the general population who are heterozygous for this trait are inferred to have a special genetic susceptibility for the effects of dietary potassium on HBP risk. More risk of hypertension would follow a low potassium diet and lower risk of HBP would follow a diet high in potassium [4].

Erythrocyte sodium–lithium countertransport (SLC)

Three independent studies have suggested segregating single-gene effects for SLC [4]. About 5% of the general population who are high SLC homozygotes had twice the rate of hypertension in cross-sectional data and 4 times the rate of hypertension in prospective follow-up [4]. They also had increased triglycerides, skinfold thicknesses and body mass index, suggesting that this genetic trait relates to metabolic factors.

Segregating high fasting insulin in NIDDM families

A 3-fold elevation in fasting insulin levels segregated as a homozygous trait among 271 normoglycemic family members in 16 large Utah pedigrees ascertained from two siblings with non-insulin-dependent diabetes mellitus (NIDDM). The high homozygotes for fasting hyperinsulinemia were also found to have lower levels of HDL-cholesterol and approximately twice the frequency of hypertension of other inferred genotypes.

Other segregating major gene traits of interest regarding hypertension include an index of body fat distribution, dense LDL subfractions, and body mass index [4]. These also relate to the plurimetabolic cluster.

Candidate loci for hypertension

Table 2 lists 22 candidate loci for hypertension. Those on the left side of the table have been connected with HBP in one or more studies of DNA markers using linkage, association, or candidate-gene sequencing as indicated in the table. Some of them deserve further discussion.

Linkage and association of AGT gene to hypertension and pre-eclampsia

Studies in Paris, Utah and Japan reported that the angiotensinogen locus on chromosome 1q42 predisposes to essential hypertension [6] and pregnancy-induced hypertension [7]. Sibship linkage found excess sharing of alleles at this locus [6]. A specific genetic variant (M235T) was observed significantly more often in hypertensive cases than in matched controls [6], in pre-eclampsia or pregnancy-induced hypertension cases than in pregnant controls [7], and in minorities (Black and Asian) than in Caucasian [6]. Persons homozygous for the AGT M235T variant gene showed angiotensinogen levels that were 20–50% higher than persons homozygous for the usual gene in Caucasians. Other, subsequent studies have consistently found linkage of HBP to the AGT locus; however, some studies have not found the M235T variant associated with hypertension.

Angiotensinogen is the rate-limiting substrate for the renal hormone renin to cleave in the production of angiotensin. Levels of angiotensinogen correlate with blood pressure and are higher in offspring of hypertensive parents. Blood pressure increases in response to angiotensinogen infusion and drops in response to antibodies to angiotensinogen. Tumors

Table 2. Candidate gene loci for hypertension

Candidate genes related to HBP in some studies			Theoretical candidates to study	
Studied genetic trait	Chromosome	Method	Other candidates	Chromosome
1. GRA hypertension	8 q 21	M	12. Kallikrein	19
2. Angiotensinogen	1 q 42	SL,A,BL	13. Kallikrein binding protein	14
3. Lipoprotein lipase deficiency	8 p 22	M	14. A-II:A-I receptor	3
4. LDL receptor	19 p 13	PL, A	15. Na$^+$H$^+$ antiporter	1
5. Insulin receptor	19 p 13	A	16. Na$^+$K$^+$ATPase	1,13
6. ACE	17 q 23	A	17. Endothelin 1,2,3	6,1,2
7. HLA	6 p 21	SL,A	18. 'SA' locus	16
8. Renin	1 q 32	A	19. VLDL receptor	9
9. MN blood type	4	L	20. Nitric oxide synthase	7
10. Haptoglobin	16 q 22	L	21. Adrenoreceptors	5,10
11. Heat shock protein	14 q 22	A	22. Fibrinogen	4

Methods for suggesting a candidate locus:
A = Genetic marker associated with cases vs. controls.
BL = Pertinent blood levels are different in persons of relevant genotypes.
M = Functional mutations sequenced for this syndrome. PL = Pedigree linkage with cosegregation.
SL = Sibship linkage with excess sharing of alleles.

found to secrete it cause hypertension, and an AGT gene can cause hypertension in transgenic mice.

Animal studies [8] suggest that much of the effect of angiotensinogen may be at a local tissue level. AGT messenger RNA and angiotensinogen levels in adipose tissue were dramatically affected by genetic obesity and overfeeding (Fig. 1). Both produced local vasoconstriction, decreased fat-pad perfusion, decreased insulin sensitivity and elevated systemic blood pressure. Fasting caused the opposite effect. These observations provide another piece of the puzzle involving salt, lipids, insulin, and hypertension.

Angiotensinogen in Adipose Tissue (Animal Studies)

Gene Effect or Diet Condition	Influence on Tissue Angiotensinogen		Local Vessel Response causes changes in Fat Perfusion & BP			
Setting	**Adipose Tissue Levels** m-RNA	Hormone ★	Flow	SBP	**Insulin Sensitivity**	**F.Acid EFFLUX**
Fasting 3 days	↓↓ (1/7)	↓↓ (1/3)	↑	↓	↑	↑
Feeding 6 days	↑↑ (2.3)	↑↑ (1.8)	↓	↑	↓	↓
ob/ob Mouse (Genetic Obesity)		↑↑ (3.4)	↓	↑	↓	↓

Frederich RC et al. Hypertension 1992; 19:339-344.
★Adipose tissue levels of angiotensinogen changed as shown while liver and plasma levels showed NO CHANGE.

Fig. 1. An animal obesity gene and overfeeding both promote high adipose tissue levels of angiotensinogen. Fasting has the opposite effect. It is interesting to note that these changes in adipose angiotensinogen are associated with changes in blood pressure, insulin sensitivity and fatty acid efflux. Perhaps these are some of the pieces in the pathophysiologic puzzle involving metabolic syndromes with hypertension. This information is summarized from a discussion presented in [8].

Direct sequencing of two candidate genes for HBP

The best documented gene for hypertension is 'Glucocorticoid Remediable Aldosteronism' (GRA). Causal mutations were sequenced [9] at a candidate locus on chromosome 8q21 that encodes for aldosterone synthase and steroid β-hydroxylase (two genes that are 95% identical). The abnormal gene induced production of high levels of abnormal adrenal steroids (18-oxocortisol and 18-hydroxycortisol). Carriers of this autosomal dominant mutation develop high-percentile blood pressures as youths, severe hypertension as young adults, and cerebrovascular accidents as middle-aged adults. GRA hypertension does not respond to ordinary antihypertensive medications but responds well to aldosterone antagonists or glucocorticoid hormone therapy.

Heterozygous lipoprotein lipase deficiency appears to be a reasonable candidate for promoting familial dyslipidemic hypertension (FDH). A variant of the lipoprotein lipase locus on chromosome 8p22 was first sequenced from the DNA of a homozygously affected person with classical type I hyperlipidemia, and this identified an amino acid substitution at residue 188 [1]. In vitro expression of this mutation demonstrated an immunologically detectable but enzymatically inactive species of lipoprotein lipase. From genealogical expansion and clinical screening of 106 individuals in this pedigree, 29 heterozygous carriers were detected [1]. Over age 40, 58% of gene carriers had triglyceride levels above the 95th percentile and HDL-cholesterol below the 5th percentile, and 68% of these gene carriers had hypertension.

A general model for genes promoting HBP

Figure 2 proposes that genes and appropriate environmental factors work together to cause several different types of hypertension. The GRA gene appears to be capable of causing

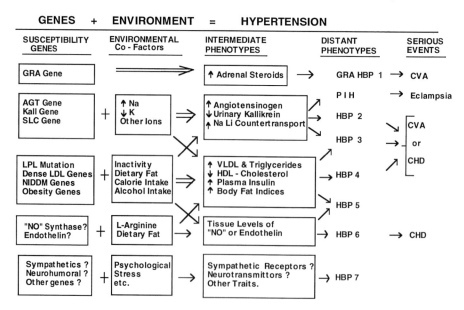

Fig. 2. A model proposing that certain genes producing susceptibility to hypertension are augmented by environmental cofactors and other genes. Measurable 'intermediate phenotypes' are thought to reflect the causal genes and environmental influences more directly. The final but nonspecific 'distant phenotype' expressions are different (but often indistinguishable) forms of hypertension and serious complications.

hypertension without environmental factors. Other genes related to cations probably interact with dietary intake of sodium, potassium and other cations to promote essential hypertension. Many persons with hypertension probably carry several predisposing genes and environmental factors. HBP may also be promoted by genes affecting lipids, obesity, and insulin balance, especially with low levels of physical activity and rich diet. Other candidate genes and environmental factors are included in Fig. 1 to suggest other mechanisms that may be involved at a local tissue and cellular level. For example, endothelin is a potent vasoconstrictor [10] and nitric oxide is a potent vasodilator [11]. Genetic factors influencing either of these two candidates could dramatically affect a person's risk of hypertension and atherosclerosis via endothelial and local effects.

Summary and recommendations

The lists of "candidate genes" for HBP has grown rapidly. In Grim and Robinson's review article 271 candidates are listed for hypertension and atherosclerosis [5]. Indeed, 240 evenly spaced anonymous markers could cover the whole human genome at about 20 cm intervals with 'shotgun linkage'. At any rate, selected environmental factors will probably have relevance for specific genetic traits (sodium with the angiotensinogen locus, potassium with the kallikrein trait, obesity and exercise with the lipoprotein lipase mutation, etc.). Powerful molecular and statistical tools now allow us to identify genetic traits accurately and begin testing for their environmental cofactors. This should lead to more effective diagnosis, prevention and treatment of hypertension.

Acknowledgements

Utah projects generating much of the data presented in this review were supported by several grants including HL21088, HL245855, HL47466, HL45325, HL45321, HL44738, and HL47651 from the National Heart, Lung and Blood Institute, Bethesda, MD. Dr Lalouel is an investigator of the Howard Hughes Medical Institute.

References

(Because of limited space, most references are review articles which in turn cite original studies too numerous to include in this brief report.)

1. Williams RR, Hopkins PN, Hunt SC, Schumacher MC, Elbein SC, Wilson DE, Stults BM, Wu LL, Hasstedt SJ, Lalouel JM. Ann Med 1992;24:469−475.
2. Selby JV, Newman B, Quiroga J et al. J Am Med Assoc 1991;265:2079−2084.
3. Lifton RP, Hopkins PN, Williams RR, Hollenberg NK, Williams GH, Dluhy RG. Hypertension 1989;13:884−889.
4. Williams RR, Hunt SC, Hopkins PN, Hasstedt SJ, Wu LL, Lalouel JM. Kidney Intl 1994;45(suppl 44):S57−S64.
5. Grim CE and Robinson MT. In: Goldbourt U, DeFaire U, Berg K (eds) Genetic Factors in Coronary Heart Disease. London: Kluwer Academic Publishers, 1994;153−177.
6. Jeunemaitre X, Soubrier F, Kotelevtsev YV, Lifton RP, Williams CS, Charru A, Hunt SC, Hopkins PN, Williams RR, Lalouel JM, Corvol P. Cell 1992;71:169−180.
7. Ward K, Hata A, Jeunemaitre X, Helin C, Nelson L, Namikawa C, Farrington PF, Ogasawara M, Suzumori K, Tomoda S, Berrebi S, Sasaki M, Corvol P, Lifton RP, Lalouel JM. Nature Genet 1993;4:59−61.
8. Frederich RC, Kahn BB, Peach MJ, Flier JS. Hypertension 1992;19:339−344.
9. Lifton RP, Dluhy RG, Powers M, Rich GM, Cook S, Ulick S, Lalouel JM. Nature 1992;355:262−265.
10. Mortensen LH, Fink GD. Hypertension 1992;19:549−554.
11. Ress DD, Palmer RMJ, Moncada S. Proc Natl Acad Sci USA 1989;86:3375−3378.

862

Atherosclerosis X.
F.P. Woodford, J. Davignon and A. Sniderman, editors.

Variants of the angiotensin converting enzyme gene are associated with high blood pressure and myocardial infarction

Herbert Schuster, Thomas F. Wienker and Friedrich C. Luft

The Franz Volhard Clinic, Rudolf Virchow University Hospitals and the Max Delbrück Center for Molecular Medicine, Free University of Berlin, Berlin, Germany

Abstract. Polymorphisms of the angiotensin converting enzyme (ACE) gene have been associated with hypertension and myocardial infarction. We studied 95 hypertensive patients and 51 control subjects. The controls had no family history of hypertension in either parent. The insertion (I) and deletion (D) alleles of the ACE gene were determined by means of the polymerase chain reaction. We found that the I allele was associated with hypertension (relative risk 2.57). We also studied 390 consecutive patients who had coronary angiography performed because of chest pain consistent with angina pectoris. Myocardial infarction was documented in 163 patients. In this group of patients with coronary disease, those with myocardial infarction had a greater prevalence of the D/D genotype than those without myocardial infarction. The association was particularly high in women. No association was found between D/D genotype and any other risk factor including high LDL, high Lp(a), low HDL, blood pressure, or body mass index. We conclude that ACE gene I/D genotypes are associated with cardiovascular disease. In the case of hypertension, the association is variable. In myocardial infarction, the D/D genotype appears to be a risk factor, particularly in those without other known risk factors.

In stroke-prone spontaneously hypertensive rats, a locus in the vicinity of the ACE gene was found to be linked to high blood pressure [1,2]. In man, Tiret et al. [3] showed that an insertion/deletion (I/D) polymorphism of the ACE gene located in intron 16 was associated with marked differences of ACE levels; the insertion-type (I) allele was associated with *lower* ACE levels than the D allele. Exactly how these intron alleles influence the expression of the structural unaltered ACE is unclear. However, neither Harrap et al. [4] nor Schmidt et al. [5] could find an association of the D allele with blood pressure per se. Hypertension is a very heterogeneous condition and cohorts are likely to differ markedly in terms of genetic characteristics. Cambien et al. [6] found that the D polymorphism was a potent risk factor for myocardial infarction. We have been interested in both hypertension and myocardial infarction as well as other risk factors. To test for associations between ACE I/D alleles, we studied patients with both conditions.

Methods

Details of our investigations have been outlined in two previous publications [7,8]. We studied 95 patients with essential hypertension, sufficiently severe to require treatment, and also identified 51 normotensive control subjects with no first-degree relatives with hypertension. We compared these individuals to a randomly obtained sample from the general population which contained about the expected prevalence of hypertension seen in Germany. We also studied 390 patients who underwent coronary angiography because

---

Address for correspondence: Herbert Schuster, Franz Volhard Clinic, Wiltberg Strasse 50, 13122 Berlin, Germany. Tel.: +49-30-948-8202. Fax: +49-30-948-8206.

of suspected coronary artery disease. Myocardial infarction was documented in 163 patients but could not be verified in the others. These two groups were compared. In all patients and controls, body mass index, blood pressure and serum lipids were determined.

The I/D polymorphism of the ACE gene was identified by means of the polymerase chain reaction using a set of oligonucleotides flanking the polymorphic site. Allele frequencies and binomial errors were determined by the gene-counting method. Genotype distributions of all groups were compared to each other and to Hardy-Weinberg expectations by χ^2 methods. Relative risks and their 95% confidence intervals (CI) were calculated by the SAS statistical program. The Fisher exact test was used to test for statistical significance.

Results and Discussion

Although no significant differences could be found between hypertensive cases and a random population which we also examined, the I allele was more common in the hypertensive subjects than in the controls without any family history of hypertension. The I allele showed a relative risk 2.57 (95% CI 1.25–5.31) which was statistically significant. The hypertensive group and the random population sample were within Hardy-Weinberg equilibrium; the normotensive control group marginally so.

While the I allele was associated with hypertension, we found the D allele to be important in risk for myocardial infarction. In the infarction and noninfarction group, the genotype distributions were within Hardy-Weinberg equilibrium. We found a significant association between the D/D genotype and infarction risk (1.59, 95% CI 1.03–2.48). The significant difference could be attributed to the high number of D/D genotypes occurring in women with myocardial infarction. This association was enhanced in low-risk individuals according to the risk factors: LDL-cholesterol, low HDL-cholesterol, Lp(a), blood pressure and body mass index. Finally, we analyzed the frequency of D/D with respect to 1, 2, or 3 vessel coronary disease. No associations with the D/D genotype and severity of coronary disease was found.

Our data confirm and extend the observations of Cambien et al. on myocardial infarction [6] with an odds ratio slightly greater than that reported in their study. They not only observed that the D/D genotype was more frequent in patients with myocardial infarction, but also found that the association was strongest among the slender and those with lower apoB values. Moreover, the D/D genotype appeared to be particularly common in women with myocardial infarction in our study. Thus, traditional risk factors appeared to operate independently of the ACE I/D polymorphism in these subjects. Superficially, these results appear contradictory; however, conceivably the influence of the polymorphism is independent of the development of atherosclerosis per se. For instance, D/D could be associated with a tendency to thrombosis.

Tiret et al. [9] assessed the ACE genotype in adults in relation to whether or not they had a parental history of myocardial infarction. They found an odds ratio of 2.6 between the D/D and I/I genotypes, and of 1.9 between the I/D and the I/I genotypes. Bohn et al. [10] reported similar results in a study of persons with a parental history of myocardial infarction, although they had not been able to confirm the data of Cambien et al. [6]. An investigation by Ludwig et al., published in abstract form, described similar findings to those reported here [11].

A linkage relationship between hypertension and the ACE gene was first observed in stroke-prone hypertensive rats [1,2]. Identification of the I/D alleles and association with cardiac hypertrophy [12] has engendered much interest. Thus far, searches to implicate

864

the D allele in human hypertension have not been successful [4,5]. However, the I allele was found to be associated with hypertension in a group of hypertensive patients from Australia [13].

The I/D genetic variation is *not* a neutral polymorphism since the D allele results in a significantly higher ACE activity in plasma; the activity is highest in DD homozygotes and lowest in II homozygotes. High ACE activity could conceivably result in an increased generation of angiotensin II, although increased levels of angiotensin II in subjects harboring the D allele have not been reported. Further, exactly how the I/D polymorphism in intron 16 of the ACE gene influences ACE activity is unknown. We believe that our finding does not necessarily speak to the pathogenesis of either hypertension or myocardial infarction.

We did not do renin profiling in our subjects; conceivably our hypertensive subjects represented some particular renin–salt subtype such as low-renin hypertension. Risk for both hypertension and myocardial infarction has been attributed to differences in renin levels at a given salt intake [14]. It is also possible that the I allele in the ACE gene on chromosome 17 is in linkage disequilibrium with a pathogenetically relevant mutation in a nearby gene.

References

1. Hilbert P, Lindpaintner K, Beckmann JS, Serikawa T, Soubrier F, Dubay C, Cartwright P, De Gouyon B, Julier C, Takahasi S, Vincent M, Ganten D, de Georges M, Lathrop GM. Nature 1991;353:521–499.
2. Jacob HJ, Lindpaintner K, Lincoln SE, Kusumi K, Bunker RK, Mao YP, Ganten D, Dzau VJ. Cell 1991;67:213–224.
3. Tiret L, Rigat B, Visvikis S, Breda C, Corvol P, Cambien F, Soubrier F. Am J Hum Genet 1992;51:197–205.
4. Harrap SB, Davidson HR, Connor JM, Soubrier F, Corvol P, Fraser R, Foy CJW, Watt GCM. Hypertension 1993;21:455–460.
5. Schmidt S, van Hooft IMS, Grobbee DE, Ganten D, Ritz E. J Hypertens 1993;11:345-348.
6. Cambien F, Poirier O, Lecerf L, Evans A, Cambou JP, Arveiler D, Luc G, Bard JM, Bara L, Ricard S, Tiret L, Amouyel P, Alhenc-Gelas F, Soubrier F. Nature 1992;359:641–644.
7. Schuster H, Wienker T, Middeke M, Holzgreve H, Luft FC. Association of angiotensin converting enzyme polymorphisms in a German hypertensive population. Hypertension 1994 (submitted).
8. Schuster H, Wienker WF, Stremmler U, Noll B, Steinmetz A, Luft FC. A variant of the angiotensin converting enzyme gene is associated with myocardial infarction, but not with risk factors or severity of coronary artery disease. Lancet 1994 (submitted).
9. Tiret L, Kee F, Poirier O et al. Lancet 1993;341:991–992.
10. Bohn M, Berge KE, Bakken A, Erikssen J, Berg K. Clin Genet 1993;44:298–301.
11. Ludwig EH, Comeli PS, Anderson JL, Marshall HW, Lalouel J-M, Ward RH. Circulation 1993;88 (suppl 2):1953 (abstract).
12. Schunkert H, Hense H-W, Holmer SR, Stender M, Perz S, Keil U, Lorell BH, Riegger GAJ. N Engl J Med 1994;330:1634–1638.
13. Morris B, See R, Ying LH, Griffiths R. Clin Sci 1993;85:189–195.
14. Alderman MH, Maddhavan S, Ooi WL et al. N Engl J Med 1991;324:1098–1014.

865

Haptoglobin polymorphism and hypertension

J. Delanghe[1], M. De Buyzere[2] and D. Duprez[2]

[1]Central Laboratory, [2]Department of Cardiology, University Hospital, 185 De Pintelaan, B-9000 Gent, Belgium

Abstract. Distributions of haptoglobin (Hp)-types in established hypertension and the reference population are similar. However, therapeutic needs and prevalence of target organ damage are higher among Hp 2-2 carriers. The effect of Hp 2-2 on therapeutic needs in hypertension is independent of the presence of coronary artery disease, body mass index and lipids. In Hp 2-2 patients, serum Hp concentration is correlated with therapeutic needs and target organ damage. In refractory hypertension, there is a strong association with Hp 2-2. The explanation of these effects is under study. Haptoglobin 2-2 molecule is a poor hemoglobin binder, which could affect the metabolism of the vasodilator nitric oxide. On the other hand, the Hp 2-2 molecule could act as a promoter of atherogenesis. Hypertensives with an Hp 2-2 type show a higher risk of developing refractory hypertension. Apart from a younger age at diagnosis, complication rate was lower in Hp 1-1 patients. In view of the higher therapeutic needs and the higher complication rate, hypertensive Hp 2-2 patients need more careful monitoring.

Treatment of essential hypertension significantly reduces blood pressure in most patients. However, it remains puzzling why a significant number of patients require more intensive treatment. Attention has been paid to possible genetic mechanisms influencing essential hypertension [1]. Haptoglobin (Hp) has been suggested as a candidate marker molecule [2]. Hp is a protein characterized by molecular variation, only present in the human species. Three types are known: Hp 1-1, 2-1, and 2-2. In normotensives, salt sensitivity has been linked to the Hp 1-1 type [3]. The aim of the study was to investigate the indices of hypertension, severity of complications and occurrence of target organ damage for the various Hp-types and their relation to therapeutic needs.

Methods

A group of 440 patients with essential hypertension (222 men, 218 women, age 61.9 ± 12.0 year) were investigated. Refractory hypertension was considered when at least two drugs were needed for treatment and when blood pressure remained above 140/90 mmHg. 187 patients (43%) were receiving diuretics, 245 (56%) β-blocking agents, 206 (47%) calcium antagonists, 112 (25%) ACE inhibitors, 56 (13%) central acting agents and 92 (21%) vasodilators. Haptoglobin typing was performed by means of starch gel electrophoresis followed by peroxidase staining [4].

Results

Table 1 summarizes clinical data for the various Hp-types. In the hypertension group, relative gene frequencies of 0.374 (Hp1) and 0.626 (Hp2) were calculated, similar to the controls (relative Hp1 gene frequency: 0.397). However, age at diagnosis was lower for the Hp 1-1 group. Patients with an Hp 2-2 type required more intensive drug treatment. Vasodilating agents were more often administered to Hp 2-2 patients than to the other patients. For the other drug classes, differences in distribution were not significant [1].

Table 2 summarizes the distribution of Hp types according to the number of administered drugs. In patients needing only one or two drugs, Hp gene distribution was

Table 1. Distribution of Hp phenotypes in essential hypertension

Variables	Hp 1-1	Hp 2-1	Hp 2-2
n	70	189	181
Men/women	34/36	103/86	93/88
SBP (mmHg)	153 ± 29	148 ± 20	150 ± 24
DBP (mmHg)	90 ± 11	87 ± 11	87 ± 11
Age at diagnosis (years)	45.6 ± 10.0[a]	49.7 ± 11.2	49.5 ± 12.1
Number of drug treatments	2.06 ± 0.91	1.88 ± 0.74	2.20 ± 0.94[b]

[a]$p < 0.05$ vs. other Hp phenotypes; [b]$p < 0.001$ vs. other Hp phenotypes.

Table 2. Drug treatment and distribution of Hp phenotypes

Patient group according to treatment	Relative Hp1 gene frequency	Hp 1-1	Hp 2-1	Hp 2-2
One drug (n = 136)	0.408	21 (14%)[a]	69 (55%)	46 (31%)
Two drugs (n = 183)	0.380	30 (17%)	79 (41%)	74 (43%)
Three drugs (n = 91)	0.341[b]	13 (11%)	36 (39%)	42 (50%)[c]
>Three drugs (n = 30)	0.283[c]	6 (6%)	5 (18%)	19 (76%)

[a]Number of patients (percentage); [b]$p < 0.05$; [c]$p < 0.01$ vs. control population (χ^2 test).

comparable to that in the controls. In those receiving more than two drugs, relative Hp1 frequency was significantly lower ($p < 0.05$), due to an overrepresentation of Hp 2-2 ($p < 0.01$).

Table 3 shows that hypertensive Hp2 gene carriers were characterized by a higher prevalence of coronary artery disease (CAD) and peripheral arterial occlusive disease (PAOD) than hypertensives carrying the Hp1 gene. In the Hp 2-2 group, prevalence of PAOD was significantly higher than expected.

In the nonrefractory group (Table 4), the relative allele frequency (Hp1) of 0.390 is similar to the Hp allele distribution in the control population. However, in the refractory group a shift towards the Hp2 allele was observed (relative allele frequencies: 0.280 (Hp1) and 0.720 (Hp2), $p < 0.05$), due to overrepresentation of the Hp 2-2 type.

Discussion

In established hypertension, distribution of Hp types is similar to the distribution in the controls. Hp 1-1 has been suggested to be a marker for salt sensitivity [2]. Blood pressure

Table 3. Target organ damage, cardiovascular disease and Hp phenotype

	Hp1 gene frequency	Hp 1-1	Hp 2-1	Hp 2-2
LVH (n = 147)	0.374	25 (36%)[a]	60 (32%)	62 (34%)
CAD (n = 177)	0.327[b]	22 (31%)[c]	72 (38%)	83 (46%)
PAOD (n = 100)	0.295[b]	11 (16%)	37 (20%)	52 (29%)[d]

LVH, left ventricular hypertrophy; CAD, coronary artery disease; PAOD, peripheral arterial occlusive disease. [a]Number of patients (percentage); [b]$p < 0.05$ vs. Hp2 gene; [c]$p < 0.05$ vs. other Hp phenotypes; [d]$p < 0.01$ vs. control population.

Table 4. Hp phenotypes in refractory and nonrefractory hypertension

Patient group	Relative Hp1 allele frequency	Hp 1-1	Hp 2-1	Hp 2-2
General Belgian population	0.397	15%	48%	37%
Nonrefractory group (n = 374)	0.390	63 (17%)	166 (44%)	145 (39%)
Refractory group (n = 66)	0.280[a]	7 (11%)	23 (35%)	36 (55%)

[a]$p < 0.05$ vs. nonrefractory group.

was similar for the three Hp types. Hp 1-1 patients were characterized by an earlier age at diagnosis, which is compatible with literature findings showing early manifestation of sodium sensitivity in Hp 1-1 subjects [3]. The patients with Hp 1-1 phenotype showed a milder evolution and a lower prevalence of complications. Despite comparable blood pressure under treatment, patients with an Hp 2-2 type needed more drug treatments than the other Hp phenotypes, mainly because of the higher need for vasodilating agents.

In the nonrefractory group, distribution of Hp phenotypes resembles the distribution observed in the reference population. In the refractory group, Hp 1 allele frequency was much lower, because of an overrepresentation of Hp 2-2 individuals. To evaluate the effect of individual parameters on therapeutic needs, we performed logistic regression analysis. Seven factors were significantly related to therapeutic needs: CAD ($p = 0.0001$), Hp 2-2 type ($p = 0.0002$), body mass index ($p = 0.0004$), left ventricular hypertrophy (LVH) ($p = 0.0004$), Hp 2-1 type ($p = 0.0009$), systolic BP ($p = 0.0062$), and HDL-cholesterol ($p = 0.047$).

Analysis of serum Hp concentration demonstrated a concentration-related effect on therapeutic needs in Hp 2-2 patients only. Frequency of PAOD was highest in the subgroup with highest Hp 2-2 concentrations. The increased occurrence of the Hp2 allele in severe hypertension and the correlation between serum Hp 2-2 values and therapeutic needs may point towards a causative role of Hp in hypertension. Hp has been described as a hemoglobin-binding molecule. Structural similarities exist between Hp, serine proteases, and the light chain of immunoglobulins. Functional differences between Hp types have been described. Hp 1-1 has higher hemoglobin-binding capacity than other Hp types. Antibody-like immunological properties have been described for the Hp 2-1 and Hp 2-2 types [5]. The same types are able to inhibit prostaglandin synthetase [6]. Distribution of Hp types differs from that of the reference population in autoimmune diseases. In acute myocardial infarction, Hp 2-2 was associated with severe infarction and left ventricular failure [7]. The worse prognosis of myocardial infarction in patients carrying the Hp 2-2 type could be explained by a deleterious effect of Hp 2-2 itself. We detected signs of ongoing inflammatory processes in Hp 2-2 patients, as evidenced by higher CRP concentrations [1]. The vascular damage in individuals carrying an Hp 2 gene is evidenced by increased prevalence of both CAD and PAOD. As free hemoglobin binds strongly to nitric oxide [8], the Hp-types could modulate the vasodilating effect of nitric oxide (endothelium-derived relaxing factor). Haptoglobin has been identified as well as an angiogenic factor in vasculitis; Hp 2-2 was associated with the most important vessel penetration [9].

Hypertensives carrying an Hp 2-2 type need more intensive treatment. The hypertensive Hp2 carrier is more likely to accumulate atherosclerotic lesions (PAOD or CAD) even when blood pressure, lipids and body mass index are similar. Further studies are required to explore the relationship between Hp polymorphism, individual response to

868

drug treatment and therapy resistance. The Hp 2-2 type is a risk factor for developing refractory hypertension and therefore needs more careful monitoring.

References

1. Delanghe J, Duprez D, De Buyzere M, Bergez B, Callens B, Leroux-Roels G, Clement D. J Hypertens 1993;11:861–867.
2. Weinberger M, Miller J, Fineberg N, Luft F, Grim C, Christian J. Hypertension 1987;10:443–446.
3. Luft F, Miller J, Grim C, Fineberg N, Christian J, Daugherty S, Weinberger M. Hypertension 1991;17 (suppl I):I-102–I-108.
4. Smithies O. Biochem J 1955;61:629–641.
5. Köhler W, Prokop O. Nature 1978;271:373.
6. Jue D, Shim B, Kang Y. Mol Cell Biochem 1983;51:141–147.
7. Chapelle JP, Albert A, Smeets J, Heusghem C, Kulbertus H. N Engl J Med 1982;307:457–463.
8. Collins P, Burman J, Chung H, Fox K. Circulation 1993;87:80–85.
9. Cid M, Grant D, Hoffman G, Auerbach R, Fauci A, Kleinman H. J Clin Invest 1993;91:977–985.

Genetics of the renin–angiotensin system and the S_A gene in hypertension

Nilesh J. Samani

Department of Medicine, University of Leicester, Leicester, UK

Abstract. Recent studies, both in rodent models of genetic hypertension and in humans, suggest that genes coding for components of the renin–angiotensin system may harbor mutations that predispose to hypertension. This paper reviews the major findings that have been made to date and discusses the caveats necessary in the correct interpretation of the data. The paper then also reviews the early observations that have been made with respect to the S_A gene, whose biochemical functions remain to be defined, but which may underlie a novel renal mechanism involved in blood pressure regulation and the tendency to hypertension.

The role played by the renin–angiotensin system in hypertension has been extensively evaluated using biochemical, physiological and pharmacological techniques. Many differences have been described. However, these approaches have all had difficulty in distinguishing any primary (causal) role played by the system from a secondary or compensatory role, especially in primary hypertension. The last decade has seen the cloning of the genes for all the major components of the renin–angiotensin cascade (renin, angiotensinogen, angiotensin converting enzyme and the angiotensin receptor). The availability of these nucleic acid sequences has allowed a new approach to studying the role of the system in hypertension, namely whether genetic variation in the genes coding for the proteins of the system influence the risk of hypertension. In the last few years all the components have been assessed in this manner in both rodent models of genetic hypertension and in human essential hypertension. This brief paper reviews and discusses the data obtained to date. While classical studies suggested that the renin–angiotensin system may be a good potential source of genetic determinants of hypertension, reverse genetic techniques have identified other, previously unknown, loci that may also play a role. The best example of this is probably the S_A gene, which may underlie a new renal mechanism through which blood pressure may be influenced. This paper also discusses the current knowledge about this novel and potentially very exciting molecule.

Genetic variation in the renin–angiotensin system and hypertension

The role of genetic variation in the genes coding for the components of the renin–angiotensin system in hypertension has been tested by cosegregation analysis in rodent models of hereditary hypertension and by a combination of association and linkage (mainly affected sibship) analysis in human essential hypertension [1]. Both positive and negative results of such studies need to be interpreted carefully. The necessary caveats are discussed below, after a brief summary of the main results that have been obtained for each component of the system.

Address for correspondence: Dr N.J. Samani, Department of Medicine, Clinical Sciences Building, Leicester Royal Infirmary, P.O. Box 65, Leicester, LE2 7LX, UK.

Renin

In 1989 Rapp et al. [2] were the first to demonstrate cosegregation of a polymorphism in the rat renin gene with increased blood pressure in a cross of the Dahl salt-sensitive (Dahl-S) rat with its normotensive control, the Dahl salt-resistant rat. Since then, linkage of the renin locus with blood pressure has been shown in crosses of several other types of genetically hypertensive rats with normotensive controls (reviewed in [1]).

In contrast to the studies in rats, studies on the renin locus in human have so far largely been disappointingly negative [1]. Several association studies have found no increased frequency of various renin gene polymorphisms in hypertensive individuals, apart from one study in which a *Bgl*II polymorphism was found to be more frequent in Afro-Caribbean hypertensives compared with normotensives [3]. Analysis of renin haplotypes in affected sib pairs and two family linkage studies have also proved negative [1].

Angiotensinogen

Angiotensinogen (AGT), the substrate for renin, has not normally been considered the rate-limiting component in the cascade. Thus, the findings in 1992 of Jeunemaitre et al. [4] of greater allele sharing at the AGT locus in affected hypertensive sibships than expected by chance, as well as the association of a particular polymorphism (met235→Thr) with hypertension, aroused considerable interest as well as debate. The linkage findings have recently been corroborated in an independent set of sibships [5] although further studies of the association of the met235→Thr polymorphism in different hypertensive populations have produced mixed results [5–7]. Nevertheless, to date, the AGT locus has the firmest evidence of the involvement of a specific locus in human essential hypertension.

The data on the AGT locus in rats have also proved interesting. In a cross of the spontaneously hypertensive rat (SHR) with the Wistar-Kyoto (WKY) rat, we have recently found the SHR allele to cosegregate with an increase in pulse pressure but not independently with systolic or diastolic pressures [8], suggesting an effect on aortic compliance, perhaps mediated through a vascular renin–angiotensin system. Pulse pressure has been shown to be an important independent determinant of cardiovascular risk. This observation therefore requires deserves further evaluation and also needs to be related to the findings being made in human hypertension.

Angiotensin converting enzyme

Recently an intronic insertion/deletion polymorphism in the angiotensin converting enzyme (ACE) gene has been associated with the risk of myocardial infarction [9] and also with other cardiac phenotypes including left ventricular hypertrophy [10]. The polymorphism, which predicates higher plasma ACE levels has, however, not so far been found to be associated with hypertension [1]. Involvement of the ACE locus has also been tested by linkage using the same sibships that proved positive for angiotensinogen. This time, no increased allele sharing was seen [11].

In rats, cosegregation of the ACE locus on chromosome 10 has been shown with blood pressure in crosses involving both the stroke-prone SHR as well as the Dahl-S rat [1]. Several other genes that could affect blood pressure lie in the vicinity of the ACE gene and the precise gene influencing blood pressure remains to be determined (see below).

Angiotensin receptors

Cloning of the genes for the angiotensin receptor subtypes (AT1A, AT1B and AT2) has been achieved only recently and extensive data on their possible genetic contribution to hypertension is not yet available. Nevertheless, one study has reported increased frequency of certain haplotypes of the AT1A receptor in hypertensives [12].

Interpretation of findings of the genetic involvement of the renin–angiotensin system in hypertension : caveats

The genetic studies discussed above suggest some exciting possibilities regarding the primary involvement of the renin–angiotensin in hypertension. On the other hand, lack of concordance between different studies (especially association studies) and the lack of correlation between the findings in rats and in humans in several cases has led to considerable debate [1]. It is therefore important to consider the several caveats that need to be borne in mind when looking at the results of these studies.

First of all, with regard to the conflicting rat and human findings e.g., for renin, there is of course no absolute reason why the genetic basis of the hypertension should be the same in the two species. It also needs to be remembered that cosegregation analysis, as performed in the various rat crosses, tests the involvement of a locus and not a specific gene. Thus, the positive cosegregation findings with some of the renin–angiotensin system polymorphisms may simply reflect the effect of a linked gene located elsewhere in the human genome. While these possibilities provide attractive explanations when the results are discordant, there are significant limitations to the human studies in excluding the involvement of a locus.

In association studies, all one can exclude is the involvement of a specific polymorphism (the one being tested) or something it is in linkage disequilibrium with. Even a large association study cannot exclude involvement of a locus [1]. While linkage studies (e.g., affected sib-pair studies) test the involvement of the whole locus, they require large numbers of subjects, as yet achieved in very few if any studies, to exclude an effect. This is especially so given the heterogeneity of hypertension and the likelihood that in only a fraction of the cohort is a particular locus likely to be important. Just as negative studies may provide only limited information, positive studies also need to be interpreted carefully. It is well known that allele frequencies for many genes vary in different ethnic groups and an association study may therefore be spuriously positive simply because of an unrecognized difference in the ethnic mixes of the hypertensive and normotensive cohorts. Similarly, many assumptions underlie the analysis of affected sibship studies, particularly where identity-by-state is used, and these can produce an artefactual result. All these various caveats need to be considered when interpreting the above results as well as the results of future studies on the renin–angiotensin system or indeed any other genes in hypertension [1].

The S_A gene and hypertension

The S_A gene was identified in 1992 by differential cloning because of its higher expression in the kidney of the SHR than in the WKY rat [13]. Interest in it has since increased considerably with the demonstration of cosegregation of a polymorphism in the gene with increased blood pressure in several crosses of hypertensive and normotensive rats [1]. The two combined — the manner of its identification and the subsequent co-segregation with blood pressure — strongly point to the S_A gene as being the causative

872

gene at the locus. In our own cross of SHR x WKY we were further able to show that the S_A locus is itself the major determinant of the level of renal S_A gene expression in these strains [14]. These data are exciting because both in rodent models of hypertension as well as in humans, the tendency to hypertension has been shown to follow the kidney after transplantation. We have proposed that the S_A gene may provide a potential genetic mechanism underlying these physiological observations [14]. It needs, however, to be noted that S_A is also expressed, albeit at lower levels, in other sites (liver and brain) through which blood pressure may also be influenced [13].

The deduced protein sequence of S_A protein does not show striking homology to any other proteins in the databases. However, there is limited but significant homology to a family of synthetic enzymes including acetyl-CoA synthetase, which suggests that it may be an enzyme, and therefore a potential target for inhibition. We have recently localized the increased S_A gene expression in the SHR kidney to the proximal tubule, so that its effects on blood pressure may be mediated through tubular mechanisms [15].

Studies on S_A in man are at an early stage. The gene is located on chromosome 16, and has been shown to be expressed in the human kidney [16]. A polymorphism in the gene has also been reported to be associated with hypertension in a Japanese population [17]. Given the caveats discussed earlier about the interpretation of association studies, further corroboration of this finding is clearly required. Nevertheless, all the data to date on S_A suggest that a novel molecule involved in blood pressure regulation has been identified, and further studies on it may provide new insights into the primary role played by the kidney in hypertension.

Acknowledgements

I am grateful to the British Heart Foundation, The Wellcome Trust and the BIOMED I program of the EEC for support.

References

1. Samani NJ. Br Med Bull 1994;50:260–271.
2. Rapp JP, Wang SM, Dene H. Science 1989;243:542–544.
3. Barley J, Carter ND, Cruickshank JK, Jeffery S, Smith A, Charlett A, Webb DJ. J Hypertens 1992;9:993–996.
4. Jeunemaitre X, Soubrier F, Koteletsev YV, Lifton RP, Williams CS, Charru A, Hunt SC, Hopkins PN, Williams RR, Lalouel JM, Corvol P. Cell 1992;71:169–180.
5. Caulfield M, Lavender P, Farrall M, Munroe P, Lawson M, Turner P, Clark AJL. N Engl J Med 1994;330:1629–1633.
6. Hata A, Namikawa C, Sasaki M, Sato K, Nakamura T, Lalouel J-M. J Clin Invest 1994;93:1285–1287.
7. Bennett CL, Schrader AP, Morris BJ. Biochem Biophys Res Commun 1993;197:833–839.
8. Lodwick D, Kaiser MA, Harris J, Vincent M, Swales JD, Samani NJ. J Hypertens 1994;12(suppl 3):S166.
9. Cambien F, Poirier O, Lecerf L et al. Nature 1992;359:641–644.
10. Schunkert H, Hense H-W, Holmer SR et al. N Engl J Med 1994;330:1634–1638.
11. Jeunemaitre X, Lifton RP, Hunt SC, Williams RR, Lalouel JM. Nat Genet 1992;1:72–75.
12. Bonnardeaux A, Davies E, Jeunemaitre X, Charru A, Cambien F, Corvol P, Soubrier F. J Hypertens 1994; 12(suppl 3):S4.
13. Iwai N, Inagami T. Hypertension 1991;17:161–169.
14. Samani NJ, Lodwick D, Vincent M, Dubay C, Kaiser MA, Kelly MP, Lo M, Harris J, Sassard J, Lathrop M, Swales JD. J Clin Invest 1993;92:1099–1103.
15. Patel HR, Thiara A, West KP, Lodwick D, Samani NJ. Increased expression of the S_A gene in the kidney of the spontaneously hypertensive rat is localised to the proximal tubule. J Hypertens (in press).
16. Samani NJ, Whitmore SA, Kaiser MA, Harris J, See CG, Callen DF, Lodwick D. Biochem Biophys Res Commun 1994;199:862–868.
17. Iwai N, Ohmichi N, Hanai K, Nakamura Y, Kinoshita M. Hypertension 1994;23:375–380.

Genetic variations in genes associated with hypertension and the risk of atherosclerosis

François Cambien

INSERM SC7, 17 rue du Fer à Moulin, 75005 Paris, France

Abstract. Identification of the genes and variants involved in the chronic and acute processes of coronary heart disease should considerably improve our understanding of the etiology and mechanisms of this disease. Several of these genes could be involved in the physiopathology of the vascular wall, but for the moment only a fraction of them have been explored. The genes coding for the component of the renin–angiotensin system have been analyzed in detail in relation to hypertension and coronary heart disease. It appears that the ACE D and Ang II AT1 [1166]C alleles are associated with an increased risk of myocardial infarction. Studies in humans suggest that these associations are more related to the effect of Ang II and/or bradykinin on vascular and cardiac hypertrophy and on vasomotricity than to their effect on atherosclerosis development. Simultaneous analysis of several alleles predisposing to coronary heart disease could provide the means of identifying high-risk individuals and to characterize groups where specific therapeutic interventions would be most effective.

The main pathologic manifestations affecting the vascular wall are tightly interconnected. They include chronic processes such as endothelial dysfunction, hypertension, atheroma, hypertrophy and remodeling and acute processes such as plaque rupture, thrombosis and vasoconstriction. Remarkable progress has been made in the characterization of the roles of the different cells involved in these processes (platelet, endothelial cells, macrophages, T lymphocytes, smooth muscle cells) and of the different molecules produced by these cells and to which these cells respond: growth factors, prostaglandins, angiotensin II (Ang II), kinins, nitric oxide, oxidized LDL and components of the intercellular matrix.

A large fraction of the genes coding for these molecules or for their precursors have been cloned. Their sequence or the sequence of the corresponding cDNA can thus be explored with the objective of finding polymorphisms that may be studied in relation to disease or intermediate phenotypes. For the moment only a few of these genes have been investigated in detail in relation to hypertension or diseases of the vascular wall. The genes already explored are mainly those coding for the components of the renin–angiotensin system; genes coding for components of the kallikrein–kinins system, for endothelins and their receptors and for nitric oxide synthases are currently being explored; and many growth factors will also be explored in the near future.

In the renin–angiotensin system, renin transforms angiotensinogen into angiotensin I, an inactive molecule, which is in turn converted into Ang II by the action of the angiotensin converting enzyme (ACE). Finally, Ang II exerts its action through angiotensin II receptors. Ang II is a very potent vasoactive molecule which plays an important role at different stages of the development and in different circumstances in several tissues and cells.

Renin

Renin is the rate-limiting enzyme of the cascade leading to Ang II formation, and was extensively studied in relation to hypertension, both in animal models and in humans. In humans various studies, including association and family studies, failed to demonstrate any association or linkage of the renin gene with hypertension [1]. These negative results do not completely eliminate the possibility that a rare allele of the renin gene could induce hypertension, but no widespread allele has a detectable effect. These studies were performed in Caucasians, and it is worth noting that in a study of Afro-Caribbeans, a difference in the allele frequency of the *Bgl* I polymorphism of the renin gene was shown between individuals in the lower quintile and the upper quintile of blood-pressure distribution [2].

As far as we know, the renin polymorphisms have not been investigated in relation to coronary heart disease. Such a study might be worthwhile since it has been suggested that a high renin profile might be associated with an increased risk of myocardial infarction [3].

Angiotensinogen

Angiotensinogen is the renin substrate and the precursor of angiotensins. Its concentration in the plasma appears critical for the kinetics of angiotensinogen I generation, even if its concentration is not limiting for generation of angiotensinogen I. Several epidemiological observations indicate a possible role of angiotensinogen in blood pressure regulation. A highly significant correlation between plasma angiotensinogen concentration and blood pressure was observed in a large epidemiological study [4], and young adults with high blood pressure born of parents with high blood pressure have higher levels of plasma angiotensinogen than young adults with low blood pressure born of low-blood-pressure parents [5].

A linkage study based on pairs of sibs affected with hypertension was performed using a highly polymorphic marker isolated on the angiotensinogen gene [6]. 215 pairs of sibs affected by essential hypertension were genotyped for this marker [7]. A significant excess of concordance of alleles was detected over the concordance expected from independent transmission of the disease and the marker. Furthermore, the linkage was stronger in hypertensives with the highest levels of blood pressure or with early-onset hypertension.

Several diallelic polymorphisms have been detected on the angiotensinogen gene by single-strand conformation polymorphism (SSCP) analysis. Polymorphisms were found along the angiotensinogen gene, on exons 2 and 3. Two of them were particularly informative, on codon 235, where a T-to-C transition changes a methionine into a threonine, and on codon 174, where a C-to-T transition changes a threonine into a methionine. The frequency of the two polymorphisms was compared in a group of normotensive controls and a group of hypertensive subjects matched for age. For both polymorphisms, the frequency of the less frequent allele (174M and 235T) was significantly higher in the hypertensives than in the normotensives.

The relationship between the plasma concentration of angiotensinogen and the marker genotypes isolated on the angiotensinogen gene was also investigated [7]. Among hypertensives, the mean plasma level of angiotensinogen was significantly different in the three genotypes defined by codon-235 variation. The highest value was found in individuals homozygous for the allele associated with hypertension in the case-control study.

A chronic moderate genotype-dependent overexpression of the angiotensinogen gene might be the source of a chronic increase in the generation of Ang II in the plasma and also in different tissues which could contribute to the development of hypertension.

The possible impact of the angiotensinogen 174M and 235T variants on the risk of coronary heart disease was also investigated in the ECTIM study (see appendix). Similar distributions of the allele frequencies of both polymorphisms were observed in patients with myocardial infarction and controls despite the association of the polymorphisms with hypertension in the control group, especially in nonoverweight subjects.

Angiotensin-I converting enzyme (ACE)

In the plasma and on the surface of endothelial cells, ACE converts the inactive decapeptide angiotensin I into Ang II. Bradykinin, the other best-known substrate of ACE, is a potent vasodilator and inhibitor of smooth muscle cells proliferation which by interacting with the bradykinin B2 receptor induces the release of endothelial factors, including nitric oxide and prostacyclin. Bradykinin is inactivated by ACE, and this could account for some of the effects associated with high ACE expression and for part of the beneficial effect of ACE inhibitors.

Repeat measurements of plasma ACE in adult humans have shown that the level of the enzyme is very stable within individuals, but differs strongly from individual to individual and is independent of a large number of environmental, metabolic and hormonal factors [8]. Plasma ACE level is strongly genetically determined. This is largely the consequence of a diallelic polymorphism (ACE S/s), situated within or close to the ACE gene, which is still uncharacterized at the molecular level. An insertion/deletion polymorphism (ACE I/D) in the 16th intron of the gene is a very good marker for ACE S/s [9]. The relationship between the ACE I/D polymorphism and plasma ACE level was studied in a sample of healthy adults. The concentration of ACE in plasma was strongly associated with the genetic polymorphism. In II homozygotes, ID heterozygotes and DD homozygotes, the mean levels of ACE were 299, 393 and 494 µg/l respectively (p < 0.001). The effect of the gene was strictly codominant and accounted for a large part of the interindividual variability of plasma ACE. ACE activity in cells expressing the enzyme is also strongly increased in presence of the D allele (p < 0.001) [10].

As a consequence of the role of ACE in the renin–angiotensin system, it was logical to hypothesize that the ACE gene could be a candidate for human hypertension. However, several association studies performed in different populations have not found any association between the ACE I/D polymorphism and blood pressure level or hypertension. A study in pairs of hypertensive siblings using a highly informative marker located close to the ACE gene has also failed to demonstrate a linkage between the ACE locus and hypertension [11].

The ACE I/D polymorphism has been identified in all human populations studied so far, but large variations in allele frequencies have been observed. The frequency of allele D is higher in populations of African origin than in European populations and lower in northern Asians than in Europeans. The frequency of several polymorphisms of candidate genes varies strongly according to population (apoE, apo(a), apoB, ACE...), and these variations could account for a non-negligible part of the differences in frequency of cardiovascular diseases between populations.

The possible association between the ACE I/D polymorphism and myocardial infarction was investigated in the ECTIM study (see Appendix). The odds ratio (relative risk) for myocardial infarction was 1.57 for DD versus II and 1.26 for ID versus II (test for trend, p < 0.003). This association was not significantly heterogeneous across populations and the frequency of the two alleles was similar in the different control groups [12]. In a low-risk group defined by absence of hyperlipidemia and obesity, the association between the ACE I/D polymorphism and myocardial infarction was highly significant and homogeneous across the populations (test for trend, p < 0.005); however, the increased risk of myocardial infarction was present only in DD individuals, the overall odds ratio comparing DD and ID+II individuals being 2.7 (p < 0.0005). Conversely, in the high-risk group, the ACE I/D polymorphism was less strongly related to myocardial infarction (p < 0.05).

In the ECTIM study the parental history of MI was carefully recorded. As expected, parental history was much more frequent in Belfast than in France (about four times). In both countries the frequency of the D allele was increased in those having a parental history [13]. Taking the II genotype as reference, very similar odds ratios for parental fatal myocardial infarction associated with the DD and ID genotypes were observed in Belfast and France, the odds ratio adjusted on population being 2.7 (p < 0.02) for DD vs. II and 1.9 (p = 0.1) for ID vs. II.

Plasma ACE activity was measured in the ECTIM study from frozen plasma samples. There was a highly significant interaction between plasma ACE and age on the risk of myocardial infarction which was due to the strong association between plasma ACE level and myocardial infarction in patients aged less than 55 (the median of age in the study) but not in the older patients. Furthermore, plasma ACE was elevated in the younger cases within each ACE I/D genotype, which indicates that this association was independent of the polymorphism [14]. In this analysis it was possible to infer the frequency and effect of the ACE S allele in cases and controls by a commingling analysis of the ACE distribution conditioned on the ACE I/D polymorphism. ACE S was more frequent in cases before than after age 55: 45 and 32% respectively (p < 0.01). This might reflect a high mortality in myocardial infarction patients carrying the D allele [15].

Since allele ACE S is associated with high plasma and cellular levels of ACE, it can be proposed that a chronic increased expression of ACE, by modulating the level of Ang II and bradykinin at specific sites, affects cardiovascular homeostasis and is responsible for the increased risk of MI. ACE probably acts locally in the coronary arteries and/or in the heart. The paracrine and autocrine effects of vascular or cardiac renin–angiotensin and kallikrein–kinin systems could explain the local action of ACE and of ACE inhibitors.

Given the important roles of Ang II and bradykinin as modulators of cellular growth and of vasomotricity, we can postulate their respective deleterious and beneficial implications at different stages of the atherosclerotic process and during the acute events leading to myocardial infarction or sudden death. Recent angiographic studies have shown that the increased risk of myocardial infarction in presence of ACE D is not the consequence of more severe atherosclerosis [16]; but in the presence of atheroma, ACE D could predispose to plaque rupture and to vasoconstriction of the coronary arteries. It has been shown that the intimal-medial thickness of the carotid artery is increased in presence of high plasma ACE levels [17]. This observation could be important in view of the strong association found in an autopsy study between the intimal thickening of coronary arteries in infants and a family history of coronary heart disease [18]. High ACE expression in the heart in presence of ACE D might also increase the local generation of Ang II and predispose to left ventricular hypertrophy [19], a strong risk factor for coronary heart disease [20]. Hence, if ventricular hypertrophy was the main consequence of ACE overexpression, the ACE polymorphism could be a risk factor for myocardial infarction and sudden cardiac death independent of atherosclerosis development. In this context, it is worth noting that patients with ischemic or idiopathic dilated myocardiopathy are more frequently ACE DD homozygous than controls [21] and that patients with hypertrophic myocardiopathy have an increased frequency of the ACE D allele, especially if there is a family history of sudden cardiac death [22].

Angiotensin II receptor of AT1 type

Ang II receptors mediate the vasoconstrictive, cell growth-promoting and salt-conserving actions of Ang II. It was then particularly important to investigate the possible effects of polymorphisms of the genes coding for these receptors on hypertension. The human Ang II type 1 receptor (AT1) gene has recently been cloned [23], and its coding sequence has been analyzed by SSCP in a group of 60 hypertensive subjects. Five silent polymorphisms were identified and three of them were studied in a larger sample of patients with hypertension (n = 206) and in controls. A common variant resulting from a A-to-C transversion at position 1166 of the coding sequence of the AT1 receptor (AT1 ^{1166}C) was more frequent in the hypertensive than in the normotensive subjects (frequency f = 0.36 versus 0.28, p < 0.01) and this association was stronger in young hypertensives (f = 0.39) and severe hypertensives (f = 0.40) [24]. This observation will have to be confirmed in independent studies. In the ECTIM study, we found that the AT1 ^{1166}C and the ACE D alleles had a strong synergistic effect on the risk of myocardial infarction, which suggests that the ACE DD genotype was associated with myocardial infarction only in the presence of the AT1 ^{1166}C allele. This interaction was particularly striking in individuals at low risk of developing a coronary heart disease (as defined by a low plasma apoB level and lack of obesity), the odds ratio for myocardial infarction associated with the ACE DD genotype being respectively 1.64, 7.03 and 13.3 in genotypes AA, AC and CC respectively (p for trend < 0.02) [25]. These results if confirmed could have clinical implications for the prevention and treatment of coronary heart disease. Screening for a genetic risk factor may indeed become worthwhile if the factor is frequent and imparts a high relative risk and if its detrimental effects can be counteracted by drugs or by other preventive means. This may be the case here, since potent drugs such as ACE inhibitors and Ang II AT1 receptor blockers are available.

The results concerning the possible synergistic effect of the ACE D and AT1 ^{1166}C alleles on the risk of myocardial infarction also raise a more general issue related to the multifactorial, multigenic nature of the disease. It suggests that the combination of several frequent genetic variants may be associated with strong increases of risk in a fairly important proportion of individuals. This is in contrast with the low relative risk generally found associated with single polymorphisms.

Appendix — the ECTIM study

The ECTIM study is a case-control study specially designed to identify genetic variants associated with MI. Four populations covered by CHD registries (WHO/MONICA [26]) were targets for study: three populations in France in the regions of Lille, Strasbourg and Toulouse, and one in Northern Ireland, in the region of Belfast. France is one of the industrialized countries where the frequency of MI is the lowest, and among middle-aged men, this disease is 3–4 times more frequent in Northern Ireland than in France. In the ECTIM study, men with definite MI aged 35–64 were recruited 3–9 months after the acute episode and during a period of 2.5 years starting at the end of 1988. Random samples of controls were recruited during the same period and in the same age range as the cases, using electoral rolls in France and general practitioner lists held by the Central Services Agency in Belfast. The participants were of Caucasian origin; parents of cases and controls had to be born in the same regions and their four grandparents had to be born in Europe.

878

References

1. Soubrier F, Jeunemaitre X, Rigat B, Houot AM, Cambien F, Corvol P. Hypertension 1990;16:712—717.
2. Barley J, Carter ND, Cruickshank JK et al. J Hypertens 1993;9:993—996.
3. Alderman MH, Madhavan S, Ooi WL, Cohen H, Sealey JE, Laragh JH. N Engl J Med 1991;324:1098—1104.
4. Walker WG, Whelton PK, Saito H, Russell RP, Hermann J. Hypertension 1979;1:287—291.
5. Watt GCM, Harrap SB, Foy CJW et al. J Hypertens 1992;10:473—482.
6. Kotelevtsev YV, Clauser E, Corvol P, Soubrier F. Nucleic Acids Res 1991;19:69—78.
7. Jeunemaitre X, Soubrier F, Kotelevtsev Y et al. Cell 1992;71:169—180.
8. Alhenc-Gelas F, Richard J, Courbon D, Warnet JM, Corvol P. J Lab Clin Med 1991;117:33—39.
9. Rigat B, Hubert C, Alhenc-Gelas F, Cambien F, Corvol P, Soubrier F. J Clin Invest 1990;86:1343—1346.
10. Costerousse O, Allegrini J, Lopez M, Alhenc-Gelas F. Biochem J 1993;290:33—40.
11. Jeunemaitre X, Lifton RP, Hunt SC, Williams RR, Lalouel JM. Nature Genet 1992;1:72—75.
12. Cambien, F, Poirier O, Lecerf L et al. Nature 1992;359:641—644.
13. Tiret L, Kee F, Poirier O et al. Lancet 1993;341:991—992.
14. Cambien F, Costerousse O, Tiret L et al. Circulation 1994;90:669—676.
15. Evans AE, Poirier O, Kee F et al. Quart J Med 1994;87:211—214.
16. Ludwig EH, Corneli PS, Anderson JL, Marshall HW, Lalouel JM, Ward RH. Circulation 1993;88(suppl):I—364.
17. Bonithon-Kopp C, Ducimetière P, Touboul PJ et al. Circulation 1994;89:952—954.
18. Kapprio J, Norio R, Pesonen E, Sarna S. Circulation 1993;87:1960—1968.
19. Schunkert H, Hense HW, Holmer SR et al. N Engl J Med 1994;330:1634—1638.
20. Kannel WB. J Hypertens 1991;9(suppl 2):S2—S9.
21. Raynolds MV, Bristow MR, Bush EW et al. Lancet 1993;342:1073—1075.
22. Marian AJ, Yu QT, Workman R, Greve G, Roberts R. Lancet 1993;342:1085—1086.
23. Takayanagi R, Ohnaka K, Sakai Y et al. Biochem Biophys Res Commun 1992;183:910—916.
24. Bonnardeaux A, Davies E, Jeunemaitre X et al. Hypertension 1994;24:63—69.
25. Tiret L, Bonnardeaux A, Poirier O et al. Lancet 1994 (in press).
26. The WHO MONICA Project. World Health Statist Annu 1989;27—149.

Atherosclerosis X.
F.P. Woodford, J. Davignon and A. Sniderman, editors.

879

Assembly and lysine binding of recombinant lipoprotein(a)

Angelika Ernst[1], Christoph Brunner[1], Attila Pethö-Schramm[1], Marion Helmhold[2], Hans-Georg Kraft[3], Gerd Utermann[3], Victor W. Armstrong[2] and Hans-Joachim Müller[1]

[1]*Boehringer Mannheim GmbH, Department of Molecular Biology, Sandhofer Straße 116, D-68305 Mannheim, Germany; [2]Georg-August Universität Göttingen, Abteilung Klinische Chemie, Robert-Koch-Straße 40, D-37075 Göttingen, Germany; and [3]Universität Innsbruck, Institut für Medizinische Biologie und Humangenetik, Schöpfstraße 41, A-6020 Innsbruck, Austria*

Abstract. Wild-type and mutant recombinant apolipoprotein(a) (r-apo(a)) species were expressed in HepG2 cells to enable us to study the structural requirements for the assembly of recombinant Lp(a) (r-Lp(a)) and the contribution of distinct apo(a) domains to the observed lysine binding of r-apo(a)/r-Lp(a). The mutants revealed the importance of both noncovalent and covalent interactions for the apo(a)/apoB association during r-Lp(a) assembly. Inhibition of this association by antibodies against apo(a) or apoB indicates that r-Lp(a) assembly occurs either at the cell surface or in the medium of transfected cells. Two functionally different lysine-binding sites were mapped to the apo(a) kringle domains 32–36 and 37, respectively.

Plasma levels of lipoprotein(a) (Lp(a)) vary more than 1,000-fold among individuals, and are determined almost exclusively by the polymorphic apolipoprotein(a) (apo(a)) gene encoding the characteristic high-molecular weight glycoprotein of Lp(a) (for review see [1,2]). Apo(a) shares homologous domains with plasminogen (Pg), the precursor of the fibrinolytic enzyme plasmin [3]. Pg comprises five disulfide-bridged structures called kringles I to V and a carboxyterminal serine protease domain. Apo(a) contains multiple tandem repeats of a kringle that shares 61–75% homology with kringle IV of Pg followed by single Pg-like kringle V and protease domains. Elevated plasma levels of Lp(a) have been identified as an independent risk factor for premature coronary heart disease [4]. The extensive homology between apo(a) and Pg gave rise to the hypothesis that Lp(a) might trigger vascular occlusion by interference with fibrinolysis. Some support for this hypothesis comes from the finding of lower plasminogen activation in the arterial wall of apo(a) transgenic mice than in normal mice [5]. In humans, accumulation of apo(a) in the arterial wall has been shown to be directly associated with Lp(a) plasma levels [6,7]. Lysine binding of Lp(a) [3] might be of critical importance for the interaction of Lp(a) with components of the arterial wall. On the basis of sequence comparisons [8] and molecular modeling [9], kringle 37, the ultimate kringle IV repeat of apo(a), has been proposed as mediating the lysine binding of Lp(a). A recently reported sequence polymorphism in this domain 4168 Met→Thr [10] has not been evaluated with respect to its possible influence on the lysine binding of Lp(a). Expression of wild-type and mutant r-apo(a) in the hepatocarcinoma cell line HepG2 allows the investigation of structure–function relationships of apo(a) [11]. After transfection with apo(a) cDNA plasmids these cells express Lp(a)-like particles (r-Lp(a)) which band between LDL and

---

Address for correspondence: Dr Hans-Joachim Müller, Boehringer Mannheim GmbH, Department of Molecular Biology, TF-MM, Sandhoferstraße 116, D-68305 Mannheim, Germany. Tel.: +49-621-759-4330. Fax: +49-621-759-6168.

880

HDL after density gradient centrifugation [11]. Here, we describe the characterization of wild-type and mutant r-apo(a) expressed in HepG2 cells. The mutants were designed in order to identify the structural domains of apo(a) which are important for the assembly and lysine binding of r-Lp(a).

Methods

Standard cloning techniques [12] were employed to derive a series of mutant plasmids (Fig. 1) from the apo(a) cDNA expression vector pCMV-A18 [11]. Samples were fractionated by reducing or nonreducing SDS-PAGE prior to immunoblotting and detection with the apo(a)-specific monoclonal antibody 1A2 as described elsewhere [11]. Cell culture supernatants containing r-apo(a)/r-Lp(a) were fractionated by lysine-Sepharose chromatography [13]. The Lp(a) content of each fraction was determined by ELISA [11].

Results and Discussion

Site of Lp(a) assembly

We have previously described the construction of the cDNA expression plasmid pCMV-A18 encoding an apo(a) isoform with 17 kringle IV repeats, a single kringle V and a protease domain [11]. In the conditioned medium of HepG2 cells which were transfected with plasmid pCMV-A18, r-apo(a) was found almost exclusively as r-Lp(a) lipoprotein

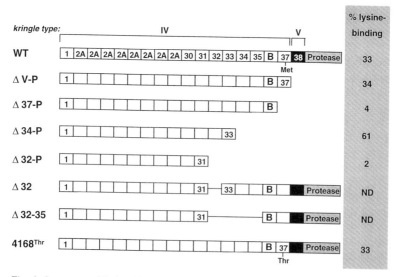

Fig. 1. Structure and lysine binding of wild-type and mutant r-apo(a)/r-Lp(a). The structure of pCMV-A18 encoded wild-type (WT) r-apo(a) containing 17 kringle IV repeats (1–37); a single kringle V domain (38) and a carboxyterminal protease domain are depicted at the top. Kringle 36 (B) contains the cysteine which is engaged in a disulfide bridge with apoB in LDL [11,15]. Carboxyterminal and internal deletion mutants and the kringle 37 variant 4168^Thr are shown below. Lysine binding of r-apo(a)/r-Lp(a) in the medium of transfected cells was determined by lysine-Sepharose affinity chromatography. The lysine-binding data (column on right) represent mean values from at least three independent determinations (ND = not determined). They reflect the portion of total r-apo(a)/r-Lp(a) which was eluted with 50 mM of the lysine analog ε-aminocaproic acid after extensive washing to remove the unbound material.

with covalently attached apo(a) and apolipoprotein B-100 (apoB) entities [11]. The site of Lp(a) assembly in vivo is still not known. It might occur in hepatocytes, at their surface, in the space of Disse or in the plasma, as suggested by the spontaneous covalent association of r-apo(a) in the plasma of transgenic mice upon infusion of human LDL [14]. Two experiments were performed to investigate where r-apo(a) is attached to apoB during the formation of r-Lp(a) particles. Lysates from HepG2 cells either untransfected or stably transfected with the pCMV-A18 plasmid were analyzed by nonreducing SDS-PAGE and subsequent immunoblotting (Fig. 2).

Lysates of untransfected cells did not show an anti-apo(a)-reactive band. In contrast, lysates of transfected cells revealed two bands: a major band representing apo(a) precursor and a minor band representing mature apo(a) glycoprotein. The absence of a band representing apoB-complexed apo(a) in the lysate of transfected cells and the predominance of this apo(a) species in the medium of the transfected cells suggested that r-Lp(a) assembly does occur outside the cells. Alternatively, rapid secretion of intracellularly assembled r-apo(a)/apoB complex might result in a low steady-state concentration of this complex inside the cells. To discriminate between these alternatives, we performed blocking experiments by adding polyclonal antibodies directed against either apo(a) or apoB to the culture medium of r-apo(a) producing HepG2 cells. As seen in Fig. 3, both reagents were able to inhibit the formation of covalent r-apo(a)/apoB complexes in a dose-dependent manner indicating that r-Lp(a) particle formation takes place at the cell surface or in the medium of transfected cells rather than inside the cells.

Identification of lysine-binding sites (LBS) in r-apo(a)

Wild-type r-apo(a) and the carboxyterminal deletion mutants ΔV-P, Δ37-P, Δ34-P and Δ32-P were compared with respect to their lysine binding. The two mutants ΔV-P and Δ37-P were found as components of r-Lp(a) particles whereas the Δ34-P and Δ32-P mutants were produced as free r-apo(a) glycoproteins (data not shown). The lysine-binding data are summarized in Fig. 1. The almost complete loss of lysine binding for the mutants

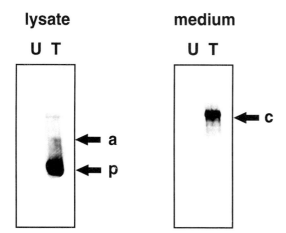

Fig. 2. Characterization of intracellular and extracellular r-apo(a) by nonreducing SDS-PAGE. Lysates and culture medium from untransfected (**U**) and pCMV-A18 transfected (**T**) HepG2 cells were fractionated by nonreducing SDS-PAGE prior to immunoblotting with apo(a)-specific monoclonal antibody 1A2. The positions of r-apo(a) precursor (**p**), mature apo(a) glycoprotein (**a**) and covalent apo(a)/apoB-complexes (**c**) are indicated.

882

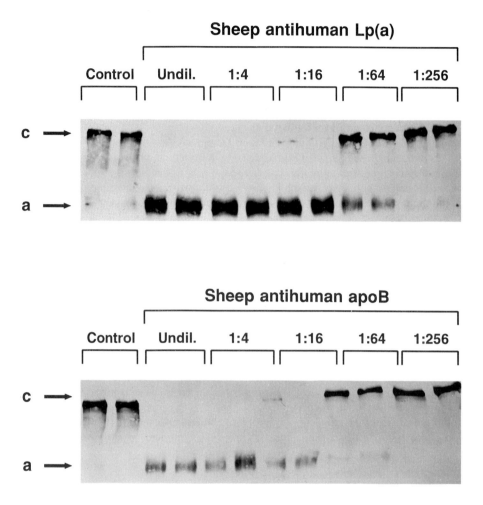

Fig. 3. Blocking of r-Lp(a) assembly by polyclonal antibodies against apo(a) and apoB. Sheep anti-human Lp(a) (Immuno) and sheep antihuman apoB (Boehringer Mannheim) sera were dialyzed against PBS. A constant volume of serial dilutions of both reagents was added to the culture medium of a stably transfected HepG2 expressing wild-type r-apo(a). Addition of PBS alone was used as a control. 24 h later, medium samples were analyzed by nonreducing SDS-PAGE and immunoblotting with apo(a)-specific monoclonal antibody 1A2. Both antisera exhibited a dose-dependent blocking of the assembly of Lp(a). The positions of free apo(a) glycoprotein (**a**) and covalent apo(a)/apoB-complexes (**c**) are indicated on the left.

Δ37-P and Δ32-P as compared to wild-type and mutant ΔV-P r-apo(a) is in agreement with the proposed existence of a single LBS in kringle 37 of apo(a) [8,9]. The increased lysine binding for the mutant Δ34-P (Fig. 1), on the other hand, is not compatible with a unique lysine-binding domain in apo(a). It rather suggests additional lysine-binding activity in kringles 32 and/or 33 of apo(a), which might be masked in Lp(a) particles. To investigate a possible role of LBS in these kringles during Lp(a) assembly we prepared two further deletion mutants, Δ32 and Δ32-35 (Fig. 1). Nonreducing SDS-PAGE and immunoblotting were used to compare wild-type, Δ32 and Δ32-35 r-apo(a)s with respect to Lp(a) assembly efficiency (data not shown). Both mutants exhibited less formation of covalent r-apo(a)/apoB complexes than wild-type r-apo(a) (>98% complex). The effect was more pronounced for the Δ32-35 mutant (9% complex) than for the Δ32 mutant (35% complex). Our data support a two-step model for the assembly of r-Lp(a) [11] in which noncovalent interactions between LBS in apo(a) and lysine residues in apoB precede the formation of an intermolecular disulfide bridge.

Met/Thr polymorphism in kringle 37 is neutral with respect to lysine binding

RT-PCR cloning from human liver polyA(+) RNA was used to obtain apo(a) cDNA subclones for the construction of the pCMV-A18 plasmid [11]. Subsequent sequencing of a cloned apo(a) cDNA fragment revealed a single nucleotide substitution in codon 4168 which results in a Met→Thr substitution in kringle 37 of apo(a). The same sequence variation occurred in four independent clones, indicating that we had identified a polymorphism rather than a cloning artifact. Site-directed mutagenesis was employed to reconstruct the published apo(a) cDNA (3) encoding a 'Met-apo(a)'. The Met/Thr polymorphism has also been observed by others [10]. In a sample of 13 persons 'Met-alleles' and 'Thr-alleles' were shown to be similarly represented. The occurrence of this sequence variation in kringle 37, the only accessible lysine-binding domain in Lp(a), might result in a different lysine binding of 'Met-Lp(a)' as compared to 'Thr-Lp(a)'. To address this question we compared r-Lp(a)s containing Met-apo(a) (WT) and Thr-apo(a) (4168^{Thr}) with respect to their lysine binding. Identical lysine-binding activity for the two variants (Fig. 1) argues against the possibility that Met-Lp(a) and Thr-Lp(a) might exhibit differential atherogenicity or thrombogenicity because of their different lysine binding.

Acknowledgements

We gratefully acknowledge the excellent technical assistance of Hildegard Kern, Gudrun Geiselmann, Gabriele Müller, Ilse Schulz and Christiane Windecker. This work was supported in part by the DFG grant AR 161/1-3.

References

1. Utermann G. Science 1989;246:904–910.
2. Gaw A, Hobbs HH. Curr Opin Lipidol 1994;5:149–155.
3. McLean JW, Tomlinson JE, Kuang W-J, Eaton DL, Chen EY, Fless GM, Scanu AM, Lawn RM. Nature 1987;300:132–137.
4. Scanu AM, Fless GM. J Clin Invest 1990;85:1709–1715.
5. Grainger DJ, Kemp PR, Liu AC, Lawn RM, Metcalfe JC. Nature 1994;370:460–462.
6. Rath M, Niendorf A, Reblin T, Dietel M, Krebber, H-J, Beisiegel U. Arteriosclerosis 1988;9:579–592.
7. Pepin JM, O'Neil JA, Hoff HF. J Lipid Res 1991;32:317–327.
8. Scanu AM, Miles LA, Fless GM, Pfaffinger D, Eisenbart J, Jackson E, Hoover-Plow JL, Brunck T, Plow EF. J Clin Invest 1993;91:283–291.
9. Guevara J Jr, Spurlino J, Jan AY, Yang C, Tulinsky A, Venkataram Prasad BV, Gaubatz JW, Morrisett JD. Biophys J 1993;64:686–700.
10. Van der Hoek YY, Wittekoek ME, Beisiegel U, Kastelein JJP, Koschinsky ML. Hum Mol Genet 1993;2: 361–366.
11. Brunner C, Kraft H-G, Utermann G, Müller H-J. Proc Natl Acad Sci USA 1993;90:11643–11647.
12. Sambrook J, Fritsch EF, Maniatis T (1989) Molecular Cloning: A Laboratory Manual. Cold Spring Harbor, NY: Cold Spring Harbor Lab.
13. Armstrong VW, Harrach B, Robenek H, Helmhold M, Walli AK, Seidel D. J Lipid Res 1990;31:429–441.
14. Chiesa G, Hobbs HH, Koschinsky ML, Lawn RM, Maika SD, Hammer RE. J Biol Chem 1992;267:24369–24374.
15. Koschinsky ML, Côte GP, Gabel B, Van der Hoek YY. J Biol Chem 1993;268:19819–19825.

884

Metabolism and atherogenicity of apo(a) in transgenic mice

F.P. Mancini[1], V. Mooser[1], J. Murata[2], D. Newland[2], R.E. Hammer[1], D.A. Sanan[2] and H.H. Hobbs[1]

[1]Department of Molecular Genetics and Biochemistry, University of Texas Southwestern Medical Center and Howard Hughes Medical Institution, Dallas, TX 75235; and [2]Gladstone Institute of Cardiovascular Disease, San Francisco, CA 94141, USA

Abstract. Apolipoprotein(a) (apo(a)) is a large glycoprotein that circulates in plasma as part of lipoprotein(a) (Lp(a)). High plasma levels of Lp(a) are associated with coronary and peripheral atherosclerosis. Transgenic mice expressing human apo(a), human apoB100, and Lp(a) have been developed to examine the metabolism and potential atherogenicity of Lp(a).

Development of apo(a) and Lp(a) transgenic mice

Apo(a) is a large glycoprotein that is attached to the apoB100 of the low density lipo-protein (LDL) by a disulfide linkage and circulates in human plasma as part of lipo-protein(a) (Lp(a)) [1,2]. Lp(a) is of medical interest because numerous cross-sectional studies [3–7] and some [8–10], but not all [11–13] prospective studies have found that high plasma levels of Lp(a) are associated with coronary atherosclerosis. Apo(a) has an unusual species distribution. It is a major cholesterol-carrying lipoprotein in the European hedgehog [14], but is not present in any other species except humans, great apes and Old-World monkeys [15]. Transgenic mice expressing apo(a) and Lp(a) have been developed to provide an easy-to-manipulate animal model in which to investigate the metabolism and the possible atherogenicity of Lp(a) [16–18]. To date, only a single mouse line has been reported that expresses a human apo(a) transgene. This transgene, which is under the control of the mouse transferrin promoter, encodes for an apo(a) glycoprotein that contains 17 tandem repeats of a cysteine-rich sequence called kringle 4 [16]. The tissue distribution of expression of apo(a) in these mice is not physiologic; there is evidence of a low level of apo(a) expression in all tissues that have been analyzed.

Apo(a) is not covalently attached to LDL in the mouse plasma [16]. When plasma from the apo(a) transgenic mice was adjusted to a density of 1.215 g/ml and subjected to ultracentrifugation, almost all the apo(a) was in the bottom fraction. Infusion of human LDL, but not mouse LDL or human HDL, into the mice resulted in the rapid, covalent association of apo(a) with the infused lipoproteins [16]. From these studies it could be concluded that there were important species-specific differences in apoB100 or LDL structure which are responsible for the failure of apo(a) to complex with mouse LDL, and it could be predicted that coexpression of a human apo(a) and human apoB100 transgenes would yield a mouse that produced Lp(a).

Development of a transgenic mouse expressing Lp(a)

In collaboration with Dr Stephen Young's laboratory (Gladstone Institute, San Francisco California), a mouse expressing human apoB100 was developed using a 79.5-kb genomic fragment that contained all the coding sequences of the human apoB100 gene, as well as 19 kb of 5′ and 17.5 kb of 3′-flanking sequences [17]. Five C57BL/6 X SJL founder animals were generated in Dallas. The levels of human apoB100 in the plasma of these mice ranged from 4.4 to 41.1 mg/dl [17]. A series of other mice were developed using the same construct [17]. A similar genomic fragment was employed by Callow et al. to make FVB expressing the human apoB100 [18]. All the transgenic mice expressed human apoB100 in the liver, with very low levels of expression in the heart, and trace amounts in the intestines. Presumably, there is a *cis*-acting sequence that is necessary for intestinal apoB expression that was not contained in the genomic fragment. Offspring of an apo(a) and apoB100 mouse, which were hemizygous for both transgenes, had Lp(a) detectable in their plasma. The plasma levels of apo(a) in the apo(a)/apoB transgenic mice were approximately twice as high as in litter-mates which expressed only the apo(a) transgene.

To test whether the higher plasma levels of apo(a) in the apo(a)/apoB mice was due to a reduced rate of removal of human apoB100, the rates of clearance of radiolabeled mouse and human LDL were compared in nontransgenic C57BL/6 X SJL mice. LDL fractions were isolated by sequential density gradient ultracentrifugation of mouse and human plasma [19] and the apoB were radiolabeled with ^{125}I by the iodine monochloride method [20]. 15 µg of either human or mouse radiolabeled LDL-apoB was injected into the external jugular vein of five mice. Plasma samples were collected at 1 min and at 1, 2, 4, 6 and 12 h. The human LDL-apoB was cleared from the plasma at a significantly slower rate than mouse LDL-apoB ($T^{1/2}$ for human and mouse apoB 4.5 and 1.3 h, respectively). These results were consistent with prior studies that showed that human LDL binds with lower affinity than mouse LDL to mouse fibroblasts [21] and suggested that the higher plasma level of apo(a) in the apo(a)/apoB transgenic mice may be due to the fact that covalent attachment of apo(a) to LDL retards its clearance by a non-LDL receptor pathway. Alternatively, the apo(a)-human apoB complex is removed from the circulation by the LDL receptor at a reduced rate because of the interspecies differences in the affinity of mouse versus human lipoproteins [21].

The LDL receptor and apo(a)

To analyze the role of the LDL receptor (LDLR) in the metabolism of apo(a), we introduced the apo(a) transgene into mice in which the LDLR had been inactivated by targeted homologous recombination (LDLR (-/-)) [22]. The plasma levels of apo(a) were about twice as high in the LDLR(-/-)/apo(a) mice as in the apo(a)/LDLR(+/+) mice. Since the apo(a) was previously shown to be localized to the nonlipoprotein plasma fraction, why would elimination of LDL receptor activity be associated with an elevation in plasma apo(a) levels? To test whether the apo(a) in these mice is associated with LDL in a noncovalent fashion, we used a polyclonal rabbit-antimouse apoB100 antibody to immunoprecipitate apoB100-containing lipoproteins from the plasma of apo(a), apo(a)/ DLR(-/-), and litter mate control mice. Immunoblot analysis of the immunoprecipitates using an antihuman apo(a)-specific antibody revealed coprecipitation of apo(a) with the mouse apoB. Thus, at least a fraction of the apo(a) that circulates in the mouse plasma is associated with mouse apoB-containing lipoproteins. If association of apo(a) with mouse LDL prolongs its residence time in plasma, the higher plasma levels of apo(a) in the apo(a)/LDLR(-/-) mice may be due to the larger pool size of LDL in these mice. Alternatively, if the apo(a) is cleared together with mouse apoB via the LDL receptor, the reduced rate of removal LDL in the LDLR(-/-) mice may be responsible for the higher plasma level of Lp(a) in these mice. Efforts are now underway to determine which of these two mechanisms is responsible for the higher plasma levels of apo(a) in the LDLR(-/-) mice.

Apo(a) expression and the development of fatty streaks

It was previously shown that the apo(a) transgenic mice developed significantly more aortic fatty streaks than control mice after a high-fat, high-cholesterol diet [23]. In order to examine the atherogenicity of apo(a), we placed 8–10-week old apo(a) transgenic mice and their litter-mate controls on a high-cholesterol, high-fat diet (1.5% cholesterol, 7.5% cocoa butter and 0.5% sodium cholate, 11% total fat) for 3.5 months. On this diet, the mean plasma cholesterol levels of the apo(a) mice (n = 19) increased from 92 ± 3 to 215 ± 16 mg/l, and from 93 ± 4 to 184 ± 10 mg/l in the control mice (n = 13).

The animals were sent to the Gladstone Institute where they were sacrificed and the heart, together with the ascending aorta, was perfused in formalin, fixed overnight and frozen in O.C.T. (Tissue-Tek O.C.T. Compound, Miles, Inc., Elkhart, IN). A total of twenty 10-μm sections were taken from a 400-μm section of the Paigen zone of the proximal aorta in 22 apo(a) transgenic (11 males, 11 females) and 19 control mice (13 males, 6 females). The Paigen zone is located downstream of the aortic sinus and beyond the coronary arteries, where the valves are reduced to small triangular cusps and the aortic profile changes from trilobate to round [23]. The sections were stained with Oil Red O and the amount of lipid was quantitated using a computerized image-analysis system. The mean lesion area in the section was calculated for the two groups of mice, and the results are shown in Fig. 1. A total of 63% of control animals and 82% of the apo(a) transgenic mice had no detectable lesions. There was no significant difference in the lesion area in the remainder of the mice (p = 0.18).

The lack of a significant difference between the amount of lipid staining is in contrast

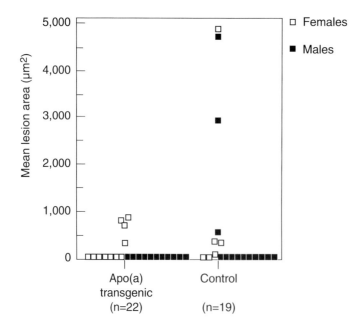

Fig. 1. Lipid-staining lesion area in mouse aortas. The mean area of lesions is shown for each of 22 apo(a) transgenic C57BL/6/SJL mice and 19 litter mate controls. Individual mice are indicated by ■ (males) and by □ (females). The mice were fed a 1.25% cholesterol, 11% total fat diet for 3.5 months before being sacrificed. The methodology used to quantitate the lipid staining is described in the text.

to what was previously reported by Lawn et al. [24]. The reason for these differences is not immediately obvious. Both groups of mice were from the same line, were fed the same diet, and housed in a similar, though not identical, facility. The mice were both maintained by crossing the apo(a) transgenic mice into C57BL/6 X SJL F_1 mice but the mice in two experiments may have subtle differences in the proportion of C57BL/6 and SJL genes. This could be important since C57BL/6 and SJL differ dramatically in their susceptibility to the development of fatty streaks. C57BL/6 is highly susceptible to the development of fatty streaks, whereas the SJL strain is very resistant [25].

The results of this study point to the need for a better model in which to examine the effect of apo(a) on the development of vascular lesions. The results of this study should not be interpreted as meaning that apo(a) is not atherogenic. Apo(a) may require additional yet-to-be-identified factors to play a role in the development of the significant atherosclerotic lesion.

Acknowledgements

This work was supported in part by the National Institute of Health (HL-20948 and HL-47619) and the Perot Family Fund. Helen H. Hobbs is an Established Investigator for the American Heart Association.

References

1. Scanu AM, Fless GM. J Clin Invest 1990;85:1709—1715.
2. Utermann G. Science 1989;246:904—910.
3. Berg K, Dahlen G, Frick MH. Clin Genet 1974;6:230—235.
4. Armstrong VW, Cremer P, Eberle E, Manke A, Schultze F, Wieland H, Kreuzer H, Seidel D. Athero-sclerosis 1986;62:249—257.
5. Sandholzer C, Boerwinkle E, Saha N, Tong MC, Utermann G. J Clin Invest 1992;89:1040—1046.
6. Dahlen GH, Guyton JR, Attar M, Farmer JA, Gotto AM. Circulation 1986;74:758—765.
7. Rhoads GG, Dahlen G, Berg K, Morton NE, Dannenberg AL. J Am Med Assoc 1986;256:2540—2544.
8. Rosengren A, Wilhelmsen L, Eriksson E, Risberg B, Wedel H. Br Med J 1990;301:1248—1251.
9. Schaefer EJ, Lamon-Fava S, Jenner JL, McNamara JR, Ordovas JM, Davis CE, Abolafia JM, Lippel K, Levy RI. J Am Med Assoc 1994;271:999—1003.
10. Cremer P, Nagel D, Labrot B, Mann H, Muche R, Elster H, Seidel D. Eur J Clin Invest 1994;24:444—453.
11. Jauhiainen M, Koskinen P, Ehnholm C, Frick MH, Manttari M, Manninen V, Huttunen JK. Atherosclerosis 1991;89:59—67.
12. Alfthan G, Pekkanen J, Jauhiainen M, Pitkaniemi J, Karvonen M, Tuomilehto J, Salonen JT, Ehnholm C. Atherosclerosis 1994;106:9—19.
13. Ridker PM, Hennekens CH, Stampfer MJ. J Am Med Assoc 1993;270:2195—2225.
14. Laplaud PM, Beaubatie L, Rall SJ Jr, Luc G, Saboureau M. J Lipid Res 1988;29:1157—1170.
15. Makino K, Scanu AM. Lipids 1991;26:679—683.
16. Chiesa G, Hobbs HH, Koschinsky ML, Lawn RM, Maika SD, Hammer RE. J Biol Chem 1992;267:24369—24374.
17. Linton MF, Farese RV Jr, Chiesa G, Grass DS, Chin P, Hammer RE, Hobbs HH, Young SG. J Clin Invest 1993;92:3029—3037.
18. Callow MJ, Stoltzfus LJ, Lawn RM, Rubin EM. Proc Natl Acad Sci USA 1994;91:2130—2134.
19. Havel RJ, Eder HA, Bragdon JH. J Clin Invest 1955;34:1345—1353.
20. Bilheimer DW, Eisenberg S, Levy RI. Biochim Biophys Acta 1992;260:212—221.
21. Corsini A, Mazzotti M, Villa A, Maggi FM, Bernini F, Romano L, Romano C, Fumagalli R, Catapano AL. Atherosclerosis 1992;93:95—103.
22. Ishibashi S, Brown MS, Goldstein JL, Gerard RD, Hammer RE, Herz J. J Clin Invest 1993;92:883—893.
23. Paigen B, Morrow A, Holmes PA, Mitchell D, Williams RA. Atherosclerosis 1987;68:231—240.
24. Lawn RM, Wade DP, Hammer RE, Chiesa G, Verstuyft JG, Rubin EM. Nature 1992;360:670—672.
25. Nishina PM, Wang J, Toyofuku W, Kuypers, FA, Ishida BY, Paigen B. Lipids 1993;28:599—605.

Reduction and oxidation of lipoprotein(a) have opposite effects on thrombo-atherogenic reactions dependent on lysine binding

Peter C. Harpel[1], Anita Hermann[1] and Neal Azrolan[2]

[1]Division of Hematology, Department of Medicine, Mount Sinai School of Medicine, New York, NY 10029; and
[2]The Rockefeller University, New York, New York, USA

Abstract. Posttranslational modification of Lp(a) significantly affects its lysine-binding site interactions. The atherogenic, sulfhydryl-containing amino acid homocysteine enhances the affinity between Lp(a) and fibrin. Lp(a) particles containing smaller apo(a) proteins may be more sensitive to reducing sulfhydryls since the total binding of various sized isoforms treated with homocysteine varies inversely with the size of the apo(a) protein. Mild oxidation of Lp(a) inhibits its binding to lysine-Sepharose and to plasmin-modified fibrin. This inhibition is associated with loss of tryptophan, a critical component of the lysine-binding pocket of apo(a) $K4_{37}$. Thus, the thrombo-atherogenic activity of Lp(a) may be influenced by its state of oxidation.

Elevated blood levels of Lp(a) are associated with carotid and coronary atherosclerosis, with reocclusion following coronary bypass surgery and angioplasty and with failure to recanalize the coronary artery in myocardial infarction survivors. Thus, Lp(a) is thrombo-atherogenic, but the underlying mechanisms are not known. Our interest in Lp(a) was stimulated by the observation that apolipoprotein(a) is partially homologous to plasminogen containing multiple copies of kringle 4, one kringle 5, and the protease region [1]. We had previously found that the binding of plasminogen to fibrin in plasma or in purified systems was increased by plasmin-induced modification of the fibrin surface [2]. Plasmin exposed new C-terminal lysyl residues in fibrin that interacted with the lysine-binding kringles of plasminogen. These results were the basis for studies showing that partial modification of the fibrin surface with plasmin enhances the binding of Lp(a) 3- to 4-fold [3]. Binding was inhibited by the lysine analog ε-aminocaproic acid (ACA), which indicates that the Lp(a)–fibrin interaction is dependent on lysine-binding site interactions. LDL failed to bind to fibrin, and plasmin treatment did not increase binding, which further implicates the apo(a) portion of Lp(a) in the interaction with fibrin. These interactions have their in vivo counterpart since extensive colocalization of Lp(a) with fibrin has been documented in human aortic atheromatous plaques [4].

Homocysteine and other sulfhydryl-containing amino acids increase Lp(a) binding to fibrin

Homozygous homocysteinuria is associated with prematurely severe atherosclerotic vascular and thromboembolic disease [5]. Individuals with moderate elevations of homocysteine also have vascular disease associated with thrombosis [6]. Several etiologic mechanisms have been proposed, but the underlying cause is not known. We have found that homocysteine, in concentrations as low as 8 μmol/l, stimulated a 20-fold increase in the affinity between Lp(a) and plasmin-modified fibrin, and a 4-fold increase with unmodified fibrin [7]. This increase in binding was also due to lysine-site interactions since ACA completely inhibited it. In contrast, after complex formation between Lp(a) and fibrin had occurred, ACA did not reverse the interaction, indicating that other binding sites were involved. Cysteine, glutathione and N-acetylcysteine also increased the binding of Lp(a) to fibrin. In addition to fibrin, Lp(a) binds to Factor XIIIa cross-linked fibrin degradation products (XFDP) [8]. Using these radiolabeled fragments as the ligand, we found that XFDP bind to immunoblotted homocysteine-treated Lp(a) as well as to the free apo(a) produced by homocysteine. In contrast, the strong reductant dithiothreitol produced apo(a) that did not bind XFDP. Thus, mild disulfide-reducing agents such as homocysteine yield highly reactive Lp(a) products whereas strong reductants inhibit functional activity.

To study the effect of homocysteine further, we purified Lp(a) from nine individuals with single-banded apo(a) phenotypes ranging from 500 to 760 kDa. No relationship was found between apo(a) size and the binding of these different isoforms to plasmin-modified fibrin. In the presence of homocysteine, however, the binding of Lp(a) was increased, and the magnitude of this increase correlated inversely with apo(a) protein mass. We studied next the effect of homocysteine on the binding to lysine-Sepharose of four different recombinant apo(a) constructs with various numbers of kringles. In the absence of homocysteine, similar molar quantities were found to bind to the lysine resin. Pre-incubation with homocysteine, however, increased total binding, and the magnitude of this increase varied inversely with the size of the apo(a) protein. Thus the reactivity of Lp(a) particles containing smaller apo(a) proteins appears to be more sensitive to reducing sulfhydryls. These studies suggest a biochemical relationship between the metabolism of sulfhydryl compounds, thrombosis, and atherogenesis.

Lipid peroxidation inhibits the binding of Lp(a) to lysine-Sepharose and to fibrin

The effects of oxidation on LDL have been extensively studied [9]. In contrast, less is known about the effects of oxidation upon the structure and function of Lp(a). Lp(a) oxidized by human mononuclear cells or by Cu^{++} showed decreased free amino groups, protein fragmentation, increased negative charge and high aggregability [10]. These particles were recognized by the macrophage scavenger receptor. We have obtained data indicating that mild oxidation has a profound effect on the lysine-binding site interactions of Lp(a). We have used 2,2'-azobis (2-amidinopropane) HCl (AAPH), a temperature-dependent free radical initiator that serves as a source of water- or lipid-soluble peroxyl radicals [11]. This agent was found to inhibit the binding of Lp(a) to lysine-Sepharose. In this study, Lp(a) incubated at 37°C for 30 and 120 min with 1 mM AAPH and subjected to gel filtration chromatography to remove the oxidizing agent was applied to lysine-Sepharose. The bound Lp(a) was eluted with ACA. Of the untreated Lp(a), 95.4% bound to the lysine column; in contrast, after 30 min of incubation with AAPH, 18.6% of the Lp(a) retained lysine-binding activity and after 120 min of incubation, only 11% of the Lp(a) was bound. These changes in lysine-binding activity were accompanied by increases in lipid hydroperoxide formation, measured as described [12], from 1.5 nmol/mg, to 34 nmol/mg at 30 min, to 71 nmol/mg at 120 min. For comparison, we incubated Lp(a) with 5 and 10 mM AAPH for different times. Maximum lipid peroxide formation occurred at 8 h; for 5 and 10 mM AAPH, values were 1,617 and 2,054 nmol/mg. Thus when less than 2% of maximum lipid peroxidation occurs, the lysine-binding capacity of Lp(a) was almost totally inhibited.

Oxidation of Lp(a) also inhibited the binding of Lp(a) to plasmin-modified fibrin. Oxidized Lp(a) also bound less well to fibrin, and this inhibition in fibrin binding increased with the time of lipid peroxidation. We have found that the binding of oxidized Lp(a) to fibrin that is not partially degraded by plasmin is similar to the binding of native Lp(a). Thus, the enhanced binding that occurs with plasmin-modified fibrin is abolished by oxidation of Lp(a). In a parallel study, we have found that lipid peroxidation of Lp(a) with 20 mM Cu^{++} causes a loss of lysine reactivity similar to that found for AAPH. These studies document that lipid peroxidation of Lp(a) is associated with an inhibition in lysine-dependent interactions. Two previous studies have found large variations in the lysine affinity-column binding activity of Lp(a) purified from different individuals [13,14]. This heterogeneity was not related to apo(a) size polymorphism. Our data raise the possibility that oxidation may be responsible for these observations.

Rhesus monkey Lp(a) binds with lower affinity to lysine-Sepharose than does human Lp(a) [15]. Modeling of monkey apo(a) kringle 37, the putative lysine-binding kringle, with kringle 4 of plasminogen showed that the Trp to Arg substitution at position 72 in the monkey significantly change the lysine-binding pocket [15]. Tryptophan is an amino acid that is susceptible to oxidative destruction and this loss of tryptophan can be measured by monitoring fluorescence (ex 280; em 340–350 nm). We have applied this technique to the oxidation of Lp(a) by AAPH. Lp(a) was incubated with different concentrations of AAPH, and the change in fluorescence continuously measured at 37°C. We documented a linear decrease in tryptophan fluorescence with time that was proportional to the concentration of the oxidizing agent added. This indicates that tryptophans in the protein portion of Lp(a) were being progressively oxidized. We propose that this destruction of tryptophan may be important in the inhibition of the lysine-binding functions of Lp(a) that posttranslational modifications of Lp(a) may profoundly influence its pathogenic potential.

Acknowledgements

This study was supported in part by U.S. Public Health Service Grant HL-18828 (Specialized Center of Research in Thrombosis).

References

1. McLean JW, Tomlinson JE, Kuang WJ, Eaton DL, Chen EY, Fless GM, Scanu AM, Lawn RM. Nature 1987;330:132–137.
2. Harpel PC, Chang T-S, Verderber E. J Biol Chem 1985;260:4432–4440.
3. Harpel PC, Gordon BR, Parker TS. Proc Natl Acad Sci USA 1989;86:3847–3851.
4. Smith EB, Crosbie L. Atherosclerosis 1991;89:127–136.
5. Mudd SH, Levy HL, Skovby F. In: Scriver CR, Beaudet AL, Sly WS, Valle D (eds) The Metabolic Basis of Inherited Disease, vol 6. New York: McGraw-Hill, 1989;693–734.
6. Clarke R, Daly L, Robinson K, Naughten E, Cahalane S, Fowler B, Graham I. N Engl J Med 1991;324:1149–1155.
7. Harpel PC, Chang VT, Borth W. Proc Natl Acad Sci USA 1992;89:10193–10197.
8. Harpel PC, Borth W. Circulation 1992;86:Abs 1341.
9. Witztum JL, Steinberg D. J Clin Invest 1991;88:1785–1792.
10. Naruszewicz M, Selinger E, Davignon J. Metabolism 1992;41:1215–1224.
11. Niki E. Methods Enzymol 1990;186:100–108.
12. El-Saadani M, Esterbauer H, El-Sayed M, Goher M, Nassar AY, Jurgens G. J Lipid Res 1989;30:627–630.
13. Armstrong VW, Harrach B, Robenek H, Helmhold M, Walli AK, Seidel D. J Lipid Res 1990;31:429–441.
14. Leerink CB, Duif PFCCM, Gimpel JA, Kortlandt W, Bouma BN, van Rijn JM. Throm Haemostas 1992;68:185–188.
15. Scanu AM, Miles LA, Fless GM, Pfaffinger D, Eisenbart J, Jackson E, Hoover-Plow JL, Brunck T, Plow EF. J Clin Invest 1993;91:283–291.

891

In vitro mutagenesis demonstrates that the catalytic triad is essential for the protease activity of recombinant apo(a)

M. Pursiainen[1], C. Brunner[2], A. Ernst[2], H.-J. Müller[2], M. Jauhiainen[1] and C. Ehnholm[1]

[1]National Public Health Institute, Department of Biochemistry, Mannerheimintie 166, SF-00300 Helsinki, Finland; and [2]Boehringer Mannheim GmbH, Molecular Pharmacology, TF-MM, Sandhoferstrasse 116, D-68305 Mannheim, Germany

Lipoprotein(a), Lp(a), is a unique lipoprotein. According to several epidemiological studies an elevated Lp(a) plasma level is an independent risk factor for coronary heart disease, but the mechanism underlying this correlation as well as the role of Lp(a) in lipid metabolism are unknown [1–3]. Lp(a) consists of a low density lipoprotein (LDL) particle linked to the glycoprotein apo(a) [4–8]. The apo(a) protein displays extensive homology with plasminogen, PLG. The serine protease zymogen PLG is composed of kringle structures and a protease domain. Apo(a) consists of several repeats of plasminogen kringle 4-like sequences, one plasminogen kringle 5, and a protease domain [9–11]. The catalytic triad characteristic of serine esterases is present in both apo(a) (His_{4350}-Asp_{4393}-Ser_{4479}) and plasminogen (His_{602}-Asp_{645}-Ser_{740}) [11]. At the site where plasminogen is cleaved to generate plasmin the arginine residue in plasminogen has been replaced by serine in apo(a). This mutation may explain why apo(a) cannot be activated by tissue plasminogen activator (t-PA) or urokinase [11].

Several studies have shown that Lp(a) expresses enzymatic activity located in the apo(a) portion of Lp(a) [12–19]. We have previously reported that recombinant apo(a) (r-apo(a)) forms a noncovalent complex with human LDL, r-Lp(a), and that this interaction results in activation of the protease domain of r-apo(a) [18,19].

Here we performed a mutational analysis of r-apo(a) in order to analyze whether the proteolytic activity of reconstituted Lp(a) is encoded in the plasminogen-like protease domain. In addition, we also explored if the introduction of a plasminogen-like activation site into r-apo(a) would result in a 'proenzyme' that could be converted into a proteolytically active enzyme by plasminogen activators. Several mutant plasmids were derived from a wild-type apo(a) expression vector encoding an apo(a) isoform with 17 kringle 4 domains, a single kringle 5 domain and a protease domain. Wild-type and mutant plasmids were transfected into 293 cells. After purification by lysine-Sepharose chromatography, r-apo(a)s were reconstituted with plasma-derived LDL. The resulting r-Lp(a) species were compared with respect to their amidolytic activity in the absence/ presence of plasminogen activators and their proteolytic activity towards LDL.

Materials and Methods

Chemicals

Lysine-Sepharose was from Pharmacia Fine Chemicals, Uppsala, Sweden. Sodium

Address for correspondence: Christian Ehnholm, National Public Health Institute, Department of Biochemistry, Mannerheimintie 166, FIN-00300 Helsinki, Finland.

[125]iodide (13–17 mCi/μg) was from Amersham International, England. Phenylmethylsulfonyl fluoride (PMSF) was from Boehringer-Mannheim, Mannheim, Germany. Chromogenic substrates, plasminogen (PLG) and tissue plasminogen activator (t-PA) were from Kabi Diagnostica, Stockholm, Sweden. L-proline, and ε-amino hexanoic acid (E-ACA) were from Fluka, Switzerland.

Preparation of lipoproteins

Human low density lipoprotein was isolated from plasma [20] and labeled with [125]I [21]. The radioactive LDL preparations had specific radioactivities of 300–450 cpm/ng protein, the proportion of TCA-soluble radioactivity being 1–2%.

Expression of recombinant apo(a)

Standard cloning methods [22] were employed to construct the three mutant plasmids pCMV-A18_37-P, pCMV-A18_4479^{Ala} and pCMV-A18_4308^{Arg} (Fig. 1). The wild-type plasmid pCMV-A18 and the three mutant plasmids were transiently transfected into 293 cells as described [23]. 72 h after transfection culture supernatants were harvested and centrifuged 10 min each at 300 × g and at 4,000 × g to remove cells and cell debris, respectively. Samples were kept on ice while shipped to Helsinki.

The mutant plasmid V-P encodes a truncated r-apo(a) which lacks the kringle 5 and the protease domain. Two further mutant plasmids 4479^{Ala} and 4308^{Arg} encode r-apo(a)s with single amino-acid substitutions either in the catalytic triad (Ser 4479→Ala) or at the activation site (4308 Ser→Arg) of the apo(a) protease domain. R-apo(a)s were isolated from the medium of transfected cells by lysine-Sepharose affinity chromatography [24].

Determination of amidolytic activity

The purified r-apo(a) preparations were preincubated for 5 min at +37°C either alone or

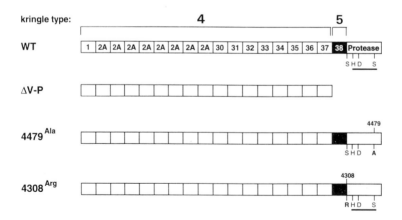

Fig. 1. Schematic representation of wild-type and mutant r-apo(a)s. The structural organization of wild-type r-apo(a) (WT) is represented at the top. It comprises 17 plasminogen kringle 4-like repeats (1,2A and 30–37), a single plasminogen kringle 5-like domain (38) and a serine-protease domain with the catalytic triad histidine (H), aspartate (D) and serine (S) shown underlined. Deletions and point mutations in the three mutants ΔV-P, 4479^{Ala} and 4308^{Arg} are indicated.

in the presence of LDL in 800 μl of 0.1 M Tris-HCl buffer, pH 8.0, after which the amidolytic activity was measured as described [16].

Analysis of r-apo(a)–LDL complex formation

Complex formation between r-apo(a) and LDL was analyzed by ultracentrifugation as described [19].

Proteolytic degradation of LDL by r-apo(a)

ELISA plates (Nunc, maxi-sorb) were coated with ^{125}I-labeled LDL, 500 ng LDL/well in phosphate-buffered saline containing 0.02% NaN_3 PBS, 100 μl/well. The plates were incubated for 2 h at +37°C and then overnight at +4°C. The wells were emptied and washed 10 times with 200 μl of PBS/well. Plates were treated with 2% BSA in PBS, and incubated for 2 h at +37°C, after which the wells were emptied and used. This coating procedure resulted in plates that contained approximately 50 ng ^{125}I-LDL/well. Different amounts of r-apo(a) were added to the wells, incubation volume was adjusted to 200 μl/well with PBS and the plates were incubated at +37°C for the times indicated. After incubation, 100 μl of the media were transferred to another plate and another 100 μl of the media was TCA-precipitated. To both plates 200 μl/well of scintillation liquid (Optiphase Hisafe 3, LKB, Wallac) was added. Radioactivity was determined using a LKB-Wallac γ-counter (Turku, Finland).

Other methods

Lp(a) was assayed using a solid-phase two-site immunoradiometric assay (Pharmacia, Uppsala, Sweden). ApoB was measured with an immunoturbidometric assay (Orion, Helsinki, Finland). Protein was quantitated by the method of Lowry et al. [25].

Results

Site-directed mutagenesis was employed to obtain three mutant plasmids from the wild-type cDNA expression vector pCMV-A18 encoding an apo(a) isoform with 18 kringle domains. Transfection of wild-type and mutant plasmids into 293 cells resulted in the secretion of free r-apo(a) glycoproteins, as these cells lack the ability to produce lipoproteins. None of the recombinant apo(a) species displayed enzymatic activity in the absence of added LDL. Upon incubation with LDL all four recombinant proteins were predominantly found in lipoprotein particles. As reported previously [19] the formation of a r-apo(a)–LDL complex resulted in activation of the protease region of the wild-type r-apo(a) and of the mutant r-apo(a)$_{Ser4308 \rightarrow Arg}$. The mutants r-apo(a)$_{del}$ and r-apo(a)$_{4479Ser \rightarrow Ala}$ did not show amidolytic activity after complex formation with LDL.

The protease domain of apo(a) is highly conserved. However, at the site where plasminogen is cleaved by its activators t-PA or urokinase to produce proteolytically active plasmin, the arginine residue is substituted by serine. To study whether restoration of the cleavage site might activate r-apo(a) we incubated wild-type r-apo(a) and mutant r-apo(a)$_{4308 \rightarrow Arg}$ in the presence and absence of t-PA (0—50 IU/ml). Upon incubation with t-PA both recombinant proteins remained enzymatically inactive. However, upon preincubation with LDL both wild-type r-apo(a) and r-apo(a)$_{4308Ser \rightarrow Arg}$ displayed amidolytic activity towards chromogenic substrates with arginine at the scissile bond (S-2765) (Fig. 2, bars 1 and 3). Neither of them cleaved the substrate S-2251 which has a lysine at the scissile bond. The addition of t-PA to the activated r-apo(a)/LDL mixtures did not result

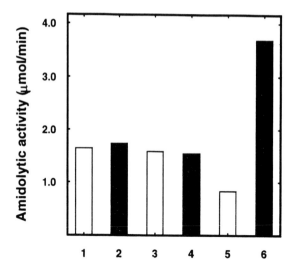

Fig. 2. Effect of tissue plasminogen activator (t-PA) on the enzymatic activity of recombinant apo(a) species and plasminogen. R-apo(a) (3 μg), r-Lp(a) (3 μg r-apo(a) + 6 μg of human LDL), or plasminogen (0.12 IU) was incubated in the presence of t-PA (50 IU/ml) and the amidolytic activity was measured using chromogenic peptide substrates S-2765 and S-2251 [16]. Bar 1: r-apo(a)$_{wild}$ + LDL with S-2765; bar 2: r-apo (a)$_{wild}$ + LDL + t-PA with S-2765; bar 3: r-apo(a)$_{4308Ser \rightarrow Arg}$ + LDL with S-2765; bar 4: r-apo(a)$_{4308Ser \rightarrow Arg}$ + LDL + t-PA with S-2765; bar 5: plasminogen with S-2251; bar 6: plasminogen + t-PA with S-2251. R-apo(a)s alone were inactive towards both substrates. R-apo(a)s with human LDL in the presence or in the absence of t-PA did not cleave substrate S-2251.

in further activation (Fig. 2, bars 2 and 4).

To study the interaction between LDL and r-apo(a), we immobilized radioactive labeled ^{125}I-LDL on polystyrene and incubated it with increasing concentrations of r-apo(a). Figure 3 illustrates one such experiment. It shows that wild-type r-apo(a) causes a dose-dependent degradation of LDL (Fig. 3, Panel A). This degradation was time-dependent (Fig. 3, Panel B) and in 24 h wild-type r-apo(a) (20 nM) degraded about 4—7% of the ^{125}I-LDL. This degradation was inhibited by the addition of excess unlabeled LDL, whereas the addition of albumin or HDL had no effect on ^{125}I-LDL degradation, which suggests that the proteolytic activity or r-apo(a) was specific for apoB (data not shown). Of the radioactive material released into the incubation medium 92—96% was TCA-soluble, indicating that the proteolysis of apoB resulted in small peptide fragments.

Neither the deletion mutant r-apo(a)$_{del}$ nor the r-apo(a) mutant carrying a single amino acid substitution in the catalytic triad at position 4479 was able to degrade immobilized LDL (Fig. 3, Panels A and B). These results clearly demonstrate that an intact catalytic triad is needed for proteolytic degradation of LDL.

Discussion

It is widely accepted that apoB100 of LDL and apo(a) are linked by a disulfide bridge in Lp(a), as recently confirmed with mutants where the critical cysteine residue in apo(a) had been substituted [23,26]. In addition to this covalent bond, noncovalent interactions have been believed to occur between human LDL and r-apo(a) [27]. The nature of these interactions and the domains involved in these interactions remain to be evaluated. Our recent results suggest that noncovalent bonding or "docking" between r-apo(a) and LDL

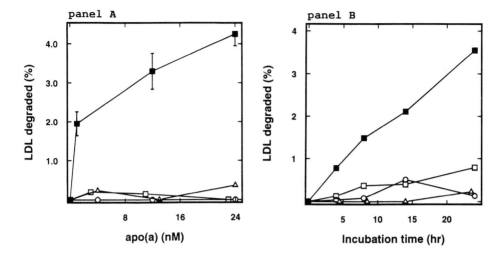

Fig. 3. Proteolysis of immobilized LDL by recombinant apo(a) species. Panel A: ^{125}I-labeled LDL was immobilized to polystyrene wells and incubated for 18 h at +37°C with increasing amounts of recombinant apo(a) species: wildtype r-apo(a), ■-■; r-apo(a)$_{del}$, O-O; r-apo(a)$_{4479Ser \to Ala}$, Δ-Δ, and with material from untransfected cells, □-□. For molar calculations a molecular weight of 250 kDa was used for r-apo(a). Values are mean ± SD of two experiments. Panel B: Immobilized ^{125}I-LDL was incubated in the presence of r-apo(a) species (20 nM) at +37°C for the times indicated. The symbols are as in panel A.

is a prerequisite for the enzyme activity of the protease region of r-apo(a).

Here we have continued the studies concerning the activation of the protease region of apo(a) by LDL. Wild-type and in vitro mutagenized apo(a) cDNA plasmids were expressed in the HepG2 cell line-293 and the r-apo(a) species expressed were purified by lysine-Sepharose affinity chromatography. We addressed three questions: 1) Are kringle 5 and the protease region of apo(a) required for noncovalent association of r-apo(a) with LDL?; 2) is an intact catalytic triad with the three invariant residues His-Asp-Ser a prerequisite for enzymatic activity?; and 3) can t-PA cause activation of apo(a) if the activation site of plasminogen is restored?

All mutant r-apo(a) species r-4479Ala, r-4308Arg and ΔV-P were able to form a noncovalent docking complex with LDL similarly to the wild-type r-apo(a). This shows that kringle 5 and the protease region are not required for the docking and suggests that factors in kringle 4 are involved in this process. Supporting evidence for this assumption comes from molecular modeling studies by Guevara et al. [28], who proposed that electrostatic interactions, hydrogen bonds and van der Waals interactions might contribute to the docking between apo(a) and apoB100 during Lp(a) particle assembly.

Employing a sensitive solid-phase LDL-degradation assay we were able to confirm our previous finding of a weak proteolytic activity associated with wild-type r-apo(a). The complete loss of enzymatic activity observed for both the deletion mutant ΔV-P (Fig. 3) and for the catalytic triad mutant 4479Ala (Fig. 3) indicates that the proteolytic activity of wild-type r-apo(a) is mediated by the plasminogen-like serine-protease domain at the carboxyterminal end of apo(a).

As the arginine residue at the site where plasminogen is activated by t-PA has been replaced by serine in apo(a), this substitution suggested that apo(a) may not be converted to an active enzyme. We therefore introduced arginine at the site where plasminogen is

896

cleaved in order to study whether this would render apo(a) activatable by plasminogen activators. Addition of tissue plasminogen activator to reconstituted Lp(a) containing either wild-type or mutant 4308^{Arg} r-apo(a) did not result in a detectable increase of amidolytic activity, which suggests that the primary sequence around the activation site might not be sufficient for activation. Kringle–kringle interactions, molecular folding of r-apo(a) or extensive glycosylation might explain why apo(a) cannot be activated by plasminogen activator.

In vivo, other activation mechanism(s) might exist to convert the proteolytic activity of r-Lp(a) described here to a more significant activity which might be related to a still unknown physiological function of Lp(a). From this we conclude that the activation mechanism for apo(a) is different from that of plasminogen.

Despite the fact that apo(a) is activated by forming a complex with apoB100, the protease activity is still low. Whether this is due to our in vitro conditions is unknown at the moment. This study illustrates the usefulness of in vitro mutated proteins in elucidating the mechanism underlying the activation of r-apo(a) proteolytic activity.

In conclusion, our mutational analysis of r-apo(a) indicates the existence and the localization of a proteolytic activity in r-apo(a) which is detectable only after reconstitution with LDL. Further studies will be needed to evaluate the physiological importance of this activity.

Acknowledgements

The authors thank Miss Tuula Lahtinen, Mrs Sirkka Metiäinen, Mrs Ritva Keva, Mrs Ritva Nurmi and Mrs Liisa Ikävalko for their expert technical assistance and Mrs Tuula Kaleva for typing the manuscript. This work was supported by Sigrid Juselius foundation, Helsinki, Finland.

References

1. Armstrong VW, Cremer P, Eberle E, Manke A, Schulze F, Wieland H, Kreuzer H, Seidel D. Atherosclerosis 1986;62:249–257.
2. Rhoads GG, Guyton JR, Attar M, Farmer JA, Katuz JA, Gotto AM. Circulation 1986;74:758–765.
3. Hoefler G, Harnoncourt F, Paschke E, Mirtl W, Pfeiffer KH, Kostner G. Atherosclerosis 1988;8:398–401.
4. Simons K, Ehnholm C, Renkonen O, Bloth B. Acta Pathol Microbiol Scand 1970;B78:459–466.
5. Ehnholm C, Garoff H, Simons K, Aro H. Biochim Biophys Acta 1971;236:431–439.
6. Utermann G, Weber W. FEBS Lett 1983;154:357–361.
7. Seman LJ, Breckenridge WC. Biochem Cell Biol 1986;64:999–1009.
8. Fless GM, Pfaffinger DJ, Eisenbart JD, Scanu AM. J Lipid Res 1990;31:909–918.
9. Kratzin H, Armstrong VW, Niehaus M, Hilschmann N, Seidel D. Biol Chem Hoppe-Seyler 1987;368:1533–1544.
10. Eaton DL, Fless GM, Kohr WJ, McLean JW, Xu Q-T, Miller CG, Lawn RM, Scanu AM. Proc Natl Acad Sci USA 1987;84:3224–3228.
11. McLean JW, Tomlinson JE, Kuang W-J, Eaton DL, Chen EY, Fless GM, Scanu AM, Lawn RM. Nature 1987;330:132–137.
12. Jürgens GM, Kostner GM, Holasek A. Artery 1977;3:13–26.
13. Salonen E-M, Jauhiainen M, Zardi L, Vaheri A, Ehnholm C. EMBO J 1989;8:4035–4040.
14. Ehnholm C, Jauhiainen M, Metso J, Salonen E-M, Vaheri A. In: Gotto AM, Smith LC (eds) Drugs Affecting Lipid Metabolism. Amsterdam: Elsevier, 1990;435–440.
15. Chulkova TM. Biochem Biophys Res Commun 1990;171:555–561.
16. Jauhiainen M, Metso J, Koskinen P, Ehnholm C. Biochem J 1991;274:491–496.
17. Chulkova TM, Tertov VV. FEBS Lett 1993;336:327–329.
18. Pursiainen MS, Jauhiainen M, Kovanen PT, Ehnholm C. Chem Phys Lipids 1994;67/68:25–33.
19. Pursiainen M, Jauhiainen M, Ehnholm C. Biochim Biophys Acta 1994 (in press).

20. Havel RJ, Eder HA, Bragdon JR. J Clin Invest 1955;34:1345–1353.
21. Bilheimer DW, Eisenberg S, Levy RI. Biochim Biophys Acta 1972;260:212–221.
22. Sambrook J, Fritsch EF, Maniatis T. Molecular Cloning: a laboratory manual. Cold Spring Harbor Lab, Cold Spring Harbor, NY, 1989.
23. Brunner C, Kraft H-G, Utermann G, Müller H-J. Proc Natl Acad Sci USA 1993;90:11643–11647.
24. Armstrong VW, Harrach B, Robenek H, Helmhold M, Walli AK, Seidel D. J Lipid Res 1990;31:429–441.
25. Lowry OH, Rosebrough NJ, Farr AL, Randall RJ. J Biol Chem 1951;193:265–275.
26. Koschinsky ML, Côté PG, Gabel B, Van der Hoek YY. J Biol Chem 1993;268:19819–19825.
27. Phillips ML, Lembertas AV, Schumaker VN, Lawn RM, Shire SJ, Zioncheck TF. Biochemistry 1993;32:3722–3728.
28. Guevara J, Spurlino JC, Jan AY, Yang C-Y, Tulinsky A, Prasad BVV, Gaubatz JW, Morrisett JD. Biophys J 1993;64:686–700.

Lp(a) and the arterial wall

M. Bihari-Varga

Second Department of Pathology, Division of Biochemistry, Semmelweis University of Medicine, Üllöi út 93, H-1091 Budapest, Hungary

Abstract. Possible mechanisms of Lp(a) penetration and arterial accumulation have been studied in vitro. 1) Lp(a), exposed to endothelial cells (EC) in culture, underwent structural alterations attributed to oxidative processes. The affinity of modified Lp(a) to serum glycosaminoglycans (GAG) was increased and it exhibited cytotoxicity to EC. 2) Lp(a) added to the culture medium of subendothelial cells stimulated their synthesizing activity and induced alterations in the pattern of excreted extracellular macromolecules; the induced alterations in the composition of proteoglycans (PG) increased their affinity to Lp(a). 3) Complex formation with PG resulted in changes in the physical structure, mobility and susceptibility to oxidation of the Lp(a) molecule and increased its recognition by macrophage receptors.

In a series of epidemiological studies in Caucasian populations a positive correlation of high serum Lp(a) levels with ischemic vascular diseases has been demonstrated. To confirm the role of Lp(a) as an independent risk factor in atherogenesis its contribution to plaque formation had to be detected. Investigations of postmortem arterial wall samples, of arterial wall biopsies obtained at bypass surgery, and of resected bypass vein grafts demonstrated the accumulation of apo(a) or Lp(a) in these tissues. Quantitative analyses found a correlation between plasma Lp(a) levels and the concentration of Lp(a) in the vascular tissues.

As to the pathophysiological processes, there are several competing hypotheses. Many reports indicate that Lp(a) either enters the arterial wall like LDL — at places of endothelial injury or by diffusion through the endothelial layer — or, due to its homology to plasminogen, displaces the latter from its binding site on endothelial cells. Traversing the endothelium Lp(a) might be trapped within the extracellular matrix of the vessel wall by binding avidly to molecules typically found in the atherosclerotic lesion such as elastin, fibronectin, collagen, fibrin, GAG and PG. It is also generally agreed that another means by which Lp(a) might accumulate in the vessel wall is inside macrophage cells; however, there is still controversy over the pathways that mediate cellular uptake of Lp(a) and might account for macrophage-derived foam cells.

In the present study we will discuss certain aspects of a) the role of structural modifications of Lp(a), caused by cell-mediated oxidation or/and by the interaction with serum GAG in the initiation of EC damage; b) the contribution of various extracellular macromolecules in retaining Lp(a) in the vascular tissue; and c) the capability of Lp(a) and its complexes to induce cholesteryl ester accumulation in macrophages.

Experimental procedures

Isolation, analysis and structural characterization of human serum lipoproteins [1,2], of serum GAG and of arterial PG, collagen and elastin [3] were described previously. EC and smooth muscle cell (SMC) culture studies, including methods for cultivation, morphological and chemical examinations, measurement of synthesizing activity and assessment of cytotoxicity were performed as published in detail [4]. Lp(a) reactivity with arterial macromolecules and the effect on foam-cell formation was investigated according to previous methods [5].

Results and Discussion

Mechanism of Lp(a) penetration: interaction with aortic EC

Our results indicate that Lp(a) exposed to EC in culture underwent certain structural alterations (Table 1). The changes might be attributed to oxidative processes and are similar to those reported previously for LDL [4]: compared to native Lp(a), oxidized particles had a greater negative charge with faster electrophoretic mobility and significantly higher concentration of thiobarbituric acid reactive substances (TBARS) and conjugated dienes. It is of interest that under the same experimental conditions Lp(a) showed a higher susceptibility to oxidation than LDL.

Our earlier work showed that soluble GAG, present in human plasma even under physiological conditions, interact with apoB-containing lipoproteins (Lp) and we suggested that Lp(a), because it reacts more strongly than LDL, might be a favored substrate for such an interaction [5]. As the negative charge of the oxidized particles is higher, it seemed likely that ionic interactions would take place to a greater extent between GAG and the modified Lp. Indeed, it could be shown that the affinity of the modified Lp molecules to serum GAG is increased: EC-incubated Lp(a) yielded a 3-fold, EC-LDL a 2-fold increase in reactivity over the relevant controls. It is of interest that HDL, which had been found to prevent LDL–GAG complex formation, also blocked the interactions between GAG and Lp(a), EC-LDL and EC-Lp(a).

On the other hand, the above studies produced evidence that structurally modified Lp might be more toxic to EC. Exposure to EC-modified Lp(a) or LDL of confluent cultures resulted in the contraction of cells and in cell detachment from the substrate. By transmission electron microscopy the presence of autophagic vacuoles and lipid droplets could be demonstrated. Incubation with media supplemented with modified Lp(a), LDL or their GAG complexes resulted in the incorporation of TBARS in the cells, accompanied by a time-dependent decrease in cell number, a marked inhibition of ^{3}H-Thy incorporation into DNA, and an increase in the release of LDH into the culture medium, an indication that the cell membrane might have been ruptured (Table 2). Signs of cell damage were most pronounced in the case of the application of EC-modified-Lp(a)–GAG complex, followed by EC-incubated-LDL–GAG complex, EC-Lp(a), EC-LDL, Lp(a] and LDL in decreasing order. The protective effect of HDL against cell injury is striking.

Extensive research provides increasing amounts of evidence that humoral or tissue

Table 1. Effect of incubation with endothelial cells on Lp(a) and LDL

Lipoprotein	Electrophoretic mobility (R_f)	TBARS (nmol MDA/mg protein)	Conjugated dienes (nmol/mg protein)	Reactivity with serum GAG (hexuranic acid/cholesterol)
Lp(a)				
Control	1.0	0.52 ± 0.08	15 ± 3	0.27
EC-incubated	1.62 ± 0.04	26.3 ± 3.1	160 ± 23	0.64
LDL				
Control	1.0	0.2 ± 0.03	12 ± 3	0.09
EC-incubated	1.43 ± 0.03	16.9 ± 2.6	90 ± 16	0.16

900

Table 2. The toxicity of Lp(a) and LDL to synchronized endothelial cells in culture

Lipoprotein	TBARS (nmol MDA/mg cell protein)	Cell number (10⁴ cells/well)	³H-Thy incorporation (10⁴ cpm/well)	LDL release (% of total)
Lp(a)				
Control	0.79	5–7	9.8	8
EC-incubated	3.17	1.8–2.9	2.6	42
LDL				
Control	0.87	5–8	9	8
EC-incubated	2.26	2.1–4	3.7	33
Lp(a)–GAG complex				
Control	1.47	4–6	6.7	8
EC-incubated	7.30	1–2	1.3	69
LDL–GAG complex				
Control	1.20	4–7	7.5	8
EC-incubated	6.40	1–3	2.8	53
HDL + EC-Lp(a)	nm	4–6	7.3	12

Nm = not measurable.

modifications of Lp play an important role in atherogenesis. Our previous and present results support the theory that Lp(a) and LDL might undergo structural alterations in the bloodstream or at the endothelial surface. Such modifications might be caused by the absorption of GAG circulating in soluble form in human plasma [6], especially in pathophysiological conditions when the concentration of GAG is increased or its composition altered, when the concentration or activity of natural inhibitors of complex formation is changed [7], or when Lp(a) level is elevated [8]. Biological modification might occur via free radical-induced peroxidation initiated by EC. EC-modified lipoproteins investigated in the present studies differ from native Lp(a) or LDL with regard to several physicochemical characteristics and their reactivity with serum GAG was also increased. Modified Lp preparations, to the greatest extent EC-Lp(a)–GAG complexes, proved to be cytotoxic to EC in culture.

It is conceivable that the vicious circle consisting of oxidation of serum Lp at the endothelial surface, interaction of the modified particles with plasma GAG, and their uptake and internalization by EC might take place in vivo as well, causing an early and persistent cell injury and initiating lipid infiltration into the arterial wall. The inhibitory effect of HDL on complex formation and its protective role in cytotoxicity might add further evidence concerning the biochemical mechanism(s) of action of HDL in preventing the development of atherosclerosis.

Mechanisms of Lp(a) accumulation

Influence of Lp(a) on the synthesis of extracellular macromolecules
The major families of arterial macromolecules synthesized by subendothelial cells are: PG, collagen, elastin, fibronectin. Their amount and composition within the vascular wall is subject to different physiological and pathological processes, including atherosclerosis. It could be shown that Lp(a) added to the medium of arterial SMC in culture was

internalized, and this stimulated the modulation of the cells from a quiescent to a proliferating condition. Since proliferating SMC are known to synthesize more extracellular macromolecules than quiescent ones, it seemed to be of interest to study the influence of Lp(a) on the synthesis of these substances. According to our results, the amount of PG, collagen and elastin within the cells was increased by 12.8, 8.6 and 14.0% respectively after incubation with Lp(a) for 7 days. The GAG composition of PG changed too: the relative amounts of chondroitin-6-sulfate and of dermatan sulfate significantly increased. The concentration of PG, collagen and elastin excreted into the culture medium increased by 16.0, 7.5 and 15.7% respectively.

Lp(a) binding to extracellular macromolecules
Immunohistochemical and biochemical evidence supports the hypothesis that PG of the intimal ground substance contribute to the deposition of LDL in atherosclerotic lesions. Our previous investigations demonstrated that Lp(a) reacts significantly more with PG than does LDL [5]. In vitro experiments, including our own studies, showed that human LDL that has been complexed to arterial PG undergoes structural alterations involving a disruption of the lipid–protein organization, as detected by low-angle X-ray analysis, differential scanning calorimetry, proton nuclear magnetic resonance and increased susceptibility to tryptic fragmentation. It has been suggested that once LDL particles enter the intima, other types of structural modifications, e.g., oxidative alteration, could take place besides those possibly induced by association with extracellular matrix components [9]. In the present study we raised the question whether the structural modifications produced in Lp(a) by the in vitro interaction with arterial PG are of the same nature and order as those occurring in LDL, and whether the complex formation could modify its susceptibility to oxidation.

Results obtained by the investigation of PG–Lp(a) complexes by temperature-dependent techniques showed changes of physical parameters characterizing the lipid domain of the Lp molecule: an irreversible phase change from liquid to liquid-crystalline took place in the core cholesteryl esters, and the spherulites formed lost their thermotropic nature. The nature and extent of physical changes of Lp(a) were similar to those described for LDL [10]. As seen in Table 3, PG-induced modifications also potentiated Cu^{2+} binding and

Table 3. Modification of copper-catalyzed in vitro oxidation of Lp(a) by arterial PG

Lipoprotein	TBARS (nmol/mg protein)	Conjugated dienes (nmol/mg protein)
Lp(a)		
Control	0.3	14
Oxidized	8.9	180
Lp(a)–PG		
Control	0.9	17
Oxidized	49.7	740
LDL		
Control	0.2	13
Oxidized	7.4	140
LDL–PG		
Control	1.6	15
Oxidized	37.3	520

902

subsequent Lp oxidation. Oxidation rate was higher for Lp(a)–PG and Lp(a) than for the relevant LDL preparations. Although the specific structural changes in the Lp(a) molecule responsible for the increased susceptibility to oxidation are not yet clarified it seems likely that the interaction with PG brought about chemical events that increased the number of binding sites for Cu^{2+}, as also suggested for LDL.

Intracellular Lp(a) accumulation

One of the initial changes seen in atherosclerosis is cellular lipid accumulation. It has been suggested that various modifications of Lp lead to their uptake by arterial cells in an unregulated fashion. In vitro studies investigated the interaction of Lp(a) with macrophages and it was found that Lp(a) behaves very similarly to LDL and possesses no higher tendency to foam-cell formation. If, on the other hand Lp(a) was oxidized, or complexed with antibodies or with dextran sulfate, foam-cell formation was observed as with complexed LDL. In our investigations the question was raised to what extent interaction with GAG or PG, known to have great affinity to Lp(a), may be involved in shuttling it into macrophages. The findings clearly showed that Lp(a)–GAG and Lp(a)–PG complexes caused a high cholesteryl ester deposition in mouse peritoneal macrophages, which was 2.3 and 5.5 times more than that found with the corresponding LDL complexes. Our findings support the hypothesis that an association between high Lp(a) levels and the risk of atherosclerosis could be related in part to modification of Lp(a) particles by GAG or PG and their effect on foam-cell formation in the arterial wall.

The results presented suggest that Lp(a), once entering the vascular wall, initiates a variety of pathological circuits. Should Lp(a) stimulate proliferation and synthesizing activity of SMC in vivo as well, the induced quantitative and qualitative alterations in the pattern of extracellular macromolecules might be shifted to one with elevated binding capacity for Lp(a). The excreted macromolecules of 'pathological' composition might initiate a feedback mechanism consisting of focal entrapment of Lp(a) in the intima and consequential changes in its physical structure, mobility and susceptibility to oxidation. All these structural modifications may have an influence on Lp(a) recognition by macrophage scavenger receptors and thus on foam-cell formation.

Acknowledgements

This study was supported by a Hungarian Scientific Research Programme grant (No. OTKA III/1070) and by a grant of the Hungarian Scientific Council on Health (No. ETT 6-266).

References

1. Bihari-Varga M et al. Int J Biol Macromol 1990;12:207–212.
2. Bihari-Varga MJ. Thermal Anal 1992;38:153–157.
3. Labat-Robert J, Bihari-Varga M, Robert L. FEBS Lett 1990;268:386–393.
4. Csonka E, Bihari-Varga M, Gruber EG. Arteriosclerosis 1993;18:103–109.
5. Bihari-Varga M et al. Arteriosclerosis 1988;8:852–857.
6. Bihari-Varga M, Sztatisz J, Gal S. Atherosclerosis 1981;39:19–23.
7. Kempen H et al. Atherosclerosis 1989;78:137–144.
8. Bihari-Varga M, Kostner G, Czinner A. Eur J Epidemiol 1992;8:33–35.
9. Camejo G et al. J Lipid Res 1991;32:1983–1991.
10. Bihari-Varga M et al. Int J Biol Macromol 1983;5:59–62.

Ranking of Lp(a) as a cardiovascular risk factor: results from a 10-year prospective study

P. Cremer[1], Dorothea Nagel[1], H. Mann[2], Barbara Labrot[2], R. Müller-Berninger[2], J. Thiery[1] and D. Seidel[1]

[1]*Institute of Clinical Chemistry, Klinikum Großhadern, Ludwig-Maximilians-Universität, Munich; and* [2]*Volkswagen AG, Gesundheitsschutz, Werk Kassel, Baunatal, Germany*

On the basis of its structural homology to plasminogen and LDL, and on several pathophysiological findings, Lp(a) has been proposed as an independent risk factor for cardiovascular disease (CVD) [1–5]. However, there are contradictory data from various epidemiological and clinical studies on this matter [6–16]. Some claim a predominant role for Lp(a) as a cardiovascular risk factor, whereas others are unable to show an association between Lp(a) serum concentration and the incidence of CVD.

This communication presents for the first time data from a large prospective cohort study, the Göttingen Risk, Incidence, and Prevalence Study (GRIPS) after a 10-year follow-up.

Participants and Methods

Details concerning the design and organization of the GRIPS study have been presented elsewhere [12,13] and will therefore be discussed only in brief.

General design

GRIPS included a total of 6,002 men aged 42–59.9 years at study entry. According to anamnestic data and noninvasive clinical examinations 5,790 of them were free of CVD at this time. At 10-year follow-up, data from 5,639 subjects (i.e., 97.4% of the total study group) were available.

Participants who developed a primary endpoint during the 10 years of follow-up are considered incidence cases for the respective disease. 4,605 subjects who remained free from any endpoint are considered the reference group.

Endpoints

787 subjects developed the following 841 primary endpoints: 299 fatal or nonfatal myocardial infarctions or sudden coronary deaths (referred to below as acute MI); 259 coronary heart disease (CHD) without acute coronary event; 101 fatal or nonfatal stroke events; 168 peripheral arterial vascular disease (PAVD); and 14 carotid stenoses (not evaluated because of the small number).

Secondary endpoints are suspect cases of cardiovascular disease (n = 34) and death from noncardiovascular causes (n = 209).

Laboratory methods

Cholesterol and triglycerides were measured by CHOP-PAP or GPO-PAP methods (Boehringer Mannheim, FRG) respectively. Lipoproteins were quantified by an analytical

Table 1. Median, 10 and 90% percentiles (PC) for Lp(a) in the reference group and the various cardiovascular incidence groups

	Reference (n = 4605)	MI (n = 299)	CHD (n = 259)	Stroke (n = 101)	PAVD (n = 168)
Lp(a)					
Median (mg/dl)	9	18	18	12	13
10% PC (mg/dl)	<5	<5	<5	<5	<5
90% PC (mg/dl)	41	58	48	47	46
p (Kolmogorov Smirnov)	–	<0.05	<0.05	NS	<0.05

The difference between reference and incidence subjects was tested for significance by the Kolmogorov Smirnov test. NS = $p \geq 0.05$: not significant.

schedule described elsewhere in detail [12,13]. Fibrinogen and apoproteins A-I and B were measured by nephelometry (Behring AG, FRG). Lp(a) was quantified as Lp(a) total mass by an ELISA technique (Immuno GmbH, FRG).

Results

The subjects of the various incidence groups revealed higher Lp(a) serum concentrations than the reference group (Table 1), and the incidence of various cardiovascular diseases was significantly higher for subjects in the 5th quintile (Q5) of the Lp(a) distribution curve than those in the 1st to 4th quintiles (Table 2).

On the basis of univariate analyses (Table 3) (relative risk of subjects in Q5 vs. those in Q1–4 for continuous variables or of subjects with vs. subjects without a categorized risk factor) the strength of the association of Lp(a) with the incidence of acute MI is less than that of LDL-cholesterol and family history for MI, similar to that of HDL-cholesterol and smoking, and stronger than that of triglycerides, age, systolic blood pressure, fibrinogen, BMI or glucose.

For chronic CHD without acute MI Lp(a) is a weaker risk factor than LDL-cholesterol, stronger than glucose, and similar to triglycerides and systolic blood pressure. For stroke, the impact of Lp(a) is stronger than that of any other plasma lipoprotein fraction, but weaker than systolic blood pressure, age, and fibrinogen. It compares with glucose, smoking, and triglycerides. For PAVD, Lp(a) is a weaker risk factor than smoking. It compares with that of LDL-cholesterol, age, and triglycerides. It is a stronger predictor than the concentration of either glucose or fibrinogen in plasma.

The ranking of risk factors for acute MI based on a multivariate logistic regression analysis (Table 4) supports the results of the univariate analyses. LDL-cholesterol proved to be the predominant risk factor, followed by family history of MI and Lp(a). Thus, the independent impact of Lp(a) on MI risk is clearly stronger than that of smoking, age,

Table 2. Relative risk of cardiovascular diseases and 95% confidence intervals (CI) for quintile 5 (≥ 29 mg/dl) vs. quintile 1–4 (<29 mg/dl) of the Lp(a) distribution curve

	Relative risk	95% CI
MI	2.3	1.9–2.9
CHD	1.9	1.5–2.4
Stroke	1.7	1.1–2.6
PAVD	2.0	1.4–2.7

Table 3. Ranking of risk factors (RF) for cardiovascular diseases based on univariate odds ratios (OR) for RF$_{pos}$ vs. RF$_{neg}$ subjects

Rank	MI (n = 299)	CHD (MI$_{neg}$) (n = 259)	Stroke (n = 101)	PAVD (n = 168)
1. OR ≥ 4 p < 0.0001	LDL-Chol (≥171 mg/dl) (cholesterol ≥ 249 mg/dl)	–	Systolic BP	–
2. OR 3—3.9 p < 0.0001	Family history for MI (yes)	LDL-Chol (cholesterol)	–	Smoking
3. OR ≥ 2—2.9 p < 0.0001	Smoking (yes) Lp(a) (≥29 mg/dl) HDL-Chol (<35 mg/dl)	Age	Age Fibrinogen	Lp(a) LDL-Chol Age Triglycerides
4. OR 1.6—1.9 p < 0.001	Triglycerides (≥196 mg/dl) Age (≥53 years) Systolic BP (≥140 mmHg) Fibrinogen (≥430 mg/dl)	Lp(a) Triglycerides Systolic BP	Lp(a) Glucose Smoking Triglycerides	Glucose Fibrinogen
5. OR <1.6 p < 0.05	BMI (≥28 kg/m^2) Glucose (≥111 mg/dl)	Glucose	–	–

systolic blood pressure, or HDL cholesterol.

As concluded earlier on the basis of 5-year GRIPS follow-up data [13], total cholesterol, apoB, apoA-I, triglycerides and body mass index did not enter either into the estimation model for MI risk in the present evaluation after a 10-year follow-up.

Based on our prediction model (Fig. 1), the MI risk derived from LDL-cholesterol is strongly influenced by other risk factors. The analysis provides evidence for the cumulative impact of multiple risk factors.

The average 10-year MI risk was 5% for the total study group. If LDL is the only risk factor in an individual and the risk profile otherwise is low, the average risk is exceeded at LDL concentrations >230 mg/dl. If, however, Lp(a) is also elevated (≥30 mg/dl) or the subject has a familial MI history, the average risk is exceeded at LDL concentrations of

Table 4. Ranking of MI risk factors (RF) based on multivariate logistic regression analyses

Category	Variable	RF-definition	Odds ratio
1. (Chi^2 ≥ 100; p < 0.0001)	LDL-Chol	+20%	2.0
2. (Chi^2 ≥ 50—99; p < 0.0001)	Family history for MI Lp(a)	Yes +30 mg/dl	3.5 2.0
3. (Chi^2 ≥ 30—49; p < 0.0001)	Smoking Age	Yes +9 years	2.3 2.0
4. (Chi^2 ≥ 20—29; p < 0.0001)	Systolic BP HDL-Chol (inverse)	+36 mmHg <35 mg/dl	2.0 2.2
5. (Chi^2 ≥ 4—10; p < 0.05)	Glucose Fibrinogen	≥150 mg/dl 250%	2.8 2.0

906

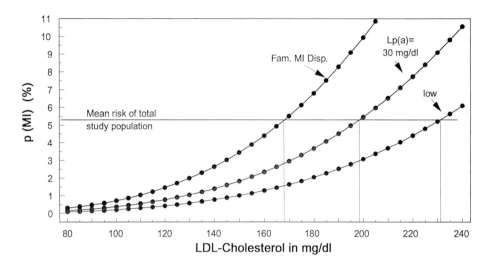

Fig. 1. Association between the LDL-cholesterol concentration and the 10-year MI risk, p (MI), as influenced by other risk factors (results based on the multivariate logistic regression model for the estimation of MI risk).

200 or 170 mg/dl respectively.

Similarly, Fig. 2 demonstrates that the impact of Lp(a) on the MI risk is strongly influenced by serum LDL concentration. The impact of Lp(a) is low if LDL-cholesterol is low (100 mg/dl), whereas it clearly augments the LDL-induced MI risk at borderline as well as at high LDL concentration levels (150 or 190 mg/dl respectively).

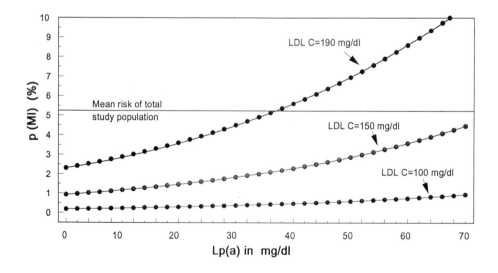

Fig. 2. Association between the Lp(a) concentration and the 10-year MI risk, p (MI), as influenced by LDL-cholesterol (results based on the multivariate logistic regression model for the estimation of MI risk).

Conclusions

1. The 10-year follow-up data of a large prospective cohort study (GRIPS) showed that LDL-cholesterol is the strongest risk factor for coronary heart disease and MI.
2. Lp(a) is an independent risk factor for myocardial infarction, with a stronger impact than HDL-cholesterol.
3. The association of Lp(a) with MI risk is strongly influenced by LDL-cholesterol concentrations.
4. There is evidence that Lp(a) is also an important risk factor for stroke and PAVD.

References

1. Kratzin H, Armstrong V, Niehaus M, Hilschmann N, Seidel D. Biol Chem Hoppe-Seyler 1987;368:1533–1544.
2. Miles LA, Fless GM, Levin EG, Scanu AM, Plow EF. Nature 1989;339:301–303.
3. Edelberg JM, Pizzo SV. Fibrinolysis 1991;5:135–143.
4. Scanu AM, Fless GM. J Clin Invest 1990;85:1709–1715.
5. Niendorf A, Rath M, Wolf K et al. Virchows Archiv Pathol Anat 1990;417:105–111.
6. Kostner GM, Avogaro P, Cazzolato G, Marth E, Bittolo-Bon G, Quinci GB. Atherosclerosis 1981;38:51–61.
7. Rhoads GG, Dahlen G, Berg K, Morton NE, Dannenberg AL. J Am Med Assoc 1986;256:2540–2544.
8. Zenker G, Költringer P, Bone G, Niederkorn K, Pfeiffer K, Jürgens G. Stroke 1986;17:942–945.
9. Armstrong VW, Cremer P, Eberle E et al. Atherosclerosis 1986;62:249–257.
10. Dahlen GH, Guyton JR, Attar M et al. Circulation 1986;74:758–765.
11. Jauhiainen M, Koskinen P, Ehnholm C et al. Atherosclerosis 1991;89:59–67.
12. Rosengren A, Wilhelmsen L, Eriksson E, Risberg B, Wedel H. Br Med J 1990;301:1248–1251.
13. Cremer P, Nagel D, Labrot B et al. Göttinger Risiko-, Inzidenz- und Prävalenzstudie (GRIPS). Heidelberg: Springer, 1991.
14. Cremer P, Nagel D, Labrot B et al. Eur J Clin Invest 1994;24:444–453.
15. Ridker PM, Hennekens CH, Stampfer MJ. J Am Med Assoc 1993;270:2195–2199.
16. Sigurdsson G, Raldursdottir A, Sigvaldason H, Agnarsson U, Thorgeirsson G, Sigfusson H. Am J Cardiol 1992;69:1251–1254.

Factors influencing the assembly of Lp(a)

Gert M. Kostner, Sasa Frank, Srdjan Durovic and Rudolf Zechner
Institute of Medical Biochemistry, University of Graz, Graz, Austria

Abstract. Recombinant apo(a)'s with different numbers of kringle-IV repeats were expressed in normal and in glycosylation-defective mammalian cells, and incubated with fresh LDL. The assembly of Lp(a) proceeded in two steps. In the first step, apo(a) forms a loose complex with LDL mediated by Lys groups on apoB and the unique kringle-IVs 30–36. This complex is dissociable by ε-aminocaproic acid and tranexamic acid. In a second step, the complex is stabilized by a disulfide bridge. The N-glycosylated sugars play no role in this assembly. The complex formation is unaffected by 10% NaCl but detergents inhibit the association. The results are compatible with an extracellular assembly of Lp(a) in vivo and might help to design Lp(a)-lowering medications.

It is generally accepted that elevated plasma concentrations of Lp(a) represent an independent risk factor for myocardial infarction and stroke [1,2]. Despite intensive investigations in recent years, the physiological function of Lp(a) remains elusive. Structurally, Lp(a) resembles a low density lipoprotein (LDL) particle with apolipoprotein (apo) B100 and apo(a) as major structural protein constituents. Apo(a) and apoB100 are linked by a disulfide bridge. A single free cysteine residue on apo(a) corresponding to Cys-4057 on the published apo(a) cDNA sequence is believed to be involved in this heterodimer formation [3]. Apo(a) is a glycoprotein with a high sialic acid content that shares extensive protein-sequence homology with plasminogen [4]. This homology includes the presence of sequences similar to kringle IV, kringle V and the protease domain of plasminogen on apo(a). There exist probably more than 50 apo(a) alleles in humans which determine proteins of different sizes, due to variation in the number of kringle IV (K-IV) repeats on apo(a). Lp(a) plasma concentrations are reported to be partially determined by the number of kringle IV repeats on the apo(a) gene [5].

Apo(a) and apoB are both produced in the liver. Metabolic studies in humans revealed that Lp(a) is not a lipolytic product of triglyceride-rich lipoprotein precursors [6]. The question of whether apo(a) forms a complex with apoB in hepatocytes or whether apo(a) binds to LDL only after its secretion to the interstitium or the plasma compartment remains open. Evidence has been found that free apo(a) can be secreted from liver cells. In transgenic mice that overexpress human apo(a), the apolipoprotein is found in the plasma of the animals in a lipid-free form. Lp(a)-like particles on the other hand were found in transgenic mice expressing human apo(a) together with human apoB [7]. Finally, several authors reported a strong binding affinity of recombinant apo(a) (r-apo(a)) or apo(a) produced in primary baboon liver cells to LDL in vitro [8].

Here we report the development of a system for the efficient expression of free r-apo(a) in cos-7 cells and different CHO cell lines. Using this system it was possible to investigate the extracellular association of r-apo(a) of various sizes with LDL, the function of the carbohydrate moiety of r-apo(a) in this process, and the influence of various substances on the assembly of Lp(a).

Address for correspondence: Gert M. Kostner, Institute of Medical Biochemistry, University of Graz, A-8010 Graz, Austria.

Material and Methods

All cell lines used were obtained from the American Type Culture Collection. Cos-7 (ATCC CRL 1651), CHO cell lines included a wild-type cell line (Pro-5-, ATCC CRL 1781), a line with blocked N-linked glycosylation (Lec 1, ATCC CRL 1735), a cell line with drastically decreased protein sialylation (Lec 2, ATCC CRL 1736), and a cell line with UDP-galactose deficiency in the Golgi apparatus (Lec 8, ATCC CRL 1737). Anti-apo(a) and anti-apoB antibodies were produced in our own laboratories [1]. Horseradish peroxidase-linked protein A and an enhanced chemiluminescent detection kit (ECL-kit) were obtained from Amersham Corp. Standard solutions for phenotyping apo(a) isoforms were purchased from Immuno AG (Vienna, Austria). Replication-defective biotinylated adenovirus (dl 312) in 40% glycerol, streptavidine-polylysine conjugate and human transferrin-polylysine conjugate in HBS buffer (20 mM HEPES, pH 7.3, 150 mM NaCl) were produced at the Institute of Molecular Pathology, Vienna.

Construction of apo(a) expression vectors

Apo(a) expression plasmids containing DNA sequences coding for 3, 5, 7, 9, 15, and 18 kringle IV-like domains, as well as the kringle V-like and protease-like domains, were assembled using several apo(a) cDNA clones reported by McLean et al. [4] (Fig. 1). Standard recombinant DNA techniques were followed. Specific apo(a) cDNA fragments (see below) were ligated into the Eco RI site of pSG 5 as described in detail previously [9,10].

Transfection of cultured cos-7 and CHO cells

Cos-7 cells were cultured in DMEM, supplemented with 10% LPDS. CHO cells (Pro 5-) and glycosylation-defective CHO cell lines (Lec 1, Lec 2, and Lec 8) were cultured in alpha MEM supplemented with 10% FCS or LPDS. Cos-7 cells were plated 24 h and CHO cells 48 h prior to DNA transfection in P60 dishes. Cell density reached approximately 300,000 cells per dish by the time of transfection. To obtain a high efficiency of transfection with the large plasmids, cells were transfected by a receptor-mediated gene delivery system [11]. Human growth hormone cDNA was cotransfected by the same method in some experiments.

Assembly of r-apo(a) with human LDL

LDL was prepared by ultracentrifugation in the density range 1.020–1.063 g/ml from

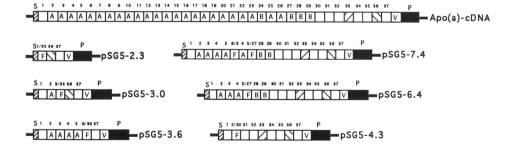

Fig. 1. Apo(a) cDNA constructs used for transfection. The numbering of K-IVs is according to McLean et al. [4]. S: Signal peptide; V: Kringle-V; P: Protease domain.

plasma obtained from healthy subjects. To avoid LDL oxidation all steps of LDL preparation were performed under nitrogen and in the presence of 0.5 mg/ml EDTA. Increasing concentrations of LDL (1, 5, 10 µg/ml of LDL-protein) were added to 0.4 ml of medium containing r-apo(a) at a concentration of 0.5 nM. Incubations were performed for 24 h at 37°C in the presence of aprotinin, leupeptin, and PMSF as protease inhibitors. Aliquots from the association incubation were removed at various times and analyzed for r-apo(a)–LDL complex formation by Western blotting. In some experiments the association mixture contained potential inhibitors of complex formation. These included iodoacetamide, detergents, ε-aminocaproic acid, and NaCl.

Analysis of recombinant apo(a) and of apo(a):apoB complexes

24 h after transfection, cell medium was harvested and incubated at various proportions with freshly prepared apo(a)-free LDL. Once the medium was aspirated a mixture of proteinase inhibitors was added to avoid r-apo(a) degradation. For analysis of r-apo(a) and complexes thereof with LDL, samples were diluted 1:1 with SDS buffer in the presence or absence of 5% β-mercaptoethanol. Samples were heated for 5 min at 100°C, cooled to room temperature and subjected to SDS agarose gel electrophoresis or SDS-PAGE followed by Western blotting using the ECL Western blotting detection reagent (Amersham). For the quantitation of free apo(a) and apo(a):apoB complexes, media incubated with LDL were analyzed by a double-antibody DELFIA using affinity-purified polyclonal anti-apo(a) for coating and anti-apo(a) or anti-apoB for detection.

Results and Discussion

Influence of the cDNA length on r-apo(a) expression and Lp(a) assembly

The cDNA constructs with 3, 5, 7, 9, 15 and 18 K-IV repeats cloned into pSG-5 were expressed in Cos-7-, CHO- and Hep-G2 cells using transferrinfection. Transfected cells were incubated for up to 72 h in DMEM and the biosynthesis was monitored. In all cases we obtained r-apo(a) concentrations between 0.5 and 1 µg/ml of culture medium. Larger apo(a) isoforms were expressed at somewhat higher concentrations than smaller ones. The r-apo(a) production reached its peak within the first 48 h, decreased markedly between 48-72 h and ceased after 96 h of cultivation. The media containing r-apo(a) were incubated with freshly prepared LDL in order to study the assembly. Time-course experiments revealed that maximal assembly was reached after 18–24 h incubation at 37°C. The assembly was studied by SDS agarose gel electrophoresis. Under nonreducing conditions cDNA constructs with more than five K-IVs, two bands were seen consisting of free r-apo(a) and r-apo(a):apoB100 heterodimers (verified by W-blotting with different antibodies). In the presence of 5% mercaptoethanol, the heterodimer complex fell apart and only free r-apo(a) and free apoB were seen. The cDNA constructs with <4.3 kB lacking the unique kringles 30–34 failed to assemble with LDL. We then quantified the relative amount of heterodimers by DELFIA. In the absence of ε-amino hexoic acid (ε-AHA) the assay measured the total amount of apoB complexed with r-apo(a), whereas in its presence, only r-apo(a):apoB heterodimers which were stabilized by disulfide bridges were recognized. As can be seen from Table 1, r-apo(a) fragments with 2.3–3.6 kB lacking the unique kringles 30–34 were unable to form complexes with LDL. The constructs with 4.3–7.4 kB associated between 64 and 72% with LDL. The addition of ε-AHA before DELFIA dissociated 14–17% of the complex; thus, only approximately 85% of the heterodimers were linked by disulfide bridges.

Table 1. Assembly of various r-apo(a) constructs (see Fig. 1) with LDL measured by DELFIA

R-apo(a)-cDNA	R-apo(a):apoB complex (%)	
	−ε-AHA	+ε-AHA
2.3 kB	<1	<1
3.0 kB	<1	<1
3.6 kB	<1	<1
4.3 kB	72	60
6.4 kB	66	56
7.4 kB	62	53

Cell media containing 0.4 µg/ml of r-apo(a) were incubated with 5 µg/ml of apo(a)-free LDL for 24 h at 37°C and the relative amount of heterodimer formation in % of total free apo(a) was measured by a double-antibody DELFIA in the absence and presence of 50 mM ε-AHA.

From these experiments we concluded that (1) an extracellular assembly of Lp(a) occurs from r-apo(a) and LDL in the absence of living cells and (2) that the unique K-IVs 30–34 are essential for this assembly.

Influence of the carbohydrate moiety on Lp(a) biosynthesis

Apo(a) is a heavily glycosylated protein, approximately 30% of the mass consisting of N- and O-glycosides. In order to study the role of sugars for the secretion and the assembly of r-apo(a), we expressed the 6.4 kB pSG-5 in wild-type (Pro 5-) as well as in the following glycosylation-defective CHO-cells: Lec-1, lack of glycosyltransferase T1; Lec-2, lack of CMP-sialic acid transport; Lec-8, lack of transport of UDP-Gal, both in the Golgi compartment. The results given in Table 2 show that r-apo(a) secretion from Lec-1 cells was reduced to approximately half; apo(a) synthesis did not appear to be changed in Lec-8 cells. Defective sialylation of apo(a) finally increased apo(a) secretion by 50%. The different glycosylation defective r-apo(a)s were incubated for 24 h at 37°C with LDL and the assembly was studied by DELFIA. In all cases we observed an assembly of 55–60%.

From these experiments we conclude that n-glycosylation of apo(a) is not essential for secretion from the cells and that the carbohydrate moiety has little if any influence on the association with LDL and the biosynthesis of native Lp(a).

Substances interfering with the Lp(a) assembly

In one experiment the free -SH groups of LDL and of r-apo(a) were blocked by

Table 2. Secretion of r-apo(a) from transfected wild-type and frm glycosylation-defective CHO-cells

Cell line	R-apo(a) (ng/ml)	R-apo(a) (%)
Pro 5- (w.t.)	733	100
Lec-1	438	56
Lec-2	1050	152
Lec-8	583	89

The 6.4 kB pSG-5 was transfected into different CHO cells and the secretion of r-apo(a) into the cell medium after 24 h was measured by DELFIA. Values are normalized to cotransfected human growth hormone and represent means from four separate experiments.

incubation with 5 mM iodoacetate. Alkylated proteins were incubated for 24 h at 37°C and the assembly was studied by DELFIA in the presence and absence of 50 mM ε-AHA. 25% of the alkylated proteins formed a loose complex which was totally dissociated by the addition of 50 mM ε-AHA. From these experiments, together with the work of others [3], we conclude that the assembly of Lp(a) proceeds in two steps: in the first, one or more K-IVs of apo(a) associated with Lys groups of apoB form a loose complex, and in the second, this complex is stabilized by a disulfide bridge.

It is known from model studies of plasmin binding to fibrin, which proceeds in a manner similar to step I of Lp(a) formation, that substances sharing structural similarities to Lys interfere with the binding. Such substances, ionic and nonionic detergents and high salt concentrations have been studied with respect to their inhibition of Lp(a) assembly (Table 3). Tranexamic acid, a known inhibitor of fibrinolysis used in humans, was 5-10 times more effective than the Lys analogue ε-AHA. The assembly was unaffected by high NaCl concentrations but sensitive to ionic and anionic detergents. We believe that our results are of relevance for strategies in the development of Lp(a)-lowering drugs.

Table 3. Effect of various substances on the Lp(a) assembly

Inhibitor	Concn	% of r-apo(a) found as heterodimer complex	% inhibition
None		61	0
ε-AHA	1 mM	60	1.5
	10 mM	34	44
	50 mM	4	93
TNX[1)]	0.1 mM	58	5
	1 mM	41	33
	10 mM	1	98.5
SDS	0.01%	33	46
	0.05%	28	54
Tween-20	0.01%	47	33
Triton X-100	0.01%	20	67
NaCl	2.00%	61	0
	10.00%	59	3

[a]TNX: Tranexamic acid.

R-apo(a) from pSG 5–7.4 was incubated with LDL for 24 h at 37°C in the presence of the indicated substances and the assembly was studied by DELFIA. The values are means of three to four experiments.

Acknowledgements

This work was supported by a grant from the Austrian Research Foundation (Grant No. S-07104). The technical assistance of Anton Ibovnik is appreciated.

References

1. Kostner GM, Avogaro P, Cazzolato G, Marth E, Bittolo Bon G. Atherosclerosis 1981;38:51–61.
2. Utermann G. Science 1989;246:904–910.
3. Brunner C, Kraft HG, Utermann G, Müller HJ. Proc Natl Acad Sci 1993;90:11643–11647.
4. McLean JW, Tomlinson JE, Kuang WE, Eaton DL, Chen EY, Fless GM, Scanu AM, Lawn RM. Nature 1987;330:132–137.
5. Kraft HG, Köchl S, Menzel HJ, Sandhofer C, Utermann G. Hum Genet 1992;90:2153–2161.
6. Krempler F, Kostner GM, Bolzano K, Sandhofer F. Biochim Biophys Acta 1979;575:63–70.

7. Callow MJ, Stoltzfus LJ, Lawn RM, Rubin, EM. Proc Natl Acad Sci 1994;91:2130–2134.
8. White AL, Rainwater DL, Lanford RE. J Lipid Res 1993;34:509–517.
9. Frank S, Krasznai K, Durovic S, Lobentanz E-M, Dieplinger H, Wagner E, Zaloukal K, Cotten M, Utermann G, Koster GM, Zecher R. Biochemistry 1994; (in press).
10. Steyrer E, Durovic S, Frank S, Gießauf W, Burger A, Dieplinger H, Zechner R, Kostner GM. J Clin Invest 1994; (in press).
11. Zatloukal K, Wagner E, Cotten M, Phillips S, Plank C, Steinlein P, Curiel TD, Birnstiel ML. Ann N Y Acad Sci 1992;660:136–153.

The fetal origins of cardiovascular disease

C.N. Martyn and D.J.P. Barker

MRC Environmental Epidemiology Unit (University of Southampton), Southampton General Hospital, Southampton SO16 6YD, UK

Abstract. To investigate links between fetal development and the later occurrence of cardiovascular disease we have followed up several thousand people born in the first half of this century in England. These people were measured at birth by midwives or health visitors and records of these measurements still survive. Both mortality from and levels of established risk factors for cardiovascular disease were higher in babies who had been small at birth or who had grown poorly during infancy. These findings suggest that reduced fetal and infant growth is an important determinant of risk of cardiovascular disease in adult life. They have implications for understanding the pathogenesis of atherosclerosis and for the prevention of cardiovascular disease.

All Western countries have adopted public health policies to prevent heart disease and stroke. These policies are aimed at altering diet, reducing the prevalence of cigarette smoking and obesity and increasing levels of physical activity. Unfortunately, enthusiasm for implementing them tends to distract attention from the fact that adult lifestyle and levels of known risk factors actually predict individual risk of cardiovascular disease rather poorly. Rose encapsulated this unwelcome truth when he pointed out [1] that the commonest cause of death for men who fell into the lowest risk groups for plasma lipid concentrations, blood pressure, cigarette smoking and presence of pre-existing symptoms of heart disease was, paradoxically, coronary heart disease.

Many features of the epidemiology of cardiovascular disease remain a puzzle. In Britain, for example, there are large geographical differences in death rates from cardiovascular disease between different parts of the country that cannot be accounted for by regional variation in the prevalence of known risk factors. And the rapid decline in rates of ischemic heart disease and stroke that has occurred in many Western countries over the past few decades has not been satisfactorily explained. While it is tempting to believe that these time trends are a result of the pharmacological treatment of risk factors such as hypertension or a reduction in case fatality due to better care of acute cases, quantitative assessments indicate that very little of the decline can be attributed to medical intervention [2].

Mortality from cardiovascular disease is linked to fetal and infant growth

Barker and Osmond's observation [3] that current mortality from ischemic heart disease showed a close geographical relation with past infant mortality gave research into the etiology of cardiovascular disease a new point of departure. This association suggested that some correlate of poor living conditions in early life had important long-term consequences for risk of cardiovascular disease. To pursue the hypothesis, it was necessary to find groups of people who were now at an age where they were at risk from cardiovascular disease and whose fetal and infant growth had been recorded. A systematic search of archives and hospitals in Britain led to the discovery of several sets of records. One set was found in Hertfordshire, a county to the north of London. From 1911 onwards, every baby born in the county was weighed at birth, visited periodically by a health visitor throughout the first year of its life, and weighed again at 1 year of age. The fact that records of these visits had survived made it possible to trace men and women born 60 and more years ago and to relate their early measurements to the later occurrence of illness and death, and to the levels of risk factors for cardiovascular disease. Similar long-term follow-up studies have also been carried out in Preston and Sheffield where, from early in the present century, unusually detailed measurements on all newborn babies were made in maternity hospitals of these cities.

The first study [4] used the records of the Hertfordshire health visitors to follow up 5,600 men born in the eastern part of the county between 1911 and 1930. The size of the sample was later increased, and Fig. 1 shows results for 8,175 men. Those who weighed 18 pounds (8.2 kg) or less at 1 year of age had death rates, shown as standardized mortality ratios (SMRs), from coronary heart disease which were almost 3 times greater than among those who weighed 27 pounds (12.3 kg) or more. Death rates fell progressively as weight at 1 year increased. There were similar, though less strong, trends with birthweight. The association between impaired early growth and risk of death from cardiovascular disease has been confirmed in a study of 1,586 men in Sheffield [5]. An important additional finding here was that mortality from cardiovascular disease was not related to duration of gestation except for a small increase in death rates for men born before 37 weeks. The inverse association of cardiovascular mortality with reduced birthweight must therefore reflect lower fetal growth and not shorter gestation.

Mechanisms

The finding of an association between mortality from cardiovascular disease in adult life and indicators of impaired fetal and infant growth immediately raises questions about mechanism. There is now evidence that levels of several established risk factors for

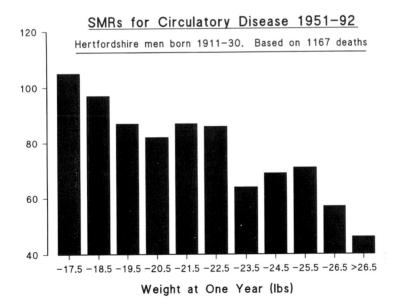

Fig. 1. Levels of systolic and diastolic blood pressure in 50-year-old men and women born in Sheffield, England, according to their weight at birth.

cardiovascular disease in adult life, including high blood pressure, impaired glucose tolerance and plasma concentrations of lipids and clotting factors, are programmed during early development. This article briefly reviews some of the evidence most relevant to the pathogenesis of atherosclerosis.

Blood pressure

Figure 2 shows systolic blood pressure in 50-year-old men and women born and still living in Sheffield. Levels of systolic and diastolic blood pressure fall progressively as birthweight increases [6]. Similar associations between birthweight and adult blood pressure have been found in a national sample of men and women born in Britain in 1946, in men and women in Preston and in Hertfordshire. These associations were independent of duration of gestation. A meta-analysis of several longitudinal studies of children and adults has demonstrated that the negative correlation between birthweight and current blood pressure becomes stronger with increasing age [7]. One interpretation of this observation is that an effect initiated in utero is slowly amplified over the lifetime of an individual.

Arterial structure

Part of the feedback mechanism that amplifies blood pressure might depend on progressive changes in the structure, physical properties and compliance of blood vessels. In humans and in animals vascular structure and compliance change with hemodynamic load. Numerous experiments have shown that a short period of hypertension in young animals induces irreversible alterations in the mechanical properties of the arterial wall. Arterial compliance determines pulse pressure, and changes in pulse pressure produce changes in the scleroprotein content of the vessel wall which, in turn, affect arterial compliance. This is one way in which adaptations in the fetal pattern of circulation could

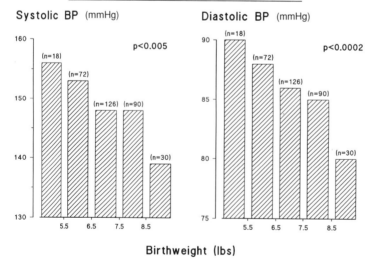

Fig. 2. Mortality from circulatory disease, shown as standardized mortality ratios (SMRs) according to weight at 1 year of age in more than 8,000 men born in Hertfordshire, England.

alter the structure of blood vessels in adults to perpetuate and amplify raised systolic blood pressure from infancy to old age.

We have estimated arterial compliance in more than 200 men and women, now aged around 50 years, using a noninvasive method that directly measures the transit time of the blood flow pulse and so allows the velocity of the pulse pressure wave to be calculated. There is a direct inverse relation between the velocity of the pulse pressure wave and the square root of the compliance of the blood vessel wall. The mean pulse wave velocity in the femoral-tibial arterial segment is consistently greater in people whose weight and abdominal circumference at birth were small [6]. Although pulse wave velocities were faster in people with higher systolic blood pressure, the relation between pulse wave velocity and measurements made at birth was still apparent after adjustment for current blood pressure. Similar, though less strong, relations were seen between pulse wave velocities in the aorta and small measurements at birth. These findings support the idea that the mechanisms that amplify raised blood pressure have their origins in fetal life and that they involve permanent structural modification of the arterial wall.

Serum lipid concentrations

Serum lipid concentrations were associated with specific patterns of impaired fetal growth in a study of middle-aged men and women in Sheffield [8]. In summary, men and women who had a small abdominal circumference at birth had raised serum concentrations of total and low-density lipoprotein cholesterol and of apolipoprotein. This association was independent of social class, current body weight, cigarette smoking and alcohol consumption. Small abdominal circumference is an indication of failure of growth of abdominal viscera in late gestation. It is possible that the mechanisms that determine adult serum cholesterol concentrations depend upon the rate of growth of the liver in the last trimester of pregnancy.

Fibrinogen

Studies of plasma fibrinogen concentration in adults have shown [9,10] that high concentrations, associated with increased risk of cardiovascular disease, are found in men who, at birth, were light in weight or whose abdominal circumferences were small. These associations are independent of factors present in the adult environment, such as cigarette smoking and obesity, that are known to influence plasma fibrinogen concentrations. As we discussed above, small abdominal circumference at birth indicates fetal growth retardation during the last trimester of pregnancy [11] − a time when the liver is undergoing a period of rapid growth. The relation between abdominal circumference at birth and increased plasma fibrinogen concentrations in adult life may therefore be a reflection of the long-term consequences of impaired development of the liver during late fetal life.

Conclusions

The relations between early growth and cardiovascular disease and its risk factors are continuous. Death rates from cardiovascular disease increase progressively up to the highest values of birthweight and weight at 1 year. If the criteria for successful fetal growth include adult health and longevity, these findings reinforce the view that babies with significant intrauterine growth retardation need not be light for their gestational age. Intrauterine growth retardation affects not just those few babies who can be recognized clinically by their unusually small size and high risk of perinatal complications and death but many babies whose birthweights are within what obstetricians would regard as the normal range.

To prevent coronary heart disease and stroke more effectively, we need to find out more about the long-term effects of intrauterine growth retardation on the different organ systems of the human fetus and to investigate how the modulation of fetal growth permanently programs its physiology and metabolism.

Acknowledgements

The studies described in this paper were supported by grants from the Medical Research Council, the Wellcome Trust and Children Nationwide.

References

1. Rose G. Int J Epidemiol 1985;14:32–38.
2. Bonita R, Beaglehole R. Lancet 1993;341:1510–1511.
3. Barker DJP, Osmond C. Lancet 1986;i:1077–1081.
4. Barker DJP, Osmond C, Winter PD, Simmonds SJ, Margetts B. Lancet 1989;ii:577–580.
5. Barker DJP, Osmond C, Simmonds SJ, Wield GA. Br Med J 1993;306:422–426.
6. Martyn CN, Barker DJP, Jespersen S, Greenwald S, Osmond C, Berry CL. Growth in utero, adult blood pressure and arterial compliance. Br Heart J 1994; (in press).
7. Law CM, de Swiet M, Fayers P, Cruddas AM, Fall CHD, Barker DJP, Osmond C. Br Med J 1993;306:24–27.
8. Barker DJP, Martyn CN, Osmond C, Hales CN, Fall CHD. Br Med J 1993;307:1524–1527.
9. Martyn CN, Meade TW, Stirling Y, Barker DJP. Plasma concentrations of fibrinogen and factor VII in adult life and their relation to intra-uterine growth. Br J Haematol 1994; (in press).
10. Barker DJP, Meade TW, Fall CHD, Lee A, Osmond C, Phipps K, Stirling Y. Br Med J 1992;304:148–152.
11. Barker DJP, Gluckman PD, Godfrey KM, Harding JE, Owens JA, Robinson JS. Lancet 1993;341:938–941.

Atherosclerosis X.
F.P. Woodford, J. Davignon and A. Sniderman, editors.

Colony-forming units and atherosclerosis

E.L. Soboleva, V.M. Popkova, O.S. Saburova, E.M. Tararak, M.G. Tvorogova and V.N. Smirnov
Department of Cell Biology, Institute of Experimental Cardiology, Moscow, Russia

Abstract. By culturing intimal cells from early lesions of human aorta in agar it is possible to demonstrate the presence of colony-forming units (CFU), able to form in vitro colonies of granulocyte-macrophages (CFU-GM), basophil-mast cells (CFU-BM) and fibroblasts (CFU-F). CFU-F were also found in blood of patients with primary hyperlipidemia (HLP) of IIa and IIb types. In these patients the percentage of stromal colonies was high, whereas in normolipidemic donors no growth of stromal colonies from blood was observed. The presence of hematopoietic and stromal CFU in atheromatous intima and the fact that stromal CFU can be also detected in blood of HLP patients suggest their likely involvement in the development of atherosclerotic lesions in humans.

By examining early atherosclerotic zones in human aorta (diffuse intimal thickening, lipid streaks and lipid fibrous plaques) we were able to show [1] focal subendothelial accumulations of blood cells where, in addition to mature cells, a number of low differentiated cell types are seen, including lymphocyte-like cells, blast cells and monocytoid cells. Seeding a mixture of intimal cells from these lesions into semisolid agar, the growth of hematopoietic colonies of granulocytes/macrophages, basophil/mast cells and of stromal colonies synthesizing fibrillar matrix [1–3].

An agar test system for CFU detection was prepared by known methods [4] with some modifications. Colonies formed in cultures from intimal cells were examined on the 14th, 17th and 21st day of growth in inverted microscope and by cytohistochemical and ultrastructural methods. By the 14th or 17th day colonies can be seen which were identified by growth characteristics, morphology, ultrastructural features and positive staining for myeloperoxidase and nonspecific esterase as granulocyte-macrophageal cells (Fig. 1A,B). The number of colonies grown from CFU-GM in agar from various types of atherosclerotic lesions varied. The highest number of CFU-GM-related colonies (2.8 ± 1.6 $/10^5$ intimal cells) were from the intima under lipid streaks (n = 9). A smaller number of colonies (1.3 ± 0.3 CFU-GM $/10^5$ intimal cells) were found in cultures from diffuse intimal thickening (n = 12) and single CFU-GM were found in intima of lipid fibrous plaques (n = 12). In cell cultures from fibrotic lesions (fibrous plaques, n = 16) no growth of hematopoietic colonies was observed. Granulocyte lineage in cultures of intimal cells (14–17th day in culture) was primarily represented by basophils and mast cells (BMC), with cytoplasm showing metachromatic granules after staining with toluidine blue. BMC were, in fact, granulocyte cells in mixed granulocyte-macrophage colonies. Colonies were also found which had exclusively basophilic cells (Fig. 2A,B). Quite often (13 out of 30 aortas) the number of cells in growing diffuse colonies increased dramatically, leading to disappearance of borders between discrete colonies and making colony counting difficult. The BMC content in these cultures was 10–50 times that of day 0. Also, by the 17th day after seeding, mast cells become dominant, as described earlier [2,3]. In addition to

---

Address for correspondence: Vladimir N. Smirnov, Department of Cell Biology, Institute of Experimental Cardiology, 3rd Cherepkovskaya str. 15A, 121552 Moscow, Russia.

920

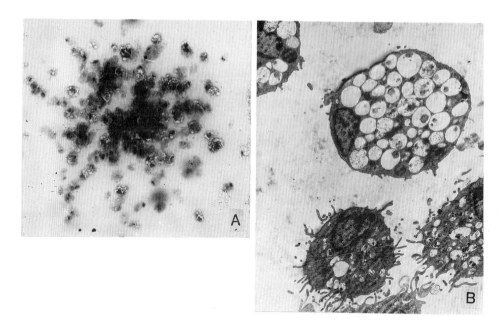

Fig. 1. Granulocyte/macrophage colony in agar cultures of intimal cells derived from a lipid streak of human aorta. 14th day in culture. A: macrophages positively stained for nonspecific esterase. Light microscopy, × 160; B: TEM. Fragment of granulocyte/macrophage colony, × 2,600.

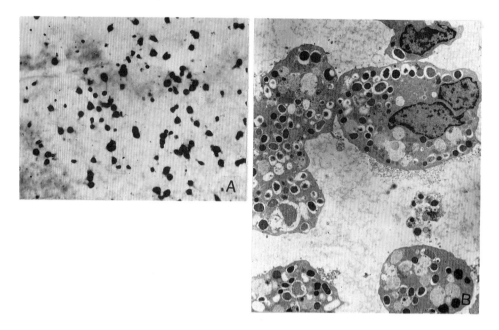

Fig. 2. Diffuse basophil colony in agar cultures of intimal cells of human aorta (lipid streak, 14th day in culture). A: basophil cells positively stained toluidine blue. Light microscopy, x 160; B: TEM. Fragment of basophil colony. Mast cells have granules of varying content of electron-dense material, ranging from lucent. Mast granules contain fibrillar material or electron-dense cores, × 2,600.

hematopoietic precursors, later (21—25th day) among intimal cells one could see precursor cells for fibroblast-like cells which formed stromal colonies synthesizing collagen (Fig. 3A,B). These colonies were dense and 100—500 nm in diameter. Ultrastructural analysis of dense colonies showed that they are formed by fibroblast-like cells with all the characteristics of actively secreting cells, having well-developed rough endoplasmic reticulum (RER), Golgi complex, numerous secretory vesicles and granules and being surrounded by typical proteoglycan and/or collagen matrix (Fig. 3B,C). In contrast to hematopoietic colonies, there was no statistically significant difference between the numbers of stromal colonies grown from the intima of diffuse intimal thickening, lipid streaks or lipid fibrous plaques (4.24 ± 1.37; 2.79 ± 1.22 and 3.12 ± 2.0 CFU-F/10^5 intimal cells, respectively). Parallel culturing of intimal cells isolated from similar lesions in liquid medium on coverslips demonstrated, in addition to fibroblast-like cells producing collagen matrix, osteogenic cells synthesizing typical osteoid matrix [3].

We also attempted to check the following hypothesis. If CFU-F found in the intimal cell population of human aorta originate from bone marrow and are able to repopulate intima, there should be some possibility of finding these CFU in blood of patients with advanced atherosclerosis. Patients were selected with primary HLP, types IIa and IIb, where the correlation between atherosclerosis progression and the degree of hyper-cholesterolemia is especially evident. Healthy volunteers with normal or moderately elevated total cholesterol formed a control group. Mononuclear cells from the peripheral blood of patients and volunteers were cultured in a semisolid test system similar to that used to culture vascular intimal cells. On the 14th day after seeding, mononuclears from normolipidemic donors gave rise only to hematopoietic colonies in culture. Growth characteristics of cells in these colonies, nuclear polymorphism, positive staining of cytoplasm for nonspecific esterase and myeloperoxidase were the markers by which the

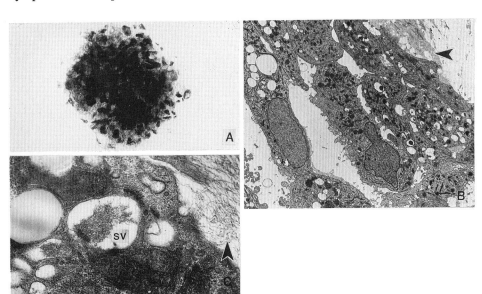

Fig. 3. Stromal colony in agar cultures of intimal cells (lipid streak of human aorta), 21st day in culture. A: staining with Wright-Giemsa. Light microscopy, × 160; B,C: fragments of stromal colony (TEM). Fibroblast-like cells surrounded by well-developed extracellular matrix (arrows). Secretory vesicles (SV) contain fibrillar matrix, × 1,600 (B), × 20,000 (C).

922

colonies could be classified as granulocyte-macrophage or granulocyte. Granulocyte lineage in these colonies was represented by neutrophils. When mononuclears from the blood of hyperlipidemic patients were cultured, it was found that in addition to hematopoietic colonies, colonies differing from hematopoietic by growth characteristics, ultrastructure and negative staining for myeloperoxidase and nonspecific esterase are also present (Figs. 4A, 5A, 6A). Ultrastructural analysis of these colonies demonstrated the correspondence of subcellular structures of the cells to classical morphological characteristics of fibroblasts at different stages of maturation [5]. This conclusion is also supported by the presence within these cells of more or less developed RER and Golgi complex.

The cellular cytoplasm contained numerous ribosomes, secretory granules, globules, dark osmiophilic bodies, lipid inclusions and microfibrils which were either randomly located or form discrete bundles (Fig. 4B, 5B). The fibrillar matrix surrounding the cells in colonies had different degrees of maturity, varying from separate collagen and proteoglycan microfibrils (Fig. 4B) to well-developed and regularly packed extracellular matrix (Fig. 5B).

The second type of stromal colonies which grew in agar from mononuclears of patients with HLP was represented by the clusters of round cells, less densely packed. After staining with Giemsa or toluidine blue, cellular cytoplasm in these colonies showed highly basophilic metachromatic granules and well-developed structure of nuclei and nucleolus. When analyzed by TEM, one could observe among cells or instead of cells a typical osteoid (bone-like) matrix seen as lamellas (Fig. 6B). When colonies were stained with

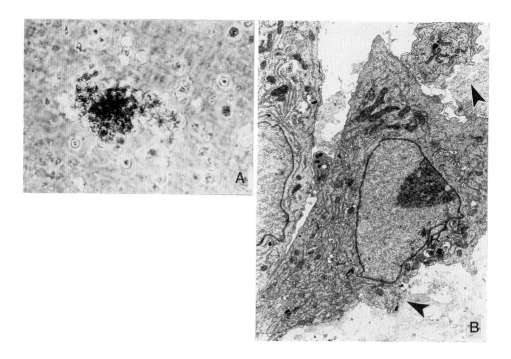

Fig. 4. Stromal colonies produced by fraction of peripheral blood mononuclears (14 days in culture) from patients with HLP type IIa. A: inverted microscopy, × 40; B: TEM of fragment of stromal colony. Fibroblast-like cell and irregular reticular matrix (arrows) have different degrees of maturity, × 1,600.

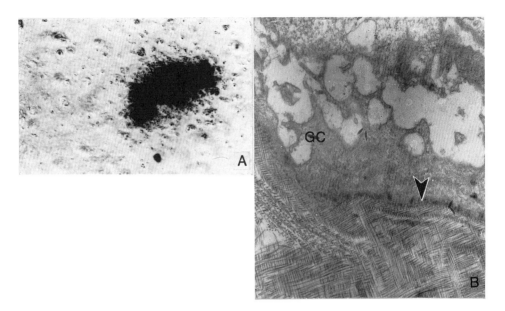

Fig. 5. Stromal colony grown from fraction of mononuclears from patients with HLP type IIb. A: inverted microscopy of "dark" dense colony in agar, × 40; B: TEM. Fragment of fibroblast-like cell: microfibrils are randomly located; a marked hyperplasia of the Golgi complex (GC) is seen. Regularly structured reticular matrix produced by cells from this colony (arrows) × 13,000.

polyclonal rabbit antibodies to human osteonectin, cells appeared osteonectin-positive (Fig. 6A). Other cell types resembling osteoclasts could also be seen (Fig. 6B). Combination of morphological, histochemical and ultrastructural characteristics of these cells in colonies grown from blood of HLP patients was sufficient to identify and quantitate stromal colonies under the inverted microscope which was required for differential counting of hematopoietic and stromal colonies.

Quantitative data on the ratio between stromal and hematopoietic colonies grown from blood mononuclears of control group of patients and the patients with high cholesterol are shown in Table 1. It is evident that in patients with HLP the percentage of stromal colonies was high (44–85%), whereas in the blood of normolipidemic donors no growth of stromal colonies was found.

Thus, the use of semisolid agar test systems to culture human intimal aortic cells isolated from various types of atherosclerotic lesions allowed us to show for the first time the presence of several types of colony-forming units in the intimal cell population (CFU-GM, CFU-BM and CFU-F). These new facts may be important in further understanding the pathogenetic mechanisms of human atherosclerosis. Firstly, hematopoietic and stromal CFU may be able to repopulate vascular intima in atherosclerosis progression. Secondly, it is possible that loci of ectopic hematopoiesis with specific microenvironment in vascular intima can be formed. It is important to note that stromal colonies from blood of HLP patients and stromal colonies from atheromatous intima grown under the same conditions in vitro look similar. In both cases colonies are formed which consist of only fibroblast-like cells or represent conglomerate colonies composed of hematopoietic and collagen-producing cells [2]. The presence of hematopoietic cells was demonstrated earlier for CFU-F colonies from bone marrow [6]. It is known that among reticular cells of bone

924

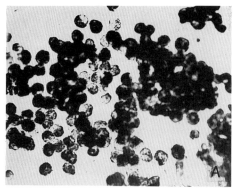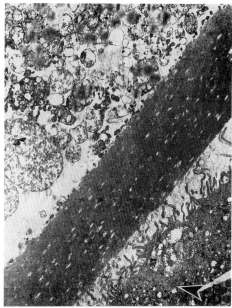

Fig. 6. Stromal colony grown from fraction of blood mononuclears from patient with HLP type IIb. A: colony of osteonectin-positive cells grow on a fibrin clot. Staining with polyclonal rabbit antibodies LF-37 to human osteonectin. PAP technique. Light microscopy, × 160; B: TEM. Osteoid matrix as bone-like lamella in the center. Numerous organelles of disintegrating cells which produce osteoid matrix. Fragment of osteoclast with numerous processes of plasma membrane (arrows), × 3300.

Table 1. Stromal growth in agar seeded with blood mononuclear cells from donors and from coronary patients with primary hyperlipoproteinemia types IIa and IIb.

Patient/donor (sex, age)			Ratio of stromal colonies to total number of colonies	Stromal colonies, % of total
1. M	48	HLP IIb	29/34	85
2. M	47	HLP IIb	9/12	75
3. F	43	HLP IIb	18/25	72
4. F	53	HLP IIb	34/77	44
5. F	37	HLP IIb	52/67	78
6. F	43	HLP IIb	44/69	64
7. M	45	HLP IIb	58/75	77
8. M	41	HLP IIb	40/54	74
9. M	30	donor	0/39	0
10. F	28	donor	0/48	0
11. M	29	donor	0/43	0
12. M	26	donor	0/46	0
13. F	32	donor	0/73	0
14. M	45	donor	0/14	0
15. M	33	donor	0/28	0
16. F	36	donor	0/26	0

Patients:		Donors:	
Total cholesterol	7.2—12.1 mmol/l	Total cholesterol	<6.2 mmol/l
LDL-C	4.9—9.8 mmol/l	LDL-C	<4.1 mmol/l
HDL-C	0.4—0.7 mmol/l	HDL-C	1.05—1.86 mmol/l
Triglycerides	2.0—6.6 mmol/l	Triglycerides	<2.0 mmol/l

marrow CFU-F are found which are able to transform in vitro into true fibroblasts with osteogenic capacity [6]. It is also important that the data on migration of CFU-F in the blood stream [7,8] correlate with our results on their presence in blood of HLP patients.

How can one explain the appearance of a significant number of progenitor cells in intima of atherosclerotic artery and their absence from noninvolved vessel? It was shown by others [9] that infusion of modified LDL to animals induced the expression of colony-stimulating factor for granulocyte/macrophages (CSF-GM and CSF-M) in endothelial cells in vitro and in vivo. This means that the activation of CSF known to occur during atherosclerosis development may play an important pathogenic role, and hyper-cholesterolemia is likely to be a key factor in CSF stimulation. It is possible that hypercholesterolemia can affect not only hematopoietic stem-cell differentiation, but may also influence stromal precursors which may be especially important in patients with advanced familial hypercholesterolemia. According to our data, a certain correlation may exist between the elevation of CFU level for stromal differentiation in blood of patients and a parallel decline in the number of hematopoietic CFU in advanced hyperlipidemia. It is thought that the level of CSF, or at least CSF-GM, in these patients should be low in spite of high blood lipids. Indirectly, this idea is supported by the data showing lowering of total cholesterol and LDL cholesterol and the decrease in luminal area covered with lesions in animals with experimental atherosclerosis after administration of recombinant CSF-GM [10,11]. Although the mechanism of cholesterol and LDL lowering by cytokines remains unknown, it is not ruled out that the administration of CSF to patients with a high level of atherogenic lipoproteins may lower LDL and decrease the number of stromal CFU appearing in blood. The presence of polypotent stroma-forming cells with osteogenic capacity in the blood of patients with HLP supports the hypothesis that at advanced stages of cholesterol-related atherosclerosis irreversible changes in myeloid tissue may take place, accompanied by the migration into blood of CFU-F capable of synthesizing reticular-like matrix and also bone-like matrix.

Acknowledgements

This research was made possible in part by Grant No MNH000 from the International Science Foundation. The authors would like to thank Prof L.W. Fisher (NIH, USA) for kindly provided antibodies LF-37 to human osteonectin.

References

1. Soboleva EL, Popkova VM. Bull Exp Biol Med (Russia) 1989;106:600–604 (English translation).
2. Smirnov VN et al. In: Stein O, Eisenberg S, Stein Y (eds) Atherosclerosis 9. Tel Aviv: R&L Creative Communications Ltd., 1992;295–298.
3. Soboleva EL et al. Abstract book 62nd EAS Congress, Jerusalem, Israel 1993;6.
4. Ash S, Detrick RA, Lanjani ED. Blood 1981;58:309–316.
5. Ross R. Biol Rev 1968;43:51–96.
6. Friedenstein AJ. In: Hursche JNM, Kanis JA (eds) Bone and Mineral Research/7. Elsevier Science Publishers B.V. (Biochemical Division), 1990;243–272.
7. Keating A et al. Nature 1982;298:280–283.
8. Piersma AH et al. Cell Tissue Kinet 1985;18:589–595.
9. Rajavashisth TB et al. Nature 1990;334:254–257.
10. Shimano H et al. J Biol Chem 1990;265:12869–12875.
11. Watanabe Y et al. 3rd Saratoga Intern Conf Atheroscler, 1993;96 (poster 65).

Role of the adventitia in atherogenesis: arterial wall vasa vasorum

S.G.E. Barker[1] and J.F. Martin[2]

[1]Department of Surgery, King's Healthcare, Denmark Hill, London SE5 9RS; and [2]Department of Medicine, King's College School of Medicine & Dentistry, Denmark Hill, London SE5 9PJ, UK

Atherosclerosis is probably initiated many years prior to its clinical manifestations, by the proliferation and migration of vascular smooth muscle cells and (macrophage) foam-cell formation between the endothelial cell layer and the internal elastic lamina. In man, the original events stimulating lesion development remain uncertain, although for more than 150 years investigators have presumed that any causative changes occur at the luminal surface of an artery and are associated with damage to the endothelium [1,2]. Accordingly, most models of atherogenesis to date have been based upon traumatizing the endothelium by physical or chemical means.

More recently, attention has been drawn to the possible role of the adventitia in atherogenesis, and both new models and a new hypothesis have been put forward in support. Whilst these new thoughts challenge the concept that morphological endothelial damage is a necessary antecedent of atherosclerotic plaque development, they do not deny that endothelial damage is a well-modelled cause.

The adventitial tunic around muscular arteries extends outwards from the media (sometimes bordered by a definite external elastic lamina) and blends into the perivascular connective tissues. It contains autonomic nerve fibers which may aid in the regulation of smooth muscle cell tone, lymphatic channels which drain fluid and contained solutes (including macromolecules), and vasa vasorum which play a vitally important role in the provision of oxygen (and possibly other nutrients) to the outer part of the media (Fig. 1).

The arterial wall of larger vessels is nourished from two directions. The inner part is well supplied by diffusion outwards from the blood circulating within the main vessel lumen, whereas the outer part is supplied by diffusion inwards from the blood within the adventitial vasa vasorum [3]. Indeed, oxygenation profiles in vivo have been mapped across the artery wall and seem to confirm that oxygen levels are highest adjacent to the intima, fall to a trough in the mid to outer media and rise again towards the adventitia [4,5]; this implies that oxygenation of the outer media is provided by the adventitial vasa vasorum.

However, the anatomical distribution of vasa vasorum varies between arteries. They have been described previously as vasa vasorum externa and vasa vasorum interna. In man, the latter are found only in the thoracic aorta and originate directly from the main vessel lumen, penetrating both the intima and inner media to supply the outer media. This anatomical type has recently been described in the rabbit carotid artery as well [6]. Vasa vasorum externa are distributed far more widely, and are present in all large, elastic and muscular arteries. They arise from arterial branching points immediately distal to their origins and divide and anastamose within the adventitial layer before penetrating down

---

Address for correspondence: Prof J.F. Martin, Department of Medicine, King's College School of Medicine & Dentistry, Denmark Hill, London SE5 9PJ, UK.

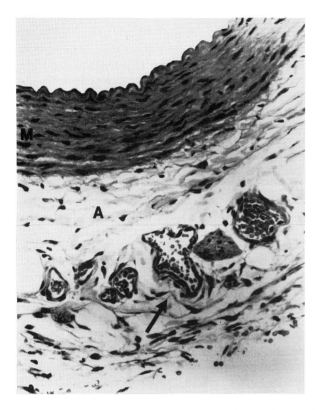

Fig. 1. Cross-section of a typical artery (rabbit carotid) showing an endothelial monolayer resting upon smooth muscle cells forming the media (M) and an adventitia (A) containing numerous vasa vasorum (arrow). (LM × 250).

into the media. Within the media they tend to be orientated axially at several branching levels.

In man, there are three relationships between the distribution of vasa vasorum and the presence of atheroma which may prove interesting. First, in general, vasa vasorum are more numerous on the anterior than on the posterior aspect of the major arteries, and their density seems to decrease from the thoracic aorta down to the abdominal aorta and the iliac arteries. Second, the vasa vasorum seem deficient in number immediately around arterial branching points [7]. This can be related to the known distribution of atheromata within the aorta, these being more prevalent in the lower abdominal aorta, posteriorly and around side-branch orifices. Third, with advancing age (and progressing atherosclerotic disease), the vasa vasorum become more numerous and perhaps more tortuous. It could be argued, therefore, that atheroma has a predilection for those zones of the arterial tree lacking an adequate distribution of vasa vasorum and hence a poor nutritional supply to the vessel wall. With disease progression, vasa vasorum proliferate upon intimal thickening in an attempt to maintain the nutrition of the vessel wall. In this scenario, the lack of oxygen able to diffuse across the arterial wall from the intimal surface may stimulate the initiation of an atheromatous lesion. In support, a profuse supply of vasa vasorum is seen in the venous adventitia of both man and dogs, which suggests that a low oxygen tension within the main vessel lumen necessitates a greater provision of oxygen from the adventitial surface.

A further important role for vasa vasorum is to clear large molecules (such as fibrinogen and low density lipoproteins) from the adventitia. Experimental damage to these vessels has been shown to result in an increased concentration of such molecules within the arterial wall, which may in turn diminish the transport of oxygen and other nutrients across the vessel wall (Baskerville, personal communication).

The essential role fulfilled by the vasa vasorum can be seen when they are obliterated experimentally. When this was first performed, by ligation of the intercostal arteries of dogs (from which the vasa vasorum to the descending aorta arise), it was noted that there was medial necrosis and subsequent fibrosis, mainly confined to the middle third of the media — i.e., at the potential 'watershed' between that part of the vessel wall supplied from the main vessel lumen and that supplied by the vasa vasorum. Furthermore, occlusion of the vasa vasorum with a thrombin and gelatin mixture into segments of the aorta and iliofemoral arteries (again of dogs) was seen for the first time to be associated with the formation of an intimal hyperplastic lesion in the corresponding areas, beneath an intact endothelium [8]. Other associations between intimal hyperplasia and adventitial manipulation have subsequently been described, including intimal lesion formation following electrical stimulation of the outside of an artery [9], the use of endotoxin-soaked thread embedded in the adventitia [10], placement of a silastic collar around the outside of an artery [11] or surgical removal of the adventitial layer from the intima and media [12].

Placement of a biologically inert silastic collar around the outside of a rabbit carotid artery (which does not seem to alter luminal blood flow) can result in the formation of an intimal hyperplastic lesion beneath an intact endothelium. Although unproven, it has been suggested that the mechanism by which such changes can be brought about is compression by the collar of the adventitial vasa vasorum at those points where the collar just touched the arterial wall. In turn, this may have promoted the development of a localized zone of arterial wall hypoxia, which as hypothesized, may be the initiating stimulus for lesion formation. Because of this model, it was considered that atherosclerosis may in fact be a disease process that can be initiated within the adventitial layer rather than at the intimal surface of an artery [13] (Fig. 2). Translating this process to man, the proposed pathophysiological mechanism by which the vasa vasorum could be occluded is plugging by platelet and fibrin aggregates. Such plugging can be seen in the adventitia of atherosclerotic coronary arteries. In turn, the plugged vasa vasorum may, of course, promote hypoxia of the outer media, inducing the release of cytokines and other growth factors from the associated lining endothelium and most importantly, from the smooth muscle cells resident in the outer media. These same smooth muscle cells might then be stimulated to proliferate and migrate. Additionally, monocytes might enter the intima from the lumen of the main vessel or from adjacent (nonplugged) vasa vasorum. In the presence of hypoxia, acyl CoA:cholesterol acyltransferase (ACAT) could be upregulated to promote cholesteryl ester formation. Intimal proliferation might then result from the combined effect of smooth muscle cell proliferation, the entry of monocytes and the subsequent formation of tissue-based macrophages in the presence of the upregulated ACAT. If such an initial lesion was then to protrude into the main vessel lumen, with altered rheology at a susceptible anatomical site, the endothelium might be sufficiently damaged to promote further lesion development through pathways previously described [1,2]. It was also conjectured that reversal of this scenario, by re- or neovascularization of the adventitia, to restore arterial wall 'normoxia' might promote lesion regression, and hence be a mechanism to allow arterial wall repair.

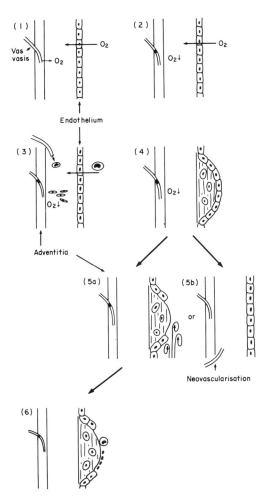

Fig. 2. Schematic representation of the hypothesis that atherosclerosis may be initiated by hypoperfusion following thrombosis of vasa vasorum. (1) Under normal conditions the oxygen tension in the outer media of many human arteries is maintained via blood in the vasa vasorum. (2) Thrombosis of a vas vasis causes hypoxia of the outer media inducing the release of cytokines from adventitial and vasa vasorum-related leukocytes. (3) Smooth muscle cells divide and migrate or migrate and divide. Monocytes enter the intima from the lumen of the vessel or from adjacent vasa vasorum. ACAT is upregulated. (4) Intimal proliferation results from the combined effect of proliferation of smooth muscle cells, the entry of monocytes and the formation of foam cells from macrophages in the presence of upregulated ACAT. (5) (a) If the lesion protrudes into the lumen and is buffeted by the hemodynamic forces in the flowing blood because of a susceptible anatomical site, endothelial damage occurs; (b) alternatively, the lesion can heal 'ad integrum' by re- or neovascularization of the adventitia. (6) Platelets and leukocytes may finally adhere to the subendothelium, releasing PDGF and other cytokines that are responsible for the formation of the advanced plaque.

There is now some support for this hypothesis. Experiments have been undertaken to analyze the relationship of the adventitia to atherogenesis. Surgical excision of the adventitia, leaving behind a morphologically intact endothelium and media, has been shown to promote the development of an intimal hyperplastic lesion, again in rabbit

930

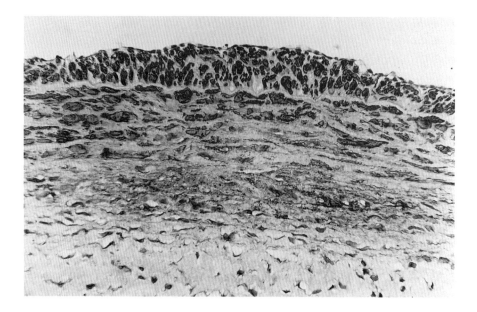

Fig. 3. Surgical excision of the arterial wall adventitia from the rabbit carotid artery promotes the development of an intimal hyperplastic lesion beneath an intact endothelium. The smooth muscle cells in the lesion are orientated longitudinally, whereas those in the media are placed circumferentially (LM × 180).

carotid arteries [12] (Fig. 3). However, it was noted that by 1 month after the initial lesion formation, the lesions began to regress. The proffered explanation was that vascular smooth muscle cells might be freely mobile between the media and the intima. Cells might move towards the intima as a response to the hypoxia resulting from loss of provision of oxygen from the vasa vasorum in the adventitial layer, along a presumed oxygen gradient maximal at the intimal surface. If the induced hypoxia could be reversed, the smooth muscle cells might migrate back towards the media where they originated. Only when this possible healing mechanism was overcome would the initial intimal lesion progress to develop, with time, into a full-blown atherosclerotic plaque.

It has been proposed earlier that regression of the intimal lesions might be due to normalization of the oxygenation gradients across the arterial wall. A technique has been devised to induce the formation of a highly vascular 'neoadventitia' around arteries from which the adventitia had been removed; this inhibited the expected lesion formation and made established lesions regress more quickly [12]. We noted in these experiments that only smooth muscle cells were 'mobile'; macrophages did not follow the same movement pattern. Once again, these experiments provide only circumstantial evidence linking hypoxia, the adventitia and atherogenesis.

Clinically, atherosclerosis is associated with a range of 'risk factors' and any conclusions drawn from laboratory-based models regarding atherogenesis and its promulgation must take these into account. How then could the provision of arterial wall oxygenation via the adventitial vasa vasorum fit in? In hypertension, there is probably a decreased blood flow via the vasa vasorum which may in turn aggravate medial hypoxia [14]. In diabetics, the vasa vasorum may be more prone to thrombotic occlusion [15] and a similar phenomenon may occur in syphilitic aortitis, where an endarteritis obliterans often involves the vasa vasorum and where a superimposed intimal hyperplastic lesion is often evident. With smoking, perhaps the major 'risk factor' for accelerating atherosclerosis, it has been recorded that overall arterial pO_2 may decline through a decreased ability of red blood cells to carry oxygen [16].

In conclusion, the real-life initiating stimulus for atherosclerotic plaque development remains unclear. Damage to or removal of the arterial adventitia containing the vasa vasorum causing arterial wall hypoxia might be responsible for initiating an early atherosclerotic lesion beneath an intact endothelium. This does not deny that endothelial damage is a potent promoter of an intimal lesion, but indicates the potential role of the adventitia in atherogenesis, to which relatively little importance has hitherto been attached and which opens up a new realm of possibilities for investigation.

Acknowledgements

S.G.E. Barker is British Heart Foundation Junior Research Fellow in Department of Surgery, King's College Hospital, London. John F. Martin is British Heart Foundation Professor of Cardiovascular Science, King's College School of Medicine & Dentistry, London.

References

1. Ross R, Glomsett JA. N Engl J Med 1976;295:369–377.
2. Ross R. N Engl J Med 1986;314:488–500.
3. Werber A, Heistad DD. Am J Physiol 1985;248:901–906.
4. Crawford DW, Back LH, Cole MA. J Clin Invest 1980;65:1498–1508.
5. Barker SGE, Talbert A, Cottam S et al. Arterioscler Thromb 1993;13:70–77.
6. Barker SGE, Causton BE, Baskerville PA et al. J Anat 1992;180:225–231.
7. Clarke JA. Br J Surg 1966;53:354–358.
8. Nakatu Y, Shionoya S. Nature 1966;212:1258–1259.
9. Betz E, Schlote E. Basic Res Cardiol 1979;74:10–20.
10. Prescott MF, McBride CK, Court M. Am J Pathol 1989;135:835–846.
11. Booth RFG, Martin JF, Honey AC et al. Atherosclerosis 1989;76:257–268.
12. Barker SGE, Tilling LC, Miller GC et al. Atherosclerosis 1994;105:131–144.
13. Martin JF, Booth RFG, Moncada S. Eur J Clin Invest 1991;21:355–359.
14. Simon BR, Kobayashi AS, Weiderheim CA, Strandrum DE. J Biomed Res 1973;6:349–359.
15. Timperley WR, Ward JD, Preston FE et al. Diabetologia 1976;12:237–243.
16. Sagone AL, Lawrence T, Balcerzak SP. Blood 1973;41:845–852.

New determinants of LDL and fibrinogen uptake by artery walls

G.V.R. Born, E.L. Cardona-Sanclemente and R. Medina

Pathopharmacology Unit, William Harvey Research Institute, St. Bartholomew's Hospital Medical College, Charterhouse Square, London EC1M 6BQ, UK

Atherosclerosis is initiated by the accumulation of atherogenic plasma proteins, predominantly low-density lipoprotein (LDL) and fibrinogen but probably also Lp(a), in the walls of coronary and other susceptible arteries. Abnormally high concentrations of LDL are associated with premature clinical manifestations of atherosclerosis, most commonly angina pectoris and myocardial infarction, which indicates that the uptake of LDL by arteries increases with its concentration in the plasma [1]. LDL promotes atherogenesis by a mechanism which does not involve the high-affinity receptor because when that is deficient or defective atherogenesis is greatly accelerated through excessive plasma LDL, experimentally in Watanabe rabbits and clinically in Type II familial hyperlipidemia. Moreover, the uptake of reductively methylated LDL, which does not bind to high-affinity receptors, by arterial walls is similar to that of native LDL [2,3]. Apparently, LDL passes through arterial endothelium by transcytosis in plasmalemmal vesicles [4,5] identical with the pinosomes in which this lipoprotein was observed by autoradiography [6]. This transcytosis has also been demonstrated with cultured endothelial cells, where it depends strongly on LDL concentration [7].

We have discovered other factors which influence the uptake of LDL and fibrinogen by large arteries in vivo in two mammalian species, viz. rabbit and rat, making it likely that these factors also operate in man, as follows: 1) the density of anionic sites on the surface of the arterial endothelium [8–10]; 2) a process which is inhibited by dihydropyridine calcium antagonists [11]; and 3) a process or processes stimulated by a variety of pressor agents. This article is limited to a discussion of the third topic.

Effect of intracarotid catecholamine administration in rabbits

Some time ago we discovered that in anesthetized rabbits the uptake of LDL, methylated to prevent recognition by high-affinity receptors, by arterial walls is accelerated by noradrenalin or adrenalin at high pathophysiological concentrations [12,13]. The principle of the experiments was to measure the vascular uptake of intravenously injected LDL labeled with radioiodine and methylated to prevent removal by high-affinity receptors. The uptake was compared in the walls of the two carotid arteries after infusing the catecholamine into the blood stream of one and saline into the other, as control. At the end of 2 or 4 h of infusion the arteries were excised and washed free of blood and their radioactivity was determined. Both catecholamines at local blood concentrations of approximately 10 nmol/l caused significant increases of LDL radioactivities in the arterial walls. Noradrenalin at the higher concentration of 100 nmol/l also increased the LDL radioactivity of the saline-infused carotid; this increase could be accounted for by increased plasma noradrenalin concentrations in that carotid to levels which increased LDL uptake in the noradrenalin-infused carotids.

Effect of systemic administration of adrenalin in rats

We then demonstrated a similar effect of adrenalin in another mammalian species, the rat, and by a very different technique in which the animals were conscious and unrestrained [14]. Osmotic minipumps (ALZET) were implanted in rats under the skin of the neck. These pumps infused either saline or adrenalin at 0.5 µl/kg·min to give plasma adrenalin concentrations of ca. 40 nmol/l for 6 days. The rise in plasma adrenalin concentration was associated with a rise in systolic blood pressure to 159 ± 3 mmHg, compared to 105 ± 5 mmHg in the saline-infused controls. Human and rat LDL prepared by sequential ultracentrifugation (Havel et al., 1955) were labeled with ^{125}I-tyramine cellobiose (^{125}I-TC-LDL). In this labeling technique the radioiodine tracer is attached to the protein via tyramine cellobiose, which is trapped intracellularly and persists in artery walls for more than 24 h while the lipoprotein itself is degraded and removed [15]. Therefore, the artery wall radioactivities represent the amounts of LDL — and of similarly labeled fibrinogen (see below) — that were present in the tissues and, therefore, a measure of the amounts of the labeled proteins that had been taken up. After 5 days of adrenalin infusion, ^{125}I-TC-LDL was injected intravenously with the infusion continued, and 24 h later the animals were killed with intracardiac pentobarbital and the thoracic aortas were prepared for radioactivity determinations. Adrenalin infused at this concentration increased the aortic radioactivities due to rat LDL by 146% (n = 11) and due to human LDL by 289% (n = 7); both these increases were highly significant.

The results confirmed that the catecholamines at high pathophysiological blood concentrations accelerate the uptake of LDL by large arteries in two mammalian species, namely rabbit and rat. These results strongly suggest that the effect is also present in Man. This discovery, therefore, appeared to contribute to an explanation for the accelerated atherosclerosis and the increased incidence of its clinical manifestations in conditions associated with elevated blood catecholamine concentrations, including the episodic increases associated with stress and with cigarette smoking [16] as well as the more persistent increases caused by pheochromocytoma. Thus there arose the possibility that the slow but continuous passage of LDL into arterial walls is influenced by the catecholamines normally present in the circulating blood.

Effect of systemic infusion of angiotensin II

The mechanism(s) underlying the accelerating effect of the catecholamines on the uptake of LDL remains uncertain. However, the most obvious possibility was that it had something to do with their hypertensive effect. For that reason another pressor agent, angiotensin II, was used in similar experiments. The results [17] showed that angiotensin II infused by implanted minipumps for 6 days into conscious unrestrained Wistar rats also significantly increased the uptake of rat or human LDL by aortic walls. In these experiments human fibrinogen labeled with ^{131}I via tyramine cellobiose was injected at the same time as the LDL labeled with ^{125}I via tyramine cellobiose. The uptake of the fibrinogen was also significantly increased. Infused angiotensin II had no significant effect on the rates of clearance of LDL and fibrinogen from the blood, so that the uptake effect of angiotensin II could not be accounted for by changes in the blood concentration of the proteins.

At the concentrations at which they were infused, both adrenalin and angiotensin II increased the blood pressure moderately and progressively. Compared to saline-infused control rats, in which the diastolic pressure gradually decreased, the increase with adrenalin became significant after 3 days and with angiotensin II after 5 days.

934

Effect of administration of an inhibitor of nitric oxide synthesis

The results so far would be compatible with the assumption that the increased uptake of LDL and of fibrinogen by artery walls caused by adrenalin and by angiotensin II is mediated by a common mechanism involving their pressor effects. This assumption appeared to be further supported by our recent finding that increases in blood pressure caused by inhibiting nitric oxide synthesis with N^G-nitro-L-arginine methyl ester (L-NAME) [18] are also associated with increased uptakes of LDL and fibrinogen by aortic walls in such rats (Cardona-Sanclemente and Born, 1994: in preparation). In these experiments the L-NAME was administered in the drinking water to the conscious, unrestrained rats over 6 days and the labeled proteins were injected, as before, so that they circulated for the last 24 h. The L-NAME caused a progressive increase in blood pressure from the control value of about 130 to about 170 mmHg after 6 days. Again, the uptake of LDL and of fibrinogen by aortic wall was significantly increased.

Discussion

Thus, moderate hypertension brought about by three different pressor agents was accompanied by increases in the uptake of two atherogenic plasma proteins into artery walls. In this respect our findings with L-NAME resembled those previously obtained with the other pressor agents noradrenalin, adrenalin and angiotensin II. Indeed, this previously observed association of uptake and blood pressure increase was a major reason for determining the effect of L-NAME as yet another means of raising blood pressure. At first sight, therefore, the results would support some direct connexion between two effects. Such a connexion is also suggested by experiments showing that the entry of ferritin into vascular endothelial cell vesicles increases with increasing intraluminal pressure [19].

Nevertheless, some of our own findings are inconsistent with such a conclusion. First, angiotensin II infused at a concentration so low as to cause only a small and temporary rise in blood pressure over about 2 days before a protein injection still produced highly significant increases in LDL and fibrinogen uptake [17]. Secondly, when similar experiments were done with spontaneously hypertensive Wistar rats of the same age, in which the diastolic blood pressure throughout the 6-day experimental period was a little higher than that produced by any of the three pressor agents, the uptake of LDL and of fibrinogen did not differ significantly from that in the control rats.

Possible mechanisms which might account for these interesting discrepancies are now under investigation. Nevertheless, considering our experimental findings in relation to human atherosclerotic disease, it is interesting that the risk of both coronary heart disease and stroke is increased more than additively when both LDL or fibrinogen and systolic or diastolic blood pressure are high [20,21] If, after all, some complex connexion between blood pressure and the accumulation of atherogenic plasma proteins in arterial walls should emerge from our work it would, at least in principle, provide an explanation for these epidemiological facts.

Acknowledgements

We wish to express grateful appreciation to the Garfield Weston Foundation and the British Heart Foundation for generous support.

References

1. Goldstein JL, Brown MS. Ann Rev Biochem 1977;46:897.

2. Mahley RW, Weisgraber KH, Innearity TL. Biochim Biophys Acta 1979;571:81.
3. Wiklund O, Carew TE, Steinberg D. Atherosclerosis 1986;5:131.
4. Vasile E, Simionescu M, Simionescu N. J Cell Biol 1983;96:1677.
5. Simionescu N, Vasile E, Lupu F, Popescu G, Simionescu M. Am J Pathol 1986;123:109.
6. Stein O, Stein Y, Eisenberg D. Z Zellforsch 1973;138:223.
7. Van Hinsbergh WM. Atherosclerosis 1984;53:113.
8. Görög P, Born GVR. Br J Exp Pathol 1982;63:447.
9. Born GVR, Palinski W. Br J Exp Pathol 1985;66:543.
10. Ludlam C, Arisawa H, Born GVR. J Physiol (London) 1991;446:220 pp.
11. Görög P, Born GVR. Arterioscler Thromb 1993;13:637.
12. Shafi S, Cusack NJ, Born GVR. Proc Roy Soc Lond B 1989;235:289.
13. Cardona-Sanclemente EL, Born GVR. Atherosclerosis 1992;96:215.
14. Cardona-Sanclemente EL, Görög P, Born GVR. J Physiol (London) 1992;452:56 pp.
15. Pittman RC, Carew TE, Glass CK, Green SR, Taylor CA, Attie AD. Biochem J 1983;212:791.
16. Cryer PE, Haymond MW, Santigo JV, Shah SD. N Engl J Med 1976;295:573.
17. Cardona-Sanclemente EL, Medina R, Born GVR. Proc Nat Acad Sci USA 1994;91:3285.
18. Moncada S, Radomski MW, Palmer RMJ. Biochem Pharmacol 1988;37:2495.
19. Moffitt H, Clough G, Michel CC. Int J Microcirc 1992;II:90.
20. Wilhelmsen L, Svardsudd H, Horsan-Bengtsen H, Larsson B, Welin L, Tibblin G. N Engl J Med 1984; 311:501.
21. Heinrich J, Balleisen L, Schulte H, Assmann G, Van de Loo J. Atheroscler Thromb 1994;14:54.

Induction of heat-shock protein 70 by oxidized LDL in human endothelial cells

Weimin Zhu[1], Paola Roma[1], Fabio Pellegatta[2] and Alberico L. Catapano[2]

[1]Institute of Pharmacological Sciences, University of Milano, Milano and [2]Ospedale S. Raffaele Milano, Italy

Abstract. Heat-shock proteins are detectable in human atherosclerotic plaques, especially in endothelial cells. In this report we demonstrate that oxidized LDL can induce the expression of hsp70 in cultured EAhy-926 cells and in human umbilical vein endothelial cells in vitro. The induction paralleled the cytotoxicity of OxLDL to the cells. Our data suggest a link between OxLDL and hsp expression in the arterial wall.

Introduction

Heat-shock (hsp) or stress proteins are a family of about 20 proteins and cognates that show a very high sequence homology among different species, from the simplest bacteria to man. Hsp expression is induced by a number of stresses including infection, high temperature, free radicals and mechanical stress, and provides cells with protection from environmental insults [1].

Increased expression of hsp65 and 70 has been observed in endothelial cells, macrophages, and smooth muscle cells from human atherosclerotic lesions. For hsp65 a role has been proposed in triggering an autoimmune response. Immunization of rabbits with bacterial hsp65 induced atherosclerotic lesions with a high expression of hsp65, and T lymphocytes isolated from lesions (either induced by immunization or cholesterol feeding) specifically responded to hsp in vitro [2,3]. In man the presence of carotid atherosclerotic lesions was related to the presence and titer of autoantibodies to hsp65, which further emphasizes the role of these proteins in determining the presence of vascular atherosclerotic lesions [4].

The possible role of other hsp like hsp70, which is expressed in high concentrations in human atherosclerotic lesions, is less studied [5,6]. Johnson et al. have suggested that hsp70 plays an important role in protecting lysosomal membrane integrity and arterial wall cell survival [6]. Indeed the amount of inducible hsp70 expressed in the rabbit myocardium relates directly to the extent of protection of the heart after anoxia [7].

In recent years lysosomal function in atherosclerosis has received much attention in view of the central role played by these organelles in controlling the traffic of lipids that enter the cell. We have recently shown that oxidized LDL (OxLDL) accumulate into lysosomes and target specifically to these organelles [8]. In view of the known cytotoxicity of OxLDL we aimed at studying the effects of OxLDL on hsp70 expression in human endothelial cells.

Materials and Methods

Cells

EAhy-926, a permanent hybrid cell line between human umbilical vein endothelial cells and human lung carcinoma cells [9], were used as a model for human endothelial cells as previously described [9]. Human umbilical vein endothelial cells (HUVEC) were cultured in M199 with the addition of 20% FCS, endothelial cell growth factor and heparin (90 µg/ml). Cells were used for experiments before the fifth passage.

Lipoproteins

LDL were isolated from human plasma by sequential ultracentrifugation in the presence of 0.01% EDTA (w/v) [10]. AcLDL were prepared according to Basu [11] and Ox-LDL were prepared in the presence of 20 µM Cu^{++}, as described [8].

Immunofluorescence

Cells were incubated at 37°C for various times in fresh medium without FCS and with or without lipoproteins, or heat shocked at 45°C (15 min), fixed with 3% paraformaldehyde at room temperature (RT) (15 min), washed with PBS and permeabilized with 0.5% Triton X-100 on ice (3 min). After blocking the nonspecific staining by an incubation in PBS with 1% BSA and 5% normal goat serum (1 h), cells were incubated in a 1:200 dilution of a mouse monoclonal antibody specific for the inducible form of hsp70 (C92F3A-5, StressGen, Canada) (RT, 1 h), washed with PBST (0.05% Tween-20 in PBS) and incubated with biotinylated anti-mouse IgG 1:250 (Amersham) (RT, 1 h), washed with PBST, then incubated with straptavidin-fluorescein 1:100 (Amersham, U.K.) (RT, 30 min), washed with PBST, mounted on microscopy slides and observed under a fluorescence microscope (Zeiss Aksioscope, Germany). Kodak Gold II (400 ASA) films were used for photographs.

[³H]Adenine release

Endothelial cell damage was estimated by [³H]adenine release as described [11].

Results

EAhy-926 cells displayed weak staining when probed with the anti-hsp70 antibody in the absence of any lipoprotein (not shown): this may be due to the low level of expression of hsp70 that has been reported for other cell types in the absence of stress [12]. After 7 h of incubation with 200 µg/ml OxLDL an intense cytoplasmic staining was observed in nonconfluent cells (Fig. 1). Staining of cells incubated with native LDL was very weak (Fig. 1). Staining of heat-shocked cells, as a positive control, indicates that after thermal stress hsp 70 mainly localizes in the nucleus, as reported for other cells [13] (not shown).

Similar results were obtained with HUVEC. In control conditions the expression of hsp70 in HUVEC was even lower than in EAhy-926 (not shown). At 7 h of incubation with OxLDL, the cytoplasm was heavily stained (Fig. 1), as observed for EAhy-926. Incubation with native LDL did not induce expression of hsp70 (Fig. 1). As observed for EAhy-926, hsp70 localized in heat-shocked HUVEC mainly within the nucleus. Since hsp synthesis is a response to toxic stimuli we aimed at verifying the linkage between the increase in hsp expression and OxLDL cytotoxicity. To test for OxLDL cytotoxicity, [³H]adenine release from labeled EAhy926 was evaluated. During incubation of cells with OxLDL, [³H]adenine release was more than twice that observed after incubation with either AcLDL, native LDL, or BSA (Table 1). Similar results were obtained with HUVEC (not shown).

Discussion

Synthesis of heat-shock proteins is a defense response triggered in cells by a variety of

938

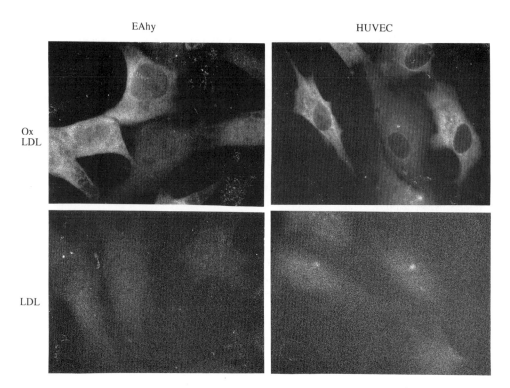

Fig. 1. Sparse monolayers of EAhy-926 and HUVEC were incubated at 37°C for the indicated times in fresh medium without FCS, containing OxLDL (200 μg/ml). Cells were then processed for immunofluorescence with anti-hsp70, examined with a fluorescence microscope and photographed.

noxious stimuli [1]. Since oxidized LDL are toxic to cells [14], we asked the question whether exposure to chemically oxidized LDL (OxLDL), a model of oxidatively modified lipoproteins, may induce hsp synthesis. Our attention was focused on endothelial cells because endothelial lining is a major target during vessel wall injury [14]; furthermore, endothelial cells can oxidize LDL [15] and oxidative events are likely to occur in the subendothelial space. In both EAhy-926 and HUVEC, increased expression of hsp70 was evident after a 7-h incubation with OxLDL. The effect of this treatment was different from that of heat shock: in fact, heat shock resulted in nuclear accumulation of hsp70 [13], while during incubation with OxLDL newly expressed hsp70 was mostly located in the cytoplasm. Stress proteins initially localize in sites of major injury [16]. In heat-

Table 1. Effect of cell density on OxLDL cytotoxicity

	[³H]Adenine release (%)			
	Ox-LDL	Ac-LDL	LDL	BSA
Sparse cells	52.4 ± 7.10	20.2 ± 0.85	21.3 ± 0.42	21.3 ± 0.10

[³H]adenine-labeled EAhy-926 cells were incubated for 24 h at 37°C with either OxLDL, AcLDL, LDL or BSA (200 μg/ml) and [³H]adenine release was measured as described in Materials and Methods. Values are the mean ± SE of three dishes and are representative of four separate experiments.

shocked cells this occurs in the nucleus. Conversely when cells take up OxLDL, cytoplasm is the first site of injury and OxLDL in particular accumulates into lysosomes; thus, hsp70 induction may be a specific response to a lysosomal damage.

Sparse endothelial cells, which actively proliferate in vitro, may be compared with an injured endothelium involved in wound repair, a characteristic of early atherosclerotic lesions. In vivo, cytoprotection afforded by stress proteins may allow cells a greater chance to survive cytotoxic events, including exposure to OxLDL. The observed expression of hsp by endothelial cells in areas of atherosclerosis is in agreement with this hypothesis [2,6]. Understanding the hsp function in this context requires further studies in vitro and in vivo, and the hybrid cell line EAhy-926 appears to be a suitable model of human endothelium for future investigation.

Acknowledgements

This work was supported in part by a grant from CNR, Progetto Finalizzato Aging, Publication No. 943458. The authors wish to thank Dr Yan Lu for supplying the HUVEC cells and Miss Maddalena Marazzini for typing the manuscript.

References

1. Hightower LE. Cell 1991;66:191–197.
2. Xu Q, Luef G, Weimann S, Gupta RS, Wolf H, Wick G. Arterioscler Thromb 1993;13:1763–1769.
3. Xu Q, Klendienst R, Waitz W, Dietrich H, Wick G. J Clin Invest 1993;91:2693–2702.
4. Xu Q, Willeit J, Marosi M, Kleindienst R, Oberhollenzer F, Kiechl S, Stulnig T, Luef G, Wick G. Lancet 1993;341:255–259.
5. Berberian PA, Myers W, Tytell M, Challa V, Bond MG. Am J Pathol 1990;136:71–80.
6. Johnson AD, Berberian PA, Tytell M, Bond MG. Exp Mol Pathol 1993;58:155–168.
7. Marber MS, Walker JM, Latchman DS, Yellon DM. J Clin Invest 1994;93:1087–1094.
9. Edgell CJS, McDonald CC, Graham JB. Proc Natl Acad Sci USA 1983;80:37834–37837.
8. Roma P, Bernini F, Fogliatto R, Bertulli SB, Negri S, Fumagalli R, Catapano AL. J Lipid Res 1992;33:819–829.
10. Havel RJ, Eder HA, Bragdon JH. J Clin Invest 1955;34:1345–1353.
11. Basu SK, Goldstein JL, Anderson RGW, Brown MS. Proc Natl Acad Sci USA 1976;73:3178–3182.
12. Welch WJ, Feramisco JR. J Biol Chem 1984;259:4501–4513.
13. Velazquez JM, Lindquist S. Cell 1984;36:655–662.
14. Balla G, Jacob NS, Eaton JW, Belcher JD, Vercelletti GM. Arterioscler Thromb 1991;11:1700–1711.
15. Janice M, Jerry SA, Gray WM, David LS. Atherosclerosis 1993;102:209–216.
16. Van Why SK, Hildebrandt F, Ardito T, Mann AS, Siegel NJ, Kashgarian M. Am J Physiol 1992;263:F769–F775.

High density lipoprotein-associated paraoxonase (apoK) and clusterin (apoJ): significance and potential functions

Richard W. James, Marie-Claude Blatter Garin, Sylvia Messmer Joudrier and Daniel Pometta

Division of Diabetology, Department of Medicine, University Hospital, Geneva, Switzerland

High density lipoproteins (HDL) have a highly beneficial impact on the atherogenic process. Whilst this is principally attributed to their role in reverse cholesterol transport and catabolism of triglyceride-rich lipoproteins [1], accumulating data suggest that HDL may have a more widespread, positive influence on vascular disease [2]. Current considerations implicate discrete HDL particles in the proposed antiatherogenic mechanisms where the functional relevance of lipoprotein particles derives from their apolipoprotein content. In consequence, identification and characterization of such particles should clarify their contribution to antiatherogenic processes as well as providing a more concise description of HDL metabolism. Recent studies from our group and other laboratories have identified two minor HDL peptide components which appear to form discrete lipoprotein particles. These studies and the potential functions of the two peptides are briefly discussed in this overview.

Clusterin (apolipoprotein J)

Clusterin is the human homologue of rat sulfated glycoprotein 2 which was identified and characterized over a decade ago [3,4]. We first demonstrated the association of clusterin with human plasma lipoproteins [5,6], an observation which was confirmed and extended by other laboratories [7,8]. Up to 50% of clusterin is complexed with plasma lipoproteins, specifically HDL [6], where it shows a high affinity for apoA-I [7]. The liver appears to be the principal source of plasma clusterin and apparently secretes the peptide as a lipoprotein complex devoid of apoA-I [9]. This would necessitate remodeling of clusterin complexes or association of apoA-I with the complex within the plasma compartment, although we have observed apoA-I in clusterin complexes isolated from HepG2-conditioned medium (S. Messmer Joudrier, unpublished observations).

Clusterin is present in a range of body fluids (plasma, cerebrospinal fluid, seminal fluid, synovial fluid, human milk), several of which do not contain apoA-I (S. Messmer Joudrier, unpublished observations). A parallel to these observations is that the peptide appears to be synthesized and secreted by a wide variety of cell types [3,4]. However, cell death and tissue differentiation figure prominently in the inventory of physiological states where clusterin expression is prominent. This has led to suggestions that it may have a protective role in the maintenance of membrane integrity [4]; its ability to modulate complement-mediated cytolytic activity would be an advantage in this context [3]. A variation on this theme is that clusterin may provide a conduit for the controlled excretion of unwanted lipids, such as those liberated from membranes during cell death. This is a seductive proposal in light of the affinity of the peptide for apoA-I/HDL. It would provide a means of directing lipids to the very elements of the lipoprotein system whose principal function appears to be controlled elimination or recycling of lipids.

Paraoxonase (apolipoprotein K)

A peptide that we originally identified and characterized as a component of human HDL [10] was subsequently shown to correspond to the enzyme paraoxonase. Paraoxonase has, in fact, long been known to associate with HDL in various species, but lack of purified preparations, antibodies and sequence data has until recently [11] hampered further characterization of the peptide, apart from its properties as an enzyme. In our recent studies, we have confirmed that the peptide is exclusively bound to HDL in human [10] and rat (M.-Cl. Blatter Garin, unpublished observations) plasma. Moreover, we have demonstrated that paraoxonase forms a discrete HDL particle composed principally of three peptides: paraoxonase, apoA-I (some 2% of total plasma apoA-I) and clusterin. This is illustrated in Fig. 1a, which shows a peptide profile of the fraction of human plasma bound by an antiparaoxonase immunoaffinity column. Its lipoprotein nature is demonstrated in Fig. 1c, which is an electron micrograph of the bound fraction. These observations have recently been confirmed by another laboratory [12].

Development of an enzyme-linked immunoassay (ELISA) has allowed us to undertake quantitative studies of human paraoxonase and its association with HDL (13). Two important conclusions have arisen from these investigations. Firstly, plasma concentrations of paraoxonase are significantly correlated with the two structural apolipoproteins of HDL, apoA-I and apoA-II (Table 1). HDL-cholesterol is also significantly correlated with the peptide in univariate analysis but not in multivariate analysis when either apoA-I or apoA-II is taken into account. These findings suggest that the structural peptides of HDL may be important determinants of plasma levels of paraoxonase, in agreement with reports of low or absent paraoxonase enzyme activity in Tangier patients who lack HDL [14,15].

The second conclusion to arise from quantitative studies of paraoxonase is that polymorphism (there exist two isoforms, A and B, which have recently been shown to

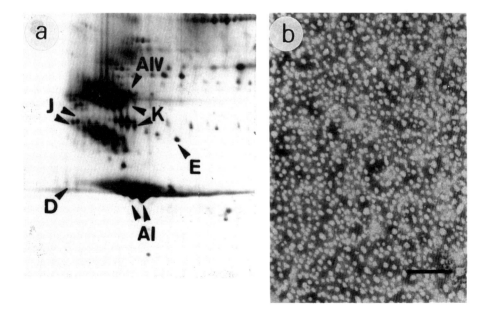

Fig. 1. Silver-stained 2-dimensional gel profile (a) and electron micrograph (b) of the fraction captured from human plasma by an antiparaoxonase immunoaffinity column.

942

Table 1. Correlations between plasma concentrations of paraoxonase and blood lipid and apolipoprotein parameters

Parameter	Correlation coefficient	Significance
ApoA-I	0.36	<0.001
ApoA-II	0.34	<0.001
HDL-cholesterol	0.30	<0.05
Cholesterol	−0.10	>0.10
Triglycerides	−0.18	>0.10
ApoB	−0.05	>0.10

arise from a single amino acid mutation [16]), appears to influence plasma concentrations of the peptide. As shown in Table 2, there are significantly higher plasma concentrations ($p < 0.05$) of the B phenotype. Whilst this polymorphism has been shown to induce activity differences with respect to paraoxon as substrate, we observed no differences in the specific activities between phenotypes with the nondiscriminating substrate phenylacetate (Table 2).

The rationale and interest for most studies of the enzyme to date have been its ability to neutralize exogenous, toxic substrates such as the organophosphate insecticide paraoxon and certain nerve gases. In contrast, the natural substrate(s) for the enzyme has not been identified. A role in lipid metabolism remains a presumption based on (i) the close association of the peptide with HDL and (ii) the apparent instability of the peptide in the absence of HDL. These argue for a function tightly linked to that of HDL. In this context, recent suggestions have attempted to make an analogy with toxic exogenous substrates of the enzyme by proposing that the physiological substrate for paraoxonase may be lipid oxidation products [17]. These are also potentially highly toxic and are thought to play a central role in vascular disease as the principal atherogenic modifications of LDL, precipitating their incorporation into fatty streaks/atherosclerotic plaques [18]. Whilst the hypothesis requires confirmation it would provide one explanation of the reported ability of HDL to protect LDL from oxidation. The proposal assumes greater significance in the context of our recent studies showing the existence of an apoA-I–paraoxonase–clusterin complex in human plasma [10]. One could imagine a role for such a complex in eliminating oxidatively modified lipids; clusterin could furnish the vehicle for transfer of such lipids (notably from sites of cell death) to paraoxonase, which would provide the means of enzymatically neutralizing them.

Acknowledgements

The studies described in this article have been supported by grants from the Fonds National de la Recherche Scientifique (No. 32-30782.91) and the Roche Research Foundation.

Table 2. Plasma concentrations and specific activity of paraoxonase as a function of phenotype

Phenotype (n)	Concentration (µg/ml)	Specific activity	
		Phenylacetate	Paraoxon
AA (52)	76.1 ± 19.5	1.30 ± 0.29	1.35 ± 0.26
AB (39)	82.2 ± 17.6	1.23 ± 0.26	2.92 ± 0.68
BB (5)	89.0 ± 17.4	0.86 ± 0.28	3.34 ± 0.85

References

1. Tall AR. J Clin Invest 1990;86:379—384.
2. Schmitz G, Lackner KJ. Curr Opin Lipidol 1993;4:392—400.
3. Jenne DE, Tschopp J. TIBS 1992;17:154—159.
4. Jordan-Starck TC, Witte DP, Aronow BJ, Harmony JAK. Curr Opin Lipidol 1992;3:75—85.
5. James RW, Hochstrasser D, Tissot J-D, Funk M, Appel R, Barja F, Pellegrini C, Muller AF, Pometta D. J Lipid Res 1988;29:1557—1571.
6. James RW, Hochstrasser A-C, Borghini I, Martin B, Pometta D, Hochstrasser D. Arterioscler Thromb 1991;11:645—652.
7. De Silva HV, Stuart WD, Duvic CR, Wetterau JR, Ray MJ, Ferguson DG, Albers HW, Smith WR, Harmony JAK. J Biol Chem 1990;265:13240—13247.
8. Jenne DE, Lowin B, Peitsch MC, Bottcher A, Schmitz G, Tschopp J. J Biol Chem 1991;266:11030—11036.
9. Burkey BF, Stuart WD, Harmony JAK. J Lipid Res 1992;33:1517—1526.
10. Blatter M-C, James RW, Messmer S, Batia F, Pometta D. Eur J Biochem 1993;211:871—879.
11. Furlong CE, Richter RJ, Chapline C, Crabb JW. Biochemistry 1991;3:10133—10140.
12. Kelos GJ, Stuart WD, Richter RJ, Furlong CE, Jordan-Starck TC, Harmony JAK. Biochemistry 1993;33:832—839.
13. Blatter Garin M-C, Abbott C, Messmer S, Mackness M, Durrington P, Pometta D, James RW. Biochem J (in press).
14. La Du BN. In: Halow W (ed) Pharmacogenetics of Drug Metabolism. New York: Pergamon Press Inc, 1992;51—91.
15. Mackness MI. Biochem Pharmacol 1989;38:385—390.
16. Adkins S, Gan KN, Mody M, La Du BN. Am J Hum Genet 1993;52:598—608.
17. Mackness MI, Arrol S, Durrington PN. FEBS Lett 1991;286:152—154.
18. Witztum JL, Steinberg D. J Clin Invest 1991;88:1785—1792.

Vaccination against cholesterol: immunologic modulation of diet-induced hypercholesterolemia and atherosclerosis in rabbits

Carl R. Alving[1], Glenn M. Swartz Jr.[1], Nabila M. Wassef[1], Edward E. Herderick[3], Renu Virmani[2], Frank D. Kolodgie[2], Gary R. Matyas[1], Jorge L. Ribas[2], Julie R. Kenner[1] and J. Frederick Cornhill[3,4]

[1]Department of Membrane Biochemistry, Walter Reed Army Institute of Research, Washington, DC 20307-5100; [2]Armed Forces Institute of Pathology, Washington, DC; [3]Ohio State University, Columbus, Ohio; and [4]Cleveland Clinic Foundation, Cleveland, Ohio, USA

Abstract. Immunization of rabbits with a protein-free formulation consisting of liposomes containing 71% cholesterol and lipid A as an adjuvant induced antibodies that recognized highly purified nonoxidized crystalline cholesterol and rabbit VLDL/IDL by ELISA. In rabbits that were fed an atherogenic diet containing 0.5–1.0% cholesterol, a markedly lower hypercholesterolemia (as much as 979 mg/dl less) was observed in the immunized animals than in nonimmunized controls. Analysis of aortic fatty streaks by automated morphometric probability-of-occurrence mapping of sudanophilia showed significantly smaller lesions in vaccinees in most areas of the aorta.

Background

Cholesterol was first proposed in 1925 as an antigenic molecule against which specific antibodies could be induced in experimental animals in the presence of heterologous proteins that served as carriers [1]. The observation of apparent antibodies to cholesterol generated a considerable early interest in lipid immunology, and some controversy, which culminated more recently in the development of specific immunoassays for a wide range of steroid hormones (reviewed in [2]). In 1988, monoclonal antibodies to cholesterol were developed by immunization of mice with protein-free liposomes heavily loaded (71 mol%) with unconjugated highly purified nonoxidized cholesterol as an antigen and lipid A, the endotoxic portion of bacterial lipopolysaccharide, as an adjuvant [3]. The antibodies recognized purified, nonoxidized, crystalline cholesterol by ELISA and immunogold electron microscopy.

After development and validation of an ELISA for detecting antibodies to purified cholesterol, naturally occurring antibodies to cholesterol were found in sera from normal humans [4] and pigs, but not guinea pigs [5]. As shown in Fig. 1, using the ELISA technique with crystalline cholesterol as an antigen, we have now assayed sera from 742 preimmunization bleedings obtained from military personnel prior to testing of an unrelated vaccine. Every sample contained easily detectable antibodies to cholesterol, thus extending our previous studies that suggested that naturally occurring IgM and IgG antibodies to cholesterol are present in virtually all normal human sera [4].

The ubiquitous presence of naturally occurring antibodies to cholesterol in sera from young adults suggested the possibility that antibodies to cholesterol might play some role in the metabolic regulation of serum cholesterol, perhaps even a hormone-like role. Several early reports showed that immunization with heterologous β-lipoproteins [6], or a heterologous protein–cholesteryl ester antigen in which cholesteryl sebacate was esterified to a heterologous protein carrier [7,8], inhibited the development of diet-induced hypercholesterolemia and aortic atherosclerosis in rabbit and cockerel models. In the present study, to test whether antibodies produced against liposomal cholesterol might

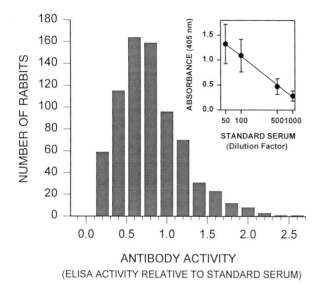

Fig. 1. Anticholesterol antibodies in normal human sera. Dilutions (1:50) of each of 742 human sera were tested in triplicate by ELISA, using mixed-affinity purified antihuman IgG, IgM and IgA (H and L chains) [3]. Titration of a standard serum used for comparison (CRA) was performed with each group of approximately 15 volunteer sera (inset shows mean ± SD of 52 assays of the standard serum). Binding was not observed when cholesterol was omitted.

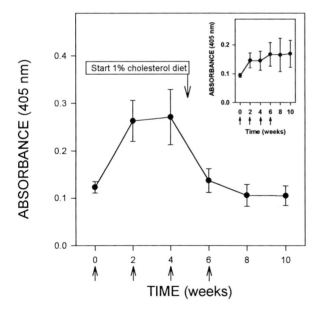

Fig. 2. Binding of rabbit IgG antibodies to cholesterol. Antibodies (mean ± SD) were detected in sera (1:100 dilution) by ELISA with highly purified nonoxidized cholesterol as an antigen [3]. Six rabbits were immunized i.m. or i.v. with liposomal cholesterol (arrows). Five weeks after initial injection, the rabbits were started on a 1% cholesterol diet. Four immunized control rabbits were maintained on a normal diet not supplemented with cholesterol (inset).

have beneficial effects, rabbits were immunized with liposomal cholesterol and then fed an atherogenic cholesterol-loaded diet.

Results

Figure 2 demonstrates increasing levels of IgG antibodies, detected by ELISA with purified crystalline cholesterol, that were induced by injection of liposomes containing 71% cholesterol and lipid A. Rabbits were injected at 0, 2, 4, and 6 weeks. At 6 weeks, 1 week after a diet containing 1% cholesterol was begun, the ability to detect antibodies

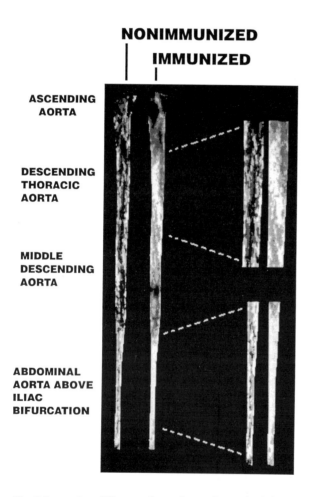

Fig. 3. Less sudanophilia on surfaces of aortas from animals immunized with liposomal cholesterol and fed a 0.5% cholesterol diet (methodological details given elsewhere [9,10]). Aortas from 40 immunized and six nonimmunized rabbits were stained with sudan IV, photographed with high-speed color film, digitized using an Eikonix 78/99 digital scanner, and transferred to an image-processing system. The stored digital images were subdivided into a mosaic of triangular subsections based on anatomical landmarks which were used to stretch individual images to remove anatomical variation among animals and produce a composite representation. Binary images were stored to form composite topographic probability-of-occurrence maps of sudanophilia at each point on the entire aortic surface. A color print showing increasing probabilities of sudanophilia through a color gradient of white-yellow-orange-brown-black was then scanned and printed to produce a black and white image.

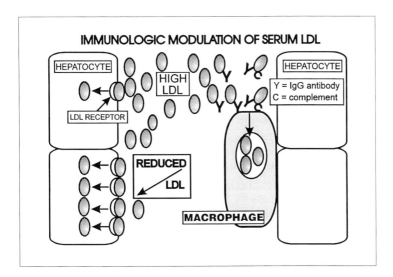

Fig. 4. Proposed mechanism of immunological modulation of diet-induced hypercholesterolemia.

in the serum was lost, presumably due to the binding of the antibodies to the VLDL/IDL that appeared in large amounts in the rabbit sera. Separate experiments demonstrated by ELISA that the antibodies did bind to purified rabbit VLDL/IDL obtained from serum of nonimmunized cholesterol-fed rabbits. Loss of the ability to detect antibodies at 6 weeks by ELISA did not occur with sera from rabbits fed a normal diet not supplemented with cholesterol (Fig. 2, inset). Similar patterns to those observed for IgG antibodies were also observed for IgM antibodies.

Although all the rabbits developed very high cholesterol levels (as high as 3,000 mg/dl in the nonimmunized animals at 12 weeks), the levels in the immunized animals were significantly and substantially lower than the nonimmunized animals (e.g., 1,770 mg/dl for immunized vs. 2,749 mg/dl for nonimmunized at 10 weeks, $p = 0.001$ by t-test).

The effect of immunization of rabbits against cholesterol on the subsequent development of aortic fatty streak lesions was determined. 40 animals were immunized monthly (0, 4, 8, and 12 weeks), and 5 weeks after completion of immunization the animals were placed on a 0.5% cholesterol diet for 12 weeks. The results showed markedly less sudanophilia in the immunized animals (Fig. 3). Although approximately 37% less sudanophilia was observed through the entire aortic surface, statistically significant less sudanophilia was demonstrated, 62 and 57% less respectively, in the descending thoracic aorta, and in the abdominal aorta (including the left and right renal arteries), both of which regions are magnified in Fig. 3.

Discussion

The results from the rabbit model demonstrate that immunization with a protein-free liposome formulation containing highly purified nonoxidized cholesterol and lipid A induces IgM and IgG antibodies that recognize both crystalline cholesterol and VLDL/IDL. The immunization procedure also provides prophylactic protection against diet-induced hypercholesterolemia and atherosclerosis. Figure 4 illustrates a mechanism that we believe can explain the experimental observations. We propose that the induced antibodies can bind to cholesterol present in circulating LDL (or VLDL or IDL), thereby opsonizing the lipoproteins for removal by scavenger macrophages, principally Kupffer cells in the liver. The reduction of serum LDL then results in an upregulation in the number of LDL receptors [11], lowering the LDL still more and causing a further amplification of the beneficial effects.

Although it is true that the rabbit model might be considered somewhat unrealistic when compared with cholesterol levels that might occur in humans, the results suggest that immunization with liposomal cholesterol has tremendous potential potency in that it was able to lower the rabbit serum cholesterol level by as much as 979 mg/dl. This suggests that the immunization procedure might be an effective means of limiting the increases in serum cholesterol induced by diet in humans.

References

1. Sachs H, Klopstock A. Biochem Z 1925;159:491–501.
2. Alving CR, Swartz GM Jr. CRC Crit Rev Immunol 1991;10:441–453.
3. Swartz GM Jr, Gentry MK, Amende LM, Blanchette-Mackie EJ, Alving CR. Proc Natl Acad Sci USA 1988;85:1902–1906.
4. Alving CR, Swartz GM Jr, Wassef NM. Biochem Soc Trans 1989;17:637-639.
5. Wassef NM, Johnson SH, Graeber GM, Swartz GM Jr, Schultz CL, Hailey JR, Johnson AJ, Taylor DG, Ridgway RL, Alving CR. J Immunol 1989;143:2990-2995.
6. Gero S, Gergely J, Jakab L, Szekely J, Virag S, Farkas K, Czuppon A. Lancet 1959;ii:6–7.
7. Bailey JM, Bright R, Tomar R. Nature 1964;201:407–408.
8. Bailey JM, Butler J. In: Di Luzio NR, Paoletti R (eds) The Reticuloendothelial System and Atherosclerosis. New York: Plenum, 1967;433–441.
9. Cornhill JF, Barrett WA, Herderick EE, Mahley RW, Fry DL. Atherosclerosis 1985;5:415–426.
10. Kolodgie FD, Wilson PS, Cornhill JF, Herderick EE, Mergner WJ, Virmani R. Toxicologic Pathol 1993; 21:425–435.
11. Brown MS, Goldstein JL. Proc Natl Acad Sci USA 1979;76:3330–3337.

The catalytic subunit of the editing enzyme is a zinc-containing cytidine deaminase with an RNA-binding motif at its active site

James Scott, Shoumo Bhattacharya, Naveenan Navaratnam, Dipti Patel and Adam L. Jarmuz
MRC Molecular Medicine Group, Royal Postgraduate Medical School, Hammersmith Hospital, London, UK

Abstract. Apolipoprotein B (apoB) is present in the circulation in two forms. In humans apoB100 is made in the liver and apoB48 in the small intestine. In the intestine apoB100 mRNA undergoes a C to U editing to generate a stop translation codon and the truncated intestinal form apoB48. The apoB mRNA editing enzyme contains a 27-kDa protein (p27) with homology to the cytidine deaminase family of enzymes. P27 is a zinc-containing cytidine deaminase that operates catalytically in a similar manner to the *Escherichia coli* enzyme that acts on monomeric substrates. However, p27 has acquired the capacity to bind to an AU sequence downstream of the editing site and this binding is required for editing. RNA binding is mediated through amino-acid residues involved in zinc coordination and proton shuttling and in forming the α-β-α structure that encompasses the active site. For full activity p27 requires other cellular components that can be found in cells such as liver that do not edit apoB mRNA. These may be involved in RNA targeting and specificity.

Apolipoprotein B (apoB) mRNA undergoes a discrete and specific C to U editing in the nucleus of certain mammalian cell types to generate apoB48 (241 kDa) [1,2]. ApoB48 is made in the enterocytes of the small intestine from the transcript of the apoB100 gene. It is required for the transport of dietary lipid in triglyceride-rich lipoproteins called chylomicrons. ApoB100 (512 kDa) is needed for the transport of lipids synthesized in the liver. The mechanism of apoB mRNA editing is a sequence-specific cytidine deamination [3,4]. The catalytic subunit of the apoB mRNA editing enzyme is a 27-kDa (p27) member of the cytosine nucleoside/nucleotide deaminase family of enzymes [5,6]. P27 is not on its own competent for apoB mRNA editing, but requires other cellular factors for RNA targeting. It is also evident that the other factors required for editing are expressed in liver cells that normally lack this function, as mixing of extracts from human liver cells with p27, transfection of liver cell lines with p27, or transduction of rabbits with p27, is sufficient to produce site-specific editing of apoB mRNA [6–8].

Results

We have previously demonstrated that the catalytic subunit (p27) of the apoB mRNA-editing enzyme is related to the cytidine deaminase family of proteins [9]. The atomic structure of the *Escherichia coli* (*E. coli*) cytidine deaminase has recently been established, and structural similarities with p27 were noted [10]. To help identify the structural motifs in p27 that are important for site-specific cytidine deamination in an oligoribonucleotide, we have identified cDNA clones for the human enzyme and compared these with the rat sequence at the proposed active site of the enzymes (Fig. 1).

Address for correspondence: James Scott, MRC Molecular Medicine Group, Royal Postgraduate Medical School, Hammersmith Hospital, Du Cane Road, London W12 0NN, UK.

Phylogenetic analysis of the amino-acid sequence at the active sites indicates that the RNA-editing cytidine-residue deaminases, the CMP/dCMP deaminases and cytidine/deoxycytidine deaminases form distinct subgroups.

The *E. coli* cytidine deaminases and the human and rat editing enzymes each contain a conserved triad of histidine and two cysteine residues that are considered to coordinate zinc, and a glutamate residue considered to act in a proton shuttle during deamination (Fig. 1). Additional residues conserved between the human and rat editing enzymes, but not found in other members of the deaminase family, are a series of phenylalanine residues that reside in the segment that links the proposed active-site residues.

We have expressed the catalytic subunit of the apoB-editing enzyme (p27) as a glutathione S-transferase (GST) fusion in *E. coli* (GST-p27). The GST fusion protein was active in the apoB mRNA-editing assay only when complemented with partially purified rat intestinal extracts that had lost intrinsic editing activity.

The homology of p27 to other deaminases has suggested residues that encompass the presumed active site [9,11]. The crystal structure of the *E. coli* cytidine deaminase complexed to the transitional-state analog 5-fluoropyrimidine-2-1-riboside indicates that the residues His102, Cys129 and Cys132 are zinc ligands and form the active site, together with Glu104, which is involved in proton transfer functions [10]. These residues correspond to His61, Cys93, Cys96 and Glu63 in rat p27 (Fig. 1).

To establish whether these conserved amino-acid residues form the active site of p27, we performed site-directed mutagenesis of GST-p27 to introduce "safe" changes at these residues [12] (Fig. 1). Replacement of His61 by Ser (H61S) or Arg (H61R), Cys93 and 96 by Ala (C93A and C96A) and Glu63 by Gln (E63Q) abolished editing activity. Mutation of the residue Val64, which is not conserved between deaminases, to Leu (V64L) had no effect on editing activity.

To investigate the proposal that p27 is a zinc-dependent cytidine residue deaminase we have used zinc-specific chelation and site-directed mutagenesis. In the first instance HA-p27 expressed in Sf9 cells was incubated with a zinc-specific chelating agent 1,10-*o*-phenanthroline. This abolished the ability of p27 to confer editing activity on partially

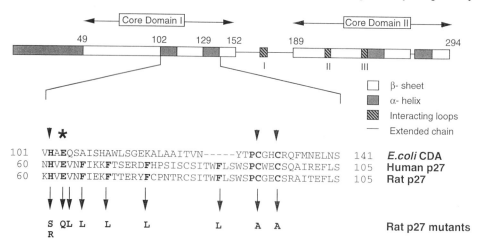

Fig. 1. Domain organization of *E. coli* cytidine deaminase and comparison of active-site primary sequence between *E. coli* cytidine deaminase and RNA-editing cytidine deaminases. Zinc-coordinating residues are indicated with vertical arrow heads. The proton-shuttling glutamate is marked with an asterisk. Conserved residues are emboldened. "Safe" changes made by site-directed mutagenesis are indicated by arrows.

purified rat intestinal extract that had lost this activity. Control incubations with either 1,7-o-phenanthroline or with the ethanol vehicle used for solubilizing this compound had no effect (results not shown). Removal of 1,10-o-phenanthroline and replacement of zinc by dialysis fully restored editing activity to HA-p27. 1,10-o-phenanthroline had no effect on the activity of the complementing, most highly purified fractions of the editing enzyme, indicating that zinc was not necessary for activity of the complementing fraction.

To evaluate the role of p27 residues His61, Cys93 and Cys96 in zinc coordination, we studied the residues for their ability to bind zinc by probing with ^{65}Zn(II). Wild-type, H61S, E63Q and V64L mutants each bound zinc. Mutations C93A and C96A abolished zinc binding. Thus, in agreement with the *E. coli* crystal structure and mutagenesis of *E. coli* cytidine deaminase, p27 binds zinc at Cys93 and Cys96 residues [10,13]. P27 is therefore a zinc-containing cytidine residue deaminase.

Phe66 is conserved between the human and rat RNA-editing deaminases whereas an aliphatic residue is found at this position in all other deaminases [11]. We therefore made the safe change of this residue to leucine. Surprisingly, F66L abolished editing. Other phenylalanines at position 70, 76 and 87 are also conserved in p27. Phe66 resides in the first active-site α-helix and Phe70, 76 and 87 in the β-sheet that links these helices (Fig. 1). Mutation of residue Phe87 (F87L) abolished editing, but mutation of Phe70 (F70L) and Phe76 (F76L) had no effect on editing. F66L, F70L, F76L and F87L each bound zinc to the same extent as wild-type.

We considered whether Phe66 and Phe87 might be involved in RNA binding and for positioning p27 for site-directed deamination of a cytidine-6666. In a variety of RNA-binding proteins RNA–protein interaction can be demonstrated by UV-cross-linking, which occurs through free radical-driven covalent linkage to aromatic residues. P27 can be specifically UV-cross-linked to its RNA substrate. GST alone does not UV-cross-link. The *E. coli* cytidine deaminase cannot be UV-cross-linked to apoB mRNA (results not shown). Mutants in the catalytic domain of p27 (H61S, H61R, E63Q and C93A) did not UV-cross-link to the RNA substrate, whereas mutants V64L and C96A did UV-cross-link to apoB mRNA. The mutants F66L and F87L also abolished UV-cross-linking to substrate RNA. Mutants F70L and F76L had no effect on cross-linking. These results indicate that p27 interacts with apoB mRNA through its active site in a highly specific manner. Phe66 and Phe87 are also involved in this interaction, as mutation of these residues also abolished editing. RNA binding by p27 is a prerequisite for apoB mRNA editing (Fig. 2).

In order to define the p27-binding site we established a series of deletion mutants encompassing the apoB mRNA-editing substrate. Wild-type and mutant F-I encompassing nucleotides 6679 to 6690 were strongly UV-cross-linked to the substrate apoB RNA. Mutant C to F also showed low-level UV-cross-linking. Other mutants that lack these nucleotides showed absent or much lower cross-linking. Thus p27 binding is localized in the region of nucleotides 6679 to 6684.

In conclusion, in this study we have shown that the catalytic subunit of the apoB mRNA-editing enzyme is a zinc-containing cytidine residue deaminase that operates by the same mechanism as the *E. coli* enzyme that acts on mononucleotides/nucleosides. The editing enzyme has evolved away from the enzymes that act on soluble substrates by binding to the edited nucleotide in an oligoribonucleotide through its active site and other residues. For editing to take place the 27-kDa catalytic subunit of the apoB mRNA-editing enzyme also needs complementing nuclear factors that are expressed in cells that do not normally express or edit apoB mRNA. Surprisingly, while p27 is not on its own competent for mRNA editing, transduction of p27 on an adenovirus vector into rabbit livers, which do not normally edit apoB mRN, confers editing on this tissue. This finding

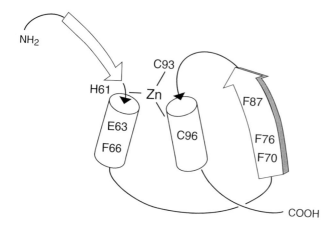

Fig. 2. Schematic representation of the active site of the RNA-editing cytidine deaminase. The diagram shows zinc coordinated by His61, Cys93 and Cys96 and the proton-shuttling glutamate Glu63. Conserved phenylalanines F66, F70, F76 and F87 are shown in the linking segment between the active site α-helices. RNA binding is mediated by His61, Glu63, Phe66, Phe87 and Cys93. This diagram is based on a cartoon in [10].

provides a tool for modulating lipoprotein levels in this experimental model.

Together, these studies illustrate how structural changes in the cytidine nucleoside/nucleotide family of enzymes have contributed to the origins of this type of editing through the adaptation of enzymatic function.

References

1. Chen S-H, Habib G, Yang CY et al. Science 1987;238:363–366.
2. Powell LM, Wallis SC, Pease RJ, Edwards YH, Knott TJ, Scott J. Cell 1987;50:831–840.
3. Bostrom K, Poksay KS, Johnson DF, Lusis AJ, Innerarity TL. J Biol Chem 1990;265:22446–22452.
4. Hodges PE, Navaratnam N, Greeve JC, Scott J. Nucl Acid Res 1991;19:1197–1201.
5. Navaratnam N, Shah R, Patel D, Fay V, Scott J. Proc Natl Acad Sci USA 1993;90:222–226.
6. Teng B, Burant CF, Davidson NO. Science 1993;260:1816–1819.
7. Giannoni F, Bonen DK, Funahashi T, Hadjiagapiou C, Burant CF, Davidson NO. J Biol Chem 1994;269:5932–5936.
8. Hughes SD, Rouy D, Navaratnam N, Scott J, Rubin EM. 67th Scientific Sessions American Heart Association November 14–17, 1994: Dallas, Texas, 1994.
9. Navaratnam N, Morrison JR, Bhattacharya S et al. J Biol Chem 1993;268:20709–20712.
10. Betts L, Xiang S, Short SA, Wolfenden R, Carter CW Jr. J Mol Biol 1994;235:635–656.
11. Bhattacharya S, Navaratnam N, Morrison JR, Scott J, Taylor WR. Trends Biochem Sci 1994;3:105–106.
12. Bordo D, Argos P. J Mol Biol 1991;217:721–729.
13. Smith AA, Carlow DC, Wolfenden R, Short SA. Biochemistry 1994;33:6468–6474.

ApoB metabolism: overview and recent advances

James Shepherd

Institute of Biochemistry, Royal Infirmary, Glasgow G4 0SF, UK

Abstract. Many individuals who succumb to early coronary heart disease have moderate hypercholesterolemia, often accompanied by an elevation of plasma triglyceride. These lipid abnormalities are associated with disturbances in the metabolism of apolipoprotein (apo) B100, the major protein associated with very low and low density lipoprotein (VLDL and LDL). The B100 protein is secreted by the liver as a constituent of triglyceride-rich VLDL which, following remodeling in the plasma through a transient intermediate density species (IDL), is ultimately converted to LDL and thereafter cleared from the circulation by receptor-mediated or other mechanisms. Endothelium-bound lipases, in conjunction with these receptor-mediated processes, control the rates of lipoprotein delipidation and metabolism. Their failure leads to hyperlipidemia of varying degree which, itself, has an impact on the structure, degree of heterogeneity and potential atherogenicity of the circulating lipoproteins. Therefore, in terms of their association with coronary risk, no lipoprotein is an island, sufficient unto itself.

The elegant complexity of the plasma lipoprotein transport system reflects the current status of a 350-million-year evolutionary process designed to facilitate the safe and efficient transport of lipids through the aqueous environment of the plasma and interstitial fluid. All body tissues make demands on this plasma lipid pool. For some it represents a reservoir of cholesterol which they use to generate hormones and bile acids, while others extract triglyceride from it as their main source of energy. Most cells are limited in their capacity to store these lipids and take steps to limit their assimilation in times of surfeit. As a consequence of this, and since the body does not possess feedback mechanisms to limit absorption, intake in excess of requirements may lead to accumulation of lipid in the circulation and the subsequent development of occlusive (and in many instances, life-threatening) atherosclerotic lesions in artery walls. Most individuals who develop these lesions exhibit only moderate hypercholesterolemia, which is often accompanied by an elevation in plasma triglyceride. Both of these lipid abnormalities can be traced back to disturbances in the metabolism of apolipoprotein B100 (apoB100), the major protein associated with very low and low density lipoproteins (VLDL and LDL).

ApoB100 is elaborated and secreted by the liver as an integral component of triglyceride-rich VLDL, which undergo intravascular lipolysis via intermediate particles (intermediate density lipoprotein, IDL) to produce LDL, a cholesterol-rich end product that is cleared from the plasma by a variety of receptor-mediated catabolic processes. The discussion below focuses on recent developments in our understanding of the metabolic cascade through which apoB100 passes from the time of its hepatic secretion until it finally succumbs to cellular catabolism.

Intravascular metabolism of apoB100 in VLDL

In the fasting state, tissue requirements for triglyceride are met by the elaboration, packaging and secretion of a spectrum of triglyceride-rich VLDL by the liver. Current evidence suggests that the size of these particles is dependent on triglyceride availability. When plasma insulin levels are low and the flux of free fatty acids to the liver high,

954

hepatic triglyceride is abundant, and the secreted VLDL is large and lipid-rich. Such particles, called by convention VLDL1, contain about 65% triglyceride by weight and have a flotation rate (Sf) of 60–400. Triglyceride-rich VLDL are metabolized by lipoprotein lipase located on the endothelial surfaces of capillary beds in adipose tissue and skeletal muscle. ApoB100 is retained on the shrinking particles, but with continuing lipolysis it undergoes a conformational change, driven by the reducing radius of curvature of the lipoprotein, and resulting in a smaller lipoprotein with increased binding affinity for LDL receptors.

The metabolism of large, triglyceride-rich VLDL is associated with alteration in both its lipid and apoprotein content. The particle loses phospholipid but gains free cholesterol and, via cholesterol ester transfer protein (CETP), cholesteryl ester. In fact $VLDL_1$ is the preferred recipient of the latter in postabsorptive plasma [1]. After the loss of sufficient triglyceride its properties change so that as a cholesterol- and apoE-enriched "remnant" it becomes susceptible to receptor-mediated clearance from the circulation [2]. The remnant population spans the range Sf 12–60 which includes VLDL2 (Sf 20–60) and IDL (Sf 12–20). How far the particle shrinks appears to depend upon the amount of cholesteryl ester acquired during its lifetime in the plasma since there is no ready mechanism to deplete VLDL of the sterol [1].

VLDL remnants have two potential fates. Some are removed by receptors and degraded, while others are converted to LDL. Those that contain excessive core cholesteryl esters are unable to follow the latter route and are more likely to be subject to direct catabolism. Results from turnover studies [3,4] indicate that approximately half of the apoB in IDL is subsequently delipidated to LDL while the remainder is catabolized, probably by the liver. It is not yet clear what directs IDL towards degradation or delipidation. LDL-receptor activity in the liver has been suggested as a primary determinant. In conditions where it is low, such as familial hypercholesterolemia or during cholesterol feeding, an increased proportion of IDL is converted to LDL [4]. Conversely, statin therapy which stimulates receptors has been shown to promote the direct catabolism of small VLDL and IDL and so reduce the flux of apoB into LDL [5].

Kinetic studies indicate that while large VLDL1 are inefficiently converted to LDL, smaller, less triglyceride-rich VLDL2 particles [3] released by the liver are the major precursors of LDL. The existence of parallel delipidation pathways leading to LDL generation had been mooted [6] for several years before evidence was obtained in man. It is now considered likely that LDL produced from different sources may exhibit different structural and metabolic features. The existence of these multiple synthetic routes helps to explain the phenomenon of LDL heterogeneity which is seen in all subjects and appears to be a primary determinant of the atherogenicity of the lipoprotein class. Formation of LDL from IDL, the final step in the delipidation cascade, is catalyzed by hepatic lipase, which acts in a complementary fashion to lipoprotein lipase [7]. The latter enzyme prefers chylomicrons and large VLDL as substrates whereas the former shows higher activity against smaller, denser lipoproteins – LDL and HDL [7]. Hepatic lipase removes triglyceride from the particle core and phospholipid from the surface by virtue of its additional phospholipase action. It is also of major importance in determining the size distribution of LDL [8]. Complete loss of HL activity blocks LDL formation, while partial inhibition of the metabolic step has been reported in homozygous FH [4] and normolipemic apoE2 homozygosity [2]. These findings suggest that all the three agents (LDL receptors, apoE and HL) interact to facilitate the conversion step. A scheme can be envisaged in which LDL receptors on the hepatocyte surface and apoE on the IDL particle anchor the particle next to the enzyme.

Metabolism of apoB100 in LDL

LDL is the main lipoprotein fraction involved in atherogenesis; hence, understanding the regulation of its concentration in the circulation is of prime importance. Across a wide range of subjects the production and catabolic rates of LDL-apoB appear to be of equal significance in determining the lipoprotein's steady-state level [9]. As described above, the pathways of LDL synthesis are complex and subject to the influence of diet, drugs and genetic variation. Catabolism of the lipoprotein occurs through one principal regulated mechanism, that of the LDL receptor, and a number of less well characterized receptor-independent routes that include macrophage scavenger activity [10,11]. In normal subjects 30–70% of LDL catabolism occurs through the receptor pathway [10,11]. Its activity can be estimated in LDL-apoB turnovers that employ dual tracers of native and chemically modified LDL [10]. The latter is generated by altering the lysine or arginine residues of apoB so that the lipoprotein is no longer recognized by cell surface receptors. A host of factors are known to influence LDL-receptor function and so alter the fractional catabolic rate (FCR) of the lipoprotein. The clearest example is the inherited disorder familial hypercholesterolemia [10,11], which is caused by a defective allele coding for the LDL receptor. Subjects homozygous for the condition have a very low LDL catabolic rate, and clearance is entirely by receptor-independent mechanisms [12]. In normal subjects receptor activity and hence LDL catabolism varies in response to dietary alterations, hormonal disturbances and the administration of pharmaceutical agents. It is also influenced by age and gender. Women are thought to have higher receptor levels as a result of estrogen stimulation of hepatic LDL receptors. Older people, on the other hand, have a lower FCR for LDL probably because expression of receptors by the liver declines during adult life. These two effects are dramatic and responsible for major variation in plasma cholesterol levels within the general population.

Expression of receptors on the surface of cells is controlled by intracellular cholesterol levels. When a cell has sufficient sterol for its needs, transcription of the receptor protein is downregulated and LDL uptake diminishes [11]. On the other hand, depletion of cellular cholesterol by inhibiting its synthesis or promoting its conversion to bile acids causes increased expression of receptors, enhanced LDL uptake and, in the whole organism, a fall in the circulating LDL concentration. This mechanism has been shown to account for the hypocholesterolemic actions of drugs such as cholestyramine and lovastatin. LDL-cholesterol reduction of up to 40% may be achieved by monotherapy with these compounds; in combination they can dramatically increase receptor-mediated catabolism of lipoproteins and generate falls of 70% in LDL – even in heterozygous FH, where only one copy of the receptor gene is functional. Most LDL receptors are located in the liver and it is the major site of LDL degradation. Most other tissues require little cholesterol and downregulate their receptors, but the liver exports gram quantities of sterol products in bile and can maintain a plasma–cell gradient in favor of LDL uptake. The influence of many lipid-lowering diets and drugs can be best understood in terms of their effects on hepatic cholesterol homeostasis.

High-affinity, receptor-mediated catabolism constitutes the variable, regulated component of LDL clearance. When circulating LDL levels are high, other mechanisms come into operation and can, in terms of the amount of LDL degraded, be quantitatively more important [10]. These alternative pathways are of critical significance because of their perceived involvement in the pathological changes that lead to atherosclerosis. Cells of the monocyte-macrophage series have been implicated as major contributors to receptor-independent LDL catabolism [13–15]. Circumstantial evidence for their participation in LDL removal comes from the finding that they are stuffed with cholesteryl esters in subjects with homozygous FH while patients with myeloproliferative disorders exhibit enhanced reticuloendothelial activity and low circulating LDL concentrations due to rapid LDL degradation [16]. Cell-culture studies demonstrate that macrophages have no particular affinity for LDL prepared from plasma by standard methods. However, if the lipoprotein is preincubated with endothelial cells or divalent metal ions such as copper, it is altered by oxidative processes to a form that is avidly taken up by macrophages [17]. Over recent years evidence has accumulated that this oxidative pathway of LDL degradation operates in vivo and has a significant role in the generation of atherosclerotic plaque. For example, experiments with Watanabe rabbits, an animal model of FH, have shown that administration of antioxidant drugs such as probucol blocks the mechanisms that damage the lipoprotein and inhibits atherogenesis.

LDL had long been considered in most normal subjects to be a homogeneous entity. However, when new high-resolution polyacrylamide gel methods were developed to measure the size distribution of LDL particles, a small number of bands were observed that indicated the presence of discrete species. Subsequent refinement of ultracentrifuge techniques led to the resolution of three major subfractions, LDL-I, LDL-II and LDL-III which are observed in virtually all subjects regardless of plasma lipid levels [18,19]. Their relative abundance has been linked to the plasma triglyceride concentration and lipoprotein lipase and hepatic lipase activities. Young females have high levels of LDL-I and virtually no LDL-III [18] whereas many patients with CHD exhibit LDL-III as the predominant subfraction [18]. The latter observation has led to the hypothesis that not all LDL species have equal atherogenic potential. When the subfractions were tested in vitro for their ability to be oxidized it became clear that LDL-III was most susceptible to this process, possibly because it carried less lipid-soluble natural antioxidant per particle [20].

The presence of small, dense LDL particles is usually accompanied by a modest elevation in plasma triglyceride, low HDL-cholesterol and an inability to clear chylomicrons efficiently. The term "atherogenic lipoprotein phenotype" has been coined to describe this dyslipidemic syndrome which is now recognized as a powerful risk factor for CHD. Its metabolic basis is yet to be discovered and it is probable that a number of aberrations give rise to the pattern. A rise in plasma triglyceride levels is probably the key event which then generates the abnormalities in the denser lipoproteins. Enhanced exchange of core lipid and subsequent action of hepatic lipase on triglyceride-enriched LDL and HDL will remove core and surface lipid and lead to the formation of smaller particles within each lipoprotein class. This process, however, cannot be solely responsible for the subfraction distribution since it does not explain the existence of multiple LDL species. Other mechanisms, including the parallel pathways of synthesis described above, must be active. Recent re-examination of LDL turnovers in normolipemic [21] and hyper-cholesterolemic subjects [22,23] has indicated that metabolic heterogeneity accompanies the structural diversity. Classically, plasma decay curves of radioiodinated LDL tracers were analyzed by mathematical methods that assumed the lipoprotein was homogeneous. However, it has been a long-standing observation [22] that when urinary excretion data are included in a model of LDL metabolism, the presence of at least two plasma species of LDL must be invoked in most subjects in order to explain the observation that the fractional degradation of plasma LDL present decreases over the period of a typical 14-day turnover study. The abundance of rapidly versus slowly metabolized LDL has been linked to the plasma triglyceride concentration [21]. When the latter is elevated, so is the proportion of slowly metabolized LDL. Furthermore, triglyceride lowering by drugs leads to a shift from the slower to the faster-removed species [24]. Available evidence suggests that the receptor pathway is responsible for the differential clearance rates of the LDL metabolic "fractions" and that drugs which were previously thought to act by stimulating receptors may actually enhance receptor-mediated removal of LDL by perturbing the nature of the ligand [24]. The precise structural features of particles that are responsible for their different clearance rates are not known. There is some evidence [25] that smaller LDL are catabolized less well than their larger counterparts. However, the link between density and metabolic properties is loose since the mass of slowly catabolized LDL cannot be restricted, for example, to the LDL-III subspecies [24].

References

1. Eisenberg S. J Lipid Res 1985;26:487–494.
2. Demant T, Bedford D, Packard CJ, Shepherd J. J Clin Invest 1991;88:1490–1501.
3. Packard CJ, Munro A, Lorimer AR, Gotto AM, Shepherd J. J Clin Invest 1984;74:2178–2192.
4. James RWB, Martin B, Pometta D, Fruchart JC, Duriez P, Puchois P, Farriaux JP, Tacquet A, Demant T, Clegg RJ, Munro A, Oliver MF, Packard CJ, Shepherd J. J Lipid Res 1989;30:159–169.
5. Gaw A, Packard CJ, Murray EF, Lindsay GM, Griffin BA, Caslake MJ, Vallance BD, Lorimer AR, Shepherd J. Arterioscler Thromb 1993;13:170–189.
6. Fisher WR. In: Berman M, Grundy SM, Howard BV (eds) Lipoprotein Kinetics and Modelling. New York: Academic Press, 1982;44–68.
7. Nicoll A, Lewis B. Eur J Clin Invest 1980;10:487–495.
8. Zambon A, Austin MA, Brown G, Hokanson JE, Brunzell JD. Arterioscler Thromb 1993;13:147–153.
9. Packard CJ, Shepherd J. In: Gotto AM, Paoletti R (eds) Atherosclerosis Reviews Vol 11. New York: Raven Press, 1983;29–63.
10. Shepherd J, Bicker S, Lorimer AR, Packard CJ. J Lipid Res 1979;20:999–1006.
11. Brown MS, Goldstein JL. Science (Washington DC) 1986;232:34–47.
12. Thompson GR, Soutar AK, Spengel FA, Jadhav A, Gavigan SJP, Myant NB. Proc Natl Acad Sci USA 1981;78:2591–2595.
13. Carew TE, Pittman RC, Steinberg D. J Biol Chem 1982;25:8001–8008.
14. Goldstein JL, Brown MS. Ann Rev Biochem 1977;46:897–930.
15. Slater MR, Packard CJ, Shepherd J. J Biol Chem 1982;257:307–310.
16. Ginsberg H, Goldbert IJ, Wang-Iverson P, Gitler E, Le N-A, Gilbert HS, Brown WV. Arteriosclerosis 1983; 3:233–241.
17. Steinberg D, Parthasarathy S, Carew TE, Khoo JC, Witztum JL. N Engl J Med 1989;320:915–924.
18. Griffin BA, Caslake MJ, Yip B, Tait GW, Packard CJ, Shepherd J. Atherosclerosis 1990;83:59–67.
19. Swinkels DW, Demacker PNM, Hendriks JCM, van't Laar, A. Arteriosclerosis 1989;9:604–613.
20. de Graaf J, Hak-Lemmers HLM, Hectors MPC, Demaker PNM, Henricks JCM, Stalenhoef AFM. Arteriosl Thromb 1991;11:298–306.
21. Caslake MJ, Packard CJ, Series JJ, Yip B, Dagen M, Shepherd J. Eur J Clin Invest 1992;22:96–104.
22. Foster DM, Chait A, Albers JJ, Faelor RA, Harris C, Brunzell JD. Metabolism 1986; 35:685–696.
23. Malmendier CL, Delcroix C, Lontie J-F. Atherosclerosis 1989;80:91–100.
24. Caslake MJ, Packard CJ, Gaw A, Murray E, Griffin BA, Vallance BD, Shepherd J. Arterioscler Thromb 1993;13:702–711.
25. Thompson GR, Teng B, Sniderman AD. Am Heart J 1987;113:514–517.

Assembly and secretion of apoB-containing lipoproteins

Sabina Rustaeus, Jan Borén, Margit Wettesten, Anders Sjöberg, Maria Andersson, Hans Lidén and Sven-Olof Olofsson
Department of Medical Biochemistry, University of Göteborg, Medicinaregatan 9, S-413 90 Göteborg, Sweden

Abstract. A cotranslational route for the assembly of lipoproteins containing apolipoprotein B100 (apoB100) is described. The nascent polypeptides take part in the assembly process after reaching 80 kDa; thereafter there is a direct relation between the size of the nascent chain and the size of the assembled particle. Our results also point to the presence of other routes to the formation of VLDL.

ApoB48 VLDL is assembled in two steps: (i) a cotranslational formation of an apoB48 HDL, (ii) the conversion of apoB48 HDL to VLDL. The possibility of a second step in the assembly of apoB100 VLDL is discussed.

Apolipoprotein B100 (apoB100) is the essential protein component of the triglyceride- and cholesteryl-ester-rich lipoproteins: very low density lipoproteins (VLDL), intermediate density lipoproteins (IDL), low density lipoproteins (LDL) and chylomicrons. ApoB exist in two forms: apoB100 and apoB48 [1]. The former consist of a unique polypeptide chain with a molecular weight of 512,000. In humans apoB100 is expressed almost exclusively in the liver [2] where it is assembled and is secreted on VLDL. ApoB48 corresponds to the N-terminal 48% of apoB100. In humans it is expressed mainly in the intestine [2] where it assembles the large triacylglycerol-rich chylomicrons. In other species, such as the rat [3], there is also a substantial expression of apoB48 in the liver, where the protein assembles VLDL-like particles.

Both forms of apoB are coded for by the same gene [4]. A posttranscriptional [5] editing converts a Gln codon in the apoB100 mRNA to an in-frame stop-codon in apoB48 mRNA [4,6]. A protein that is essential for the editing process has recently been cloned [7].

Results from electron microscopy of rat livers [8] indicate that the assembly of VLDL occurs in the smooth termini of the rough ER, i.e., there is a separation between the site of assembly and the site of translation of the protein. In addition, results from HepG2 cells indicate that the assembly of the apoB100-containing lipoproteins occurs in the ER, in particular in regions which are poor in ribosomes but rich in the enzyme diacylglycerol:acyltransferase, i.e., regions involved in the biosynthesis of triglycerides [9].

Results from studies of HEPG2 cells

ApoB100 is bound to different lipid surfaces in the endoplasmic reticulum (ER)

ApoB100 is bound to the ER membrane and occurs on at least two types of lipoproteins that are present in the ER lumen [10]: (i) particles that are secreted from the cell (i.e., mainly triglyceride-rich particles with the size and density of large LDL. We will refer to these mature lipoproteins produced by the HepG2 cells as the LDL-VLDL); and (ii) dense particles (referred to as "HDL-like"), that are not secreted from the cell [10].

The facts that the signal sequence of the membrane-bound apoB100 is cleaved and the protein is glycosylated indicate that the membrane-bound apoB100 is at least partially translocated to the ER lumen [10]. Several authors have presented evidence that a relatively large portion of apoB100 is present on the cytoplasmic surface of the ER membrane [11,12]. This conclusion is mainly based on the observation that the membrane-bound apoB100 is accessible to exogenous proteases, but also on results from experiments with monoclonal antibodies. Taken together, the obtained results suggest that apoB100 spans the ER membrane. This conclusion is countered by the fact that apoB100 lacks a typical membrane-spanning sequence. The presence of apoB100 on the cytoplasmic surface of the ER has been seriously questioned by several authors [13,14] and there are no obvious ways at present to reconcile these diverging observations into a hypothesis for the interaction between apoB100 and the ER membrane.

A cotranslational route for the assembly of LDL-VLDL in HepG2 cells

Results from pulse-chase studies in HepG2 cells [15] indicated that apoB100 nascent polypeptides that had reached a size of 80–100 kDa were engaged in assembly of lipoproteins. Moreover the longer the nascent polypeptide had grown, the larger and more triglyceride-rich lipoprotein it had assembled (Fig. 1A–C). Our results thus demonstrated the presence of a cotranslational route for the assembly of apoB100-containing lipoproteins (Fig. 1). The results were confirmed by other authors [16].

Recent results by other investigators indicate that the assembly process could be activated by incubation with oleic acid at periods longer than the expected time needed for the elongation of the nascent polypeptides [17]. Such observations clearly point to the presence of alternative pathways for the assembly of apoB100-containing lipoproteins. This will be discussed below in conjunction with the assembly of apoB48-containing VLDL.

The HDL-like particles with apoB100 were also formed cotranslationally. The amount of apoB100 that is translocated onto mature LDL-VLDL particles depends on the rate of triglyceride biosynthesis. Thus when this biosynthesis is increased most of the apoB100 forms LDL-VLDL particles and when the triglyceride biosynthesis is low apoB100 forms HDL-like particles. We have suggested that the HDL-like particle is the result of partial lipidation of apoB100 (Fig. 1D,E).

Posttranslational degradation of apoB100

It is well established that variation in the secretion of apoB100 is not coupled to variations in the transcription of the gene or to the amount of apoB100 mRNA [18,19]. Rather, this secretion appears to be regulated posttranscriptionally, involving a posttranslational degradation (see for example [10,20,21]). As discussed above, an increased formation of secretable LDL-VLDL is induced when HepG2 cells are incubated with oleic acid. This in turn leads to decreased formation of the apoB100-containing HDL-like particles [10]. Since such particles appear to be degraded in the cell, the oleic acid must stabilize apoB100 and decrease the posttranslational degradation of the protein. In addition, apoB100 that is tightly bound to the ER membrane appears to be a target for degradation [10,21].

In our view apoB100 behaves very much like other secretory proteins or membrane proteins that are regulated posttranslationally, i.e., only the proteins that acquire the correct structure will be allowed to exit from the ER while all other proteins are retained by chaperones and eventually degraded [22]. In the case of apoB100, the protein that is incorporated into the surface of a mature lipoprotein with a diameter of 250 Å or more could be expected to fold correctly. If the particle is too small, as is the case with HDL-

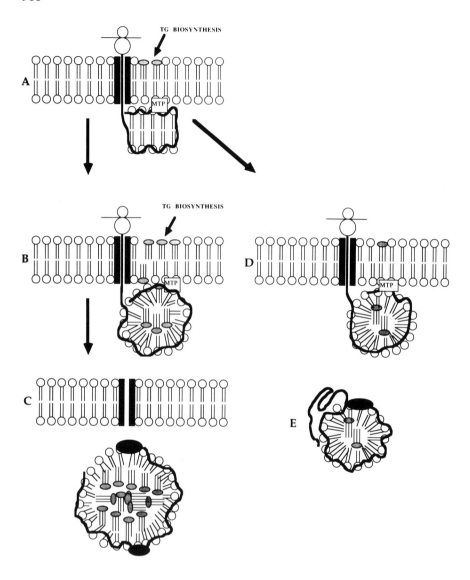

Fig. 1. A schematic representation of the suggested cotranslational route to the formation of the different apoB100-containing lipoproteins identified in the endoplasmic reticulum (ER). During the translation/translocation, apoB100 is lipidated (A). We propose that the microsomal transfer protein (MTP) [27] has a key role in this lipidation, moving phospholipids from the luminal leaflet of the ER membrane to the growing nascent polypetide as it protrudes into the ER lumen. In this way an amphipathic surface is formed that could be the target for an MTP-mediated transfer of triacylglycerol (B). If the size of the assembled particle is large enough (C), apoB100 can fold properly in the lipoprotein surface, allowing the particle to be secreted. If, on the other hand, the assembly product is an HDL-like particle (D and E), apo-B100 cannot fold correctly in the particle surface and the particle will be retained in the cell and eventually degraded.

like particles, it is not likely that apoB100 will find enough room on the surface to acquire its correct structure. This model would imply that a truncated form of apoB100 could be secreted on HDL-like particles; work from our group and others clearly indicates that this is so. Moreover, apoB48 assembles HDL-size particles that can be secreted (see below).

It is also likely that the tertiary structure of apoB100 that is integrated into the ER membrane differs from that of apoB100 that is present in a LDL-VLDL particle.

Results from studies of McA RH 7777 cells

VLDL are assembled in close connection with the translation of apoB100

Pulse-chase studies [23] revealed that VLDL was the first apoB100-containing lipoprotein that could be detected in the lumen of the secretory pathway. Pulse-labeling experiments demonstrated that labeled apoB100 VLDL could be detected as early as 3-min after incubation with [^{35}S]-methionine. This incubation time corresponds to 1/5 of the estimated transit time for a ribosome on the apoB100 mRNA [24]. Together the results demonstrated that the apoB100-containing VLDL are assembled in close connection with the translation of the protein. The close coupling between the assembly and translation processes is also underlined by the observed effects of cycloheximide on the assembly process [23]. Thus the assembly of apoB100 VLDL was acutely and completely blocked by cycloheximide added after the pulse. If, however, a 15-min chase was introduced between the pulse and the incubation with cycloheximide, there was no inhibition of the assembly and secretion of apoB100 VLDL. A 15-min chase allows the apoB100 nascent polypeptides to be elongated to full-length apoB100. The assembly of apoB48-containing VLDL was not influenced by such a chase period between the pulse and the treatment with cycloheximide.

Almost all of the pulse-labeled apoB100-containing lipoproteins disappeared from the secretory pathway during a 180-min chase, while radioactive apoB100 was still present in the ER membrane [23]. Pulse-labeled cells that had been chased for 180 min secreted only traces of apoB100 VLDL during a new chase period of 180 min. If, however, the first chase was carried out in the presence of cycloheximide, i.e., conditions when the elongation of the labeled nascent polypeptides was blocked, substantial amounts of apoB100-containing VLDL were assembled and secreted during the next chase (carried out in the absence of cycloheximide). Again no effects of the cycloheximide were seen on the assembly and secretion of apoB48 VLDL.

We observed the expected increase in the amount of assembled apoB100 VLDL during the first 15-min chase [23]. However, the increase in the amount of apoB100 VLDL continued for 10–15 min after the 15 min needed to complete the nascent polypeptides. This observation indicated that not all apoB100 VLDL could be formed during the elongation of apoB100 nascent chains but that other precursors could be recruited to the assembly process. Examples of such possible precursors are the HDL- and LDL-like particles. A comparison between the kinetics for the turnover of apoB100 in the HDL-LDL particles and for the formation of VLDL could suggest a possible precursor–product relation. Thus, in spite of the rapid assembly of apoB100 VLDL during the leading part of the pulse (see above) the process may in fact involve two or more steps. In order to address this possibility we investigated the assembly of apoB48 VLDL.

Different kinetics for the assembly of apoB48 and apoB100 VLDL

Pulse-labeling and pulse-chase studies [23] clearly indicated that the formation of apoB48 VLDL was slower than that of apoB100 VLDL and that the first apoB48-containing lipoprotein detectable in the secretory pathway was instead an HDL-like particle (referred to as apoB48 HDL). This apoB48 HDL appeared to be assembled cotranslationally.

962

Indeed, our previous results [25] indicate that apoB48 is only able to assemble an HDL-size particle during the translation/translocation. This apoB48 HDL is to a certain extent secreted, particularly if the cells are grown in the absence of oleic acid. Incubation with oleic acid was essential for the assembly of apoB48 VLDL; in the absence of the fatty acid only apoB48 HDL is formed. Pulse-chase studies carried out in the presence of oleic acid showed that the apoB48 HDL-like particle decreases with time while at the same time there was an increase in apoB48 VLDL.

The turnover of the apoB48 HDL in the cell was slower than that of the other apoB-containing particles. Thus, after a 90–120-min chase there were substantial amounts of apoB48-containing HDL left in the microsomal lumen, while almost all other pulse-labeled apoB-containing particles had disappeared. The apoB48-containing HDL-like particle could be converted into apoB48 VLDL; thus, if cells that had been pulse-labeled and then chased for 120–180 min were incubated with oleic acid, most of the apoB48 HDL was converted into apoB48 VLDL and only a small amount was recovered in the HDL density range. In the absence of oleic acid, only small amounts of apoB48 VLDL were formed and the dominating amount of apoB48 secreted from the cells occurred on HDL-like particles. These observations clearly demonstrate that apoB48 VLDL is assembled in at least two steps, i.e., first the formation of the HDL-like particle (a process that probably occurs cotranslationally) and second the conversion of this particle to VLDL (a schematic presentation is given in Fig. 2).

The formation of apoB48 VLDL was inhibited by the addition of cycloheximide late in the assembly process, i.e., during the second step. Thus this "second step" depends on a continuation of protein biosynthesis.

Is the signal for the second step present in apoB48? Implications for the assembly of apoB-containing lipoproteins

The results obtained for the assembly of apoB48-containing VLDL indicate that a

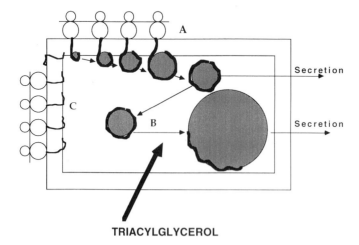

TRIACYLGLYCEROL

Fig. 2. Schematic representation of the assembly of apoB48-containing VLDL in the endoplasmic reticulum (ER). During the translation/translocation of apoB48, an HDL-like lipoprotein particle is assembled (A). This particle is to some degree secreted from the cell. However, it could also, depending on the rate of the biosynthesis of triglyceride, be converted into a VLDL particle in a second assembly step (B). ApoB48 is also bound to the ER membrane (C).

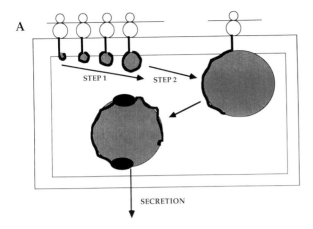

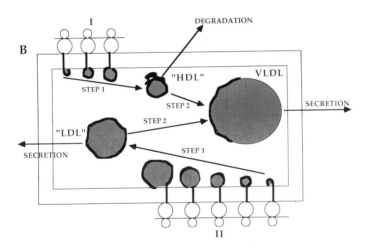

Fig. 3. Possible mechanism for the recruitment of apoB100 for the assembly of VLDL through a two-step model. On the basis of the results from the studies on the assembly of apoB48 VLDL, we propose that the information for the assembly of a triglyceride-rich VLDL particle resides within the apoB48 portion of apoB100. We also propose that this portion of apoB100 must have a correct tertiary structure for secretion. It is possible that three different forms of apoB100 could be used for the assembly process. A: ApoB100 could be recruited during the translation/translocation, provided that the B48 portion has been completed and optimally lipidated. Thus the first step would be the cotranslational formation of an HDL-like particle, containing the apoB48 part of apoB100 [1]. The second step would be an addition of triglycerides to the growing particle, forming the VLDL-size particle. This particle could then acquire the growing apoB100 (which is still attached to the ribosome). B: Another possibility is that the apoB100-containing particles that are released to the secretory pathway could be used as precursors for the formation of VLDL. This involves all particles that contain a correctly folded (lipidated) apoB48 portion of apoB100. This could be the case for both the HDL ("HDL")- and the LDL ("LDL")-like particles that are formed cotranslationally (I and II respectively).

sufficiently lipidated apoB48 HDL could be recognized by a mechanism that in a second step transfers lipids to the particle to form a VLDL particle. Results from electron microscopy [8] suggest the presence of preformed lipid droplets that fuse with apoB in the ER. Such lipid droplets could obviously explain the conversion of the HDL-like particle to a VLDL particle without a significant amount of intermediates (compare the results from the pulse-chase studies). The second step depends on continuing protein biosynthesis, which in turn suggests that this step depends on the expression of gene(s) that could facilitate the addition of the major triglyceride load to the particle. Such genes could be candidate genes for the so-called chylomicron retention disease [26].

The information for the assembly of the triglyceride-rich lipoproteins appears to exist within apoB48, i.e., in the N-terminal half of apoB100. It is possible that the C-terminal half of apoB100 has relatively little to do with this assembly but rather confers other biological activities on the particle, such as binding to the LDL receptor. Thus it is possible, but not certain, that apoB100 could be recruited for the formation of full-size VLDL once an apoB48 portion with the correct tertiary structure has been translocated to the ER lumen. This may occur during the translation/translocation of apoB100 (a schematic presentation is shown in Fig. 3A). It is also possible that the apoB48 portion of apoB100 in the HDL- and LDL-size particles may have the correct structure to interact with the mechanism of the second step. The proposed model takes into account the results from the pulse-chase studies, suggesting that the assembly of apoB100 VLDL continues after the completion of the apoB100 nascent chains. Moreover, a second assembly pathway involving precursor particles in the ER lumen may explain the observation made by other authors that the secretion of apoB100-containing particles could be stimulated after the time needed for the completion of the apoB100 nascent chains (a schematic presentation of the possible second pathway to assemble apoB100 VLDL is seen in Fig. 3B).

It should, however, be pointed out that if there is a second step in the assembly of apoB100, the mechanism behind it is not identical to that for apoB48. The assembly of apoB100 VLDL occurs much faster, and closer to the translation of the protein. Moreover, the second step in the assembly of apoB48 VLDL is inhibited by cycloheximide, which is not so for apoB100.

Acknowledgements

We thank Anita Magnusson for excellent technical assistance. This paper was supported by grant 7142 from the Swedish Medical Research Council, by grants from the Swedish Heart and Lung foundation, the Oleo-Margarine foundation for Nutritional Research, King Gustav V:s Foundation, Novo Nordisk Foundation, Ulf Widenbergs Foundation, the Göteborg Medical Society and AB Hässle.

References

1. Kane JP, Hardman DA, Paulus HE. Proc Natl Acad Sci USA 1980;77:2465–2469.
2. Glickman RM, Rogers M, Glickman JN. Proc Natl Acad Sci USA 1986;83:5296–5300.
3. Sjöberg A, Oscarsson J, Boström K, Innerarity TL, Edén S, Olofsson S-O. Endocrinology 1992;130:3356–3364.
4. Powell LW, Wallis SC, Pearse RJ, Edwards YH, Knott TJ, Scott J. Cell 1987;50:831–840.
5. Lau PP, Xiong W, Zhu H-J, Chen S-H, Chan L. J Biol Chem 1991;266:20550–20554.
6. Chen S-H, Habib G, Yang C-Y, Gu Z-W, Lee BR, Weng S-A, Silberman SR, Cai S-J, Deslypere JP, Rosseneu M, Gotto AM Jr, Li W-H, Chan L. Science 1987;238:363–366.
7. Teng BB, Burant CF, Davidson NO. Science 1993;260:1816–1819.
8. Alexander CA, Hamilton RL, Havel RJ. J Cell Biol 1976;69:241–263.
9. Borén J, Wettesten M, Sjöberg A, Thorlin T, Bondjers G, Wiklund O, Olofsson S-O. J Biol Chem 1990; 265(18):10556–10564.
10. Borén J, Rustaeus S, Wettesten M, Andersson M, Wiklund A, Olofsson S-O. Arterioscler Thromb 1993; 13(12):1743–1754.

11. Davis RA, Thrift RN, Wu CC, Howell KE. J Biol Chem 1990;265:10005–10011.
12. Dixon JL, Chattapadhyay R, Huima T, Redman CM, Banerjee D. J Cell Biol 1992;117:1161–1169.
13. Pease RJ, Harrison GB, Scott J. Nature 1991;353:448–450.
14. Shelness GS, Morris-Rogers KC, Ingram MF. J Biol Chem 1994;269(12):9310–9318.
15. Borén J, Graham L, Wettesten M, Scott J, White A, Olofsson S-O. J Biol Chem 1992;267:9858–9867.
16. Spring DJ, Chen-Liu LW, Chatterton JE, Elovson J, Schumaker VN. J Biol Chem 1992;267:14839–14845.
17. Sakata N, Dixon WX jL, Ginsberg HN. J Biol Chem 1993;268(31):22967–22970.
18. Boström K, Borén J, Wettesten M, Sjöberg A, Bondjers G, Wiklund O, Carlsson P, Olofsson S-O. J Biol Chem 1988;263(9):4434–4442.
19. Pullinger CR, North JD, Teng B-B, Rifici VA, Ronhild de Brito AE, Scott J. J Lipid Res 1989;30:1065–1077.
20. Dixon JL, Furukawa S, Ginsberg HN. J Biol Chem 1991;266:5080–5086.
21. Thrift RN, Drisko J, Dueland S, Trawick JD, Davis RA. Proc Natl Acad Sci USA 1992;89:9161–9165.
22. Helenius A, Marquardt T, Braakman I. Trends Cell Biol 1992;2:227–231.
23. Borén J, Rustaeus S, Olofsson S-O. J Biol Chem 1994 (in press).
24. Boström K, Wettesten M, Borén J, Bondjers G, Wiklund O, Olofsson S-O. J Biol Chem 1986;261(29): 13800–13806.
25. Borén J, White A, Wettesten M, Scott J, Graham L, Olofsson S-O. Prog Lipid Res 1991;30:205–218.
26. Levy E, Marcel Y, Deckelbaum RJ, Milne R, Lepage G, Seidman E, Bendayan M, Roy CC. J Lipid Res 1987;28:1263–1274.
27. Wetterau JR, Aggerbeck LP, Bouma M-E, Eisenberg C, Munck A, Hermier M, Schmitz GG, Rader DJ, Gregg RE. Nature 1992;258:999–1001.

HyperapoB — an update

Peter O. Kwiterovich Jr. and Mahnaz Motevalli

Departments of Pediatrics and Medicine, Johns Hopkins University Medical School, Baltimore, Maryland, USA

Hyperapobetalipoproteinemia, or hyperapoB, a disorder common in coronary artery disease (CAD), is characterized by an increased number of small, dense low density lipoprotein (LDL) particles; the plasma triglyceride (TG) level is normal or elevated [1]. Small, dense LDL particles are also present in those with familial combined hyperlipidemia (FCHL), LDL subclass pattern B, familial dyslipidemic hypertension, and syndrome X [1]. The small, dense LDL syndromes cluster in families with premature CAD, are probably inherited as an autosomal dominant, and are genetically heterogeneous [1].

Two metabolic defects have been described in hyperapoB patients (Fig. 1). First, there is an overproduction of VLDL apoB in liver, which leads to overproduction of LDL apoB [1]. Small, dense LDL may result from increased transfer of core TG from VLDL to LDL in exchange for cholesteryl ester. The TG in the cholesteryl ester-depleted LDL is hydrolyzed by lipoprotein lipase (LPL), producing a small, dense LDL particle. Both in vivo and in vitro studies indicate that LDL-receptor activity is normal in hyperapoB [1]; however, the affinity of small, dense LDL particles for the LDL receptor is decreased [2]. Small, dense LDL may be more susceptible to oxidation, perhaps because of depletion of fat-soluble antioxidants in its core [1].

The second metabolic abnormality in hyperapoB concerns the abnormal clearance of postprandial TG-enriched lipoproteins (Fig. 1). This defect may involve LPL [3]; or the faulty transfer of its cofactor apoC-II from HDL to chylomicrons, perhaps due to an abnormal apoA-IV [4]; or the antipolytic effects of an increased level of apoC-III [4]; finally, as shown by Sniderman and colleagues [5], the uptake by adipocytes of free fatty acids (FFA) derived from the hydrolysis of TG may be decreased in hyperapoB, because of a deficiency in the cell's response to the stimulation of intracellular TG synthesis by the acylation stimulatory protein (ASP) [6], also called basic protein I or BP I [7]. If the rate of FFA uptake into adipose tissue is reduced, this may result in an increased flux of FFA to liver, leading to increased hepatic VLDL apoB overproduction (Fig. 1). Another serum basic protein, BP II, abnormally stimulates cholesteryl ester production in hyperapoB cells [7]. Its role in the pathogenesis of hyperapoB is unresolved. These basic proteins appear to mediate their effect through a high-affinity, receptor-mediated mechanism [7,8].

Nine candidate genes have been proposed for the small, dense LDL syndromes [1]. These include APOB, transDNA binding protein for APOB, LPL gene, APOC-III, APOA-IV, ATHS on chromosome 19, insulin-receptor gene, the genes for serum basic proteins and their putative "basic protein receptor". Recent evidence indicates that the APOB gene [1] and the LPL gene [3] are not common causes of hyperapoB and FCHL, although the APOB gene may be involved in some families [9]. Recent evidence indicates that an apoD DNA polymorphism is significantly associated with three components of syndrome X,

Address for correspondence: Lipid Research Atherosclerosis Unit, Departments of Pediatrics and Medicine, Johns Hopkins University Medical School, 600 N. Wolfe Street/CMSC 604, Baltimore, MD 21287-3654, USA.

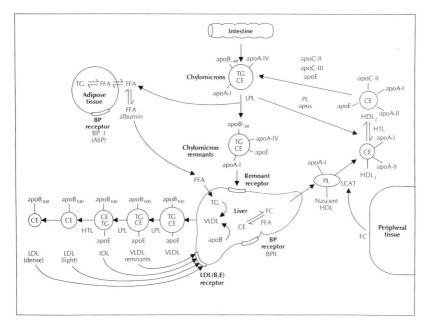

Fig. 1. Schematic diagram of hypothetical pathways that may be involved in the pathogenesis of hyperapoB and FCHL. TG — triglyceride; FFA — free fatty acids; CE — cholesteryl esters; PL — phospholipids; LPL — lipoprotein lipase; LCAT — lecithin:cholesterol acyl transferase; HTL — hepatic triglyceride lipase; BP — serum basic proteins; ASP — acylation stimulatory protein. Reproduced with permission [1].

hyperinsulinism, obesity and non-insulin-dependent diabetes [10]. This update focuses upon studies related to BP I (or ASP), BP II and their postulated receptor(s) (Fig. 1).

Two possible general mechanisms for the effect of the serum basic proteins will be discussed. The first general hypothesis is related to the high-affinity binding, internalization and intracellular transport of the basic proteins to microsomes, where they may act as a direct cofactor for an enzyme. The second general hypothesis concerns the high-affinity binding of the basic proteins resulting in intracellular effects via second-messenger pathways.

Direct intracellular effects of basic proteins

In Fig. 2, we have schematically summarized the effect of ASP on triglyceride synthesis and glucose transport, on the basis of a series of important papers published by Dr Sniderman and colleagues from Montreal. First, Cianflone and co-workers [11] showed that ^{125}I-ASP bound with high affinity to normal cultured fibroblasts, that the stimulation of TG synthesis was proportional to the degree of binding, and that this process was defective in hyperapoB fibroblasts.

Yasruel and co-workers [12] examined the effect of ASP on adipose tissue microsomal enzymes of the TG synthetic pathway (Fig. 2). They found that ASP did not stimulate acyl CoA synthetase. However, ASP significantly stimulated the activities of GPAT (by 30%) and DGAT (by 90%) [12] (Fig. 2). No significant effect of ASP on the hydrolysis of phosphatide by PAPH was found. ASP increased the V_{max} but not the K_m of GPAT and DGAT, which indicates that ASP was primarily having a direct effect on enzyme activity rather than increasing delivery of substrate.

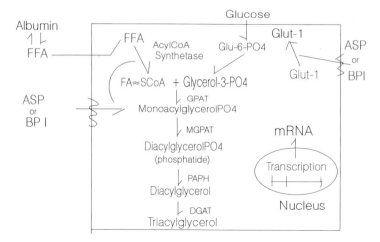

Fig. 2. Effect of ASP on TG synthesis and glucose transport.

Germanario and co-workers [13] subsequently examined the effect of ASP on both fatty acid transport (Fig. 2, upper left corner) and glucose transport (Fig. 2, upper right corner). There was no direct effect of ASP on FFA transport across the cell membrane. Using either 2-deoxyglycose or 3-O-methyglucose in cultured fibroblasts, ASP about doubled hexose transport, an effect that was time- and concentration-dependent; this effect of ASP appeared to be carrier-mediated, since it was blocked by cytochalasin. The increase in V_{max}, with no change in K_m, further suggested that ASP might increase a sugar transporter, a tenet that was supported by an increase in the glucose transporter, Glut1, from the intracellular membranes to the plasma membrane (Fig. 2).

More recently, evidence has been presented by Baldo and co-workers [14] that ASP is homologous to C_{3a} desarg, a basic protein generated from three components of complement: B, C_3 and D (adipsin). In Fig. 3, we have summarized schematically the adipsin–ASP system in adipocytes, based on the work of Cianflone and co-workers [15], reviewed in detail elsewhere in this symposium. Differentiated adipocytes process messenger RNA for three complement factors, C_3, B, and D (adipsin). Adipsin, a

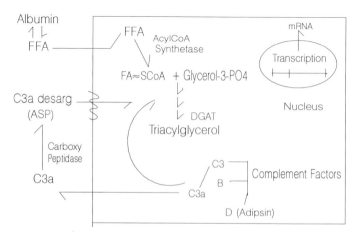

Fig. 3. Adipsin–ASP system in adipocyte.

proteolytic enzyme, generates C_{3a} from C_3 (Fig. 3). C_{3a} may have a direct intracellular effect on TG synthesis. However, as the TG content of adipocytes increases, enhanced secretion of C_{3a} into the medium occurs. After C_{3a} is released from a cell, a carboxypeptidase may generate C_{3a} desarg (or ASP) which then binds to the surface of the adipocyte and has its intracellular effect (Fig. 3). Such stimulation by ASP of TG synthesis may facilitate the clearance of postprandial FFA.

Indirect effects of basic proteins via signal transduction

In normal fibroblasts, BP I doubled the mean mass of triglycerides, whereas there was significantly less stimulation in hyperapoB cells [16]. The increase in the mass of cell cholesteryl esters seen in normal cells with BP I was also significantly reduced in hyperapoB cells [16]. In contrast, BP II abnormally stimulated the mass of cell cholesteryl esters 6-fold in hyperapoB cells [16]. To address whether these effects of BP I and BP II may be mediated by second messengers, we performed a series of experiments that are depicted in Fig. 4 for BP I, and in Fig. 5 for BP II.

BP I (or ASP) may bind to a transmembrane receptor containing tyrosine-kinase catalytic domains (here depicted as boxes) (Fig. 4). Such high-affinity interaction phosphorylates the receptor which in turn phosphorylates a variety of proteins, including PLC (or phospholipase C) γ, an enzyme associated with transmembrane tyrosine-kinase receptors [17]. Activation of PLC γ initiates the hydrolysis of PIP_2, producing IP_3 and diacylglycerol (DG) (Fig. 4). DG activates PKC (protein kinase C). Either PKC, or the transmembrane tyrosine-kinase receptor, may phosphorylate proteins that have enzymatic activity.

Transcription factors may also be phosphorylated by the tyrosine-kinase receptor, leading to enhanced transcription of messenger RNA. For example, this might lead to an increase in DGAT mRNA. Dephosphorylation can also result from this cascade, activating DGAT.

In Fig. 5, the possible effects of BP II on cholesterol metabolism via second messenger pathways are depicted. We again hypothesized pleiotrophic effects of a transmembrane tyrosine-kinase receptor, including the phosphorylation and dephosphorylation of a family of proteins. This process may effect the production of cholesterol through HMG-CoA reductase, the esterification of cholesterol by ACAT, or the hydrolysis of esterified

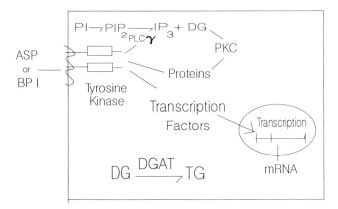

Fig. 4. Role of basic proteins in second-messenger pathways.

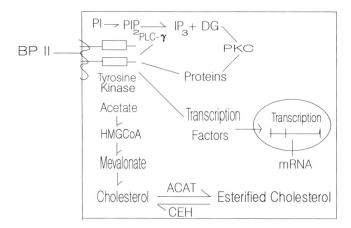

Fig. 5. Role of basic proteins in second-messenger pathways.

cholesterol by CEH. As a result of this cascade, BP II may also affect the mRNAs for these enzymes of cholesterol metabolism.

Effect of inhibition of PKC. The effects of both BP I on TG synthesis and BP II on cholesterol esterification were blocked by H-7 (1-C5-isoquinoline-sulfonyl)-2-methyl piperozine dihydrochloride), an inhibitor of PKC, in a concentration-dependent fashion, in both normal and hyperapoB fibroblasts [16].

Effect of stimulation of PKC. We next stimulated PKC, using C:8, an analogue of diacylglycerol which activates PKC (Fig. 4). When normal fibroblasts were incubated in F-12 medium without basic proteins, C:8 stimulated TG production about 5-fold over baseline; BP I doubled this effect in both control and C:8-treated normal cells [16]. In the hyperapoB cells, the addition of C:8 to F-12 medium alone stimulated TG formation 7-fold; when BP I was added to C:8 in the hyperapoB cells, there was much less additional stimulatory effect of BP I than occurred in normal cells [16]. These data suggested that the intracellular component of the phosphatidylinositol pathway is normal in hyperapoB cells, and that the cellular defect resides in a deficient response to BP I.

In normal cells, BP II stimulated the formation of esterified cholesterol only a small amount and the addition of C:8 to medium containing either F-12 or BP II did not stimulate cholesteryl ester formation [16]. In hyperapoB cells, the greater than normal stimulation of cholesteryl ester formation by BP II was markedly accentuated by C:8, suggesting that the abnormal response of hyperapoB cells to BP II may be modulated by this pathway.

Effect of inhibition of tyrosine kinase. Genistein, a highly specific inhibitor of protein tyrosine kinase [18], was used to determine if the effects of BP I and BP II were mediated through tyrosine phosphorylation, and if there was a deficiency in such a process in hyperapoB fibroblasts. The effect of genistein was time- (6 h max) and concentration-dependent (25 µg/ml medium, nadir) [19]. Genistein inhibited significantly the effect of BP I on the mass of TG in normal cells, but not in hyperapoB cells [19]. BP II abnormally stimulated cholesterol production in hyperapoB cells, an effect that was inhibited by genistein [19]. In distinct contrast, genistein + BP II markedly stimulated the mass of cholesteryl esters in normal cells, but inhibited it in hyperapoB cells. This "crossover" effect of genistein + BP II produced about a 30-fold difference in mass of cholesteryl esters between normal and hyperapoB cells. Tyrosine kinase phosphorylation mediates the effect of BP I and BP II in normal cells, and appears deficient in hyperapoB cells.

Summary

The basic proteins modulate both intracellular triglyceride and cholesterol metabolism. These effects appear to involve a high-affinity, receptor-mediated mechanism, resulting in either a direct effect of the basic proteins on intracellular enzymes, or an indirect effect through signal transduction. HyperapoB cells manifest a defect in this pathway; the precise molecular defects remain to be elucidated.

Acknowledgements

This work was supported by the following grants from the National Institutes of Health 1 P50 HL47212-03 (Specialized Center of Research in Arteriosclerosis), HL31497, National Institutes of Health, 1 R01 DH3219301, General Clinical Research Center Program, RR-52, RR-35 and CLINFO. We thank Pauline Gugliotta for preparation of this manuscript.

References

1. Kwiterovich PO Jr. Curr Opin Lipidol 1993;4:133—143.
2. Galeano NR, Miles R, Marcell YL et al. J Biol Chem 1994;269:511—519.
3. Nevin DN, Brunzell TD, Deeb SS. Arterioscler Thromb 1994;14:869—873.
4. Wojciechowski AP, Farrall M, Cullen P et al. Nature 1991;349:161—164.
5. Sniderman AD, Brown, Stewart FF et al. Curr Opin Lipidol 1992;3:137—142.
6. Cianflone KM, Sniderman AD, Walsh MJ et al. J Biol Chem 1989;264:426—430.
7. Kwiterovich PO Jr, Motevalli M, Miller M. Proc Natl Acad Sci USA 1990;87:8980—8984.
8. Kwiterovich PO Jr, Motevalli M, Miller M et al. Clin Chem 1991;37(3):317—326.
9. Laing AE, Amos Ci, DeMeester C et al. Genet Epid 1994;11:29—49.
10. Vijayarajhvan S, Hitman GA, and Kopelman PG. J Clin Endocrin Metabol 1994;79:568—570.
11. Cianflone KM, Maslowska MH, Sniderman AD. J Clin Invest 1990;85:722—730.
12. Yasruel Z, Cianflone K, Sniderman A et al. Lipids 1991;26:495—499.
13. Germinario R, Sniderman AD, Manuel S et al. Metabolism 1993;40:574—580.
14. Baldo A, Sniderman AD, St-Luce S et al. J Clin Invest 1993;92:1543—1547.
15. Cianflone K, Roncari DAK Maslowska M et al. Biochemistry 1994;33:9489—9495.
16. Kwiterovich PO Jr, Motevalli M, Miller M. Arterioscler Thromb 1994;14:1—7.
17. Bolen JB. Oncogene 1993;8:2025—2031.
18. Yarden Y. Ann Rev Biochem 1988;57:443—477.
19. Kwiterovich PO and Motevalli M. Inhibition of tyrosine kinase phosphorylation differentially alters the effects of serum basic proteins in normal and hyperapoB fibroblasts. Circulation 1994; (abstr) (in press).

The adipsin–Acylation Stimulating Protein pathway and hyperapobetalipoproteinemia

Katherine Cianflone

McGill Unit for the Prevention of Cardiovascular Disease, McGill University, Montreal, Canada

Abstract. HyperapoB (hyperapobetalipoproteinemia) is common among patients with premature coronary artery disease and is characterized by an increased number of LDL particles in plasma [1]. This increase in LDL, easily measured through determination of plasma apoB100, is due to an increased hepatic secretion of apoB-containing lipoproteins [2]. What causes this increased secretion? Our results, and those of others, in in vitro human cell systems, have shown that an increased substrate load to the hepatocytes results in increased apoB lipoprotein secretion [3,4]. Our central hypothesis in hyperapoB is that an increased substrate load to the liver has a direct effect on the secretion of apoB-containing lipoproteins, and that this increased flux is a direct consequence of reduced adipose tissue efficiency of fatty-acid uptake and storage [5]. The adipsin-Acylation Stimulating Protein pathway is a recently described pathway which plays a role in regulation of adipose tissue triglyceride synthesis, and dysfunction of this pathway appears to be involved in the pathogenesis of hyperapoB [6].

Hepatic substrate response and hyperapoB

HyperapoB is that group of dyslipoproteinemias characterized by overproduction of hepatic apoB100 lipoproteins. This overproduction leads to an increased LDL particle number in plasma, the common theme being an elevated plasma apoB. The lipid phenotype is variable, not only from one individual to the next, but from time to time in the same individual. There are probably several reasons for the overproduction of hepatic B100 lipoproteins, but we have focused on one possible explanation: namely, that the increased secretion of these lipoproteins is a response to increased lipid (fatty acid and cholesterol) flux into the liver [5]. A number of in vitro studies have demonstrated in HepG2 cells that an increased flux of fatty acids or cholesterol, either in free or lipoprotein form, results in increased apoB100 secretion by these cells [3,7–11]. In contrast, an increased flux of carbohydrate in the form of glucose causes increased triglyceride secretion from the cells, but does not affect apoB100 secretion [12]. This fits well with the results of in vivo studies in humans which have shown that carbohydrate feeding in normals [13] or familial hypertriglyceridemia is characterized by increased hepatic triglyceride secretion, but not increased secretion of apoB100.

Although it has not been directly demonstrated that increased fatty acid or cholesterol flux to the liver causes increased apoB100 hepatic production, there are a number of lines of evidence to support this in vivo. We have shown in patients with hyperapoB a greater postprandial increase in fatty-acid levels than in normals [14]. Moreover, Cabezas et al. have demonstrated [15] that patients with hyperapoB have a marked and sustained postprandial elevation of free fatty acids and increased numbers of triglyceride-enriched remnant particles. Patsch showed that circulating fatty-acid levels correlate with LDL levels [16]. Similarly, the correlation of LDL-cholesterol to preheparin lipoprotein lipase [17] suggests that displacement of active lipoprotein lipase from endothelial binding sites may mark triglyceride-rich lipoproteins or their remnants for metabolic pathways that lead to LDL. This is also supported by recent studies that show a correlation between postprandial lipoprotein lipase levels and diet-generated plasma FFA levels [18].

Free fatty acids and lipoprotein lipase

Why are there increased free fatty acid levels? The consensus has been that triglyceride synthesis in adipose tissue is not rate-limiting but acts as an endless free fatty acid acceptor and that the plasma enzyme lipoprotein lipase responsible for generation of free fatty acid is the rate-limiting step. But is this consensus correct? Olivecrona has reviewed the evidence relating triglyceride clearance to lipoprotein lipase, the step that has been thought to be rate-limiting, and shown that the correlation is poor [19,20]. Moreover, the correlation between local lipoprotein lipase activity and corresponding triglyceride synthesis in different adipose tissue sites is also poor [21,22]. It appears, therefore, that the amount of lipoprotein lipase present is well in excess of normal requirements [19]. Taken together, these data suggest that tissue uptake of free fatty acid is a key step and that failure of free fatty acid uptake to proceed at the necessary rate will result in secondary inhibition of lipoprotein lipase activity in a number of ways. Saxena and Goldberg have demonstrated that free fatty acids can cause lipoprotein lipase to detach from its endothelial cell attachment site [23]. Free fatty acids also cause product inhibition of lipoprotein lipase and displace the cofactor apoC-II needed for effective catalytic action. In vivo, fatty acid infusion results in release of lipoprotein lipase into the circulation both in the free form and attached to lipoproteins. As lipoprotein lipase is normally cleared from the liver, uptake of the lipoprotein lipase attached to a triglyceride-rich particle through the LRP receptor or other receptor mechanism may even enhance substrate delivery to the liver. In this way, hyperapoB may be associated with a decreased activity of lipoprotein lipase, without there being any specific gene defect in lipoprotein lipase itself.

HyperapoB, postprandial triglyceride clearance and adipose tissue triglyceride synthesis

We have examined postprandial triglyceride clearance and adipose tissue triglyceride synthesis in hyperapoB subjects [14], in whom there was a marked delay in postprandial clearance of triglyceride and remnants, this delay being associated with reduced HDL2. Cabezas and colleagues have also demonstrated a delayed clearance of triglyceride and remnants postprandially in hyperapoB subjects [15]. It is unlikely that this is due to a limitation of the enzyme lipoprotein lipase, as in both cases plasma free fatty acid levels rose markedly and were much higher than those in control patients.

However, reduced efficiency of adipose tissue fatty acid uptake and triglyceride synthesis could explain these results. Studies by Walldius [24,25] and Teng [26] have demonstrated that FFA incorporation into adipose tissue does, in fact, vary and Teng et al. have shown that patients with hyperapoB incorporate fatty acids into adipose tissue triglyceride more slowly [26]. To examine this directly, using human skin fibroblasts as a cell model of peripheral tissue, we studied triglyceride synthesis in hyperapoB vs. normolipidemic subjects. Our initial studies showed no difference in triglyceride synthesis between normal and hyperapoB cells cultured in a serum-free medium, but when the cells were supplemented with a lipoprotein-deficient human serum, the normal cells had a markedly higher capacity for triglyceride synthesis [27]. On the basis of these results, we postulated the existence of a serum protein which stimulated triglyceride synthesis and to which the hyperapoB cells were not responding. We then set out to purify this protein.

Regulation of triglyceride synthesis in adipose tissue

Although the individual enzymatic steps involved in synthesizing a triglyceride molecule have been identified for some time, none of these enzymes has been isolated or cloned, and the regulation of triglyceride synthesis has yet to be described at a molecular level. Until recently there was little evidence to suggest a regulator of this pathway in adipocytes other than insulin. Although insulin does influence triglyceride synthesis, by far its greatest effects are to increase glucose transport and inhibit lipolysis rather than on FFA esterification. ASP (Acylation Stimulating Protein) is a small basic protein that has now been isolated from human plasma. ASP has been shown to stimulate triglyceride synthesis in human skin fibroblasts [28], a finding which has been confirmed independently by other investigators [29]. Experiments on primary isolated subcutaneous adipocytes from obese subjects have shown that ASP also stimulates fatty acid incorporation and esterification in adipocytes [30]. In fact, this stimulation is much greater than that seen in fibroblasts (on average a 5-fold increase in adipocytes vs. a 2- to 3-fold increase in fibroblasts).

Acylation stimulating protein

We have recently shown that ASP is identical to C3adesArg, a biologic fragment of human complement factor C3 [31]. C3a is generated through the proximal step of the alternative complement pathway by the initiating action of the specific serine-protease enzyme complement factor D [32]. Reconstitution experiments with complement factors B, C3 and D (the components necessary to generate ASP), incubated under the appropriate conditions, produce C3a and stimulate triglyceride synthesis, confirming the identity of ASP and C3a. A series of studies by Spiegelman and his colleagues are also relevant in this regard [33–36]. They first demonstrated that murine 3T3 adipocytes, on differentiation, express large amounts of a message for a protein which they named adipsin which had considerable homology to human factor D [33]. They subsequently showed that human adipsin was identical with human factor D and that it was predominantly expressed in human fat tissue [35]. Building on and extending this work, we have shown that human adipocytes are competent to produce ASP in their microenvironment, and respond appropriately to stimulation by ASP [37]. In fact, we have shown that human adipocytes demonstrate the capacity to synthesize and secrete the three proteins necessary to generate C3a: adipsin, factor B and factor C3 [37], and that this is a differentiation-dependent process (unpublished observations). It should be noted that human C3adesArg has no previously characterized functional activity in the complement pathway, and no human cell receptor has as yet been identified or characterized. ASP, therefore, appears to be the final effector molecule generated by a novel regulatory system which modulates the rate of triglyceride synthesis in adipocytes.

How does ASP increase triglyceride synthesis? Studies with Dr. R. Germinario have shown that ASP increases triglyceride synthesis through a coordinate effect on both the V_{max} for the enzymes of triglycerol synthesis and through an increase in the V_{max} of glucose transport [38]. That is, ASP does not increase substrate delivery (K_m) but increases the enzymatic rate of these two processes. The increase in glucose transport is achieved through translocation of intracellular glucose transporters to the plasma membrane, in a manner similar to insulin, but additive to insulin. ASP appears to achieve these effects through cellular interaction and generation of a second-messenger signal, probably mediated through a protein kinase C pathway (unpublished observations).

Taken together, these results suggest that the rate at which triacylglycerols are cleared from plasma depends not only on the activity of lipoprotein lipase but also on the rate of fatty acid uptake and esterification in key peripheral tissues such as adipose tissue. With respect to hyperapoB, in contrast to the normal triglyceride-stimulating response of human skin fibroblasts to ASP, human skin fibroblasts from patients with hyperapoB showed a lower response to ASP for both triglyceride synthesis [39] and glucose transport (K. Cianflone, R. Germinario, unpublished observations) and this appears to be related to the number of binding sites on the plasma membrane. This reduced response to ASP in hyperapoB may help to explain the lower rate of synthesis of triacylglycerol in their adipose tissue and the delayed clearance of postprandial triglyceride in these subjects.

References

1. Teng B, Thompson GR, Sniderman AD, Forte TM, Krauss RM, Kwiterovich PO Jr. Proc Natl Acad Sci USA 1983;80(21):6662−6666.
2. Teng B, Sniderman AD, Soutar AK, Thompson GR. J Clin Invest 1986;77(3):663−672.
3. Cianflone K, Yasruel Z, Rodriguez MA, Vas D, Sniderman AD. J Lipid Res 1990;31(11):2045−2055.
4. Sniderman AD, Cianflone K. Arterioscler Thromb 1993;13(5):629−636.
5. Sniderman AD, Brown BG, Stewart FF, Cianflone K. Curr Opin Lipid 1992;3(2):137−142.
6. Sniderman AD, Baldo A, Cianflone K. Curr Opin Lipid 1992;3(3):202−207.
7. Pullinger CR, North JD, Teng B, Rifici VA, Ronhild de Brito AE, Scott J. J Lipid Res 1989;30:1065−1077.
8. Moberly JA, Cole TG, Alpers DH, Schonfeld G. Biochim Biophys Acta 1990;1042:70−80.
9. Fuki IV, Preobrazhensky SN, Misharin AY, Bushmakina NG, Menschikov GB, Repin VS, Karpov RS. Biochim Biophys Acta 1989;1001:235−238.
10. Kosykh VA, Preobrazhensky SN, Fuki IV, Zaikina OE, Tsibulsky VP, Repin VS, Smirnov VN. Biochim Biophys Acta 1985;836:385−389.
11. Dashti N. J Biol Chem 1992;267:7160−7169.
12. Cianflone K, Dahan S, Monge JC, Sniderman AD. Arterioscler Thromb 1992;12(3):271−277.
13. Abbott WGH, Swinburn B, Routolo G, Hara H, Patti L, Harper I, Grundy SM, Howard BV. J Clin Invest 1990;86:642−650.
14. Genest J, Sniderman AD, Cianflone K, Teng B, Wacholder S, Marcel YL, Kwiterovich PO Jr. Arteriosclerosis 1986;6(3):297−304.
15. Cabezas CM, de Bruin TWA, de Valk HW, Shouldus CC, Jansen H, Erkelens DW. J Clin Invest 1993;92:160−168.
16. Patsch JR, Miesenbock G, Hopferwieser T, Muhlberger V, Knapp E, Dunn JK, Gotto AM Jr, Patsch W. Arterioscler Thromb 1992;12:1336−1345.
17. Glaser DS, Yost TJ, Eckel RH. J Lipid Res 1992;33(2):209−214.
18. Karpe F, Olivecrona T, Walldius G, Hamsten A. J Lipid Res 1992;33:975−984.
19. Olivecrona T, Bengtsson-Olivecrona G. Curr Opin Lipidol 1990;1:222−230.
20. Peterson J, Bihain BE, Bengtsson-Olivecrona G, Deckelbaum RJ, Carpenter YA, Olivecrona T. Proc Natl Acad Sci USA 1990;87:909−913.
21. Marin P, Rebuffé-Scrive M, Bjorntorp P. Eur J Clin Invest 1990;20:158−165.
22. Julius U, Leonhardt W, Noack D, Schulze J, Nikulcheva NG, Jaross W, Hanefeld M. Exp Clin Endocrinol 1989;94:187−193.
23. Saxena U, Witte LD, Goldberg IJ. J Lipid Res 1992;33:975−984.
24. Walldius G, Rubba P. Scand J Clin Lab Invest 1976;36:357-369.
25. Carlson LA, Walldius G. Eur J Clin Invest 1976;6(3):195−211.
26. Teng B, Forse A, Rodriguez MA, Sniderman AD. Can J Physiol Pharmacol 1988;66:239−242.
27. Cianflone K, Rodriguez MA, Walsh M, Vu H, Sniderman AD. Clin Invest Med 1988;11(2):99−107.
28. Cianflone K, Sniderman AD, Walsh MJ, Vu H, Gagnon J, Rodriguez MA. J Biol Chem 1989;264:426−430.
29. Kwiterovich PO Jr, Motevalli M, Miller M. Proc Natl Acad Sci USA 1990;87:8980−8984.
30. Walsh MJ, Sniderman AD, Cianflone K, Vu H, Rodriguez MA, Forse RA. J Surg Res 1989;46:470−473.
31. Baldo A, Sniderman AD, St-Luce S, Kohen R, Maslowska M, Hoang B, Monge JC, Bell A, Mulay S, Cianflone K. J Clin Invest 1993;92(3):1543−1557.
32. Schreiber RD, Muller-Eberhard HJ. J Exp Med 1978;148:1722−1727.
33. Cook KS, Min HY, Johnson D, Chaplinsky RJ, Fler JS, Hunt CR, Spiegelman BM. Science 1987;237:402−405.

34. Cook KS, Groves GL, Min HY, Spiegelman BM. Proc Natl Acad Sci USA 1985;82:6480–6484.
35. White RT, Damm D, Hancock N, Rosen BS, Lowell BB, Usher P, Flier JS, Spiegelman BM. J Biol Chem 1992;267:9210–9213.
36. Choy LN, Rosen BS, Spiegelman BM. J Biol Chem 1992;267:12736–12741.
37. Cianflone K, Roncari DAK, Maslowska M, Baldo A, Forden J, Sniderman AD. Biochemistry 1994; (accepted).
38. Germinario R, Sniderman AD, Manuel S, Pratt S, Baldo A, Cianflone K. Metabolism 1993;42(5):574–580.
39. Cianflone K, Maslowska M, Sniderman AD. J Clin Invest 1990;85:722–730.

977

LDL subfractions: properties and functions

M.J. Chapman[1], S. Lund-Katz[2], M.C. Phillips[2], R. Prassl[3], P Laggner[3], C. Flament[1], S. Goulinet[1], F. Nigon[1], M. Rouis[1], P.M. Laplaud[1], M. Guérin[1], E. Bruckert[1] and P.J. Dolphin[4]

[1]*INSERM Unit 321 and Service d'Endocrinologie-Métabolisme, Hôpital de la Pitié, Paris, France;* [2]*Biochemistry Department, Medical College of Pennsylvania, Philadelphia, PA, USA;* [3]*Institute of Biophysics, Austrian Academy of Sciences, Graz, Austria; and* [4]*Dalhousie University, Halifax, Canada*

Elevated circulating levels of low-density lipoproteins (LDL) have long been linked to the premature development of atherosclerotic disease. It is only recently, however, that the relationship of the qualitative features of LDL particles to coronary artery disease has attracted considerable interest [1].

LDL particles are markedly heterogeneous in their physical and chemical properties, which include particle size, buoyant density, chemical composition (lipid subclasses and apoproteins), surface electrical charge and hydrodynamic behavior [2]. Indeed, several subpopulations of LDL particles have been identified on the basis of their hydrated density by isopycnic density gradient ultracentrifugation and on the basis of particle size by electrophoresis in nondenaturing polyacrylamide gradient gels [2,3]. Major questions remain, however, regarding several aspects not only of the structural variations between distinct LDL subpopulations, but also concerning the biological functions of individual particle subspecies. In an attempt to shed further light on the structural and metabolic heterogeneity of LDL particles, we have developed an ultracentrifugal density gradient methodology which allows reproducible differentiation of up to 15 LDL subspecies, whose hydrated densities differ by increments of only ~0.003 g/ml or less. While the overall decrement in particle diameter from the lightest (d 1.02–1.03) to the densest (d 1.04–1.06) LDL subspecies in normolipidemic subjects is only of the order of 1 nm, the volume of light LDL is some 12% greater than that of dense LDL (Fig. 1); in addition, each light LDL particle contains some 30% more cholesterol molecules (in free and esterified form) than dense LDL. All LDL particles contain a single copy of apoB100 [2]. When considered together, the size and compositional properties of LDL subspecies are reflected in marked differences in particle molecular weights; light LDL are of the order of 3×10^6, while those of dense LDL are some 23% less (~2.3×10^6) [2]. How then are such distinct physicochemical properties reflected in the functions of LDL?

The major cellular pathway for tissue catabolism of LDL particles is that of the LDL receptor [4]. We therefore evaluated whether discrete LDL subspecies from normolipidemic subjects might differ in their binding affinities and rates of degradation by the cellular LDL-receptor pathway. We used a homologous system of human U.937 monocyte-like cells, which express large numbers of LDL receptors. Both direct binding and displacement studies showed LDL of intermediate density (d 1.030–1.036 g/ml) to display the highest binding affinity (K_d ~5 mM) and degradation rates [5]. By contrast, dense LDL were of lowest affinity (K_d ~7 nM) and were degraded at rates some 60% lower than the intermediate subspecies. Light LDL displayed binding affinities and degradation rates which were intermediary between those of intermediate and dense subspecies [5].

These investigations led us to propose that the conformation of apoB100 for LDL-receptor recognition and binding is optimal in LDL of intermediate density (d 1.03–1.036

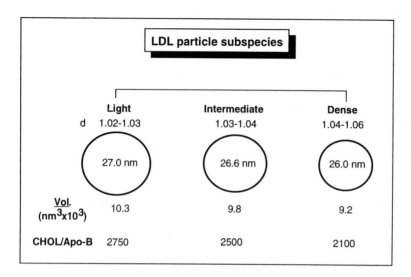

Fig. 1. Major physicochemical characteristics of the three principal subpopulations of LDL particles in normolipidemic subjects. CHOL : no. of cholesterol molecules (in free and esterified forms) per particle.

g/ml). To evaluate this hypothesis, we employed ^{13}C-nuclear magnetic resonance (NMR) spectroscopy and ^{13}C-isotope enrichment to compare the microenvironments of lysine residues in surface-exposed domains of apoB100 in discrete LDL subspecies [6]. The proportions of active (pK 8.9) and normal (pK 10.5) lysines in apoB100 of light, intermediate and dense LDL particles were compared to those in a mixture of total LDL (d 1.019–1.063 g/ml) as a reference. As shown in Table 1, the number of active (pK 8.9) lysine residues in apoB of intermediate density LDL was maximal, and distinct from those of LDL subspecies of lower and of higher density, in which lower numbers of active lysines were detected despite the higher overall degree of ^{13}C-labeling. Comparison of apoB100 conformation in individual subspecies by circular dichroism showed that the α-helical content (~40%) was the same, within experimental error, in all subclasses (S. Lund-Katz, M.C. Phillips and M.J. Chapman, unpublished studies). These findings therefore support the hypothesis that while the overall conformation of apoB100 may be indistinguishable in discrete LDL subspecies, differences in protein domains and conformation may be detected at the level of local microenvironments. Since active (pK 8.9) lysine residues are thought to be particularly involved in the apoB100–LDL receptor interaction

Table 1. Content of normal and active lysine in apoB of LDL and its subspecies isolated by density gradient ultracentrifugation

LDL fraction	% lysine ^{13}C-labeled	No. ^{13}C-labeled lysine residues[a]	
		Active (pK 8.9)	Normal (pK 10.5)
Total[b]	15	21	31
Light[c]	23	21	63
Intermediate[d]	15	28	24
Dense[e]	30	24	84

[a]Derived by integration (±10%) of [[13]CH$_3$]$_2$Lys resonances in NMR spectra; [b]LDL, d 1.019–1.063 g/ml; [c]LDL, d 1.0244–1.0271 g/ml; [d]LDL, d 1.0327–1.0358 g/ml; [e]LDL, d 1.0358–1.0393 g/ml.

[6], these data are consistent with the proposal that intermediate LDL subspecies are the optimal ligand for the LDL receptor.

X-ray diffraction studies of protein crystals allow precise definition of three-dimensional structural domains. We have therefore undertaken the crystallization of highly defined LDL subspecies by a hanging-drop vapor diffusion technique. Crystals of LDL prepared by this procedure possess two minimal and one long axis and an elongated, thrombic-type appearance; they are birefringent and thus optically active. Electron micrographs of thin sections of fixed and embedded crystals show a regular hexagonal arrangement of spherical particles with the characteristic dimensions of LDL. The optical diffraction pattern exhibits a first-order hexagonal packing with center–center distances of 17 nm (R. Prassl, P. Laggner and M.J. Chapman, unpublished studies). High-resolution X-ray diffraction studies of these crystals will afford new insight into the domain structure of apoB100 in LDL.

Earlier studies have shown that LDL subpopulations differ markedly in their capacity to resist oxidative stress in vitro [7,8]. Indeed, intermediate LDL exhibit an elevated degree of resistance to copper-mediated oxidation in vitro, as judged by the duration of the lag phase of conjugated diene formation [8]. The efficient removal of intermediate LDL by the LDL receptor suggests that these particles may be of lower atherogenic potential than dense LDL, the latter exhibiting both low resistance to oxidation and poor affinity for the LDL receptor.

Intermediate LDL subspecies thus fulfill a major function in cholesterol homeostasis. Moreover, recent studies of the transfer of cholesteryl esters (CE) from HDL to apoB-containing lipoproteins show that intermediate LDL subspecies are targeted as major CE acceptors by CETP [9]. In this context the CETP (CE transfer protein) appears to play a protective rather than a proatherogenic role in normolipidemic subjects.

In conclusion, structural and metabolic studies of physicochemically defined LDL subspecies clearly differentiate light, intermediate and dense subpopulations on the basis of their biological functions and potential atherogenicity.

Acknowledgements

The authors are indebted to Mlles V. Soulier and L. Bonheur for production of the typescript.

References

1. Slyper AH. J Am Med Assoc 1994;272:305–308.
2. Chapman M, Laplaud PL, Luc G, Forgez P, Bruckert E, Goulinet S, Lagrange D. J Lipid Res 1988;29: 442–458.
3. McNamara JR, Campos H, Ordovas JM, Peterson J, Wilson PWF, Schaefer EJ. Arteriosclerosis 1987;7: 483–490.
4. Brown MS, Kovanen PT, Goldstein JL. Science 1981;212:628–635.
5. Nigon F, Lesnik P, Rouis M, Chapman MJ. J Lipid Res 1991;32:1741–1753.
6. Lund-Katz S, Ibdah JA, Letizia JY, Thomas MJ, Phillips MC. J Biol Chem 1988;263:13831–13838.
7. De Graaf J, Hak-Lemmers HLM, Hectors MPC, Demacker PNM, Hendriks JCM, Stalenhoef AFH. Arterioscler Thromb 1991;11:298–306.
8. Dejager S, Bruckert E, Chapman MJ. J Lipid Res 1993;34:295–308.
9. Guerin M, Dolphin PJ, Chapman MJ. Arterioscler Thromb 1994;14:199–206.

Genetic and metabolic influences on LDL subclasses

Ronald M. Krauss[1], Jerome I. Rotter[2] and Aldons J. Lusis[3]

[1]Life Sciences Division, Lawrence Berkeley Laboratory, University of California, Berkeley, California; [2]Division of Medical Genetics, Departments of Medicine and Pediatrics, Cedars-Sinai Medical Center, and University of California, Los Angeles, California; and [3]Department of Medicine, Department of Microbiology and Molecular Genetics, and Molecular Biology Institute, University of California, Los Angeles, California, USA

Abstract. Genetic and environmental factors influence LDL particle size and density, and expression of an atherogenic lipoprotein phenotype (ALP) characterized by predominance of small, dense LDL particles. Linkage of ALP to the LDL receptor locus has been reported previously. Quantitative sib-pair and relative-pair linkage methodologies were used to test for linkage of LDL particle size to candidate loci in 25 large pedigrees with familial coronary artery disease. Linkage to the LDL receptor gene locus was confirmed (p = 0.008). Evidence was also obtained for linkage to the genes for apoC-III, cholesteryl ester transfer protein, and manganese superoxide dismutase. The results suggest several genetic determinants of LDL particle size that may involve different metabolic mechanisms giving rise to small, dense LDL and increased atherosclerosis risk.

LDL subclasses and atherogenic lipoprotein phenotype

An LDL subclass pattern characterized by a predominance of small, dense LDL particles, principally LDL_3 [1], has been identified using both non-denaturing gradient gel electrophoresis [2] and analytic ultracentrifugation (Miller BD, Haskell WL, Alderman EL, Fair J, Krauss RM, unpublished data). The prevalence of this trait, which has been designated LDL subclass pattern B, is 30—35% in adult men, but is much lower in males <20 yr and in premenopausal women (5—10%) [2], and is intermediate (15—25%) in postmenopausal women [2—4]. Individuals with subclass pattern B have been shown to have higher levels of triglyceride-rich lipoproteins and remnants, reduced levels of HDL_2 [2] and a greater degree of resistance to insulin-stimulated glucose uptake than subjects with predominantly larger LDL (pattern A) [5]. Levels of plasma and LDL apoB are higher in pattern B than pattern A subjects, indicative of larger numbers of LDL particles, but total LDL-cholesterol is minimally if at all higher [2], consistent with the shift toward denser, more lipid-depleted LDL particles.

The evidence that individuals with small, dense LDL have a number of interrelated metabolic features associated with increased risk of coronary artery disease led to the designation of pattern B as an atherogenic lipoprotein phenotype (ALP) [2]. Case-control studies of subjects with acute myocardial infarction [6] and angiographically documented coronary artery disease [7,8] have shown up to a 3-fold or greater [9] increase in risk associated with a predominance of small, dense LDL. However, a high degree of intercorrelation among the features of ALP has made it difficult to determine the extent to which individual components of the syndrome contribute to disease risk.

Address for correspondence: Ronald M. Krauss, MD. Lawrence Berkeley Laboratory, University of California, Donner Laboratory, Room 465, One Cyclotron Road, Berkeley, CA 94720, USA.

Genetic influences on LDL particle distribution

Heritability of LDL particle size, as assessed by relative concordance in monozygotic vs. dizygotic twins, has indicated that genetic factors account for 30—50% of the variation in LDL particle size in both men [10] and women [4], with the remainder due to nongenetic or environmental influences. Several such influences have been identified, including abdominal adiposity [11], noninsulin-dependent diabetes mellitus [12], use of progestin-containing oral contraceptives [13], and dietary fat and carbohydrate intake [14].

Complex segregation analyses in healthy families [15] and in families of probands with familial combined hyperlipidemia [16] have indicated that LDL subclass pattern B, as assessed by gradient gel electrophoresis, is under the influence of a major gene or genes, each with transmission consistent with autosomal dominant inheritance, and an additional polygenic or additive component. More recent studies, in which the small, dense LDL phenotype was assessed by density gradient ultracentrifugation [13] and by measurement of LDL particle size as a continuous parameter [17], have confirmed a major gene effect. The frequency of the allele(s) responsible for pattern B in these studies, which involved four different study populations, ranged from 0.1 to 0.3, consistent with the prevalence of the trait as assessed by population studies. It is of interest that in the familial combined hyperlipidemia families, the distribution of apoB levels in pattern B but not pattern A subjects was bimodal [18], which raised the possibility of a second major gene responsible for apoB elevations that is fully expressed only in the genetic background of pattern B.

Linkage of pattern B to candidate gene loci chromosome 19p has been reported previously [19]. On the basis of both two-point and multipoint linkage analyses, the maximal LOD (log odds ratio) score for linkage to the LDL-receptor locus was 4.43 at a recombination fraction of 0.05, assuming 100% penetrance of ALP. Weaker linkage was observed with the insulin-receptor locus on chromosome 19p (LOD score 1.78 at a recombination fraction of zero). Utilizing nonparametric quantitative sib-pair and relative-pair linkage methodologies, we have tested for linkage of a gene or genes determining LDL particle size to the LDL-receptor locus and other candidate gene loci in 278 members of 25 pedigrees in whom the proband and at least one other blood relative had coronary artery disease. We obtained evidence for linkage of a locus controlling LDL particle size to a three-allele marker within the LDL-receptor gene locus (p = 0.008). With relative-pairs, significant evidence for linkage (p = 0.001—0.007) was also observed for the apoC-III gene on chromosome 11, the gene for cholesterol ester transfer protein on chromosome 16p, and the manganese superoxide dismutase gene locus on chromosome 6q. No linkage was observed for other candidate loci tested: apoB, apoA-II, apo(a), apoE-CI-CII, lipoprotein lipase, and HDL-binding protein.

Although these genetic loci have been identified by polymorphic DNA markers that do not indicate the presence of causative mutations in the respective genes, it is intriguing that their protein products have connections to metabolic pathways that may be involved in the generation of the pattern B phenotype. Small, dense LDL have been shown to have reduced affinity for the LDL-receptor [20], and, conceivably, altered LDL-receptor function or regulation could result in further impairment of plasma clearance of these LDL or their metabolic precursors. Variation in insulin-receptor function or regulation could be responsible for the insulin resistance associated with increased triglyceride, reduced HDL, and small, dense LDL [5].

It has been demonstrated that apoC-III gene haplotypes are associated with variation in plasma triglyceride levels [21], which in turn could affect levels of small, dense LDL [22]. It is also of interest that some investigators have demonstrated association [23] and linkage [24] of polymorphisms in the AI/CIII/AIV cluster to familial combined hyperlipidemia.

In the case of CETP, there is evidence for polydispersity and increased mass of small, triglyceride-rich LDL particles in patients with homozygous CETP deficiency [25], and that in vitro incubation of LDL with CETP results in conversion to a larger and more uniform size distribution [26]. On the other hand, CETP may facilitate lipolytic conversion of larger to smaller LDL particles by promoting triglyceride transfer into the LDL core [27]. A possible mechanistic association of lipoprotein metabolism with MnSOD activity is much more speculative, but it is noteworthy that in vitro susceptibility of LDL to copper-induced oxidation increases as a function of decreasing LDL particle size [28].

Other candidate mechanisms for the small, dense LDL phenotype include those that result in overproduction and/or impaired clearance of triglyceride-rich lipoproteins. These particles could include precursors of small, dense LDL, or could promote their formation by cycles of triglyceride exchange and lipolysis as described above. There is evidence for reduced exogenous triglyceride clearance in pattern B subjects, independent of fasting triglyceride level [12], as well as recent evidence from stable isotope kinetic studies for lower fractional catabolism of VLDL and IDL fractions than in pattern A subjects (Krauss RM, La Belle M, Blanche PJ, Shames D, and Hellerstein M, unpublished observations). While pattern B subjects have been found to have reduced levels of heparin-releasable lipoprotein lipase activity [29,30], and patients with heterozygous lipoprotein lipase deficiency have a lipoprotein phenotype that appears similar to that found in subjects with pattern B [31], the prevalence of genetic lipoprotein lipase deficiency appears to be much lower than that of pattern B, and LDL particle size was not linked to the lipoprotein lipase gene locus in the present study. However, it remains possible that other genetically influenced factors resulting in retardation of catabolism of triglyceride-rich lipoproteins or their remnants, such as increased levels of apoC-III as suggested above, may have an etiologic or contributory role in many subjects with the small, dense LDL phenotype.

The findings described above have led to the hypothesis that several different genetic loci contribute to the expression of the small, dense LDL phenotype, that these genes cumulatively influence the prevalence of the trait in the general population, and that in any family one or more of the loci are responsible for the major gene and additive effects identified by complex segregation analyses. Moreover, the results suggest that different genetically determined metabolic mechanisms may give rise to ALP, and that these differences, as well as gene–environment and gene–gene interactions, may result in variability of metabolic and pathologic manifestations among affected individuals.

Acknowledgements

This work was supported by the National Institutes of Health Program Project Grants HL 18574 and HL 28481 from the National Heart, Lung, and Blood Institute, a grant from the National Dairy Promotion and Research Board and administered in cooperation with the National Dairy Council, and the Cedars-Sinai Board of Governor's Chair in Medical Genetics, and was conducted in part at the Lawrence Berkeley Laboratory through the U.S. Department of Energy under Contract No. DE-AC03-76SF00098.

References

1. Krauss RM, Blanche PJ. Curr Opin Lipidol 1992;3:377–383.
2. Austin MA, King MC, Vranizan KM, Krauss RM. Circulation 1990;82:495–506.

3. Campos H, Blijlevens E, McNamara JR, Ordovas JM, Posner BM, Wilson PWF, Castelli WP, Schaefer EJ. Arterioscler Thromb 1992;12:1410−1419.
4. Austin MA, Newman B, Selby JV, Edwards K, Mayer EJ, Krauss RM. Arterioscler Thromb 1993;13:687−695.
5. Reaven GM, Chen Y-DI, Jeppesen J, Maheux P, Krauss RM. J Clin Invest 1993;92:141−146.
6. Austin MA, Breslow JL, Hennekens CH, Buring JE, Willett WC, Krauss RM. J Am Med Assoc 1988;260:1917−1921.
7. Campos H, Genest JJ Jr, Blijlevens E, McNamara JR, Jenner JL, Ordovas JM, Wilson PWF, Schaefer EJ. Arterioscler Thromb 1992;12:187−195.
8. Coresh J, Kwiterovich PO Jr, Smith HH, Bachorik PS. J Lipid Res 1993;34:1687−1697.
9. Griffin BA, Freeman DJ, Tait GW, Thomson J, Caslake MJ, Packard CJ, Shepherd J. Atherosclerosis 1994;106:241−253.
10. Lamon-Fava S, Jimenez D, Christian JC, Fabsitz RR, Reed T, Carmelli D, Castelli WP, Ordovas JM, Wilson PWF, Schaefer EJ. Atherosclerosis 1991;91:97−106.
11. Terry RB, Wood PD, Haskell WL, Stefanick ML, Krauss RM. J Clin Endocrinol Metab 1989;68:191−199.
12. Feingold KR, Grunfeld C, Pang M, Doerrler W, Krauss RM. Arterioscler Thromb 1992;12:1496−1502.
13. de Graaf J, Swinkels DW, de Haan AFJ, Demacker PNM, Stalenhoef AFN. Am J Hum Genet 1992;51:1295−1310.
14. Dreon DM, Fernstrom HA, Miller B, Krauss RM. FASEB J 1994;8:121−126.
15. Austin MA, King MC, Vranizan KM, Newman B, Krauss RM. Am J Hum Genet 1988;43:838−846.
16. Austin MA, Brunzell JD, Fitch WL, Krauss RM. Arteriosclerosis 1990;10:520−530.
17. Bu X, Krauss RM, Puppione D, Gray R, Rotter JI. Am J Hum Genet 1992;51:A336.
18. Austin MA, Horowitz H, Wijsman E, Krauss RM, Brunzell J. Atherosclerosis 1992;92:67−77.
19. Nishina PM, Johnson JP, Naggert JK, Krauss RM. Proc Natl Acad Sci USA 1992;89:708−712.
20. Nigon F, Lesnik P, Rouis M, Chapman MJ. J Lipid Res 1991;32:1741−1753.
21. Dammerman M, Sandkuijl LA, Halaas JL, Chung W, Breslow JL. Proc Natl Acad Sci USA 1993;90:4562−4566.
22. Krauss RM. Am Heart J 1987;113:578−582.
23. Tybjærg-Hansen A, Nordestgaard BG, Gerdes LU, Færgeman O, Humphries SE. Atherosclerosis 1993;100:157−169.
24. Wojciechowski AP, Farrall M, Cullen P, Wilson T, Bayliss JD, Farren B, Griffin BA, Caslake MJ, Packard CJ, Shepherd J, Thakker R, Scott J. Nature 1991;349:161−164.
25. Sakai N, Matsuzawa Y, Hirano K, Yamashita S, Nozaki S, Ueyama Y, Kubo M, Tarui S. Arteriosclerosis 1991;11:71−79.
26. Lagrost L, Gandjini H, Athias A, Guyard-Dangremont V, Lallemant C, Gambert P. Arterioscler Thromb 1993;13:815−825.
27. Lagrost L, Gambert P, Lallemant C. Arterioscler Thromb 1994;14:1327−1336.
28. Tribble DL, Holl LG, Wood PD, Krauss RM. Atherosclerosis 1992;93:189−199.
29. Jansen H, Hop W, Van Tol A, Bruschke AVG, Birkenhäger JC. Atherosclerosis 1994;107:45−54.
30. Campos H, Dreon DM, Krauss RM. Associations of hepatic and lipoprotein lipase activities with changes in dietary intake and low density lipoprotein subclasses. J Lipid Res (in press).
31. Miesenböck G, Hölzl B, Föger B, Brandstätter E, Paulweber B, Sandhofer F, Patsch JR. J Clin Invest 1993;91:448−455.

984

Angiographic assessment of atherosclerosis progression and regression

G.B. John Mancini

Vancouver Hospital and Health Sciences Centre, University of British Columbia, Vancouver, Canada

Abstract. This paper reviews the basic aspects of atherosclerosis progression and regression that complicate the interpretation of angiographic changes in clinical trials. The fundamental difficulties arise from the diffuse and mural nature of the process and the ability of the vascular tree to remodel to retain luminal cross-sectional area during early atherosclerosis progression. There is no single, angiographic parameter that can reflect all of these processes and changes induced by interventions and, therefore, a comprehensive analysis strategy is required when planning an angiographic trial. Moreover, there are processes not reflected by angiographic changes that are perhaps even more important than the morphologic changes themselves in determining the impact, both early and late, on clinical outcome. For example, effects on plaque stabilization, normalization of endothelial function, effects on platelet–thrombin interactions, viscosity, collaterals and other mechanisms can only be inferred from the results of angiographic trials. For some of these mechanisms, the importance of changes in mild/moderate lesions and in new lesion formation provides an angiographic bridge or linkage between morphology and physiology, but it is an imperfect one. Accordingly, carotid and intravascular ultrasound, nuclear studies, computed tomography and magnetic resonance imaging are important adjuncts to angiographic trials. Even so, it is recommended that such trials continue to be of a sufficient size to allow conclusions about clinical events which will remain of overriding importance and which may not always be strongly linked to morphologic changes.

What are the processes underlying atherosclerosis progression and regression?

There are three fundamental concepts of atherosclerosis development that must be appreciated when envisaging an angiographic study of progression/regression. The first is that the process has two rates of progression: a slow rate (related to accumulation of foam cells, creation of a fatty streak, transformation of lipoid accumulation to crystalline cholesterol and accumulation of cellular components such as smooth muscle cells and fibroblasts) and a rapid rate (related to plaque fissuring and/or hemorrhaging leading to platelet-rich thrombus accumulation). The second is that in the early stages, the process affects the wall, not the lumen, and generally induces a form of compensatory remodeling of the external elastic lamina and muscular wall that allows preservation of the luminal conduit for blood flow [1]. This compensatory remodeling appears to be effective in some patients [2] until 40–45% of the overall cross-sectional area of the artery is occupied by atheroma. Luminal encroachment, and hence angiographic detection of the so-called "new" or "minimal" lesion, will be evident only once atheroma build-up has exceeded this capacity to remodel by outward expansion of the arterial wall. The third concept is that the process is diffuse, thereby rendering invalid the jargon of angiography that refers to "the normal reference segment" and to "discrete lesions". More properly, the former should be called simply a "reference segment" and there can truly be no such thing as a "discrete lesion". Moreover, it is important to recognize that reference segments should conceptually be considered to represent "pre-new" or "pre-minimal" lesions. This framework helps to bridge the gap between pathologists' perception and angiographers' perception of the atherosclerotic process. It also helps solidify the link that we now understand between the pathogenesis of clinical events and angiographic findings, a linkage that has led to the concept of plaque stabilization and a refocus on early atherosclerosis, particularly "new" lesions and mild stenoses. Implicit in these fundamental concepts is that the morphologic appearance of atherosclerosis is altered in a complex fashion over time and this complexity applies throughout the entire coronary tree.

So far, the known mechanisms of regression of atheroma are limited to mobilization of lipids from either lipid pools or cholesterol crystals or out of foam cells and to intrinsic fibrinolysis of spontaneously formed clot. The sclerotic components of atheroma rarely if ever regress [3,4].

What aspects of these processes are we trying to measure in progression/regression trials?

Schwartz et al. have succinctly summarized the goals of current progression/regression trials [5]. They are to demonstrate a) slowing of the natural progression rate, b) regression of established disease, c) prevention of initiation of disease, and d) stabilization of plaque. The first two goals were the main ones of the earliest studies. The concept of plaque stabilization [6,7] has come to light only as a result of the unexpected, early improvement in clinical events noted in many of the most recent angiographic trials. Linked to this new concept is the goal of demonstrating prevention of disease, which to the angiographer is relegated to the demonstration of prevention of "new" or "minimal lesions" or demonstration of specific salutary effects on mild lesions. The realization of changes in clinical events early in the course of angiographic trials that were statistically powered only to show morphologic changes has mandated a rethinking of the advisability of planning studies with small numbers of patients.

What are the technical aspects of angiography that must be met to achieve successful measurement of these processes?

The prime goal of angiography in these trials is to be able to provide a reliable gauge of atherosclerosis progression and regression and to be able to provide insight into differential, topographical effects of therapy. Because this gauge is intended to represent the overall effect on a given patient, aggregate indexes are needed to indicate a net change in a given patient even though disparate changes may occur throughout the coronary tree.

Most studies have broken down the analysis of angiograms segmentally and these segments generally are the proximal and largest segments of the coronary tree, generally delimited by branch points. Although the atherosclerotic process obviously spans segments, it is practical and convenient to undertake analyses in this segmental fashion [8] and then to average net changes over time by taking into account the number of segments undergoing analysis. It has been our convention to designate the segment showing total occlusion as having a 100% diameter stenosis and 0 mm of mean, maximum and minimum diameters (as well as reference diameter and distal reference diameters) and to ignore all segments distal to this segment.

The parameter to be measured within segments remains the subject of continued controversy. Unfortunately, most of this controversy is based on trying to "guess" which parameter is likeliest to show a significant P value at the termination of the study. Instead, this controversy should focus on the fundamental concepts noted above and the specific question that one wishes to answer. It is suggested that the angiographic analyses to date have only begun to demonstrate the complexities of vascular remodeling in response to interventions such as aggressive cholesterol lowering and that all studies should provide data in as comprehensive a fashion as possible in order to allow the academic community the best opportunity to learn how interventions affect coronary remodeling. A good example of this is provided by the comprehensive reporting of Gould et al. [9] which provides data on the proximal, stenotic and distal segments of lesions. However, given the importance of "mild lesions" and "new" lesion formation, it is important not to constrain analyses only to segments showing visually apparent luminal encroachment [10].

The minimum diameter is the most commonly used parameter and can be justified because it is most directly related to the hemodynamic significance of a given stenosis. A secondary reason for its popularity is that it is the most commonly reported parameter that shows significance in angiographic trials. The percent diameter stenosis measurement has similar qualities and it is also so entrenched in clinical jargon that its measurement and reporting should not be abandoned. But it is more variable in its measurement *as well as in its interpretation*. For example, basic work suggests that almost all interventions aimed at modifying or preventing atherosclerosis should be most efficacious in the earliest stages of the process [3,5]. If, as noted above, the reference segment is truly more likely to have characteristics of early atheroma than areas of luminal encroachment, then regression of atheroma in this area without a comparable degree of regression within the area of luminal encroachment would lead to the calculation of a worsened percent diameter stenosis and the loss of an opportunity really to understand what the intervention is inducing [9].

Although the minimum diameter and the percent diameter stenosis are well justified on the basis of their relationship to the hemodynamic significance of coronary disease, an additional and major goal of angiographic trials is to determine the effects of interventions on the *extent* of atheroma in the entire coronary tree. In this regard, the mean segmental diameter is the most commonly proposed measurement parameter. This parameter has the added advantage of being more reproducible than either the minimum diameter or the percent diameter stenosis [11–13]. Within a segment, an area of minor luminal encroachment may progress more than an area showing more luminal encroachment in the baseline study. The mean diameter measurement would reflect the overall change and would not require subjective decisions as to which areas of minimal narrowing should be compared between baseline and follow-up films. The parameter per se, however, is not as sensitive to changes induced by interventions. One of the reasons for this is that the mean diameter is really being proposed as a surrogate for atheroma volume. If one were to calculate the overall atheroma volume differences implied by a net change in mean diameter, then one would be conveying more correctly the information on atheroma *extent* that justified proposing its measurement in the first place. It can easily be shown that given the same magnitude of measured change in either the minimum diameter or the mean diameter, the latter would imply more than 500 times the atheroma bulk in a given patient than would the change in minimum diameter measurement. This results from converting the diameter changes to volume changes and is principally determined by the fact that the mean diameter is measured over a length that is about 500 times greater than the length over which the minimum diameter is measured. Another reason for including mean diameter measurement in analysis plans of angiographic trials is that this measurement is related to the overall resistance of the coronary tree. We should not lose sight of the fact that the apparently small changes in percent diameter stenosis and minimum diameter seem difficult to relate to improvements in functional capacity noted in some studies. The latter may be the result of yet to be established changes in blood viscosity, improvements in endothelial function and alterations in collateral flow recruitment. But the evidence would also suggest that major changes in the extent of atheroma, as reflected crudely by the mean diameter measurements, must be considered a prime mechanism for the long-term improvements in functional capacity that have been noted.

With respect to the goal of demonstrating prevention of initiation of disease, angiography is extremely limited because early atherosclerosis is a mural process, not a luminal one, that induces centrifugal remodeling that prevents luminal encroachment and angiographic visualization. However, if analyses are *absolute* (not limited to percent diameter stenosis), if they include specific measures of changes in reference areas within segments, and if they include all segments irrespective of whether visually apparent focal, luminal encroachment is present, then the angiographer will have contributed as best as s/he can to demonstrating whether the intervention has had an effect on early atherosclerosis. It must be stated, however, that although it is clear that the natural and slow progression of atherosclerosis induces remodeling that, up to a certain point, compensates to maintain luminal cross-sectional area, it is not clear whether the expansile processes reverse, and whether they reverse at the same pace as the more rapid (over the course of 1–3 years) morphological changes in luminal atheroma that have been induced by aggressive cholesterol-lowering therapy. If the expansile processes reverse in parallel with regression of luminal atheroma, then the arteriogram is rendered even less useful in assessing early atherosclerosis. If this is not the case, however, then an increase in lumen diameter or cross-sectional area measured in short-term studies would be a valid indication of atherosclerosis regression. Indeed, the STARS trial showed significant changes in overall mean diameter measurements suggesting that "reverse remodeling", if it occurs, does not proceed as rapidly as the regression induced by short-term interventions [14].

The final issue, that of plaque stabilization, has grown out of the demonstration that the morphologic, angiographic motivation to undertake progression/regression trials, i.e., the "plumbers' view" of improving the coronary conduits, was overly simplistic. Based on current knowledge, there are two ways in which angiographic trials can contribute to demonstrating plaque stabilization. The lesser of the two, but still highly important, is to ensure that the analyses of less obviously diseased areas of the tree are analyzed and that "new" lesions or effects on "moderate" lesions are explicitly incorporated into analysis plans [15–17]. The more important of the two deals with the sample size of angiographic trials. While there are numerous technical and statistical ways to decrease the theoretical sample size of angiographic trials [13,18], in my view this will diminish the impact of angiographic trials and will diminish the opportunities to learn more explicitly about the true effects of our interventions on coronary disease. More effort should be expended on improving tools for measuring "softer" but nevertheless crucial endpoints and ensuring that angiographic trials are adequately powered to allow for conclusions on clinical events that can then be related to the underlying morphological findings or that may stimulate consideration of new mechanisms of efficacy.

What have the angiographic trials shown us so far?

The trials to date have shown us that cholesterol lowering in males with high or moderately high cholesterol can increase the odds of stabilizing angiographic disease and inducing regression of disease. The risk of progressing is significantly diminished. These morphologic changes are most consistently predicted by lowering LDL-cholesterol [19–21]. The specific sites of morphologic efficacy remains unsettled, with two recent trials [15–17] showing dominant effects on new lesion formation and prevention of

988

progression of modest lesions, in contrast to earlier trials suggesting dominant effects on severe lesions. There is evidence that quantitative angiographic parameters [22] and changes in these have prognostic importance [23].

The effects on women and elderly populations or cohorts with other risk factors such as diabetes is not as well established. The ideal patient that should be targeted for such therapy is not well defined beyond the general recommendation that high-risk patients, especially those who have already manifested coronary disease, should benefit not just angiographically but also clinically. Roussow [21] has demonstrated, through meta-analysis of angiographic trials, a decreased coronary heart disease mortality. Current angiographic trials provide only indirect evidence to support the current LDL target of 100 mg/dl (2.4 mmol/l) [24].

What are the limitations of angiographic trials and what role will alternative imaging approaches play?

As noted above, angiography is very limited in assessment of the mural aspects of atherosclerosis, especially in the early and most important stages. The functional importance of interventions on exercise capacity and other parameters is not easily extrapolated from angiographic data. Accordingly, it is important to anticipate a greater utilization of complementary techniques. The most important of these today are carotid B-mode ultrasound and stress perfusion imaging. Whether intracoronary ultrasound, magnetic resonance and electron beam computed tomography can be developed for such purposes is the subject of intense investigation at this time.

References

1. Glagov S, Weisenberg E, Zairns CK et al. N Engl J Med 1987;316:1371–1375.
2. Clarkson TB, Prichard RW, Morgan TM, Petrick GS, Klein KP. J Am Med Assoc 1994;271:289–294.
3. Small DM, Bond MG, Waugh D, Prack M, Sawyer JK. J Clin Invest 1984;73:1590–1605.
4. Blankenhorn DH, Alaupovic P, Wickham E et al. Circulation 1990;81:470–476.
5. Schwartz CJ, Valente AJ, Sprague EA et al. Circulation 1992;86(suppl 3):III117–III123.
6. Brown BG, Yue-Qiao Z, Sacco DE et al. Circulation 1993;87:1781–1791.
7. Falk E. Circulation 1992;86 (suppl III):III30–III42.
8. The CASS Principal Investigators: The National Heart, Lung, and Blood Institute Coronary Artery Surgery Study (CASS). Circulation 1981;63(suppl I):I1–I39.
9. Gould KL, Ornish D, Kirkeeide R et al. Am J Cardiol 1992;69:845–853.
10. Crouse JR, Thompson CJ. Circulation 1993;87(suppl II):II17–II33.
11. Ellis S, Sanders W, Goulet C et al. Circulation 1986;74:1235–1242.
12. de Cesare NB, Williamson PR, Moore NB, DeBoe SF, Mancini GBJ. Am J Cardiol 1992;69:77–83.
13. Selzer RH, Hagerty C, Azen SP et al. J Clin Invest 1989;83:520–526.
14. Watts GR, Lewis B, Brunt JNH et al. Lancet 1992;339:563–569.
15. Waters D, Higginson L, Gladstone P et al. Circulation 1994;89:959–968.
16. Pitt B, Ellis SG, Mancini GBJ et al. Am J Cardiol 1993;72:31–35.
17. Pitt B, Mancini GBJ, Ellis SG et al. J Am Coll Cardiol 1994;131A (Abst).
18. Gibson CM, Sandor T, Stone PH et al. Am J Cardiol 1992;69:1286–1290.
19. Vos J, de Feyter PJ, Simmoons ML et al. Prog Cardiovasc Dis 1993;35:435–454.
20. Superko HR, Krauss RM. Circulation 1994;90:1056–1069.
21. Roussouw JE, Lewis B, Rifkind BM. N Engl J Med 1990;323:1112–1119.
22. Mancini GBJ, Bourassa MG, Williamson PR et al. Am J Cardiol 1992;69:1022–1027.
23. Waters D, Craven TE, Lesperance J. Circulation 1993;87:1067–1075.
24. Stewart BF, Brown BG, Zhao X-Q et al. J Am Coll Cardiol 1994;23:899–906.

©1995 Elsevier Science B.V. All rights reserved.
Atherosclerosis X.
F.P. Woodford, J. Davignon and A. Sniderman, editors.

Ultrasound assessment of atherosclerosis progression and regression

John Wikstrand and Inger Wendelhag
Wallenberg Laboratory for Cardiovascular Research, Göteborg University, Sahlgrenska Hospital, Gothenburg, Sweden

Abstract. It is now possible to study noninvasively the morphology of large, superficially located arteries such as the carotid and femoral arteries, though not deep-seated arteries like coronaries. The atherosclerotic process can be followed over time by repeated imaging of the arterial wall, so that data from several observational and interventional studies have recently been presented. However, further studies need to be done to clarify if and when a reduced progression or regression of intima-media thickness or cross-sectional intima-media area of the superficial arteries also involves a favorable prognosis regarding coronary atherosclerosis and coronary events.

With the development of the B-mode ultrasound technique it has become possible to study noninvasively the morphology of large, superficially located arteries such as the carotid and femoral arteries [1,2]. The atherosclerotic process can be followed over time by repeated imaging of the arterial wall; data from several observational and interventional studies have recently been presented [3—6]. We discuss here some fundamental principles of the ultrasound method and briefly comment on how to evaluate results from prospective ultrasound studies.

Comments on anatomical limitations

Atherosclerosis is a disease affecting the intima leading to intimal thickening but there is no method available at present which can measure only intima thickness in vivo. Intima-media thickness may be measured with ultrasound, but noninvasively only in large superficially located arteries and not in the coronary arteries.

The anatomical location of a biological structure is always defined by the leading edge of an echo, and the thickness of a structure as the distance between the leading edges of two different echoes. In spite of the similarity of the near and far wall images, it is only in the far wall position that the intima-media thickness may be accurately measured, see Fig. 1 [1,2]. It may therefore be concluded that until more experience is gathered, main outcome variables in ultrasound studies of atherosclerosis should preferably be from the far wall. If analyses of the near wall are performed they ought to be separately presented. If lumen diameter is measured (which may be necessary for a valid judgement, see below), this measurement ought to be read from the leading edge of the intima-lumen interface of the near wall as illustrated in Fig. 1.

Common carotid, carotid bulb and internal carotid artery

The development of atherosclerosis typically begins with an increased intima thickness in the bifurcation area, i.e., in the proximal part of the internal carotid artery and the carotid bulb, and the intima-media complex is often thicker here than in the straight part of the common carotid artery. To be able to make a correct comparison of the results from different laboratories, it is therefore important to report where the measurements were performed.

990

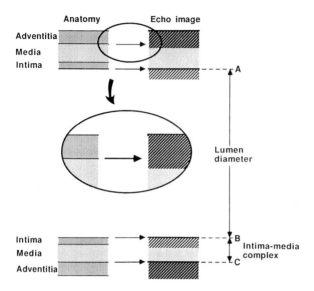

Fig. 1. Illustration of the anatomical correlates to echoes that may be recorded from an artery. Observe that all measurements are performed on leading edges of the different echoes, that any thickness of an echo is of no interest, and that the thickness of an anatomical entity (e.g., the intima-media complex) is defined by the distance between the leading edges of two different echoes. The figure also illustrates that the near wall adventitia-media interface cannot be identified in the ultrasound image (circled). From [2], by permission.

Good-quality multiple scans of the far wall of the straight part of the common carotid artery may be achieved in nearly every case. The percentage of missing images is so high from the internal carotid artery that it is not meaningful to try to perform quantitative measurements of intima-media thickness in the internal carotid artery in all subjects. If measurements are routinely performed in the carotid bulb, which we would recommend, it should be noted that the bulb of the internal carotid artery is not always located in the far wall position. It might be advisable to note the topographical location of the arteries in the far wall position and also to analyze if there are any differences between different topographical situations.

The judgement of plaques

Irrespective of the location of plaques in the carotid arteries, i.e., internal, external or common carotid artery or carotid bulb, it may be of value to record all plaques in both the near and far wall position [7,8]. Further studies are needed to define the usefulness of any quantification of plaques (area, base, height, etc.), especially in prospective studies [2]. One important question to be addressed is how blindness should be preserved if one wants to return to the same plaque in prospective studies.

Not all atherosclerotic plaques are the same even if they are similar in size and location. Some plaques may stabilize, like an inactive volcano. For others, plaque formation may continue with complications such as sclerosis, calcification, inflammation, hemorrhage or necrosis, that can alter the vulnerability of plaques to disruption. It would be highly desirable to develop methods with the possibility of identifying plaques with different qualitative characteristics. Calcification gives intense echoes and often also an echo shadow. However, although work is continuing the possibility of identifying plaques with different qualitative tissue characteristics in vivo seems to be limited at present [1,2].

Recording and analysis techniques

We recognize at the present time several differences in the recording and analysis routines between different laboratories. Some investigate only the common carotid artery, others the common carotid, the carotid bulb and the internal carotid artery, and still others both the carotid and femoral arteries. Some perform measurements of just a single maximal intima-media thickness, some on several locations in the carotid artery region and present scores from these measurements, while others do measurements along a predefined section of the artery of interest and from these measurements calculate means and maximum values. If the sum of several measurements from different sections of the carotid artery is used to define a score, it is important to report also the separate means or maximum values from each section of the artery, otherwise it will be hard to compare study results from different research groups. There is at present no consensus on whether and how these scores should be formed and used.

It may be recommended that analyses are performed on images frozen via ECG-triggering (top of R-wave) to minimize variability due to changes in intima-media thickness and lumen diameter during the cardiac cycle. Our experience indicates that real-time recordings may simplify the judgement of what the frozen images show. Furthermore, we believe that the best quality of analysis is achieved if the responsible technologist masters both registration and analyses.

Clinical relevance

We see an increasing use of the ultrasound method in the evaluation of preventive measures in randomized clinical trials. In the interpretation of results from these trials several important issues should be addressed: a) How should changes in intima-media thickness directly dependent on changes in lumen diameter be handled? b) How should missing data be handled? c) Is intima-media thickness measured by ultrasound in carotid or femoral arteries an appropriate surrogate variable for coronary atherosclerosis?

Changes in lumen diameter

Suppose a randomized trial compares two drugs, one of which causes lumen contraction, while the other does not affect lumen diameter. Other things being equal, wall thickness must increase after the first drug but not after the second. Cross-sectional area will, however, be unchanged. In the recently presented large-scale Multicenter Isradipine/Diuretic Atherosclerosis Study (MIDAS) [6], comparing a thiazide diuretic with a calcium antagonist (isradipine) in patients with hypertension, a difference in intima-media thickness was recorded after 6 months, with a greater intima-media thickness in those randomized to the diuretic. Lumen diameter was not investigated in this study. However, theoretical calculations show that the results regarding the thicker intima-media complex in the diuretic group could be explained by a mere 3% decrease in lumen diameter. Thus, small changes in lumen diameter may lead to significant changes in the thickness of the intima-media complex that are unrelated to the atherosclerotic process. Therefore, we would recommend monitoring lumen diameter also in ultrasound studies of atherosclerosis. Cross-sectional area of the intima-media complex may then be calculated as an important surrogate endpoint.

992

Subjects lost to follow-up

Subjects inevitably get lost to follow-up in long-term, prospective, randomized trials. Often it cannot be excluded that treatment may have affected the disease process negatively in those lost to follow up, which may introduce a bias in interpretation. One way of handling this problem is to compare treatment groups using a nonparametric scoring test in which the highest score is given to all patients lost to follow-up. This method of analysis should be stated prospectively in the study protocol [1,2].

The value of surrogate endpoints

Is it possible to use intima-media thickness in the carotid artery as a surrogate variable for coronary atherosclerosis? As yet, there is no clear answer to this question and the answer may also partly depend on which surrogate variable is used. We cannot take for granted that measurements performed in the common carotid artery bring the same information as measurements performed in the carotid bulb or in the internal carotid artery. At present we cannot even with certainty claim that an increased thickness of the intima-media complex in the carotid artery indicates atherosclerosis at the location where the measurement was performed. It is unlikely that simple surrogate ultrasound endpoints from the carotid or femoral artery can substitute for measurements of coronary atherosclerosis and for hard endpoints such as myocardial infarction, stroke and cardiovascular death. There are many examples in the literature where results from surrogate variables have been misleading, e.g., the Cardiac Arrhythmia Suppression Trial (CAST), the International Nifedipine Trial on Atherosclerotic Therapy (INTACT) and recently results from MIDAS [1,6]. In the latter study there was a trend towards significantly more cardiovascular complications after 3 years in those randomized to isradipine than in those randomized to diuretics, in spite of a favorable trend in intima-media thickness in the former group (see above) [6].

The results from four ultrasound trials in which the effect of cholesterol lowering has been studied have recently been presented. A study in patients with prior coronary bypass surgery, the Cholesterol Lowering Atherosclerosis Study (CLAS), reported a significant reduction in carotid intima-media thickness after 2 and 4 years of treatment with colestipol–niacin plus dietary advice [3]. Preliminary results from the study Pravastatin, Lipids, and Atherosclerosis in the Carotid arteries (PLAC II) showed a significant reduction in carotid intima-media thickening in coronary patients given pravastatin as cholesterol-lowering therapy (Furberg CD, personal communication) [4]. Results from another randomized double-blind placebo-controlled ultrasound study with lovastatin in asymptomatic high-risk individuals, the Asymptomatic Carotid Artery Plaque Study (ACAPS), besides a decrease in carotid intima-media thickness also indicated that the combined event rate of coronary deaths, nonfatal acute myocardial infarctions and strokes was lower in the lovastatin-treated group than in the placebo group (Furberg CD, personal communication) [5]. A group of patients with familial hypercholesterolemia were examined with B-mode ultrasound before and after 3 years of intensified cholesterol-lowering therapy in our own laboratory (pravastatin, cholestyramine or a combination). The results showed a significant decrease in mean carotid intima-media thickening in comparison with a control group. There was also a significant decrease in common carotid cross-sectional intima-media area, with no difference between the groups in lumen diameter [9]. However, no corresponding decrease was recorded in common femoral intima-media thickening in the hypercholesterolemic group, but on the contrary significant increase. There is at present no explanation for this negative finding; the results may indicate that atherosclerosis in the femoral artery may be difficult to retard by intervention in lipid metabolism. However, there is a series of consistent ultrasound data showing a decrease in intima-media thickening in carotid arteries during lipid-lowering treatment. The morphological basis for this reduction cannot be deduced from available data.

Conclusion

The ultrasound method is a promising technique, with a great potential for refined, computerized analyzing techniques. However, atherosclerotic lesions are complex structures and, therefore, difficult to measure. Thus, there is a need for improved interaction between pathologists and researchers who use different methods to measure atherosclerosis in vivo, to increase our understanding of what the recordings show. In addition, agreement about standardized measurement routines and endpoints should be reached. This will simplify comparisons between different studies and aid interpretation of results. More studies are also needed to clarify the relation between the thickness of the intima-media complex in large arteries (surrogate endpoints) and coronary athero-sclerosis and coronary heart disease. Hard endpoints like myocardial infarction and sudden death are usually due to a combination of an underlying atherosclerotic disease and triggering or precipitation factors such as left ventricular electrical instability, plaque instability, or a disturbed thrombogenesis-fibrinolysis balance. It might be advisable, therefore, to combine different surrogate variables (for both the underlying atherosclerotic disease and triggering or precipitation mechanisms) to obtain a broader perspective of the disease process. An intervention may or may not be effective in treating the condition of interest but could be harmful in other respects. Therefore, total mortality should be considered, as well as cause-specific fatal and nonfatal events, in addition to the primary surrogate variables whenever possible. Nevertheless, ultrasound evaluation of vascular disease looks increasingly promising as a noninvasive, cost-effective method for the future [10].

References

1. Wikstrand J, Wiklund O. Arterioscler Thromb 1992;12:114–119.
2. Wikstrand J, Wendelhag I. J Int Med 1994;236:565–570.
3. Blankenhorn DH, Selzer RH, Crawford DW, Barth JD, Liu C-r, Liu C-h, Mack WJ, Alaupovic P. Circulation 1993;88:20–28.
4. Furberg CD, Crouse JR, Byington RP, Bond MG, Espeland MA. J Am Coll Cardiol 1993;21:71A.
5. Furberg CD, Byington RP for the ACAPS group. Circulation 1993;88(suppl):I–386.
6. McClellan K. Weekly Inpharma 1994;932:4.
7. Wendelhag I, Wiklund O, Wikstrand J. Arterioscler Thromb 1993;13:1404–1411.
8. Suurküla M, Agewall S, Fagerberg B, Wendelhag I, Widgren B, Wikstrand J, on behalf of the Risk Intervention Study (RIS) group. Arterioscler Thromb 1994;14:1297–1304.
9. Wendelhag I, Wiklund O, Wikstrand J. Atherosclerosis 1994;109:293–294 (abstract).
10. Lees RS. Curr Opin Lipidol 1993;4:325–329.

Noninvasive management of coronary artery disease by reversal of coronary atherosclerosis

K. Lance Gould

University of Texas Health Science Center, Houston, Texas, USA

For diagnosis of coronary artery disease, current cardiovascular practice focuses principally on ECG exercise testing, stress perfusion imaging and coronary arteriography. For treatment, current cardiovascular practice focuses principally on antianginal and antiplatelet drugs, percutaneous transmural coronary angioplasty (PTCA) or bypass surgery. An alternative approach is the comprehensive, noninvasive management of coronary artery disease using PET perfusion imaging for definitive diagnosis and vigorous risk-factor modification aimed at regression of coronary atherosclerosis and stabilization of plaque to prevent the clinical events of myocardial infarction, sudden death and unstable coronary syndromes requiring PTCA or bypass surgery [1].

In recent randomized trials [2–15], vigorous cholesterol lowering by moderate low-fat diet and cholesterol-lowering drugs or by intensive lifestyle change resulted in stopping progression or partial reversal of coronary artery disease in up to 80% of treated subjects. The regression in these recent trials was only modest, 3–10% diameter stenosis units, depending on stenosis severity at baseline, but was consistently observed and statistically significant. There was a proportionately larger, major decrease in clinical events of myocardial infarction, death, bypass surgery or balloon angioplasty in up to 80% of the treatment groups undergoing vigorous cholesterol lowering compared to control groups in several of these studies [2,6,9,10,13–18]. The reason for proportionately greater clinical benefit than extent of anatomic regression appears to be due to plaque stabilization and reduction in the risk of plaque rupture which leads to acute unstable coronary syndromes, particularly at sites of relatively mild narrowing in diffusely atheromatous coronary arteries [16–22]. There is also a marked decrease in angina pectoris in parallel with decreased coronary events. Therefore, dietary and pharmacologic cholesterol lowering and control of other risk factors, in conjunction with antianginal and antiplatelet drugs, is an alternative approach to the treatment of coronary atherosclerosis that substantially reduces the necessity for balloon angioplasty or bypass surgery.

The combination of low-fat diet of less than 10% fat as calories combined with cholesterol-lowering drugs has a more profound cholesterol-lowering effect than either of these treatment approaches alone and readily decreases cholesterol to 140 mg/dl or below in most patients, even with modest doses of an HMG-CoA reductase inhibitor (statin) as the only drug. For individuals with low HDL, the addition of stopping smoking, adequate dietary protein, exercise and/or Lopid or niacin is used to normalize HDL.

In patients with coronary artery disease and relatively normal levels of cholesterol at baseline, lowering cholesterol to well below normal ranges has substantial benefit [2,14–17], probably more than in patients with very high cholesterol levels [17]. In the correlation of coronary-related deaths to cholesterol levels in the 10-year follow-up of 361,662 men screened for the MRFIT program, mortality decreased continuously with decreasing cholesterol down to levels of 140 mg/dl [14]. On the basis of these reports and the author's personal experience, achieving lean body mass and a total cholesterol of 140 mg/dl or below with an HDL of 45 mg/dl or greater using a very low-fat diet and lipid-altering drugs increases to over 90% the probability of partial regression or no progression of disease and absence of clinical events. Partial reversal of coronary artery stenosis and protection from clinical events occurs even in patients with initially normal cholesterol levels if these targets are reached [2,14–17].

Despite the current widespread use of PTCA there are no randomized trials of elective PTCA in stable coronary artery disease compared to medical antianginal or reversal treatment. Furthermore, in long-term follow-up, coronary bypass surgery does not appear to decrease incidence of myocardial infarction or death [23]. Therefore, on balance in the literature, there are more trials showing decreased coronary events by reversal treatment than reports on decreased coronary events after elective PTCA or bypass surgery in stable coronary artery disease. Accordingly, in the author's practice reversal treatment has replaced virtually all invasive procedures in the treatment of stable coronary artery disease.

With the modest changes in anatomic severity of coronary artery stenoses after lipid lowering, the commonly used term 'regression' or 'reversal' might be questioned. The process of atherosclerosis in the coronary arterial wall consists of a complex mix of cholesterol deposition, cellular proliferation, inflammation and calcification. With vigorous cholesterol lowering, lipid content and inflammatory cells in the wall decrease [16,17,18,20,24–31] but cellular and fibrotic elements remain with calcification. The lumen becomes somewhat larger due in part to diminution of lipids and inflammation and in part to structural remodeling of the artery [27], which remains scarred and smaller than normal [26]. With diminution of lipids and inflammation, plaque stabilization occurs with a decrease in unstable coronary syndromes or coronary events [16–21]. These pathologic correlates with coronary events or lack of events parallel the clinical observation that progression of stenosis severity on arteriograms is associated with subsequent coronary events, whereas stabilization or partial regression by arteriography are associated with low risk of coronary events [16–18,22,28,29]. Thus, the term reversal or regression as used clinically incorporates the spectrum of beneficial changes in plaque composition and pathology, compensatory arterial structural changes, arteriographic severity, vasomotor function, flow capacity, symptoms and prognosis. Certainly, regression back to normal in all of these processes does not occur. However, these terms appropriately characterize the cumulative benefits seen clinically as a symptom-free individual at low risk of coronary events with continuing lifelong risk-factor modification.

Figure 1 illustrates a clinical pathway or algorithm relying principally on noninvasive PET and reversal treatment for the comprehensive management of coronary artery disease. For patients who do not choose reversal treatment or prefer the immediate results of PTCA or coronary artery bypass surgery, or if the reversal program is not successful, these invasive procedures are backup alternatives in this clinical algorithm. This approach parallels conclusions of the CASS study demonstrating the appropriateness and safety of antianginal medical treatment with deferral of invasive revascularization [30]. However, in this algorithm, the principally antianginal treatments used in the CASS study are augmented by reversal regimens that stabilize plaque, partially reverse stenoses and prevent myocardial infarction, sudden death and unstable coronary syndromes requiring bypass surgery or PTCA.

A firm diagnosis of coronary artery disease is essential as the basis for undertaking a vigorous, lifelong reversal regimen, as for example documentation by prior myocardial infarction, coronary arteriography, previous PTCA or coronary artery bypass surgery. For individuals without an established diagnosis of coronary artery disease, cardiac positron

996

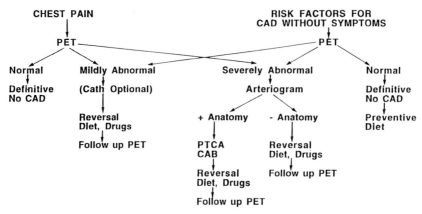

Fig. 1. Diagnosing and managing the cardiovascular patient with cardiac PET.

emission tomography (PET) detects coronary artery disease and assesses its severity with a diagnostic sensitivity and specificity of 95% as shown in Table 1, thereby providing a noninvasive, reliable diagnosis of coronary artery disease as the basis for reversal treatment. PET identifies which coronary arteries are involved [31,32], and the quantitative severity of disease [31–35], is as accurate in asymptomatic as in symptomatic subjects in one study [35], and in our experience is as good or better than arteriography for following changes in stenosis severity [31,36]. Since myocardial perfusion reflects the integrated effects of single or several stenoses, diffuse atherosclerosis and vasomotor dysfunction on coronary flow [5,31–40], quantitative PET imaging indicates severity of coronary artery disease beyond a single dimension (percent stenosis) of a single localized coronary arterial narrowing by arteriography. In addition, since perfusion is related to lumen radius raised to the fourth power, small changes in arteriographic lumen diameter that are difficult to see or measure on an arteriogram produce proportionately greater changes in perfusion that are visually obvious and easily quantified on a PET scan [31]. Finally, improved myocardial perfusion by PET is observed as early as 90 days after starting vigorous lipid lowering before anatomic regression occurs, thereby reflecting early improvement in vasomotor responses probably mediated by the favorable influence of cholesterol lowering on endothelial function [41].

Table 1. Sensitivity and specificity of cardiac PET

Sensitivity	Specificity	Number of patients	Reference
94%	95%	193	Demer Circ 79:825,1989
94%	95%	48	Gupta AHJ 122:293, 1992
98%	93%	208	Williams J Myo Isch 2:38, 1990
95%	82%	132	Go JNM 31:1899, 1990
95%	100%	50	Gould JACC 7:775, 1986
84%	88%	81	Stewart AJC 67:1303, 1991
98%	100%	51	Tamaki JNM 29:1181, 1988
97%	100%	32	Schelbert AJC 49:1197, 1982
97%	100%	60	Yonekura AHG 113:645, 1987
95%	95%	855	Average

Conclusion

Current knowledge and practical experience suggest that the comprehensive noninvasive management of coronary artery disease based on PET and reversal treatment is a valid, safe and effective alternative to traditional invasive approaches for diagnosing and treating coronary heart disease at substantial cost reductions compared to standard cardiology practice emphasizing coronary arteriography, balloon dilation and bypass surgery.

References

1. Gould KL. Circulation 1994;90:1558—1571.
2. Brown GB, Albers JJ, Fisher LD, Schaefer SM, Lin JT, Kaplan CA, Zhao XQ, Bisson BD, Fitzpatrick VF, Dodge HT. N Engl J Med 1990;323:1289—1298.
3. Ornish DM, Scherwitz LW, Brown SE, Billings JH, Armstrong WT, Ports TA, McLanahan SM, Kirkeeide RL, Brand RJ, Gould KL. Lancet 1990;336:129—133.
4. Kane JP, Malloy MJ, Ports TA, Philips NR, Diehl JC, Havel RJ. J Am Med Assoc 1990;264:3007—3012.
5. Gould KL, Ornish D, Kirkeeide R, Brown S, Stuart Y, Buchi M, Billings J, Armstrong W, Ports, Thomas, Scherwitz L. Am J Cardiol 1992;69:845—853.
6. Watts GF, Lewis B, Brunt JN, Lewis ES, Coltart DJ, Smith LD, Mann JI, Swan AV. Lancet 1992;339:563—569.
7. Schuler G, Hambrecht R, Schlierf G, Grunze M, Methfessel S, Hauer K, Kubler W. J Am Coll Cardiol 1992;19:34—42.
8. Schuler G, Hambrecht R, Schlierf G, Niebauer J, Hauer K, Neumann J, Hoberg E, Drinkmann A, Bacher F, Grunze M, Kubler W. Circulation 1992;86:1—11.
9. Buchwald H, Vargo RL et al. N Engl J Med 1990;323:946—955.
10. Singh RB, Rastogi SS, Verna R et al. Br Med J 1992;304:1015—1019.
11. Blankenhorn DH, Nessim SA, Johnson RL, Sanmarco ME, Azen SP, Cashin-Hemphill L. J Am Med Assoc 1987;257:3233—3240.
12. Cashin-Hemphill L, Mack WJ, Pogoda JM, Sanmarco ME, Azen SP, Blankenhorn DH. J Am Med Assoc 1990;264:3013—3017.
13. Haskell WL, Alderman EL, Fair JM, Maron JD, Mackey SF, Superko HR, Williams PT, Johnstone IM, Champagne, MA, Krauss RM, Farquhar JW. Circulation 1994;89:975—990.
14. Second Report of the Expert Panel on Detection, evaluation, and treatment of high blood cholesterol in adults (adult treatment panel II), National Cholesterol Education Program. Circulation 1994;89:1329—1445.
15. Blankenhorn DH. Coronary Artery Dis 1991;2:875—879.
16. Brown BG, Zhao XQ, Sacco DE, Albers JJ. Circulation 1993;87:1781—1791.
17. Stewart BF, Grown BG, Zhao XQ, Hillger LA, Sniderman AD, Dowdy A, Fisher LD, Albers JJ. J Am Coll Cardiol 1994;23:899—906.
18. Fuster V, Badimon L, Badimon JJ, Chesebro JH. N Engl J Med 1992;326:242—318.
19. Loree HM, Kamm RD, Stringfellow RG, Lee RT. Circ Res 1992;71:850—858.
20. van der Wal AC, Becker AE, van der Loos CM, Das PK. Circulation 1994;89:36—44.
21. Richardson PD, Davies MJ, Born GVR. Lancet 1989;2:941—944.
22. Ambrose JA, Tannenbaum MA, Alexopoulos D et al. J Am Coll Cardiol 1988;12:56—62.
23. The VA Coronary Artery Bypass Surgery Cooperative Study Group. Circulation 1992;86:121—130.
24. Benzuly KH, Padgett RC, Kaul S, Piegors DJ, Armstrong ML, Heistad DD. Circulation 1994;89:1810—1818.
25. Small DM, Bond MG, Waugh D, Prack M, Sawyer JK. J Clin Invest 1984;73:1590—1605.
26. Armstrong ML, Heistad DD, Marcus ML, Piegors DJ, Abboud FM. J Clin Invest 1983;71:104—113.
27. Glagov S, Weisenberg E, Zarins CK et al. N Engl J Med 1987;316:1371—1375.
28. Buchwald H, Matts JP, Fitch LL, Campos CT, Sanmarco ME, Amplatz K, Castaneda-Zuniga WR, Hunter DW, Pearce MB, Bissett JK et al. J Am Med Assoc 1992;268:1429—1433.
29. Waters D, Craven TE, Lesperance J. Circulation 1993;87:1067—1075.
30. CASS Principal Investigators and Their Associates. Circulation 1983;68:939—950.
31. Gould KL. Coronary Artery Stenoses. A textbook of coronary pathophysiology, quantitative coronary arteriography, PET perfusion imaging and reversal of coronary artery disease. New York, Amsterdam, London: Elsevier Scientific Publishing Company, 1991;7—135.
32. Gould KL. J Nucl Med 1991;32:579—606.

998

33. Demer LL, Gould KL, Goldstein RA, Kirkeeide RL. Circulation 1989;79:825–835.
34. Gould KL, Goldstein RA, Mullani N, Kirkeeide R, Wong G, Smalling R, Fuentes F, Nishikawa A, Matthews W. J Am Coll Cardiol 1986;7:775–792.
35. Gould KL. Circulation 1991;84(Suppl I):I-22–I-36.
36. Gould KL, Ornish D, Brown S, Edens RB, Hess MJ, Mullani, N, Bolomey L, Dobbs F, Merritt T, Sparler S, Scherwitz L, Billings J. Changes in myocardial perfusion abnormalities by positron emission tomography at five years in the lifestyle heart trial. Circulation (abstract in press, AHA Scientific meeting November 1994, Dallas, Texas).
37. Seiler C, Kirkeeide RL, Gould KL. Circulation 1992;85:1987–2003.
38. Gould, KL, Kirkeeide RL, Buchi M. J Am Coll Cardiol 1990;15:459–474.
39. Gould KL, Lipscomb K, Hamilton GW. Am J Cardiol 1974;33:87–94.
40. Gould KL. Am J Cardiol 1978;41:267–278.
41. Gould KL, Martucci JP, Goldberg DI, Hess MJ, Edens RP, Latifi R, Dudrick SJ. Circulation 1994;89: 1530–1538.

Gamma camera imaging of atherosclerotic lesions

Robert S. Lees[1,3] and Ann M. Lees[2,3]

[1]*Harvard/MIT Division of Health Sciences and Technology,* [2]*Harvard Medical School and* [3]*Boston Heart Foundation, Cambridge, Massachusetts, USA*

Abstract. A major challenge in the treatment of patients with atherosclerosis is the detection of unstable atherosclerotic plaques before they occlude the blood supply to vital organs. We have used the techniques of nuclear medicine to work towards a practical solution to this important problem. Using the planar gamma camera, with radiolabeled low density lipoproteins as the radiopharmaceutical, a virtually noninvasive technique, we have made considerable progress in detecting unstable lesions. Recently we have developed labeled plaque-seeking synthetic peptides, and have shown that they provide even better resolution of active atheromatous lesions.

Atherosclerosis is a relapsing and remitting disease characterized by bursts of active lesion growth followed by periods of healing and fibrosis [1]. Catastrophic arterial occlusion usually occurs when minimally stenotic, metabolically active plaques, rather than hemodynamically significant, metabolically quiescent stenoses, undergo rupture or intramural hemorrhage and produce sudden luminal obstruction [2–3]. The active plaque is full of foam cells, monocytes and other leukocytes, necrotic debris and newly grown thin-walled blood vessels [2]. The foam cells in the shoulders of the lesion cause mechanical weakness, which predisposes to plaque rupture and thrombotic occlusion, while the thin-walled blood vessels in the plaque are prone to break and cause intramural hemorrhage and mechanical occlusion as the plaque is pushed into the lumen by the growing intramural clot [2].

Current diagnostic methods cannot assess plaque stability. Unstable plaques usually cause less than 50% diameter stenosis and therefore do not cause turbulent blood flow at the site, or diminished end-organ perfusion. Thus, the patient suffers no warning symptoms and there is no audible bruit at the site, if a peripheral vessel is involved.

We have approached this problem over the last dozen years by taking advantage of the plaque's metabolic activity in order to detect its presence. The profound changes which atherosclerosis produces in the vessel wall are accompanied by equally great changes in its metabolism. In 1983 we observed that healing experimental arterial lesions in the rabbit showed marked accumulation of ^{125}I-labeled low-density lipoproteins (^{125}I-LDL) [4]. In the same year we showed that human carotid atheromas could also be imaged and localized with ^{125}I-LDL and the clinical gamma scintillation ("Anger") camera [5]. However, since ^{125}I was not a satisfactory isotope for external imaging, we set out to find a better one. This led to the synthesis of ^{99m}technetium-labeled LDL (^{99m}Tc-LDL) and to the demonstration that this radiopharmaceutical could be used to image experimental rabbit arterial lesions [6] as well as receptor-mediated adrenal LDL uptake in rabbits [7]. We followed with a clinical study in which ^{99m}Tc-LDL was shown to image unstable human atherosclerosis [8]. In human studies, however, the long plasma half-life of LDL diminished the sensitivity of the method, since the persistence of ^{99m}Tc-LDL in the human

Address for correspondence: Boston Heart Foundation, 139 Main Street, Cambridge, MA 02142, USA.

blood pool produced an increased background which hindered visualization of lesion LDL uptake. These studies made it clear that we could detect active plaque with much greater accuracy and sensitivity if we could design an agent that would rapidly enter athero-sclerotic lesions, and simultaneously leave the blood pool rapidly.

We made the assumption that LDL is directed into the arterial wall by its protein rather than its lipid moiety, since the protein, apolipoprotein B (apoB) is unique to LDL, VLDL (very-low-density-lipoproteins) and chylomicrons, which are also atherogenic, while the lipids are similar to those in the antiatherogenic lipoprotein, HDL, as well as most body tissues. We made one other assumption, supported by experimental data [9], that the LDL receptor was not involved in LDL accumulation in the arterial wall, since patients with total absence of that receptor develop severe premature atherosclerosis. Taking advantage of the then recently published primary structure of apoB, we synthesized a peptide representing a surface domain [10] of apoB in the non-receptor-binding region of the molecule, labeled it with ^{125}I, and tested its accumulation in experimental rabbit lesions [11]. As a control, we also made a peptide which represented the LDL-receptor-binding domain of apolipoprotein E (apoE). The non-receptor-binding apoB peptide ("SP-4") accumulated rapidly at high concentration in the rabbit lesions, while the receptor-binding apoE peptide ("SP-2") accumulated diffusely in the surrounding de-endothelialized areas [11].

We and our collaborators [12] showed that ^{125}I-labeled SP-4 allowed experimental rabbit arterial lesions to be imaged, much as was accomplished with whole LDL, despite the much smaller size of the peptide (~2.2 kDa) in comparison to LDL (~2,500 kDa). The small, radiolabeled peptide was removed from the blood pool with a half-time of a few minutes, in striking comparison to that of LDL, which is about 20 h in the rabbit.

In collaboration with Drs Richard T. Dean and John Lister-James at Diatech Incorporated, two similar ^{99m}Tc labeled analogs of SP-4 were synthesized. They, too, allowed ready imaging of experimental rabbit atheromas as well as spontaneous lesions in Watanabe rabbits [12,13]. One of these agents is now in a multicenter US clinical trial. Although in its early stages, the trial suggests that active human arteriosclerotic plaques may be imaged with the ^{99m}Tc-peptide with a very low blood pool background, since both plaque uptake and radiopharmaceutical disappearance from the blood pool seem to be very rapid, just as in the rabbit. The role of plaque-imaging radiopharmaceuticals in diagnosis of unstable atherosclerotic plaques and their value in directing therapy to avoid myocardial infarction and stroke remains to be seen when the current study is completed and wider clinical testing is undertaken.

Acknowledgements

The authors are grateful for the valuable insight of their many collaborators in this work. Drs Robert and Ann Lees have a direct and indirect equity interest, respectively, in Diatech Incorporated.

References

1. Forrester JS et al. Circulation 1987;75:505–523.
2. Davies MJ, Thomas AC. Br Heart J 1985;53:363–373.
3. Fuster V et al. Circulation 1990;82 (suppl 2):47–59.
4. Roberts AB, Lees AM, Lees RS, Strauss HW, Fallon JT, Taveras J, Kopiwoda S. J Lipid Res 1983;24:1160–1167.
5. Lees RS, Lees AM, Strauss HW. J Nucl Med 1983;24:154–156.

6. Lees RS, Garabedian HD, Lees AM, Schumacher DJ, Miller A, Isaacsohn JL, Derksen A, Strauss HW. J Nucl Med 1985;26:1056—1062.

7. Isaacsohn JL, Lees AM, Lees RS, Strauss HW, Barlai-Kovach M, Moore TJ. Metabolism 1986;35:364—366.

8. Lees AM, Lees RS, Schoen FJ, Isaacsohn JL, Fischman AJ, McKusick KA, Strauss HW. Arteriosclerosis 1988;8:461—470.

9. Fischman AJ, Lees AM, Lees RS, Barlai-Kovach M, Strauss HW. Arteriosclerosis 1987;7:361—366.

10. Forgez P, Gregory H, Young JA, Knott T, Scott J, Chapman MJ. Biochem Biophys Res Commun 1986; 140:250—257.

11. Shih I-L, Lees RS, Chang MY, Lees AM. Proc Natl Acad Sci USA 1991;87:1436—1440.

12. Hardoff R, Braegelmann F, Zanzonico P, Herrold E, Lees RS, Lees AM, Dean R, Lister-James J, Borer J. J Lipid Res 1993;33:1039—1047.

13. Dean RT, L-James J, Lees RS, Lees AM, Vallabhajosula S, Goldsmith SJ. In: Martin-Comin J (ed) Radiolabeled Blood Elements. New York: Plenum Press, 1994;195—199.

Three- and four-dimensional visualization of the coronary artery tree from standardized magnetic resonance angiography by interactive computer tools and volumetric holography

Justin D. Pearlman

Harvard Medical School and Department of Radiology, Beth Israel Hospital, Boston, MA 02215, USA

Abstract. Four approaches for performing 3D and 4D submillimeter-resolution magnetic resonance angiography (MRA) of the coronary arteries are presented. In all cases, images are collected using either progressive tip-angle turboFLASH with standard imaging planes, or echo-planar imaging. The techniques to be presented allow a complete examination to be performed on a clinical MRI system in less than 30 min and do not require operator knowledge of the coronary anatomy. The advantages and tradeoffs of each of four approaches are discussed. Novel computer and holographic methods for image postprocessing and display improve the visualization of coronaries over conventional and selective MIP techniques. The techniques presented make standardized acquisition MRA of the major epicardial coronary arteries suitable for trial clinical applications.

Introduction

Imaging of human coronary arteries by X-ray angiography began in 1945 [1] and is now pervasive, with over 500,000 catheterizations performed per year in the United States, at a cost of $1.8 billion/year. Magnetic resonance imaging (MRI), developing rapidly over the past 2 decades, initially was noted to show only small segments of the coronary arteries [2]. Computer reconstruction of long segments by dark-blood angiography showed that MRI could quantify the severity of stenosis in the proximal coronary arteries with good sensitivity and specificity [3]. Relatively recent improvements in MRI enable bright-blood angiography by magnetic resonance angiography (MRA) making artery segments bright whether they lie in the imaging plane or perpendicular to it [4,5]. Bright-blood coronary MRA can now be performed readily on standard clinical systems [6]. This has been applied clinically [7] with image planes selected by experts in cardiovascular anatomy. The goals of this study were to simplify the data collection to a method that requires no knowledge of the coronary anatomy, and to reconstruct the entire coronary artery tree rather than selected segments.

Methods

Data were collected using progressive tip angle turboFLASH with fat saturation, a fast magnetic resonance imaging (MRI) technique [8] that uses a rapid series of radiowave excitations to collect the magnetic resonance data needed in a dozen heartbeats or less. Four different strategies were compared. (1) SEQUENTIAL STATIC GRAPHIC PRESCRIPTION: 1–3 parallel images were acquired in a single breath-hold, ECG triggered to cover the last 150 ms of diastole, 10 datalines per heartbeat for 14–16 heartbeats or seven datalines per heartbeat for 18 heartbeats, producing a single image with 3-mm slice thickness and an in-plane resolution of 0.85 × 1.4 mm. On the basis of an initial transverse view, additional views are taken to identify the origin of the right and left coronary arteries in the aortic root. The results were used to prescribe a stack of six parallel slices that capture, substantially in-plane, the proximal and middle right coronary as it runs from its origin around in the atrioventricular groove to the posterior septum. A similar stack encompassing the septum shows the left-anterior descending, and a third stack shows the left circumflex, including its connection to the left main. The entire series of images requires 30 min. (2) STANDARDIZED STATIC STACK: 40–72 parallel overlapping slices (3 mm thick, 1 mm overlap, 0.85×1.4 mm in-plane resolution) were obtained during successive end-expiratory 18 s breath-holds, triggered to the diastasis period in mid-diastole. The number of slices required varies according to the size of the heart. Images are acquired either one or three slices at a time in a stack of either transverse or left-anterior oblique orientation. (3) BREATH-HOLD DYNAMIC STANDARDIZED STACK: shared centric reordered data are acquired for 12 successive heartbeats resulting in 24 movie frames of each slice. The total imaging time is the same as method 2, but produces a time-series volumetric stack instead of just diastolic images. (4) BREATH-HOLD STATIC 3D: the entire stack is obtained by sequential 3D phase-encoded echoplanar imaging (EPI) [8,9] in a single 24-s breath-hold, using fast-switching gradients. This produces eight slices (65 ms each) with a 128×256 matrix and 3/4 rectangular field of view, resulting in $3 \times 1.1 \times 1.7$ mm resolution (P. Wielopolski, unpublished).

In all 2D cases, the tip-angle ranged from 15 to 40°, starting low to avoid saturation of blood signal that remains in-plane, so that blood vessels appear bright whether flow is in the image planes or crosses through perpendicular to the imaging plane.

Images were presented as a movie, as maximal intensity projections through selected image planes that include the target artery (selective MIP), and by novel processing involving recognition and automated removal of obstructing blood pools from the data treated as 3D or 4D stacks [10] to produce unobstructed views of the coronary arteries. (A 4D stack is a time series of 3D stacks). Recognition of an overlying right atrioventricular blood pool, for example, was trained for the entire stack by a single click of a mouse button while pointing to a border of that blood pool (Fig. 1). A second click marked it for removal from the 3D stack, while interactive movie and arbitrary angle projections showed the immediate results, to ensure that only obstructing blood pool was removed and not any vessel branches. Fat saturation facilitated this because it results in a black zone around the epicardial vessels, separating them from blood-pool signal.

Volumetric holography was achieved by performing the image processing to remove the blood pools, followed by multiple exposure of X-ray film to each image layer in the stack. Each image layer presents an interference pattern between a reference laser beam and a beam reflected off a screen showing a particular imaging plane at its mechanically shifted slice location, using Voxel equipment (Voxel, Inc., Laguna Hills, CA). After multiple exposures the entire 3D dataset, not just a surface rendering, is displayed in the volumetric hologram.

Results

Figure 2 shows a comparison of selective MIP and object removal applied to right coronary images obtained by method 1. The techniques that make the coronary arteries bright also make other cardiac blood bright, and the locations of these blood pools interfere with projections, even when they are selectively limited to views that contain the target coronary artery (left). The object-removal technique circumvents this problem, revealing a much greater length of the coronary arteries in a single composite view (right).

Figures 3 and 4 show composite projections of the entire coronary artery tree using method 2 to obtain a transverse stack (Fig. 3) or a 40° left anterior oblique (LAO) stack

1004

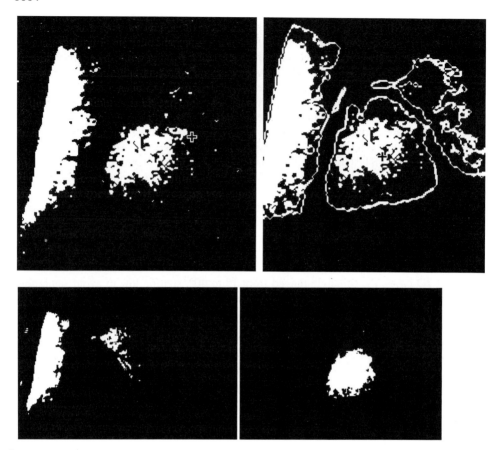

Fig. 1. (A, upper left): A single image frame from a stack of images encompassing the proximal right coronary. (B, upper right): Demarcated points have the same discriminant power as the training point for right ventricular blood-pool border definition. (C, lower left): all points outside the selected region. (D, lower right): points inside the selected region.

The computer learns what border you want from a single button click, for example with the mouse cursor (cross mark) at the border of the right ventricular blood and inter-ventricular septum. The computer examines statistically the signal intensities and distribution in the vicinity, defines a border by minimizing misclassification of in as out and vice versa, promptly and automatically marking all borders with similar characteristics, for the entire 3D stack of images. Removal of the selected region (by a second mouse button click) prevents right ventricular blood pool from obstructing the view of underlying segments of the right coronary artery when the remaining data are viewed as a 3D dataset.

(Fig. 4). The transverse stack required 72 overlapping slices, while the LAO stack required only 48 slices to cover the entire heart; each was completed in less than 30 min. Both the straight transverse and the oblique standardized stacks provided good visualization of the coronary tree. The straight transverse stack provided a better cranial view. It revealed small branch vessels not seen by method 1, including the right atrial branch of the right coronary artery as well as significant distal branches such as the acute marginal and the posterior descending. Anterior projections from the transverse stack are relatively coarse because they rely on out-of-plane resolution and data from separate breath-holds. Examination of selective projections and movie loops allowed rapid

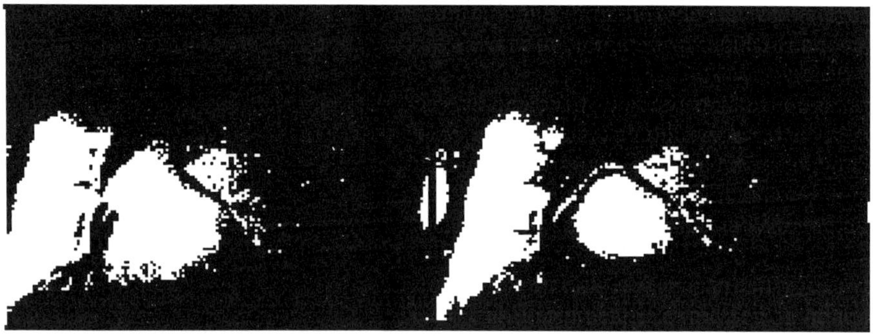

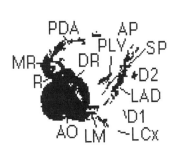

Fig. 2. Right coronary artery visualized by selective MIP (left) and by selective MIP after removal of obscuring blood-pools from individual images (right).

correction for misregistration, which ranged from 0 to 3 pixels. The LAO stack, which was faster to obtain because it required fewer images, provides better anterior views. Acquiring the stack of slices three slices at a time instead of one at a time increased the bandwidth per pixel by a factor of 3 and thus lowered the signal-to-noise ratio (SNR) by a factor of √3.

Volumetric holography [11] summarized the findings effectively in a single 3D view of the coronary arteries. The 3D myocardium can be used as an overlay to show the relation of vessel branches to the muscle supplied. The LAO stack was most effective for the holography, again because of the benefits of in-plane resolution for anterior projections.

The single breath-hold 3D avoids the problem of misregistration between breath-holds, at a sacrifice of SNR. Although the major coronary arteries can be identified, the resulting 3D data are lower in quality than that from the other methods and will require improved coil design to be reliable.

The 4D data facilitate image registration, at a sacrifice of SNR. The individual images

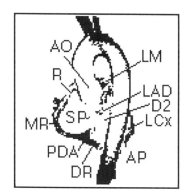

Fig. 3. 3D reconstructed coronary artery tree obtained from transverse stack. Key to labels appears below.

Fig. 4. 3D reconstructed coronary artery tree obtained from 40° LAO stack. Key to labels appears below.

AO = aortic root, AP = apex, LM = left main, LAD = anterior descending, LCx = circumflex, D1 = first diagonal, D2 = second diagonal, SP = septal perforator, R = right coronary, MR = midright, PDA = posterior descending, DR = distal right, PLV = posterior left ventricular extension of right coronary.

in the centric-shared movies have less than 70% of the SNR of the images by methods 1 and 2, but multiple time frames can be combined to a single improved view, or the 3D coronary maps can be produced for each time frame, resulting in a dynamic movie loop of 3D reconstructions.

Discussion

This study shows that MRA can produce good-quality 3D coronary angiograms completely noninvasively, without injection of a contrast agent. Furthermore, it shows that the data for the 3D angiograms can be easily collected in a standardized manner by a technologist without knowledge of the coronary anatomy. Reconstruction using special software to remove obstructing blood pools is effective and reliable, and volumetric holography is an effective means of presenting the results on a single sheet of film. Comparison of 2D, 3D and 4D methods shows that image quality at the target resolution (1 mm or smaller in-plane) is the primary determinant of the quality of the results, for subjects who can follow instructions for sequential 20-s end tidal breath-holds and who can lie still for 25 min. The single breath-hold 3D method requires less cooperation but requires optimized cardiac coils and fast gradient switching. The level of cooperation needed is not strikingly different from that required for X-ray selective angiography. Thus for the purpose of mapping out the anatomy of the major epicardial coronary arteries, standardized-acquisition 3D MRA is now suitable for trial clinical applications.

Although there has been much effort devoted to quantification of the severity of stenoses, treatment planning often combines clinical evidence of the severity of ischemia or risk by history, perfusion and stress tests with knowledge of the coronary anatomy to identify suitable implant sites for bypass grafts or accessibility of lesions for angioplasty and other catheter-based interventions. Thus coronary anatomy alone can provide useful data, independent of the assessment of lesion severity.

MRA is not without significant limitations. The bore of the magnet eliminates the extremely obese and the claustrophobic. The magnetic field eliminates those with pacemakers. The techniques that require several heartbeats to represent similar cardiac position have difficulties with cardiac dysrhythmia. The use of vascular clips and stents can produce image artifacts that impair the usefulness of MRA. Nevertheless, a large patient population is suited for the techniques presented, and can benefit from virtually zero-risk examination of their coronary anatomy.

If magnetic resonance angiography (MRA) can supplant X-rays for screening or for select follow-up, it could reduce the risk and possibly facilitate earlier detection of problems. Although the risk of X-ray angiography is low, it is still undesirable for screening asymptomatic subjects with low a priori risk. As half the coronary artery disease cases in the Framingham study [12] presented as sudden death, improved detection of silent disease is highly desired.

Three-dimensional data are harder to present than two-dimensional images, but the 3D data convey holistic information that is difficult if not impossible to garner from lower dimensions. A variety of computer methods were employed for visualization, relying on movie sequences to simulate motion parallax, shading and obstruction to indicate depth. Special devices allow inclusion of binocular disparity (different images presented to each eye, representing slightly different viewpoints) but volumetric holography supplants these with a more natural interaction that includes virtually all depth cues because information is in fact reconstructed in three dimensions. Thus the entire stack of image planes is reproduced on a single film, including views not possible by X-ray angiography such as the superior–inferior view shown with computer shading for depth in Figs. 3 and 4. Volumetric holography can in principle present the 4D data as well, as a series of volumetric holograms presented successively as a movie, but that has yet to be implemented, so we rely on computer-generated movies to review the data as depth-shaded images in a movie loop, with epicycles of rotation to show the data from different views.

Conclusion

The 3D coronary artery anatomy can be delineated by MRA. Using the image processing techniques presented here, a technologist without knowledge of the coronary anatomy can acquire all the information needed for visualization of the coronaries using a standardized acquisition. Features of MRA that are desirable for this achievement are: submillimeter resolution, SNR > 20, acquisition during breath-hold, effective fat saturation, and bright signal from coronary arteries whether they lie in-plane or cross through the image sections. The use of sequential breath-holds at comfortable end-tidal diaphragm position provided reasonably good image registration (less than three pixel shift, substantially corrected by software). Obtaining a movie at each level greatly increases the amount of data, but allows both 4D presentation (rendered on the computer screen), and selective combinations of views to improve SNR and optimize image registration for changes in timing. Completion of the entire 3D acquisition in a single breath-hold is possible by segmented EPI, but at a 3-fold loss in SNR or the equivalent increase in size of the resolution elements. The coronary arteries are visible by the 3D single breath-hold technique, and use of specialized cardiac coils may improve the SNR sufficiently to make that technique clinically valuable. Currently, the most reliable and effective visualization was achieved by sequential breath-hold parallel slice coverage of the heart in left anterior oblique orientation, using segmented turboFLASH.

References

1. Radner S. Acta Radiol 1945;26:497.
2. Paulin S, von Schulthess GH, Fossel ET, Krayenbuehl HP. Am J Radiol 1987;148:665–670.
3. Pearlman JD. In: Sideman S, Beyar R (eds) Image Analysis and Simulation of the Cardiac System. Proc 5th Henry Goldberg Workshop on Analysis and Simulation of the Cardiac System. London: Freund Publishing House, 1990;451–464.
4. Atkinson DJ, Edelman RR. Radiology 1991;178:357–360.
5. Chien D, Edelman RR. Magn Reson Q 1991;7:31–56.
6. Edelman RR, Mattle HP, Atkinson DJ, Hoogewoud HM. J Roentgenol 1990;154(5):937–946.
7. Manning WJ, Li W, Edelman RR. N Engl J Med 1993;328(12):828–832.
8. Pearlman JD, Edelman RR. In: Radiologic Clinics of North America. Philadelphia: W.B. Saunders, 1994; 593–612.
9. Edelman RR, Wielopolski P, Schmitt F. Radiology 1994;192(3):600–612.
10. Pearlman JD, Li W, Chuang ML. J Mag Res Img 1994;4(P):81.
11. Pearlman JD, Chuang ML, Schulz RA, Geil G. In: Boehme JM, Rowberg AH, Wolfman NT (eds) Computer Applications to Assist Radiology, Proceedings of S/CAR-94, Carlsbad CA: Symposia Foundation, 1994;775–776.
12. Gordon T, Costelle W, Hjortland M. Am J Med 1977;62:701–714.

Accurate quantitation of atheroma inside arterial walls by ^{1}H-NMR

J.D. Pearlman and Y. Gazit

Harvard Medical School and Department of Radiology, Beth Israel Hospital, Boston, MA 02215, USA

Abstract. Magnetic resonance (MR) techniques can identify lipid signals from arteries of human subjects. Two very similar lipid signals are found; one, inside the wall, can lead to heart attack and stroke (the atheroma lipid) and the other, just outside the vessel wall, does not (perivascular fat). Since the spatial resolution of typical MR systems is of the order of the size of the vessel wall itself, these systems fail to distinguish completely the atheroma signal from that of perivascular fat. Consequently, a major focus of our investigations has been a) to characterize the signal differences, b) to distinguish between the two similar signals and c) to quantify the atheroma content. We have successfully measured chemical information about early atherosclerosis in human artery walls using noninvasive magnetic resonance techniques on patient volunteers. The chemical information provides a quantitative estimate of the accumulation of atheroma lipid that causes atherosclerosis within the blood vessel wall. We have developed analytic techniques that can differentiate between the MR signals generated by atheroma and fat. These techniques may assess wall-active treatments to liquefy and expel atheroma deposits from the arterial wall, and monitor atheromatous disease at very early stages. These results offer clinically useful techniques to diagnose, characterize and quantify atherosclerosis at early reversible stages of its development.

There is no clinical technique available to identify the onset and progression of atherosclerosis until it has progressed to a point of impinging on obstruction of a blood vessel. Blood tests do not assess the severity of the disease within the vessel wall, but only indicate an indirect risk factor. Problematically, severe disease may occur with normal blood cholesterol levels and vice versa. The unavailability of a diagnostic technique to detect and monitor the progress of atherosclerosis during the early stages of the disease inhibits the ability of the clinician to halt progression, prevent the catastrophic consequences of atherosclerosis (stroke, heart attack, and kidney failure) and potentially avoid invasive procedures that would be needed at later stages of the disease. NMR offers a noninvasive method for measuring the amount of atheroma in blood vessel walls. We sought to develop techniques that measure the small amounts of atheroma that are present during the early stages of the disease. Such techniques can help the clinician to detect and monitor the progress of the disease under dietary and drug-therapy regimens.

Two problems inhibit the utilization of current MR imaging methods for the assessment of atheroma deposits in blood vessel walls. First, the basic resolution of the clinical methods is of the order of the target size, i.e., the vessel wall thickness, making it difficult to obtain useful information on a clinical system that is based on location [1–3]. Second, the MR spectral peaks of perivascular fat and atheroma are similar, which makes it difficult to differentiate between them. As perivascular fat and atheroma are both present in the vessel vicinity it is essential to develop methods that distinguish between their contributions to the MR signal. Three new methods based on T1, T2 and relative intensity measures were investigated. Spectral analysis of fat and atheroma show that the greatest difference in T1 (spin-lattice relaxation time) occurs at the secondary methyl peak. While the measured signal intensities can be modeled with double exponentials we find that the resulting errors are too great given the amount of data that can be collected in a clinical examination. We developed a new method, termed the "effective T1" method, which uses a simple model to characterize the data, and produces an accurate one-to-one relationship with the fraction of atheroma in the mixture.

Methods

Studies were performed both in human volunteers and ex vivo for validation of accuracy. The noninvasive human studies were performed first on a GE Signa, then on a Siemens Vision prototype, at 1.5 tesla. An open bird-cage receive coil with Q = 300 was constructed to optimize signal detection. Scout magnetic resonance images of the target artery (carotid or popliteal) were obtained for localization, and the target region was designated by graphics prescription. For carotid studies, the region of interest was centered on the carotid bifurcation. For the popliteal artery, the region of interest was centered in the popliteal fossa, and reference distances along the vessel to branch points were recorded, so that the same area could be identified for future comparison studies. The target region for spectroscopy was then designated by graphics prescription. The chemical spectrum of the material within the designated voxel was measured either by STEAM [4] or by RME [5,6]. STEAM is readily implemented on convention MRI systems but at a minimum echo time of 10 ms. This was problematic because the T2 values of interest are shorter than 10 ms [7]. RME provides relaxivity-corrected excitation with effectively zero echo time and the target can be set as small as 1 mm^3 with <2% signal from outside the specified region [6]. Inversion recovery spectra are obtained with 12 different TI values, TR = 2 s, TE = 0 or 10 ms, 1024 points. Water suppression of 1000:1 was achieved by applying a modified CHESS preparation [8] with four selective excitations and a geometric progression of spoilers (8–10).

For controlled evaluation of accuracy, a series of ex vivo samples containing varying ratios of synthetic atheroma and human perivascular fat were prepared. The human perivascular fat was stripped from the aorta and from mesenteric arteries fresh at autopsy. Atheroma lipids from early atheromatous lesions were extracted in methanol [11], characterized spectroscopically [7] and chemically by thin-layer chromatography, trans-esterification and high-pressure gas–liquid chromatography [12], and then simulacra were prepared to supply several identical samples with the composition and physical state representative of the *early stages* of atherosclerosis.

Synthetic atheromata were prepared with 35.3% cholesteryl linoleate, 27.0% cholesteryl oleate, 27.8% cholesterol and 9.8% triolein. Spectra from this simulacrum matched the spectral and chemical characteristics of human atheroma [7,12,13]. Samples were housed in an NMR tube of 10 mm diameter together with an insert comprising an 8-mm diameter outer tube with a clay plug at the bottom and an inner tube of 3 mm diameter, flushed with nitrogen (to prevent oxidation), sealed, and refrigerated. With every batch of samples an extra sample, having the same geometry but filled with saline, was prepared and used for shimming the magnet. 24 h before the experiment the samples were brought to room temperature. At least 2 h before the experiment samples were placed in a 37°C thermal bath for equilibration to body temperature.

The ex vivo experiments were conducted on a Bruker 9.4T MSL-400 Imaging Spectrometer, using a VT1000 temperature control unit. The temperature control was set to 37°C with an accuracy of ±1°C.

The spin-lattice relaxation time (T1) measurements were performed using the inversion recovery sequence: 180°-τ-90°. A series of twelve inversion times was used for each sample. The dwell time was 50 μs; the acquisition delay 30 μs; TR 10 s; the 90° pulse was typically 19 μs. Sixteen scans were obtained for each inversion time. The intensity values for each peak were then fitted to an exponential inversion recovery curve of the form:

$$I = I_0(1-B \cdot e^{\frac{-t}{T1}})$$ (1)

to obtain an estimate of T1. The fit was performed using the nonlinear regression Marquardt method [14]. A three-parameter inversion recovery curve was used. Including the B parameter corrects for B1 inhomogeneity and potential inaccuracies in the flip angles [15,16].

Both single- and double-exponential inversion recovery curves were fit to the data from fat–atheroma mixtures. Use of the single exponential model on mixtures results in a single value of T1, termed the *effective T1*. The *effective T1* and its error are used to estimate the fractional content of atheroma in the mixture by each of two methods.

Method 1 relies on a priori knowledge of:
- T1 of pure fat (determined by analyzing a region of fat) and its standard error.
- T1 of atheroma (determined by ex vivo measurements) and its standard deviation.
- The coefficient, B, of the inversion recovery curve,

$$I = I_0(1-B \cdot e^{\frac{-t}{T1}})$$

which reflects inaccuracies in the tip angles and the B1 inhomogeneity.

These constants were used to generate a data set that matches the fractional content of atheroma with the *effective T1* and its error. For each of the twelve *inversion times*, T1 values of atheroma and fat are chosen randomly from normal populations using the known means and standard deviations. Each set of twelve data points is analyzed by a nonlinear regression algorithm to determine the *effective T1*. This process is repeated 1,000 times for each fractional value. The resulting 1,000 values of *effective T1* are then analyzed to determine their mean and standard deviation.

Method 2 assumes that if a value of **t** existed for which the equation:

$$1-B \cdot e^{\frac{-t}{T1_{eff}}} = f(1-B \cdot e^{\frac{-t}{T1_{ath}}}) + (1-f)(1-B \cdot e^{\frac{-t}{T1_{fat}}})$$ (2)

held for every value of the fractional content of atheroma lipid by weight, f, the percentage could be calculated by using the formula:

$$f = \frac{e^{\frac{-t}{T1_{fat}}} - e^{\frac{-t}{T1_{eff}}}}{e^{\frac{-t}{T1_{fat}}} - e^{\frac{-t}{T1_{ath}}}}$$ (3)

However, we know that a different value of f will yield a different value of **t** as the solution. Nevertheless, it will be shown that we will not jeopardize our accuracy at all by using a single value of **t** for all calculations, namely the *effective T1* for a 50:50 mixture of atheroma and adipose tissue.

Both methods were applied to a series of $T1_{eff}$ values ranging from 760 ms to 1150 ms with an increment of 10 ms and $\delta T1_{eff} = 10$ ms.

Results

Figure 1 shows a scout image of the popliteal fossa of a human volunteer, and Fig. 2 shows graphic prescription of a 1-cm^3 volume encasing the popliteal artery for spectroscopy. Fig. 3C shows the ^{1}H spectrum obtained in 64 s (TR = 2 s, NA = 32). For comparison, Fig. 3A shows the ex vivo ^{1}H spectrum of a sample of pure fat (human adipose) and Fig. 3B shows the ^{1}H spectrum of just the atheroma lipids extracted at necropsy. In all three, water signal is suppressed >1000:1. The human popliteal spectrum is a hybrid of perivascular fat and atheroma lipid. Relative heights differ, but the chemical shifts (position along the horizontal axis) of the peaks are similar, as this is primarily determined by the electron cloud due to the immediate chemical neighborhood. The chemical assignments corresponding to the prominent peaks in these spectra are shown in Table 1. Table 1 also shows the T1 values for those peaks, which distinguish fat from atheroma.

T1 of the spectral peaks in fat and atheroma

While the spectra of fat and atheroma exhibit essentially the same peaks (Fig. 3) they can still be differentiated by their T1 relaxation times. Typical values of T1 for the four most prominent peaks in these spectra, at 9.4 tesla, are listed in Table 1. Since the greatest difference in T1 of fat and atheroma occurs at the secondary methyl peak, we rely on this peak to differentiate between the two components. Consequently, in the following discussion T1$_{fat}$ and T1$_{ath}$ refers to the T1 at the secondary methyl peak in the spectra of fat and atheroma, respectively.

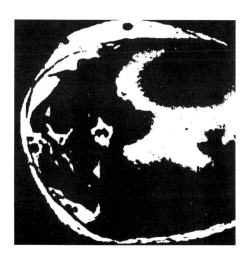

Fig. 1. MR image of a human knee. In this axial scout image of a human knee the popliteal artery is identified and located for further spectroscopic analysis. This artery is selected since it is near the surface and will readily respond to external thermotropic changes. This will allow the characterization of the physical state of atheroma as a function of temperature.

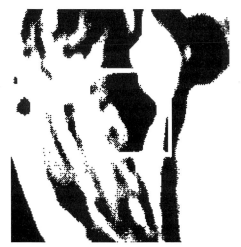

Fig. 2. Localization of 1-cm^3 voxel for spectroscopic analysis. A 1-cm^3 volume element (voxel) is defined to include the interior of the artery and the vascular walls.

Table 1. Principal chemical assignment of the major spectral peaks and their T1 relaxation times

Peak	Location (ppm)	$T1_{fat}$ (ms)	$T1_{ath}$ (ms)
Vinyl (=CH-)	5.28	940	850
Allylic methylene (=CH-CH₂)	1.99–2.18	560	680
Aliphatic methylene ((CH₂)ₙ)	1.27	615	655
Secondary methyl (CH₃)	0.87	1200	750

Double-exponential fit

The inversion recovery experimental data points, which originate from two separate components of different T1 (perivascular fat and atheroma), can be fit to the double exponential inversion recovery curve

$$I = I_1(1 - B \cdot e^{\frac{-t}{T1_{fat}}}) + I_2(1 - B \cdot e^{\frac{-t}{T1_{ath}}})$$ (4)

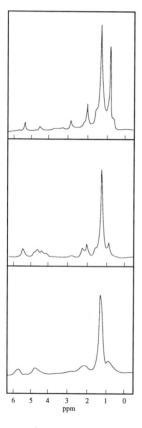

Fig. 3. ¹H-NMR spectra from the popliteal artery of a patient, and from ex vivo samples of perivascular fat and purified atheroma lipid. TOP: pure atheroma (total lipid extract from the medial wall of the artery, ex vivo). MIDDLE: pure adipose (ex vivo spectrum of microdissected perivascular fat). BOTTOM: in vivo spectrum from the popliteal artery of a patient. The in vivo spectrum includes fat and atheroma lipid signals, which are distinguished by T1 analysis.

which requires identification of five independent parameters from twelve data points.

Defining the fractional atheroma content as:

$$f = \frac{I_2}{I_1 + I_2} \tag{5}$$

the error in the fractional content estimate is

$$\Delta f = \sqrt{(\frac{I_1}{(I_1+I_2)^2} \Delta I_2)^2 + (\frac{I_2}{(I_1+I_2)^2} \Delta I_1)^2} \tag{6}$$

where $\Delta I_{1,2}$ are the standard errors of I_1 and I_2, respectively.

The results of the analysis based on the five-parameter fit exhibit large error bounds ($\Delta f = 0.43 \pm 0.23$). We concluded that a different approach to the T1 mixture analysis needs to be taken to reduce the errors in the fractional content estimates.

Effective T1 methods

The fractional content calculations using T1 measurements were performed using two methods, both of which employ the effective T1, $T1_{eff}$, as their input.

Method 1

The data from known mixtures of fat and atheroma fit a second-order polynomial:

$$f = -0.004800 \cdot T1_{eff} + 0.000001321 \cdot T1_{eff}^2 + 3.843 \tag{7}$$

where f is the fractional atheroma content and $T1_{eff}$ is the *effective T1* in ms, with $r^2 = 0.999942$, and is plotted in Fig 4.

The standard deviation data fit a second-order polynomial:

$$SDT1_{eff} = -0.342 \cdot T1_{eff} + 0.000175 \cdot T1_{eff}^2 + 189.2 \tag{8}$$

where $SDT1_{eff}$ is the standard deviation of the effective T1 (in ms), with $r^2 = 0.941935$. A measured value of effective T1 ($T1_{eff}$) can be substituted into the above equations to determine the fractional content of atheroma. The error is much smaller than that for double exponential fit. Figure 4 shows the fractional content of atheroma vs. effective T1, based on method 1. For example the effective T1 of 1,140 ms for the spectrum from a patient's popliteal artery indicates that 10% of the lipid in the sampled region was atheroma.

Method 2

Regression determined the slope of true fractional content vs. the calculated fractional content as m = 1.0055 ± 0.0019 with $r^2 = 0.9999$. Paired *t*-test showed the mean difference is –0.00041 between the true fractional content and the calculated fractional content, with a standard deviation of 0.00080. The difference is not significant ($p > 0.5$). Use of a fixed **t** (i.e., the zero crossing for 50:50 mixture) for all Method 2 calculations provides a simple technique without significant loss of accuracy. Comparison of Method

1014

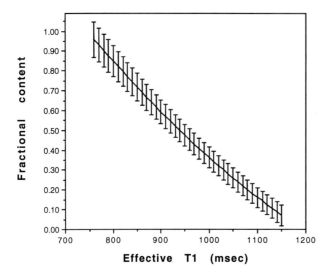

Fig. 4. Fractional content of atheroma vs. effective T1 by Method 1. The fractional atheroma content and its error were calculated for a series of effective T1 values using Method 1, with error in effective T1, $\delta T1_{eff} = 10$ ms.

1 to Method 2 by paired *t*-test detected no significant difference between methods (p > 0.74). Figure 5 shows the dependence of fractional atheroma content on effective T1 as produced by method 2 for

$$T1_{fat} = 1188 \pm 32 \quad T1_{atheroma} = 750 \pm 30 \quad \delta T1_{eff} = 10 \ ms.$$

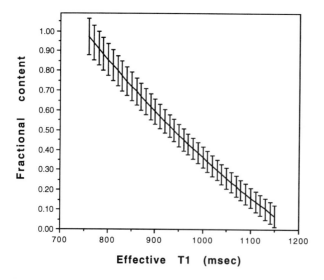

Fig. 5. Fractional content of atheroma vs. effective T1 by Method 2. Results of simulation based on real data, assuming the error in effective T1 is $\delta T1_{eff} = 10$ ms. The fractional atheroma content and its error were calculated for a series of effective T1 values using Method 2 for T1 analysis. The resemblance to Fig. 4 demonstrates that the simpler calculation of Method 2 yields comparable value and confidence limits to results from Method 1.

Weight calibration

The fractional content estimates derived by the methods described above are based on intensity measurements and reflect the fractional content of the atheroma signal rather than the fractional content of the atheroma weight. This discrepancy is due to the fact that the MR visibility of atheroma is different from that of perivascular fat for a given set of acquisition parameters. To calibrate the fractional atheroma content estimate by weight we note that the fractional weight content f_w is related to the fractional signal content f by:

$$f_w = \frac{\alpha \cdot I_2}{\alpha \cdot I_2 + I_1} \tag{9}$$

where α is a constant accounting for the relative difference in MR visibility between the materials.

Inverting the above equation we get:

$$\frac{1}{f_w} = 1 + \frac{1}{\alpha} \cdot \frac{I_1}{I_2} \tag{10}$$

and since $I_1/I_2 = (1-f) / f$, Equation (10) becomes

$$\frac{1}{f_w} = 1 + \frac{1-f}{f} \cdot \frac{1}{\alpha} \tag{11}$$

The parameter α can be estimated by calibrating mixtures where the partial weights are known.

Accuracy of T1 method

A series of seven samples of varying mixtures as well as pure samples were studied. Each component of these samples was preweighed so that the exact fractional content by weight was known. Calibration was performed using the two data points of the lowest and highest atheroma signal content, and gave $\alpha^{-1} = 4.83$. The estimates obtained by the T1 method and the two-point weight calibration agree with the true fractional content values. The true values all fall within the boundaries of the error estimates, as shown in Fig. 6. By paired *t*-test the difference between the calculated fractional weight content and the true fractional weight content was 0.0016 ± 0.0045.

Discussion

We have shown that we can obtain spectra from human arteries that reveal the atheroma content within the arterial wall. The signal is contaminated by a contribution from perivascular fat, but we have shown that assessment of the *effective T1* of the methyl peak allows accurate estimation of the atheroma content by weight.

We have analyzed the measurement error both in terms of fractional content and atheroma content by weight. The method is insensitive to shimming (magnetic field uniformity) because it is determined by T1 relaxivity, not T2. It is important that the acquisition method has a short echo time (<<10 ms) because echo times near to or greater than the atheroma T2 values (7–9 ms) attenuate atheroma signal excessively [7,12]. RME [13,14] provides effectively zero echo time, it can localize down to 1 mm³ (1 µl), and it

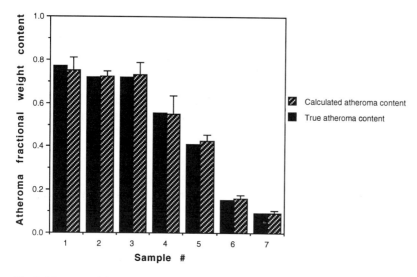

Fig. 6. Atheroma weight constant estimates and true values. The calculated fractional weight content of atheroma is displayed next to the true weight content, in a series of seven known mixtures.

generates the maximum available signal, so it is particularly well suited to these measurements.

These results establish that we can observe atheroma lipids inside the wall of human arteries noninvasively. Direct observation of atheroma lipid content in the arterial wall has an advantage over measurements of blood cholesterol levels which identify a population risk factor, but do not accurately indicate whether atheroma is accumulating inside the arteries of an individual. The magnetic resonance method is harmless, so it should be useful for screening and for monitoring the response to treatments. It should be especially valuable in assessing the benefit of wall-active agents such as probucol or antioxidant regimens that may reduce the build up of atheroma in artery walls without affecting the blood lipid levels. The method provides a direct measurement of the disease, even when no stenosis has developed.

Conclusion

We have developed methods to measure atheroma lipid content inside the arteries of patients, based on magnetic resonance signals of atheroma and fat mixtures. The "effective T1" methods are reliable and accurate when applied to both simulation data and experimental data. The agreement between the measured and the preweighed values of the fractional atheroma content is strong.

References

1. Asdente M, Pavesi L, Oreste PL, Colombo A, Kuhn W, Tremoli E. Atherosclerosis 1990;80:243–253.
2. Herfkens RJ, Higgins CB, Hricak H et al. Radiology 1983;148:161–166.
3. Pearlman JD, Southern JF, Ackerman JL. Angiology 1991;42:726–733.
4. Haase A, Frahm J, Matthaei D, Hanicke W, Bomsdorf H, Kunz D, Tischler R. Radiology 1986;160:787–790.
5. Pearlman JD, Wieczorek TJ. Relaxivity corrected response modulated excitation (RME): a T2-corrected technique achieving specified magnetization patterns from an RF pulse and a time-varying magnetic field. Mag Reson Med (in press).

6. Pearlman JD, Wieczorek TJ. Excitation of a 1 mm diameter beam using response modulated excitation. Soc Mag Reson Med Dallas Texas 1994 (abstract).
7. Pearlman JD, Zajicek J, Carman CS, Merickel M, Ayers CR, Brookeman JR, Brown MF. Mag Reson Med 1988;7(3):262–279.
8. Haase A, Frahm J, Hanicke W, Matthaei D. Phys Med Biol 1985;30(4):341–344.
9. Emid S, Konijnedijk J, Smidt J. J Mag Res 1980;37:509–513.
10. Kroon PA. J Biol Chem 1981;256:5332–5339.
11. Folch J, Lees M and Stanley G. J Biol Chem 1957;226:497–508.
12. Pearlman JD. Nuclear magnetic resonance spectral signatures of liquid crystals in human atheroma as basis for multidimensional digital imaging of atherosclerosis. PhD dissertation, School of Engineering and Applied Science, University of Virginia, August 1986.
13. Smith EB. J Atheroscler Res 1965;5:224–240.
14. Marquardt D. J Soc Ind Appl Math 1963;11:431–441.
15. Kowalewski J, Levy G, Johnson L, Palmer L. J Mag Res 1977;26:533–536.
16. Sass M, Ziessow D. J Mag Res 1977;25:263–276.

Identification of patients at risk for coronary artery disease using electron-beam CT

Robert S. Schwartz, John A. Rumberger, Patrick F. Sheedy II, Rachel Kaufmann and Patricia Peyser

Mayo Clinic and Foundation, Rochester, MN 55905, USA and Department of Epidemiology, University of Michigan, Ann Arbor, MI 48109, USA

Abstract. Clinicians currently lack accurate methods to detect asymptomatic coronary atherosclerosis. Functional tests rely on the physiological consequences of coronary stenosis such as myocardial ischemia or differences in flow to detect disease, yet recent data suggest that non-flow-limiting lesions may be responsible for catastrophic clinical events through plaque rupture and subsequent thrombosis. Coronary artery calcification occurs in regions of atherosclerotic plaque, and is easily detected by electron-beam CT (EBCT). The advantage of this method is that it is anatomically rather than functionally based, fast, and noninvasive. Recent studies have shown that calcification detected by EBCT is a more potent predictor of angiographic coronary artery disease than all traditional risk factors. Moreover, this technology can detect angiographic coronary artery disease with a sensitivity of 82%, specificity 85%, and overall accuracy 83%. The ability of EBCT to determine prognosis is yet to be established, although suggestive data are emerging. Further study of this method will be required to determine its final place in the clinical arena for detecting, quantitating, and predicting prognosis in coronary atherosclerosis.

Early detection of coronary artery disease remains an unsolved challenge for the cardiology community. Nearly 300,000 Americans die suddenly and unexpectedly from occult coronary artery disease each year. There are roughly 1.5 million myocardial infarctions yearly in the United States, and the American male today has a 20% likelihood of developing coronary artery disease before the age of 60.

The benefits to detecting asymptomatic coronary artery disease, while theoretically appealing, are uncertain since this capability has never been realized. The clinician currently has no accurate method to detect coronary atherosclerosis in its silent or preclinical stage. Virtually all "screening" tests available, including exercise treadmill, radionuclide thallium (and sestamibi), and stress echo rely on detecting the secondary effects of coronary stenosis manifested in myocardial ischemia.

These functional tests cannot be used to detect coronary stenoses that are not severe enough to cause myocardial ischemia. Functional tests thus exhibit substantially lower performance in the general (asymptomatic) population than in clinical populations. The frequent occurrence of false-positive tests imposes emotional concern, and may result in the risk and expense of invasive procedures being imposed on individuals without coronary artery disease. The sensitivity of these tests in the asymptomatic population is also lower than in clinical populations.

A test that is anatomically based and has high sensitivity could theoretically detect coronary artery disease in its earlier stages. Evidence is increasing that subcritical stenoses

Address for correspondence: Robert S. Schwartz, MD. Division of Cardiovascular Diseases, E-16B, Mayo Clinic, Rochester, MN 55905, USA. Tel.: +1-507-284-4389. Fax: +1-507-284-5470.

are quite important since they may rupture and cause thrombus, consequent myocardial infarction and/or sudden death.

Coronary atherosclerosis: detection via calcification

A common feature of atherosclerotic plaque is calcification. Coronary artery calcification is common in patients with known coronary artery disease and is strongly related to age, increasing dramatically after 50 years. McCarthy studied 65 consecutive autopsy-derived hearts (death not necessarily of cardiac causes) and found 63% to have some coronary artery calcification, nearly always associated with some degree of luminal coronary artery disease at the calcified location [1]. 94% of coronary arteries from patients older than 60 years had some degree of calcification present. In a series of 360 (living) patients undergoing cardiac catheterization, Bartel found a 43% prevalence of calcification by coronary fluoroscopy, and roughly 60% of patients over age 60 had some calcification noted with fluoroscopic examination. In living patients referred for noncardiac reasons, the prevalence of calcification is reported to be roughly 20%.

Coronary calcification may have use in detecting coronary artery disease, for instance through fluoroscopic detection [2,3]. An earlier study, using fluoroscopic detection of coronary artery calcification to screen 1,466 asymptomatic US Air Force aviators (mean age 42.5 years, range 28–62) for coronary artery disease [4], showed the performance of coronary fluoroscopy to be similar to or better than both treadmill exercise testing and planar thallium-201 scintigraphy [5,6]. The positive predictive value of treadmill testing, planar thallium-201 scintigraphy, and coronary fluoroscopy were 42, 63 and 72% respectively. The negative predictive value of planar thallium-201 testing was 71 vs. 90% for coronary fluoroscopy.

The amount and location of calcification is correlated with stenosis severity. For example, in the autopsy series mentioned above, significant stenosis and/or occlusion was virtually certain if calcification longer than 1 cm was present. This relation has been borne out by other studies. Hamby [7] found that 81% of patients with angiographic two- or three-vessel disease had coronary artery calcification.

A strong relation between the presence of coronary arterial calcification and prognosis has also been shown. Margolis et al. [8] reported that 5-year survival with and without coronary arterial calcification detected fluoroscopically was 58 and 85% respectively in a selected patient population [8]. More recently, Detrano and colleagues prospectively studied 1,461 asymptomatic patients for coronary events related to risk factors, exercise testing, and coronary artery calcification detected by fluoroscopy [3]. One-year follow-up showed that coronary calcification indicated a risk ratio of 2.6 for the aggregate endpoints of angina pectoris, death from coronary heart disease, nonfatal myocardial infarction, or myocardial revascularization. The detection of coronary calcium independently predicted at least one of these endpoints after controlling for age, gender and all other risk factors. Fluoroscopic calcium was not associated with coronary death or silent myocardial infarction when considered as separate endpoints since three cardiac deaths and one nonfatal myocardial infarction occurred in the 768 patients without detectable calcium. These results are consistent with earlier studies of coronary calcium and prognosis in patients with known coronary disease [8,9]. However, cardiac fluoroscopy does not offer the possibilities of quantification or exact localization of calcification. These problems are solved when coronary calcification is imaged using EBCT.

Noninvasive detection of coronary calcification by electron-beam CT

EBCT of the coronary arteries is a newer computed tomographic imaging technology available for clinical and research applications. This device can image the beating heart with rapid sequential acquisition of tomographic data (up to eight tomographic levels in 224 ms) and image reconstruction. Calcific deposits in arterial walls have high CT numbers (typically >200 Hounsfield units) provided the deposit is larger than 1 voxel in size. These deposits are quite visible even to untrained observers.

EBCT has been used for several years to study calcification in the coronary arteries [10,11]. An early study from hearts derived by autopsy showed that EBCT is an excellent method to measure the total calcified volume within the epicardial coronary arteries [12]. In this study, 39 coronary arteries from 13 hearts were sectioned into 522 segments perpendicularly to the vessel long axes. A direct relationship was found between the amount of atherosclerotic plaque determined histopathologically and by the degree of calcium measured by EBCT scans of the intact necropsy hearts. Generally, more extensive calcification was associated with more atheromatous plaque. This relationship was general only; specific lesion sites were not well correlated with calcification detected at that site. This study also demonstrated that the absence of calcification at coronary artery sites did not establish absence of atherosclerosis at the site. However, the absence of calcification within a segment was associated with a lack of stenosis >50%, with a negative predictive value of 97.5%. If an entire vessel was negative for coronary calcification by EBCT, the negative predictive value for significant stenosis was 100%, since in all segments without calcification no severe stenoses occurred. The overall sensitivity and specificity for segments containing calcification by EBCT were 59 and 90% for corresponding amounts of *any* atherosclerotic plaque. The positive predictive value of calcification by EBCT was 87% for detecting *any* disease. Receiver operating characteristic curves have shown an excellent relationship between the EBCT data and corresponding pathologically determined calcification (Fig. 1) [13]. This analysis of calcification by EBCT as a measure of angiographic coronary artery disease indicates excellent performance, with sensitivity 82%, specificity 85%, and accuracy of 83%. The high sensitivity of the test may be a problem, since even mild angiographic disease is detected. Studies are underway to determine how quantitation of calcific area can improved detection of severe angiographic disease. The value best associated with discriminating mild from severe disease was 18 mm^2 of calcific area by EBCT. In view of the minimally and/or atypically symptomatic status of these patients, the utility of EBCT appears to be substantial, and may be independent of gender [14–16].

By definition, calcification within a coronary artery implies atherosclerosis. The evidence that EBCT can reliably detect coronary artery calcification implies that this method can detect even small amounts of atherosclerosis in the living patient. Current studies are evaluating the relationship between EBCT-detected calcification and coronary atherosclerosis in patients undergoing coronary arteriography. These studies permits a better understanding of the relationship between angiographic coronary artery disease and calcification detected noninvasively by the EBCT scan [17–21]. In one such study, 160 patients (143 males) underwent coronary arteriography. The mean age was 48.5 years. In this study 33% had no coronary disease by angiography, 24% had "mild" disease (greatest angiographic diameter stenosis less than 50%), and 43% had significant disease. Excluding calcification, the most significant predictor of calcific area was age, followed by male sex and total/HDL cholesterol. Smoking history (pack-years) and family history of coronary artery disease predicted presence of calcium, but not quantity. The most important

EBCT vs. Pathologic Stenosis

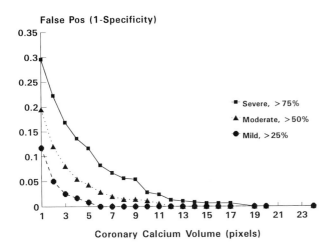

Fig. 1. False-positive rate for determining histopathologic coronary stenosis by EBCT calcification in pixels. Relationships for three discrete categories of histopathologic disease are shown.

predictors of angiographic coronary artery disease were age, male sex, and total/HDL cholesterol ratio. These three variables accounted for only 24% of the variability in maximal stenosis when calcification by EBCT was not considered. However, calcific area alone accounted for 56% of the variability in maximal stenosis. These data strongly suggest that calcific area is more strongly related to severity of angiographic disease than all other conventional atherosclerosis risk factors combined.

To assess the use of EBCT to study the prevalence of asymptomatic coronary athero-sclerosis in the general population, we have embarked on a cross-sectional study of asymptomatic patients [22]; 772 subjects have been taken as a sample of the general population in and around Olmsted County, Minnesota. The prevalence of calcification in this asymptomatic cohort is shown in Fig. 2. For a given age, females had less calcifi-cation than male counterparts. These data are consistent with those published by other groups. Calcification is remarkably prevalent in this general population. Calcification was strongly related to age, as expected.

Conclusion

The relevance of detecting calcification will be its ability to differentiate patients with good and poor prognoses. Many asymptomatic patients have much coronary calcification, and few of these will ever suffer a clinical coronary event during their lifetime. The likelihood that asymptomatic coronary atherosclerosis will cause morbidity or mortality is unknown, but could be quite low, given the high disease prevalence and low event incidence. Might subclinical coronary atherosclerosis and calcification be a "benign" condition? Is EBCT too sensitive in diagnosing subclinical coronary disease, since few identified patients will suffer clinical problems? Long-term follow-up of many patients will be required to answer these thorny questions.

Can EBCT identify patients at risk for coronary atherosclerosis? The answer appears

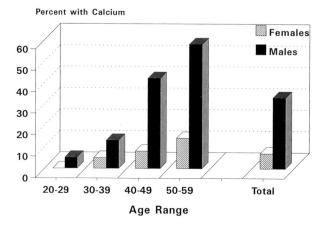

Calcium Prevalence by Age
Asymptomatic Subjects

Fig. 2. Prevalence of coronary artery calcification determined by EBCT in a cohort of asymptomatic subjects grouped by age. Males have substantially more calcification than females, and in both sexes calcification is a strong function of age. The high prevalence of calcification (and thus atherosclerosis) in the asymptomatic population may be problematic for this method.

to be a resounding "yes". The principal remaining questions concern how best to use this new information in the clinical setting.

Acknowledgements

This work was supported in part by NIH Grant HL46292.

References

1. McCarthy JH, Palmer FJ. Br Heart J 1974;36(5):499–506.
2. Schwartz R. J Am Coll Cardiol 1994;24:359–361.
3. Detrano R, Wong N, Tang W et al. J Am Coll Cardiol 1994;24:354–358.
4. Loecker TH, Schwartz RS, Cotta CW, Hickman JRJ. J Am Coll Cardiol 1992;19(6):1167–1172.
5. Schwartz RS, Jackson WG, Celio PV, Richardson LA, Hickman JR. Circulation 1992;87:165–172.
6. Detrano R, Simpfendorfer C, Day K et al. Am J Cardiol 1985;56:434–440.
7. Hamby RI, Tabrah F, Wisoff BG, Hartstein ML. Am Heart J 1974;87(5):565–570.
8. Margolis JR, Chen JT, Kong Y, Peter RH, Behar VS, Kisslo JA. Radiology 1980;137(3):609–616.
9. Hudson NM, Walker JK. Clin Radiol 1976;27(4):545–547.
10. Agatston AS, Janowitz WR, Hildner FJ, Zusmer NR, Viamonte MJ, Detrano R. J Am Coll Cardiol 1990; 15(4):827–832.
11. Janowitz WR, Agatston AS, Viamonte MJ. Am J Cardiol 1991;68(1):1–6.
12. Simons DB, Schwartz RS, Edwards WD, Sheedy PF, Breen JF, Rumberger JA. J Am Coll Cardiol 1992; 20(5):1118–1126.
13. Rumberger J, Schwartz R, Simons D, Sheedy PI, Edwards W, FItzpatrick L. Am J Cardiol 1994;74:1169–1173.
14. Rumberger J, Schwartz R, Simons D, Edwards W, Sheedy P, Fitzpatrick L. Circulation 1993;88(4):I638 (abstract).
15. Rumberger J, Schwartz R, Simons D, Edwards W, Sheedy PI, Fitzpatrick L. Circulation 1993;88:I639 (abstract).
16. Rumberger J, Schwartz R, Breen J, Sheedy PI, Stanford W. Circulation 1993;88:I15.

17. Bielak L, Kaufmann R, Moll P, McCollough C, Schwartz R, Sheedy PI. Radiology 1994;192:631–636.
18. Breen JF, Sheedy PF2, Schwartz RS et al. Radiology 1992;185(2):435–439.
19. Kajinami K, Takekoshi N. Circulation 1993;88:I–638 (abstract).
20. Georgiou D, Budoff M, Kennedy J et al. Circulation 1993;1993(4):I638 (abstract).
21. Georgiou D, Kennedy J, Brody A et al. J Am Coll Cardiol 1994;Feb 94:179A (abstract).
22. Kaufmann R, Sheedy PI, Maher J et al. Quantity of coronary artery calcium detected by electron beam CT in asymptomatic subjects and angiography patients. Mayo Clin Proc 1994 (in press).

1024

Gene induction in vessel wall injury: implications for restenosis after angioplasty

Mark B. Taubman, Michael Poon, Jonathan D. Marmur and Stephen D. Wax

Mount Sinai School of Medicine, Box 1269, One Gustave L. Levy Place, New York, NY 10029, USA

Abstract. Vascular smooth muscle cell (VSMC) proliferation is central to the development of atherosclerosis and of restenosis following percutaneous transluminal coronary angioplasty (PTCA). We have employed cultured VSMC and rat arterial balloon injury to identify genes that are activated in proliferating VSMC. *JE* and *KC* encode secretory glycoproteins that function as monocyte- and neutrophil-specific chemotactic factors, respectively. Their induction in the vessel wall may play a role in recruiting leukocytes to the site injury. The early induction in medial and neointimal VSMC of tissue factor (TF), the initiator of coagulation, may play a role in thrombus formation accompanying vessel injury. SM-20 is a recently identified novel growth-factor-responsive gene, whose expression is induced by vessel injury and limited to the VSMC of the media and neointima. SM-20 may provide a smooth-muscle-specific target for mediating the response to injury in the vessel wall.

Percutaneous transluminal coronary angioplasty (PTCA) is widely used for the treatment of symptomatic coronary artery disease, with over 300,000 procedures performed yearly in the United States alone. Despite an initial success rate of ≈90%, the utility of PTCA remains limited by the high rate of restenosis, ≈30–45%, occurring within 6 months of the procedure. A plethora of clinical trials have failed to demonstrate an impact on the rate of restenosis by any of the currently available drugs, including nitrates, β-blockers, calcium channel blockers, antiplatelet agents, anticoagulants, angiotensin converting enzyme inhibitors, etc. These studies suggest that a more complete understanding of the molecular events associated with restenosis will be necessary before effective treatments can be designed.

The development of intimal hyperplasia following vessel injury and the resultant stenosis is a complex process occurring in several phases [1,2]. The first 48 h is characterized by an inflammatory response, involving the recruitment of leukocytes to the site of injury, and by the development of the platelet-thrombus. The second phase, beginning 24–48 h after injury, is characterized by the proliferation of vascular smooth muscle cells (VSMC) in the vessel media and the migration of these cells into the intima, where they continue to proliferate. The stimulus for VSMC migration and proliferation is thought to be growth factors and cytokines derived from the platelet-thrombus, from leukocytes recruited to the site of injury, and from cellular elements of the vessel wall. The third phase, beginning within weeks of injury and persisting for months, involves the secretion of extracellular matrix by the VSMC comprising the neointima and results in the progressive expansion of the lesion. The regrowth of the endothelium over the neointima may be critical to inhibiting further smooth muscle proliferation and migration and may attenuate the secretion of extracellular matrix.

In order to develop new modalities for treatment of restenosis, it is necessary to elucidate the molecular events associated with the development of intimal hyperplasia. Among the many questions which need to be answered, two have provided the focus for considerable investigation. What are the factors (i.e., growth factors, vasoconstrictor agonists, cytokines) responsible for initiating the changes in VSMC which lead to their proliferation and migration? What are the genetic programs activated in the VSMC by these factors?

Our laboratory has employed two model systems for elucidating genes that are activated in VSMC in association with injury: 1) cultured VSMC derived from human and rat aorta; and 2) rat arterial (aortic and carotid) balloon injury. Using these systems, we have examined the expression in the injured arterial wall of genes (*JE*, *KC*, and tissue factor) with known functions relevant to vascular injury and have also identified a novel growth-factor-responsive gene (SM-20), expressed specifically in the VSMC of the arterial wall.

Leukocyte chemoattractants, *JE* and *KC*

JE and *KC* encode secretory glycoproteins that function as monocyte- and neutrophil-specific chemotactic factors, respectively. Quiescent VSMC constitutively express low levels of both *KC* and *JE* mRNA. When these cells were exposed to 10% calf serum, there was a rapid accumulation of *KC* mRNA above constitutive levels, beginning within 15 min, peaking at 1 h, and falling to below baseline after 4 h [3]. Levels of *JE* mRNA also markedly increased 1 h after serum treatment and remained elevated for $\approx$ 9 h. The induction of mRNA was accompanied by a marked secretion of JE protein into the culture medium [4]. In VSMC culture, the regulation of *KC* is ubiquitous: angiotensin II, α-thrombin, and PDGF all induce similar levels of mRNA. Unlike *KC* and other early growth-related genes such as c-*fos* and c-*myc*, *JE* mRNA induction appears to be specific for PDGF in cultured VSMC.

JE and *KC* mRNA are barely detectable in normal rabbit aorta. After balloon injury, levels of *JE* increased rapidly, peaking at approximately 4 h and returning to near baseline by 8 h [4]. A similar induction of *KC* mRNA occurred following balloon injury [3]. The acute inflammatory response which follows vessel injury is characterized by the accumulation of monocytes and the activation of neutrophils. Monocytes may serve as a source of growth factors and cytokines, and may be responsible for the foam cells seen in atherosclerotic lesions. Although neutrophils have rarely been demonstrated within the vessel media in models of acute injury, neutrophil activation does occur following PTCA. Neutrophil activation may play an important role in injury by releasing growth factors, proteolytic enzymes and cytokines, and by activating platelets.

Tissue factor

Tissue factor (TF) is a cell-surface glycoprotein that initiates the clotting cascade by binding to circulating factor VII/VIIa, resulting in the conversion of factors IX and X to IXa and Xa respectively [5]. TF mRNA is not detected in quiescent rat aortic VSMC. PDGF induced a rapid and marked rise in TF mRNA levels, beginning at $\approx$20 min and peaking between 60 and 90 min. The induction of TF mRNA was short-lived, with levels returning to baseline within 3–4 h [6]. TF mRNA was induced to similar levels and with a similar time course by serum, angiotensin II, α-thrombin and basic fibroblast growth factor. Minimal TF activity was measured in untreated, quiescent VSMC. In contrast, after induction with 10% calf serum or other agonists, there was a 10- to 15-fold increase in TF activity, beginning at $\approx$1 h, peaking at 2–8 h, and then slowly returning to baseline.

TF was also induced in the vessel wall by balloon injury [7]. TF mRNA was not detected in medial preparations from normal aorta, but was markedly induced 2 h after rat aortic balloon injury. The induction was followed by a rapid decline in mRNA levels. To localize the expression of TF mRNA, we performed in situ hybridization using ^{35}S-labeled TF cRNA probes. High levels of TF mRNA were detected in the adventitia of normal vessels, whereas essentially no TF mRNA was found in the media or intima. After balloon injury, high levels of TF mRNA were detected both in the adventitia and the media. TF activity was very high in uninjured adventitia and remained so following balloon injury. In contrast, TF activity was minimal in uninjured medial preparations, but rose markedly within 2 h of injury. TF activity remained elevated for up to 48 h.

Unlike human coronary arteries, which are usually severely diseased in acute myocardial infarction or unstable angina or after PTCA, most experimental animal models are based on normal arteries. In addition, injury models employing normal rodent arteries are usually not associated with macroscopic thrombosis, but are characterized by the deposition of platelets and minimal amounts of fibrin. To examine TF induction in a model that may be more representative of human coronary artery disease, we employed rat arterial double injury, similar to that reported in rabbits [8]. In this model, an initial balloon injury is performed as usual and the rats are allowed to recover. Two weeks later, a second injury is performed at the same site. TF activity was minimal in aortic media and intima 2 weeks after the initial injury. High levels of TF activity were measurable within 30 min of a second injury. Peak levels were reached within 1 h and were ≈3-fold those found 1 h after single injury. By in situ hybridization, we deduced that TF mRNA had been induced in both the media and neointima, as well as in the adventitia. To examine this further, we stained aortic sections with anti-rat-fibrinogen antibodies. In single injury, no staining was detectable on the luminal surface any time after injury (1 h–2 weeks). In contrast, fibrin(ogen) staining of the luminal surface was detectable within 1 h after a second injury and increased for at least 24 h. These results suggest that the doubly injured vessel provides a more thrombogenic surface. In contrast to single injury, the rapidity with which TF activity is induced by the second injury is consistent with a role for this induction in the initiation of thrombosis.

Identification of growth-factor-responsive genes in VSMC

While the above genes may be important in the initial response to vessel injury, they represent only a small percentage of the number of genes induced in association with injury. We have thus attempted to identify other growth-factor-responsive genes in VSMC using differential screening [9] of cDNA libraries from PDGF-stimulated cells and injured rat aorta. Using this approach, we have isolated five clones representing PDGF-responsive genes. Four encode known proteins: the muscle isoform of lactate dehydrogenase (LDH), thrombospondin, osteopontin, and lysyl oxidase. LDH plays an important role in cell metabolism and in the regulation of lactic acid. Thrombospondin induces platelet aggregation and has been shown previously to be regulated by growth factors in VSMC. Osteopontin has recently been identified in VSMC by Giachelli et al. using a different screening strategy and shown to be induced in the vessel wall in response to injury [10]. Recent studies have suggested that osteopontin may play a role in regulating the adhesion and migration of VSMC. Lysyl oxidase has several activities, including the cross-linking of collagen, the production of free radicals, and enhancement of leukocyte–endothelial interactions. These activities may all play a role in the response of the blood vessel to injury.

A fifth cDNA clone, SM-20 [9], encodes an ≈2.8 k mRNA whose derived amino acid sequence is novel (not found in national databases). Levels of SM-20 mRNA were induced ≈3-fold within 1 h of treatment with growth factors and returned to baseline within 3 h. SM-20 mRNA is expressed in all types of muscle cells and in brain, but not in liver, spleen, testes, or other nonmuscle tissues. Most significantly, SM-20 mRNA is not found in rat fibroblasts or endothelial cells. Antibodies raised against the SM-20 protein expressed in *E. coli* have demonstrated SM-20 protein in the cytoplasm of cultured human and rat VSMC which is apparently not secreted. Using this antibody, we detected SM-20 antigen in the media of normal rat arteries, but not in the endothelium or adventitia. After balloon arterial injury, staining for SM-20 antigen persisted in the media, but was most prominent in the neointimal VSMC.

SM-20 thus encodes a novel growth-factor-responsive gene whose expression in the vessel wall is limited to the VSMC and is enhanced in the neointima. The function of SM-20 protein remains to be elucidated. The specificity of SM-20 makes it a useful marker for VSMC in the vessel wall and raises the possibility that this protein could provide a VSMC-specific target.

In summary, VSMC have long been thought to play a critical role in restenosis by proliferating and migrating from the vessel media to the intima, resulting in intimal hyperplasia. Recently, it has been suggested that the VSMC may play an earlier role in the events leading to restenosis, for example through the production of PDGF. The work described here suggests that the VSMC may mediate both the early inflammatory and thrombotic responses associated with vessel injury. Thus the VSMC may act as a pluripotent cell involved in all phases of vascular injury, including thrombosis, inflammation, and intimal hyperplasia. Additional work will be necessary to elucidate fully the programs activated in VSMC in response to growth and migratory factors. The recent advances in recombinant DNA technology provide the hope that this will lead to novel approaches to attenuate the response of this pluripotent cell to injury.

Acknowledgements

This manuscript summarizes work funded in part by National Institutes of Health Grants HL43302 and HL29019, by a Grant-in-aid from the American Heart Association, New York Affiliate, and from awards from the Irma T. Hirschl-Monique Weill-Caulier Charitable Trusts and the Heart Research Foundation, New York. The authors would also like to acknowledge the contribution of the following investigators to the work summarized above: Billie S. Fyfe, Arabinda Guha, Milton Mendlowitz, Yale Nemerson, Claire-Lise Rosenfield, Maria Rossikhina, Singanallore V. Thiruvikraman and Lana Tsao of Mount Sinai School of Medicine, New York, and Barrett J Rollins, Harvard Medical School, Boston, MA.

References

1. Clowes AW, Clowes MM, Fingerle J, Reidy MA. J Cardiovasc Pharm 1989;14:S12—S15.
2. Steele PM, Chesebro JH, Stanson AW, Holmes DR Jr, Dewanjee MK, Badimon L, Fuster V. Circ Res 1985;57:105—112.
3. Marmur JD, Poon M, Rossikhina M, Taubman MB. Circulation 1992;86:III-53—III-60.
4. Taubman MB, Rollins BJ, Poon M, Marmur J, Green RS, Berk BC, Nadal-Ginard B. Circ Res 1992;70: 314—325.
5. Nemerson Y. Blood 1988;71:1—8.
6. Taubman MB, Marmur JD, Rosenfield C-L, Guha A, Nichtberger S, Nemerson Y. J Clin Invest 1993;91: 547—552.
7. Marmur JD, Rossikhina M, Guha A, Fyfe B, Friedrich V, Mendlowitz M, Nemerson Y, Taubman MB. J Clin Invest 1993;91:2253—2259.
8. Groves HM, Kinlough-Rathbone RL, Richardson M, Jorgensen J, Moore S, Mustard JF. Lab Invest 1982; 46:605—612.
9. Wax SD, Rosenfield C-L, Taubman MB. J Biol Chem 1994;269:13041—13047.
10. Giachelli CM Bae N, Almeida M, Denhardt DT, Alpers CE, Schwartz SM. J Clin Invest 1993;92: 1686—1696.

Cyclo-oxygenase-2, a potential target for treatment

Julio A. Rimarachin, Shiao Pan, Timothy A. McCaffrey and Babette B. Weksler
Department of Medicine, Division of Hematology and Oncology, Cornell University Medical College, New York, NY 10021, USA

Abstract. Cyclo-oxygenase-2 (prostaglandin endoperoxide synthase-2, Cox-2), is induced after vascular injury and mediates production of prostaglandins that modulate vasomotor tone, thrombosis, and smooth muscle proliferation. Endothelial cells express basal levels of Cox-2 upregulated by serum, phorbol ester, or IL-1. Smooth muscle cells normally do not express Cox-2 but the enzyme is rapidly and strongly induced by injury, mitogens, vasopressors and cytokines. In human atherectomy lesions Cox-2 is abundant. Modifying the expression and/or activity of Cox-2 has potential important therapeutic application because of its several roles during vascular response to injury.

The arterial wall is the main target of diseases like atherosclerosis, hypertension, and diabetes, processes frequently complicated by inflammation and thrombosis. Blood vessels respond to injury by activation of their major cellular components, smooth muscle cells (SMC) and endothelial cells (EC). This process is mediated by cytokines, growth factors, products of coagulation, lipids and shear stress. EC activation involves production of cytokines, increases in fibrinolytic factors, and early upregulation of Cox-2. SMC activation involves cell migration and proliferation, especially in the presence of dysfunctional EC. Activated SMC also rapidly upregulate Cox-2, as well as nitric oxide synthase. These responses are important elements in outcome: vascular occlusion vs. maintenance of blood flow.

Cyclo-oxygenase, the rate-limiting enzyme in prostaglandin synthesis, has two forms, the constitutive Cox-1 and the inducible Cox-2, homologous proteins governed by separate but related genes. First demonstrated in fibroblasts [1], Cox-2 induction has now been observed to be an early response to injurious stimuli in many cell types. In vascular cells, Cox-2 is an early component of EC activation by IL-1 and phorbol ester (PMA) [2], rheumatoid synovial microvascular cells [3], and SMC [4]. It is also induced in macrophages, mastocytoma cells, synoviocytes and chondrocytes and neurons [5]. It is associated with cell-cycle entry in rat intestinal epithelium. Furthermore, increased Cox-2 expression occurs in brain with ischemia or seizures [5], and may be implicated in the control of fever [6].

Cox-2 is also a major component of activation of both EC and SMC. Cox-2 is readily induced by a variety of stimuli in EC and SMC. Cox-2 is induced in HUVEC by IL-1 and PMA [2] and in SMC by mitogens [4].

The central role of Cox-2 in inflammatory pathology processes has made development of specific enzyme inhibitors of interest. Existing cyclo-oxygenase inhibitors are not specific. Indomethacin, piroxicam, and sulindac sulfide inhibit mostly the constitutive enzyme Cox-1 (the only Cox isoform in platelets). Ibuprofen and meclofenamate inhibit both Cox-1 and 2, and 6-methoxy-2-naphthylacetic acid inhibits preferentially Cox-2. Aspirin has a unique pattern since it irreversibly inactivates Cox-1 but shifts the enzymatic activity of Cox-2 to produce 15-hydroxy-eisosatetraenoic acid (15-HETE) rather than PGH2 [7]. Inhibitors specific for Cox-2 seem only to affect inflammatory sites and not constitutive Cox-1-dependent prostaglandin release in some tissues such as stomach [8].

We have investigated the role of Cox-2 induction in vascular injury, in vitro and in vivo, and have examined the presence of Cox-2 in human coronary artery atherectomy lesions and cells derived therefrom, since responses of the vessel wall to mediators of injury are particularly pertinent in the coronary circulation in angina, angioplasty or restenosis. In these conditions, dysfunctional EC and hyperreactive SMC are thought to play important roles.

Results

Expression of Cox-2 in EC
Endothelial cells express low levels of Cox-2 constitutively. In vivo, Cox-2 protein can be demonstrated by immunochemistry in EC of both large and small vessels in humans and rats. In vitro, cultured EC show a basal level of Cox-2 that is readily increased in the presence of cytokines PMA or serum. Messenger RNA for Cox-2 is rapidly induced in human EC by thrombin (in preparation). This increase in mRNA is followed by an increased in Cox-2 protein demonstrable by Western blotting as well as increased production of PGI2 and PGE2.

Expression of Cox-2 in SMC
Induction of Cox-2 mRNA. Cox-2 behaves as an early response gene in vascular SMC, being induced at the G_0/G_1 transition and superinduced by cycloheximide. Figure 1 shows that Cox-2 mRNA is absent from synchronized SMC in G_0, while addition of serum rapidly and transiently induces Cox-2 mRNA with a peak between 1.5 and 3 h. This

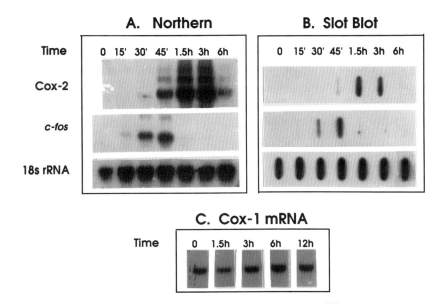

Fig. 1. Quiescent vascular smooth muscle cells were stimulated with 20% serum and total RNA was harvested at the indicated time points. Panel A shows a Northern blot, panel B the same sample in a dot blot. Cox-2 mRNA is rapidly and transiently induced, peaking between 1.5 and 3 h. c-fos is a marker for cell-cycle entry and 18S rRNA a control for loading. Panel C shows Cox-1 mRNA levels detected with a riboprobe because of the weakness of the signal using a cDNA probe. Cox-1 mRNA does not significantly change with cell cycle entry ([4], reproduced with permission from Arteriosclerosis and Thrombosis, as are Figs. 2–4).

Time   0 15' 30' 45' 1.5h 3h 6h 9h 12h

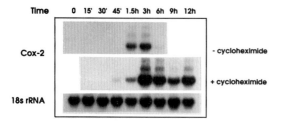

Cox-2   - cycloheximide

                                                   + cycloheximide

18s rRNA

Fig. 2. Northern blot showing Cox-2 mRNA induction in the absence (upper panel), and presence of cycloheximide (10 μg/ml). Cycloheximide significantly increases and prolongs the expression of Cox-2 mRNA. Lower panel is the 18S rRNA loading control ([4], reproduced with permission).

induction is slightly slower than that of c-fos. Superinduction in the presence of cycloheximide, suggesting stabilization of mRNA, is shown in Fig. 2.

Certain mitogens, used at concentrations that give optimal growth effects, stimulate Cox-2 expression in synchronized, quiescent SMC; other mitogens are weak inducers. In Fig. 3, PDGF, EGF, thrombin and PMA strongly induce Cox-2 mRNA, whereas the fibroblast growth-factor family (basic and acidic FGF) show minimal effects.

Expression of Cox-2 protein. Western blotting and immunofluorescence were utilized to demonstrate the appearance of Cox-2 following stimulation. Antibodies used were raised against the unique carboxy-terminal peptide of Cox-2 that is not present in Cox-1 [4]. In Western blots (Fig. 4) Cox-2 is not demonstrable at time zero but reaches a peak 3—6 h after addition of serum and starts to disappear again after 12 h. Both rat and human SMC respond to serum and thrombin in this way. Indeed, the tethered thrombin peptide alone can elicit Cox-2 protein expression (in preparation). Immunofluorescence confirms these kinetics of Cox-2 induction and shows striking initial subcellular localization of Cox-2 in the nucleus with a gradual shifting to the cytoplasm by 6 h (Fig. 5). In addition, increased prostaglandin production by SMC parallels the protein expression, as demonstrated by enzyme-linked immunoassay of secreted prostaglandins.

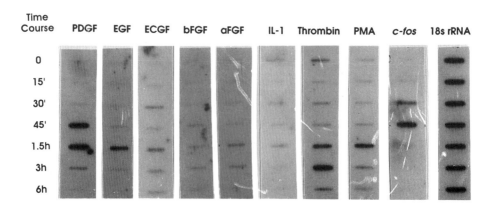

Fig. 3. Stimulation of Cox-2 mRNA by different mitogens. PDGF, EGF, bFGF, aFGF, IL-1 α (10 ng/ml). ECGF (200 μg/ml), thrombin (1 U/ml), PMA (50 ng/ml). This slot blot demonstrates that PDGF, EGF, thrombin and PMA induce Cox-2 strongly while aFGF, bFGF ECGF, and IL-1a are weak inducers. Parallel samples were tested for *c-fos* and 18S rRNA ([4], reproduced with permission).

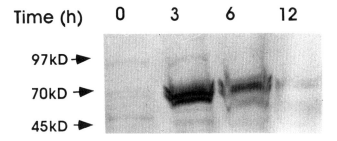

Time (h)   0   3   6   12

97kD ►

70kD ►

45kD ►

Fig 4. Western blot of cyclooxygenase-2 induction in SMC. Quiescent SMC showed almost no presence of immunoreactivity for Cox-2 protein. Upon stimulation with 20% serum, Cox-2 is rapidly expressed as a protein doublet of 70 kD, maximal at 3 h fading gradually at 12 h. ([4], reproduced with permission).

Stimulation by vasoconstrictor agents. Vasoconstrictors comprise another group of substances that activate Cox-2 expression in SMC. Angiotensin II, catecholamines,

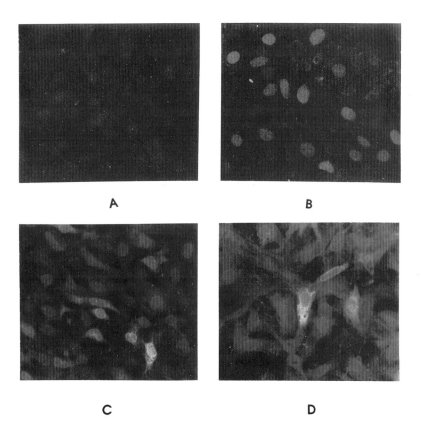

A   B

C   D

Fig. 5. Immunofluorescence of SMC stimulated with 20% serum, using specific anti-Cox-2 antibodies and fluorescein-labeled second antibody. Unstimulated cells show no immunoreactivity (panel A). At 3 h, nuclear staining is visible (Panel B). At 6 h most cells show strong staining in a perinuclear, granular cytoplasmic pattern. In panel D, some cells at 12 h still show positive staining.

serotonin and thromboxane A2 were evaluated for effects on Cox-2 mRNA, protein, and prostaglandin production. Angiotensin II is a strong inducer of Cox-2 expression in SMC.

In vivo demonstration of Cox-2 expression. Cox-2 is induced in models of vascular injury such as balloon angioplasty of the rat aorta. As shown in Fig. 6A, specific Cox-2 immunoreactivity is observed in the injured vessel but none is detected in the contralateral control vessel (Fig. 6B). Immunoreactivity was present from 12 h after injury and continues for 2 weeks, especially in the developing intimal proliferative lesion.

Activation of Cox-2 in human atherosclerosis
Cox-2 is prominently expressed in lesions of human coronary arteries. Atherectomy specimens obtained from angiographically demonstrated obstructive lesions were immunostained with antibody specific for Cox-2. Both primary and restenotic (post-angioplastic) lesions were positive for Cox-2.

Discussion

We have shown that Cox-2 is induced in vascular SMC by a variety of SMC activators including mitogens and vasoconstrictors. In vitro, Cox-2 induction follows the pattern of a primary response gene and is followed by markedly increased production of prostaglandins. In vivo, Cox-2 induction rapidly follows injury but persists much longer, at least during the phase of intimal proliferation, where there may be continued stimulation by cycling SMC. In addition, the positive reaction of vascular cells from atherectomy specimens suggests continuing activation of this gene in ongoing atherosclerotic disease not marked by rapid cell proliferation. These findings suggest that Cox-2 expression is part of SMC activation and of the SMC proliferative response, and constitutes a marker of SMC activation. Whether the increased Cox-2 expression and concomitant increase in prostaglandin production is protective or possibly injurious (for example, providing a protracted source of lipid peroxides) remains to be determined. Activation of Cox-2 in vitro as well is not always linked to cell-cycle entry, as shown by vasopressor-mediated induction in SMC and thrombin- or cytokine-mediated induction in EC, which suggests several pathways for its induction.

Cox-2 expression is part of the reaction of the vessel wall to injury, resulting in enhancement of eicosanoid formation. Prostaglandins in the normal vessel wall are mainly

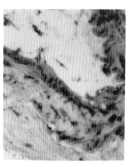
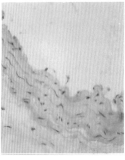

A   B

Fig 6. Balloon injury of the rat carotid. Panel A, injured carotid. 12 h after injury, medial SMC expresses Cox-2 protein strongly, while the noninjured contralateral control (panel B) is negative.

vasodilatory and antiproliferative. In this sense, prostaglandins may exert a useful role during injury by preventing vasoconstriction and mitogenesis. It is well known that prostaglandins can enhance the production and function of nitric oxide, another vascular-derived vasodilator. However, evidence from hypertension and angina pectoris point to a defect in vascular function in those conditions, an overreaction to vasopressor stimuli that occurs in particular when the endothelium is dysfunctional or defective. Eicosanoid intermediates derived from induced Cox-2 activity in injured vessels could be shunted to vasopressor products (such as thromboxane) instead of forming PGI2 or PGE2. In this regard, specific suppression of Cox-2 would become a desired goal as it has been in inflammation. Indeed, the limitations on beneficial effects of aspirin in preventing occlusive vascular disease could reflect the capacity of that drug to shift Cox-2 activity to production of 15-HETE, since its immediate precursor 15-HPETE is a known inhibitor of prostacyclin synthase.

Acknowledgements

This work was supported by NIH SCOR in Thrombosis grant HL-18828. T.A.M is supported by NIH, PO1 HL46403 and R29 HL42606.

References

1. Kujubu DA, Fletcher BS, Varnum BC, Lim RW, Herschmann HR. J Biol Chem 1991;266:12866−12872.
2. Habib A, Creminon C, Frobeert Y, Grassi J, Pradelles P, Maclouf J. J Biol Chem 1993;268:23448−23454.
3. Szczepanski A, Moatter T, Carlet WW, Gerritsen ME. Arthr Rheumat 1994;37:495−503.
4. Rimarachin JA, Jacobsen JA, Szabo P, Maclouf J, Creminon C, Weksler BW. Arteriosclerosis 1994;14: 1021−1031.
5. Yamagata K, Andreason KI, Kaufmann WE Barnes CA, Worley P. Neuron 1993;11:371−386.
6. Kennedy BP, Chan CC, Culp SA, Cromlish WA. Biochem Biophys Res Commun 1993;197:494−500.
7. Lecomte M, Laneuville O, Ji C, DeWitt DL, Smith WL. J Biol Chem 1994;269:13207−13215.
8. Masferrer JL, Weifel BS, Manning T, Hauser SD, Leahy KM, Smith WG, Isakson PC, Seibert K. Proc Natl Acad Sci USA 1994;91:3228s−3232s.

Direct drug control of the vascular wall

Rodolfo Paoletti, Franco Bernini, Alberto Corsini and Maurizio Soma

Institute of Pharmacological Sciences, Via Balzaretti 9, 20133 Milan, Italy

Reduction of the major potentially modifiable cardiovascular risk factors (hypertension, hypercholesterolemia, cigarette smoking) with nonpharmacological methods and with drugs has, during the last 2 decades, dominated the field of cardiovascular prevention. However, some difficulties can be foreseen for this approach. First of all, risk factors are often combined in the same individual, particularly in the aging population of the industrialized countries; secondly, each risk factor is best controlled by a plurality of drugs with a complex and often uncontrollable increase of side effects during prolonged treatments. A third difficulty is represented by the long-time treatment of risk factors, particularly dyslipoproteinemias and hypercholesterolemias, in order to obtain clinically significant results in primary prevention.

For these reasons, more attention should be paid to the development and clinical use of drugs acting directly on the arterial wall.

Primary and secondary prevention of coronary heart disease (CHD)

Myocardial infarction (MI) is the commonest cause of death in most industrialized countries. In the USA 6.3 million people have coronary heart disease in spite of a 32% decline in death rate [1].

Smoking induces CHD at a much earlier age than controls [2], and smoking cessation reduces by 50% the incidence of CHD [2]. The risk of MI increases in a dose–response fashion with the number of cigarettes smoked [3]. Cigarette smoking induces coronary spasm and vasoconstrictive response to intracoronary muscarinic drugs (acetylcholine) [4,5]. *Hypertension*, from systolic values of 130–139 mmHg upwards, is also closely related to increased CHD mortality [6]. According to a review by Stamler [6] of the MRFIT data (Multiple Risk Factor Intervention Trial), prevention of hypertension in the general population could reduce by 36% the 11.6-year CHD. Antihypertensive drug therapy results in a modest reduction of the CHD risk, with a 16% reduction in CHD morbidity and mortality according to a recent meta-analysis [7]. Increased left ventricular mass (LVM) is a stronger predictor of CHD death than hypertension [8] and responds positively to drug therapy [9].

Total plasma cholesterol levels have also declined from 280 to about 205 mg/dl during the last 3 decades [10], in spite of the high frequency of LDL-C (low density lipoprotein-cholesterol) above 130 mg/dl [11]. Secondary prevention trials subjected to a recent meta-analysis [12] suggest a 36% lower risk of progression and an odds ratio of 2.13 for atheroma regression; in the last paper by Blankenhorn the MARS study (Monitored Atherosclerosis Regression Study), a group treated with lovastatin showed decreases of total and LDL-cholesterol of 32 and 38% [13], with doubling of the frequency of regression. Waters [14] recently showed a 2.3-fold decrease in risk of CHD morbidity and mortality after 44 months. Total mortality is, however, not decreased in primary prevention trials with drugs or diet, since meta-analyses show increased noncardiovascular deaths [15,16].

Triglycerides (TG) and *decreased HDL* (high density lipoproteins) are correlated with CHD, at least in univariate studies. The PROCAM study (Prospective Cardiovascular Munster Study) showed a strong risk for CHD in subjects with a high LDL/HDL ratio (>5) [17] and elevated TGL. The same subtype of patients responded to the lipid-lowering drug gemfibrozil in the Helsinki Heart Study [18]. For these reasons measurement of plasma TG levels, HDL concentration and HDL subfractions may be recommended and, when dietary and lifestyle changes are insufficient, lipid-lowering drugs should be used [19,20]. Lowering of LDL-cholesterol remain the primary goal of therapy [21], with special emphasis in secondary prevention. In postmenopausal women low HDL-cholesterol is a powerful predictor of death, further increased by hypertriglyceridemia [22]. In postmenopausal women hormonal replacement therapy (HRT) should precede lipid-lowering drugs; this reduces carotid artery thickness [23] and in some studies cardiovascular events (−40%) and death (−80%) [24].

Direct arterial protection

The nondefinitive results of the commonest preventive drug treatments of CHD and MI have prompted the study of drugs preventing the formation of plaques even in the presence of one or several risk factors.

Several mechanisms are involved in atheroma formation, with an important role for endothelial injury, intimal lipid accumulation and extracellular matrix synthesis which may result from a reaction to endothelial injury and may involve a number of cytokines and vasoactive molecules. All the cells involved in the atherogenic process (endothelium, smooth muscle cells, macrophages and platelets) may release these mediators [25]. Understanding of the mechanisms involved in atherogenesis has only recently opened the way to developing new antiatherosclerotic drugs.

Antioxidants, long-lasting ACE (angiotensin converting enzyme) inhibitors, lipophilic calcium antagonists and lipophilic statins are potential drugs acting directly on the arteries. In the present study calcium antagonists and statins are discussed.

Calcium antagonists

The calcium antagonists show several important antiatherosclerotic activities in vitro and in vivo. In cultured cells these drugs protect arterial smooth muscle cells (SMC) against cholesterol deposition and control cellular proliferation. In addition, matrix synthesis by SMC is reduced. In in vivo models calcium antagonists protect against lesions induced by cholesterol feeding, endothelial injury and experimental calcinosis [26].

The antiatherosclerotic effect of calcium antagonists does not involve a reduction of plasma cholesterol or blood pressure, and we deduce a direct effect on the arterial wall [26]. In a series of animal experiments the influence of calcium antagonists on calcium deposition within the vessel wall and on the development of artificially induced atherosclerosis proved to be favorable [27–29]. Two randomized, placebo-controlled studies [30,31] have reported on the effects of calcium antagonists on atheroma in the coronary arteries. The first study is the International Nifedipine Trial of Anti-atherosclerotic Therapy (INTACT). 425 patients were controlled and randomized to treatment with nifedipine. The study lasted for 3 years. No regression, or lack of progression, was reported, but a 28% reduction in the number of new lesions could be recorded. In the second study, by Waters et al. [31], 383 patients were randomized to treatment with nicardipine. The study lasted for 2 years and the findings were essentially the same of those reported in the INTACT study: no effect on established coronary lesions, but a reduction in the number of small or new lesions. In both studies the inhibitory effect on appearance of new lesions was accomplished without a corresponding effect on blood lipid levels. The results of these studies indicate that some as yet unidentified biological processes in the early development of atheromatous lesions are sensitive to calcium antagonists. While the efficacy of calcium antagonists as coronary and peripheral vascular dilators can be accounted for in terms of their inhibitory effects on calcium influx throughout the voltage-sensitive calcium channels, their ability to act as antiatherosclerotic agents is less understood. Several calcium-dependent processes contribute to atherogenesis, including lipid infiltration and oxidation, endothelial injury, action of chemotactic and growth factors, smooth muscle cell migration and proliferation.

Proliferation of vascular smooth muscle cells is an early and key event in the formation of an atherosclerotic lesion. Smooth muscle cells accumulate in the intima under atherogenic conditions. In response to experimental arterial injury, SMC migrate from the media into the intima, where they proliferate and secrete large amounts of extracellular matrix. This reaction results in rapid neointimal hyperplasia and provides a convenient means of studying the kind of proliferative atherosclerotic lesions and stenotic processes that are frequently observed in patients undergoing percutaneous transluminal coronary angioplasty (PTCA) [32].

An in vivo model for the study of SMC in the carotid walls of rabbits has been used in our laboratory to characterize the antiatherogenic activity of the new calcium antagonist lacidipine. We studied the effect of this drug on the atherosclerotic response of the hyper-cholesterolemic rabbit carotid artery 14 days after perivascular manipulation of the vessel. This model, described by Booth et al. [33], allows direct monitoring in vivo and independently of other factors, of the effect of a drug on arterial myocyte proliferation in normotensive hypercholesterolemic rabbits. The results with lacidipine, a lipophilic dihydropyridine, clearly indicates the possibility of using this, and similar, calcium antagonists as protective agents against lesions of the arterial wall (Table 1).

The availability of quantitative procedures to assess in man the thickening of the carotid arterial walls in pathological condition also opens the way for clinical studies leading to the protection of the carotid artery in presence of one or more major risk factors, not only in hypertensive patients.

Direct arterial effects of statins

The 3-hydroxy-3-methylglutaryl coenzyme A (HMG-CoA) reductase inhibitors (vastatins) are potent pharmacological agents that are active in reducing plasma total and LDL-C levels in subjects with primary hypercholesterolemia [34]. Recent studies in animals and humans [35] have documented a reduction in the severity of arterial lesions and

Table 1. Effect of lacidipine (3 mg/kg/day) on proliferative lesions induced by perivascular manipulation of hypercholesterolemic normotensive rabbit carotid arteries

Treatment	I:M	SD	% of control	p value
Control	0.56	0.11	100	—
Sham	0.03	0.02	5	—
Lacidipine	0.32	0.10	57	0.01

Ten rabbits each in the control and lacidipine treatment groups; 20 rabbits in the sham group. I:M = intimal:medial thickness ratio (mean ± SD); SD = standard deviation; p value = lacidipine vs. control treatment.

cardiovascular diseases after treatment with lovastatin or simvastatin. The antiatherosclerotic effect of these drugs has been linked to their hypolipidemic properties [36–38], and it has been suggested that the hypolipidemic effect is the main mechanism for preventing the development of atherosclerosis.

Vastatins competitively inhibit intracellular synthesis of mevalonate, a precursor of nonsterol compounds (such as geranylgeraniol and farnesol) involved in cell function and proliferation [39,40]. For this reason these drugs have received increasing attention as pharmacological tools for controlling abnormal cell growth in pathological conditions such as tumors [41] and hyperplasia of vascular smooth muscle cells (myocytes) under athero-genic conditions. Pharmacological approaches using vastatins to inhibit SMC proliferation have already been tried. Simvastatin inhibits growth in vitro [42]. Aggressive lipid-lowering treatment with lovastatin prevented restenosis after balloon angioplasty in hyper-cholesterolemic rabbits [43] and humans [44]. However, no correlations between serum cholesterol and restenosis were found in PTCA patients.

Several vastatins have been tested in our laboratory in order to establish if they directly affect neointimal formation in the carotid arteries of normocholesterolemic rabbits independent of the lowering of plasma cholesterol concentration. For this purpose, we have used a scheme for the drug-treatment regimen that did not modify the plasma cholesterol level in normolipemic rabbits. Intimal thickening was induced by inserting a flexible extra-arterial collar around the common carotid artery.

The effect of vastatins was evaluated 14 days after collar insertion. The sham-operated contralateral arteries showed no thickening of the intima either in positive control or drug-treated rabbits (Table 2). A marked increase in intimal thickness (mostly cellular) was evident in the carotid arteries with the collar applied to otherwise untreated animals (positive control group). The mean value of intimal carotid thickening in the positive control group, expressed as the I:M ratio, was 12 times greater than in the contralateral sham-operated carotid artery (Table 2). The levels of total plasma cholesterol measured before surgery and at the time the animals were killed (14 days later) did not change, and the values were similar in positive control and vastatin-treated animals throughout the study (Table 3).

Figure 1 reports the effect of the different vastatins on thickening induced in the carotid intimas of rabbits: all drugs at the dose of 20 mg/kg body wt per day limited the increase of the I:M ratio seen with the positive control group. Fluvastatin was the most effective drug in this regard, followed by simvastatin, lovastatin, and pravastatin in decreasing order. Differences vs. positive controls were statistically highly significant for all drugs with the exception of pravastatin (Table 2). In all rabbits treated with vastatins,

Table 2. Effect of different vastatins on intimal thickening induced by perivascular manipulation of rabbit carotid arteries after 2 weeks

Treatment	I:M (mean)	SD	Percentage of control	p
Positive control	0.36	0.04	100	–
Sham	0.03	0.02	3	–
Pravastatin	0.32	0.03	89	NS
Lovastatin	0.24	0.03	67	0.001
Simvastatin	0.20	0.03	56	0.001
Fluvastatin	0.17	0.03	47	0.001

I:M = intimal:medial thickness ratio; SD = standard deviation; NS = not significant (n = 12). The sham value is the mean ± SD of all 60 rabbits.

Table 3. Total plasma cholesterol levels throughout the study in control and vastatin-treated groups

Treatment	Total cholesterol before surgery	Total cholesterol at sacrifice
Positive control	28.4 ± 3.6	31.5 ± 4.2
Pravastatin	26.5 ± 4.8	24.6 ± 6.3
Lovastatin	29.6 ± 5.2	27.8 ± 6.4
Simvastatin	29.7 ± 12.5	31.1 ± 7.8
Fluvastatin	32.6 ± 7.7	28.9 ± 5.5

Values are in mg/dl and are mean ± SD.

the inhibition of hyperplasia resulted in fewer layers of intimal cells.

The inhibition of SMC proliferation induced by statins is totally abolished by local infusion of mevalonate (Table 4). These in vivo data correlate with in vitro results published by us [42] indicating that the inhibition of SMC proliferation by statins is related to the inhibition of intracellular synthesis of mevalonic acid with consequent depletion of the isoprenoids geranylgeraniol and farnesol. This novel mechanism of control of cell multiplication indicates that even statins may act directly on the arterial walls, with the exception of the hydrophilic pravastatin.

Conclusions

The examples of two classes of drugs which protect arterial walls even in the presence of risk factors or after endothelial and smooth muscle cell damage indicate new ways to prevent atherosclerosis and its cardiovascular consequences. New approaches using quantitative and repeated observations of arterial wall thickness and the progression and regression of plaques in man are needed to study newly developed drugs clinically. Combinations of drugs (such as a calcium antagonist and a vastatin) may be tested in human subjects with a variety of risk factors (hypertension, dyslipoproteinemias and diabetes). This new approach is needed to avoid the proliferation of drugs which affect individually each risk factor without a well-demonstrated global impact on the atherosclerotic disease.

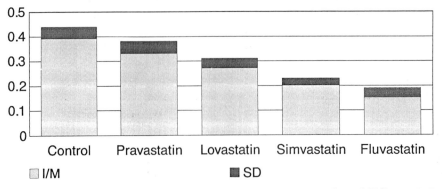

Intimal / Medial tissue

*p < 0.05 Duncan test

Fig. 1. Bar graph of vastatins' effect on neointimal formation induced by perivascular manipulation of normocholesterolemic rabbit carotid arteries. Vastatins were administered for 3 weeks mixed with food at a daily dose of 20 mg/kg body weight starting on the day of collar placement.

Table 4. Effect of mevalonate on arterial SMC proliferation inhibited by fluvastatin

	Control	Fluva	Fluva + MVA
I/M	0.22	0.12	0.20
LI	3.6	1.6	3.1

FLUVA = Fluvastatin 5 mg/kg/day intraperitoneally for 5 days. MVA = Sodium mevalonate 8 mg/kg/day (local delivery) for 5 days. I/M = Intima/medial thickness ratio. LI = labeling index (INTIMA/MEDIA).

References

1. American Heart Association: Heart and Stroke Facts: 1994 Statistical Supplement. Dallas: American Heart Association, 1993.
2. Jonas MA, Oates JA, Ockene JK, Hennekens CH. Circulation 1992;86:1664–1669.
3. Negri E, Franzosi MG, La Vecchia C, Santoro L, Nobili A, Tognoni G. Br Med J 1993;306:1567–1570.
4. Sugiishi M, Takatsu F. Circulation 1993;87:76–79.
5. Nitenberg A, Antony I, Foult JM. Am J Med 1993;95:71–77.
6. Stamler J, Stamler R, Neaton JD. Arch Int Med 1993;153:598–615.
7. Herbert PR, Moser M, Mayer J, Glynn RJ, Hennekens CH. Arch Int Med 1993;153:578–581.
8. Devereux RB, Roman MJ. J Hypertens 1993;11(suppl 4):S3–S9.
9. Carr AA, Prisant LM, Houghton JL. Am J Hypertens 1993;6:271S–276S.
10. Johnson CL, Rifkind BM, Sempos CT, Carroll MD, Bachorik PS, Briefel RR, Gordon DJ, Burt VL, Brown CD, Lippel K, Cleeman JI. J Am Med Assoc 1993;269:3002–3008.
11. Brown SA, Hutchinson R, Morrisett J, Boerwinkle E, Davis CE, Gotto AM, Patsch W. Arterioscler Thromb 1993;13:1139–1158.
12. Vos J, de Feyter PJ, Simoons ML, Tijssen JGP, Deckers JW. Prog Cardiovasc Dis 1993;35:435–454.
13. Blankenhorn DH, Azen SP, Kramsch DM, Mack WJ, Cashin-Hemphill L, Hodis HN, DeBoer LWV, Mahrer PR, Masteller MJ, Vailas LI, Alaupovic P, Hirsch LJ, and the MARS Research Group. Ann Int Med 1993;119:969–976.
14. Waters D, Craven TE, Lesperance J. Circulation 1993;97:1067–1075.
15. Muldoon MF, Manuck SB, Manhews KA. Br Med J 1990;301:309–314.
16. Smith GD, Song F, Sheldon TA. Br Med J 1993;306:1367–1373.
17. Assman MD, Schulte H. Am J Cardiol 1992;70:733–737.
18. Manninen V, Tenkanen L, Koskinen P, Huttunen JK, Maenttaeri M, Heinonen OP, Frick MH. Circulation 1992;85:37–45.
19. NIH Consensus Development Panel on Triglyceride, High-Density Lipoprotein and Coronary Heart Desease. J Am Med Assoc 1993;269:505–510.
20. Kreisberg RA. Am J Med 1993;94:1–6.
21. Expert Panel on Detection, Evaluation, and Treatment of High Blood Cholesterol in Adults. J Am Med Assoc 1993;269:3015–3023.
22. Stensvold I, Tverdal A, Urdal P, Graff-Iversen S. Br Med J 1993;307:1318–1322.
23. Manolio TA, Furberg CD, Shemanski L, Psaty BM, O'Leary DH, Tracy RP, Bush TL. Circulation 1993;88:2163–2171.
24. Grady D, Rubin SM, Petitti DB, Fox CS, Black D, Ettinger B, Ernster VL, Cummings SR. Ann Int Med 1992;117:1016–1037.
25. Ross R. Nature 1990;362:801.
26. Raiteri M, Corsini A, Soma MR, Donetti E, Bernini F, Fumagalli R, Paoletti R. In: Catapano AL, Gotto AM Jr, Smith LC, Paoletti R (eds) Dordrecht: Kluwer Academic Publishers, 1993;317–331.
27. Schmitz G, Hankovitz J, Kovacs EM. Atherosclerosis 1991;88:109.
28. Fronek K. Cardiovasc Drug Rev 1990;8:229.
29. Scheneider W, Kober G, Roebruck P, Noack H, Alle M, Cieslinski G, Reifart N, Kaltenbach M. Eur J Clin Pharmacol 1990;39:S17.
30. Lichtlen PR, Hugenholtz PG, Hecker H, Jost S, Deckers JW. Lancet 1990;335:1109.
31. Waters D, Lesperance J, Francetich M, Causey D, Theroux P, Chiang YK, Hudon G, Lemarbre L, Reitman M, Joyal M, Gosselin G, Durda I, Macer J, Havel RJ. Circulation 1990;82:1940.
32. Popma JJ, Califf RM, Topol EJ. Circulation 1991;84.1426–1436.
33. Booth RGF, Martin JF, Honey AC, Hassall DG, Beesley JE, Moncada S. Atherosclerosis 1989;76:257–268.

34. Hunninghake DB. Curr Opin Lipid 1992;3:22–28.
35. Zhu BQ, Sievers RE, Sun YP, Isemberg WM, Parmley WW. J Cardiovasc Pharmacol 1992;19:246–255.
36. Kobayashi M, Ishida F, Takahashi T, Taguchi K, Watanabe K, Ohmura I, Kamei T. Jpn J Pharmacol 1989;49:125–133.
37. Blankenhorn DH. Curr Opin Lipidol 1991;2:2324–2329.
38. Watanabe Y, Ito T, Shiomi M, Tsujita Y, Kuroda M, Arai M, Fukami M, Tamura A. Biochim Biophys Acta 1988;960:294–302.
39. Maltese WA. FASEB J 1990;4:3319–3328.
40. Habenicht AJR, Glomset JA, Ross R. J Biol Chem 1980;255:5134–5140.
41. Soma MR, Pagliarini P, Butti G, Paoletti R, Paoletti P, Fumagalli R. Cancer Res 1992;52:1–9.
42. Corsini A, Raiteri M, Soma MR, Fumagalli R, Paoletti R. Pharmacol Res 1991;23:173–180.
43. Gellman J, Ezekowitz MD, Sarembock IJ, Azrin A, Nochomowitz LE, Lerner E, Haudenschild CC. J Am Coll Cardiol 1991;17:251–259.
44. Sahhi R, Maniet AR, Voci G, Banka VS. Am Heart J 1991;121:1600–1608.

Antagonism of platelet integrins and specific thrombin inhibition: the human pharmacology of antithrombotic drugs

Domenico Pratico, Francesca Catella and Garret A. FitzGerald

Center for Experimental Therapeutics, University of Pennsylvania, Philadelphia, Pennsylvania, USA

Aspirin has been shown, in placebo-controlled trials, to prevent myocardial infarction, stroke and vascular deaths in patients who have previously suffered such events [1,2]. It is perhaps surprising that a drug which inhibits formation of just one platelet agonist should have an effect sufficiently large to be detected in clinical trials, given the redundancy in the process of platelet activation. It is thought that this may result from the role played by thromboxane (Tx) A_2 as an amplifying signal for platelet activation by primary agonists, such as thrombin [3]. Although the case for aspirin in the primary prevention of vascular occlusive events remains to be made, its success in secondary prevention served, for a time, as a deterrent to the clinical development of theoretically superior antiplatelet drugs, particularly those configured on preventing Tx-dependent platelet activation, such as thromboxane antagonists. Enthusiasm for drug development in this area has been restored by the recent results of the EPIC (Evaluation of 7E3 for the Prevention of Ischemic Complications) study. This showed that the probability of periprocedural ischemic complications was reduced in patients undergoing coronary angioplasty by infusion of a novel antiplatelet agent, the 7E3 monoclonal antibody, directed against the platelet integrin $\alpha_{IIb}\beta_3$ [4]. This review will consider issues relevant to the further development of drugs of this class and the implications of the results of EPIC for other antithrombotic drugs in development.

Inhibition of platelet $\alpha_{IIb}\beta_3$

Integrin activation

Current understanding of the biochemistry and molecular biology of the $\alpha_{IIb}\beta_3$ complex in platelets has recently been reviewed [5]. Briefly, the configuration of the complex in resting platelets has low affinity for its primary ligand, the adhesive macromolecule fibrinogen. Fibrinogen binding occurs via Arg-Gly-Asp (RGD) motifs and residues 400–410 (HHLGGAKQAGDV) of the γ-carboxyl terminal of fibrinogen.

The 7E3 antibody and peptides containing the RGD or related motifs are thought to act as competitive inhibitors for fibrinogen at the corresponding sites in the integrin. However, it is also appreciated that such ligands possess the potential to function as partial agonists. Ginsberg et al. demonstrated that synthetic peptide ligands could activate the integrin either in situ or when purified and soluble [6]. No obvious manifestation of such a property has been apparent in the limited clinical experience to date. It is possible that indices of platelet activation, such as urinary excretion of thromboxane metabolites, might allow detection of compounds which function as partial agonists in preclinical models.

Address for correspondence: Dr G.A. FitzGerald, Center for Experimental Therapeutics, 909 Biomedical Research Building-1, 422 Curie Blvd., University of Pennsylvania, Philadelphia, PA 19004, USA.

Most early clinical studies of such inhibitors have involved their use with aspirin, because of a pragmatic approach to clinical trial design. However, it is unknown how precisely these drugs might interact with each other. It would seem illogical, at first glance, to expect aspirin to add to the efficacy — or indeed risk — of an integrin inhibitor, as Tx-dependent platelet activation would culminate in transformation of $\alpha_{IIb}\beta_3$ and enhanced fibrinogen binding. However, there are several ways in which the drugs might interact. For example, interindividual differences in pharmacokinetics are likely to result in some patients failing to achieve the degree of receptor occupancy to completely inhibit fibrinogen binding, and such patients might benefit from additional aspirin. Secondly, liver blood flow is sensitive to prostaglandin inhibitors, and small-molecule integrin inhibitors subject to high first-pass metabolism might undergo a clinically important interaction resulting from altered clearance due to concomitant aspirin.

Thirdly, we are beginning to appreciate that binding of ligand to $\alpha_{IIb}\beta_3$ may transmit signals from the outside to the inside of the cell as well as undergoing transformations which communicate signals within the cell to the outer membrane [7]. Tyrosine phosphorylation of a variety of platelet proteins results from stimulation of platelets via G protein-coupled receptors by agonists such as thrombin and epinephrine [8]. Indeed, the integrin itself is tyrosine-phosphorylated.

One interesting substrate is the pp125^{FAK} (Focal Adhesion Kinase) which appears to play a role in the focal clustering of integrins and their association with the membrane skeleton [9]. Phosphorylation of this particular substrate is associated with the formation of large platelet aggregates and requires the coordinate action of "outside-in" signaling by ligand occupancy of the integrin and activation of G protein-coupled receptors in platelets. Studies with Tx antagonists and other pharmacological probes suggest that the latter component is largely attributable to Tx-dependent activation of protein kinase C and elevation of $[Ca^{++}]_i$ resulting in antecedent cytoskeletal reorganization [10]. RGD-based peptides do not result in tyrosine phosphorylation of pp125^{FAK} or other platelet substrates and it is possible that aspirin might alter the dose–response relationships for such antagonists by preventing amplification of pp125^{FAK} phosphorylation by Tx-dependent mechanisms. Finally, it is unknown whether $\alpha_{IIb}\beta_3$ is acetylated by aspirin.

Clarification of the potential mechanisms of interaction between these classes of drugs would be helpful as they are often empirically combined in practice and because of the potentially confounding effect of unstructured aspirin usage in clinical trials of integrin antagonists.

Bleeding

This is the most common side effect of $\alpha_{IIb}\beta_3$ antagonists. The EPIC results afforded considerable encouragement in that clinical efficacy was demonstrable without an excess of strokes in patients who received 7E3, despite concomitant aspirin and heparin. Bleeds elsewhere, mostly at the site of catheter insertion, but also in the retroperitoneum, did occur with greater frequency in these patients than in the control group [4]. The most commonly employed surrogate measure of bleeding risk in clinical studies is the template bleeding time. However, the factors which lead to its prolongation are poorly understood and we do not know how this relates to bleeding risk. Does a drug-induced prolongation of bleeding time to 30 min have the same implications of risk as a similar bleeding time due to uremia?

The approach in the EPIC study was to be guided by clinical response rather than adjusting dose in response to the bleeding time. Given the very steep dose–response relationship between 7E3 and the bleeding time, this was probably integral to detecting the efficacy of this compound. However, the recent interruption of two trials of the thrombin inhibitor hirudin because of an excess of strokes [11,12] serves as a caution against too cavalier an approach. One is mindful that in volunteers taking aspirin, a 2-fold increase in the dose of 7E3 caused average bleeding time to increase from about 10 min to un-recordable at 30 min. Interindividual differences of more than 2-fold are well documented in steady-state plasma levels achieved after standard doses of many approved drugs.

When monomeric cell-recognition peptides derived from fibrinogen bind to $\alpha_{IIb}\beta_3$ they induce expression of epitopes which may be detected by FACS analysis in vitro or ex vivo. Such an approach may discriminate between the interaction of the integrin with one functional antagonist vs. another. For example, differential expression of the D_3 binding site [13] has been observed with structurally distinct small-molecule inhibitors. We have failed to observe a difference in the effectiveness of compounds which do and do not lead to expression of D_3 when used as adjuvant therapy with rt-PA in a canine model of thrombolysis (Fitzgerald DJ et al., unpublished).

We have recently utilized FACS analysis of D_3 ex vivo in a study of an integrin inhibitor in patients with chronic stable angina [14]. Interestingly, disappearance of the signal was highly correlated with recovery of the response of platelets to aggregating agonists ex vivo after the infusion was terminated, which suggests that it was a good measure of receptor occupancy.

Dose–response studies indicated that there was an unanticipated degree of inter-individual variability in both prolongation of the bleeding time and inhibition of platelet aggregation ex vivo. While these two indices correlated poorly with each other during the infusion, there was a striking correlation between the length of the bleeding time and D_3 expression, both within and between patients. This observation needs to be explored further with a structurally distinct antagonist that induces exposure of the D_3 epitope, but it raises the possibility that construction of an "epitope profile" of potential inhibitors might allow detection of induced conformational changes in the integrin that might relate to bleeding risk.

Vascular proliferation

The design of the EPIC study addressed the hypothesis that a potent platelet inhibitor would prevent periprocedural events due to thrombotic vascular occlusion in patients undergoing coronary angioplasty. The precedent on which this hypothesis was based was the proven efficacy of aspirin in this setting. Upwards of 30% of patients undergoing this procedure develop angiographic appearances of restenosis by 6 months after angioplasty. Although the relative contributions of intimal hyperplasia and smooth muscle cell proliferation to this process as well as the technical aspects of estimating minimal luminal diameter are debated [15,16], there is at the very least intense interest in trying to prevent this outcome. The most dramatic results have been obtained with antisense oligonucleo-tides directed against oncogenes thought relevant to cell cycling. Thus, Rosenberg et al. demonstrated that perivascular application of anti c-myb virtually prevented the proliferative lesion that complicates catheter injury to the rat carotid [17]. Similarly, Shi et al. and Ebstein et al. have demonstrated that anti c-myc inhibits proliferation of human and rat vascular smooth muscle cells [18,19]. Although antisense technology is still at the formative stage [20,21], such an approach is currently being evaluated in the treatment of human cancer and it is possible that it may find a use in cardiovascular surgery.

Although prevention of restenosis was not a primary endpoint in the EPIC study and

7E3 was given only as a periprocedural bolus with or without a short-term infusion, the actual incidence of angiographic restenosis on follow-up was lower in the groups who had received 7E3 [22]. If this is a real effect, the mechanism by which it occurs is unclear. Prevention of restenosis has not been apparent in trials of aspirin and other platelet inhibitors [23], and biochemical evidence of platelet activation during angioplasty suggests that it is transient [24]. It is, of course, possible that an intense period of platelet–wall interactions may trigger a chronic cascade of events in the vasculature, culminating in proliferation. Interestingly, 7E3 has also been shown to prevent the development of a vascular proliferative lesion in a canine model of chronic platelet activation in the coronary circulation. Perhaps these observations reflect an action of 7E3 other than on $\alpha_{IIb}\beta_3$. The results of similar studies [25] with integrin antagonists which exhibit higher specificity than 7E3 will be of particular interest in this regard.

Pharmacokinetic considerations

Little attention has been paid to the implications of interindividual differences in response to integrin antagonists. This may prove to be an important factor with this class of drugs, particularly given their steep dose–response relationships with aggregation and the bleeding time. Studies with an array of structurally distinct antagonists suggest that roughly 80% receptor occupancy represents the top of the dose–response curve for inhibition of aggregation ex vivo. Such relationships with the bleeding time are more imprecise, and observation of this parameter is usually terminated at 30 min. There is no information yet published on potential differences in response based on gender or ethnicity.

The merits of a short half-life are arguable. Drugs are currently being developed for relatively short-term usage and will be administered as infusions. It would seem desirable, under these circumstances, for a drug to possess a short half-life, allowing for rapid termination of action if bleeding becomes a problem. A more prolonged half-life would be desirable for chronic oral usage, as would continuity of therapy with the same molecule. Clearly, controlled-release oral preparations may allow for such dual purposes to be served. The implications for development of an oral analog are quite different from those for the present parenteral preparations. Given the established efficacy and relative safety of chronic dosage with aspirin in the secondary prevention of vascular death [1,2], it will perhaps be more difficult to establish a niche for a more potent platelet inhibitor than was the case in acute situations. Even though we do not understand the implications of the bleeding time, it might also be difficult to persuade practitioners to administer a drug which caused marked prolongation of this index during chronic dosing.

The potential drug interactions of $\alpha_{IIb}\beta_3$ inhibitors with concomitant medication, even in the acute cardiovascular setting, have scarcely been addressed. It would be expected that they might add to the efficacy of thrombin inhibitors [26]. These latter compounds are effective in animal models in which heparin fails to prevent arterial thrombosis. Specific thrombin inhibitors such as hirudin, hirulog and argatroban are effective in such models, perhaps because of their greater access to the prothrombinase complex on activated platelets [27]. Limited data suggest that their effects will be additive with inhibitors of $\alpha_{IIb}\beta_3$ [28]. Experimental data also raise the possibility that thrombin inhibition might also modify vascular proliferation [29,30]. Interestingly, the progress of drugs in both classes towards approval may well be similar, although difficulties with dose titration for hirudin and, more recently, hirulog, may retard the progress of the thrombin inhibitors. Approval of an integrin antagonist in combination with heparin at roughly the same time as a specific thrombin inhibitor is shown to be superior to heparin in the same clinical condition. It is not only for this reason that exploration of the comparative effects of heparin and specific thrombin inhibitors on the dose–response relationships of integrin inhibitors is timely. It is possible that the lack of effect of the specific inhibitors on platelets, their greater effectiveness in prevention of arterial thrombosis (this is true, at least in animal models) and their failure to prolong the bleeding time at equally anticoagulant doses may allow for safer combination of integrin antagonists with these drugs than with heparin.

Finally, the combination of integrin antagonists with thrombolytic drugs must be evaluated with the utmost caution. Platelet activation is marked during thrombolysis, and aspirin and streptokinase are additive in preventing death in the first 35 days after myocardial infarction [31,32], so the rationale for their usage exists. However, doses of integrin antagonists which have limited effects on the bleeding time in a canine model cause it to prolong markedly when they are administered with a thrombolytic drug [33]. Given the evaluation of these compounds in unstable angina and the potential translation of this syndrome into acute myocardial infarction, the desirability of a short-acting compound which allows for dose adjustment before administration of a thrombolytic is obvious.

Summary

The demonstrable effectiveness of a clinically tolerated dose of a monoclonal antibody to the $\alpha_{IIb}\beta_3$ integrin in the prevention of platelet-dependent acute complications of coronary angioplasty has prompted widespread interest in this class of drugs; peptide and small-molecule inhibitors are under investigation [25,34,35]. However, we incompletely understand how to evaluate the relative merits and safety profiles of such candidates for development. The potential implications of partial agonism, integrin selectivity and conformational effects on the integrin complex are poorly understood. Given the steep dose–response relationships of these drugs to inhibition of aggregation and the bleeding time [35], the effects of differences in pharmacokinetics on the comparative safety and efficacy of such inhibitors merit detailed investigation.

Other antiplatelet and anticoagulant drugs

Specific thrombin inhibitors may be superior to heparin as antithrombotic drugs in the arterial circulation, as discussed above. Potential advantages include more direct access than the bulky thrombin–antithrombin III complex to the prothrombinase complex as it is being assembled on platelet membranes, inability to be neutralized by heparin inhibitors such as platelet factor 4, lack of direct effects on platelets and relative serine protease specificity for thrombin. These theoretical advantages have translated into a more potent antithrombotic effect in a variety of animal models at similar anticoagulant doses as heparin [37] and into a failure to prolong the bleeding time in patients compared to heparin at doses which prolong the aPTT to a similar degree [38]. The relative advantage, if any, of thrombin-receptor antagonists [39] over direct inhibitors remains to be explored. Some of the inhibitors have been shown to have an antiproliferative effect at high doses. However, given at high enough doses these compounds will also prolong the bleeding time and they appear to cause bleeding complications in humans, as inferred from the interruption of clinical trials with hirudin recently. Despite a large number of phase II clinical trials which provide data on outcomes, the first clinical trial with these compounds, adequately sized to assess clinical outcome and safety, remains to be reported. Oral analogs of these drugs are in the early stages of clinical development and will ultimately compete with oral anticoagulants such as warfarin.

Two interesting classes of compounds are inhibitors of Factor (F) Xa and inhibitors of Gp 1b [40,41]. F Xa plays a pivotal role in clot formation [41], and its inhibition has theoretical appeal as an even more efficient approach than inhibition of thrombin [42]. Inhibitors of F Xa have been shown to be more effective than specific thrombin inhibitors in some animal models. Although small-molecule inhibitors have been developed, there are no data as to their efficacy from clinical trials. Gp1b is critical to adhesive interactions between platelets and vascular cells [40]. Several antibodies directed against this integrin have been developed and found to be effective in animal models of thrombosis [40,43]. There is a reasonable theoretical basis to the assumption that inhibitors of Gp1b and $\alpha_{IIb}\beta_3$ might act synergistically [44]. Both F Xa and GpIb inhibitors have minimal or no effects on the bleeding time at effective antithrombotic doses in animal models.

Given our focus on the differing mechanisms of action of these compounds, it is perhaps worth considering that a leech F Xa inhibitor antistasin, the leech thrombin inhibitor hirudin and two $\alpha_{IIb}\beta_3$ inhibitors, discorsin and ornatin, conserve the same structural motif, despite marked differences in primary sequence [45]. The use of different binding epitopes to influence diversely the hemostatic process from a common protein scaffold is provocative, as we consider how molecules might be engineered to limit the risk of bleeding.

Ticlopidine has been shown to be as effective as aspirin in the secondary prevention of stroke [46]. Its comparative cost and association with an apparently reversible neutropenia in about 1% of cases has, with reports of hypercholesterolemia, tended to diminish enthusiasm for the drug [47]. It appears that ticlopidine and its derivative, clopidogrel, interfere with the activation of platelets by ADP [48], although its precise mechanism of action remains to be defined. Clopidogrel is currently the subject of a large-scale study of its efficacy in the prevention of cardiovascular events.

Although dipyridamole was promoted as a phosphodiesterase inhibitor, the concentrations achieved after oral dosing in humans were unimpressive and it has been difficult to establish its clinical efficacy [49]. A large-scale controlled evaluation of its utility in the prevention of stroke is currently under way. More specific and potent phosphodiesterase inhibitors are in development [50]. Similarly, oral prostacyclin analogs, activated protein kinase C and thromboxane antagonists/synthase inhibitors are currently the subjects of continuing clinical investigation.

Conclusion

There is perhaps more evidence for the efficacy of aspirin in the secondary prevention of cardiovascular events than there is for any drug in any aspect of clinical medicine. This very success deterred the development of theoretically superior antithrombotic drugs until recently. The results of the EPIC study have prompted widespread interest, not only in inhibitors of $\alpha_{IIb}\beta_3$, but also in other antithrombotic drugs. It is likely that the complexity of the human pharmacology of these compounds is prone to underestimation in the rush to phase III clinical trials. Recent experience of adverse effects and lack of anticipated efficacy in phase III trials of distinct thrombin inhibitors seem attributable to inappropriate dose selection. Antithrombotic drugs merit a careful investment of effort to identify properties which discriminate efficacy from risk.

References

1. Patrono C. N Engl J Med 1994;330:1287–1294.

2. Antiplatelet Trialists' Collaboration. Br Med J 1994;308:81–106.
3. FitzGerald GA. Am J Cardiol 1991;68:11B–15B.
4. The EPIC Investigators. N Engl J Med 1994;330:956–961.
5. Smyth SS, Joneckis CC, Parise LV. Blood 1993;81:2827–2843.
6. Xiaoping D, Plow EF, Frelinger III AL, O'Toole TE, Loftus JC, Ginsberg MH. Cell 1991;65:409–416.
7. Haimovich BH, Lipfert L, Brugge JS, Shattil SJ. J Biol Chem 1993;268:15868–15877.
8. Furman MI, Grigoryev D, Bray PF, Dise KR, Goldschmidt-Clermont PJ. Circ Res 1994;172–180.
9. Kornberg L, Earp HS, Parsons JT, Schaller M, Juliano RL. J Biol Chem 1992;267:23439–23442.
10. Shattil SJ, Haimovich B, Cunningham M, Lipfert L, Parsons JT, Ginsberg MH, Brugge JS. J Biol Chem 1994;269:14738–14745.
11. Antman EM. Circulation 1994;90:1624–1630.
12. Neuhaus KL, Essen Rv, Tebbe U, Jesel A, Heinrichs H, Maurer W, Doring W, Harmjanz D, Kotter V, Kalhammer E, Simon H, Horacek T. Circulation 1994;90:1638–1642.
13. Jennings LK, Fox CF, Kouns WC, McKay CP, Ballou LR, Schultz HE. J Biol Chem 1990;265:3815–3822.
14. Moran N, Delanty N, Maker M, Jennings SL, Catella F, FitzGerald GA, Fitzgerald DJ. Antagonism of the Gp IIb/IIIa receptor. J Am Coll Cardiol 1994 (in press).
15. Glagov S. Circulation 1994;89:2888–2891.
16. Isner JM. Circulation 1994;89:2937–2941.
17. Simons M, Edelman ER, DeKeyser J-L, Langer R, Rosenberg RD. Nature 1991;359:67–70.
18. She Y, Hutchinson HG, Hall DJ, Zalewski A. Circulation 1993;88:1190–1195.
19. Epstein SE, Speir E, Finkel T. Circulation 1993;88:1351–1353.
20. Davis AR. Trends Cardiol Med 1994;4:51–55.
21. Albert PR, Morris SJ. Trends Pharmacol Sci 1994;15:250–254.
22. Topol EJ, Califf RM, Weisman HF et al. Lancet 1994;343:881–886.
23. Schwartz L, Bourassa MG, Lesperance J et al. N Engl J Med 1988;318(26):1714–1719.
24. Braden G, Knapp HR, FitzGerald GA. Circulation 1991;84:679–685.
25. Mousa SA, Bozarth JM, Forsythe MS et al. Circulation 1994;89:3–12.
26. Rydel TJ, Ravichandran A, Tulinsky WB et al. Science 1990;249:277–280.
27. Swords NA, Mann KG. Arterioscler Thromb 1993;13:1602–1612.
28. Nicolini FA, Philmo L, Rios G, Kottke-Marchant K, Topol EJ. Circulation 1994;89:1802–1809.
29. Edelman ER, Karnovsky MJ. Circulation 1994;89:770–776.
30. Hedin U, Frebelius S, Sanchez J, Dryjski M, Swedenborg J. Arterioscler Thromb 1994;14:254–260.
31. FitzGerald DJ, Catella F, Roy L, FitzGerald GA. Circulation 1988;77:142–150.
32. Ridker PM, Hebert PR, Fuster V, Hennekens CH. Lancet 1993;341:1574–1577.
33. FitzGerald DJ, Hanson M, FitzGerald GA. J Clin Invest 1991;88:1589–1595.
34. Roux SP, Tschopp TB, Kuhn H, Steiner B, Hadvary P. J Pharmacol Exp Ther 1992;264:501–508.
35. Peerlinck K, De Lepeleire I, Goldberg M, Farrell D, Barrett J, Hand E, Panebianco D, Deckmyn H, Vermylen J, Arnout J. Circulation 1993;88:1512–1517.
36. Gold HK, Gimple LW, Yasuda T, Leinbach RC, Werner W, Holt R, Jordan R, Berger H, Collen D, Coller BS. J Clin Invest 1990;86:651–659.
37. Yoshimi I, Stassen J-M, Collen D. J Pharmacol Exp Ther 1992;261:895–898.
38. Kerins DM, Williams K, Fitzgerald DJ, FitzGerald GA. Clin Res 1992;40:272A.
39. Vu T-K, Hung DT, Wheaton VI, Coughlin SR. Cell 1991;64:1057–1068.
40. Ruggeri ZM. Circulation 1992;86:III26–III29.
41. Eisenberg PR, Siegel JE, Abendschein DR, Miletich JP. J Clin Invest 1993;91:1877–1883.
42. Krishnaswamy S, Field KA, Edgington TS, Morrissey JH, Mann KG. J Biol Chem 1992;267:26110–26120.
43. Yao S-KY, Ober JC, Garfinkel LI, Hagay Y, Ezov N, Ferguson JJ, Anderson HV, Panet A, Gorecki M, Buja LM, Willerson JT. Circulation 1994;89:2822–2828.
44. Savage B, Shattil SJ, Ruggeri ZM. J Biol Chem 1992;267:11300–11306.
45. Krezel AM, Wagner G, Seymour-Ulmer J, Lazarus RA. Science 1994;264:1944–1947.
46. Bellavance A, and the TASS Investigators. Stroke 1993;24:1452–1457.
47. FitzGerald GA. Circulation 1990;82:296–298.
48. Mills DCB, Puri R, Hu C-J et al. Arterioscler Thromb 1992;12:430–436.
49. FitzGerald GA. N Engl J Med 1987;316:1247–1257.
50. Saitoh S, Tomiyoshi S, Otake A et al. Arterioscler Thromb 1993;13:563–570.

1048

The POSCH Trial: 13-year follow-up and disease-free interval analysis

Henry Buchwald[1], Christian T. Campos[2], James R. Boen[3], Phoung Nyugen[1], and Stanley E. Williams[1] for the POSCH Group

[1]Department of Surgery, University of Minnesota, Minneapolis, Minnesota; [2]Division of Cardiothoracic Surgery, New England Deaconess Hospital and Harvard Medical School, Boston, Massachusetts; and [3]School of Public Health, University of Minnesota, Minneapolis, Minnesota, USA

Abstract. The Program on the Surgical Control of the Hyperlipidemias (POSCH) has provided clear and convincing evidence of the benefits of secondary intervention by effective lipid modification in a postmyocardial infarction population. Utilizing partial ileal bypass as the intervention modality, this trial demonstrated a highly significant reduction in the incidence of the combined endpoint of coronary heart disease (CHD) mortality and confirmed nonfatal myocardial infarction ($p < 0.001$). The total number of invasive coronary artery procedures (coronary artery bypass grafting (CABG), percutaneous transluminal coronary angioplasty (PTCA), and heart transplantation) was 2.6 times greater in the control group ($p < 0.001$). POSCH provided up to 10 years of sequential coronary arteriographic assessments and showed less atherosclerosis progression ($p < 0.001$) and more atherosclerosis regression ($p < 0.01$) in the intervention group. The POSCH findings have also been translated for the clinician into the number of years of freedom gained for a given endpoint by the intervention group.

POSCH was a randomized, prospective, secondary, atherosclerosis intervention trial designed to test whether the marked lipid changes induced by the partial ileal bypass operation would favorably affect CHD. The primary endpoint of POSCH was death due to any cause. A specific objective of the study was to assess the validity of the use of changes observed on sequential coronary arteriograms as surrogate endpoints for clinical atherosclerosis events. The study population consisted of 838 patients in four clinical centers (University of Minnesota, Minneapolis; University of Arkansas, Little Rock; University of Southern California, Los Angeles; and the Lankenau Hospital and Research Center, Philadelphia). There were 417 patients in the diet-treated control group and 421 in the diet plus partial ileal bypass-treated surgery group, both men and women, who had survived a single myocardial infarction. Formal trial closure occurred on July 19, 1990 with a mean follow-up of 9.7 years, a minimum follow-up of 7 years, and a maximum follow-up of 14.8 years [1]. Detailed descriptions of the design and methods of the POSCH trial [2], of the recruitment experience [3], of the 5-year lipid results [4], of the analysis of changes in sequential coronary arteriograms and their correlation with subsequent coronary events [5], and of the findings in the women in POSCH [6] have been published. The POSCH disease-free interval analysis has been presented as an abstract [7] and submitted for publication. POSCH is currently in an extended follow-up phase.

Methods

Patients were eligible for the trial if they were between the ages of 30 and 64 years and

---

Address for correspondence: Henry Buchwald MD, PhD, Box 290 UMHC, University of Minnesota, Minneapolis, MN 55455, USA.

had survived a single myocardial infarction, documented by electrocardiographic and enzymatic changes, that had occurred between 6 and 60 months before the date of randomization. Before randomization, all patients received instruction in the American Heart Association Phase II diet. The patients taking hypocholesterolemic drugs were asked to discontinue this treatment at least 6 weeks before baseline lipid measurement, and all patients were encouraged not to resume or start taking hypocholesterolemic medications during their participation in the trial. Patients were required to have a total plasma cholesterol level of at least 5.69 mmol/l (220 mg/dl) or a low density lipoprotein (LDL) cholesterol level of at least 3.62 mmol/l (140 mg/dl) if their total plasma cholesterol level was between 5.17 and 5.66 mmol/l (200 and 219 mg/dl), after they had followed the Phase II diet for a minimum of 6 weeks.

Most of the potentially confounding major risk factors for atherosclerosis (e.g., hypertension, diabetes, or obesity) were criteria for exclusion, with the exception of cigarette smoking. Patients with a ≥75% stenosis of the left main coronary artery or with no measurable coronary-artery stenosis on the baseline arteriogram were excluded. The intervention modality, partial ileal bypass, was performed according to a standard protocol, and one surgeon was responsible for the procedures at each participating institution [2]. The lipid analyses were performed in the POSCH lipid laboratory, following procedures that had been standardized and certified by the lipid standardization laboratory of the Centers for Disease Control in Atlanta, GA. The assessments of the sequential coronary arteriograms were made by two-member panels utilizing an evaluation protocol similar to that employed by the Cholesterol Lowering Atherosclerosis Study (CLAS) [8]. Peripheral arteriograms were read in blinded fashion by a single reader. Resting and exercise electrocardiograms were obtained at each follow-up visit. After March of 1981, the peripheral pulse pressures were determined by Doppler ultrasonography at each clinic visit, and the ankle–arm index was calculated for sequential comparisons. All patients were followed by means of clinic visits and telephone contacts, according to a uniform protocol [2]. Follow-up coronary and peripheral arteriograms were obtained at 3, 5, and at either 7 years (in patients enrolled on or after 1 June 1980) or 10 years (in patients enrolled before 1 June 1980).

Statistical analyses were based on randomization assignment (intention-to-treat). The specific statistical tests utilized have been reviewed in prior POSCH publications. A two-sided p value less than 0.05 was considered to indicate statistical significance.

Results

Study population

The average age of the patients at randomization was 51 years. Of the 838 patients, 90.7% were men and 97.9% were Caucasian. The baseline mean total plasma cholesterol level was 6.49 mmol/l (250 mg/dl), with an average LDL-cholesterol level of 4.62 mmol/l (179 mg/dl). The mean interval between the qualifying myocardial infarction and entry into the trial was 2.2 years. Detailed baseline patient characteristics have been presented elsewhere [9]. Of the 421 patients assigned to the surgery group, 22 refused the operation and 23 underwent reversal, primarily for diarrhea, during the trial. They were all, however, included in the surgery group for statistical assessment. There were no immediate, in-hospital deaths after partial ileal bypass. The side effects of partial ileal bypass included diarrhea, kidney stones, gallstones, late symptoms of bowel obstruction, and a mean weight loss of 5.3 kg (p < 0.0001). There were 28 neoplasms in the control group and 32 in the surgery group (p = NS). No patient has been lost to follow-up.

Lipid results

At 5 years, the surgery group, as compared with the control group, had a 23.3 ± 1.0% (mean ± SE) lower total plasma cholesterol level (p < 0.0001), a 37.7 ± 1.2% lower LDL-cholesterol level (p < 0.0001), a 4.3 ± 1.8% higher HDL-cholesterol level (p = 0.02), an 18.3 ± 7.5% higher VLDL-cholesterol level (p = 0.02), a 19.8 ± 6.5% higher triglyceride level (p = 0.003), a 37.8 ± 2.8% higher ratio of HDL-cholesterol to total plasma cholesterol (p < 0.001), a 71.8 ± 4.3% higher ratio of HDL-cholesterol to LDL-cholesterol (p < 0.0001), and significantly higher levels of the HDL_2 subfraction (p < 0.0001) and of apolipoprotein A-I (apoA-I) (p < 0.0001) and a significantly lower level of apoB100 (p < 0.0001).

Clinical endpoint results

For the combined endpoint of CHD mortality and confirmed nonfatal myocardial infarction, there was a highly significant 35.0% risk reduction in the surgery group (125 vs. 82 events; 95% confidence interval, 9.1 to 52.8; p < 0.001). The addition of suspected nonfatal myocardial infarction and unstable angina events to either CHD mortality or overall mortality further widened the difference between groups and increased the level of significance. There was a reduction in peripheral vascular disease in the surgery group by clinical (p = 0.038), Doppler ultrasonographic (p < 0.01), and arteriographic (p = 0.09 at 10 years) criteria. The total number of cardiac interventions (CABG, repeat CABG, PTCA, or heart transplantation) was 2.6 times greater in the control group (p < 0.0001), 137 control and 52 surgery patients undergoing a first CABG (p < 0.0001), and 33 control and 15 surgery patients undergoing a first PTCA (p = 0.005). On 19 July 1990, there had been 62 deaths in the control group and 49 in the surgery group (149 per 1,000 vs. 116 per 1,000), thus a 21.7% risk reduction (95% confidence interval, −17.0 to 47.6, p = 0.164). Concurrently, CHD mortality was reduced by 28.0%, 44 (106 per 1,000) deaths in the control group and 32 (76 per 1,000) deaths in the surgery group (95% confidence interval, −16.1 to 55.3; p = 0.113). In a data-derived, subgroup analysis, patients with an ejection fraction ≥50% had a 36.1% decrease in overall mortality (95% confidence interval, −9.4 to 62.9; p = 0.052 by Mantel-Haenszel test, and p = 0.021 by Gehan test). By 1992, the incidence levels for overall mortality (28.8% risk reduction, p = 0.052) and CHD mortality (34.1% risk reduction, p = 0.058) were approaching statistical significance (data submitted for publication). It is planned to present follow-up clinical event data every 2 years.

Sequential coronary arteriographic results

POSCH provided the largest and longest (3, 5, 7, and 10 years) sequential assessments of coronary arteriograms of any reported lipid intervention trial. Consistently, all interval analyses showed less atherosclerosis progression (p < 0.001) [1] and more atherosclerosis regression (p < 0.001) [10] in the intervention group. The rates of progression were control group vs. surgery group: 41.4 vs. 28.1% at 3 years, 65.4 vs. 37.5% at 5 years, 77.0 vs. 48.1% at 7 years, and 85.0 vs. 54.7% at 10 years. Comparable results were found in the cohort of women in POSCH [6]. Assessment of the relationship between changes in sequential coronary arteriograms and subsequent clinical coronary events showed a statistically compelling (p < 0.01) relationship for overall mortality and CHD mortality [5].

Disease-free interval analysis

In a recent analysis (submitted for publication), the POSCH data were subjected to disease-free interval assessment, an evaluation not traditionally found in the reporting of lipid intervention trials and possibly of great relevance to clinicians. An overall mortality of 10% occurred at 6.7 years in the control group and at 9.5 years in the intervention group, for a gain in this disease-free interval of 2.8 years in the intervention group (p = 0.054). A CHD mortality of 8% occurred at 7.2 years in the control group and at 11.3 years in the intervention group, for a gain in this disease-free interval of 4.1 years in the intervention group (p = 0.029). 20% of the patients demonstrated the combined endpoint of CHD mortality and confirmed nonfatal myocardial infarction at 5.9 years in the control group and at 11.7 years in the intervention group, for a gain in this critical disease-free interval of 5.8 years in the intervention group (p < 0.001). 25% of the patients underwent either a CABG, a PTCA or a heart transplant at 5.4 years in the control group and at 13.0 years in the intervention group, for a gain in this disease-free interval of 7.6 years in the intervention group (p < 0.001).

Discussion

The original publication of the POSCH results in October of 1992 [1] has been cited approximately 200 times in the scientific literature. Organ et al. stated "This study provides the strongest evidence yet of a link between the modification of the lipid profile and reduction of atherosclerotic progression" [11]. Vos et al. wrote "POSCH is the only trial that presents data on the long-term effects of lipid lowering" [12]. In a paper on how to put findings of recent trials to practical use, Kahn stated "Of the recent randomized studies examining the potential for reversing coronary atherosclerosis with lipid-lowering methods, the Program on Surgical Control of the Hyperlipidemias (POSCH) may provide the most irrefutable evidence of success" [13]. Gotto described the relevance of POSCH in stating, "The benefit of cholesterol-lowering intervention in patients with established coronary disease was clearly shown in the recently reported Program on the Surgical Control of the Hyperlipidemias (POSCH)" [14]. And Blankenhorn and Hodis, in 1993, ended their review of the POSCH trial with the statement "This study remains a landmark" [15].

Indeed, POSCH has had a major impact on putting the so-called lipid controversy to rest and in establishing the validity of the lipid/atherosclerosis theory. POSCH has shown benefits of secondary intervention clinically and arteriographically, and it has given substance and statistical credence to the use of sequential coronary arteriography as a surrogate endpoint for clinical atherosclerosis events. This demonstration justifies trials of CHD employing sequential coronary arteriography in lieu of clinical event analyses and, thereby, substantially reducing the number of patients, the time, and the costs of these trials. POSCH was one of the few CHD intervention trials to recruit women and to demonstrate parallel lipid results in women, thus allowing for the conjecture that effective treatment of high blood cholesterol levels is indicated in the management of atherosclerosis in women as well as in men. The 62% reduction in invasive coronary artery procedures demonstrated in the intervention group in POSCH can, if translated into monetary terms, lead to a significant reduction of the annual cost attributable to CHD in the health-care budgets of the western nations. The ongoing extended follow-up analysis of the POSCH patients may provide evidence of a statistically significant reduction by lipid intervention in overall and CHD mortality.

1052

Acknowledgements

Supported by Grants R01-HL-15265 and R01-HL-49522 from the National Heart, Lung, and Blood Institute, NIH.

References

1. Buchwald H, Varco RL, Matts JP, Long JM, Fitch LL, Campbell GS, Pearce MB, Yellin AE, Edmiston WA, Smink RD Jr, Sawin HS Jr, Campos CT, Hansen BJ, Tuna N, Karnegis JN, Sanmarco ME, Amplatz K, Castaneda-Zuniga WR, Hunter DW, Bissett JK, Weber FJ, Stevenson JW, Leon AS, Chalmers TC, and the POSCH Group. N Engl J Med 1990;323:946–955.
2. Buchwald H, Matts JP, Fitch LL, Varco RL, Campbell GS, Pearce M, Yellin A, Smink RD Jr, Sawin HS Jr, Campos CT, Hansen BJ, Long JM, and the POSCH Group. J Clin Epidemiol 1989;42:1111–1127.
3. Buchwald H, Matts JP, Hansen BJ, Long JM, Fitch LL and the POSCH Group. Controlled Clin Trials 1987;8:94S–104S.
4. Campos CT, Matts JP, Fitch LL, Speech JC, Long JM, Buchwald H and the POSCH Group. Surgery 1987;102:424–432.
5. Buchwald H, Matts JP, Fitch LL, Campos CT, Sanmarco ME, Amplatz K, Castaneda-Zuniga WR, Hunter DW, Pearce MB, Bissett JK, Edmiston WA, Sawin HS, Weber FJ, Varco RL, Campbell GS, Yellin AE, Smink RD, Long JM, Hansen BJ, Chalmers TC, Meier P, Stamler J, and the POSCH Group. J Am Med Assoc 1992;268:1429–1433.
6. Buchwald H, Campos CT, Matts JP, Fitch LL, Long JM, Varco RL, and the POSCH Group. Ann Surg 1992;216:389–400.
7. Buchwald H, Campos CT, Boen JR, Nyugen P, Williams SE, and the POSCH Group. J Am Coll Cardiol 1994;23:389A.
8. Blankenhorn DH, Johnson RL, Nessim SA, Azen SP, Sanmarco ME, Selzer RH. Controlled Clin Trials 1987;8:356–387.
9. Matts JP, Buchwald H, Fitch LL, Campos CT, Varco RL, Campbell GS, Pearce MB, Yellin AE, Edmiston WA, Smink RD Jr, Sawin HS Jr, Hansen BJ, Long JM, and the POSCH Group. Controlled Clin Trials 1991;12:314–339.
10. Campos CT, Buchwald H, and the POSCH Group. Cardiovasc Risk Factors 1992;2:261–275.
11. Organ CH, Henderson VJ. J Am Med Assoc 1991;265:3172–3175.
12. Vos J, de Feyter PJ, Simoons ML, Tijssen JGP, Deckers JW. Prog Card Dis 1993;35:435–454.
13. Kahn JK. Postgrad Med 1993;94:50–65.
14. Gotto AM Jr. Am J Med 1994;91(suppl 1B):1B–31S.
15. Blankenhorn DH, Hodis HN. Western J Med 1993;159:172–179.

In memoriam

Memorials of leading atherosclerosis
researchers who died between the
IXth and Xth International
Symposia on Atherosclerosis

David H. Blankenhorn (1924–1993)

On 9 May 1993, Dr David H. Blankenhorn, professor of medicine at the University of Southern California, died at age 68 from prostate cancer. He is greatly missed by all who knew him.

David was born in Cleveland, Ohio in 1924. He was a graduate of Dartmouth College and the University of Cincinnati Medical School. After 2 years in the army, where he served as Chief of Medicine at the US Army Hospital in Vienna, Austria, he embarked upon what would become his life's work, studying lipid and cholesterol metabolism at the Rockefeller Institute.

In 1957 he joined the faculty of the University of Southern California Medical School in Los Angeles. From 1963 until 1980 he directed the division of cardiology. During this time he received a Specialized Center of Research (SCOR) grant to study progression and regression of atherosclerotic plaques in patients. At the same time, Robert H. Selzer, of

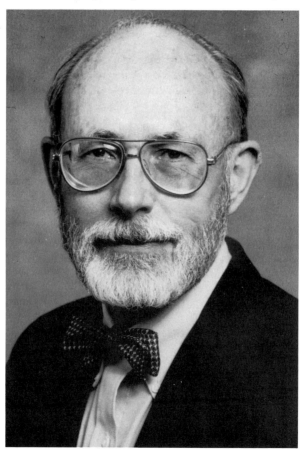

NASA's Jet Propulsion Laboratory in Pasadena, was developing computer image-processing programs to remove noise encountered during transmission of photographs from planetary space craft. Learning of Robert's work, David immediately recognized the applicability of this technology to the quantitation of atherosclerosis. A 23-year friendship and collaboration began between the two men, and quantitative angiography was born. In 1977, David and Robert published the first study which used computer image processing to show regression of femoral atherosclerosis as a result of diet and drug therapy. Skepticism, however, remained strong.

1980 was a watershed year — the year David dedicated himself full-time to clinical research, and began his NIH-funded Cholesterol Lowering Atherosclerosis Study (CLAS). The results, published in 1987, made atherosclerosis research history. For the first time, it was conclusively demonstrated that the progress of this "degenerative" disease could be slowed, halted, and even reversed. Not content to rest on his laurels, David followed up the CLAS trial with the Monitored Atherosclerosis Regression Study (MARS). This trial, which tested monotherapy with lovastatin, produced results similar to those of CLAS and was published after his death in November of 1993.

His lifetime accomplishments were recognized by various awards including an honorary doctorate from the University of Uppsala, the Daniel Drake medal for achievement in medicine from his alma mater, the University of Cincinnati Medicine School, and the presentation of the George Lyman Duff Memorial Lecture at the 1992 AHA Scientific Sessions.

His life will be remembered as one of enthusiastic inquiry and creative energy. His many friends and associates also recall his dry sense of humor and his personal concern and empathy. He is survived by his wife Anne, four children, David, Mary, Susan and John, and four grandchildren.

Linda Cashin-Hemphill

Thomas E. Carew (1943–1993)

Tom Carew had all the qualities of a true scientist. He had the youthful, joyous curiosity about things and how they worked. He loved to come up with that critical experiment that yields an unambiguous solution (at least in theory!). He also looked at data with a healthy skepticism and he was just as skeptical about his own data as he was about other people's. He was a very good scientist.

Tom had a formidable background in bioengineering and biomathematics (BA, Johns Hopkins University, 1965 Biophysics; MSE, The Catholic University of America, 1967 Biomedical Engineering–Physiology program; PhD, The Catholic University of America, 1971 Biomedical Engineering–Physiology Program) and then learned atherogenesis research with Don Fry. When he joined our group in La Jolla, he quickly picked up the techniques of cell biology and became a real triple-threat man.

When Tom started working with our group the accepted dogma was that LDL must be removed entirely by the liver, otherwise there would be progressive buildup of cholesterol in the peripheral tissues. Working with Alan Sniderman, Tom tested the dogma and found it wanting. Even after hepatectomy, LDL continued to disappear from the plasma of swine. Later studies, using residual labeling, showed that in fact only about half of the LDL removal takes place in the liver. Those studies showed that there must be an active reverse cholesterol transport system.

Arguably the most important paper Tom published was his 1987 PNAS article with Dawn Schwenke showing that an antioxidant can markedly slow the progression of atherosclerosis in LDL receptor-deficient rabbits. That paper, along with the paper from Kita's laboratory, published at the same time, was of pivotal importance in the field. It stimulated a rapid increase in the pace of research on the oxidative modification hypothesis.

Tom was a very good friend and colleague. He was wonderfully witty and wise. He loved to take the Devil's Advocate position and challenge whatever the current politically current position might be — whether in science or in politics. It was always a joy to exchange ideas with him. He loved a good laugh and he provided many. Some of you will remember his famous rabbit slide. Without comment, in the course of a serious scientific presentation, he would flash on the screen this ordinary white laboratory rabbit — ordinary *except* that its eyes were covered by a solid, black rectangle, like the photos of patients found in medical textbooks! It usually took just a beat for the delicious incongruity of this slide to sink in and then everyone dissolved into helpless laughter, including Tom.

Tom, the good scientist and good friend, will be remembered by all who were privileged to know him.

Daniel Steinberg

Christos Cladaras (1951–1994)

Dr Christos Cladaras was born on 1 August 1951 in Alexandroupolis in northern Greece. At the age of 16, his family moved to Thessaloniki where he completed his high-school education. Following a stiff entrance exam, he was admitted to the Department of Biological Sciences of the University of Thessaloniki. Chris received his BS in Biology in 1974, and remained for an additional 2 years as a research fellow in the Department of Genetics of the same University.

His natural inclination and genuine interest for science led him to pursue graduate education abroad. Chris was admitted in 1976 to the University of Texas Southwestern Medical School and received his PhD in Biochemistry in 1980 under the direction of Dr L. Cottam. He received additional training in biochemistry and molecular biology, initially at the Department of Biochemistry of the University of Chicago, 1981–1982 (in the laboratory of Dr K. Agarwal) and then at the Institute of Molecular Virology of the

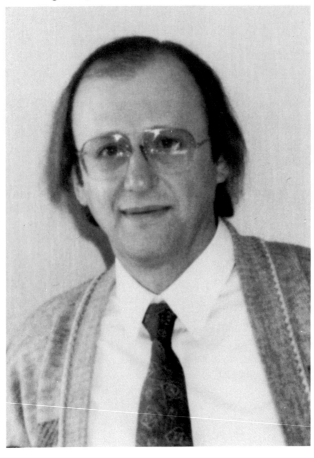

University of St. Louis Medical School, 1982–1984 (in the laboratory of Dr W. Wold). His thesis topic was the regulation of the synthesis of pyruvate kinase, and his postdoctoral work dealt with the biochemistry and molecular biology of the adenovirus E3 and E1B genes.

Dr Cladaras and I met by chance at the Federation Meetings in June 1984 in St Louis; a few months later he joined as an instructor in the newly formed Section of Molecular Genetics at Boston University. This was the great era of gene cloning and Dr Cladaras very quickly lived up to the challenge. During 1984–1986 he was the driving force in determining the structure of human apoB100. This classic scientific contribution was published in the December issue of the EMBO Journal (vol. 5, pp. 3495–3507). Having won a competitive battle, Dr Cladaras took a 1-year leave of absence to work on the posttranscriptional regulation of HIV1 genes by the Rev protein at the Frederick Cancer Research Institute of the National Institutes of Health (in the laboratory of Dr G. Pavlakis). Upon his return to Boston, he was promoted to Assistant Professor in 1988 and was provided independent laboratory space and facilities to develop his research. In 1988, Dr Cladaras entered a new, exciting era dealing with the regulation of expression of the human apolipoprotein genes.

As a result of his original and independent scientific contributions and initiatives, he was awarded an Established Investigatorship Award of the American Heart Association in 1988, a First Award by the National Institutes of Health in 1990, and a Grant-In-Aid Award by the American Heart Association in 1990. He also received numerous local awards and research support as a Co-Principal Investigator and was promptly promoted to Associate Professor of Medicine and Biochemistry at Boston University in 1992. Dr Cladaras was one of the most valuable faculty members of the Section of Molecular Genetics. He was an intelligent, innovative and fiercely independent scientist. He stood up to all the challenges he was confronted with and he always came up a clear winner. Throughout the years he played a key role in the training and supervision of graduate students and postdoctoral fellows. The thesis work completed by Dimitris Kardassis was characterized as an outstanding piece of work by the faculty of the Department of Biochemistry and was a reflection of Christos' diligent supervision and guidance. It will not be an exaggeration to say that Christos' love for science ranked as high as his devotion to his family.

It is ironic that Dr Cladaras succumbed unexpectedly to a massive heart attack, on 10 August 1994 – the very same condition he devoted his scientific career to prevent. He leaves behind his wife Margarita Hadzopoulou-Cladaras, who is an Assistant Professor in the Section of Molecular Genetics in the Department of Medicine at Boston University, and his son George Cladaras, age 9, who reside in Needham, Massachusetts. He also leaves behind his parents George and Margarita Cladaras and his sister Litsa and niece Maria Soulakidou, who live in Thessaloniki, Greece. His family, his friends, his colleagues and the scientific community are all going to miss him very dearly.

Vassilis I. Zannis

André Crastes de Paulet (1929–1994)

On 3 October 1994, during a mountain excursion, our friend André Crastes de Paulet, professor of biochemistry of the Faculty of Medicine of Montpellier University, died suddenly and discreetly. We all suffered a great emotional blow but we were left rich with the many memories that each of us keeps of his warm friendship, of his luminous smile, of his communicative joy, of his lively intelligence, of his apparently boundless activity, of his very full life. Thanks to his great qualities of the heart, his energy always put to the service of others and his inquiring nature, he remains a model to all researchers.

Born 28 January 1929 in the sunny region of Béziers, France, he was indelibly marked with the imprint of the Midi. A very good student, was admitted at the age of only 16 to Montpellier University in 1945 where he undertook brilliant studies in sciences and medicine. In 1951, he graduated in Science and in 1953 he became a doctor of medicine! In 1949, he had joined the Laboratory of Biochemistry and Toxicology of the Faculty of Medicine of Prof P. Cristol, where he studied under the direction of the young Prof

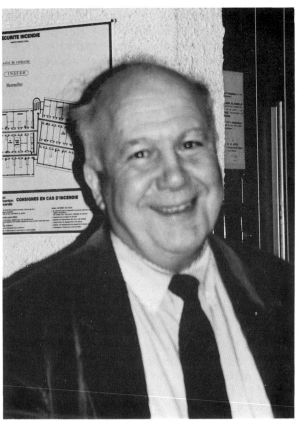

Christian Bénézech, was named head of the laboratory in 1950 and Director of Research 1952–1958. It was his training in physical and organic chemistry that give him a taste for structural biochemistry and reactive mechanisms. He succeeded Prof Bénézech, who had opted for a chair in biophysics, as chairman of the biochemistry department in 1966. It is to A. Crastes de Paulet, who was the soul of the department, that we owe its brilliance and its remarkable development of medical biochemistry at Montpellier. As a member of an important team of researchers which make up an INSERM unit that is recognized as one of the best in France, he contributed to the renown of research at Montpellier in biochemistry and nutrition. He also worked to establish his region as a European center for studies in nutrition.

His research was principally directed at the biosynthesis of cholesterol, oxysterols, the peroxidation of lipids, free radicals and antioxidants, the metabolism of unsaturated fatty acids and lipid metabolism. In all of these areas, his work has yielded more than 300 publications of very high caliber. In the biology of steroidal hormones, especially of estrogens, one mainly notes his work on action mechanisms and estrogen receptors, on the synthetic analogs of estradiol and on the relations between structure and activity of its derivatives. His chapter on the stereochemical biosynthesis of sterols and the poly-isoprene precursors in the Treatise of General Biochemistry is a classic of enduring value.

Having developed an enzymatic method to measure steroids, he created a general method of enzymatic amplification which provides numerous micro-assays, from that of NADH to those of androgens and bile acids. After the development of immunoenzymatic techniques, he made them more sensitive by using bioluminescence. With his team of researchers, he developed the luminescence techniques to study the metabolism of oxidative free radicals and the regulation mechanisms of gene expression (with the luciferase gene as reporter gene). Other contributions, too numerous to detail, were in the fields of sterol biosynthesis and catabolism, polyunsaturated fatty acids and their prostanoid derivatives, and the role of prostaglandins in fetoplacental activity, in osteo-arthritis and in asthma.

His interest in research on nutrition led him to collaborate with other French and Mediterranean centers. The last publication that he presented to the National Academy of Medicine this year was on the favorable effects of supplementation of milk formulas with α-linolenic acid for premature infants.

Always ready to embark on new research projects, he clearly displayed a communica-tive dynamism and an insatiably curious nature. His devotion and the quality of his work led him to accept directorial responsibilities on university, regional, INSERM and other national fronts. In the context of the IAS, I mention only his presidency of the French Society of Clinical Biology, and his active membership of the Study and Research Group on Lipids and Lipoproteins of the French Society of Biochemistry and Molecular Biology, and of the Research Commission of the Association for Research into Cholesterol and Cardiovascular Diseases.

He was a Knight of the National Order of Merit and he was an elected correspondent of the National Academy of Medicine. He always had the support of his wife Pierrette Crastes de Paulet, who is also a biochemist. He had a large team of students and collaborators to whom he passed on his love of research, his scientific rigor, his great sense of biochemistry and his enthusiasm for new ideas. All those who had the privilege of working with him are deeply saddened and will want to continue all he had undertaken in the same spirit.

Jacques Polonovski

1062

Giancarlo Descovich (1937–1993)

Professor Giancarlo Descovich was born at Fiume on 2 March 1937. He married Angiola in 1965 and had five children.

He graduated at Bologna in 1962 in Medicine and Surgery with a thesis entitled "Hemodynamic effects in intraventricular septal defects". From the start of his academic career he concentrated on scientific research under the guidance first of Prof Sotgiù and then of Prof Lenzi. He achieved significant academic goals in a short time — Senior Lecturer in 1971, Assistant 1st Medical Clinic University of Bologna, Associated Professor in 1980, Full Professor in 1986, Director of the Bologna Center and of the Italian Study Groups on Dysmetabolic Diseases and Atherosclerosis in 1986, Head of the Gerontology Department, Bologna — and also professional goals — specialty boards in General Medicine 1967, Endocrinology 1969, Cardiology 1970, Physiotherapy and Rehabilitation 1977.

In the 30 years of his scientific career he organized and chaired several meetings on atherosclerosis and cardiovascular diseases. He was president of the Italian Society of Epidemiology and Preventive Medicine and was responsible for countless CNR research

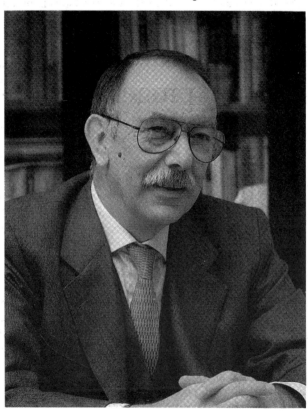

programs. In particular he was responsible for devising and organizing the Brisighella Heart Study, one of the most important epidemiological studies in the field of prevention and identification of risk factors for cardiovascular diseases. This study, which began in 1972, required the commitment and constant dedication of the researchers as well as students of numerous specializations (physicians, biologists, biochemists, mathematicians, physicists), and they all continue to work today even without the guidance of their sadly missed leader. The results of this intense research activity have led to decisive contributions to the progress of medicine and in particular to the understanding of the role of catecholamines in IMA (1964—1966), to the evaluation of circadian rhythms of certain adrenal hormones (1967—1968, 1972—1974), to the definition of the epidemiology of metabolic and nonmetabolic cardiovascular risk factors (1977—1985), and recently arriving at a complete definition of the concept of community medicine and its organizational, practical and social implications.

He was the author of countless publications, teaching texts for students in geriatrics, gerontology and internal medicine, and his contribution in the field of epidemiology has placed Italy in a leading position throughout the world.

Antonio Gaddi

Sándor Gerö (1904–1992)

Sándor Gerö was born in Budapest on 12 April 1904. He gained his medical degree from the Semmelweis University of Medicine and practiced medicine for more than 6 decades at the Szabolcs Street Hospital and the Semmelweis University of Medicine, from 1959 to 1974 as head of the Third Department of Medicine. In 1973 he formed an independent research team studying the pathogenesis of atherosclerosis, and led this research team until his death.

He was the founding member of the Hungarian Atherosclerosis Society, president of the society for 10 years, and honorary president until his death. He was a leading member of the Gerontology Society. He was also a member of the American College of Cardiology (Washington), the Royal Society of Medicine (London), the Société d'Athérosclérose (Paris) and honorary member of the Polish Cardiology Society. He was a leading member of the European Atherosclerosis Society. For years he was on the editorial board of *Atherosclerosis*.

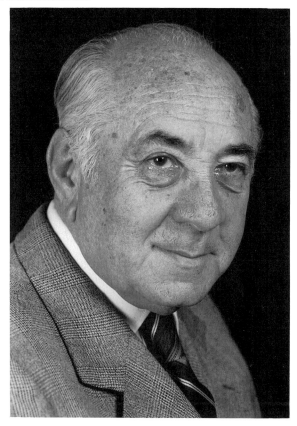

His main scientific interests were in theoretical and clinical problems associated with atherosclerosis. He received international acclaim in this field. His main conclusions can be divided into three groups:

1. In contrast to the lipid conception of atherosclerosis which was dominant at that time he proved that the primary mechanism involved connective tissue changes.
2. His team showed the production of specific complexes between mucopolysaccarides and a β-lipoprotein after damage to the basic material in the vessel wall.
3. He was the first to draw attention to the immunological factors involved in changes to the aorta and vessel walls.

Over his career he published more than 200 papers, most of them in international periodicals. Perhaps the best recognition of his work and research lies in the fact that his theories are quoted widely in the medical literature.

Albert Császár

Jacky Larrue (1942–1993)

Dr Jacky Larrue, Director of the Cardiology Research Unit, INSERM, left us on a chilly afternoon in November 1993, aged only 51. His death plunged us into disarray and sadness.

His career, which was exemplary in many ways, was that of a master. Already at a very young age, he obtained his PhD. Then, 21 years ago, he entered INSERM, and his great talent was to succeed in an early push forward with diversification of the life sciences. Despite stiff competition, he was appointed Director of Research, then Director of INSERM Unit 8, one of the few cardiology units of its kind in France.

His brio, dynamism and talents were manifested in his membership of several scientific associations. As a life member of the French Society of Cardiology, though not himself a doctor (an exceptional fact), and as a most respected General Secretary of the French Society of Atherosclerosis, Jacky Larrue's gifts were recognized in several ways:

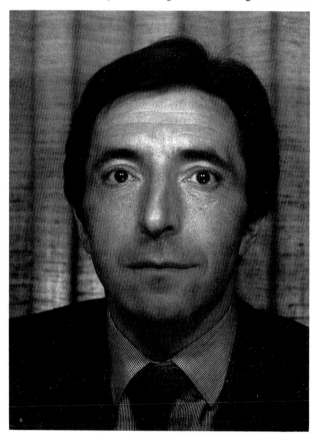

- he was called upon by the Ministry of Higher Education and Research to sit on various scientific commissions, and was named a member of the Medical Section of the National Council for Universities;
- he was elected to the Scientific Council of the University of Bordeaux II;
- having been a driving force in developing the "Pole Régional Médicament" in Aquitaine, he was elected President of the Regional Scientific Council of INSERM in Aquitaine, and was a member of the Consultative Committee for Technological Research and Development; and
- he was a much respected expert on behalf of NATO and the CNRS.

The numerous scientific conferences and meetings he attended and his many publications bear witness to the vitality with which he conducted his own research and helped others in theirs, and to his tenacious attachment to an open-minded approach. Through his doctoral teaching, it was clear to all that Jacky Larrue was a fine communicator and mentor, a gift that his many students over the years always cherished. To have accomplished so much in such a short time, both in his professional and personal life, Jacky Larrue must have been a truly exceptional man, with exceptional qualities that he never ceased to develop in a career cut off in its prime:

- a profound illuminating intelligence that you could read in his laughing eyes, and a lucidity and solidity in his understanding of himself, of others, of the quintessence of life;
- an acute vision of things to come;
- intellectual rigor and a critical mind;
- constant open-mindedness, and an uncommon generosity of heart and mind.

Respected and loved by all who knew him, Jacky Larrue leaves behind him an immense void.

Henri Bricaud

Atherosclerosis X.
F.P. Woodford, J. Davignon and A. Sniderman, editors.

Iwan S.F. Ranti (1923–1988)

Members of the Indonesian Cardiovascular Society (ICS) were very grieved when Dr Ranti suddenly left us forever in St Carolus Hospital, Jakarta in 1988.

He was born in 1923 in Jakarta. He went to high school and medical school in The Netherlands, where he graduated in 1955. He then studied child health in Amsterdam. In 1957 he returned to Indonesia, and studied further at the Department of Child Health of the University of Indonesia in Jakarta. He became a pediatric cardiologist, but his main interest always remained atherosclerosis.

As head of the National Cardiology Institute in Jakarta, which he became in 1967, Dr Ranti was one of the pioneers of modern cardiology in Indonesia, together with others like Dr R.I.S. Santoso (a cardiothoracic surgeon) and Dr T.B. Gan (an adult cardiologist). He was therefore an obvious choice for chairman when the Indonesian Cardiovascular Society was established in 1980, and indeed was so elected by the 17 founding members. He was not only a scientist, but also a good leader, and under his influence the membership of the ICS expanded to more than 100 members and extended over the whole of Indonesia, whose population is now 180 million. Under Dr Ranti's influence and guidance, ICS became an active member of the IAS in the 1980s.

His widow, formerly E. Muller, unfortunately also passed away (in 1990). Their four children will always retain fond memories of their beloved father and mother.

Y. Risyanto

Daniel A.K. Roncari (1937–1994)

Dan Roncari passed away on 28 May 1994 in Toronto. Members of the Canadian Athero-sclerosis Society will all remember Dan's diligent and hard work as President of the Society despite his many other responsibilities.

Dan had a distinguished scientific career at the Universities of Calgary and Toronto. He was formerly the Director of the Institute of Medical Science at the University of Toronto (1980–1983), the first Julia McFarland Professor of Diabetes Research a Chair of the Research Unit at the University of Calgary (1983–1987) and the first Professor of Investigative Medicine at Sunnybrook Health Science Centre and its former Physician-in-Chief (1988–1993).

He was extremely well regarded for his research on precursors of adipocyte cells and on adipocyte metabolism. His research on adipocyte differentiation helped to revise concepts of fat-tissue growth. Dan was a committed and dedicated scientist and caring physician. He possessed a strong commitment to fundamental scientific research. He was always interested and supportive of research that had a precise hypothesis and a very good model to test the hypothesis. He will be sorely missed in the Canadian scientific community.

We extend our sincere sympathies to his wife Luba and his three young children.

W. Carl Breckenridge

Index of authors

Keyword index